CONTENTS IN BRIEF

i

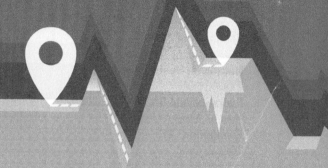

ELEVENTH EDITION

11

TOWARD HEALTHY AGING

Human Needs and Nursing Response

Theris A. Touhy, DNP, CNS, DPNAP

Emeritus Professor
Christine E. Lynn College of Nursing
Florida Atlantic University
Boca Raton, Florida

Kathleen Jett, PhD, GNP-BC, DPNAP

Gerontological Nurse Practitioner
Memphis, Tennessee

ELSEVIER

Elsevier
3251 Riverport Lane
St. Louis, Missouri 63043

TOWARD HEALTHY AGING:
HUMAN NEEDS AND NURSING RESPONSE, ELEVENTH EDITION   ISBN: 978-0-323-80988-7

Notice

Practitioners and researchers must always rely on their own experience and knowledge in evaluating and using any information, methods, compounds or experiments described herein. Because of rapid advances in the medical sciences, in particular, independent verification of diagnoses and drug dosages should be made. To the fullest extent of the law, no responsibility is assumed by Elsevier, authors, editors or contributors for any injury and/or damage to persons or property as a matter of products liability, negligence or otherwise, or from any use or operation of any methods, products, instructions, or ideas contained in the material herein.

Previous editions copyrighted 2020, 2016, 2012, 2008, 2004, 1998, 1994, 1990, 1985, and 1981

Content Strategist: Sandra Clark
Content Development Manager: Lisa Newton
Content Development Specialist: Andrew Schubert
Publishing Services Manager: Julie Eddy
Senior Project Manager: Cindy Thoms
Design Direction: Renee Duenow

Printed in the United States of America

Last digit is the print number: 9 8 7 6 5 4 3 2 1

Working together
to grow libraries in
developing countries

www.elsevier.com • www.bookaid.org

For Danny
You touched your family and so many others in your social work practice
with your presence, caring, deep love, and your music.
Your gentle spirit lives on.

To all the students who read this book: I hope each of you will improve the
journey toward healthy aging through your competence and compassion.

To all of my students who have embraced gerontological nursing as their specialty
and are improving the lives of older adults through their practice and teaching.

To the older adults I have been privileged to nurse, and their caregivers,
thank you for making the words in this book a reality through your
caring and for teaching me how to be a gerontological nurse.

Theris Touhy

To the older adults in my personal and professional life who have
taught me the most important things to share with students.

To my husband, Steve, and our wonderful children and grandchildren, who never
cease to remind me that the best part of life and aging is the love we share.

To my mother-in-law, Gloria Jett, one of the many victims of the
COVID-19 pandemic. Through her illness and my caregiving, I
discovered that I really do know how to be a gerontological nurse and
how many ways the knowledge found within this text can be used.

Kathleen Jett

Theris A. Touhy, DNP, CNS, DPNAP, has been a clinical specialist in gerontological nursing, nurse practitioner, and nursing educator for more than 40 years. Her expertise is in the care of older adults in long-term care and those with dementia. Dr. Touhy received her BSN degree from St. Xavier University in Chicago, a master's degree in care of the aged from Northern Illinois University, and a Doctor of Nursing Practice from Case Western Reserve University. She is an emeritus professor in the Christine E. Lynn College of Nursing at Florida Atlantic University, where she has served as Assistant Dean of Undergraduate Programs and taught gerontological nursing and long-term, rehabilitation, and palliative care nursing in the undergraduate, graduate, and doctoral programs. Her research is focused on spirituality in aging and at the end of life, caring for persons with dementia, caring in nursing homes, and nursing leadership in long-term care. Dr. Touhy was the recipient of the Geriatric Faculty Member Award from the John A. Hartford Foundation Institute for Geriatric Nursing, is a two-time recipient of the Distinguished Teacher of the Year at the Christine E. Lynn College of Nursing at Florida Atlantic University, and received the Marie Haug Award for Excellence in Aging Research from Case Western Reserve University. Dr. Touhy was inducted into the National Academies of Practice in 2007. She is co-author with Dr. Kathleen Jett of *Gerontological Nursing and Healthy Aging* and co-author with Dr. Priscilla Ebersole of *Geriatric Nursing: Growth of a Specialty.* In addition to her professional activities, Dr. Touhy and her husband of 54 years are blessed with a loving family of three sons, two grandsons, and one granddaughter. Being a grandparent is the greatest adventure and joy of growing older!

Kathleen Jett, PhD, GNP-BC, DNAP, brings more than 40 years of gerontological nursing practice to this text. Her clinical experience is broad, from her roots in public health to leadership in long-term care, assisted living, hospice, and gerontological education, to her work as a researcher and advanced practice nurse as both a clinical nurse specialist and a nurse practitioner. Dr. Jett received her bachelor's, master's, and doctoral degrees from the University of Florida, where she also holds a graduate certificate in gerontology. In 2000 she was selected as a Summer Scholar by the John A. Hartford Foundation—Institute for Geriatric Nursing. In 2004 she completed a Fellowship in Ethno-Geriatrics through the Stanford Geriatric Education Center. Dr. Jett has received several awards, including recognition as an Inspirational Woman of Pacific Lutheran University in 1998 and 2000 and for her excellence in undergraduate teaching in 2005 and Distinguished Teacher of the Year at the Christine E. Lynn College of Nursing at Florida Atlantic University. A board-certified gerontological nurse practitioner, Dr. Jett was inducted into the National Academies of Practice in 2006. She has taught an array of courses, including public health nursing, women's studies, advanced practice gerontological nursing, and undergraduate courses in gerontology. She has coordinated two gerontological nurse practitioner graduate programs and an undergraduate interdisciplinary gerontology certificate program. Most of her research has been in the area of reducing health disparities experienced by older adults. The thread that ties all of her work together has been a belief that nurses can make a difference in the lives of older adults. She is currently retired and enjoys putting her skills to use through volunteer work in service to vulnerable older adults.

CONTRIBUTORS AND REVIEWERS

CONTRIBUTORS

Lenny Chiang-Hanisko, PhD, RN
Associate Professor
Christine E. Lynn College of Nursing
Florida Atlantic University
Boca Raton, Florida

Priscilla Ebersole, PhD, RN, FAAN
Professor Emerita
San Francisco State University
San Francisco, California

Debra Hain, PhD, ARNP, ANP-BC, GNP-BC, FAANP
Associate Professor/Lead Faculty AGNP Program
Christine E. Lynn College of Nursing
Florida Atlantic University
Boca Raton, Florida
Nurse Practitioner, Department of Hypertension/Nephrology
Cleveland Clinic Florida
Weston, Florida

María de los Ángeles Ordóñez, DNP, ARNP/GNP-BC
Director
Louis and Anne Green Memory and Wellness Center
Florida Atlantic University
Boca Raton, Florida
Assistant Professor
College of Nursing
Florida Atlantic University
Boca Raton, Florida
FAU Memory Disorder Clinic Coordinator
Louis and Anne Green Memory Disorder Clinic
Department of Elder Affairs
Boca Raton, Florida

REVIEWERS

Cynthia R. Becker, MSN, RN
Professor
Black Hawk College
Moline, Illinois

Keisha Butler, MSN, RN
Instructor of Nursing
Tennessee Technological University
Cookeville, Tennessee

Jacqueline M. Garland, MSN, RN, LMT
Assistant Professor of Nursing
Rockford University
Rockford, Illinois

Deborah S. Petty, DNP, APRN, ACNS-BC
Clinical Assistant Professor
Louise Herrington School of Nursing
Baylor University
Dallas, Texas

Debra D. Rapaport, MSN, RN
Nursing Faculty, Tenured
Helena College
University of Montana
Helena, Montana

PREFACE

In 1981, Dr. Priscilla Ebersole and Dr. Patricia Hess published the first edition of *Toward Healthy Aging: Human Needs and Nursing Response,* which has been used in nursing schools around the globe. Their foresight in developing a textbook that focuses on health, wholeness, beauty, and potential in aging has made this book an enduring classic and the model for gerontological nursing textbooks. In 1981, few nurses chose this specialty, few schools of nursing included content related to the care of older adults, and the focus of care was on illness and problems. Today, gerontological nursing is a strong and evolving specialty with a solid theoretical base and practice grounded in evidence-based research. Dr. Ebersole and Dr. Hess set the standards for the competencies required for gerontological nursing education and the promotion of healthy aging. Many nurses, including us, have been shaped by their words, their wisdom, and their passion for care of elders. We thank these two wonderful pioneers and mentors for the opportunity to build on such a solid foundation in the multiple editions of this book we have co-authored since their retirement. We hope that we have kept the heart and spirit of their work, for that is truly what has inspired us, and so many others, to care for older adults with competence and compassion.

We are very excited to have been able to offer a timely and completely revised 11th edition of this text guided by the National Council of State Boards of Nursing (NCSBN) model of clinical judgment. In 2019, the NCSBN identified the need to enhance the clinical judgment skills of entry-level nurses and, in a few years, the Next-Generation NCLEX® Examination for nursing licensure will be based on the new model of clinical judgment. *The Essentials: Core Competencies for Professional Nursing Education* (American Association of Colleges of Nursing, 2021) identifies clinical judgment as one of the key attributes of professional nursing. Clinical judgment refers to the process by which nurses make decisions based on nursing knowledge (evidence, theories, ways, and patterns of knowing), other disciplinary knowledge, critical thinking, and clinical reasoning (Manetti, 2019). This process is used to understand and interpret information in the delivery of care. Clinical decision making based on clinical judgment is directly related to care outcomes for nursing at all levels.

Enhancing clinical judgment skills is especially relevant to guide the design of nursing actions in care of older adults. Older adults are complex, and their responses to illness are often subtle and may not meet standard diagnostic criteria seen in younger individuals. Cues to impending health concerns are often missed or blamed on age, leading to unnecessary disability, complications, and compromised quality of life. Nurses are key to recognizing and analyzing cues leading to the prioritization of hypotheses needed to generate solutions, take action, and evaluate outcomes to enhance the healthiest aging while dealing with the most common challenges facing an aging population. This text provides comprehensive information to guide the development of competent clinical judgment in nursing practice with older adults across the continuum of care.

Toward Healthy Aging is a comprehensive gerontological nursing text. The framework is holistic, addressing body, mind, and spirit along a continuum of wellness, within the context of culture, and grounded in caring and respect for older adults. Within the covers, the reader will find gerontological nursing actions based on the latest evidence-based practice guidelines available. This fosters the provision of the highest level of care to adults in settings across the continuum. The content is also consistent with the Recommended Baccalaureate Competencies and Curricular Guidelines for the Nursing Care of Older Adults, the Hartford Institute for Geriatric Nursing Best Practices in Nursing Care to Older Adults, and content relevant to the gerontological nursing and adult-gerontological nurse practitioner certification exams. Although *Toward Healthy Aging* is written with baccalaureate and graduate students in mind, it also can be used in associate degree programs or as a reference for interprofessional care teams, care facilities, and nurses' libraries. The text makes an ideal supplement to health assessment, medical-surgical, community, and psychiatric and mental health textbooks in programs that do not have a freestanding gerontological nursing course.

ORGANIZATION OF THE TEXT

Toward Healthy Aging has 35 chapters, organized into 5 sections.

Section 1 begins with foundational information from demographics to long-term care structure. It includes information about the roles and responsibilities of contemporary gerontological nurses in making timely, sound, evidence-based clinical judgments to optimize wellness.

Section 2 provides the reader with foundational information needed to make clinical judgments to inform nursing actions. This section includes details about the cues nurses use to recognize and analyze maximize overall outcomes for older adults. This ranges from optimizing communication, to recognizing the cues needed for a comprehensive assessment, to ensuring safe medication use.

Section 3 provides information to enable nurses to recognize and prioritize functional needs that may be overlooked when caring for older adults, such as vision, physical activity, and safety and security. Prevention is emphasized to decrease the risk for unnecessary frailty, morbidity, mortality, and development of multidimensional geriatric syndromes.

Section 4 addresses the most common chronic disorders seen in later life. Content includes the recognition of cues, development of hypotheses, and nursing actions leading to optimal outcomes. The emphasis is on the interplay between the disorder, aging, and living with chronic disease.

Section 5 steps beyond health conditions and functional needs to consider the older adult within the greater context of relationships, ethical dilemmas, loss, and finding meaning in life.

KEY COMPONENTS OF THE TEXT

A Student Speaks/An Older Adult Speaks: Introduces every chapter to provide perspectives of older adults and nursing students on chapter content.

Using Clinical Judgment to Promote Healthy Aging: Special headings detailing pertinent cues, nursing actions, and outcomes.

Key Concepts: Concise review of important chapter points.

Clinical Judgment and Next-Generation NCLEX® Examination–Style Questions: Practice examples designed to assist students in the recognition of key cues, hypotheses, and the identification of essential nursing actions to maximize outcomes to ensure safety in care delivery.

Nursing Studies: Accompanying select chapters, these provide short nursing studies to help students see content put into practical use.

Critical Thinking Questions and Activities: Assist students in developing critical thinking related to chapter and nursing study content and include suggestions for in-classroom activities to enhance learning.

Research Questions: Suggestions to stimulate thinking about ideas for nursing research related to chapter topics.

Boxes: Key Essential Learning is Highlighted

Safety Tips: Safety issues related to care of older adults.

Research Highlights: Summary of pertinent current research related to chapter topics.

Resources for Best Practice: Suggestions for further information for chapter topics and tools for practice.

Tips for Best Practice: Summary of evidence-based nursing actions for practice.

Healthy People 2030: Reference to the goals cited in *Healthy People 2030*.

A Student Speaks

An Older Adult Speaks

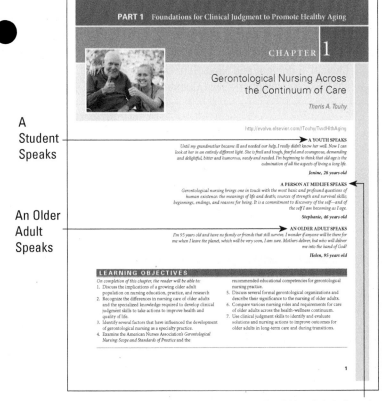

An Older Adult Speaks

Healthy People Box

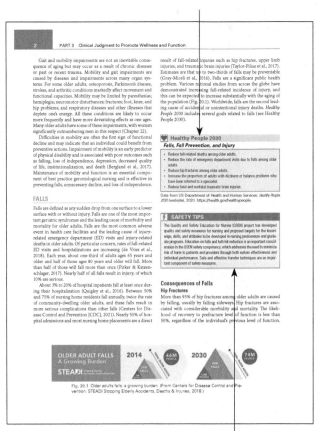

Safety Alert Box

Research Highlights Box

Tips for Best Practice Box

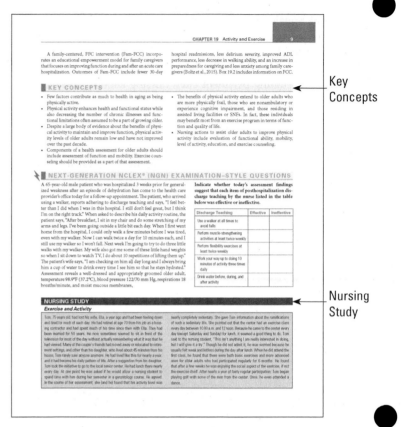

Key Concepts

Nursing Study

Resources for Best Practice Box

Clinical Judgment and Next-Generation NCLEX® Examination–Style Questions

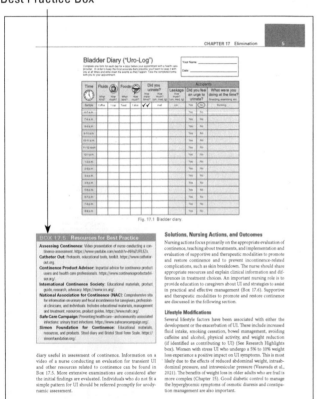

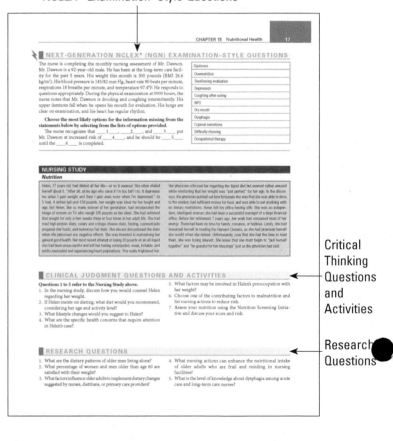

Critical Thinking Questions and Activities

Research Questions

EVOLVE ANCILLARIES

Instructors

Test Bank: Hundreds of questions with rationales to use in creating exams

PowerPoint: Lecture slides for each chapter, including integrated audience response questions

Teach for Nurses Lesson Plans: Detailed listing of resources available to instructors for their lesson planning, also including unique case studies and class activities that can be shared with students

Next-Generation NCLEX® (NGN) Examination–Style Case Studies: Most of the chapters contain Next-Generation NCLEX® Examination–Style Case Studies, which provide opportunities for students to develop clinical judgment skills in care of older adults as well as prepare for the NCLEX

Answers to Nursing Studies and Clinical Judgment Questions and Activities (in the Print Book)

Answers to Next-Generation NCLEX® (NGN) Examination–Style Questions (in the Print Book)

Answers to Student Review and Critical Thinking Questions

Image Collection: More than 75 illustrations and photos that can be used in a presentation or as visual aids

Students

Student Review and Critical Thinking Questions: Open-ended study questions covering nearly every element of each chapter

Case Studies: Accompanying select chapters, these provide short case studies with questions to help students see content put into practical use

NCLEX® Examination-Style Review Questions: More than 150 questions organized by chapter

ACKNOWLEDGMENTS

This book would not have been possible without the support and guidance of the staff at Elsevier. Special thanks also to Sandra Clark, Content Strategist; Andrew Schubert, Content Development Specialist; and Cindy Thoms, Senior Project Manager. We also acknowledge our reviewers and contributors, because without their efforts this edition would not have been possible. Finally, we acknowledge the past and future readers who, we hope, will provide us with enough feedback to keep us honest and relevant in any future writing.

Theris A. Touhy
Kathleen Jett

CONTENTS

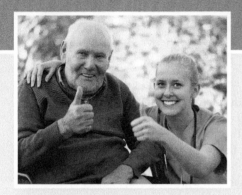

CHAPTER 1

Gerontological Nursing Across the Continuum of Care

Theris A. Touhy

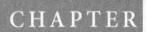

http://evolve.elsevier.com//Touhy/TwdHlthAging

A YOUTH SPEAKS

Until my grandmother became ill and needed our help, I really didn't know her well. Now I can look at her in an entirely different light. She is frail and tough, fearful and courageous, demanding and delightful, bitter and humorous, needy and needed. I'm beginning to think that old age is the culmination of all the aspects of living a long life.

Jenine, 28 years old

A PERSON AT MIDLIFE SPEAKS

Gerontological nursing brings one in touch with the most basic and profound questions of human existence: the meanings of life and death; sources of strength and survival skills; beginnings, endings, and reasons for being. It is a commitment to discovery of the self—and of the self I am becoming as I age.

Stephanie, 46 years old

AN OLDER ADULT SPEAKS

I'm 95 years old and have no family or friends that still survive. I wonder if anyone will be there for me when I leave the planet, which will be very soon, I am sure. Mothers deliver, but who will deliver me into the hand of God?

Helen, 95 years old

LEARNING OBJECTIVES

On completion of this chapter, the reader will be able to:

1. Discuss the implications of a growing older adult population on nursing education, practice, and research
2. Recognize the differences in nursing care of older adults and the specialized knowledge required to develop clinical judgment skills to take actions to improve health and quality of life.
3. Identify several factors that have influenced the development of gerontological nursing as a specialty practice.
4. Examine the American Nurses Association's *Gerontological Nursing: Scope and Standards of Practice* and the recommended educational competencies for gerontological nursing practice.
5. Discuss several formal gerontological organizations and describe their significance to the nursing of older adults.
6. Compare various nursing roles and requirements for care of older adults across the health-wellness continuum.
7. Use clinical judgment skills to identify and evaluate solutions and nursing actions to improve outcomes for older adults in long-term care and during transitions.

CARE OF OLDER ADULTS: A NURSING IMPERATIVE

Healthy aging is now an achievable goal for many. It is essential that nurses have the knowledge and skills to help people of all ages, races, and cultures to achieve this goal. Older adults today are healthier, are better educated, and expect a much higher quality of life as they age than did earlier generations. Enhancing health in aging requires attention to health throughout life, as well as expert care from nurses. Most nurses care for older adults during their careers, and estimates are that up to 75% of nurses' time is spent with older adults. In addition, the public will look to nurses to have the knowledge and skills needed to assist people to age in health. Every older adult should expect care provided by nurses with competence in gerontological nursing. Knowledge of aging and gerontological nursing is core knowledge for the profession of nursing.

The terms *geriatric nursing* and *gerontological nursing* are both used in the literature and in practice to describe the specialty of caring for older adults. Although both terms are used in the text, we prefer *gerontological nursing* because this reflects a more holistic approach encompassing both health and illness.

Who Will Care for an Aging Society?

By 2040, the number of older adults in the world will be at least 1.3 billion. The increase in the older adult population will far outpace growth in other age groups. It is a critical health and societal concern that gerontological nurses, other health professionals, and direct care workers be prepared to deliver care in all settings across the globe. The eldercare workforce is in shortage in most of the developed world, and the increased aging population is posing challenges for many countries to meet the expanding need for care services for older adults. Developing countries are experiencing the most rapid growth in numbers of older adults, and at the same time they lack systems of care and services.

The eldercare workforce shortage also presents a looming crisis for the 43.5 million unpaid family caregivers providing care for someone age 55 years or older. Without improvement in the eldercare workforce, even more stress will be placed on family and other informal caregivers. With smaller family sizes, the rising divorce rate, and the increase in geographical relocation, the next generation of older adults may be less able to rely on families for caregiving (Chapter 32). Will there be enough care workers to assist families in the care of loved ones?

In the United States, eldercare is projected to be the fastest growing employment sector in health care. Despite demand, the number of health care workers who are interested and prepared to care for older adults remains low (Institute of Medicine [IOM], 2008). Less than 1% of registered nurses (RNs) and less than 3% of advanced practice nurses (APNs) are certified in geriatrics. "We do not have anywhere close to the number of nurses we need who are prepared in geriatrics, whether in the field of primary care, acute care, nursing home care, or in-home care" (Christine Kovner, RN, PhD, FAAN, as cited in Robert Wood Johnson Foundation, 2013).

Geriatric medicine faces similar challenges, with about 7000 prepared geriatricians, 1 for every 2546 older Americans—and

 HEALTHY PEOPLE 2030
Older Adults Workforce

> Increase the proportion of the health care workforce with geriatric certification.

Data from US Department of Health and Human Services, Office of Disease Prevention and Health Promotion: *Healthy People 2030* (website), 2020. https://health.gov/healthypeople.

this number is falling, with the trend predicted to be less than 5000 geriatricians by 2040 (IOM, 2008). Other professions such as social work, physical therapy, and psychiatry have similar shortages. It is estimated that by 2030, nearly 3 million additional health care professionals and direct care workers will be needed to meet the care needs of a growing older adult population. *Healthy People 2030* has addressed this concern.

DEVELOPMENT OF GERONTOLOGICAL NURSING

Historically, nurses have always been in the frontlines of caring for older adults. They have provided hands-on care, supervision, administration, program development, teaching, and research and to a great extent are responsible for the rapid advancement of gerontology as a profession. Gerontological nurses have made significant contributions to the body of knowledge guiding best practice care of older adults. Gerontological nursing has emerged as a circumscribed area of practice only within the past 6 decades. Before 1950, gerontological nursing was seen as the application of general principles of nursing to the older adult with little recognition of this area of nursing as a specialty similar to obstetric, psychiatric, or surgical nursing. Whereas most specialties in nursing developed from those identified in medicine, this was not the case with gerontological nursing because health care of the older adult traditionally was considered within the domain of nursing.

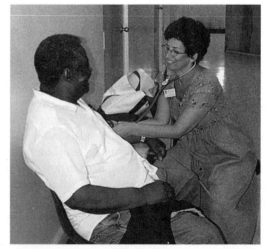

Gerontological nurses provide care in a number of settings (© iStock.com).

The foundation of gerontological nursing as we know it today was built largely by a small cadre of nurse pioneers, many

Mary Opal Wolanin, Gerontological Nursing Pioneer

"I believe that one of the most valuable lessons I have learned from those who are older is that I must start with looking inside at my own thinking. I was very guilty of ageism. I believed every myth in the book, was sure that I would never live past my seventieth birthday, and made no plan for my seventies. Probably the most productive years of my career have been since that dreaded birthday, and I now realize that it is very difficult, if not impossible, to think of our own aging." (From interview data collected by Priscilla Ebersole between 1990 and 2001.)

Terry Fulmer, President of The John A. Hartford Foundation

"I soon realized that in the arena of caring for the aged, I could have an autonomous nursing practice that would make a real difference in medical outcomes. I could practice the full scope of nursing. It gave me a sense of freedom and accomplishment. With older patients, the most important component of care, by far, is nursing care. It's very motivating." (From Ebersole P, Touhy T: *Geriatric nursing: growth of a specialty*, New York, 2006, Springer, p 129.)

Jennifer Lingler, PhD, CRNP, Professor, Vice Chair for Research, Health and Community Systems, University of Pittsburgh

"When I was in high school, a nurse I knew helped me find a nursing assistant position at the residential care facility where she worked. That experience sparked my interest in older adults that continues today. I realized that caring for frail elders could be incredibly gratifying, and I felt privileged to play a role, however small, in people's lives. At the same time, I became increasingly curious about what it means to age successfully. I questioned why some people seemed to age so gracefully, while others succumbed to physical illness, mental decline, or both. As a Building Academic Geriatric Nursing Capacity (BAGNC) alumnus, I now divide my time serving as a nurse practitioner at a memory disorders clinic, teaching an ethics course in a gerontology program, and conducting research on family caregiving. I am encouraged by the realization that as current students contemplate the array of opportunities before them, seek counsel from trusted mentors, and gain exposure to various clinical populations, the next generation of geriatric nurses will emerge. And, I am confident that in doing so, they will set their own course for affecting change in the lives of society's most vulnerable members." (As cited in Fagin C, Franklin P: Why choose geriatric nursing? Six nursing scholars tell their stories, *Imprint* 5[4]:72–76, 2005.)

of whom are now deceased. The specialty was defined and shaped by those innovative nurses who saw, early on, that older adults had special needs and required the most subtle, holistic, and complex nursing care. This history is similar to that of pediatric nursing and the recognition that pediatric nursing is "not med-surg nursing on little people" (Taylor, 2006, p. E128), and nurses need special skills to care for children. In examining the history of gerontological nursing, one must marvel at the advocacy and perseverance of nurses who have remained committed to improving the care of older adults despite struggling against great odds over the years. Box 1.1 presents the views of some of the geriatric nursing pioneers, as well as those of current leaders, on the practice of gerontological nursing and the reasons they are attracted to this specialty.

Nursing was the first of the professions to develop standards of gerontological care and the first to provide a certification mechanism to ensure specific professional expertise through credentialing. The most recent edition of *Gerontological Nursing: Scope and Standards of Practice* (American Nurses Association [ANA], 2018) provides a comprehensive overview of the scope of gerontological nursing, the skills and knowledge required to address the full range of needs related to the process of aging, and the specialized care of older adults as a group and as individuals. The document also identifies levels of gerontological nursing practice (basic and advanced) and standards of clinical gerontological nursing care and gerontological nursing performance. Box 1.2 presents some of the early history of gerontological nursing.

Current Initiatives

The most significant influence in enhancing the specialty of gerontological nursing has been the work of the Hartford Institute for Geriatric Nursing, established in 1996 and funded by the John A. Hartford Foundation. Initiatives in nursing education,

nursing practice, nursing research, and nursing policy have addressed enhancement of geriatrics in nursing education programs through curricular reform and faculty development, creation of the National Hartford Center of Gerontological Nursing Excellence, predoctoral and postdoctoral scholarships for study and research in geriatric nursing, and clinical practice improvement projects to enhance care for older adults (http://www.hartfordign.org). The National Hartford Center of Gerontological Nursing Excellence offers a Distinguished Educator in Gerontological Nursing Program as well as Leadership Conferences on Aging. Another resource is Sigma Theta Tau's Center for Nursing Excellence in Long-Term Care, which sponsors the Geriatric Nursing Leadership Academy (GNLA) and offers a range of products and services to support the professional development and leadership growth of nurses who provide care to older adults in long-term care (LTC). Box 1.3 provides additional resources.

GERONTOLOGICAL NURSING EDUCATION

Essential educational competencies and academic standards for care of older adults have been developed by national organizations such as the American Association of Colleges of Nursing (AACN) for both basic and advanced nursing education. Comprehensive competencies and curricular guidelines for baccalaureate programs were published in 2010 by the AACN and the Hartford Institute of Geriatric Nursing. In addition, gerontological nursing competencies for advanced practice graduate programs have been developed. All of these documents can be accessed from the AACN website. There are also competencies for gerontological nursing educators published by the National Hartford Center of Gerontological Nursing Excellence (Skemp & Wyman, 2019). There has been some improvement in the

BOX 1.2   Highlights of Early History of Gerontological Nursing

1906   First article is published in *American Journal of Nursing* (AJN) on care of the elderly.

1925   AJN considers geriatric nursing as a possible specialty in nursing.

1950   Newton and Anderson publish first geriatric nursing textbook.

1966   American Nurses Association (ANA) creates the Division of Geriatric Nursing.

   First master's program for clinical nurse specialists in geriatric nursing developed by Virginia Stone at Duke University.

1970   ANA establishes *Standards of Practice for Geriatric Nursing.*

1974   Certification in geriatric nursing practice offered through ANA; process implemented by Laurie Gunter and Virginia Stone.

1975   *Journal of Gerontological Nursing* published by Slack; first editor, Edna Stilwell.

1976   ANA begins certifying geriatric nurse practitioners.

   Nursing and the Aged, edited by Burnside and published by McGraw-Hill.

1979   *Education for Gerontic Nursing,* written by Gunter and Estes; suggested curricula for all levels of nursing education.

1980   *Geriatric Nursing* first published by AJN; Cynthia Kelly, editor.

1983   Florence Cellar Endowed Gerontological Nursing Chair established at Case Western Reserve University, first in the nation; Doreen Norton, first scholar to occupy chair.

   National Conference of Gerontological Nurse Practitioners established.

1984   National Gerontological Nurses Association established.

1989   ANA certifies gerontological clinical nurse specialists.

1992   Terry Fulmer of the John A. Hartford Foundation founds a major initiative to improve care of hospitalized older patients: Nurses Improving Care for Healthsystem Elders (NICHE). NICHE is an international nursing education and consultation program designed to improve geriatric care in health care organizations.

1996   John A. Hartford Foundation establishes the Institute for Geriatric Nursing at New York University under the direction of Mathy Mezey.

2007   Atlantic Philanthropies provides a grant of $500,000 to the American Academy of Nursing to improve care of older adults in nursing homes by improving the clinical skills of professional nurses (Nursing Home Collaborative).

   American Association for Long-Term Care Nurses formed.

2008   *Research in Gerontological Nursing* launched by Slack Inc; Dr. Kitty Buckwalter, editor.

   Institute of Medicine publishes *Retooling for an Aging America: Building the Health Care Workforce* report and addresses the need for enhanced geriatric competencies for the health care workforce.

   Consensus Model for Advanced Practice Registered Nurses (APRN) Regulation: Licensure, Accreditation, Certification & Education designates adult-gerontology as one of six population foci for APRNs

BOX 1.3   Resources for Best Practice

American Association of Managed Care Nurses: Certification, educational resources. http://www.aamcn.org/

American Geriatrics Society: CoCare: HELP (formerly Hospital Elder Life Program): Model of hospital care designed to prevent both delirium and functional decline. https://help.agscocare.org/About_AGS_CoCare_program_help.

American Nurses Credentialing Center: Nursing Case Management Certification (CMGT-BC): https://www.nursingworld.org/our-certifications/nursing-case-management/.

American Nurses Credentiality Center: Geriatric Nursing Certification: https://www.nursingworld.org/our-certifications/gerontological-nurse/.

APRN Gerontological Specialist–Certified (GS-C) Exam: https://www.gapna.org/certification.

CARES Dementia-Friendly Hospitals: Online training program to improve care of individuals with dementia in acute care. https://hcinteractive.com/hospitals.

Case Management Society of America: Standards of practice, certification, educational resources. https://www.cmsa.org/.

Core Competencies for Gerontological Nurse Educators: https://www.nhcgne.org/core-competencies-for-gerontological-nursing-excellence.

End of Life Nursing Education Consortium (ELNEC): Education programs for end-of-life care. https://www.aacnnursing.org/ELNEC.

Hartford Institute for Geriatric Nursing: Try This Series: assessment tools for best practices of care for older adults. https://hign.org/consultgeri-resources/try-this-series.

Hospice & Palliative Nurses Association: Education, research, certification examination (Certified Hospice and Palliative Nurse). https://advancingexpertcare.org/.

National Hartford Center of Gerontological Nursing Excellence: https://www.nhcgne.org/.

National Hospice and Palliative Care Organization: https://www.nhpco.org/.

amount of geriatrics-related content in nursing school curricula, but it is still uneven across schools and hampered by lack of faculty expertise in the subject.

The vast majority of schools have no faculty members certified in gerontological nursing by the American Nurses Credentialing Center. There is a critical need for nurses with master's and doctoral preparation and expertise in the care of older adults to assume faculty roles. Most schools still do not have freestanding courses in

the specialty that are similar to courses in maternal/child or psychiatric nursing. This means that a substantial number of graduating nurses have not had the education needed to competently meet the needs of the burgeoning number of older adults for whom they will care. "In the past, nursing education has been dogged about assuring that every student has the opportunity to attend a birth, but has never insisted that every student have the opportunity to manage a death, even though the vast majority of nurses are more likely to practice with clients who are at the end of life" (AACN, 2007, p. 7). Best-practice recommendations for nursing education include provision of a stand-alone course, as well as integration of content throughout the curriculum so that care of older adults is valued and considered an integral part of nursing care.

Curriculum and clinical experiences have to be inspirational and so do faculty and clinical mentors teaching students.

Care of older adults now covers a 50-year span of ages 60 to 110 and older, so there need to be practice experiences in a variety of settings, including the community and LTC (Kydd et al., 2014). Experiences with well older adults in the community and opportunities to focus on health promotion should be the first experience for students. This will assist them to develop more positive attitudes, understand the full scope of nursing practice with older adults, and learn nursing responses to enhance health and wellness. Practice in rehabilitation centers, subacute and skilled nursing facilities (SNFs), and hospice settings is suited for more advanced students and provides opportunities for leadership experience, nursing management of complex problems, interprofessional teamwork, and research application (Sherman & Touhy, 2017).

ORGANIZATIONS DEVOTED TO GERONTOLOGY RESEARCH AND PRACTICE

The Gerontological Society of America (GSA) demonstrates the need for interdisciplinary collaboration in research and practice. The divisions of Biological Sciences, Health Sciences, Behavioral and Social Sciences, Social Research, Policy and Practice, and Emerging Scholar and Professional Organization include individuals from myriad backgrounds and disciplines who affiliate with a section based on their particular function rather than their educational or professional credentials. Nurses can be found in all sections and occupy important positions as officers and committee chairs in the GSA.

This mingling of the disciplines based on practice interests is also characteristic of the American Society on Aging (ASA). Other interdisciplinary organizations have joined forces to strengthen the field. The Association for Gerontology in Higher Education (AGHE) has partnered with the GSA, and the National Council on Aging (NCOA) is affiliated with the ASA. These organizations and others have encouraged the blending of ideas and functions, furthering the understanding of aging and the interprofessional collaboration necessary for optimal care. International gerontology associations, such as the International Federation on Ageing and the International Association of Gerontology and Geriatrics, also have interdisciplinary membership and offer the opportunity to study aging internationally.

Organizations specific to gerontological nursing include the National Gerontological Nursing Association (NGNA), Gerontological Advanced Practice Nurses Association (GAPNA), National Association of Directors of Nursing Administration in Long Term Care (NADONA/LTC) (also includes assisted living RNs and licensed practical/vocational nurses [LPNs/LVNs] as associate members), American Association of Directors of Nursing Services (AADNS), American Assisted Living Nurses Association (AALNA), and Canadian Gerontological Nursing Association (CGNA).

RESEARCH ON AGING

Inquiry into and curiosity about aging is as old as curiosity about life and death itself. Gerontology began as an inquiry into the characteristics of long-lived people, and we are still intrigued by them. Anecdotal evidence was used in the past to illustrate issues assumed to be universal. Only in the past 60 years have serious and carefully controlled research studies on aging flourished. The impact of disease morbidity and impending death on the quality of life and the experience of aging have provided the impetus for much of the study by gerontologists. Much that has been thought about aging has been found to be erroneous, and early research was conducted with older adults who were ill. As a result, aging has been inevitably seen through the distorted lens of disease. However, we are finally recognizing that aging and disease are separate entities, although frequent companions.

Aging has been seen as a biomedical problem that must be reversed, eradicated, or controlled for as long as possible. The trend toward the medicalization of aging has influenced the general public as well. The biomedical view of the "problem" of aging is reinforced on all sides. A shift in the view of aging to one that centers on the potential for health, wholeness, and quality of life, and the significant contributions of older adults to society, is increasingly the focus in research, popular literature, the public portrayal of older adults, and the theme of this text.

The National Institute on Aging (NIA), National Institute of Nursing Research (NINR), National Institute of Mental Health (NIMH), and Agency for Healthcare Research and Quality (AHRQ) continue to make significant research contributions to our understanding of older adults. Research and knowledge about aging are strongly influenced by federal bulletins that are distributed nationwide to indicate the type of research most likely to receive federal funding. These are published in requests for proposals (RFPs). Ongoing and projected budget cuts are of concern in the adequate funding of aging research and services in the United States.

Nursing Research

Nursing research draws from its own body of knowledge, as well as from other disciplines, to describe, monitor, protect, and evaluate the quality of life while aging and the services more commonly provided to the aging population, such as hospice care. Nurses have generated significant research on the care of older adults and have established a solid foundation for the practice of gerontological nursing. Research with older adults receives considerable funding from the NINR, and its website (http://www.ninr .nih.gov) provides information about results of studies and funding opportunities. Gerontological nurse researchers publish in many nursing journals and journals devoted to gerontology, such as *The Gerontologist* and *Journal of Gerontology* (GSA), and there are several gerontological nursing journals, including *Journal of Gerontological Nursing, Research in Gerontological Nursing, Geriatric Nursing,* and the *International Journal of Older People Nursing.*

Knowledge about aging and the lived experience of aging has changed considerably and will continue to change in the future. Past ideas and current practices will not be acceptable to present and current cohorts of older individuals. Nursing research will continue to examine the best practices for care of older adults who

BOX 1.4   Suggestions for Gerontological Nursing Research

- Staffing patterns and the most appropriate staffing mix to improve care outcomes in long-term care settings
- Strategies to increase preparation in gerontological nursing and increase recruitment into the specialty
- Gay, lesbian, bisexual, transgender couples, families, and relationships
- Dementia as a chronic illness and staying well with the disease
- Interventions for drug and alcohol abuse and mental health problems of current and future generations of older adults
- Integration of current best practice protocols into settings across the continuum in cost-effective and care-efficient models
- Health promotion and illness management interventions in the assisted living setting; role of professional nurses and advanced practice nurses in this setting
- Development of models for end-of-life care in the home and nursing home
- Aging in developing countries
- Older adults in the context of natural disaster management

are ill and living in institutions, but increasing emphasis will be placed on strategies to maintain and improve health while aging. In 2021, Young stressed the critical need for gerontological nursing research to address: "1) the growing heterogeneity of older adults with three generations older than 65 with a wide range of priorities, strengths, and abilities; 2) the growing diversity of the aging population, with increases in the proportion of Latinx, African American, and LGBTQ older adults; and 3) the invisible family workforce of caregivers who provide the majority of long-term care for older adults" (Young, 2021, p. 2) (Chapter 32).

Other research priorities include a focus on community and home care resources, primary and acute care provided to older adults, improving quality of life for individuals with chronic illness, end-of-life and palliative care, translational research, interprofessional studies, and societal and policy issues affecting older adults. The urgent need for gerontological nursing research has been amplified by the "triple pandemic of COVID-19, racism, and ageism. The pandemic has revealed health inequities and systemic racism. The pandemic has also prompted a faster pace of change and invention, as communities, health systems, and academic settings respond to new demands" (Young, 2021, p. 2). Schutte (2020) suggests the following goals for a research agenda focused on the health of older adults during the COVID-19 pandemic: (1) mitigating harms during the expected ongoing waxes and wanes of the current pandemic; and (2) preventing harm in future large-scale disruptions (whether infectious disease outbreaks, natural disasters, or other rapid change). Other suggestions for nursing research are provided in Box 1.4.

GERONTOLOGICAL NURSING ROLES

Gerontological nursing roles encompass every imaginable venue and circumstance. The opportunities are limitless because we are a rapidly aging society. Specialized knowledge in gerontological nursing is essential for nurses to fulfill these emerging roles. In 2019, the National Council of State Boards of Nursing (NCSBN) identified the need to enhance the clinical judgment skills of entry-level nurses, and the National Council Licensure

Examination (NCLEX) will be modified toward a greater focus on clinical judgment. Using the NCSBN Clinical Judgment Measurement Model and Action Model, our emphasis in the text is on use of the six cognitive skills identified as essential for nurses to make appropriate clinical judgment in the care of older adults: Recognize Cues, Analyze Cues, Prioritize Hypotheses, Generate Solutions, Take Action, Evaluate Outcomes.

The Essentials: Core Competencies for Professional Nursing Education (AACN, 2021) identifies clinical judgment as one of the key attributes of professional nursing. Clinical judgment refers to the process by which nurses make decisions based on nursing knowledge (evidence, theories, ways or patterns of knowing), other disciplinary knowledge, critical thinking, and clinical reasoning (Manetti, 2019). This process is used to understand and interpret information in the delivery of care. Clinical decision making based on clinical judgment is directly related to care outcomes.

Increasing client age and acuity, as well as changes in health care, make this especially important for nurses who care for older adults. The dearth of curricular content, as well as inadequate faculty preparation and interest in care of older adults, makes improvement of clinical judgment skills in the care of older adults challenging. Older adults are complex, and their responses to illness may not meet standard diagnostic criteria and are often missed, leading to unnecessary disability, complications, and quality-of-life issues. Nurses are key to recognizing and analyzing cues and taking action to improve outcomes of care. The text provides comprehensive information to guide the development of competent clinical judgment in nursing practice with older adults across the continuum of care.

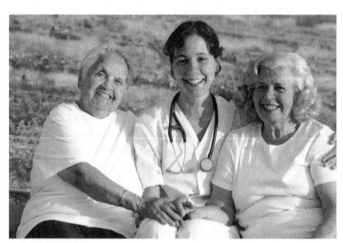

Gerontological nursing is important in our rapidly aging society. (© iStock.com/DianaHirsch.)

A gerontological nurse may be a generalist or a specialist. The generalist functions in a variety of settings (primary care, acute care, home care, post–acute and LTC, and the community), providing nursing care to individuals and their families. National certification as a gerontological nurse is a way to demonstrate one's special knowledge in the care of older adults and should be encouraged (https://www.nursingworld.org/our-certifications/gerontological nurse/#:~:text=The%20ANCC%20Gerontological%20Nursing%20board,specialty%20after%20initial%20RN%20licensure) (see Box 1.3). The gerontological nursing specialist has advanced preparation at the master's level and performs all the functions of a generalist but has developed advanced clinical expertise as well as an understanding of health and social policy and proficiency in planning, implementing, and evaluating health programs.

Specialist Roles

Under the Consensus Model for APRN Regulation, advanced practice registered nurses (APRNs) must be educated, certified, and licensed to practice in a role and a population. APRNs are educated in one of four roles, one of which is adult–gerontology. This population focus encompasses individuals from age 13 years (adolescent) to older adults. Titles of APRNs educated and certified across both areas of practice include Adult–Gerontology Acute Care Nurse Practitioner, Adult–Gerontology Primary Care Nurse Practitioner, and Adult–Gerontology Clinical Nurse Specialist. Certification is available for all these levels of advanced practice; in most states this is a requirement for licensure. The APRN Gerontological Specialist–Certified (GS-C) is also available to APRNs and recognizes expertise at the proficient level in managing complex older adults (see Box 1.3).

Advanced practice nurses with certification in adult–gerontology will find a full range of opportunities for collaborative and independent practice both now and in the future. Direct care sites include geriatric and family practice clinics, LTC, acute care and post–acute care facilities, home health care agencies, hospice agencies, continuing care retirement communities, assisted living facilities, managed care organizations, and specialty care clinics (e.g., Alzheimer's disease, heart failure, diabetes). Gerontological nursing specialists are also involved with community agencies such as local Area Agencies on Aging, public health departments, and national and worldwide organizations such as the Centers for Disease Control and Prevention and the World Health Organization. They function as care managers, eldercare consultants, educators, and clinicians.

One of the most important advanced practice nursing roles that emerged over the last 40 years is that of the gerontological nurse practitioner (GNP) and the gerontological clinical nurse specialist (GCNS) in SNFs. Nurse practitioners have been providing care in nursing homes in the United States since the 1970s, in Canada since 2000, and only recently in the United Kingdom. Recommendations from expert groups in the United States and Canada have called for a nurse practitioner in every nursing home, but numbers remain small and there is a need for continued attention at the policy and funding level for increased use of nurse practitioners with expertise in the care of older adults in LTC settings (Chapter 6). This role is well established, and there is strong research to support the impact of advanced practice nurses working in LTC settings (Campbell et al., 2019, 2020) (Box 1.5).

An encouraging trend is that the number of doctors and advanced practitioners in the United States who focus on providing care to individuals in skilled care facilities is increasing. The skilled nursing facility (SNF) provider is similar to the hospitalist role in acute care. This suggests the rise of a significant new specialty in medical and nursing practice that will affect patient outcomes. The Society for Post-Acute and Long-Term Medicine provides educational programs for this role (Morley, 2017).

BOX 1.5   Outcomes of Advanced Practice Nurse Working in Long-Term Care Settings

- Improvement in or reduced rate of decline in incontinence, pressure ulcers, aggressive behavior, and loss of affect in cognitively impaired residents
- Lower use of restraints with no increase in staffing, psychoactive drug use, or serious fall-related injuries
- Improved or slower decline in some health status indicators, including depression
- Improvements in meeting personal goals
- Lower hospitalization rates and costs
- Fewer emergency department visits and costs
- Improved satisfaction with care

Data from Ploeg J, Kaasalainen S, McAiney C, et al: Resident and family perceptions of the nurse practitioner role in long term care settings, *BMC Nurs* 12(1):24, 2013; Campbell T, Bayly M, Peacock S: Provision of resident-centered care by nurse practitioners in Saskatchewan long-term care facilities: qualitative findings form a mixed methods study, *Res Gerontol Nurs* 13(2):73–81, 2020.

Generalist Roles

Acute Care

Older adults often enter the health care system with admissions to acute care settings. Older adults comprise 60% of the medical-surgical patients and 46% of the critical care patients. Acutely ill older adults frequently have multiple chronic conditions and comorbidities and present many challenges. Hospitals can be dangerous for older adults. Despite almost two decades of research to counter harmful iatrogenic problems, iatrogenic complications occur in as many as 29% to 38% of hospitalized older adults, a rate three to five times higher than that seen in younger patients (Inouye et al., 2000; Parke & Hunter, 2014). Thirty-four percent of Medicare patients who were hospitalized experienced functional decline resulting in readmission (AARP, 2021). Older adults may be admitted for heart failure or pneumonia, and during their stay the condition improves; however, the person who came in walking and able to perform activities of daily living on their own often leaves unable to function (Box 1.6) (Chapter 19). In most cases, iatrogenic complications can be prevented.

Common iatrogenic complications associated with hospitalization include functional decline, pneumonia, delirium, new-onset incontinence, malnutrition, pressure ulcers, medication reactions, and falls. Many of these are geriatric syndromes that require prevention and treatment to prevent untoward consequences for older adults. The geriatric syndromes (also called geriatric giants) are discussed in Chapter 8 and in Chapters 12 to 20.

Older adults with dementia have higher rates of hospitalizations compared to their age-matched counterparts without dementia and have worse outcomes and longer hospital stays, resulting in higher costs of care than for patients without dementia (Fogg et al., 2018). Acute care hospitals generally are not equipped to provide best care to individuals with dementia (Chapter 26; Healthy People 2030 box). The CARES Dementia-Friendly Hospitals program provides dementia training in acute care settings. The online program consists of 16 video-based modules that include real-life video footage illustrating the effects of common and best practices to improve care of individuals with dementia in the acute care setting (see Box 1.3). All acute care

---

BOX 1.6 Example: The Spiral of Iatrogenesis

An 84-year-old man lives alone and has no family. He has osteoarthritis and hypertension and wears bilateral hearing aids and glasses for reading. He is independent in activities of daily living (ADLs) and instrumental activities of daily living (IADLs) and takes care of his small home. He avidly reads the newspaper, watches sports, drives, and participates in a water aerobics class at the local YMCA. He is admitted to the hospital after a fall on the sidewalk in front of his home. Neighbors called an ambulance, and he was admitted through the emergency department (ED). X-rays revealed no fractures, but he has pain in the left leg and in his back. Unfortunately, he was not wearing his hearing aids when admitted, so communication has been problematic. He often appears distracted and does not always respond readily.

He was unable to participate in the brief cognitive assessment and has been labeled confused on the chart. He has been agitated at night and not sleeping, so a benzodiazepine was ordered. An indwelling catheter was inserted in the ED, and he is being given narcotics for pain. Oral intake is poor, and he has not had a bowel movement in the 3 days since admission. He has been maintained on bedrest and identified as a high fall risk. When the catheter is removed, he is unable to hold his urine and is placed in adult briefs. His mental status has deteriorated further, and he is dehydrated, in a negative caloric balance, incontinent, and constipated. He is unable to ambulate and is considered unsafe to return home, so plans are being made to discharge him to an assisted living facility.

---

facilities need to have education, training, and institutional support for improving care of individuals with dementia (Hobday et al.,2017; Murray et al., 2019; Yates et al., 2018). *Healthy People 2030* addressed acute care of individuals with dementia.

 HEALTHY PEOPLE 2030

Older Adults: Dementias

Reduce the proportion of preventable rehospitalizations in older adults with dementia

Data from US Department of Health and Human Services, Office of Disease Prevention: *Healthy People 2030* (website), 2020. https://health.gov/healthypeople.

Recognizing the impact of iatrogenesis, both on patient outcomes and on the cost of care, the Centers for Medicare and Medicaid Services (CMS) has instituted changes that will reduce payment to hospitals relative to these often-preventable outcomes (https://www.cms.gov/medicare/medicare-fee-for-service-payment/hospitalacqcond/hospital-acquired_conditions.html). The changes target hospital-acquired conditions (HACs) that are high cost or high volume, result in a higher payment when present as a secondary diagnosis, are not present on admission, and could have reasonably been prevented through the use of evidence-based guidelines. Targeted conditions include several of the common geriatric syndromes, such as catheter-associated urinary tract infections, pressure ulcers, and falls.

To improve acute care of older adults, it is essential that all health care professionals (hospitalists, primary care providers, members of the interprofessional team, and nurses) are knowledgeable about care of older adults. "Acute care nursing specialty knowledge alone is not enough to ensure quality hospital care for older adults. Important nursing care actions are overlooked when gerontological expertise is absent from medical and surgical inpatient units. Acute care nursing of older adults must reflect a sense of responsibility for functional outcomes, not just carrying out interventions associated with biomedical concerns. Nursing care of hospitalized older adults requires integration of acute care specialty knowledge with gerontological nursing knowledge and skill" (Parke & Hunter, 2014, pp. 1574, 1579).

Roles for nurses caring for older adults in hospitals include direct care provider, care manager, discharge planner, care coordinator, transitional care, and leadership and management positions. Many acute care hospitals are adopting new models of geriatric and chronic care to meet the needs of older adults and maintain cognitive and physical function when hospitalized. These include geriatric emergency departments and specialized units such as acute care for the elderly (ACE), geriatric evaluation and management (GEM) units, and transitional care programs. These new models of care have been successful in coordinating care, maintaining physical and cognitive function, preventing iatrogenesis, and reducing the risk of delirium (Chapter 26). The American Geriatrics Society CoCare: HELP (formerly Hospital Elder Life Program) is a well-studied, effective, and innovative model of hospital care designed to prevent both delirium and functional decline. The program provides a successful intervention geared toward helping older adults maintain cognitive and physical functioning that includes early mobilization with walking and exercises (Lach, 2021) (see Box 1.3).

ACE units are distinct areas of a hospital specifically designed to reduce the incidence of functional disability of older adults occurring during hospitalization for acute medical illness (Palmer, 2018) by proactively identifying and managing geriatric syndromes to help maintain the patient's function (Box 1.7). Three randomized clinical trials and systematic review of ACE or related interventions demonstrate reduced functional disability, reduced risk of nursing home admission, and lower costs of hospitalizations. ACE principles could improve care of older adults

---

BOX 1.7 Characteristics of Acute Care for the Elderly (ACE) Units

- Patient-centered as opposed to disease-centered care
- Comprehensive geriatric assessment with emphasis on functional abilities
- Transition planning from beginning of a patient's stay
- Involvement of patient and all caregivers from physicians to family in care planning
- Interdisciplinary teams (geriatrician, nurse coordinator, nurses, physical and occupational therapists, pharmacists, dietitians, social workers) making daily rounds
- Environmental modifications such as handrails in patient rooms, bathrooms, hallways; contrasting colors to aid people with vision loss and other safety features
- Promotion of self-care activities
- Homelike atmosphere, common rooms where patients can gather to socialize and engage in cognitive stimulation and therapeutic activities

Data from Cowan-Lincoln M: *10 things geriatricians want hospitalists to know* (website), 2015. https://www.the-hospitalist.org/hospitalist/article/122103/10-things-geriatricians-want-hospitalists-know; Palmer R: The acute care for elders unit model of care, *Geriatrics* 3(3):59, 2018.

in any acute setting, and future designs of medical units for older adults should resemble the ACE unit (Palmer, 2018).

Other initiatives include Nurses Improving Care for Health-system Elders (NICHE), a program developed by the Hartford Geriatric Nursing Institute in 1992 and designed to improve outcomes for hospitalized older adults (http://www.nichepro-gram.org). NICHE-LTC recently was developed to enhance quality of care delivered to older adults in long-term and residential care facilities and is designed around the CMS Five-Star Quality Rating System (Greenberg et al., 2018) (Chapter 6). NICHE offers many opportunities for new roles for acute and LTC nurses, such as the geriatric resource nurse (GRN). The GRN role emphasizes the pivotal role of the bedside nurse in influencing outcomes of care and coordination of interprofessional activities. NICHE-LTC also uses certified geriatric nursing assistant roles to promote geriatric expertise among frontline staff. These types of initiatives will increase the need for well-prepared geriatric professionals working in interprofessional teams to deliver needed services.

Community-Based and Home-Based Care

Nurses will care for older adults in hospitals and LTC facilities, but the majority of older adults live in the community. Care will continue to move out of hospitals and LTC institutions into the community because of rapidly escalating health care costs and the person's preference to "age in place" (Chapter 21). Community-based care occurs through home and hospice care provided in persons' homes, independent senior housing complexes, retirement communities, residential care facilities such as assisted living facilities, hospice facilities, and adult day health centers. It also takes place in primary care clinics and public health departments.

Nurses in the home setting provide comprehensive assessments, including physical, functional, psychosocial, family, home, environmental, and community assessments. Care management and working with interprofessional teams are integral components of the home health nursing role. Nurses may provide and supervise care for older adults with a variety of care needs (including chronic wounds, intravenous therapy, tube feedings, unstable medical conditions, and complex medication regimens) and for those receiving rehabilitation and palliative and hospice services. Hospice care is provided in residential hospices, long-term and skilled facilities, and acute inpatient hospice units. However, most hospice care is provided in the individual's home.

Nurses are leaders in hospice care and assume roles as team leaders and direct caregivers. It is a very rewarding role, and the ability to form caring relationships with patients and families, similar to nursing in LTC settings, is a rewarding component of hospice nursing practice. Nurses described "working with the dying as an honour, as life affirming, and as encouraging them to appreciate their own lives more fully" (Ingebretsen & Sagbakken, 2016). However, nursing education in palliative care is limited, and this lack of education can be a source of moral distress for nurses working with individuals who are dying (Wolf et al., 2019). Schools of nursing must increase education and practice experiences for nursing students in home- and community-based care as well as hospice and palliative care (Research

Highlights A box). Chapter 34 discusses hospice and palliative care in greater depth.

🔬 RESEARCH HIGHLIGHTS A

Palliative Care and Moral Distress: An Institutional Survey of Critical Care Nurses

Purpose

To examine critical care nurses' perceived knowledge of palliative care, their recent experiences of moral distress, and possible relationships between these variables.

Method

The Palliative Care Competencies of Registered Nurses survey and the Moral Distress Thermometer instrument were mailed to 517 critical care nurses across 17 intensive care units at an academic health center.

Results

One hundred and sixty-seven completed questionnaires were analyzed. Age of respondents were 22 to 35 years, with fewer than 5 years of nursing practice experience. Most respondents perceived palliative care as a highly important competency but fewer than 40% of respondents reported being highly competent in any palliative care domain. Most had little palliative care education, and most reported moral distress during the study period.

Conclusions

Many critical care nurses do not feel prepared to provide palliative care and experience moral distress when palliative care is perceived as inadequate. Palliative care education must be provided to nursing students and practicing nurses to reduce barriers to palliative care.

Data from Wolf A, White K, Epstein E, et al: Palliative care and moral distress: an institutional survey of critical care nurses, *Crit Care Nurse* 39(5):38–48, 2019.

Case management and care management roles. Nurses are especially well suited for roles as case managers and care managers. There are increasing opportunities for these roles both in the care of individuals with chronic illnesses and in transitional care (discussed later in the chapter). Although the terms *case manager* and *care manager* have slightly different connotations, in practice the roles are seldom that clear and there is much overlap. Both roles include that of advocate, broker, leader, manager, counselor, negotiator, administrator, and communicator. Ideally the care manager follows the person through the entire continuum of care. Care managers must be experts regarding community resources and understand how these can best be used to meet the person's needs. They are expected to make appropriate referrals within the person's expectations and abilities and to monitor the quality of arranged services. The care or case manager is a resource person whom the older adult or caregiver can seek out for advice and counsel and for brokering (negotiating, arranging) the flow of services. As a gatekeeper, the care or case manager controls the entrances and exits to services to make sure that the individual gets what is needed without wasting resources.

Care managers usually are paid privately. Those who cannot afford the out-of-pocket expenses of purchased care management services must rely on services available through Medicaid-managed care plans or nonprofit community agencies, such as Catholic Senior Services, if available. Access to publicly funded programs varies by state and areas within the state and is dependent on state, county, and agency budgets and priorities. Hospitals, SNFs, and insurance agencies also use care or case managers. Care that is well managed is believed to be a solution to both the spiraling costs and the fragmentation of care often experienced by older individuals with multiple needs. The care manager works to optimize the resources and outcome for the client and the agency or community in which the person resides. Standards of Practice and certifications are available for care or case manager roles (see Box 1.3).

Certified Nursing Facilities

Certified nursing facilities, commonly called nursing homes, have evolved into a significant location where health care is provided across the continuum, part of long-term and postacute care (LTPAC) services. The old image of nursing homes caring for older adults in a custodial manner is no longer valid. Today, most facilities have postacute care units that more closely resemble the general medical-surgical hospital units of the past. Postacute care in nursing facilities will continue to grow with health care reform, and many new roles and opportunities for professional nursing exist in this setting (Chapter 6).

Roles for professional nursing include nursing administrator, manager, supervisor, charge nurse, educator, infection control nurse, Minimum Data Set (MDS) coordinator (Chapter 9), case manager, transitional care nurse, quality improvement coordinator, and direct care provider. Professional nurses in nursing facilities must be highly skilled in the complex care concerns of older adults, ranging from postacute care, to rehabilitation, to end-of-life care. The nurse in this setting needs specialized knowledge to be able to recognize and analyze the complexity of cues unique to individuals and families in this setting. Excellent assessment skills; ability to work with interprofessional teams in partnership with residents and families; skills in acute, rehabilitative, and palliative care; and leadership, management, supervision, and delegation skills are essential.

Practice in this setting requires independent decision making and is guided by a nursing model of care because fewer physicians and other professionals are on-site at all times. In addition, stringent federal regulations governing care practices and greater use of licensed practical nurses and nursing assistants influence the role of professional nursing in this setting. Many new nurses will enter this setting upon graduation, so it is essential to provide education and practice experiences, particularly leadership and management skills, to prepare them to function independently in this setting. The opportunity to form long-term relationships with individuals and families is valued by nurses and cited as one of the most rewarding aspects of practice in LTC facilities (Box 1.8). LTC and home-based care share similar role responsibilities and rewards for nurses. Chapter 6 provides in-depth information on LTC.

NURSING ROLES IN TRANSITIONS OF CARE ACROSS THE CONTINUUM

Care transition refers to the movement of patients from one health care practitioner or setting to another as their condition and care needs change. Older adults may have complex health care needs and often require care in multiple settings across the health-wellness continuum. This makes them and their families and/or caregivers vulnerable to poor outcomes during transitions. Despite efforts to streamline care transitions, the journey from hospital to home remains hazardous and frustrating for many patients and caregivers (Mitchell et al., 2018). An older adult may be treated by a family practitioner or internist in the community and by a hospitalist and specialists in the hospital; discharged to a postacute care setting and followed by another practitioner; and then discharged home or to a less care-intensive setting (e.g., assisted living facilities, residential care settings) where their original providers may or may not resume care.

The lack of coordinated care often contributes to serious consequences and frequent readmissions. Approximately 1 in 4 patients experiences an adverse event from medical mismanagement within 3 weeks of discharge from the hospital; 66% of those events are drug related (Jusela et al., 2017). Most health care providers practice in only one setting and are not familiar with the specific requirements of other settings. Each setting is seen as a distinct provider of services, and little collaboration exists (Jones et al., 2017) (Chapter 6). The purpose of health care reform initiatives (accountable care organizations, medical homes, bundled care) is to improve coordination and communication among providers so that the individual receives the most appropriate care in the most appropriate setting.

Readmissions: The Revolving Door

Avoidable readmissions are one of the leading problems facing the US health care system. Hospital readmission is a critical event for both the patients and the health care system, with extraordinary associated costs. One in four Medicare patients is readmitted to the hospital within 30 days of discharge. Approximately 1 in 5 emergency department visits by individuals over the age of 65 years result in readmission, even when the initial visit is for something minor (AARP, 2021). Readmissions have been a critical quality indicator for more than two decades because they cost the health care system money and they indicate incomplete discharge planning (Horney et al., 2017; Jones et al., 2017).

To address the concern of hospital readmission, the Hospital Readmissions Reduction Program (HRRP) was established in 2013 as a permanent component of Medicare's inpatient hospital payment system. The HRRP requires Medicare to reduce payments to hospitals with relatively high readmission rates for selected conditions for patients in traditional Medicare (Box 1.9). Under the HRRP, hospitals with readmission rates that exceed the national average are penalized by a reduction

---

BOX 1.8   Caring Nurse and Resident Relationships in Long-Term Care (LTC)

"The residents become our friends and surrogate family. Nowhere else in healthcare are relationships formed the way they are in LTC. I would say that we have more value for our residents as people and patients than they are given elsewhere in healthcare."

From Sherman R, Touhy T: Unpublished data from a study of nurse leader challenges and opportunities in nursing home settings, 2017.

- Acute myocardial infarction
- Heart failure
- Pneumonia
- Total hip and knee replacement
- Chronic obstructive pulmonary disease
- Coronary artery bypass surgery

in payments from the CMS across all of their Medicare admissions, not just those that resulted in readmissions.

Since the HRRP, readmission rates for the selected conditions have dropped nationwide, and the HRRP has been the impetus for many hospitals to institute—system-wide interventions to prevent readmissions that also have contributed to the decline in readmission rates. Readmission concerns have encouraged the development of closer alliances (e.g., accountable care organizations) and communication between hospitals and posthospital care providers, including SNFs, home health, and primary care. Hospital readmission rates are posted on the CMS Hospital Compare website (Boccuti & Casillas, 2017).

In addition, 30-day readmissions to acute care for patients at SNFs are common and preventable. Medicare patients discharged to an SNF have a 25% likelihood of readmission within 30 days, with a quarter readmitted to the hospital in the first week (Mendu et al., 2018). Individuals with dementia are an especially high-risk group for readmissions. Challenges unique to this population include the need for dementia care expertise among the team, the reliance on the caregiver as an essential member of the team, the need for caregiver education and preparation, and the challenges of behavioral symptom management (Hirschman & Hodgson, 2018).

Interventions to Reduce Acute Care Transfers (INTERACT) is an exemplary program for reducing the frequency of transfers to acute care hospitals from SNFs. INTERACT is a quality improvement program with communication tools, care paths or clinical tools, and advance care planning tools to assist nursing homes in identifying and managing acute changes in condition without hospital transfer when safe and feasible (https://pathway-interact.com/). Other successful interventions include the use of nurse practitioners working as part of collaborative teams with physicians, standardized admission assessments, palliative care consultations for residents with recurrent hospitalizations, and interprofessional case conferences. A decision aid based on nursing research, *"Go to the hospital or stay here?"* (Tappen et al., 2020), has been found to help families make decisions about whether to have a family member stay in the nursing home or transfer to acute care when there is a change in condition (Box 1.10).

Multiple factors contribute to poor outcomes during transitions: patient, provider, and system (Boxes 1.11 and 1.12). Coordination and communication between settings contribute to poor outcomes during transitions (especially between acute care and SNFs), as does medication management. Contributing factors related to medication management include complex medication regimes, a lack of recognition by health professionals of

the medication activities performed by families, haphazard and disorganized medication plans of care, and a lack of shared decision making (Manias et al., 2019).

BOX 1.12   Clinical Judgment: Transitional Care

Story of Mr. Jordan

Mr. Jordan is a 68-year-old retired farm laborer who was readmitted for heart failure 10 days after hospital discharge. He lives alone in a rural community, has no friends or family to assist in his care, and was not given a referral for home health care follow-up. His medical records document teaching about medication usage and his ability to repeat back the instructions correctly. On his first postdischarge medical visit, he brought all his pill bottles in a bag; all the bottles were full, not one had been opened. When questioned why he had not taken his medication, he looked away and began to cry, explaining that he had never learned to read and could not read the instructions on the bottles.

Suggested Solutions and Nursing Actions

Adequate discharge planning is essential upon hospital discharge. Risk factors for this man's readmission include low literacy, living alone, and complex chronic illness. Suggested interventions are 1) assessment of literacy and adaptations of health teaching; 2) collaboration with a pharmacist to develop a person-centered plan of care for medication administration, medication reconciliation; 3) determination of the most appropriate setting for posthospital care; 4) informing the patient about symptoms that should be reported after discharge; and 5) social work collaboration to identify community resources and other forms of assistance and support (e.g., Meals on Wheels, transportation).

Adapted from Center for Patient Safety: *Hot topics in healthcare: transitions of care: the need for a more effective approach to continuing patient care* (website), 2020. https://www.centerforpatientsafety.org/resource/hot-topics-in-healthcare-transitions-of-care-the-need-for-a-more-effective-approach-to-continuing-patient-care/. Accessed January 2020.

BOX 1.13   Factors Associated With Readmission Risk

- The presence of complex comorbidities
- Sensory impairment
- Functional decline
- Cognitive dysfunction
- Poor communication between disciplines and across sites of care
- Inadequate discharge planning and involvement of caregivers
- Increasing acuity of patients in skilled nursing facilities (SNFs)
- Inadequate reimbursement for postacute care and staff shortages
- Shorter hospital stays
- Increasing acuity of patients in SNFs
- Scarcity of geriatric trained professionals
- Inadequate knowledge and use of evidence-based protocols for geriatric care
- Social concerns (e.g., isolation, living situation, lack of caregiver support, socioeconomic factors)
- Language and literacy
- Culture
- Place of residence and health care available
- Inadequate end-of-life planning or advance directives

Other factors contributing to poor outcomes identified in the literature are presented in Box 1.13. The importance of feeling cared for and cared about has been found to be a desired outcome of excellent transitional care in studies with patients and caregivers (Research Highlights B box).

RESEARCH HIGHLIGHTS B

Care Transitions From Patient and Caregiver Perspectives

Purpose

The aims of this study were to (1) describe patient and caregiver experiences during care transition and (2) characterize patient and caregiver desired outcomes of care transitions and the health services associated with them.

Method

Interviews with 138 patients and 110 family caregivers recruited from 6 health networks in the United States. Forty-four focus groups were conducted, and audio transcripts were transcribed and analyzed using principles of grounded theory to identify themes and the relationship between them.

Results

Patients and caregivers identified three desired outcomes of care transition services: (1) to feel cared for and cared about by medical providers; (2) to have accountability from the health care system; and (3) to feel prepared and capable of implementing care plans. Five care transition services deemed important to achieving the outcomes were: (1) using empathic language and gestures; (2) anticipating patient needs to support self-care at home; (3) collaborative discharge planning; (4) providing actionable information; and (5) providing uninterrupted care with minimal handoffs.

Conclusion

Clear accountability, continuity of care, and caring attitudes across the care continuum are important outcomes for patients and caregivers. When these outcomes are achieved, care is perceived as trustworthy and excellent. Otherwise the care transition is experienced as unsafe and leaves patients and caregivers feeling abandoned by the health care system.

Data from Mitchell S, Laurens V, Weigel G, et al: Care transitions from patient and caregiver perspectives, *Ann Fam Med* 16(3):225–231, 2018.

Using Clinical Judgment to Promote Healthy Aging: Transitional Care

Solutions, Nursing Actions, and Outcomes

Transitional care "refers to a broad range of time-limited services to ensure health care continuity, avoid preventable poor outcomes among at-risk populations, and promote the safe and timely transfer of these patient groups from one level of care (e.g., acute to subacute) or setting (e.g., hospital to home) to another" (Naylor, 2012, p. 116). National attention to improving patient safety during transfers and preventing avoidable readmissions is increasing, and a growing body of evidence-based research provides data for design of care to improve transition outcomes.

Nurse researchers Dorothy Brooten and Mary Naylor, along with their colleagues, have significantly contributed to knowledge in the area of transitional care and the critical role of nurses in transitional care improvement. The Transitional Care Model (TCM) is a rigorously tested, comprehensive advanced practice model of care that starts in the hospital and continues through SNFs and back to the community. The TCM focuses on person-centered care; education and promotion of self-managed care; and continuity, collaboration, and care coordination with all members of the interprofessional team. The TCM has been one of the most rigorously studied transitional care approaches and has demonstrated reductions in preventable hospital readmissions, improvements in health outcomes, improved care transitions for individuals with dementia and their caregivers, enhancement in patient satisfaction, and reductions in total health care costs (Garcia, 2017; Hirschman & Hodgson, 2018).

Nurses in acute and long-term care are uniquely positioned to play a lead role in transitional care to improve outcomes and form a "bridge across settings" (Jones et al., 2017, p 18). This will require closer collaboration and knowledge of the settings and valuing of the different nursing practice roles. In addition to roles as care managers and transition coaches, nurses play a key role in many of the elements of successful transitional care models, such as medication management, patient and family caregiver education, comprehensive discharge planning, and adequate and timely communication between providers and sites of service.

The nursing role in discharge planning and patient and family education is critical. Engaging patients and families in learning about care required after discharge contributes to improved outcomes. Teaching must be based on a complete assessment of the unique needs of the individual and adapted to ensure understanding (Chapter 8). Patients who lack the knowledge, skills, and confidence to manage their own care after discharge have nearly twice the rate of readmissions as patients with the highest level of engagement (Kangovi et al., 2014; Schneidermann & Critchfield, 2012–13). Box 1.14 gives tips for best practice in preventing readmissions.

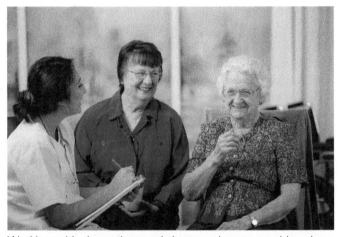

Working with the patient and the caregiver to provide education to enhance self-care abilities and to facilitate linkages to resources is important to promote safe discharges and transitions to home and other care settings. (©iStock.com/Pamela Moore.)

BOX 1.14   Tips for Best Practice
Nursing Role in Preventing Readmissions

- Identify patients at high risk for poor outcomes (e.g., low literacy, living alone, frequent or recent hospitalizations, complex chronic illness, cognitive impairment, socioeconomic deprivation).
- Adapt patient teaching for health literacy, language, culture, cognitive function, and sensory deficits.
- Determine most appropriate setting for posthospital care and educate discharge planners and family about capacity of skilled nursing facility (SNF) to care for high-risk patients (see Chapter 6, Box 6.13).
- Timely transfer of accurate information between hospital and SNF, including direct communication of time-sensitive information critical to care of high-risk patients (phone, secure text, or other form of protected health information technology).
- More intensive monitoring of high-risk patients upon admission to SNF (more frequent vital signs, including weight in patients with congestive heart failure, and pulse oximetry in patents at risk for hypoxia, and specific monitoring for high-risk conditions in this patient population, including volume depletion, bleeding, and hypoglycemia or hyperglycemia in adults with diabetes.
- Discussion of goals of care and advance directive status; palliative or hospice care consultations as appropriate.
- Provide a complete and updated medication record; explain purpose of all medications, side effects, correct dosing, and how to obtain more medication. Evaluate barriers to successful medication management (delirium, financial, transportation).
- Perform a medication reconciliation.
- Assist in establishing a regimen for proper administration of medication (consider patient's usual routine when developing a plan of care).
- Discuss symptoms that should be reported after discharge and how to contact provider; provide follow-up plan for how outstanding diagnostic tests and follow-up appointments will be completed.
- Coach patient and family in self-care skills and encourage active involvement in care.

New roles for nursing are emerging in the era of health care reform and heightened attention to improved patient outcomes. Nursing education must prepare graduates to develop the clinical judgment skills to practice effectively in roles across the continuum and work collaboratively to improve care outcomes, particularly during times of transition. We can no longer work in our individual "silos" and not be concerned with what happens after the patient is out of our particular unit or institution. Nurses are well positioned "to create services and environments that embrace values that are at the core of this profession—patient/caregiver centered care, communication and collaboration, and continuity" (Naylor, 2012, p. 140).

KEY CONCEPTS

- Older adults are complex, and their responses to illness may not meet standard diagnostic criteria and are often missed, leading to unnecessary disability, complications, and quality-of-life issues. Nurses are key to recognizing and analyzing cues and taking action to improve outcomes of care through competent clinical judgment.

- The major changes in health care delivery and the increasing number of older adults have resulted in numerous revised, refined, and emergent roles for nurses in the field of gerontological nursing. There is a critical shortage of nurses and nurse educators with expertise in care of older adults.

- Nursing has led the field of gerontology, and nurses were the first professionals in the United States to be certified as geriatric specialists.
- Advanced practice role opportunities for nurses are numerous and seen as potentially cost-effective in health care delivery while facilitating more holistic care.
- Professional nursing involvement is an essential component in models to improve transitions of care across the continuum.

NEXT-GENERATION NCLEX® (NGN) EXAMINATION–STYLE QUESTIONS

The registered nurse (RN) at a long-term care agency is providing orientation and education to new assistive personnel (AP) who have limited experience working with older adults. All of the new AP are eager to learn and to provide assistance to the residents. After the orientation, the RN asks if there are any questions or comments from the AP before they begin working on a care unit.

From the following list, select three statements made by new AP that require the RN to provide further education.

1. "When caring for older adults, we may have patients who are age 50 and older."
2. "We should report any new or unusual resident behavior to the nurse promptly."
3. "It sounds like residents with dementia are at high risk for hospital readmissions."
4. "Forming professional relationships with residents on hospice is important to me."
5. "I might be called upon by the nurse to provide teaching to the resident and family."
6. "The older adult population will continue to increase in number in the coming years."
7. "An Adult-Gerontology Nurse Practitioner can provide primary care for our residents."
8. "I worked with children in my previous job, so caring for older adults will be very similar."

CLINICAL JUDGMENT QUESTIONS AND ACTIVITIES

1. Discuss your clinical education experiences and reflect on how they have influenced your views about care of older adults and gerontological nursing.
2. Reflect on the Recommended Baccalaureate Competencies and Curricular Guidelines for the Nursing Care of Older Adults (Appendix 1.1). Which have you had the opportunity to encounter in your nursing program?
3. Review one of the gerontological nursing journals (*Geriatric Nursing, Journal of Gerontological Nursing, Research in Gerontological Nursing*) and choose a research study of interest to you. How could you use the findings of the study in your clinical practice with older adults?
4. You are asked to write a small proposal for a research project related to care of older adults. What would be the focus of your research and why?
5. Based on your experience in the acute care setting, what would you suggest to improve transitions to other care settings? Discuss any experience you or your friends and family may have had with transitions after hospital discharge.

RESEARCH QUESTIONS

1. Which aspects of gerontological nursing roles do practicing nurses find most rewarding and which do they find most challenging?
2. Why do so few students choose gerontological nursing as an area of practice? What factors might encourage more interest in the specialty?
3. What is the actual amount of time in the curricula of baccalaureate nursing schools spent on content and practice experiences related to the care of older adults?
4. How do nurses perceive their role in transitional care?

REFERENCES

AARP: Explaining post-hospital syndrome, *AARP Bulletin* April:32, 2021.

American Association of Colleges of Nursing: *White paper on the education and role of the clinical nurse leader* (website), 2007. https://www.aacnnursing.org/Portals/42/AcademicNursing/pdf/Essentials-2021.pdf. Accessed February 2021.

American Association of Colleges of Nursing: (2021): The essentials: core competencies for professional nursing education of baccalaureate education for professional nursing practice, https://www.aacnnursing.org/Portals/42/AcademicNursing/pdf/Essentials-2021.pdf. Accessed February 4, 2022.

American Nurses Association: *Gerontological nursing: scope and standards of practice*, ed. 2, Silver Springs MD, 2018, Nursebooks.org.

Boccuti C, Casillas G: *Aiming for fewer hospital U-turns: the Medicare hospital readmission reduction program, issue brief* (website), 2017. https://www.kff.org/medicare/issue-brief/aiming-for-fewer-hospital-u-turns-the-medicare-hospital-readmission-reduction-program/. Accessed June 2021.

Campbell T, Bayly M, Peacock S: Provision of resident-centered care by nurse practitioners in Saskatchewan long-term care facilities: qualitative findings from a mixed methods study, *Res Gerontol Nurs* 6:1–9, 2019.

Campbell T, Bayly M, Peacock S: Provision of resident-centered care by nurse practitioners in Saskatchewan long-term care facilities, *Res Gerontol Nurs* 13(2):73, 2020.

Fogg C, Griffiths P, Meredith P, et al.: Hospital outcomes of older people with cognitive impairment: an integrative review, *Int J Geriatr Psychiatry* 33(9):1177–1197, 2018.

Garcia C: A literature review of heart failure: transitional care interventions, *Am J Accountable Care* 5(3):21–25, 2017.

Greenberg S, Greenberg SA, Gilmartin M, et al.: NICHE (nurses improving care for healthsystem elders) program: long-term care, *JAMDA* 19(3):PB12–PB13, 2018.

Hain D, Tappen R, Diaz S, et al.: Characteristics of older adults rehospitalized within 7 and 30 days of discharge: implications for nursing practice, *J Gerontol Nurs* 38(8):32–44, 2012.

Hirschman K, Hodgson N: Evidence-based interventions for transitions in care for individuals living with dementia, *Gerontologist* 58(Suppl. 1):S129–S140, 2018.

Hobday J, Gaugler J, Mittelman M: Feasibility and utility of online dementia care training for hospital staff: the CARES dementia-friendly-hospital program, *Res Gerontol Nurs* 10(2):58–65, 2017.

Horney C, Capp R, Boxer R, et al.: Factors associated with early readmission among patients discharged to post-acute care facilities, *J Am Geriatr Soc* 65(6):1199–1205, 2017.

Ingebretsen L, Sagbakken M: Hospice nurses' emotional challenges in their encounters with the dying, *Int J Qual Stud Health Well-being*, 11, 2016.

Inouye S, Bogardus S, Baker D, et al.: The Hospital Elder Life Program: a model of care to prevent cognitive and functional decline in older hospitalized patients, *J Am Geriatr Soc* 48(12):1697–1706, 2000.

Institute of Medicine, National Academies: *Retooling for an aging America: building the health care workforce* (website), 2008. http://www.nationalacademies.org/hmd/reports/2008/retooling-for-an-aging-america-building-the-health-care-workforce.aspx/. Accessed February 2021.

Jones J, Lawrence E, Ladebue A, et al.: Nurses' role in managing "the fit" of older adults in skilled nursing facilities, *J Gerontol Nurs* 43(12):11–19, 2017.

Jusela C, Struble L, Gallagher N, et al.: Communication between acute care hospitals and skilled nursing facilities during care transitions: a retrospective chart review, *J Gerontol Nurs* 43(3):19–28, 2017.

Kangovi S, Barg F, Carter T, et al.: Challenges faced by patients with low socioeconomic status during the post-hospital transition, *J Gen Intern Med* 29(2):283–289, 2014.

Kydd A, Engstrom G, Touhy T, et al.: Attitudes of nurses, and student nurses towards working with older people and to gerontological nursing as a career in Germany, Scotland, Slovenia, Sweden, Japan and the United States, *Int J Nurs Educ* 6(2):33–40, 2014.

Lach H: Home sweet home: resources for promoting mobility for aging in place across settings, *J Gerontol Nurs*, 47(5), 2021.

Manetti W: Sound clinical judgment in nursing: a concept analysis, *Nurs Forum* 54(1):102–110, 2019.

Manias E, Bucknall T, Hughes C, et al.: Family involvement in managing medications of older patients across transitions of care, *BMC Geriatrics*, 19(95), 2019.

Mendu M, Michaelidis C, Chu M, et al.: Implementation of a skilled nursing facility readmission review process, *BMC Open Quality*, 7(3):e000245, 2018.

Mitchell S, Laurens V, Weigel G, et al.: Care transitions from patient and caregiver perspective, *Ann Fam Med* 16(3):225–231, 2018.

Morley J: The future of long-term care, *J Am Med Dir Assoc* 18:1–7, 2017.

Murray M, Shee A, West E, et al.: Impact of the Dementia Care in Hospitals program on acute hospital staff satisfaction, *BMC Health Serv Res* 19:680, 2019.

Naylor M: Advancing high value transitional care: the central role of nursing and its leadership, *Nurs Admin Q* 36(2):115–126, 2012.

Palmer R: The acute care for elders unit model of care, *Geriatrics* 3(3):59, 2018.

Parke B, Hunter K: The care of older adults in hospital: if it's common sense why isn't it common practice? *J Clin Nurs* 23:1573–1582, 2014.

Robert Wood Johnson Foundation: *The revolving door: a report on U.S. hospital readmission*, (website), 2013. http://www.rwjf.org/content/dam/farm/reports/reports/2013/rwjf404178. Accessed February

Schneidermann M, Critchfield J: Customizing the "teachable moment": ways to address hospital transitions in a culturally conscious manner, *Generations* 36(4):94–97, 2012–13.

Schutte D: Research goals during and beyond the COVID-19 pandemic: reframing older adults as essential and priceless, *Res Gerontol Nurs* 13(3):118–119, 2020.

Sherman R, Touhy T: An exploratory descriptive study to evaluate Florida nurse leader challenges and opportunities in nursing homes settings, *SAGE Open Nurs* 3:1–7, 2017.

Skemp L, Wyman J: Promoting quality instruction in the care of older adults: core competencies for gerontological nurse educators, *J Gerontol Nurs*, 45(10), 2019.

Tappen R, Worch S, Newman D, et al.: Evaluation of a novel decision guide "Go to the Hospital or Stay Here?" for nursing home residents and families: a randomized trial, *Res Gerontol Nurs* 13(6):309–317, 2020.

Taylor M: Mapping the literature of pediatric nursing, *J Med Libr Assoc* 92(2 Suppl):E128–E136, 2006.

Tong M, Thomas J, Patel S, et al.: Nursing home medication reconciliation: a quality improvement initiative, *J Gerontol Nurs* 43(4):9–14, 2017.

Wolf A, White K, Epstein E, et al.: Palliative care and moral distress: an institutional survey of critical care nurses, *Crit Care Nurse* 39(5):38–48, 2019.

Yates M, Watts J, Bail K, et al.: Evaluating the impact of the Dementia Care in Hospitals Program (DCHP) on hospital-acquired complications: study protocol, *Int J Environ Res Public Health* 15(9):1878, 2018.

Young H: The inflection point: increased urgency for high impact gerontological nursing research, *Res Gerontol Nurs* 14(1):2–3, 2021.

Recommended Baccalaureate Competencies and Curricular Guidelines for the Nursing Care of Older Adults
Gerontological Nursing Competency Statements

1. Incorporate professional attitudes, values, and expectations about physical and mental aging in the provision of patient-centered care for older adults and their families.
2. Assess barriers for older adults in receiving, understanding, and giving of information.
3. Use valid and reliable assessment tools to guide nursing practice for older adults.
4. Assess the living environment as it relates to functional, physical, cognitive, psychological, and social needs of older adults.
5. Intervene to assist older adults and their support network to achieve personal goals, based on the analysis of the living environment and availability of community resources.
6. Identify actual or potential mistreatment (physical, mental, or financial abuse, and/or self-neglect) in older adults and refer appropriately.
7. Implement strategies and use online guidelines to prevent and/or identify and manage geriatric syndromes.
8. Recognize and respect the variations of care, the increased complexity, and the increased use of health care resources inherent in caring for older adults.
9. Recognize the complex interaction of acute and chronic comorbid physical and mental conditions and associated treatments common to older adults.
10. Compare models of care that promote safe, quality physical and mental health care for older adults such as PACE, NICHE, Guided Care, Culture Change, and Transitional Care Models.
11. Facilitate ethical, noncoercive decision making by older adults and/or families/caregivers for maintaining everyday living, receiving treatment, initiating advance directives, and implementing end-of-life care.
12. Promote adherence to the evidence-based practice of providing restraint-free care (both physical and chemical restraints).
13. Integrate leadership and communication techniques that foster discussion and reflection on the extent to which diversity (among nurses, nurse assistive personnel, therapists, physicians, and patients) has the potential to impact the care of older adults.
14. Facilitate safe and effective transitions across levels of care, including acute, community-based, and long-term care (e.g., home, assisted living, hospice, nursing homes), for older adults and their families.
15. Plan patient-centered care with consideration for mental and physical health and well-being of informal and formal caregivers of older adults.
16. Advocate for timely and appropriate palliative and hospice care for older adults with physical and cognitive impairments.
17. Implement and monitor strategies to prevent risk and promote quality and safety (e.g., falls, medication mismanagement, pressure ulcers) in the nursing care of older adults with physical and cognitive needs.
18. Use resources/programs to promote functional, physical, and mental wellness in older adults.
19. Integrate relevant theories and concepts included in a liberal education into the delivery of patient-centered care for older adults.

NICHE, Nurses Improving Care for Healthsystem Elders; *PACE*, Programs of All-Inclusive Care for the Elderly.
From American Association of Colleges of Nursing, Hartford Institute for Geriatric Nursing, New York University College of Nursing: *Recommended baccalaureate competencies and curricular guidelines for the nursing care of older adults* [supplement to *The essentials of baccalaureate education for professional nursing practice*], September 2010. https://www.pogoe.org/NursingCompetencies. Accessed July 2021.

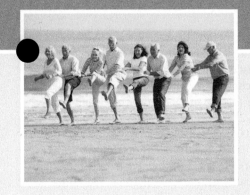

CHAPTER 2

Aging, Health, and Wellness in a Global Community

Kathleen Jett

http://evolve.elsevier.com/Touhy/TwdHlthAging

A STUDENT SPEAKS

I was so surprised when I went to the senior center and saw all those old folks doing tai chi! I feel a bit ashamed that I don't take better care of my own body.

Maggie, age 24

AN OLDER ADULT SPEAKS

Just a change in perspective! I can choose to be well or ill under any situation. I think, too often we feel like victims of circumstance. I refuse to be a victim. It is my choice and I have control.

Maria, age 86

LEARNING OBJECTIVES

On completion of this chapter, the reader will be able to:

1. Compare and contrast the historical events influencing the health and wellness of those ages 60 and older.
2. Discuss the implications of the wide range of life expectancies of older adults in different parts of the world.
3. Describe a wellness-based model that can be used to promote the health of an aging global community.
4. Discuss the multidimensional nature of wellness and its implications for healthy aging.
5. Define and describe the three levels of prevention and how each relates to nursing actions intended for older adults.
6. Develop health-promoting strategies at each level of prevention that are consistent with the wellness-based model for healthy aging.

From the perspective of Western medicine, health is defined as the absence of physical or psychiatric illness. It is measured in terms of accepted "norms," such as blood pressure readings, laboratory test results, or the absence of established signs and symptoms of illness. When any of the parameters negatively affect the ability of the individual to function independently, debility is assumed.

The measurement of a population's health status has been inferred almost entirely from life expectancy, morbidity, and mortality statistics. Although the numbers are informative, health-related quality of life and wellness of the population cannot be determined easily. Adding the examination of the common causes of death and the expectation of healthy years of life can be helpful as we move toward health promotion, disease prevention, and understanding the needs of persons with functional limitations now and in the future.

Caring for persons who are aging is a practice that touches nurses in all settings: from pediatrics involving grandparents and great-grandparents; to the residents of skilled nursing facilities and their spouses, partners, and children; to nurses providing relief support inside and outside of their own countries. The core knowledge of gerontological nursing is important for all members of the profession and is not limited to any one individual nursing specialty.

As we move forward in the 21st century, the way in which nurses respond to our aging society will determine our character; we are no greater than the health of the country and the world in which we live. Gerontological nurses can help shape the world so that persons can grow old and thrive, not merely survive. They have unique opportunities to facilitate wellness in those who are recipients of care. This text is written using a wellness-based model to guide the reader in maximizing strengths, minimizing limitations, facilitating adaptation, and encouraging growth along the continuum of health and across the continuum of care. It is about helping people move *Toward Healthy Aging.*

AGING

American physician Ignatz Nascher proposed the term *geriatrics* in recognition that the needs and medical care of persons in later life differed from that of other population groups, such as pregnant women or children. In 1914, he authored the first medical textbook on treatment of the "old" in the United States (Nascher, 1914). Aging was reflected in his eyes as it was in society—as a problem that must be reversed, eradicated, or held at bay for as long as possible.

How Old Is Old?

Each culture has its own definition of when and who is "old." Some of the terms used to name such persons are the elderly, senior citizens, elders, grannies, older adults, and tribal elders. In some cultures, elderhood is determined *functionally* when one is no longer able to perform one's usual activities (Jett, 2003). *Social aging* is often determined by changes in roles, such as retirement from one's usual occupation, appointment as a wise person of the community, or at the birth of a grandchild. Transitions may be marked by special rituals, such as birthday and retirement parties, invitations to join groups such as AARP, eligibility for age-related pensions or income, or qualifying for "senior discounts" (Box 2.1).

Biological aging is a complex and continuous process involving every cell in the body (Chapter 3). The physical and biological traits by which we identify one as "older" (e.g., gray hair, wrinkled skin) are referred to as the aging phenotype, the external expression of one's individual genetic makeup and internal changes.

Chronological aging may be used alone or combined with functional, social, or biological aging. In most developed and developing areas of the world, chronological late life is recognized as beginning sometime between 50 and 65 years of age. These arbitrary numbers had been set with the expectation that persons are in the last decade or two of their lives.

There is an ongoing controversy among demographers and gerontologists regarding the use and accuracy of chronological aging. In 1800, only 25% of men in Western Europe lived to the age of 60, yet in 2008, 90% of these men lived to the age of 90 (Sanderson & Scherbov, 2008). Elderhood now has the potential to span 40 years or more, attributable in a large part to increased access to quality health services, improved sanitation, and an emphasis on improving public health. In 1800 was one "old" at age 40? Is "old age" today delayed until age 70? How will we define old age in the future? How will the definitions, meaning, and perception of aging change as the health and wellness of individuals, communities, and nations change after the COVID-19 pandemic? How will nursing roles and responsibilities change? How can we promote wellness in those who have a much greater chance of living to age 100 and older?

THE YEARS AHEAD

In 2020, the number of persons at least 60 years of age across the globe was just over 1 billion, or 13.5% of the total global population. This number is 2.5 times greater than it was in 1980 and is expected to more than double to 2.1 billion by 2050; the majority of these older adults live or will live in middle-income countries (World Health Organization [WHO], 2020). It is expected that the number of Americans at least 65 years of age will reach 95 million by 2060 and make up 23% of the population (Mather et al., 2019). During this same period, the older population is also expected to become more ethnically and racially diverse: 45% of older adults are expected to identify with groups other than non-Hispanic White.

However, these figures may change considerably between this writing and the end of the COVID-19 pandemic, which has disproportionately affected older adults, especially those with concomitant noninfectious diseases. As of May 2021, 8 in 10 COVID-19 deaths have been among adults 65 years old and older (Centers for Disease Control and Prevention [CDC], 2021).

In 2018, the overall life expectancy at birth in the United States was 78.7 years. This represents a decrease of 0.2 and 0.1 years in the life expectancy of men and women, respectively, since 2014 after a slow increase in the years since 2000. However, there have been notable variations by racial group and gender and further variations for expectancy at different ages (Fig. 2.1) (Arias & Xu, 2020).

Unfortunately, by the fall of 2020, life expectancy at birth had dropped to 77.48 years. It has been projected that the life expectancy at the age of 65 in the United States would have been 19.4 years without COVID-19 but is expected to decline somewhere between 0.75 and 0.94 year overall. The loss of expected years is most notable for Whites at least 75 years of age, Blacks 65 to 85 years of age, and Latinx 65 to 75 years of age (Andrasfay & Goldman, 2021).

With limited data available, this decrease in longevity due to the associated increase in excess mortality (deaths that would

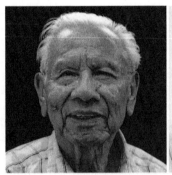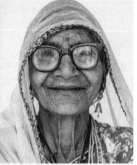

The aging phenotype. (©iStock.com/LPETTET; Mlenny.)

BOX 2.1   Becoming a "Senior"

A few years ago, I stopped coloring my hair, which is almost completely silver now. It was quite a surprise to me the first time the very young movie theater clerk assumed I was 65 and automatically gave me the "senior discount." My husband's hair is only fading to a dull brown. When he goes alone, they tentatively ask, "Do you have any discounts?"

Kathleen, at age 60

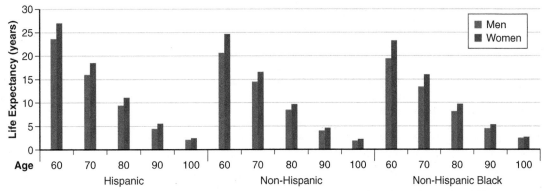

Fig. 2.1 Expectation of years of life remaining by age and sex, for Hispanic and non-Hispanic populations, United States, 2018 (pre–COVID-19).

not have occurred ordinarily). As of September 2021, the number of deaths from COVID-19 in the United States exceeded those that occurred during the Spanish flu pandemic of 1918 (Gamillo, 2021). The excessive number of deaths due to COVID-19 includes those related to untreated underlying conditions due to the overburdened health care system, decreased access to preventive health care due to unemployment and loss of health insurance, and the collateral deaths of survivors. It has been further predicted that the declines in life expectancy will most significantly affect Black and Latinx populations (Fig. 2.2). The Black-White discrepancy will have increased from 3.6 years to 5 years (38% gain), and the 3-year survivor advantages that Latinos have had (compared to Whites) will decrease from 3 years to 1 year (70% loss) (Andrasfay & Goldman, 2021). Those most at risk from COVID-19 have been older adults already in late life. This means that the change in life expectancy at birth will be less important than life expectancy at 60, 70, 80, or 90 years of age.

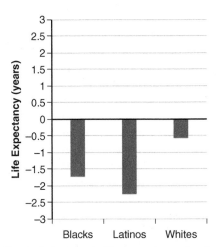

Fig. 2.2 Estimated changes in life expectancy for those at least 65 years old related to the COVID-19 pandemic, February 2, 2021. (From Andrasfay T, Goldman N: Reductions in 2020 U.S. life expectancy due to COVID-19 and the disproportionate impact on the Black and Latino population, *Proc Natl Acad Sci USA* 118(5):e2014746118, 2021.)

Although healthy aging will again become an achievable goal for many in developed and developing regions, it will still be only a distant vision for those living in less developed areas of the world, where lives are shortened by persistent communicable diseases, inadequate sanitation, and lack of both nutritious food and health care/immunizations. It is essential that nurses across the globe have the knowledge and skills necessary to help people of all ages achieve the highest level of wellness possible. Some of the questions that must be asked include the following: How can global conditions change for those who are struggling? How can the years of healthy elderhood be maximized and enriched to the extent possible, regardless of the conditions in which one lives?

Since the 1950s and 1960s, four generational subgroups have emerged: supercentenarians, centenarians, baby boomers, and those in between. The following discussions are only overviews; there is no "typical older person."

The Supercentenarians

The supercentenarians are those who live until at least 110 years of age. Their ages were first verified (to the extent possible) in the 1960s. The exact number of these very long-lived persons is unknown, but it is estimated that there may be between 150 and 600 alive today, the majority of whom are women (Aging Analytics, 2020). As of February 1, 2021, the oldest known person was 118-year-old Kane Tanaka of Fukuoka, Japan, born January 2, 1903. The second oldest, Sister André of France, a COVID-19 survivor, turned 117 years old on February 11, 2021. Although some questions have arisen, the person who is still thought to have lived the longest was France's almost 122-year-old Jeanne Calment (Allard et al., 1999) (Box 2.2).

Many of the fathers and older siblings of the oldest of this cohort fought and died in World War I (WWI; 1914–18). Most were involved with World War II (WWII; 1939–46) in some way. If they lived in Eastern Europe during the war, a supercentenarian of today may be a survivor of the Holocaust or German-occupied Europe.

In most developed countries, especially in non-tropical areas, there were no new cases of yellow fever after 1905, missing most of the supercentenarians, but cholera and typhoid still occurred during their childhoods. Many were children during the 1916

BOX 2.2 A Well-Known Supercentenarian

Mme Calment of Arles, France, was born in 1875 and died in 1997 at 122 years and 4.5 months old. When she was 90 years old, her lawyer recognized the value of the apartment in which she lived and owned and made her what turned out to be the deal of a lifetime. In exchange for the deed to the apartment, he would pay her a monthly "pension" for life, and she could live in the apartment the rest of her life. Over the next 32 years she was paid more than double the apartment's value. She also outlived the lawyer; her husband of 55 years; her daughter; and her only grandson. An active woman, she took up fencing at 85 and was still riding a bike at 100. She smoked until she was 117 and preferred a diet rich in olive oil.

From Allard M, Robine JM, Calment J: *Jeanne Calment: from Van Gogh's time to ours, 122 extraordinary years*, Waterville, ME, 1999, Thorndike Press.

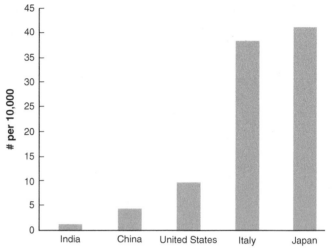

Fig. 2.3 Numbers of persons at least 100 years of age per 10,000 persons in the population (select countries). (From Stepler R: *World's centenarian population projected to grow eightfold by 2050 (website)*, 2016. https://www.pewresearch.org/fact-tank/2016/04/21/worlds-centenarian-population-projected-to-grow-eightfold-by-2050/)

polio epidemic in the United States. The sheer numbers affected by this and other communicable diseases of the early 1900s changed the view of science and the acceptance of government's role in protecting the public's health.

All supercentenarians survived the influenza pandemic of 1918 to 1919, which killed an estimated 20 million to 40 million people, or up to one-fifth of the world's population at the time. Referred to as the "Spanish flu" or "La Grippe," this outbreak began in the United States, Europe, and a small part of Asia. It spread worldwide almost overnight. The virulence was such that the period between exposure and death could be a matter of hours. In 1 year, the life expectancy in the United States dropped by 10 to 12 years, far more than is likely to occur by the end of the COVID-19 pandemic.

Several researchers who have studied supercentenarians report that most functioned independently until after age 100, with no signs of frailty until about the age of 105. They were found to be remarkably homogeneous. They rarely had cancer, stroke, or cardiovascular disease. Few had been diagnosed with dementia (Young & Kroczek, 2020). They have been found to have higher levels of endogenous cardioprotective factors and inflammatory mediators and thereby reduced sensitivity to the cellular oxidation and inflammation associated with aging (Chapter 3). One would expect to find higher concentrations of NT-proBNP (N-terminal pro-B-type natriuretic peptide), a potential surrogate for hemodynamic stress in late life, but this is not so for supercentenarians (Hirata et al., 2020).

Arai et al. (2017) found that those who were physically independent at age 100 were the most likely to live beyond age 110. While the number of supercentenarians alive today is small, it is predicted to grow as the centenarians behind them live longer and healthier lives.

The Centenarians

Centenarians are between 100 and 109 years of age, the majority of whom are between ages 100 and 104 (Meyer, 2012). Most of the men fought in WWII, when approximately 55 million of their contemporaries died. It was projected that there would be more than 570,000 persons worldwide at least 100 years of age in 2021. While the United States has the highest overall number of centenarians simply due to its large population overall, Japan

has more than double the number relative to their population (Buchholz, 2021) (Fig. 2.3).

Centenarians in the United States are overwhelmingly White women living in urban areas of the Southern states. Along with the rapidly expanding numbers in this cohort, there is an exponential increase in biological and genetic research to attempt to better understand their exceptional longevity and the underpinnings of morbidity that is compressed toward the end of their lives (Giuliani et al., 2017; Karasik & Newman, 2015). Although centenarians still carry genetic markers within their chromosomes for any number of health problems, for unknown reasons these are not "activated" until much later, if at all, when compared with other persons (Sebastiani & Perls, 2012). The relatively low number of centenarians (and supercentenarians) with dementia of any kind may be explained by the presence of some type of genetic neuroprotective factors (Takao et al., 2016). While most people have normal age-related declines in immune functioning and increases in a state of chronic inflammation, this does not appear to be the case for this group of long-lived people (Iannitti & Palmieri, 2011).

Centenarians were teenagers or young adults at the time of the Great Depression (approximately 1929–40). Jobs were scarce, and poverty and malnutrition were rampant. In areas where the water lacked natural fluoride, children's teeth were soft and cavity prone. "Pigeon chest," a malformation of the developing rib cage caused by lack of vitamin D, was common. Goiter and myxedema were less common but were present regionally because of unrecognized iodine deficiencies. Smallpox had been a threat to centenarians for more than half of their lives. Many centenarians had the "childhood" diseases of measles, mumps, chickenpox, and/or whooping cough; some had polio as children.

Those in Between (Born 1921–46)

There is a unique cohort born in the 30 years between the baby boomers (discussed in the next section) and the centenarians: the septuagenarians (70-year-olds), octogenarians (80-year-olds), and nonagenarians (90-year-olds). The number of persons between the ages of 70 and 99 is growing at an exponential rate as the baby boomers begin to join their ranks.

The oldest in this cohort were born between WWI and WWII. They may have fought in WWII, but many others fought in the Korean War or were drafted or volunteered to serve in the Vietnam War. They came of age during tumultuous times. Some witnessed or had personal experience with the American Civil Rights Movement (1955–68) or the assassination of President John F. Kennedy (1963). The Cold War was felt as the tensions between the United States and the former Soviet Union reached a fever pitch. Others lost friends and family to the global AIDS epidemic before the human immunodeficiency virus (HIV) was isolated in France and the United States in 1983. If born between about 1929 and 1939, they were children during the Great Depression. They have survived any number of childhood illnesses. They have also survived several communicable disease outbreaks and influenza pandemics (Table 2.1). As well, they have been most at risk for COVID-19 mortality.

Polio infection was a major fear for this cohort, and for some, either they or their friends were affected. A vaccine was not available to children in the United States until 1955, providing the most benefits to the youngest of the "in-betweeners." Penicillin, first discovered in 1928 by Alexander Fleming, became usable in humans in 1936 and likely prevented many infection-related mortalities since that time (Markel, 2013).

The Baby Boomers

The youngest of the "older generation" are referred to as "baby boomers" or "boomers." They were born somewhere between approximately 1946 and 1964. In the United States, the first to become baby boomers turned 65 years old in 2011; the last will do so in 2029. More babies were born in the United States in 1946, the year after the end of WWII, than in any other year—3.4 million, or 20% more than were born in 1945. These numbers increased every year until they tapered off in 1964. In just 18 years, 76.4 million babies had been born, making up 40% of the US population (History, 2021).

The differences in the life experiences between those born in the late 1940s and early 1960s are quite significant. For example, the eldest had mothers and fathers who had served in WWII, and as young adults they may have been drafted into the Vietnam War, obtained a "college deferment," or volunteered to serve in the military. The youngest in this cohort may have had only a childhood recollection, if any, of that period.

Each day another 10,000 boomers turn 65 years old (US Census Bureau, 2020). More than any previous cohort, baby boomers have had better access to medication and other preventive treatment regimens as they were growing up. They will nevertheless live longer with chronic illness than any of their predecessors (Chapter 22).

Many current chronic illnesses are related to tobacco use as they were growing up. For example, in the 1950s and 1960s smoking was not only condoned but considered a sign of status. Candy cigarettes were popular with children. Work and public places and homes were filled with smoke, affecting both the

smokers themselves and those who were exposed to second-hand smoke. The use of cigarettes peaked in 1963, near the end of the baby boom. There has been a very slow but steady decline in tobacco use since then, from 21 out of 100 adults in 2005 to 14 out of 100 in 2019. This includes 8 out of 100 adults at least 65 years of age (CDC, 2020).

Cigarette smoking is the number one cause of preventable deaths in the United States, especially from cardiovascular disease and stroke. Both have been the top causes of

TABLE 2.1 A Sampling of Events That Occurred During the Lives of Today's Older Adults

1914–18	World War I (WWI)
1915	First cross-country telephone service
1916	New York City polio epidemic
1918–19	The Spanish flu (La Grippe) H1N1 kills 20 million worldwide (500,000 in the United States)
1920	Women are "granted" the right to vote
1927	Charles Lindbergh makes the first solo transatlantic flight in the *Spirit of St. Louis*
1929–40	Great Depression; creation of the Civilian Conservation Corps to provide jobs
1932–72	Tuskegee syphilis experiment is conducted
1935	Social Security is created
1939–45	World War II (WWII)
1941	Japanese bomb Pearl Harbor, Hawaii
1942	Penicillin becomes available to the public
1945	United States drops atomic bombs on Hiroshima and Nagasaki, Japan, and WWII ends
1946	Immunization against influenza becomes available
1950–53	Korean War between Communist and non-Communist forces
1952–54	*Brown v. Board of Education*: US Supreme Court rules that segregation in public schools is unconstitutional
1955	Polio vaccine available to the public
1955–68	US Civil Rights Movement
1955–75	Vietnam War
1957–60	Asian flu H2N2 pandemic
1960	Birth control pill becomes available
1961	Alan Shepard commands first spaceflight
1963	Assassination of President John F. Kennedy
1965	Medicare and Medicaid are established
1968	My Lai massacre: US troops kill 300 Vietnamese villagers
1968	Assassination of Dr. Martin Luther King, Jr.
1968–69	Hong Kong flu H3N2 pandemic
1969	Astronauts Neil Armstrong and Buzz Aldrin walk on the moon
1973	*Roe v. Wade*: US Supreme Court rules on the legality of abortions in the first trimester
1980	World Health Organization (WHO) declares the world "smallpox free"
1981	AIDS epidemic is recognized
1983	The HIV virus, which causes AIDS, is identified
1983	First pneumococcal vaccine becomes available
2009–10	Swine flu H1N1 pandemic
2011	Second pneumococcal vaccine becomes available
2017	Highly effective Shingrix vaccine for shingles becomes available
2020	First case of COVID-19 coronavirus identified in the United States; WHO declares a COVID-19 pandemic emergency First supply of COVID-19 vaccine becomes available

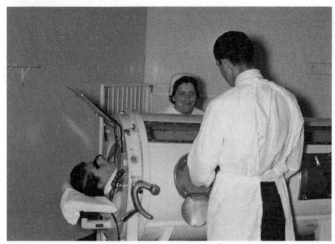

Hospital staff examining a patient in an iron lung during the Rhode Island polio epidemic, 1960. (From the Centers for Disease Control and Prevention Public Health Image Library.)

From Office of Disease Prevention and Health Promotion (ODPHP): *Healthy People 2030 framework* (website), 2020. https://www. healthypeople.gov/2020/About-Healthy-People/Development-Healthy-People-2030/Framework

> **BOX 2.3   Overarching Goals of *Healthy People 2030***
>
> - Attain healthy, thriving lives and well-being, free of preventable disease, disability, and premature death.
> - Eliminate health disparities, achieve health equity, and attain health literacy to improve the health and well-being for all.
> - Create social, physical, and economic environments that promote attaining full potential for health and well-being for all.
> - Promote healthy development, healthy behaviors, and well-being across the lifespan.
> - Engage leadership, key constituents, and the public across multiple sectors to take action and design policies that improve the health and well-being of all.

noncommunicable death worldwide for more than 15 years, accounting for 20% of deaths in the United States (CDC, 2020).

Like their older cohorts, most boomers born in the 1950s contracted at least several of the childhood diseases of measles, mumps, rubella, and chickenpox. Scarlet fever was also common. The younger boomers in developed countries have had the benefit of the availability of immunizations against more and more communicable diseases, including polio. The social emphasis today on healthier lifestyles will go far to help the older adults of the future reach higher levels of wellness, but for many of today's older adults the challenges to healthy aging are significant.

Significant Events That Occurred During the Lives of Today's Older Adults

To provide the best, most sensitive care for older adults, it is necessary to have some knowledge of the historical context in which they have lived their lives. At the same time, this would require a course in history covering at least 117 years. Instead, a list of some if the major world events that may be significant to those at least 65 years old is provided in Table 2.1. The nurse is encouraged to learn the effect that any of these events have or had on the life experience of the older adult.

The gerontological nurse also has a role in fostering wellness from a macro perspective. This includes facilitating the movement toward overarching goals set forth in *Healthy People: The Surgeon General's Report on Health Promotion and Disease Prevention* (Box 2.3). These goals have evolved from the first iteration, *Healthy People 1990*, which was published in 1979 and has been updated every 10 years since, with the most recent version published in 2020 as *Healthy People 2030* (Office of Disease Prevention and Health Promotion [ODPHP], 2020).

The outcomes and solutions appropriate to healthy older adults will differ from those for very frail older adults or those with a limited life expectancy. When select preventive actions are questionable, the nurse can contribute to health care conversations leading to the best decision for any one person. Primary

prevention strategies are those which are intended to prevent the development of a disease or illness, such as using immunizations. Secondary prevention, that is, early illness detection, such as health screening is generally not recommended for the most impaired or those with very short life expectancies, but some primary and all tertiary prevention is appropriate. For those nearing the end of life or with advanced neurocognitive impairments, the burden and benefit of lifestyle recommendations must be considered carefully. It is the responsibility of the skilled gerontological nurse to design and implement appropriate interventions for persons all along the wellness continuum: from the very active, to those with advanced cognitive impairments, to those approaching death.

A WELLNESS-BASED MODEL

The burgeoning population of persons entering their last 20 to 40 years of life presents the nurse with opportunities to make a difference in promoting wellness and stemming the tide of prolonged life that is accompanied by chronic disease and disability, especially for the baby boomers. In this text we provide basic information that can lead to the development of nursing solutions and actions to promote health in the face of the most common health challenges to late life. This is done from the perspective that a state of relative wellness can be an ongoing expectation.

We use a broad view of wellness to provide nurses with a framework for addressing the needs of our aging population. A wellness-based model encompasses the idea that health is composed of multiple dimensions. Wellness and health are expressed in functional, environmental, psychological, spiritual, social, and biological dimensions of the human experience within the context of culture. These dimensions are juxtaposed on myriad other factors, including normal changes of aging, income, education, sexual orientation, gender identity, gender, race, religion, ethnicity and country of origin, place of residence, life opportunities, and access to health care. The challenge to both living and dying in wellness is to balance each of these dimensions to the extent possible. The dimensions are like overlapping petals on a flower, anchored together at the center (Fig. 2.4). Wellness

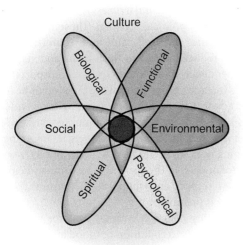

Fig. 2.4 Wellness model.

TABLE 2.2 Promoting Health and Wellness: Three Levels of Prevention With Examples of Associated Solutions and Nursing Actions			
Level	**Outcome**	**Solutions**	**Nursing Action**
Primary	Prevention of occurrence or worsening of chronic condition	Immunization Healthy diet Never smoke or stop smoking Regular exercise Stress management	Organize offerings and administer vaccinations Culturally appropriate nutritional education Lead and facilitate smoking prevention and cessation programs Role model and help person find a program that works for them Teach management techniques
Secondary	Early detection of new problem Early detection of exacerbation of chronic condition	Health screening (e.g., mammogram) Seek care in timely fashion	Monitor need for and facilitate availability of screening Educate relative to side effects, signs of changes in condition, most healthful response
Tertiary	Treatment and/or rehabilitation for acute and chronic conditions	Participate in rehabilitation Complete course of treatment	Provide active rehabilitative care Provide information regarding treatment plan

involves each of these singularly and in interaction making a fuller, richer whole.

A wellness-based model, derived from a holistic paradigm, is one in which health is viewed on a continuum. At one end there is either an absence of disease as we know it or the presence of chronic diseases that are controlled to the point where their damaging effects are minimized (e.g., a person's blood pressure reading or blood glucose level are within normal limits). At the other end of the continuum is the point when an acute episode or multiple concurrent conditions result in approaching death but one in which suffering of all kinds is minimized to the extent possible (Chapter 22). Age and illness influence the ease with which one moves along the continuum but do not define the individual.

The concept of healthy aging from a wellness perspective is uniquely defined by each individual and changes over time. The subcomponents within the wellness model particularly applicable to healthy aging are functional independence, self-care management of chronic illness and disability, positive outlook, personal growth, social contribution, and activities that promote one's health. The gerontological nurse has the opportunity and the responsibility when working with persons all along the continuum, including at the time of death, to promote wholeness and wellness as defined by the individual at any point in time.

USING CLINICAL JUDGMENT TO PROMOTE HEALTHY AGING

The gerontological nurse can use the wellness-based model to promote healthy aging across the continuum of wellness and care settings and at all levels of health promotion and disease prevention (Table 2.2). However, determining the best candidate for each level of prevention, especially health screening, depends on several key factors. Will *knowing* that one has a disease or condition change the course along the continuum and projected timing of death? Is aggressive treatment such as radiation or surgery, or even tight glycemic control, reasonable for someone with dementia or a short life expectancy (Box 2.4)? Although one

BOX 2.4 Primary Prevention in Question
A breast mass was found in a patient in a skilled nursing facility. The nurse was adamant that she should have a mammogram. Although the 85-year-old woman was still quite mobile and cheerful, she also had very advanced dementia. My inclination was to not pursue any further exam (secondary prevention). In conversation with her only living child, we agreed that the mammogram would most likely lead to a diagnosis of breast cancer but would be a hardship for her mother because she would not understand what was being done to her. If cancer was indeed diagnosed, questions about radiation, chemotherapy, and so on would need to be addressed. It was agreed that under the circumstances the harm of the screening procedure exceeded the potential benefits. She could neither understand the diagnostic procedure nor withstand any treatment, both of which would negatively affect her current quality of life. The woman did not receive the mammogram and died of an acute myocardial event about 3 months later.

cannot entirely compensate for a lifetime of lifestyle choices that were detrimental to one's health, many small health-promoting changes can ameliorate their impact in later life.

Nurses foster *biological wellness* at all levels of prevention by promoting regular physical activity such as playing tennis, participating in wheelchair bowling, or sitting upright for intervals throughout the day. Healthy lifestyles are encouraged: healthy eating and adequate and restful sleep; achieving control over acquired health problems such as hypertension or diabetes; and avoiding tobacco, tobacco products, and exposure to smoke and other pollutants.

Meeting basic biological needs, especially food and health care, may be difficult for some, especially those facing health inequities or discrimination for whatever reason. The nurse can observe for cues related to biological integrity and, if necessary, facilitate the older adults or family to obtain support services (e.g., food stamps or food commodities, home-delivered meals, Medicaid) that are possible and appropriate. Fostering maximal biological wellness means advocating for the person to secure the highest quality of medical care when it is needed (Box 2.5). The implementation of evidence-based care and cutting-edge research is an expectation, not an option.

Nursing actions to promote *social wellness* include facilitating activities in which desired interactions with others, pets, or both are possible. Ongoing social interactions have been found to have a significantly positive effect on cognition, memory, and mood (Chapter 32). Through social interaction, persons can be recognized with inherent value as men and women, regardless of age or functional ability (Box 2.6).

Nursing actions to promote *functional wellness* occur across the continuum of care and roles. The bedside nurse ensures that the physical environment is one that promotes healing and encourages the person to remain active and engaged at the highest level possible. For example, it is not appropriate to help someone out of a chair who is able to do so unassisted, albeit slower. This type of "help" negatively affects both muscle tone and self-esteem.

Addressing *environmental wellness* is individual to the person but often includes political activism. Those living in the inner city may be facing increased crime and victimization, exposure to pollution, reduced access to fresh fruits and vegetables, and greater dependence on dwindling public transportation. Nursing actions include engagement in the creation of healthy living spaces by advocating for adequate funding for a wide range of resources such as street lighting, community gardens, or aging-related services including local Area Agencies on Aging (https://www.usaging.org/) or EUROFAMCARE (https://www.uke.de/extern/eurofamcare/). The gerontological nurse helps develop communities respect and support an environment in which healthy aging is possible.

Addressing *psychological wellness* calls for identifying cues suggestive of threats to cognition or mood and developing solutions to optimize outcomes. Promoting psychological wellness includes accepting the older adult as someone of value regardless of that person's health status (Box 2.7). The nurse is often the one to challenge the view held by both persons themselves and health care providers—that declines in mental and cognitive health are "normal changes with aging." In many cases, depression is misdiagnosed as dementia (Chapter 30). The nurse can take the lead in addressing these misconceptions and helping persons who are wrestling with new or lifelong psychiatric or psychological challenges as they age.

Spiritual wellness may be described as a sense that one's life has meaning. This may be a relationship with a greater source (e.g., God, Allah, The Great Spirit, Wakan Tanka, Gitche Manitou), a relationship with others, or the sense of the community or world. The nurse fosters the spiritual dimension of the person through openness to how others view and express their spirituality. This may be done by ensuring that the person's spiritual rituals are considered when scheduling medical appointments or procedures or even when taking vital signs in the hospital setting. It also means that the nurse and the rest of the health care team respect and account for dying and death rituals as appropriate (Chapter 34).

The nurse promotes wellness in all dimensions within the context of the person's *culture*. When nurses address needs within a a person's perspective, they are respecting culture regardless of what it is and the form it takes. It may be ensuring that the appropriate food is provided, such as a serving of pasta or rice with each meal, or facilitating the inclusion of an indigenous healer in the care team.

BOX 2.5 Promoting Biological Wellness and Tertiary Prevention

About 9 months ago Helen suffered a stroke that left her partially paralyzed on the right side. With extensive rehabilitation she was able to regain independent ambulation with the help of a cane and functional use of her affected hand with a brace. Her left shoulder had become quite tender due to a combination of chronic arthritis and overuse, as she relied on it to remain mobile. She came to the clinic requesting a referral for physical therapy. There she was taught how best to use her cane, taught stretching exercises, and received heat and massage therapy. She has now returned to her usual activities, until she needs another "dose" of tertiary prevention.

BOX 2.6 Promoting Social Wellness in Long-Term Care

The staff of a long-term care facility consistently interacted with the residents, regardless of their functional or cognitive status. For many residents, the staff was all the family they had left. One of the younger residents had been there a long time and would likely spend the rest of his life there because of brain damage from uncontrollable seizures. Although communication was difficult, he got much pleasure in "flirting" with the staff. One day a nurse was observed stopping by his chair and commenting on a new baseball cap he had been given. She remarked, "You're smokin' in that cap, there!" His smile could not have been broader, and they each went in their separate directions.

BOX 2.7 Promoting Psychological Wellness in the Face of Death

Mrs. Heinz was coming very close to the end of her life. Her symptoms were well controlled, but during what turned out to be my last home visit she seemed very agitated. When asked if there was anything I could do, she was remarkably frank: "I know I have very little time left. My sister-in-law insists she wants to see me before it is 'too late.' I have never liked her and have no desire to spend one minute of my remaining time in the company of someone I do not like. Please discuss this with my husband; he doesn't seem to understand what I want and why." Mr. Heinz was my patient that day, and after many tears he agreed to respect his wife's wishes. She died peacefully in his arms several days later.

The nurse's role across the globe is to facilitate the creation of political, economic, social, and physical environments that enhance the opportunity for persons to move toward wellness through the promotion of healthy lifestyles, timely health screening, and the ability to participate in tertiary prevention at every stage of life. The wellness-based approach is perhaps the most equitable in supporting the individual's potential for maximal health and functioning at all levels. By listening closely, nurses can hear what is most important to persons and what can be done to promote their wellness.

KEY CONCEPTS

- Wellness is a multidimensional concept. It is human adaptation at the most individually satisfying level in response to existing internal and external conditions.
- COVID-19 has presented long-term challenges to the aging population, especially for those in underrepresented groups.
- For the first time in history an individual and that person's parent and grandparent may all be of the same socially described "generation" of older adults.
- The definition of who is "old" and "elder" or a "senior citizen" is changing rapidly; this is expected to change even further as more and more of the "baby boomers" live longer.
- Health status is now recognized in unique and specific ways as noted in the US document *Healthy People 2030*.
- By using a wellness perspective as a basis of practice, the gerontological nurse can promote health regardless of where a person is on the health continuum.
- A nurse with a wellness focus designs nursing actions to promote optimal outcomes, enhance healthy aging, and maximize quality of life.

NEXT-GENERATION NCLEX® (NGN) EXAMINATION–STYLE QUESTIONS

Mrs. Parsons recently celebrated her 95th birthday with many family and friends attending from far and near. She shared, "That was the best day of my life! I was married twice, but none of the weddings were as exciting as this. I never have thought I would live to be this old. Yes, life has been a struggle. My first husband died in the Second World War right after we were married; my second husband was not very nice to me, but I hung in there until he died last year. He developed Alzheimer's and I cared for him for 6 years and now I am very tired. My children sometimes wonder how I have managed. They live in another state and are not able to visit due to their own health problems. I believe I have lived so long because of my ability to persevere."

Mrs. Parsons is frail and thin, regularly takes acetaminophen to treat the discomfort from advanced osteoarthritis and eats sparingly but likes almost all foods and is concerned about good nutrition. Until last year she walked two brisk miles a day. Three months ago, she broke her hip after slipping on an acorn, has not regained her full strength, has more pain than in the past, and is frustrated that she cannot continue her usual activities. She is hoping that with enough exercise in the gym she will make it to her next birthday.

If Mrs. Parsons is injured again, she is at __Option 1___ risk for a poor outcome. You base this analysis on the following biological cues (Option 2): _____ _____ _____.
The most important set of cues from option 3 is: _____.
Which social and psychological cues will influence her outcome the most (Option 4): _____ _____.

Option 1	Option 2	Option 3	Option 4
high	95 years old	95 years old	Best day of my life
average	Tired	Tired	Long-term caregiver
low	Frail and thin	Frail and thin	Frustrated
	Has pain		Children live in another state
	Recent hip fracture		
	Has not regained past strength		

CLINICAL JUDGMENT QUESTIONS AND ACTIVITIES

1. Construct a personal definition of health that incorporates the dimensions of the wellness-based model.
2. Looking into the future, consider which decade you expect will be your last. In what state of health do you expect to be?
3. There are three levels of prevention. As science advances, so does our knowledge of which solutions are effective in promoting health and in preventing illness and which are not. Think of a strategy you use or have heard of and believe to be effective. Then look in scientific literature (not the newspaper or Wikipedia) to see what the evidence is at this time.

RESEARCH QUESTIONS

1. What factors are the most significant influences of health in aging?
2. What are the factors that indicate one is in a state of "wellness"?
3. What are the perceptions of younger people about the possibility of healthy aging?
4. How can nurses enhance wellness for older adults in various stages across the continuum?

REFERENCES

Aging Analytics: *Supercentenarians landscape overview* (website), 2020. http://data.longevity.international/Supercentenarians-Landscape-Overview-Report.pdf.

Allard M, Robine JM, Calment J: *Jeanne Calment: from Van Gogh's time to ours, 122 extraordinary years*, Waterville, ME, 1999, Thorndike Press.

Andrasfay T, Goldman N: Reductions in 2020 life expectancy due to COVID-19 and the disproportionate impact on the Black and Latino populations, *Proc Natl Acad Sci USA*, 2021 118(5):e201476118.

Arai Y, Sasaki T, Hirose N: Demographic, phenotypic, and genetic characteristics of centenarians in Okinawa and Honshu, Japan: part 2 Honshu, Japan, *Mech Ageing Dev* 165(Pt B):80–85, 2017.

Arias E, Xu J: United States life tables, 2018, *Natl Vital Stat Rep* 69(12):2020.

Buchholz K: *Where 100 is the new 80* (website), 2021. https://www.statista.com/chart/14931/where-100-is-the-new-80/.

Centers for Disease Control and Prevention (CDC): *Current cigarette smoking among adults in the United States* (website), 2020. https://www.cdc.gov/tobacco/data_statistics/fact_sheets/adult_data/cig_smoking/index.htm.

Centers for Disease Control and Prevention (CDC): *COVID-19: older adults* (website), 2021. https://www.cdc.gov/coronavirus/2019-ncov/need-extra-precautions/older-adults.html. Accessed June 1, 2021.

Gamillo E: COVID-19 surpasses 1918 flu to become deadliest pandemic in American history, *Smithsonian Magazine* September 24, 2021.

Giuliani C, Pirazzini C, Delledonne M, et al.: Centenarians as extreme phenotypes: an ecological perspective to get insight into the relationship between the genetics of longevity and age-associated diseases, *Mech Ageing Dev* 165(Pt B):195–201, 2017.

Goldstein JR, Lee RD: Demographic perspectives on the mortality of COVID-19 and other epidemics, *Proc Natl Acad Sci USA* 117(36):e22035–e22041, 2020.

Hirata T, Arai Y, Yuasa S, et al.: Associations of cardiovascular biomarkers and plasma albumin with exceptional survival to the highest ages, *Nat Commun* 11(1):e3820, 2020.

History: Baby boomers (website), 2021. http://www.history.com/topics/baby-boomers.

Iannitti T, Palmieri B: Inflammation and genetics: an insight in the centenarian model, *Hum Biol* 83(4):531–559, 2011.

Jett KF: The meaning of aging and the celebration of years, *Geriatr Nurs* 24(4):290–293, 2003.

Karasik D, Newman A: Models to explore genetics of human aging, *Adv Exp Med Biol* 847:141–161, 2015.

Markel, H. The real story behind penicillin, 2013 (website). www.pbs.org/newshour/health/the-real-story-behind-the-worlds-first-antibiotic

Mather, M, Scommegna, P., Kilduff, L.

Fact sheet: Aging in the United States, 2019. www.prb.org/resources/fact-sheet-in-the-united-states/

Meyer J: *Centenarians: 2010: 2010 Census special reports (Report no. C2010SR-03)*, Washington, DC, 2012, United States Census Bureau, US Government Printing Office.

Nascher I: *Geriatrics*, Philadelphia, 1914, P. Blakiston's Son & Co.

National Prevention Council: Healthy aging in action (website), 2016. https://www.surgeongeneral.gov/priorities/prevention/about/healthy-aging-in-action-final.pdf.

Office of Disease Prevention and Health Promotion (ODPHP): Healthy people 2030 (website), 2020. https://www.healthypeople.gov/2020/About-Healthy-People/Development-Healthy-People-2030/Framework.

Sanderson W, Scherbov S: Rethinking age and aging, *Popul Bull* 63(4):3–16, 2008.

Sebastiani P, Perls TT: The genetics of extreme longevity: lessons from the New England centenarian study, *Front Genet* 3:277, 2012.

Takao M, Hirose N, Arai Y, et al.: Neuropathology of supercentenarians—four autopsy cases, *Acta Neuropathol Commun* 4(1):97, 2016.

US Census Bureau: *By 2030, all baby boomers will be age 65 or older* (website), 2020. https://www.census.gov/library/stories/2019/12/by-2030-all-baby-boomers-will-be-age-65-or-older.html.

World Health Organization (WHO): *Decade of healthy aging: baseline report* (website), 2020. https://www.who.int/publications/m/item/decade-of-healthy-ageing-baseline-report.

Young RD, Kroczek WJ: Validated living worldwide supercentenarians 112+, living and recently deceased: February 2020, *Rejuvenation Res* 23(1):65–67, 2020.

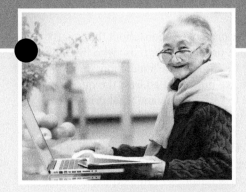

CHAPTER 3

Theories of Aging

Kathleen Jett

http://evolve.elsevier.com/Touhy/TwdHlthAging

A STUDENT SPEAKS

Until I started learning about the science of aging, I had no idea how complicated it could be. We seem to have learned so much but still have so much more to learn.

Helena, age 23

AN OLDER ADULT SPEAKS

When I was a young girl, Einstein was proposing the theory of matter and energy and we had only heard of DNA or genetics. Now I hear that scientists believe genetics strongly influence what has been happening to me as I age. I really hope they find out more before I die.

Beatrice, age 92

LEARNING OBJECTIVES

On completion of this chapter, the reader will be able to:

1. Describe the evolving knowledge regarding the biological theories of aging.
2. Compare and contrast the major psychosocial theories of aging.
3. Describe the cultural and economic limitations of the current psychosocial theories associated with successful aging.
4. Use at least one psychosocial theory of aging to support commonly provided social services for older adults living in the community.
5. Create theory-based solutions to foster the highest level of wellness while aging.

A theory is an attempt to explain phenomena, to give a sense of order, and to provide a framework from which one can interpret reality (Einstein, 1920). The current research on biological theories of aging focuses on the genetic and cellular changes within organisms over time. In some cases, the associations between biological processes and common diseases in later life have been described (Stanić & Matić, 2019). Psychosocial theories of aging focus on the psychological and social adaptations to aging. Although they are more subjective and may be ethnocentric, they can still provide potential context for aging and social behavior.

This chapter provides the reader with an overview of several prominent biological and psychosocial theories of aging. The nurse can use the biological theories to help understand the physical changes of aging and the genetic underpinnings of some of the most common disorders. The nurse can use the psychosocial theories to develop nursing actions that promote healthy and successful aging. Taken together, the nuances of aging and the individual can provide guidance in developing nursing actions to enhance wellness.

BIOLOGICAL AGING

Biological aging, referred to as *senescence,* is an exceedingly complex, nonlinear, but universal process of change, resulting in decreased physiological compensatory reserves, an increased rate of cellular deterioration, unrepaired damage, and increased vulnerability to disease (Bektas et al., 2018; Fougère et al., 2019). Aging changes are made visible in what is referred to as the aging phenotype.

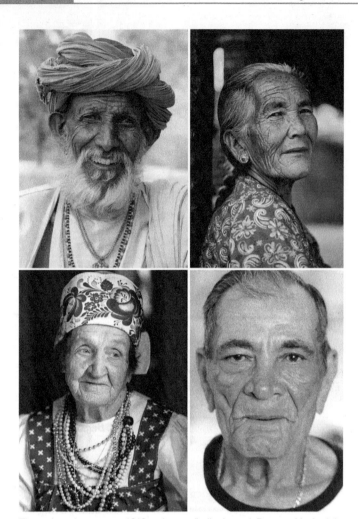

The aging phenotype. (©iStock.com/kailash soni; Bartosz Hadyniak; De Visu; ProArtWork.)

The genome or genetic components of each cell (DNA and RNA) lie within its nucleus and in the mitochondria, which direct cellular metabolism and serve as templates for cellular reproduction. Maintaining the integrity of the genome is the most important function of the cell; this includes regulation of reproduction, repair of damaged DNA, and senescence (MacRae et al., 2015). Survival of an organism depends on successful cellular reproduction (mitosis). If reproduction were always perfect, the organism would never age. Instead, the ability of some cells to reproduce decreases, errors occur in the process, and ultimately the ability to reproduce ceases altogether.

Although there is a growing body of knowledge about the genomics of aging, complex questions remain. What triggers the changes at the cellular or organ level? Are the changes orderly and predictable or random and chaotic? What are the roles of cellular mutation and epigenetics, that is, the effect of the environment on the RNA? What are the effects of lifestyle choices, and how do they influence the aging phenotype? If aging is universal, why are there such broad differences from person to person?

Evolution and Aging

Evolution theories are recognized as important tools in understanding the genetic influence on cellular aging and longevity.

These theories draw heavily on conversations about the concept of "natural selection," which presumes that those who live long enough to procreate are the fittest of a population. Since we become less fit as we age, we now must address the questions of why some persons live to very late life, and what genetic and cellular factors influence who survives and who does not.

The most developed evolution-based theory of aging is that of the "disposable soma [cell]." Growth is viewed in terms of the use of metabolic resources. These are spent either in the preparation for and the production of offspring or in "keeping … going from one day to the next" (Kirkwood, 2017, p. 23). Theoretically, those whose metabolic resources are spent almost entirely on procreation die earlier than those with fewer offspring. During procreation fewer metabolic resources are available to meet metabolic needs and repair naturally occurring cellular damage (Box 3.1). The organism dies when metabolic needs are not met. Studies have shown that longevity is proportionate to an organism's ability to balance its somatic systems and metabolic needs (Kirkwood, 2017).

Free Radicals

Free radicals are molecules within the cell that are physiologically unstable (missing an electron). Reactive oxygen species (ROS) are also found in the cell, some of which are already free radicals or cause their formation. Both are formed spontaneously during cell metabolism. While both free radicals and ROS are necessary for some cellular activities, they are also capable of damaging lipids, proteins, and other macromolecules (Speakman & Selman, 2011). They have been found to cause mutations within the mitochondrial DNA (mtDNA) (Lai et al., 2017; Pomatto & Davies, 2018).

The number of ROS is increased by several external factors, such as pollution and cigarette smoke, and by internal factors, including inflammation (Dato et al., 2013). A dramatic rise in the level of ROS, referred to as oxidative stress, has been well documented to lead to cell damage and an accumulation of senescent (aging) cells. These cells have been found to be associated with a number of diseases (Kirkland, 2017; Speakman & Selman, 2011) (Box 3.2). The damage from oxidative stress appears to be random and unpredictable, varying from one cell to another and from one person to another (Speakman & Selman, 2011).

The free radical theory of aging has its origins in the 1950s when scientists were studying the effect of radiation following

---

BOX 3.1   Examples of Somatic Maintenance Needs

Ability to repair damaged DNA
Ability to remove antioxidants
Ability to control stress proteins
Ability to accurately replicate DNA and proteins
Ability to suppress tumor growth
Ability to maintain a healthy immune system

Adapted from Kirkwood TB: Evolution theory and the mechanisms of aging. In Fillit H, Rockwood K, Young JB, editors: *Brocklehurst's textbook of geriatric medicine and gerontology*, ed 8, Philadelphia, 2017, Elsevier, pp 22–26.

the use of atomic weapons by the United States in Japan. It was discovered that the extensive damage done by the radiation was primarily caused by free radicals' damage to the body's macromolecules (e.g., DNA, proteins, lipids). Subsequently the paradigm emerged that the molecular damage seen in aging was from the same source, free radicals. It was postulated that any actions that increase the protection against free radicals or decrease oxidative damage would slow aging and hence prolong life (Speakman & Selman, 2011).

For many years it has been promoted in the popular press that the consumption of some dietary *supplements* can delay or minimize the effects of aging by counteracting the oxidative stress and free radicals. However, some antioxidant supplements such as beta-carotene and vitamins C and E have been found to be potentially harmful (Box 3.3). High doses of beta-carotene supplements may increase the risk for lung cancer in smokers, and high doses of vitamin E may increase the risk for hemorrhagic stroke and prostate cancer. At the same time, evidence has been consistent that *diets* high in the antioxidants found in fruits and vegetables and Mediterranean diets rich in red wine and olive oil may prevent or delay some cell damage and several diseases. It is not yet known if this is the effect of the antioxidants themselves or something else, such as lifestyle (National Center for Complementary and Integrative Health [NCCIH], 2013).

As research has become more sophisticated, this theory has been called into question when considered alone but becomes more robust when considering the role of free radicals in the ability to maintain homeostasis (Pomatto & Davies, 2018). Using animal models, decreasing cellular protection by decreasing oxidative damage has not been shown to affect longevity, but it does seem to negatively affect the development of "age-related disease," those conditions found most commonly in later

life, especially degenerative disease conditions (Speakman & Selman, 2011).

Mitochondrial Dysfunction

Mitochondrial DNA, or mtDNA, is key to the production of adenosine triphosphate (ATP), the precursor to the energy needed for physiological processes (Fig. 3.1). mtDNA is also necessary for the reproduction of the mitochondria themselves. Damage results in mutations and consequential errors during replication (Kirkland, 2017; Lagouge & Larsson, 2013; Wang et al., 2013). Such mutations have been found in both normal aging cells and those associated with neurodegenerative disorders such as Alzheimer's disease (Chapter 25) (Fougère et al., 2019).

Telomeres and Aging

Telomeres are sequences of DNA wrapped in proteins found at the end of each chromosome (Fig. 3.2). Initial telomere length has been found to be determined by genetic factors. They shorten as they reproduce, and when a critical shortening is reached, the cell dies. The rate of shortening is influenced by multiple psychosocial, environmental, and behavioral factors (Starkweather et al., 2014) (Boxes 3.4 and 3.5). Shortened telomeres have been associated with decreased longevity and several chronic diseases, including cardiovascular disease, hypertension, diabetes, and dementia (Fougère et al., 2019; Turner et al., 2019). There is also evidence associating shortening with oxidative stress and chronic inflammation. The enzyme telomerase prevents telomere shortening but is present only in human stem cells, reproductive cells, and cancer cells. Length is considered a reliable measure of age (Vaiserman & Krasnienkov, 2020).

Inflammation

It has been well documented that aging is accompanied by chronic, low-level, subclinical inflammation and an increase in mediators such as cytokines. This is referred to as "inflammaging" and is theorized to accelerate biological aging, reduce immunity, and increase the risk for a number of "age-related" diseases and cellular senescence (Fougère et al., 2019; Ray & Yung, 2019) (Box 3.6). The inflammatory response is exacerbated by oxidative stress and impaired antioxidant defense. It is likely that the reduced immune function associated with age-related chronic inflammation is a factor in the high mortality from COVID-19 among older adults (Smorenberg et al., 2021). Although some of the effects of chronic inflammation are well known, others remain theoretical.

USING CLINICAL JUDGMENT TO PROMOTE HEALTHY AGING: BIOLOGICAL THEORIES

As we apply our growing knowledge of biological aging, it appears reasonable to expect that slowing or reducing cellular damage may have the potential to promote healthy aging. Helping persons reduce external factors (e.g., pollutants in the environment such as secondhand smoke) that are known to increase the development of ROS may decrease vulnerability to disease. Facilitating optimal nutrition may be found to reduce

BOX 3.3 Tips for Best Practice

High doses of supplemental antioxidants have been found to be harmful. Some studies have shown that high-dose beta-carotene supplements increase the risk for lung cancer in smokers and high doses of vitamin E increase the risk for stroke. There are also many potential and actual drug-supplement interactions; for example, the interaction between warfarin and vitamin E increases the risk for bleeding. Check to make sure that the multivitamin used does not exceed the daily recommended requirement. Encourage people to avoid those products advertised as "mega-vitamins."

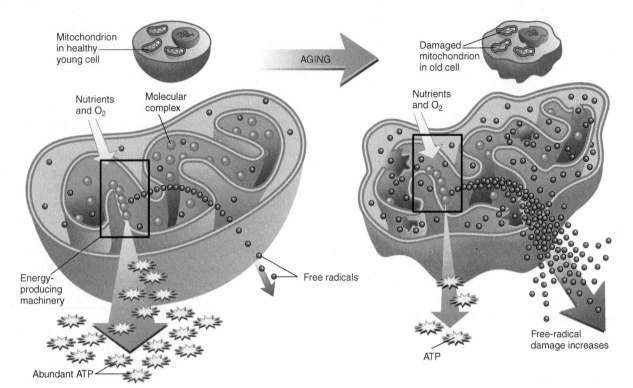

Fig. 3.1 Mitochondria in young and old cells. *ATP*, Adenosine triphosphate. (From McCance KL, Huether SE: *Pathophysiology: the biologic basis for disease in adults and children,* ed 6, St Louis, 2010, Mosby.)

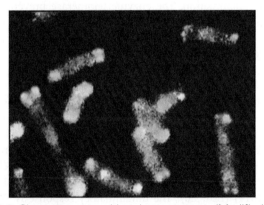

Fig. 3.2 Chromosomes with telomere caps. (Modified from Jerry Shay and the University of Texas Southwestern Medical Center at Dallas, Office of News and Publications, 5323 Harry Hines Blvd, Dallas, TX 75235.)

BOX 3.4   Telomeres, Aging, and Longevity

Telomere length decreases at a rate of 24.8 to 27.7 base pairs per year. A number of lifestyle factors can increase the rate of shortening. Smoking one pack of cigarettes a day for 40 years is associated with the loss of five additional base pairs a year, or 7.4 years of life. Obesity also causes accelerated telomere shortening, resulting in 8.8 years of life lost. Excessive emotional stress results in the release of glucocorticoids by the adrenal glands. They have been shown to reduce antioxidants and thereby increase oxidative and premature shortening of telomeres. Shorter telomeres are suggested as greatly increasing one's vulnerability to early onset of age-related health problems such as heart disease.

From Shammas MA: Telomeres, lifestyle, cancer and aging, *Curr Opin Clin Nutr Metab Care* 14(1):28–34, 2011.

BOX 3.5   Examples of Factors That Have Been Suggested to Accelerate Telomere Shortening

Chronic stress (perceived)
Pessimism
Inter-partner violence
Long-term caregiving (e.g., in Alzheimer's disease)
≤6 hours of sleep a night
Self-reported poor quality of sleep
Higher body mass index and lack of exercise
History of childhood neglect or adverse events
Smoking
Major depressive disorder

Data from Astuti Y, Wardhana A, Watkins J, et al: Cigarette smoking and telomere length: a systematic review of 84 studies and meta-analysis, *Environ Res* 158:480–489, 2017; Starkweather AR, Alhaeeri AA, Montpetit A: An integrative review of factors associated with telomere length and implications for biobehavioral research, *Nur Re* 63(1):36–50, 2014.

---

the speed of telomere shortening and prolong life (Box 3.7). Levels of *naturally* occurring antioxidants can be increased by encouraging regular exercise and a healthy diet (NCCIH, 2013). Because we have realized the deleterious effects of supplemental antioxidants such as vitamin E, the gerontological nurse can use this knowledge to encourage persons to abandon long-held habits and beliefs and replace these with the skills needed to make judicious use of herbs and dietary supplements (Chapter 11).

BOX 3.6 Diseases Associated With Excessive Inflammation (Increased Cytokines)

Dementia
Parkinson's disease
Atherosclerosis
Type 2 diabetes
Sarcopenia
Rheumatoid arthritis
Osteoporosis
Osteoarthritis
Frailty syndrome
High risk of morbidity and mortality

Adapted from Fougère B, Boulanger E, Nourhashèmi F, et al: Chronic inflammation: accelerator of biological aging, *J Gerontol A Biol Sci Med Sci* 72(9):1218–1225, 2016; Ventura MT, Casciaro M, Gagem S, et al: Immunosenescence in aging: between immune cells depletion and cytokines up-regulation, *Clin Mol Allergy* 15(21), 2017.

BOX 3.7 Tips for Best Practice

Finding ways for all persons to have access to nutritious food is an important nursing intervention. This includes political actions to decrease the number of "food deserts" in the community, that is, geographic areas where reasonable-priced quality food and fresh fruits and vegetables are unavailable.

Of significant importance in the clinical setting is inflamm-aging and implications for its increased susceptibility to infections, autoimmune disorders, and cancers with aging. Observing for early signs and symptoms of infections in older adults is a particularly important contribution that nurses can make to facilitate a return to wellness (Chapter 1).

With an understanding of the changes in immunity, the conscientious nurse can take an active role in promoting specific preventive strategies such as the use of immunizations (especially for COVID-19, influenza, zoster, and pneumococcal disease), frequent handwashing, and avoiding exposure to others with infections. The nurse observes for cues of an inflammation response (i.e., erythema, edema, and pain) and promptly develops solutions to improve health outcomes.

PSYCHOSOCIAL THEORIES OF AGING

A person is not just a biological being but a multidimensional whole (Chapter 2, Fig. 2.4). Only when life is considered in its totality can we begin to truly understand aging. Here we discuss a selection of psychosocial theories of aging, which attempt to explain and understand the adaptation in late life necessary for successful aging. As with the biological theories of aging, there has not been an agreement on one overarching paradigm.

Psychosocial theories began appearing in the gerontological literature in the 1950s. Most were based on little research and primarily on "face validity," that is, emerging from the personal and professional experience of scientists and appearing to be reasonable explanations of their perceptions of successful aging. Potential answers to questions are proposed regarding how life circumstances affect late life, how support systems develop and change, the appropriate role of community and government in responding to the needs of older persons, how society perceives older adults and how older adults perceive the world around them, and the hallmarks of successful aging (Kolb, 2014).

Role Theory

Role theory, an approach drawn from sociology and social psychology, was one of the earliest propositions of what it means to age successfully (Biddle, 1979). According to this theory, self-identity is defined by one's role in society (e.g., nurse, teacher, banker, parent). As individuals evolve through the various stages of life, so do their roles. Successful aging means that as one role is completed, it is replaced by another one of comparative personal and societal value. For example, the wage-earning work role is replaced by that of a volunteer, or a parent becomes a grandparent. The ability of an individual to adapt to changing roles is a predictor of successful aging. Resistance to change is seen as a harbinger of difficulty at the end of life.

Role theory is operationalized in the phenomenon of age norms otherwise referred to as *social stereotypes.* These are culturally constructed expectations of what is deemed acceptable behavior and are internalized by the individual. Age norms are based on the assumption that chronological age and gender, in and of themselves, imply roles; for example, one may hear, "If only they would act their age," or "You are too old to do/say/behave like that." Although beliefs in age- and gender-segregated roles are still present, contemporary challenges began with the socially controversial but popular television show *Maude* (1972–78) and continued with *The Golden Girls* (1985–93). In both of these shows, the characters behaved in ways that challenged long-established age norms for White middle-aged and older women. While older men have long served as role models (albeit unrealistic ones) in movies and television, role models are now becoming available to women, such as those performed by Dame Judi Dench (born in 1934), Dame Helen Mirren (born in 1945), and Meryl Streep (born in 1949). With the aging of the baby boomers (Chapter 2), popular culture is challenging age norms; for example, older persons are now depicted as still sexually active in advertisements for genital lubricants and medications to treat erectile dysfunction. These images replace the historical view that persons become asexual as they age, or so their children hope!

Activity Theory

Based on data from the Kansas City Studies of Adult Life, Havinghurst and Albrecht (1953) proposed that continued activity and the ability to "stay young" were indicators of successful aging. It is expected that the productivity and activities of middle life are replaced with equally engaging pursuits in later life (Maddox, 1963). The theory assumes that it is better to be active (and young) than inactive (Havinghurst, 1972). Further, increased activity leads to a greater sense of well-being due to a higher level of satisfaction (Heinz et al., 2017). *Activity theory* is consistent with Western society's emphasis on work, wealth, and productivity and therefore continues to influence the perception of both successful and unsuccessful aging (Wadensten, 2006).

Continuity Theory

Continuity theory has similarities to both activity and role theories. Atchley (1999) proposed that individuals develop and maintain a consistent pattern of behavior over a lifetime. Aging, as an extension of earlier life, reflects a *continuation of the patterns* of roles, responsibilities, and activities. Personality influences the roles and activities chosen and the level of satisfaction drawn from these. Successful aging is associated with one's ability to maintain and continue previous behaviors and roles or demonstrate adaptation by finding suitable replacements (Kolb, 2014).

Disengagement Theory

Disengagement theory contrasts with both role and activity theories. Cumming and Henry (1961) proposed that in the natural course of aging the individual does, and should, slowly withdraw from society to allow the transfer of power to younger generations. The transfer is viewed as necessary for the maintenance of social equilibrium and beneficial to the older adult (Hooyman et al., 2018; Wadensten, 2006). A belief in the appropriateness of disengagement provides the basis of age discrimination when an older employee is replaced by a younger one. Although this practice has been overtly outlawed in the workplace (in the United States), it is still present covertly but challenged socially and legally. An older adult's withdrawal is no longer considered an indicator of successful aging. It is not *necessarily* a good thing for society and does not consider the needs of the individual or culture in which one lives. Disengagement theory is no longer widely accepted in gerontological science but maintains a foothold in society.

Social Exchange Theory

Social exchange theory conceptualizes aging from an economic perspective. The presumption is that as one ages, one has fewer and fewer economic resources to contribute to society. This paucity results in loss of social status, self-esteem, and political power (Dowd, 1975; Hooyman et al., 2018). Only those who can maintain control of their financial resources have the potential to remain fully participating members of society and experience successful aging. Although this may have some applicability in the communities in the world that have been able to develop a stable economy for its citizens, this theory marginalizes those in communities and countries who struggle for the barest necessities now and into the foreseeable future (World Health Organization [WHO], 2021).

Modernization Theory

Although not usually associated with social exchange theory, *modernization theory* can be used to consider nonmaterial aspects of exchange. This theory is an attempt to explain the social changes that have resulted in devaluing the contributions of older adults (Cowgill & Holmes, 1972). Material and political resources were controlled by the older members of society in the United States before about 1900 (Achenbaum, 1978). The resources included their knowledge, skills, experience, and wisdom (Fung, 2013). In agricultural cultures and communities, the oldest members held power through property ownership and the right to make decisions related to food distribution. Older men and women often held valuable religious and cultural roles of instructing youth and controlling ceremony (Sokolovsky, 2020).

According to modernization theory, successful aging would mean that older adults maintain status, their skills are valued, and kinship groups remain intact. In contemporary society, the status and value of older adults may be lost, labors no longer valued, and kinship networks dispersed (Hendricks & Hendricks, 1986). Modernization has had a notable effect on cultures such as those in China and Japan where filial duty predominated as an underlying construct of eldercare (Fung, 2013). Conflicts between traditional values mount as more and more adult children enter the marketplace or emigrate for social or economic reasons (see *The Bonesetter's Daughter* by Amy Tan [2001]). It is proposed that these changes are the result of advancing technology, urbanization, and mass education (Cowgill, 1974).

Gerotranscendence Theory

Gerotranscendence theory is similar to that of disengagement theory, yet the reason for the withdrawal is not for societal needs but to give the person time for self-reflection, contemplation of the meaning of life, and movement away from the material world (Chapter 35) (Tornstam, 1989, 2000, 2005; Wadensten, 2007). Aging is viewed as movement from birth to death and maturation toward wisdom, an ever-evolving process that alters one's view of reality, sense of spirituality, and meaning beyond the self. Inasmuch, gerotranscendence implies achieving wisdom through personal transformation. With aging, time becomes less important, as do superficial relationships.

Transcendence is considered a marker of successful aging and the highest goal any person can achieve. This theory is based on a highly ethnocentric approach to aging. It is less likely to be applicable in cultures based on the quality of interpersonal relationships (Chapters 4 and 32). It also does not account for differences in economic resources, which may or may not provide the individual with the "luxury" of time for introspection.

Socioemotional Selectivity Theory

Carstensen (1992) proposed that as people age, they become increasingly selective with their emotions, goals, and activities. Relative to younger adults, older adults reported a preference for positive over negative information and relationships; time is spent with those persons who share a history of rewarding relationships. Called the "positivity effect," there is the potential for successful aging and improved emotional well-being (e.g., happiness) by selectively choosing positive rather than negative memories (Reed & Carstensen, 2012).

When one's life expectancy is viewed as limited, as it is in late life, the focus is present-oriented; life goals are prioritized and become focused on making the most of the "time left," such as by spending time with valued others, rather than on the distant future (Barber et al., 2016; Carstensen et al., 1999).

Selective Optimization and Compensation Theory

The *selective optimization and compensation (SOC) theory* is a model of behavior leading to successful aging and happiness.

Successful aging and daily happiness are viewed as the ability to adapt and cope with the common losses in late life by focusing on strengths; compensatory strategies are used when challenges occur (Baltes & Baltes, 1993). Success has been found to be influenced by the degree to which an individual (1) electively selects goals, (2) modifies this selection in the presence of resource loss, (3) enhances or acquires resources to achieve the new goal, and (4) compensates by using new resources to achieve the goals and therefore promotes individual function and happiness (Steptoe, 2019).

Teshale and Lachman (2016) found that individuals who used SOC regularly were the happiest and that following a time of distress, SOC could subsequently restore a sense of well-being. However, using SOC to adapt in the face of very limited resources could make the management of these limitations difficult. The losses associated with age-related changes may be able to be buffered. Persons with multiple chronic conditions who use SOC to cope with and adapt to potential alterations in their quality of life were found to report fewer symptoms, increased ability to perform activities of daily living (ADLs), more subjective reports of well-being, fewer falls and sick days, and use of fewer pain medications. Taken together, health outcomes were optimized (Carpentieri et al., 2017; Zhang & Radhakrishnan, 2018).

Some of the psychosocial theories of aging have been criticized because of their limited applicability, problems with intersubjectivity of meaning, and inability to be tested. They fail to consider social class, education, health, and economic and cultural diversity as influencing factors (Hooyman et al., 2018; Marshall, 1994). However, this may be simply consistent with the historical period of their development. Nonetheless, the expressions of how successful aging is defined may prove useful (Table 3.1).

USING CLINICAL JUDGMENT TO PROMOTE HEALTHY AGING: PSYCHOSOCIAL THEORIES

Psychosocial theories of aging provide the gerontological nurse with useful information to serve as context in the development of solutions and nursing actions. Although these theories have been neither proved nor disproved, they have stood the test of time and may have applicability in the promotion of healthy aging. They have been used as the rationale for many nursing and social actions, from the creation of senior activity centers to laws regulating employment. However, nurses have a unique opportunity to work with multiple approaches to understanding aging. In doing so, they can have an important voice in testing, modifying, and discussing psychosocial theories and how they apply to worldwide diversity.

Many questions about late life development remain unanswered. Do biological differences exist between persons of different races and ethnicities, and how does this influence the aging of the human body and the psyche? How do people change in the later years? What is the reason for and purpose of aging? What is the meaning of aging, and can this ever be generalized? What is successful aging? These are not new questions, but they still beg answers.

TABLE 3.1 Psychosocial Theories of Aging, the Meaning of Successful Aging, and Examples of Nursing Actions Consistent With Theories

Theory	Successful Aging	Nursing Action
Role theory	As one role is completed, it is replaced by another one of comparative value to the individual and society	Discuss how roles have changed and how each can be or is valued
Activity theory	Ability to maintain an active lifestyle	Become aware of exercise opportunities designed for older adults in your community
Continuity theory	The ability to maintain and continue previous behaviors and roles or to find suitable replacements. Productivity and activities of middle life are replaced with equally engaging pursuits in later life	Provide activities in your Memory Unit that resemble persons' previous activities
Social exchange theory	Ability to maintain control of their financial resources in order to remain fully participating members of society	Refer to financial counselors and other professionals to maximize independence
Modernization theory	Status is maintained, skills remain valuable, and kinship groups remain intact	Become aware of continuing education programs teaching new skills which are available to older adults in the community
Gerotranscendence theory	To achieve wisdom through personal transformation	Offer and encourage participation in meditation and spiritual growth for those living in long-term care facilities
Socioemotional selectivity theory	Selectively choosing positive rather than negative memories, companions, and activities	Ask persons residing in a nursing home to have photos and other mementos available that have special memories
Selective optimization with compensation theory	The ability to adapt and cope with the common losses in late life by focusing on strengths; compensatory strategies are used when challenges occur	Encourage persons to draw on previous strengths and coping and apply them to current situations

KEY CONCEPTS

- The timing of when one begins to have features that are identified as "old" is significantly affected by one's genetic makeup and both exogenous and endogenous stressors experienced over a lifetime.
- There is no longer one exclusive explanation for biological aging or for psychosocial adaptation to aging.
- Regardless of the theory, biological aging results in damage within the cell itself, resulting in a decrease in or loss of its ability to function or reproduce.

- The increased incidence of many chronic diseases in later life can be explained by biological theories of aging.
- Although the psychosocial theories in use today apply to some populations, this applicability is limited by socio-economic, educational, and cultural factors.

CLINICAL JUDGMENT QUESTIONS AND ACTIVITIES

1. What is meant by the phrase "later life is culturally and socially determined"?
2. Consider the psychosocial theories of aging and discuss how each would or would not apply to the oldest person with whom you most commonly interact.
3. Identify at least two "older persons" among your family or friends and ask them their own theories of why the body ages and how their perceptions of the world today compare to that when they were younger. In a classroom discussion, compare their responses to the current state of the science of biological aging.

4. Discuss the meanings and the thoughts triggered by the student's and older adult's viewpoints as expressed at the beginning of the chapter. How do these vary from your own experience?
5. Imagine yourself at 90 years old and describe the lifestyle you will have and the factors you believe will account for your long life.
6. Organize a debate in which each student attempts to convince others of the logic of one particular psychosocial theories of aging.

RESEARCH QUESTIONS

1. What environmental factors have the potential to affect longevity?
2. What factors in relationships have the potential to contribute to survival?

3. What factors have been associated with extreme longevity?

REFERENCES

Achenbaum WA: *Old age in a new land*, Baltimore, 1978, Johns Hopkins University Press.

Atchley RC: *Continuity and adaptation in aging: creating positive experiences*, Baltimore, 1999, Johns Hopkins University Press.

Baltes PB, Baltes MM: *Successful aging: perspectives from the behavioral sciences*, Cambridge, UK, 1993, Cambridge University Press.

Barber SJ, Opitz PC, Martins B, et al: Thinking about a limited future enhances the positivity of younger and older adults' recall: support for socioemotional selectivity theory, *Mem Cognit* 44:869–882, 2016.

Bektas A, Schurman SH, Sen R, et al: Aging, inflammation and the environment, *Exp Gerontol* 105:10–18, 2018.

Biddle BJ: *Role theory: expectations, identities, and behaviors*, New York, 1979, Academic Press.

Carpentieri JD, Elliott J, Brett CE, et al: Adapting to aging: older people talk about their use of selection, optimization, and compensation to maximize well-being in the context of physical decline, *J Gerontol B Psychol Sci Soc Sci* 72(2):351–361, 2017.

Carstensen LL: Motivation for social contact across the life span: a theory of socioemotional selectivity, *Nebr Symp Motiv* 40:209–254, 1992.

Carstensen LL, Isaacowitz DM, ST Charles: Taking time seriously: a theory of socioemotional selectivity, *Am Psychol* 54(3):165–181, 1999.

Cowgill D: Aging and modernization: a revision of the theory editor. In Gubrium JF, editor: *Late life communities and environmental policy*, Springfield, IL, 1974, Charles C Thomas.

Cowgill DO, Holmes LD: *Aging and modernization*, New York, 1972, Appleton-Century-Crofts.

Cumming E, Henry W: *Growing old, the process of disengagement*, New York, 1961, Basic Books.

Dato S, Crocco P, D'Aquila P, et al.: Exploring the role of genetic variability and lifestyle in oxidative stress response for healthy aging and longevity, *Int J Mol Sci* 14:16443–16472, 2013.

Dowd J: Aging as exchange, *J Gerontol* 30:584–594, 1975.

Einstein A: *Relativity: the special and the general theory*, New York, 1920, Henry Holt.

Fougère B, Boulanger E, Nourhashèmi F, et al.: Retraction to chronic inflammation: accelerator of biological aging, *J Gerontol A Biol Sci Med Sci* 72(9):1218–1225, 2019.

Fung HH: Aging in culture, *Gerontologist* 53(3):369–377, 2013.

Havinghurst RJ: *Developmental tasks and education*, New York, 1972, David McKay.

Havinghurst RJ, Albrecht R: *Older people*, New York, 1953, Longmans, Green and Co.

Heinz M, Cone N, da Rosa G, et al.: Examining supportive evidence for psychosocial theories of aging with the oral history narratives of centenarians, *Societies* 7(8):1–21, 2017.

Hendricks J, Hendricks CD: *Aging in mass society: myths and realities*, Boston, 1986, Little, Brown.

Hooyman NR, Kawamoto KS, Kiyak HA: *Social gerontology: a multidisciplinary perspective*, ed 9, New York, 2018, Pearson.

Kirkland JL: Cellular mechanisms of aging. In Fillit HM, Rockwood K, Young J, editors: *Brocklehurst's textbook of geriatric medicine and gerontology*, ed 8, Philadelphia, 2017, Elsevier, pp 47–52.

Kirkwood TB: Evolution theory and the mechanisms of aging. In Fillit HM, Rockwood K, Young J, editors: *Brocklehurst's textbook of geriatric medicine and gerontology*, ed 8, Philadelphia, 2017, Elsevier, pp 22–26.

Kolb P: *Understanding aging and diversity: theories and concepts*, New York, 2014, Routledge.

Lagouge M, Larsson NG: The role of mitochondrial DNA mutations and free radicals in disease and ageing, *J Int Med* 273:529–543, 2013.

Lai CQ, Parnell LD, Ordovás JM: Genetic mechanisms of aging. In Fillit HM, Rockwood K, Young J, editors: *Brocklehurst's textbook of geriatric medicine and gerontology*, ed 8, Philadelphia, 2017, Elsevier, pp 43–46.

MacRae SL, Croken MM, Calder RB, et al.: DNA repair in species with extreme lifespan differences, *Aging* 7(12):1171–1182, 2015.

Maddox G: Activity and morale: a longitudinal study of selected elderly subjects, *Soc Forces* 42:195–204, 1963.

Marshall VW: Sociology, psychology, and the theoretical legacy of the Kansas City studies, *Gerontologist* 34(4):768–774, 1994.

National Center for Complementary and Integrative Health (NCCIH): *Antioxidants: in depth* (website), 2013. https://www.nccih.nih.gov/health/antioxidants-in-depth.

Pomatto LC, Davies KJA: Adaptive homeostasis and the free radical theory of ageing, *Free Radic Biol Med* 124:420–430, 2018.

Ray D, Yung R: Immune senescence, epigenetics, and autoimmunity, *Clin Immunol* 196:59–63, 2019.

Reed AE, Carstensen LL: The theory behind the age-related positivity effect, *Front Psychol* 3:339, 2012.

Smorenberg A, Peters EJG, van Daele PLA, et al.: How does SARS-CoV-2 target elderly patients? A review on potential mechanisms increasing disease severity, *Eur J Intern Med* 83:1–5, 2021.

Sokolovsky J: *The cultural context of aging: worldwide perspectives*, 4th Ed., Santa Barbara, CA, 2020, Praeger.

Speakman JR, Selman C: The free-radical damage theory: accumulating evidence against a simple link of oxidative stress to ageing and lifespan, *Bioessays* 33(4):255–259, 2011.

Stanić MS, Matić SL: The biology and theories of aging, *Theor Biol Forum* 112(1–2):79–89, 2019.

Starkweather AR, Alhaeeri AA, Montpetit A, et al: An integrative review of factors associated with telomere length and implications for biobehavioral research, *Nurs Res* 63(1):36–50, 2014.

Steptoe A: Investing in happiness: the gerontological perspective, *Gerontology* 65(6):634–639, 2019.

Tan A: *The bonesetter's daughter*, New York, 2001, Random House.

Teshale SM, Lachman ME: Managing daily happiness: the relationship between selection, optimization and compensation strategies and well-being in adulthood, *Psychol Aging* 31(7):687–692, 2016.

Tornstam L: Gerotranscendence: a meta-theoretical reformulation of the disengagement theory, *Aging Clin Exp Res* 1:55–64, 1989.

Tornstam L: Transcendence in later life, *Generations* 23:1014, 2000.

Tornstam L: *Gerotranscendence: a developmental theory of positive aging*, New York, 2005, Springer.

Turner KJ, Vasu V, Griffin DK: Telomere biology and human phenotype, *Cells* 8(1):73, 2019.

Vaiserman A, Krasnienkov D: Telomere length as a marker of biological aging: state-of-the-art, open issues, and future perspectives, *Front Genet*, 2020 11:630186.

Wadensten B: An analysis of psychosocial theories of ageing and their relevance to practical gerontological nursing in Sweden, *Scand J Caring Sci* 20:347–354, 2006.

Wadensten B: The theory of gerotranscendence as applied to gerontological nursing—part 1, *Int J Older People Nurs* 2:289–294, 2007.

Wang CH, Wu SB, Wu YT, et al: Oxidative stress response elicited by mitochondrial dysfunction: implication in the pathophysiology of aging, *Exp Biol Med* 238:450–460, 2013.

World Health Organization (WHO): *Global financial crisis and the health of older people* (website), 2021. http://www.who.int/ageing/economic_issues/en.

Zhang W, Radhakrishnan K: Evidence on selection, optimization, and compensation strategies to optimize aging with multiple chronic conditions: a literature review, *Geriatr Nurs* 39(5):534–542, 2018.

Providing Cross-Cultural Care

Kathleen Jett

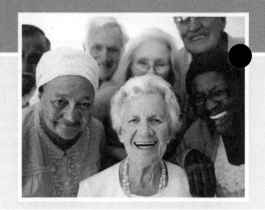

http://evolve.elsevier.com/Touhy/TwdHlthAging

A STUDENT SPEAKS

We are trying to do our work with the patient, but her daughter keeps getting in the way and saying things like "it is not the way we do things." I don't understand, we are just trying to do what we were taught to do.

Sandy, age 19

AN OLDER ADULT SPEAKS

It seems like I do not fit in anywhere anymore. My children do their best, but they must work, and my grandchildren don't have the same respect for me that I had for my grandparents. I know they love me, but it is just not the same.

Yi Liu, age 87

LEARNING OBJECTIVES

On completion of this chapter, the reader will be able to:

1. Compare the major paradigms of health and illness.
2. Identify solutions and actions one might take to move toward cultural proficiency in the delivery of cross-cultural care.
3. Accurately identify situations in which expert interpretation is essential.
4. Be prepared to work with interpreters effectively.
5. Formulate analyses and solutions that lead to culturally sensitive nursing actions when caring for older adults.
6. Demonstrate clinical reasoning to develop gerontological nursing solutions and actions aimed at reducing health disparities and inequities.

CULTURE, AGING, AND HEALTH CARE

Culture is most often referred to in terms of the shared and learned values, beliefs, and expectations of a group of people. Culture guides thinking; decision making; and beliefs about aging, health and health seeking, illness, treatment, and prevention (Jett, 2003; Spector, 2017). Cultural values influence health care delivery any time the "seeker" and "giver" meet. The "seekers" determine the perceived seriousness of the problem. The "givers" determine the problems that are present (if any), the treatments that are appropriate, and the way they expect seekers to respond. In turn, seekers decide if they agree with the problems the givers have identified, the value of the treatment, if they will accept the "prescription," and if they will act on it (e.g., get the "prescription" filled, take medication as instructed).

Culture guides individuals as they interact with family and friends within the same group and outside of their group, such as during health care encounters. Culture allows members of the group to predict each other's behavior and respond in ways that are considered appropriate. Cultural beliefs are passed down from one generation to another through *enculturation* and involve the family, the community, and even the political and structural aspects of an environment, such as where they live.

In contrast, *acculturation* is the process by which persons from one culture adjust to another culture. There has been much concern about immigrants who moved to their adopted country in later life. Adjustments needed to find late life satisfaction may be significant. Different degrees of acculturation and assimilation between generations create a communication gap between young and older immigrants as they join their families in new countries where the language and customs may be unknown to them. This may cause isolation and estrangement between the oldest and youngest generations. Enculturated and acculturated expectations may clash (see any of the books by author Amy Tan). In marginalized groups of older adults, illness, poverty, and migration are destroying the insulation previously afforded by the family and community (Jett, 2006). Members of minorities in any community are extremely vulnerable as they age. They may experience triple jeopardy when devalued because of age, race, and ethnicity.

Some aspects of acculturation are more critical to functional adaptation than others. For example, outward adaptations that incorporate language and dress are expressions of cultural identity, but many have less importance than beliefs about aging, health, illness and treatment, the use of time, and interactions with others (Fung, 2013; Spector, 2017). The level of acculturation is influenced by age at immigration, socioeconomic status, and educational level. These factors, as well as degree of exposure to the dominant health care system, influence health literacy.

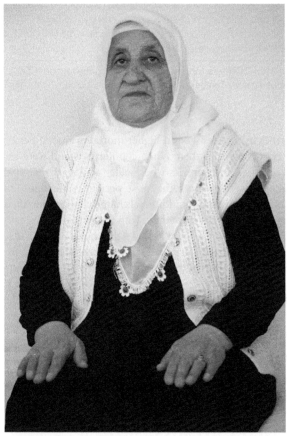

Common attire of Muslim women as expressions of culturally expected modesty. (©iStock.com/Reddiplomat)

This chapter provides an overview of cross-cultural health care, diversity, inequity, and the aging adult. It is important to note that an encyclopedic approach is not used. The reader will not find lists of "what term is used to refer to a German elder," and so on. Many texts devoted solely to culture can serve as resources for this, if desired. Instead, larger concepts that may be used by more than any "group" of people, such as health belief systems, are discussed.

Strategies are provided to help the gerontological nurse respond to the changing face of older adults, regardless of their backgrounds, but particularly those with beliefs and values that

differ from those of the nurse. The goal of cross-cultural caring is to move toward cultural proficiency and thereby optimize health outcomes and promote healthy aging.

DIVERSITY

Extending the idea of culture is that of *cultural diversity* or simply the existence of more than one group that is different from one another. Countries vary greatly in the level of diversity of all kinds. For example, the Philippines is an archipelago composed of more than 7000 islands inhabited by 175 different ethnolinguistic groups, with different cultural identities, health beliefs, and practices (Abad, 2014). This is dramatically different from Argentina, where most of the citizens are White (of European descent) and Roman Catholic, and Spanish is their primary language. Canada is the only "Western" country in the top 20 in terms of diversity. The United States ranks near the middle (World Population Review, 2021).

Diversity in the United States usually refers to two ethnic groups: Hispanic/Latinx or non-Hispanic/Latinx and five racial groups: Black or African American, Asian, Native Hawaiian/Pacific Islander, American Indian/Alaskan Native, or White. Other persons consider themselves "multiracial" or "some other race" (Marks & Jones, 2020). Of note: most of the older adults referred to as African American are descendants of persons who were brought to the United States against their will as slaves in the 17th century (Spector, 2017). Other persons who identify as Black have immigrated since that time.

The relative percentage of persons who identify as either non-White or Hispanic/Latinx is growing rapidly (Fig. 4.1). The immigration policies of a country significantly affect who, when, and where persons immigrate. Some experienced horrific events in their home country or during their immigration process and hold a unique and perhaps lifelong concern for safety and security. Other older immigrants today arrived in the United States late in life when joining their children who had become naturalized citizens.

It is important to note that within any one group, culturally similar or disparate, there is diversity of education, religion, gender, power, socioeconomic status, sexual orientation, gender identity, and an untold number of other factors. These factors

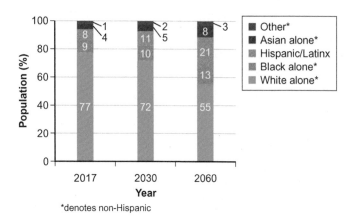

Fig. 4.1 Projected percent distribution of the US population ages 65 and older by race and ethnicity.

greatly influence the delivery and receipt of health care in all places in the world.

HEALTH INEQUITIES AND DISPARITIES

The terms *health inequities* and *health disparities* are often used interchangeably. Although they are somewhat different, both have implications for health care outcomes. *Health disparities* is the term used in discussions of the results of health inequities (Braveman, 2014). A current and significant health disparity is exemplified by the rate of COVID-19 infections and immunizations, timing and outcomes of hospitalizations, and number of deaths between non-Hispanic Whites and persons of color (Artiga et al., 2020a) (Table 4.1).

The term *health inequalities* refers to differences in avoidable, unnecessary, and unjust differences in health outcomes between advantaged and disadvantaged groups, such as many older adults. This inequity results in higher rates of both morbidity and mortality. Race is being used as a marker for disparities in the number of underlying health problems, hence increased risk for COVID-19-related mortality (Centers for Disease Control and Prevention [CDC], 2021). It most often is the result of unequal distribution of wealth and status; one group holds the power and influence in a community, including control of a resource such as health care (Box 4.1).

In 2002 the Institute of Medicine published the landmark report of the state of the science of health disparities in the United States, titled *Unequal Treatment: Confronting Racial and Ethnic Disparities in Health Care* (Smedley et al., 2002). Previous research had demonstrated an irrefutable differential in access to health care between White Americans and all others. Hence researchers were charged with determining the state of care in recognition of this disparity.

Among the results of the study were that health care treatment in and of itself was unequal (Smedley et al., 2002). The barriers were found regardless of insurance status, intensity of symptoms, geographical location, age, gender, and sexual orientation. Disparities occurred in all clinical settings, including public hospitals, private hospitals, and teaching hospitals. Most notable was that the

---

BOX 4.1   The Tuskegee Experiment

Among some older African Americans today there remains mistrust of White health care providers, especially those conducting research. This distrust will continue at some level until the memory of the infamous "Tuskegee Experiment" fades. In 1932 a study to understand the "natural history of syphilis" was conducted. Nearly 600 Black men from Macon County, Mississippi, were recruited to participate in a study conducted jointly by the US Public Health Service and the Tuskegee Institute. About half of the men had documented syphilis and were told they were being treated for "bad blood," a phrase with several meanings in the US Southern dialect. The men were never treated, even when penicillin became the evidence-based practice in 1947. Although concerns were raised in 1968, the study was not discontinued until 1972 when it was deemed to be ethically unjustified for being misleading and for failing to inform the subjects of the risks of participation. In 1973 a class action suit was filed, and in 1974 $10 million was awarded to the survivors and surviving families. In 1997 President Clinton apologized on behalf of the nation, and not long afterward, strict rules on the conduct of research were created. The last participant died on January 16, 2004. The last widow died on January 27, 2009. It is believed that this "experiment" is a major factor in the lack of trust that many Black Americans have in the health care system in the United States.

Adapted from Centers for Disease Control and Prevention (CDC): *The Tuskegee timeline* (website), 2017. http://www.cdc.gov/tuskegee/timeline.htm.

---

disparities in care resulted in higher mortality among persons of color compared with their White counterparts and were exacerbated with age. In countries where older adults are marginalized simply because of their age, they are especially vulnerable to health disparities. If a person has additional characteristics that differentiate that person further from those with power and status (e.g., skin color, religion, sexual orientation), the disparities are amplified.

In the years since *Unequal Treatment* was published, the US Agency for Healthcare Research and Quality (AHRQ) has produced an annual *National Healthcare Quality and Disparities Report* to track the prevailing trends of key indicators of health care quality and access for vulnerable populations, especially those who are statistical minorities, including a number of indicators that are highly significant to older adults (AHRQ, 2021). The World Health Organization (WHO, 2021) contributes to this knowledge base by monitoring special needs groups such as migrants, migrant workers, and asylum seekers.

OBSTACLES TO CROSS-CULTURAL CARING

Both overt and covert barriers to care include ageism, racism, ethnocentrism, and stereotyping; all can lead to significant conflict and decreased quality of care. Conflict can occur in the nursing situation any time one person interacts with another whose beliefs, values, customs, languages, behavior patterns, or expectations differ from their own. Hesitancy about the receipt of immunizations, lack of usual care, and logistical barriers (e.g., lack of transportation) remain obstacles to the acceptance and receipt of COVID-19 immunizations (Ndugga et al., 2021). African Americans have the least trust of vaccines of any subgroup within the US population (Artiga et al., 2020b). Black residents of long-term care facilities are the least likely to receive immunizations of any kind (Bardenheier et al., 2020) (Box 4.2).

TABLE 4.1   COVID-19 Hospitalization and Death by Race/Ethnicity, Ratio Compared to Non-Hispanic Whites

	American Indian/ Alaskan Native	Asian American	Black, Non-Hispanic	Hispanic/ Latinx
Cases	1.9×	0.7×	1.1×	1.3×
Hospitalization	3.7×	1.1×	2.9×	3.2×
Death	2.4×	1.0×	1.9×	2.3×

From Centers for Disease Control and Prevention (CDC): *COVID-19 hospitalization and death by race/ethnicity* (website), 2021. https://www.cdc.gov/coronavirus/2019-ncov/covid-data/investigations-discovery/hospitalization-death-by-race-ethnicity.html. Accessed February 12, 2021.

BOX 4.2 Disparity in Influenza Immunizations

Between 2018 and 2019 the Black-White disparity in influenza immunization rates increased from 7.1 to 9.9% (76.2% among White residents and 66.3% among Black residents). Vaccination rates were the highest in facilities with no Black residents and lowest in facilities with at least 50% Black residents. Standing orders improved the rate, but differences were attributed to higher refusal rates among Black residents.

From Bardenheier BH, Baier RR, Silva JA, et al.: Persistence of racial inequalities in receipt of influenza vaccination among nursing home residents in the United States, *Clin Infect Dis*, September 29, 2020 (epub ahead of print). doi:10.1093/cid/ciaa1484.

BOX 4.3 Intercultural Conflicts in Nursing Care

A newly immigrated Korean nurse is instructed to ambulate an 80-year-old male patient. He says that he is tired and wants to remain in bed. The Korean nurse does not insist that he ambulate. The White nurse manager reprimands the nurse for not getting the patient out of bed. The Korean nurse says to another Korean nurse: "Those Americans do not respect their elders; they treat them as if they were children." The nurse manager complains to another nurse: "Those Asian nurses allow patients to walk all over them." Both the manager and the Korean nurse were reacting to the other by applying stereotypes, leading to conflicts in the care setting.

Gerontological nurses will have to find ways to overcome these obstacles in their workplaces and communities to promote healthy aging while crossing cultures (NCCC, n.d.a.).

Ethnocentrism

Ethnocentrism is an expression of the belief that one ethnic or cultural group is superior to that of another. This belief may be acquired through enculturation learned at an early age or acculturation later in life. In the Western system of health care, it is expected that seekers adapt to the rules of the givers: for example, to be on time for appointments and to listen and follow the directions that are given. Following the "rules" is believed to result in improved health outcomes. Those who "choose" to disobey the rules are regarded as noncompliant. In an institutional setting, acculturated older adults will accept the type, frequency, and timing of such things as bathing and personal grooming and sleep and rest schedules. Older adults knowledgeable and accepting of the culture of an institution in which they find themselves are less likely to experience conflict with the health care staff. Meals are eaten when provided, even if the food does not look or taste like what the person is accustomed to. A "compliant" non-English-speaking resident will accommodate the staff, with or without the help of an interpreter.

Stereotyping

Stereotyping is the application of limited knowledge of a race, ethnic group, age, or culture to an individual. The nurse may hear or say something about what "all old people are like." While the specific stereotype may be either complimentary or derogatory, it prevents the nurse from getting to know the person as a unique individual and member of a tribe, clan, family, community, or even workplace (Box 4.3). Identification of the heterogeneity *within* the group is not recognized. However, due to the fast-paced health care that is expected today, the use of some stereotypes can be a helpful starting point. For example, a common stereotype about Latinx older adults is that they live in a multigenerational home and that a male in the family is the decision maker. If the nurse simply assumes this to be true, it could have a negative outcome, such as fewer referrals for support (e.g., home-delivered meals). On the other hand, a potentially positive stereotype can be used to shortcut the assessment. In discussing discharge plans, the non-Hispanic nurse may say, "I have always understood that many Latinx older adults live with family members. Is this the case for you, and if so, is anyone at home to help you if you need help?" This same approach would be appropriate for most racial or ethnic groups and must be done with utmost tact and respect to shield the patient from embarrassment if the stereotype does not apply.

MOVING TOWARD CULTURAL PROFICIENCY

Providing cultural and linguistically appropriate services and care in a way that reduces disparities in the health care setting is no longer an option (The Joint Commission, n.d.). Gerontological nurses can learn to do this more expertly as they move along a continuum from cultural destructiveness to cultural proficiency beyond cultural competence (Fig. 4.2). This requires a willingness to become more self-aware of subtle bias, to learn to know others from their perspectives (i.e., "where they are

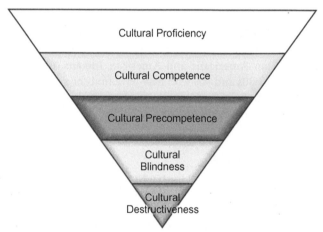

Fig. 4.2 A model for cross-cultural caring. (Adapted from Cross T, Bazron B, Dennis K, et al.: *Toward a culturally competent system of care,* vol 1, Washington, D.C., 1989, CASSP Technical Assistance Center, Center for Child Health and Mental Health Policy, Georgetown University Child Development Center; Goode TD: *Cultural competence continuum,* revised ed., Washington, D.C., 2004, National Center for Cultural Competence, Georgetown University Center for Child and Human Development, University Center for Excellence in Developmental Disabilities; and Lindsey R, Robins K, Terrell R: *Cultural proficiency: a manual for school leaders,* Thousand Oaks, CA, 2003, Corwin Press.)

BOX 4.4   **Moving Toward Cultural Proficiency and Healthy Aging**

- Become familiar with your own cultural perspectives, including beliefs about disease etiology, treatments, and factors leading to outcomes.
- Examine your personal and professional behavior for signs of bias and the use of negative stereotypes.
- Remain open to viewpoints and behaviors that are different from your expectations.
- Appreciate the inherent worth and dignity of all persons from all groups.
- Develop the skill of attending to both nonverbal and verbal cues in communication.
- Develop sensitivity to the communication, indicating the paradigm from which they face health, illness, and aging.
- Learn to negotiate, rather than impose, solutions to healthy aging consistent with the beliefs of the persons to whom we provide care.

coming from"), and finally, to apply new solutions skillfully and more effectively work with individuals to support rather than hinder their cultural strengths (Box 4.4).

Cultural Destructiveness

Cultural destructiveness is the systematic elimination of the culture of another. There are many well-known examples of this: the genocide of the Jews in Eastern Europe (1933–45) and of the Hutu in Rwanda (1994). In Canada, Australia, and the United States, cultural destructiveness occurred when indigenous children were forced from their homes and sent to boarding schools where the language, dress, and food expressive of their heritages were forbidden (Australian Human Rights Commission, n.d.; Bear, 2008; Pember, 2020; Little, 2018). American Indian healing ceremonies, performed by tribal elders, were forbidden. Practices referred to as "traditional" or "folk" healing were and continue to be discounted. Suspiciousness of Western medicine is still present among many African Americans and American Indians, especially those in their 80s and 90s who may have first- or secondhand knowledge of the cultural destruction inflicted by Whites in power (Grandbois et al., 2012).

Cultural Blindness

It is hoped by this point that the reader has begun to understand that there are multiple cultures coexisting in countries and continents and that such things as skin color and socioeconomic, political, and educational power affect the health care experience. Yet some people, including health care providers, state that they see a person's difference (such as age) and value but still harbor negative stereotypes and bias that interfere with good gerontological nursing practice, such as "all old people fall" or "what can they except at that age?" Some are blind to the fact that life experiences such as prejudice, historical trauma, social trauma, and ageism influence both the pursuit and the receipt of health care (Feagin & Bennefield, 2014). Cultural blindness prevents the nurse from providing sensitive and, more importantly, effective care. It prevents even the possibility of reducing health disparities and inequities.

Cultural Precompetence

The development of cultural precompetence begins in the cross-cultural setting with self-awareness of one's personal biases, prejudices, attitudes, and behaviors toward persons different from oneself. For persons whose culture or status places them in a position of power, such as nurses in the US health care system, cultural awareness is realizing that this alone often means special privilege and freedoms (Box 4.5). Achieving cultural precompetence requires a willingness to learn how health is viewed by others. It means playing an active role to combat ageism in society.

Cultural Competence

Nurses who move beyond cultural precompetence are able to step outside of their biases and accept that others bring a different set of values and priorities to the health care setting. Nurses who are able to provide competent cross-cultural care accept that all persons are deserving of respect. Nurses are expected to recognize that they need some knowledge of other cultures, particularly those they are most likely to encounter in the health care setting. Cultural knowledge is both what the nurse brings to the caring situation and what the nurse learns from others (Fung, 2013).

Cultural Knowledge

Cultural knowledge has the potential to minimize frustration and conflict between older patients and other health care providers (Kirmayer, 2012). It is expected that cultural knowledge will allow the nurse to provide care more appropriately and effectively and improve health outcomes (Campinha-Bacote, 2011; Kirmayer, 2012).

Definitions of terms. Cultural knowledge includes the appropriate use of terms, especially *race* and *ethnicity*. While often used interchangeably, each has a separate meaning. *Race* is a phenotype as expressed in observable traits, such as eye color, facial structure, hair texture, and skin tones. *Ethnicity* refers to the cultural group with which one self-identifies. Persons may share a common nationality, migratory status, language or dialect, religion, or even geographical location (e.g., rural versus urban). Traditions, symbols, literature, folklore, food preferences, and dress are often expressions of ethnicity. Persons from a specific ethnic group may

BOX 4.5   **Unrecognized Privilege and Racism in the Health Care Setting**

A gerontological nurse responded to a call from an older patient's room. While she was with the patient, he repeatedly, and without comment, dropped his watch on the floor. She calmly picked it up, handed it back to him, and continued talking. One time an aide walked into the room as the patient dropped the watch. The aide picked it up and handed it back to him just as the nurse had done. The patient immediately started yelling and cursing at the aide for attempting to steal his watch. When telling this story, the nurse thought the whole situation odd but not too remarkable.

The patient and nurse were White, and the aide was Black. The nurse did not realize that the behavior of the patient was grounded in racism and culturally destructive until the nurse learned of the concepts while taking a formal class on cross-cultural health care; this treatment of Black staff had become culturally acceptable behavior in the health care setting.

not share a common race. For example, persons who identify as Hispanic/Latinx may be from any race and from multiple countries. It is most appropriate to ask an older adult to self-identify ethnicity rather than to make assumptions (Box 4.6).

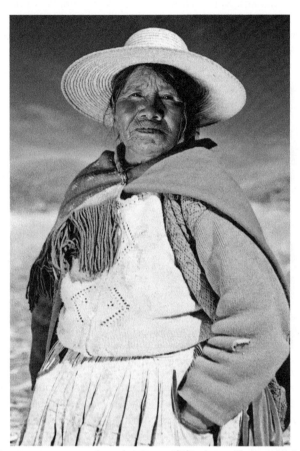

Dress as an expression of culture. (©iStock.com/Bartosz Hadyniak)

Orientation to family and self. Family support is highly variable between groups, social classes, and subcultures, yet the nuclear or extended family is the chief avenue of transmitting cultural values, beliefs, customs, and practices. The family may provide stability and sanctuary to the aging individual. Useful concepts in providing cross-cultural health care to older adults include knowing their orientation to self and family. Many of those of northern European descent place great value on personal autonomy and individuality (Fung, 2013). In a classic study, Rathbone-McCune (1982) found that the residents of a segregated ("White") retirement community went to great lengths and lived with significant discomforts rather than ask for help. To seek or receive help was considered a sign of weakness and dependence, something to be avoided at all costs.

BOX 4.6   The Problem With Assumptions

I was collecting data for a study while in the home of a woman with black skin and no accent. As I began with the demographics page, I said simply, "I assume you are African American?" With her head held high, she declared, "No ma'am, I am an American!" I will never make that mistake again.

Kathleen

The importance of autonomy and individualism in the US health care system stems from the writing of the Constitution and was institutionalized in health care when the Patient Self-Determination Act was enacted in 1991. Individuals were recognized as the sole decision makers regarding their health. Without the person's explicit permission, health care providers are now legally bound to restrict access to health care information only to the patient.

This behavior is the antithesis of a collectivist or interdependent culture, a norm in most parts of the world, including Japan, Germany, and Canada. It is the responsibility of each citizen to contribute to the care of others (Kubba, 2020). In the Latinx culture this has been referred to as "familismo" (Savage et al., 2016). Self-identity is drawn from family ties (broadly defined) rather than the individual. The "family" (e.g., extended family, tribe, clan) is traditionally of primary importance; decisions are made by the group or designee. Within families, the exchange of help and resources has been both expected and commonplace. In many African American families, fictive kin (persons considered family but not related by blood or marriage) are equally as important. The cultural beliefs and behaviors around families is particularly significant for health in aging because it relates to eldercare and health-related and end-of life decision making. The cultural value of collectivism is also important in response to pandemic precautions where multigenerational living is the norm and social distancing is not always possible. This becomes complicated in places like the United States where those whose focus has been on others also have to deal with a history of personal persecution (Kubba, 2020).

When a nurse from a culture in which independent decision making is expected cares for an older adult whose dominant value is interdependence, or vice versa, the potential for cultural conflict and poor outcomes is great (Box 4.7).

Orientation to time. Orientation to time is often overlooked as a cultural construct that influences the use of health care and the attitudes toward preventive practices (Belgrave & Allison, 2014). Time orientations are culturally described as future, past, or present (Box 4.8).

BOX 4.7   Opportunities for Cultural Conflicts: Independent Versus Interdependent Health Care Decision Making

An older Chinese woman is seen in her home by a European American public health nurse and found to have a blood pressure reading of 210/100 mm Hg and a blood glucose level of 380 mg/dL. The nurse insists on calling the patient's nurse practitioner and arranging for immediate transportation to an acute care hospital. The woman insists that she must wait until her son-in-law and daughter return home from work so that she can discuss the matter with them before any decisions are made. They will decide if, where, and when she will go for treatment. She is concerned about the welfare of the family and wants to ensure that income is not lost and that the family can afford a health care provider's visit and possible hospitalization. They would need to make alternate arrangements for childcare and meal preparation. The nurse's main concern is the health of the individual elder, and the elder's main concern is her family. The nurse is operating from the value that says an individual is independent and responsible for personal health care decisions, inconsistent with the value of this older adult.

A **past orientation** to health and health problems views both as dependent on the actions in one's past (such as in a past life or earlier in this life) or on events or circumstances of one's ancestors. For example, dishonoring ancestors by failure to perform certain rituals or having poor interactions with others earlier in one's life may result in illness today. Illness today may be considered punishment for past deeds, and it may be prevented by living an honorable life.

A **present orientation** means that when a health care problem occurs, immediate treatment is needed. Future treatment is considered potentially too late for a positive outcome. The success of freestanding "immediate care centers" or those associated with pharmacy and grocery chains in the United States may be a reflection of a present orientation. In general, preventive actions for future health are not consistent with a present orientation toward illness and need for treatment.

Future time orientation is consistent with a belief that when one is ill today, a health care appointment can be made for the future (e.g., the "next available" appointment). The health problem and its treatment can "wait." The problem will still be there, and the delay will not necessarily affect the outcome. Prevention is important because of its effect on future health days, years, and even decades (e.g., weight control).

Conflicts between future-oriented Westernized medical care and those with past- or present-time orientations are many. Patients are likely to be labeled as *noncompliant* for failing to keep an appointment set tomorrow for a health problem of today, for failing to participate in preventive measures such as a "turning schedule" for a bed-bound patient to prevent a (future) pressure injury, or for failing to receive immunizations to prevent a potential future infection. Members of present-oriented cultures are often accused of overusing hospital emergency departments in the United States, when in fact it may be considered the only reasonable option available for today's treatment of today's problem (Belgrave & Allison, 2014).

Beliefs about health, illness, treatment, and prevention. The increasing diversity of the global community increases the potential for clashes between health beliefs. Aging itself further increases diversity due to long-held beliefs about normal changes with aging and potentially extensive experience related to illness and treatment of self, family, and others. In most cultures, older adults are likely to treat themselves and others for familiar or chronic conditions in ways they have found successful in the past, practices that are referred to as *domestic medicine,* folk medicine, or folk healing. Folk medicine is, and always has been, based on beliefs regarding the appropriate treatment for the symptoms and presumed diagnoses. Only when self-treatment fails will a person consult with others known to be knowledgeable or experienced with the problem, such as an older family member, neighbor, community member, or indigenous healer. If this fails, people may (or may not) seek help within a formal system of health care.

The culture of nursing and health care in the United States is one that advocates what is called the *Western* or *biomedical model.* The health care providers within this model usually consider it to be superior to all other models, a highly ethnocentric viewpoint. However, many of the world's people have different beliefs, such as those based on *personalistic* (magico-religious) or *naturalistic* (holistic) models (Table 4.2). Each model includes beliefs and

attitudes about disease prevention, disease causation, acceptable treatment, and definitions of health. It is not uncommon for an older adult from any ethnic group to adhere to beliefs other than those in the biomedical approach used by most nurses in "Westernized" nations. Nonetheless, nurses who are familiar with the range of health beliefs and realize their importance will be able to provide more sensitive and appropriate care. In the absence of understanding, the potential for conflict is great.

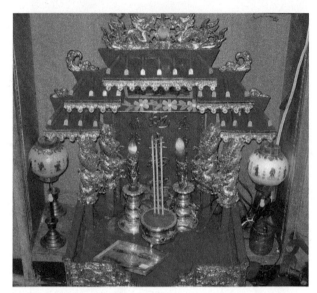

Buddhist shrine. (Courtesy Rachel E. Spector, 2006)

Eye contact. Eye contact is a highly culturally constructed behavior. For some, direct eye contact is believed to be a sign of honesty and trustworthiness. Nursing students in the United States are taught to establish and maintain eye contact when interacting with patients, but this behavior also may be misinterpreted. Some persons avoid eye contact, not as a sign of deceit but as a sign of respect. A more traditional American Indian elder may not allow the nurse to make eye contact, moving the eyes slowly from the floor to the ceiling and around the room. During a health care encounter, in most Asian cultures, direct eye contact is considered disrespectful. Making eye contact implies equality; therefore older adults may avoid eye contact with physicians and nurses if health professionals are viewed as authority figures or those with higher status (eDiplomat, 2016). In other cultures, direct eye contact between men and women is considered a sexual advance. The gerontological nurse can follow the lead of older adults by being open to eye contact but neither forcing it nor assigning any inherent value to it.

A handshake is the customary and expected greeting in most of North America. A firm handshake is thought to be a sign of good character and strength, yet this is not always possible or desired. Arthritis may affect the hands, making a grasp painful. The types of acceptable physical contact vary widely. Traditional American Indian elders may interpret firm or vigorous handshakes as signs of aggression. Their handshakes instead may be more of a passing of the hand with a light touch as a sign of respect rather than of weakness. In the Muslim culture, cross-gender physical contact (including handshakes) may be considered highly inappropriate or even forbidden. Before a nurse makes physical contact with an

TABLE 4.2   Comparison of Health Belief Models

Model	Illness Causation	Assessment and Diagnosis	Treatment	Prevention	Health
Western (biomedical)	Invasion of germs or genetic mutation identified as a "disease"	Objective identification of pathogen or process May include consultation with a health practitioner identified as a specialist in the subcategory of disease (e.g., oncologist)	Remove or destroy invading organism; repairing, modifying, or removing affected body part	Avoidance of pathogens, chemicals, activities, and dietary agents known to cause abnormalities	Absence of disease
Personalistic (magico-religious)	The actions of the supernatural, such as gods, deities, or nonhuman beings (e.g., ghosts, spirits) A punishment for a breach of rules, breaking a taboo, or displeasing or failing to please the source of power	Consultation with a health practitioner specializing in the subcategory of practice (e.g., minister, curandero)	Religious practices, such as praying, meditating, fasting, wearing amulets, burning candles, and "laying of the hands"	Making sure that social networks with their fellow humans are in good working order Avoid angering family, friends, neighbors, ancestors, and gods	A blessing or reward of God
Naturalistic (holistic)	Physical, psychological, or spiritual imbalance resulting in disharmony	Consultation with a health practitioner specializing in the specific subcategory of practice (e.g., Chinese physician, herbalist)	Dependent on the submodel (e.g., hot/cold practices of treating a hot illness with a cold treatment)	Life practices that maintain balance	Balance (e.g., the right amount of exercise, food, sleep)

older adult of any culture, the nurse should ask the person's permission or follow the person's lead, such as an outstretched hand. In a number of East Asian cultures, especially China and Japan, the handshake is used in the business setting, but it is expected to be slight and accompanied by a slight bow (eDiplomat, 2016). In nonbusiness settings a bow is expected, especially when greeting a person older than oneself. The depth of the bow is an expression of the status afforded each other. A deep bow at the waist is usually expected when greeting an elder.

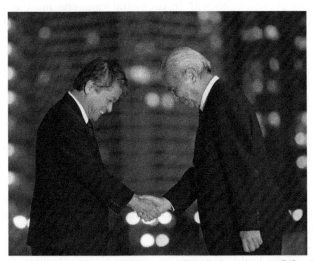

The bow is a gesture of respect in many East Asian cultures. (©iStock. com/stockstudioX)

The use of silence. The value, use, and interpretation of silence also varies markedly from one culture to another and between persons of different ages. In many Eastern cultures, especially those in which the Confucian philosophy is embraced, silence is highly valued. It is expected of young family members and those with less authority. Silence may be considered a sign of respect for the wisdom of an elder. In traditional Japanese and Chinese families, silence during a conversation may indicate that the speaker is giving the listener time to ponder what has been said before moving on to another idea. In traditional American Indian cultures, it is believed that one learns self-control, courage, patience, and dignity from remaining silent. In contrast, Western cultures place much importance on verbal communication. French, Spanish, and older adult immigrants from the former Soviet Union may interpret silence as a sign of agreement (Purnell & Paulanka, 2008).

Spoken communication. If the nurse and the older adults share the same spoken language, communication may be inappropriately assumed. Expert communication requires that the nurse use words and phrases that are understood and at the appropriate level of health literacy. This expertise is especially important due to the large role that nurses play in education, witnessing consents, giving directions (e.g., related to assessment techniques), and making requests.

Interpretation is the processing of one *spoken* language into another in a manner that preserves the meaning and tone of the original language without adding or deleting anything. The job of the interpreter is to work with two different linguistic codes in a way that will produce equivalent messages without adding meaning or opinion. The interpreter acts as a culture broker to ensure that the world of the provider and the world of the older adult are mutually respected and understood (National Center for Cultural Competence [NCCC], n.d.b.). Interpretation and translation are needed when different languages are spoken (Box 4.9).

It is ideal to engage those who are trained in medical interpretation and who are adults and of the same culture and gender. Unfortunately, too often children or even grandchildren are called on to fulfill this role. When they are not available, secretaries or housekeepers may be asked. When depending on lay interpreters, the nurse must realize that either the interpreter or the older adult may "edit" comments because of cultural restrictions about the content by deciding what is or is not appropriate to speak about to, or in front of, an elder, parent, child, or stranger. When there are no other reasonable options, "interpreter lines" via the telephone or computer are used. Due to the frequency of hearing loss in aging, the use of high-quality headphones or visual imaging of the speaker will maximize the accuracy of the communication. Closed captions are an option for those who have the necessary visual acuity and reading level, especially for those who are hearing impaired. Regardless of the type of communication assistance used, there are guidelines available to maximize the quality and acceptability of these methods (Box 4.10).

Written communication. *Translation* is the exchange of one *written* language for another, such as in the translation of printed patient education materials. It is recommended that a "back translation" be done for accuracy. The material is first translated into the language needed and then translated back to the original language in which it was written to ensure accuracy. There are many patient education materials in multiple languages available on the internet and through professional organizations. However, it is essential that the nurse remember that many older adults across the globe have low or no literacy. Many of the oldest persons in the southern United States, especially if African American, have only a third-grade education due to limited access to school when growing up or for financial or political reasons.

To provide the best care to all persons regardless of age, race, ethnicity, or culture, it is now expected that the nurse demonstrate at least cultural competence but can go further and move toward cultural proficiency (see Fig. 4.2).

BOX 4.9   When a Professional Interpreter Is Needed

An interpreter is needed any time the nurse and the patient speak different languages, when the elder has limited proficiency in the language used in the health care setting, or when cultural tradition prevents the elder from speaking directly to the nurse. The more complex the decision making, the more important are the interpreter and his or her skills. In gerontological nursing these circumstances are many, such as when discussions are needed about the treatment plan for a new condition, the options for treatment, advanced care planning, or even preparation for care after discharge from a health care institution. The use of a specially trained interpreter is even more important if the elder has limited health literacy.

BOX 4.10   Guidelines for Working With Interpreters

- Before an interview or session with a client, meet with the interpreter to:
  - Explain the purpose of the session.
  - Instruct the interpreter to use the person's own words and avoid paraphrasing.
  - Instruct the interpreter to avoid inserting his or her own ideas or omitting any information.
- Look and speak directly to the person, not the interpreter.
- Be patient. Interpreted interviews take more time because of the need for three-way communication.
- Use short units of speech. Long, involved sentences or complex discussions create confusion.
- Use simple language. Avoid technical terms, professional jargon, slang, abbreviations, abstractions, metaphors, and idiomatic expressions.
- Listen to the person and watch nonverbal communication (facial expression, voice intonation, body movement) to learn about emotions regarding a specific topic.
- Clarify the person's understanding and the accuracy of the interpretation by asking the person to tell you in his or her own words what the person understands, facilitated by the interpreter.

Modified from Lipson JG, Dibble SL, Minarik PA, editors: *Culture and nursing care: a pocket guide*, San Francisco, 1996, UCSF School of Nursing Press.

Cultural Proficiency

The culturally proficient nurse can move smoothly between two worlds for the promotion of healthy aging. Culturally proficient care to older adults is that which is respectful, compassionate, and relevant. It includes the recognition of factors beyond culture, such as the effect of past and current trauma, social status and bias, poverty, and education leading to health disparities and inequities. The nurse providing proficient cross-cultural health care can work with and build relationships with members from a variety of cultural groups as a natural part of daily practice. The relationship building results in the ability to communicate effectively and sensitively assess the individual's state of health, negotiate mutually acceptable goals, and support solutions and actions that are culturally acceptable and empowering.

To provide proficient cross-cultural care, one must enter into an unknown conceptual world in which time, space, tradition, and wellness are expressed through a unique language that conveys the perceived nature of health, illness, and humanity. It requires a sensitive and effective search for cues and the setting of mutual goals that are possible within the limitations of available resources.

USING CLINICAL JUDGMENT TO PROMOTE HEALTHY AGING

Communication is a foundational skill in any nursing practice but particularly important in gerontological nursing due to the complexity of decision making that is often needed and the frequency of end-of-life conversations. Cross-cultural care increases the complexity significantly, and the increasing diversity of the health care workforce provides even further challenges. When the nurse or aide speaks with an accent or uses tones and phrases reflective of their background, communication may be difficult with older adults who speak a different language. Most people with presbycusis (normal age-related hearing loss) depend on lip reading to some extent to augment what they are hearing. The words may be the same, but the physical (oral) way they are spoken differs, making understanding difficult. Medical jargon should be used only when addressing a patient who is another health care professional from the same health belief paradigm.

The nurse uses all the skills that may be needed to facilitate communication with older adults (e.g., good lighting, hands away from face, facing the person at eye level) (Chapters 7 and 13). Yet miscommunication is common. The LEARN model (Box 4.11) (Berlin & Fowkes, 1983; Ladha et al., 2018) serves as a guide to overcome this problem to the extent possible and can lead to the opportunity for improved clinical reasoning and judgment care delivery.

L—Listen

Promoting healthy aging and providing the highest quality of cross-cultural care for older adults requires the ability to communicate in new and expert ways. Communication begins long before a word is spoken. As soon as the nurse observes the patient, the recognition of cues begins. The nurse attends not just to the words spoken but also to movement, evidence of comfort, and nonverbal expressions. If the person communicates verbally, it includes attention to idiom, style, jargon, voice tone, and inflection. Communication means first and foremost listening carefully for cues that indicate the person's perception of the situation and what is most important. It includes the identification of the availability of culturally appropriate and sensitive resources, including those in the person's community. When working with older adults, resources also may include indigenous healers, priests, monks, rabbis, or ministers, if their presence is desired or believed to be helpful. The nurse recognizes relevant data when asking about the person's use of time, who is involved in decision making, and the health belief paradigm or paradigms that are the most meaningful to the individual and significant others (Box 4.12).

If the person is nonverbal due to any condition, most cues will come from attention to body language. In many cultures the unspoken message may be as or more important than what is said, and the nurse should recognize this.

BOX 4.11 LEARN Model

L Listen carefully to what the person is saying. Listen to the perception of the person's situation, desired goals, and ideas for treatment (see Kleinman model, Box 4.12).

E Explain your perception of the situation and the problems.

A Acknowledge and discuss both the similarities and the differences between your perceptions and goals and those of the elder and their significant others or decision makers as appropriate.

R Recommend a plan of action that takes both perspectives into account.

N Negotiate a plan that is mutually acceptable and possible.

Adapted from Berlin E, Fowkes W: A teaching framework for cross-cultural health care: application in family practice, *West J Med* 139:934–938, 1983.

BOX 4.12 Kleinman's Explanatory Model for Culturally Sensitive Assessment

1. How would you describe the problem that has brought you here? (What do you call your problem; does it have a name?)
   a. Who is involved in your decision-making processes about health concerns?
2. How long have you had this problem?
   a. When do you think it started?
   b. What do you think started it?
   c. Do you know anyone else with it?
   d. Tell me what happened to that person when dealing with this problem.
3. What do you think is wrong with you?
   a. How severe is it?
   b. How long do you think it will last?
4. Why do you think this happened to you?
   a. Why has it happened to the involved part?
   b. What do you fear most about your sickness?
5. What are the chief problems your sickness has caused you?
6. What do you think will help this problem? (What treatment should you receive, and what are the most important results you hope to receive?)
   a. If specific tests or medications are listed, ask what they are and do.
7. Apart from me, who else do you think can make you feel better?
   a. Are there therapies that make you feel better that I do not know about? (Maybe in another discipline?)

Modified from Kleinman A: *Patient and healers in the context of culture: an exploration of the borderland between anthropology, medicine, and psychiatry*, Berkeley, CA, 1980, University of California Press.

E—Explain

The gerontological nurse recognizes the cues and completes an analysis of them, including differentiating normal age-related changes from potential pathology. Cross-cultural gerontological nursing takes a further step when conducting the analysis in the context of the person's culture. The priorities that the nurse has assigned to the problem are communicated to the individual using language, phrasing, and body language that is culturally acceptable. The nurse shares the tentative priorities and realizes that the final decision lies with the individual and not the health care provider.

A—Acknowledge

Nurses acknowledge where their analyses differ from the person with whom they are talking and convey clearly that this is the *starting* point for further discussion. This is a demonstration of valuing the individual and the person's perceptions as important and unique. It is a way of moving away from the model of care "seeker" and care "giver" to one of joint collaborators in pursuit of healthy aging outcomes.

R—Recommend

Only after the different perspectives are acknowledged can the nurse move on to begin to recommend solutions and actions to address the mutually identified and acceptable health care needs and the perspective of both the older adult and family and the nurse and health care system.

N—Negotiate

Negotiation begins when the nurse and the older adult (and caregiver as appropriate) work toward an agreement of the

BOX 4.13   **Speaking to the Wrong Person**

Madame DuBois came to the clinic for a checkup related to her diabetes and hypertension, both of which were out of control. She spoke no English. At the first visit the nurse spent a long time reviewing ideal outcomes and explaining the appropriate strategies to reach these through an interpreter, making the interaction especially time-consuming for the patient, the nurse, the interpreter, and the person accompanying Mme DuBois. No questions were asked. A different person accompanied Mme DuBois at her next visit and asked questions that had been addressed in the first visit. The nurse then discovered that the woman at the second visit was the person who helps Mme DuBois. The person at the first visit was a neighbor who happened to have time to accompany Mme DuBois and thought it was impolite to question the nurse.

BOX 4.14   **Cross-Cultural Caring**

Determine the following about the older adult:
- Preferred cultural, ethnic, and racial identity
- Expectations concerning formality of the encounter
- Expectations concerning use of names, titles, addressing the patient and the nurse
- Preferred language
- Level of health and reading literacy and availability of assistance if needed
- Past personal experience with the Western health care model
- Level of acculturation, adherence to traditional approaches, and openness to new approaches
- Factors influencing decision making: who, how, when, and what

prioritization of the recognized needs (Box 4.13). As solutions and subsequent actions are explored, the person must feel welcome to voice dissent at any time. Failure to encourage and recognize this will result in a failure to achieve even apparently negotiated outcomes. The nurse who has listened carefully to social cues will realize that setting up a future appointment for a frail elder will not necessarily mean that the person can keep it unless the value of this is agreed upon and negotiations are made with both the older adult *and* the caregiver or source of transportation.

The study of aging is one of the most complex and intriguing opportunities of our day. Realistically, it will be almost impossible to become familiar with the whole range of clinically relevant cultural differences of older adults one may encounter. Attempting to provide care holistically and sensitively is the most challenging opportunity leading to personal growth for both the nurse and the person receiving care.

Today's nurse is expected to provide culturally proficient care to persons regardless of their age, health beliefs, experiences, values, and styles of communication (Box 4.14). This means that clinical reasoning is based on what has the *most* value to the individual and finding ways to work with it rather than expecting conformity to the cultural model in which the health care is provided.

Cross-cultural communication is especially important because of the inherent complexity of health while aging and the combination of generational and cultural differences between the older adult and the gerontological nurse. The nurse will need to communicate effectively regardless of the languages spoken. Communication may depend on limited verbal exchanges and attend more to facial and body expressions, postures, and gestures and knowledge about when an interpreter is needed and how to work with one. Effective gerontological nurses providing cross-cultural care engage in clinical thinking that uses the cultural knowledge and skills needed to optimize communication and make effective and appropriate clinical judgments.

To skillfully recognize cues in an unbiased manner, nurses must develop cultural proficiency through awareness of their own ethnocentricities. Skillful cross-cultural nursing means developing a sense of mutual respect between the nurse and the person. A sense of caring is conveyed in gestures of personal recognition. It involves working "with" the person rather than "on" the person, and in doing so the person's self-esteem and quality of life and health are enhanced to the extent possible. Health disparities and inequities can begin to be reduced, and movement toward healthy aging can be facilitated. Unbiased caring can surmount cultural differences.

KEY CONCEPTS

- Global population diversity is rapidly increasing and will continue to do so. This suggests that nurses will be caring for a greater number of older adults from a broader number of cultural backgrounds and that older adults will encounter caregivers from a greater number of cultures as well.
- Research has shown that significant disparities and inequities in the outcomes of health care persist. Those who bear the greatest burden of morbidity and mortality are those who are the most marginalized from those in control of health care resources; this includes older adults, especially those who are frail. This has become more obvious during the COVID-19 pandemic.
- Nurses can contribute to the reduction of health disparities and the promotion of social justice by increasing their own cultural awareness, knowledge, and skills.
- Cultural proficiency and sensitivity require awareness of issues related to age, culture, race, social class, and economic situations.

- Stereotyping can mask heterogeneity within cultural groups.
- Health beliefs of various groups emerge from three general belief systems: biomedical (allopathic), magico-religious, and naturalistic. Older adults may adhere to one or more of these systems.
- Providing effective cross-cultural care to older adults includes skills related to both verbal and nonverbal communication.
- The more complex the decision making, the more important is the quality of communication. For those with limited English proficiency, expert interpretation is especially needed whenever serious decisions are required (e.g., end-of-life care, treatment changes).
- The use of family, children, or support staff as interpreters is not recommended and may result in censored interpretation because of rules of cultural etiquette that may be unknown to the nurse.
- The LEARN model provides a useful framework for working to reach mutually agreeable and possible health care goals.

NEXT-GENERATION NCLEX® (NGN) EXAMINATION–STYLE QUESTIONS

Ms. Yazzie is a 64-year-old woman who has just moved to a long-term care facility. Her mother belonged to the Mescalero Apache Tribe in New Mexico. Her father was White. Her mother gave her up at birth, hoping she would be adopted, but she spent her childhood in foster care. She performed low-earning odd jobs to support herself, had few friends, never married, and had no children. She did not have health insurance, and as a result her health care was sporadic. When she was about 62 years old, she was raped and severely beaten, resulting in severe posttraumatic stress disorder (PTSD), and could no longer work. She has a history of hypothyroidism, hypertension, multi-infarct dementia, and osteoarthritis with chronic pain, limiting her ability to walk. She has a 66 pack-year history of smoking. Prior to entering the facility, she drank 8 to 10 ounces of liquor each night but is no longer allowed to do so. She is 5′5″ tall and weighs 110 pounds (BMI 18.30 kg/m²). She becomes very frightened when male staff approach her and only allows female nurses, assistive personnel, and staff to work with her. She is no longer ambulatory. However, she wheels herself around the facility and can often be heard crying and repeatedly asking, "Do you love me?" She engages in conversation, stops crying when prompted, talks about her childhood.

Highlight the data that provide cues to health disparities. Underline factors that place Ms. Yazzie at the highest risk for poor health outcomes at this point.

CLINICAL JUDGMENT QUESTIONS AND ACTIVITIES

1. Define the terms *culture, ethnicity, ethnocentricity,* and *cultural proficiency.*
2. Identify several personal values or beliefs that are derived from your ethnic roots.
3. Privately list your biases and "ethnocentrisms" for various ethnoracial cultural groups and explore the basis of these beliefs (e.g., taught, fear, experience, lack of knowledge).

Then consider what you can do to limit their effect on your practice.

4. Describe the advocacy role of nurses to reduce health disparities.
5. What are the primary difficulties in providing nursing care for individuals from a different background than one's own?

RESEARCH QUESTIONS

1. How is culture influencing a community's response to the COVID-19 epidemic?
2. What are the enduring cohort differences that are unlikely to change throughout life?

3. What are the outcomes of an integrated cultural approach versus a separate-culture approach in a curriculum?

REFERENCES

Abad PJB, Tan ML, Baluyot MMP, et al.: Cultural beliefs on disease causation in the Philippines: challenge and implications in genetic counseling, *J Community Genet* 5(4):399–407, 2014.

Agency for Healthcare Research and Quality (AHRQ): 2021 *National healthcare quality and disparities report* (website), 2021. *https://www.ahrq.gov/research/findings/nhqrdr/nhqdr19/index.html.*

Artiga S, Corallo B, Pham O: *Racial disparities in COVID-19: key findings from available data and analysis* (website), 2020a. https://www.kff.org/racial-equity-and-health-policy/issue-brief/racial-disparities-covid-19-key-findings-available-data-analysis/.

Artiga S, Michaud J, Kates J, et al.: *Racial disparities in flu vaccination: implications for COVID-19 vaccination efforts* (website), 2020b. https://www.kff.org/policy-watch/racial-disparities-flu-vaccination-implications-covid-19-vaccination-efforts/.

Australian Human Rights Commission: *Track the timeline: the stolen generation. History of separation of Aboriginal and Torres Strait Islander children from their parents* (website), n.d. https://www.humanrights.gov.au/timeline-history-separation-aboriginal-and-torres-strait-islander-children-their-families-text.

Bardenheier BH, Baier RR, Silva JB, et al.: Persistence of racial inequalities in receipt of influenza vaccination among nursing home residents in the United States, *Clin Infect Dis,* 2020 ciaa1484.

Bear C: *American Indian boarding schools haunt many* (website), 2008. http://www.npr.org/templates/story/story.php?storyId=16516865.

Belgrave FZ, Allison K: *African American psychology: from Africa to America,* Thousand Oaks, CA, 2014, Sage.

Berlin EA, Fowkes WC Jr: A teaching framework for cross-cultural health care: application in family practice, *West J Med* 139:934–938, 1983.

Braveman P: What are health disparities and health equity? We need to be clear, *Public Health Rep* 129(Suppl 2):5–8, 2014.

Campinha-Bacote J: Delivering patient-centered care in the midst of a cultural conflict: the role of cultural competence, *Online J Issues Nurs* 16(2):5, 2011.

Centers for Disease Control and Prevention (CDC): *COVID-19 hospitalization and death by race/ethnicity* (website), 2021. https://www.cdc.gov/coronavirus/2019-ncov/covid-data/investigations-discovery/hospitalization-death-by-race-ethnicity.html. Accessed February 12, 2021.

eDiplomat: *Japan* (website), 2016. http://www.ediplomat.com/np/cultural_etiquette/ce_jp.htm#topnav.

Feagin J, Bennefield Z: Systematic racism and U.S. healthcare, *Soc Sci Med* 103:7–14, 2014.

Fung HH: Aging in culture, *Gerontologist* 53(3):369–377, 2013.

Grandbois DM, Warne D, Eschiti V: The impact of history and culture on nursing care of Native American elders, *J Gerontol Nurs* 38(10):3–5, 2012.

Jett KF: The meaning of aging and the celebration of years among rural African-American women, *Geriatr Nurs* 24:290–293, 2003.

Jett KF: Mind-loss in the African American community: dementia as a normal part of aging, *J Aging Stud* 20(1):1–10, 2006.

The Joint Commission: *The Joint Commission stands for racial justice and equity* (website), n.d. https://www.jointcommission.org/resources/news-and-multimedia/the-joint-commission-stands-for-racial-justice-and-equity/.

Kirmayer LJ: Rethinking cultural competence, *Transcult Psychiatry* 49(2):149–164, 2012.

Kubba S: *The importance of culture in societal response to COVID-19* (website), 2020. https://harvardpolitics.com/culture-response-covid-19/.

Ladha T, Zubairi M, Hunter A, et al.: Cross-cultural communication: tools for working with families and children, *Paediatr Child Health* 23(1):66–69, 2018.

Little B: *How boarding schools tried to "kill the Indian" through assimilation* (website), 2018. http://www.history.com/news/how-boarding-schools-tried-to-kill-the-indian-through-assimilation.

Marks R, Jones N: *Collecting and tabulating ethnicity and race responses in the 2020 census* (website), 2020. https://www2.census.gov/about/training-workshops/2020/2020-02-19-pop-presentation.pdf.

National Center for Cultural Competence (NCCC): *What is the role of cultural brokers in health care delivery?* (website), n.d. https://nccc.georgetown.edu/culturalbroker/2_role/index.html.

National Center for Cultural Competence (NCCC): Self-assessments. (website), n.d.a. https://ncc.georgetown.edu/assessments/.

Ndugga N, Hill L, Artiga S, et al.: *Latest data on COVID-19 vaccinations, race/ethnicity* (website), 2021. https://www.kff.org/coronavirus-covid-19/issue-brief/latest-data-on-covid-19-vaccinations-by-race-ethnicity/.

Pember MA: Healing by "revealing the truth", *Indian Country Today,* 2020 Nov 26.

Purnell L, Paulanka B: *Guide to culturally competent health care,* (2nd Ed.), Philadelphia, 2008, FA Davis.

Rathbone-McCuan E: *Isolated elders: health and social intervention,* Rockville, MD, 1982, Aspen.

Savage B, Foli KJ, Edwards NE, et al.: Familism and health care provision to Hispanic older adults, *J Gerontol Nurs* 42(1):21–29, 2016.

Smedley B, Stith AY, Nelson AR, editors: *Unequal treatment: confronting racial and ethnic disparities in health care,* Washington, D.C., 2002, National Academy Press.

Spector RE: *Cultural diversity in health and illness,* 9th Ed., New York, 2017, Pearson.

World Health Organization (WHO): *Migration and health* (website), 2021. https://www.euro.who.int/en/health-topics/health-determinants/migration-and-health.

World Population Review: *Most diverse countries* (website), 2022. https://worldpopulationreview.com/country-rankings/most-diverse-countries.

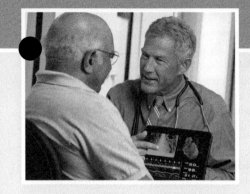

CHAPTER 5

Economics and Health Care in Late Life

Kathleen Jett

http://evolve.elsevier.com/Touhy/TwdHlthAging

A STUDENT SPEAKS

We went on a home visit with our preceptors today. I could hardly stand it. The house was almost bare. The only food was left over from the "home-delivered meals" he gets from the local service organization. The preceptor said that he was doing the best he could with what he had.

Evelyn, age 19

AN OLDER ADULT SPEAKS

When I was growing up, life was hard. We were so poor we couldn't do much but to hold on tight. When I was lucky, I could get work plowing a field for $1 an acre. You work hard, and you make do. There were not such things as going to a doctor or hospital; you just pray you don't get sick. . . . Then when I turned 65, I got a little check from the government and a red, white, and blue Medicare [insurance] card. The check [SSI] isn't much, about $550 a month, but I consider myself blessed and much better off than ever before. And now I don't worry about my health; I will be taken care of, praise the Lord.

Aida, age 94

LEARNING OBJECTIVES

On completion of this chapter, the reader will be able to:

1. Briefly explain the history of Social Security, Supplemental Security Income, Medicaid, and Medicare.
2. Explain how health care is financed in the United States.
3. Compare the types of health care services available under Medicare.
4. Describe the role of the nurse advocate in relation to the health and economic issues of concern to older adults.

ECONOMICS IN LATE LIFE

Social Security Income

Considered by many to be one of the most successful federal programs in the United States, Social Security was established in 1935 by President Franklin Delano Roosevelt during the depths of the Great Depression (Chapter 2). The primary function was to prevent or minimize the financial burden on younger members of society by providing monetary benefits to older retired workers (National Archives, 2010). Social Security was established as an "age-entitlement" based on the societal belief that older adults were uniformly poor in relation to younger adults. This means that eligible individuals (beneficiaries) could receive a monthly monetary benefit simply because of their age, regardless of their actual financial need (Box 5.1). However, the benefits were and are limited to those who have paid Social Security taxes on a requisite amount of income prior to receiving them (Box 5.2).

The program is funded by what is called a pay-as-you-go system. In most cases Social Security taxes are collected from a percentage of one's income and matched by employers. Although individually deposited, the funds are not reserved for any one person (i.e., no one has an account set aside in one's name). The funds not immediately paid out to beneficiaries are "borrowed" by the federal government for regular operating expenses. If the amount of the combined workers' and employers' contribution exceeds that paid to beneficiaries, the program, as designed, cannot remain solvent. There continues be concern that the program will no longer be viable at some point in the future. This is potentially a serious threat to the millions who depend on Social Security as their sole source of income. To delay this problem, legislation was passed in 1983 to gradually increase

TABLE 5.1 Full Retirement Age

Year of Birth[a]	Full (Normal) Retirement Age
1937 or earlier	65
1938	65 and 2 months
1939	65 and 4 months
1940	65 and 6 months
1941	65 and 8 months
1942	65 and 10 months
1943–1954	66
1955	66 and 2 months
1956	66 and 4 months
1957	66 and 6 months
1958	66 and 8 months
1959	66 and 10 months
1960 and later	67

[a]If you were born on January 1, you should refer to the previous year.
From Social Security: *Retirement benefits* (website), n.d. https://www.ssa.gov/OACT/quickcalc/earlyretire.html.

the age when one could reach "full retirement" and therefore be eligible to receive Social Security (Table 5.1).

In 2020 more than 69 million Americans received over $1 trillion in benefits. About 84% of those at least 65 years of age receive Social Security benefits; 55% of these are women. At least 50% of married couples and 59% of those unmarried depend on Social Security for 50% of their income, and an estimated 25% of all persons (2014 figures) depend on it for 90% of their income (Dushi et al., 2017). In 2020 the average monthly income from Social Security was $1503 for those who had reached the "age of full retirement." The monthly payment increases every year one *delays* receiving the benefit between their full retirement age and the age of 70, at which time the maximum benefit was $3895 in 2021. Beneficiaries may receive

an annual cost-of-living adjustment (COLA), depending on the state of the country's economy and measured by the Consumer Price Index for the previous year. The COLA for 2021 was 1.3%.

Supplemental Security Income

Not all older people living in the United States have income from any source that is adequate to provide even the most basic necessities of life. This is especially true for persons who have spent their lives employed in the agriculture industry, in the food industry, or as domestic workers and were paid very low wages or on a cash basis. Supplemental Security Income (SSI) was established in 1965 to provide a minimal level of economic support to eligible persons age 65 or older, blind or disabled adults, and children. Although the population over age 65 has the highest percentage of persons who live below the poverty level, they make up the smallest percentage of those receiving SSI. SSI either provides "total support" or supplements a low Social Security benefit (Box 5.3).

Other Late Life Income

Finally, late life income may come from private retirement investments and/or employer pensions. These monies are held for the beneficiary until such a time when they must begin to withdraw some portion of this (required minimum distribution, or RMD), at the age determined by the fund but no later than 70½ years of age if this was reached before January 1, 2020. The RMD does not begin until the age of 72 for those reaching 70½ years of age in 2020 or later (Internal Revenue Service [IRS], 2020).

Some private retirement plans offer several choices for receipt of funds. Retirees can elect to take their pensions in one lump sum or in a monthly amount based on their life expectancy alone or based on the life expectancy of the retiree and a spouse or partner. They may establish a plan so that all or most of the benefit is received during their *expected* lifetime rather than providing for any survivor benefit. Notification of the potential survivor is now required but was not always so in the past. This still may affect some of the oldest survivors (Box 5.4).

HEALTH CARE DELIVERY

Before the industrial revolution of the late 1800s people in most countries and cultures worked until they were no longer physically able to do so. In many cases the type of work changed as they aged, but the expectation was that the person would continue to contribute to the family or the community until shortly before death (Fleming et al., 2003). Family members, friends,

BOX 5.4 A Surprising Change of Income

Mrs. Jones lived in a small rural community. Her husband had worked for the same company from the time he was 18 years old until he died. He had a limited but adequate pension to meet the couple's day-to-day needs, but nothing extra. His Social Security benefit was small due to his lifelong low wages. When Mr. Jones died suddenly, Mrs. Jones was informed that she would no longer receive support from his pension. He had opted for the "no survivor benefit" when he enrolled, meaning that all benefits would cease upon his death.[a] Because she had never worked outside of the home, Mrs. Jones was dependent solely on her husband's survivor Social Security benefit. She was in danger of losing her home because she could not afford her taxes.

[a]This is no longer legal without the express permission of the potentially surviving spouse.

and the community provided care to those who were no longer able to care for themselves. While this is still the case in some cultures, as countries industrialized the care of members of the family with diminished capacity became problematic in both social and economic terms. As younger family members joined the urban workforce, many older adults stayed behind in agricultural areas of the country with less social and caregiving support (Achenbaum & Carr, 2014).

Almshouses and poor houses emerged in the early 19th and 20th centuries to provide care for the indigent who did not have family available and were unable to care for themselves. Most of these facilities were initially supported by charitable groups, especially religious organizations. Governments eventually became involved when the primary population of these homes was frail older adults and the disabled; they became public nursing institutions. In some communities, public monies replaced or supplemented charitable offerings. Local governments were authorized to purchase land and erect facilities through taxes to others. The care of indigent older adults was considered a public responsibility; however, because of the long-held social belief in personal responsibility, those residing in such care facilities were required to contribute any property they owned and most or all of their income to help cover the expenses related to their care (Achenbaum & Carr, 2014; Social Security, n.d.).

Economic factors are always driving forces in the delivery of health care in the United States, regardless of who pays for it and where it is provided. Whereas some higher income countries are struggling to keep up with the escalating costs of technology, persons in low-income countries may not receive even the most rudimentary care. In countries with universal health care, it is supported to a large extent by significant payroll taxes, and the financial risk is shared between all citizens where some level of health care is available to all those living in the country. The expectation is that all people can use services while being protected from associated financial hardship. However, currently there is a very wide variation in who is eligible for "universal health care" and if it even exists within any one country. It has been especially difficult to implement in low- and middle-income countries. Ensuring the provision of safe primary and ambulatory care has been the focus of the World Health Organization in the past (Slawomirski et al., 2018). However, the

ravages of the COVID-19 pandemic and addressing the health care needs of their populations has been a challenge to all countries regardless of their previous health standing.

With few exceptions health care has always been a purchased service in the United States. In most cases it is not considered a right. The federal government is the major purchaser of health care through its insurance plans (Medicare, Railroad Medicare, Medicaid, and TRICARE) or provided directly through the US Department of Veterans Affairs (VA). Medicare is the major insurance plan available to and used by eligible disabled US citizens and those at least 65 years of age. Those with very low incomes also may be eligible for Medicaid, an insurance plan that is jointly funded by state and federal resources.

Changes in Health Care for Older Adults

When Social Security was proposed in 1934, President Roosevelt also proposed a universal health insurance plan, but because of the opposition to it, he removed it from the proposal to avoid losing Social Security (Corning, 1969). The American Medical Association was part of the opposition of any nationalized program of health insurance, believing it to be "socialized medicine," and successfully prevented its implementation (Goodman, 1980). *Fortune* magazine polled the American public in 1942 and found that 76% of those questioned opposed government-financed medical care (Cantril, 1951).

In the early 1960s President Lyndon Johnson recognized that the numbers of poor children, those with serious disabilities, and older persons were significantly increasing and were vulnerable to little access to health services of any kind. Although opposition continued, President Johnson proposed amendments to the Social Security Act to address this widespread public health problem. In Senate and House hearings, some legislators described the amendments as steps that would continue to destroy independence and self-reliance and would tax the poor and middle classes to subsidize the health care of the wealthy (Social Security, n.d.a.). Nonetheless, legislation was passed in 1965 and 1966 to expand the Social Security system by establishing Medicare and Medicaid.

A short time after implementation of these plans, millions more people could receive health care, and the associated costs escalated rapidly. Prescription drug coverage (Medicare Part D) was added in 2006 by President George W. Bush's administration. The Affordable Care Act of President Barack Obama's administration (2010) contained several provisions with the potential to further improve health care in general and services for older adults, especially coverage for preventive services (Table 5.2).

Medicare

Medicare is the insurance plan specifically designed to provide health care for those eligible for Social Security. It is administered by a special entity, the Centers for Medicare and Medicaid Services (CMS). Medicare is made up of three components: the age-entitlement Medicare A, the purchased Medicare B or the alternative commercial Advantage plans (Medicare C), and the purchased commercial Prescription Drug Plan (PDP) (Medicare D). Commercial supplemental insurance is also available for uncovered expenses.

TABLE 5.2   Major Components of the Affordable Care Act That Affect Older Adults

Component	Description
Primary care	Incentives to health care providers based on quality and not just quantity of care ("evaluation of quality-based indicators")
Bundled payments	Payment to hospitals for an entire "bundle of care," which includes both the hospital stay and the medical needs for a period of time after discharge
Five-star programs	Yearly evaluation and ranking of all Medicare-related commercial products
Decreasing out-of-pocket costs for prescription medications	Reduce current size of the donut hole and decrease the copay in the donut hole from 100% to 25%
No copays for those preventive services with most evidence of usefulness	Increased access to preventive services

BOX 5.5   The "Welcome to Medicare" Exam

Must be obtained within 12 months of enrolling in Medicare Part B and must include the following:

- Review of medical record, including family history, current health conditions, prescriptions
- Review of social history related to person's health
- Education and counseling about preventive services
- Health screenings, immunizations, or referrals for other care as needed
- Height, weight, and blood pressure measurements
- Calculation of body mass index
- Simple vision test
- Review of risk for depression and level of safety
- An offer to discuss advance directives
- Written preventive health plan
- Making sure person is up to date on recommended cancer screens and immunizations

BOX 5.6   Yearly "Wellness Visits"[a]

Completion of a "Health Risk Assessment"

- A review of medical and family history, including medications, herbs, and dietary supplements taken
- Developing or updating a list of current health care providers
- Height, weight, blood pressure, and other routine measurements
- Screening for any cognitive impairment or indications of depression
- Screening for potential functional impairments or safety risks
- Personalized health advice related to assessment, including health risks identified, and treatment options
- A screening schedule for appropriate preventive services

[a]First one at least 12 months after "Welcome to Medicare" visit. Cannot include a physical exam of any kind.
See https://www.medicare.gov/coverage/yearly-wellness-visits to determine coverage, copay, and eligibility for screenings.

As soon as a person is 65 years old (or meets special disability requirements, including end-stage renal disease), the person is expected to apply for no-cost Medicare A. The choices associated with Medicare Parts B or C, D, and supplements are selected based on personal preference, regional availability, and ability to pay. In most cases selection and enrollment must take place during a 6-month period beginning 3 months before and ending 3 months after a person's 65th birthday to avoid late enrollment penalties and higher premiums. It is effective on the first day of the 65th birthday month unless an equivalent insurance is provided by an employer or past employer through a pension benefit (Social Security Administration, n.d.b). More than 60 million persons received Medicare in 2020. Over 50 million of these were at least 65 years of age (NCPSSM, 2021).

At the time of this writing, two comprehensive no-cost health-promoting services are available to older adults. A one-time "Welcome to Medicare" visit (Box 5.5) and annual "Wellness Visits" beginning 12 months after the initial exam (Box 5.6). These services are both specifically designed to promote healthy aging through primary and secondary prevention (Chapter 2, Table 2.2).

Like Social Security, Medicare was designed as a pay-as-you-go system; taxes collected from employees are used for the payment of specific health-related expenses of current beneficiaries. The funds are not earmarked for any particular taxpayer's future medical expenses but used as they are needed. Although the federal government pays most of the health-related costs covered by Medicare, the beneficiaries contribute in the form of premiums and copayments (copays). All commercial plans are evaluated annually using a five-star rating from worst (0) to best (5). The results are posted on the CMS website and useful when one is considering changing plans or selecting a service such as a long-term care facility (Medicare.gov, n.d.). Established by the Affordable Care Act, this is an attempt to hold these plans more accountable for the quality of the product they provide, including pricing and patient safety.

Medicare Part A

Medicare Part A is a hospital insurance plan covering acute care, short-term rehabilitation in a skilled nursing facility or at home, and most of the costs associated with hospice care (Box 5.7). There is no premium for eligible beneficiaries, and the program is administered directly by CMS. Others may purchase Part A coverage and pay a monthly premium. Individual must enroll in Part A at the time of their 65th birthday to avoid penalty.

Medicare Part B

Medicare B (referred to as *Original Medicare*) provides insurance coverage for medical services provided on an outpatient basis and some durable medical equipment (Box 5.8). This plan is also administered directly by CMS. The premium for Medicare B increases annually and is based on one's income as reported to the IRS. For persons with incomes of $91,000 or less (individual tax return) or $182,000 or less (joint tax return), the standard monthly premium was $170.00 per person in 2022, up from $148.50 in 2021. The significant increase was the result of

---

BOX 5.7   Health Services Provided Through Medicare Part A

Designed to partially cover the costs of acute hospitalization semiprivate rooms and any necessary medical services and supplies; care as listed below:

1. There is a deductible for days 1 to 60 (each stay).
2. Days 60 to 120 copay amounts increase over time.
3. There is no coverage after 150 days.
4. Deductibles and copays increase every year.
5. Deductibles and copays are either paid out-of-pocket or reimbursed by Medicaid or Medigap policies.

Skilled rehabilitative nursing care in a health care facility (only when care by a licensed nurse or physical or occupational therapist is needed):

1. Only after a minimum of 72-hour acute care hospital admission (not observation).
2. The first 20 days are covered at 100% if skilled care is needed the entire time.
3. Days 21 to 100 have a daily copay of more than $100.
4. No coverage after 100 days.
5. Coverage ceases on the day skilled care is no longer needed.

Home health services requiring skilled care (only when care by a licensed nurse or physical or occupational therapist is needed):

1. Intermittent skilled care for the purpose of rehabilitation provided in the home.
2. The person must be ill enough to be considered homebound.
3. Medicare may pay 80% of the approved amount for durable medical equipment and supplies (e.g., hospital bed).

Hospice care is provided for terminally ill persons expected to live less than 6 months who elect to forgo traditional medical treatment for the terminal illness:

1. Possible copay of ≤$5 for each prescription drug or similar item for pain relief or symptom control.
2. Possible copay of 5% for limited respite or pain management stays.
3. Replaces Medicare Parts A and B for all costs associated with the terminal condition.

Inpatient psychiatric care:

1. Limited coverage of 190 days in a lifetime.
2. Partial payment.
3. Other significant restrictions apply.

BOX 5.8   Health Services Provided Through Medicare Part B

Designed to cover some of the costs associated with outpatient or ambulatory services. Deductibles and copays are required in most cases:

1. Physician, nurse practitioner, or physician assistant medically necessary services
2. Limited prescribed supplies
3. Medically necessary diagnostic tests
4. Physical, occupational, and speech therapy for the purpose of rehabilitation
5. Limited durable medical equipment if prescribed by a physician and for documented medical necessity. Copay and deductible apply.
6. Outpatient hospital treatment, blood, and ambulatory surgical services
7. Some preventive services (many with no copay or deductible)
8. Diabetic supplies and services (excluding insulin and other medications)

---

the approval of a new, very expensive medication that became available for select persons with Alzheimer's disease. Most elect to have the premium withheld from their monthly Social Security benefit.

Advantages of *Original* Part B are choice of the primary care provider and referrals are not necessary. Providers who "accept assignment" have agreed to charge only an "allowable fee" that Medicare determines annually. The physician receives 80% of this amount from Medicare, and the patient is responsible for the remaining 20% and any annual deductible. This same amount is paid to the physician for the work done by the nurse practitioner if it is done "incident to" or as a part of the physician's usual care. If a nurse practitioner provides the service independently, the reimbursement rate is 85% of the 80% (Medicare Payment Advisory Commission [MedPAC], 2019).

A health care provider who does not accept assignment may charge the patient up to 15% more than the total allowable charge. The combination of an increasing number of wealthy older adults and fewer primary care providers has spawned an industry of "boutique" services, including physician practices. For an additional "membership," "convenience," or "surcharge," patients are eligible for a wide range of special services such as immediate access to the provider (e.g., via private cell phone).

Medicare Part C

When enrolling in or changing Medicare plans, one selects either *Original* Medicare Part B or Medicare Part C. Otherwise referred to as a Medicare Advantage Plan (MAP), Medicare Part C uses a prospective payment system and includes traditional health maintenance organizations (HMOs) and other similar programs; all are managed by commercial companies. All traditional services covered by *Original* Medicare Parts A and B must be provided while the MAP is receiving monthly payments (capitation) for every person on the plan regardless of the expenses. Additional services, copays, and deductibles are predetermined by the MAP; prescription drug benefits (MAP-DP) may or may not be provided. Not all MAPs are offered at all locations in the United States; premiums vary depending on location and range of services. In some cases, no premium is charged to the member and is paid directly by the federal government.

MAPs may provide a cost savings to the member and extra benefits in comparison to the *Original* Medicare plan. However, special rules must be followed, including the requirement that care is obtained only with a referral from an assigned primary care provider. The provider serves as a "gatekeeper" in an effort to ensure that only the highest quality medical care and that which is deemed "medically necessary" is received. Should a member obtain services without a referral, there is no coverage, and all costs are "out-of-pocket," i.e., at the consumer's expense.

Alternatives to Medicare C

Several programs have emerged as health care finance is changing in the United States. These include Medicare Cost Plans and Medicare Savings Plans available in some areas of the country and subject to the annual five-star rating.

Medicare Part D

The Medicare Modernization Act of 2003 established Medicare Part D, a Prescription Drug Plan (PDP) for eligible recipients of Medicare (Box 5.9). It is an *elective* plan with associated out-of-pocket premiums and copays and is offered by

---

BOX 5.9   Medicare Prescription Drug Plans

Most Prescription Drug Plans (PDPs) are set up in a similar way with deductibles and copays; however, to be a provider in Medicare Part D, the insurance plan must meet the following specific guidelines:

1. Annual deductible as low as zero
2. Copay of medications dependent on plan
3. After having spent a set amount in any one year, person receives what is called "catastrophic coverage," and all medications are at a minimum amount or percentage

---

Medicare-approved commercial companies. Which medications are covered (a formulary) and their associated costs depend on the plan selected and where the prescriptions are filled. Electronic prescriptions are recommended. Effective January 1, 2021, a 30-day supply of insulin can cost no more than $35 if it is on the plan's formulary.

All persons with Medicare, except those in MAP-PD programs, are eligible to voluntarily purchase a PDP. However, if one chooses to do so, the same rules and timing related to enrollment and incurring of penalties seen in Medicare B apply. People can change their plans only during the "open enrollment" periods each year without penalty or when they have a change of circumstances, such as entering a long-term care facility. Help with the associated costs is available for persons with low incomes. A Medication Therapy Management program is available to accompany Medicare D.

Supplemental Insurance (Medigap)

Because of potentially high deductibles and copays, people who have the financial resources often purchase Medicare supplement insurance plans, referred to as Medigap. They are purchased from a company that provides coverage in specific geographic areas. Premiums vary by company depending on location and range of services and can increase at any time the company chooses. While Medicare Parts A and B remain the "primary" insurance and therefore are billed first, the Medigap plan serves as a "secondary insurance" and is billed second. The copays and deductibles are dependent on the plan purchased. When enrolling in a plan at the same time as enrolling in Medicare Part B, all applicants must be automatically approved. Although changes can be made at a later time, they are subject to review.

Persons searching for an appropriate plan can be referred to the Medicare website or request a printed copy of the standard plans (available at https://www.medicare.gov/supplements-other-insurance). They will then need to contact the company and arrange payment for the premium. Help in selecting one of twelve different plans from a host of insurers is available from most states' aging services programs. In 2021 monthly premiums ranged from $52 to $1548 depending on the age, sex, and health status of the person when the plan is purchased and the benefits that are provided. The premium increases annually.

Medicaid

Medicaid was established in 1965 at the same time as Medicare as part of the revisions to the Social Security Act. It is a health insurance program jointly funded by federal and state governments using tax dollars. CMS administers the program at the federal level, and a state agency administers it at the state level.

Medicaid covers the costs of health services for low-income children, pregnant women, those who are permanently disabled, and persons age 65 or older. Eligibility is determined by the state and is based on income and assets, categorical need, and lack of ability to afford any insurance premiums, including those associated with Medicare. Only a limited number of people can receive Medicaid regardless of their situation due to their state's fiscal health and political priorities.

Medicaid covers all Medicare premiums, copays, and deductibles and may provide additional health benefits. Persons who are dually eligible for both Medicare and Medicaid are frequently required to enroll in MAP-PD plans. Federal law requires that states provide a certain minimal level of service and may add other coverage such as for vision care, dentures, prostheses, case management, and other medical or rehabilitative care provided by a licensed health care practitioner. Medicaid pays for most of the care provided in nursing homes in the United States. This includes "nonskilled" care such as bathing and medication administration.

Consistent with the early expectations in the almshouses, if institutional long-term care is needed, people are expected to be fiscally responsible for their own care to the extent possible before depending on the tax support of the community. They are required to use personal income and their own assets (e.g., Social Security) first to pay for care. When assets are no longer (or ever) available or they are inadequate, then Medicaid (funded through taxes) provides a "safety net" to ensure that the poorest, most disabled, and frailest persons receive care.

For a person who requires the financial support of Medicaid for a nursing home stay and has a spouse who is able to remain in the community, the spouse is protected from "spousal impoverishment." Depending on the spouse's income, only a percentage of the joint assets are counted as belonging to the patient and used to determine eligibility, and the spouse's percentage of the assets are not expected to be used to pay for the patient's care. On the death of a community-living spouse, it is expected that the amount that Medicaid has spent on the care (and only up to that point) be reimbursed with any remaining funds in the couple's shared estate (Medicaid, n.d.).

In the past, some people who believed they would soon need nursing home care transferred their assets to others to be able to meet Medicaid eligibility and thereby avoid using their own funds to pay for their care. Although some transfers to a spouse or a disabled, dependent child are permitted, any other transfer (i.e., to another person or to a trust) is considered Medicaid fraud. When a person applies for Medicaid, a "look-back period" is done to determine if funds that would normally be available to the applicant have been transferred. If transfers were made, Medicaid support will not begin until the costs incurred equal the amount of the transfer. For example, a person may be eligible for Medicaid due to low monthly income but has assets of $100,000. If the person had transferred these assets to someone else during the "look-back period" and is in a nursing home where the monthly rate is $10,000, the person would not be eligible for Medicaid for 10 months. This is known as "spend-down." These regulations attempt to ensure that individuals pay what they can for the care they need but still provide a safety net when funds are exhausted.

Most of the Medicaid funds are used to provide extended long-term, day-to-day nursing home care for poor older and disabled adults, but persons who are near-poor and without assets and who have monthly incomes greater than the "low income" limit set by the state are not eligible for assistance through Medicaid. In the absence of the availability of informal caregivers, providing for those who need assistance continues to be a major social and public health problem in the United States.

Other Health Care Delivery Services

In some parts of the country (and for some persons), alternative plans have been developed to both finance and provide for health needs while aging.

Indian Health Service

The Indian Health Service (IHS) is a federal health program for American Indians and Alaskan Natives (https://www.ihs.gov/). Services are provided both at the tribal level and through Urban Indian Health Programs. The provision of health services is complex among this population. For American Indians who are also military veterans, care obtained from IHS is paid for by the VA. Retired workers are most likely eligible for Medicare, and if low income, they also may qualify for Medicaid but not IHS care. Traditional IHS care ensures that all documented members of one of the many Indian Nations have care. There are a number of programs in development, and implementation is intended to promote health among American Indians of all ages, ranging from those who are aging healthfully to those caring for aging and debilitated older adults (https://www.ihs.gov/medicalprograms/eldercare/index.cfm?module=longtermcare).

In 2020 IHS formed a Critical Care Response Team to provide urgent care for life-threatening conditions as needed during the COVID-19 crisis. As in other communities of color, the average positivity rate has been high and variable by community and tribe, ranging from only 3.3% for those living in Alaska to 22.9% for those in Oklahoma City (as of January 10, 2021) (IHS, 2021). As elsewhere, older adults of color have borne the greatest burden of virus-related mortality.

Care for Veterans

The US Department of Veterans Affairs (VA) has long held a leadership position, conducted research, and developed innovations in gerontological care. The VA system has been a forerunner of the various continua of care providers now in place. Since early on, VA-administered nursing homes, home care and community-based programs, respite care, blindness rehabilitation, and mental health services are available to veterans.

In the past, veterans' hospitals and services were available on an as-needed basis for anyone who had served in the uniformed services at any time and for any length of time. It was not necessary for individuals to use their Medicare benefits. However, this system has undergone significant change as the number of veterans increased and the needs of older veterans became more complex. One of the first changes was a restriction on the use of veterans' hospitals and services. Instead of coverage of any health problem, priorities were set for those health problems that are deemed "service connected" in some way, that is, the health care problem began during active duty.

The older veteran is now expected to obtain and use Medicare for non-service-connected health problems. They are responsible for copays and deductibles the same as those for other Medicare beneficiaries. An outcry among veterans and veteran groups resulted in the development of a free Medigap policy known as TRICARE For Life (TFL).

For those veterans at least 65 years old who are disabled and receive a military pension, monetary support is available if personal assistance is needed for themselves or their spouses. These funds can be used for home care, nursing home, and assisted living facilities. The program is referred to Aid and Attendance (A&A). There is also a "Housebound" program that increases the monthly pension for those who are substantially confined to home due to a permanent disability (VA, 2017). The range of program services and eligibility criteria are complex. The reader is referred to https://www.benefits.va.gov/persona/veteran-elderly.asp.

TRICARE for Life

TRICARE For Life (TFL) is an automatic insurance program for select military persons, their dependents, and retirees who receive Social Security or a pension from the Railroad Retirement Board. It is provided by the US Department of Defense. For those who are eligible for Medicare, Part B must be purchased, and TRICARE serves as a free Medigap policy. It is not necessary to purchase Medicare D, as TFL covers the costs for prescription medicines obtained through the VA. It is expected that most persons with TFL receive non-service-connected health care from a community provider. Dependent parents or parents-in-law may be eligible for pharmacy benefits if they turned age 65 on or after April 1, 2001, and are also enrolled in Medicare Part B. For more information about this, see https://www.tricare.mil/Plans/Eligibility/MedicareEligible.

Long-Term Care Insurance

Additional insurance for potential future long-term care needs may be purchased by those with the financial means to do so. Ideally these policies would cover the expenses related to copays for long-term care and coverage for help with day-to-day needs and custodial care. Traditionally these policies were limited to care in long-term care facilities and provided a flat-rate reimbursement to residents for their costs. However, these policies have become more creative and innovative, and some plans cover home care costs instead of or in addition to care in long-term care facilities. To offer assistance to older adults, nurses can refer persons to the websites provided by the Administration on Aging (https://act.gov/ltc) or the American Association for Long-Term Care Insurance (http://www.aaltci.org).

The premiums for these policies are based on the age at the time of purchase, the maximum amount the plan will pay, the maximum number of days or years covered, and the types of care desired. Optional benefits can be added to the policy for additional fees.

The purchaser of a long-term care policy is cautioned to read the policy carefully and understand all details, limitations, and exclusions, to ensure that the plan covers the amount and type of service the person anticipates needing. It is advisable to suggest that persons speak to an independent financial advisor and refer to reviews of the chosen insurance company before purchasing a policy.

KEY CONCEPTS

- The Social Security system in the United States provides a guaranteed income for eligible persons who have paid a requisite amount into the system earlier in their lives.
- Both Social Security and the Medicare insurance programs are based on a "pay-as-you-go" arrangement, with funds from current workers used to support current retirees.
- Social Security provides income for the majority of older persons in the United States.
- Medicare is a health insurance plan for eligible persons who are age 65 or older, blind, or permanently disabled or who have end-stage renal disease.
- Medicare is composed of Parts A, B, C (Medicare Advantage Plans), and D. There is no premium for Medicare Part A, which covers hospitalization. There are considerable differences between Parts B and C, which must be selected at the age of eligibility to avoid late penalties. Advantage plans (Medicare C) and Medicare D drug plans are purchased from commercial providers.
- Medigap policies can be purchased from commercial providers to cover the out-of-pocket costs associated with Medicare.
- Medicaid provides coverage for the out-of-pocket medical expenses of poor Medicare beneficiaries.
- TRICARE For Life and the Indian Health Service provide health care or insurance coverage for select populations.

CLINICAL JUDGMENT QUESTIONS AND ACTIVITIES

1. Ask a person who is insured under Medicare what is most helpful about the plan. What is least helpful?
2. How would older adults like to see Medicare changed?
3. What are the prevalent attitudes of a person at least 65 years of age with whom you are acquainted regarding that person's economic future? Has this attitude been affected by the COVID-19 pandemic?

RESEARCH QUESTIONS

1. Whom do older adults most frequently contact when they need economic advice?
2. How many older adults feel secure about their economic future?
3. What are the current average out-of-pocket costs for health care when combining Medicare and Medigap policies?
4. How do people feel about the rationing of health care based on age or survivability?
5. How will the COVID-19 pandemic affect the solvency of the Social Security trust funds?

REFERENCES

Achenbaum WA, Carr LC: A brief history of aging services in the United States, *Generations* 38(2):9–13, 2014.

Cantril H: *Public opinion 1935–1946*, Princeton, NJ, 1951, Princeton University Press.

Corning P: *The evolution of Medicare: from idea to law* (Research report no. 29), Washington, D.C., 1969, US Department of Health, Education and Welfare, Social Security Administration, Office of Research and Statistics, US Government Printing Office.

Dushi I, Iams HM, Trenkamp B: *The importance of Social Security benefits to the income of the aged population* (website), 2017. https://www.ssa.gov/policy/docs/ssb/v77n2/v77n2p1.html.

Fleming KC, Evans JM, Chutka DS: A cultural and economic history of old age in America, *Mayo Clin Proc* 78(7):914–921, 2003.

Goodman JC: *The regulation of medical care: is the price too high?* (Cato public policy research monograph no. 3), San Francisco, 1980, Cato Institute.

Indian Health Service (IHS): *Coronavirus (COVID-19)* (website), 2021. https://www.ihs.gov/coronavirus/.

Internal Revenue Service (IRS): *Retirement plan and IRA required minimum distributions FAQs* (website), 2020. https://www.irs.gov/retirement-plans/retirement-plans-faqs-regarding-required-minimum-distributions.

Medicaid.gov: *Spousal impoverishment* (website), n.d. www.medicaid.gov/medicaid/eligibility/spousal-impoverisment/index.html.)

Medicare.gov: *5-star special enrollment period* (website), n.d. https://www.medicare.gov/sign-up-change-plans/when-can-i-join-a-health-or-drug-plan/5-star-special-enrollment-period.

Medicare Payment Advisory Commission (MedPAC): *Improving Medicare's payment policies for advanced practice registered nurses and physician's assistants* (website), 2019. http://www.medpac.gov/-blog-/the-commission-recommends-aprns-and-pas-bill-medicare-directly-/2019/02/15/improving-medicare's-payment-policies-for-aprns-and-pas.

National Archives: *Social Security marks 75th anniversary, August 14* (website), 2010. http://www.archives.gov/press/press-releases/2010/nr10-128.html.

National Committee to Preserve Social Security and Medicare (NCPSSM): *Medicare, 2021,* (website), WWW.NCPSSM.org/our-issues/medicare/medicare-fast-facts.

Slawomirski L, Auraaen A, Klazinga N: *The economics of patient safety in primary and ambulatory care: flying blind* (website), 2018. https://www.oecd.org/health/health-systems/The-Economics-of-Patient-Safety-in-Primary-and-Ambulatory-Care-April2018.pdf.

Social Security: *Historical background and development of Social Security* (website), n.d.a. https://www.ssa.gov/history/briefhistory3.html.

Social Security Administration: Medicare benefits (website), n.d.b, https://ssa.gov/benefits/medicare/.

US Department of Veterans Affairs (VA): *Elderly veterans* (website), 2017. https://www.benefits.va.gov/persona/veteran-elderly.asp.

Promoting Excellence in Long-Term Care

Theris A. Touhy

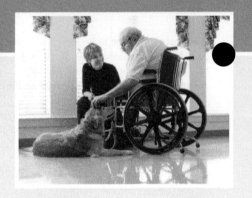

http://evolve.elsevier.com/Touhy/TwdHlthAging

A STUDENT SPEAKS

I feel so depressed when I see all the older people in nursing homes. I don't know how families can put loved ones into a nursing home, and I have promised my parents that I will never do that to them.

John, age 25

AN OLDER ADULT SPEAKS

This nursing home is my home now. We are all like a family, and I will die here. The girls that help me during the day, we treat one another like family members. We have some days when we are grumpy, some days when we are happy, and we don't hold our feelings back, just like you would do with your own family at home.

Helen, age 88

LEARNING OBJECTIVES

On completion of this chapter, the reader will be able to:

1. Discuss long-term care (LTC) as a component of the health care system.
2. Describe factors influencing the provision of long-term care.
3. Compare the major features, advantages, and disadvantages of several residential options available to the older adult.
4. Describe the role of skilled nursing facilities in the provision of subacute care.
5. Understand the role of nursing in quality improvement and culture change in LTC facilities.
6. Use clinical judgment skills to identify and evaluate solutions and nursing actions to improve outcomes for older adults in LTC.

The term *long-term care* (LTC) is often associated only with nursing homes and with care of older adults, but LTC describes a variety of services, including medical and nonmedical care, provided on an ongoing basis to people of all ages who have a chronic illness or a physical, cognitive, or developmental disability. LTC can be provided informally or formally in a range of environments, from an individual's home to the home of a friend or relative, an adult day health center, independent and assisted living facilities (ALFs), continuing care retirement communities (CCRCs), skilled nursing facilities, and hospice.

Long-term services and supports (LTSS) consist predominantly of assistance with or supervision of activities of daily living (ADLs), such as bathing, dressing, toileting, or eating, or with instrumental activities of daily living (IADLs), such as shopping or cleaning. Older adults receive the majority of LTSS (80%) on a yearly basis, but children and younger adults also receive this type of care. Children younger than age 18 are a small percentage of the total population requiring LTSS but can have substantial needs that will last a lifetime. Most people with LTSS needs live in their own home, with family, friends, and volunteers (as well as hired personnel) providing most of the care. However, the bulk of LTC throughout the developed world is informal, unpaid care provided by friends and relatives. The nature of family caregiving is changing as more individuals are discharged early from acute settings with increasingly complex medical care needs to be met in the home. Without family caregivers, the present level of LTC could not be sustained (Chapter 32).

FUTURE PROJECTIONS

The number of older adults needing LTSS is dramatically increasing year after year, and the challenge of ensuring the quality and financial stability of care provision is one faced by governments in both developed and developing countries. Estimates are that 56% of Americans who reach age 65 at some point will develop a disability serious enough to require LTC services, although most will need assistance for less than 3 years. Experts estimate that 1 in 6 Americans provide billions of dollars' worth of unpaid care to a relative or friend age 50 or older in their home (Zuraw & Rodriguez, 2021). In the coming years, most families will have a member with a need for LTSS. However, with shrinking family sizes, there will be fewer potential caregivers, and reliance on formal care services can be expected to expand.

COSTS OF LONG-TERM CARE

The total LTC spending in the United States is currently financed through a mixture of Medicaid, Medicare, out-of-pocket spending, private LTC insurance, and appropriations from the Older Americans Act (Chapter 5). LTSS is expensive and becoming more expensive; costs have outpaced inflation since 2003 (Table 6.1). Estimates are that spending on LTSS will increase fivefold by 2045 in the United States. An American turning 65 years old today will incur $138,000 in costs on future LTC services. The cost of LTSS continues to be much higher than what most people can afford, and only people in the wealthiest 10% to 20% of older adult households have savings that could absorb the risks of high LTSS spending (Reinhard et al., 2017).

Finding a way to pay for LTC is a growing concern for people of all ages, especially older adults, individuals with disabilities, and their families. Most people have not planned for their LTC needs and are not knowledgeable about existing resources. Many people still believe that Medicare and Social Security protect them from the costs of LTC, until "they discover otherwise when their first family member needs long-term care. Then they realize that Medicaid is their safety net, but Medicaid requires

both severe poverty and substantial illness and disability, and often provides less appealing nursing homes" (Lynn, 2019).

Funding for Long-Term Care
Medicaid
Medicaid is the primary payer for LTSS for people who have low incomes and who deplete their personal savings to pay for medical expenses and LTC. Medicaid accounts for more than 62% of national LTC spending in the United States. Of this amount, about 47% is for institutional care and 53% is for home and community-based services (HCBS) (Nguyen, 2017). Without affordable private insurance options or public insurance alternatives, such as a national LTC insurance system or expanded coverage for Medicare beneficiaries, there will be continued reliance on the Medicaid program. The Medicaid program is administered by the states, and there is wide variation in support of LTSS funding. Where you live really matters because there are huge differences across the states in how well they are doing in expanding and funding LTSS. Although some states are developing innovative, coordinated, and accessible LTSS systems, a recent report found that most states are not doing a great job of helping people who need such care (Fig. 6.1).

Proposals to reduce Medicaid spending further jeopardize the availability and affordability of LTSS. Medicaid is the primary payer for nursing homes, covering more than 60% of all nursing home residents and approximately 50% of costs for all LTC services. However, Medicaid reimbursements cover only 70% to 80% of the actual cost of nursing home care. National and state initiatives are being directed toward changing the bias from institutional care to more HCBS that can be less expensive and reflect the desires of people to "age in place." While progress has been made, it is not adequate to meet the needs of aging baby boomers and beyond. Recommendations from experts suggest that the pace of change needs to triple or quadruple to meet the needs of an aging population (Reinhard et al., 2017).

Medicare
Medicare is not designed to provide coverage for LTC services and only covers acute and postacute medical care for people 65 years of age and older and for younger populations who qualify for Social Security because of disability. Medicare only pays for limited coverage for short-term skilled nursing facility stays and home health services for postacute rehabilitation care (Chapter 5). Medicare does not cover the costs of care in chronic, custodial, and LTC units or for care in the home that does not require skilled services. If an older adult was admitted to a nursing home because of a dementia diagnosis and the need for assistance with ADLs and maintenance of safety, Medicare would not cover the cost of care unless some skilled care was needed.

Private Long-Term Care Insurance
LTC insurance covers many types of LTC and benefits, including palliative and hospice care. The exact coverage depends on the type of policy purchased and what services are covered. Policies cover nursing home care only or can be more comprehensive and cover both facility and home care. Relatively few people

TABLE 6.1 **Monthly Costs of US Long-Term Care Services and Support Programs**	
Service	Cost
Homemaker services	$4,481 $23.50/hour
Home health aide	$4,576 $24.00/hour
Adult day health	$1,603
Assisted living facility (Private, One bedroom)	$4,300
Nursing home care Semi-Private Room Private Room	$7,756 $8,821

Monthly costs for homemaker/home health aide vary depending on hours needed/day.
Data from Genworth Cost of Care Survey (2020). From: Genworth Cost of Care Survey (2020). https://www.genworth.com/aging-and-you/finances/cost-of-care.html.

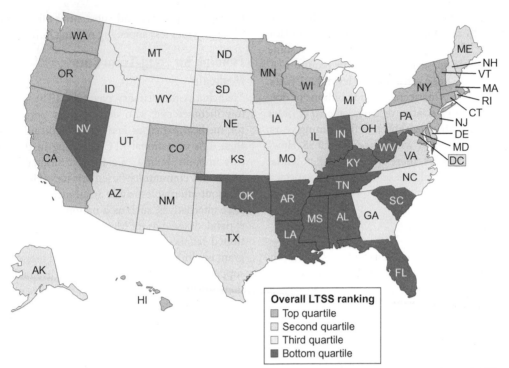

Overall LTSS ranking
- Top quartile
- Second quartile
- Third quartile
- Bottom quartile

Fig. 6.1 2020 Long-term services and supports *(LTSS)* state scorecard. (Adapted from AARP: *Long-term services & supports state scorecard* [website], 2020. http://www.longtermscorecard. org/~/media/Microsite/Files/2020/LTSS%202020%20Reference%20Edition%20PDF%209.)

have purchased this type of insurance. Barriers to the purchase of LTC insurance include the inability of many people to afford coverage, the belief that LTC is covered by their general policies or by Medicare, and the reluctance of private insurers to write policies for those in poor health (the individuals most likely to require LTC services). Some new and more cost-effective options for LTC insurance are emerging, as are proposed reforms to encourage more individuals to obtain coverage.

Out-of-Pocket Spending

For those who do not qualify for Medicare or Medicaid benefits, the costs of LTC are paid out-of-pocket. Individual and family out-of-pocket spending pays for as much as 40% of all paid care. LTC expenses, such as for nursing homes and assisted living, are the number one category of out-of-pocket spending, followed by home care (Cubanski et al., 2019).

LONG-TERM CARE AND THE US HEALTH CARE SYSTEM

The US health care system has been focused on delivering acute care services and addressing time-limited and specific illnesses or injuries as they occur in episodes, driven by the restrictions of Medicare, Medicaid, and private insurance. Traditionally, health care has been made up of two sectors: acute care and ambulatory care. Each setting has been viewed as an independent entity with little coordination or recognition of LTSS as an integral part of the continuum of care.

Such a system does not address the increasingly complex and long-term needs of people with chronic conditions who need acute and long-term services and support systems. Healthy

People 2030 addresses the need for supports and services for older adults.

Today, the total spectrum of care has been expanded to include long-term and postacute care (LTPAC) services, which includes nursing homes, ALFs, home care, and hospice (Fig. 6.2). However, in the United States today, the LTPAC system is complex and fragmented, isolated from other service providers, and poorly funded; it also is confusing and difficult for the individual and the caregiver to access and negotiate. Access to services is dependent on funding governed by a mix of federal, state, and local rules and procedures. Separate agencies have unique eligibility rules, intake, and assessment processes. When individuals need LTSS, they and their families must find and arrange for services on their own, sometimes on short notice when the need arises from a medical event or with a change in the individual's functional capacity.

There is no comprehensive approach to care coordination in the LTC system. As a result, services and supports may not be provided in the most appropriate setting by the most appropriate provider, the individual's needs and preferences may not be met, and caregivers may experience substantial stress trying to arrange for or provide care. This fragmented, provider- and setting-centered approach (as opposed to a person-centered

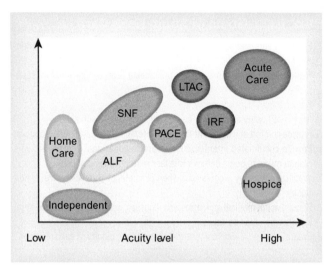

Fig. 6.2 Long-term and postacute care spectrum of care. *ALF,* assisted living facility; *IRF,* inpatient rehabilitation facility; *LTAC,* long-term acute care facility; *PACE,* Programs of All-Inclusive Care for the Elderly; *SNF,* skilled nursing facility. (From John F. Derr, JD & Associates Enterprises, Inc. https://www.jd-associatesenterprises.com/ltpac-health-it-collaborative.html.)

BOX 6.1 One Woman's Story

Myra is an 86-year-old woman who lives in her own condominium apartment in Florida. Her diagnoses include osteoarthritis and hypertension. She is a widow with no children or close relatives. She has about $80,000 in savings and is very careful in living on a limited income monthly budget. Her hands are so deformed by arthritis that she cannot dress herself or turn the knob on her kitchen stove. She is very alert but is having increasing difficulty living alone. Friends and neighbors have been helping as much as they can. She has been on a waiting list for home and community-based services for a month. Due to her savings, she is not eligible for assistance with in-home care under Medicaid, and the cost of a homemaker or aide is more than she can afford. Her savings make her ineligible for Medicaid, and she would have to spend down to $2000 to qualify.

She visits her primary care provider for her annual exam and asks about how she can get care services so that she can stay in her own home. Her primary care provider tells her she is not safe to live alone, and she is given a list of nursing homes. She is shocked to discover that a nursing home can cost up to $90,000 yearly and is not covered by Medicare unless she has a skilled care need. If she became ill and was discharged to a nursing home, Medicare would pay for a short-term nursing home stay (full coverage for 20 days and partial coverage for up to 80 days if she had a prior 3-day hospital admission) and skilled care needs. Upon discharge from the nursing home, if she still required skilled care, she could receive part-time home health care (registered nurse [RN] supervision, therapy, home health aide a couple of hours per day for personal care) for a limited time.

---

approach) results in unmet needs, risk for injuries, and adverse outcomes (Box 6.1). There is also a critical shortage of well-prepared health care professionals and direct care staff to provide LTSS, putting the individual who needs this care at further risk of poor outcomes (Chapter 1).

The disastrous consequences of the COVID-19 pandemic highlighted many areas that need attention to make LTC an integral component of the health care system. Individuals living in nursing homes and assisted living facilities (0.62% of the U.S. population)

accounted for 42% of all deaths from COVID-19 (Roy, 2020). However, an estimated 43.7 % of COVID-19 cases and 40% of COVID-19 related deaths prior to May 24, 2020, were not reported to the CDC's tracking system. This may demonstrate a widespread inability of nursing homes to reliably collect data early in the pandemic or that pressures to report fewer cases and deaths were common across facilities of all types. Although current measures of COVID-19 prevalence and mortality reflect a devastating public health crisis, it is likely that even more lives were impacted that will never be fully captured in existing data. As a result, it is not possible to make conclusions about the role of different facility characteristics and state or federal policies in explaining COVID- 19 outbreaks in nursing homes (Shen et al., 2021).

Nursing homes serving higher proportions of racial and ethnic minority residents were especially hard hit. COVID-19 deaths at nursing homes where more than 40% of residents were Black or Hispanic were about 3.3 times higher than those in nursing homes with the highest proportion of White residents (Gorges and Konetza, 2021). Compared with Whites, racial/ethnic minorities tend to be cared for in nursing homes with limited clinical and financial resources, low nurse staffing levels, and a relatively high number of care deficiency standards (Harrington et al., 2020). Even the best quality homes had a substantial number of COVID cases and deaths but the average number of cases was lower in facilities with higher quality ratings and more total staff and registered nurses. However, COVID-19 infections in nursing homes reflected the extent of spread in the surrounding community.

Ouslander and Grabowski (2020) stated: "The combination of a vulnerable population in nursing homes and assisted living facilities that manifests nonspecific and atypical presentations of COVID-19, staffing shortages due to viral infection, inadequate resources for and availability of rapid, accurate testing and personal protective equipment, and lack of effective treatments for COVID-10 among nursing home residents created a 'perfect storm' in our country's LTC facilities". The major response to the pandemic was focused on acute care facilities and the overwhelming number of admissions of individuals with COVID-19 to hospitals. Inadequate attention was paid to discharges from acute care to LTC for patients with COVID-19, and statistics initially did not include the number of deaths from the virus in LTC. Even fewer data are available for assisted living facilities.

Additionally, nursing homes are a congregate living setting, and despite social distancing measures, including no group dining or activities, most nursing homes have a majority of rooms with more than one occupant and shared bathrooms. Care includes close activities such as bathing, dressing, and toileting that do not allow for social distancing. Many residents in nursing homes and ALFs have dementia and cannot cooperate with social distancing and mask wearing. Staff and clinicians who come in and out of the building, many of whom work in multiple facilities, can be presymptomatic or asymptomatically shedding the virus while passing screening questionnaires and temperature recordings. To combat spread, facilities did not allow visitors, and this contributed to social isolation and decline for many individuals who were accustomed to having family present frequently.

Residents and staff in nursing homes were in the first priority group to get vaccinated against COVID-19. Health protocols

---

BOX 6.2   Focus of Acute and Long-Term Care

Acute Care Orientation

- Illness
- High technology
- Short term
- Episodic
- One-dimensional
- Professional
- Medical model
- Cure

Long-Term Care Orientation

- Function
- High touch
- Extended
- Interdisciplinary model
- Ongoing
- Multidimensional
- Paraprofessional and family
- Care

BOX 6.3   Goals of Long-Term Care

1. Provide a safe and supportive environment for chronically ill and functionally dependent people.
2. Restore and maintain the highest practicable level of functional independence.
3. Preserve individual autonomy.
4. Maximize quality of life, well-being, and satisfaction with care.
5. Provide comfort and dignity at the end of life for residents and their families.
6. Provide coordinated interdisciplinary care to subacutely ill residents who plan to return to home or move to a less restrictive level of care.
7. Stabilize and delay progression, when possible, of chronic medical conditions.
8. Prevent acute medical and iatrogenic illnesses, and identify and treat them rapidly when they do occur.
9. Create a homelike environment that respects the dignity of each resident.

---

such as masking, social distancing, and hand hygiene have been in place at LTC facilities throughout the crisis, and federal guidelines require testing staff and residents for COVID-19 regularly when there is an outbreak on site. Since vaccinations began in December 2020, the number of new COVID-19 cases among nursing home staff members fell by 83% and infections among residents fell by 89% (Bailey & Dubnow, 2021). Infection control prevention and control practices and programs have been enhanced, and further attention will be paid to these efforts. Strategies that will help nursing homes of all sizes to improve infection control and prevention, including intensive education and the requirement of a full-time infection prevention specialist, will help prevent the devastation that was experienced by the pandemic (Ouslander & Grabowski, 2020).

Many aging experts believe that the COVID-19 disaster presents an opportunity to reimagine the role of nursing homes and health care for older adults and to develop creative strategies to provide LTC. Gerontological nursing expert Terry Fulmer, PhD, RN, FAAN, president of the John A. Hartford Foundation, says, "COVID-19 gives us the chance to accelerate the change we want to see. We have a mandate—ethical, moral, and clinical—to get things right going forward" (Fulmer et al, 2020). The federal government has allocated more than $15 billion to assist nursing homes to support increased testing, staffing, and personal protective equipment (PPE) needs, but industry experts suggest that much more is necessary to help support ongoing efforts (Gerontological Society of America, 2021).

Health care professionals who have not had experience in the LTC system are often unaware of the many differences between acute care and LTC. Unless they have experienced the need for LTC in their own families, they may be unaware of the challenges associated with obtaining quality care for individuals with long-term needs. It is important for health care professionals, especially nurses, to understand the total spectrum of care and the differences between acute care and LTC (Boxes 6.2 and 6.3). "Without addressing the obstacles discussed above,

we will continue to move forward with a partial view of older adults—one seen through an acute and medical lens, rather than seeing a person with a story, a family system, and a community" (Golden & Shier, 2012–13, p. 11).

GLOBAL APPROACHES TO LONG-TERM CARE

Most countries are facing increasing challenges surrounding LTC for the growing numbers of older adults. Many of the developed countries have been preparing for big increases in their older populations and the associated growth in the need for LTC services for many years. Every developed country in the world, except for the United States and the United Kingdom, has some system for universal LTC. The United States and the United Kingdom (excluding Scotland) are the only developed countries that still operate a means-tested system (Medicaid in the United States). Most governments have established collectively financed systems for personal and nursing home care cost. It may be social insurance (e.g., Germany, Japan, Korea), a personal care benefit (e.g., paying informal caregivers in cash or in-kind for services; e.g., France, Italy, Australia), or fully integrated social care (e.g., Sweden, Norway) (Box 6.4).

All nations need to take steps to prepare for the growing numbers of older adults by creating sustainable financing systems, developing better ways to support informal caregivers, and focusing efforts on prevention and chronic care management. By sharing best practices, nations can learn from one another in designing systems of care that support the health and well-being of their citizens. As the United States looks to improve the LTC system, there is a slow shift away from a solely acute medical model and more emphasis on prevention, managing chronic disease and LTC while lowering costs and preserving quality.

SOLUTIONS, NURSING ACTIONS, AND OUTCOMES: IMPROVING LONG-TERM CARE SUPPORTS AND SERVICES

We know we can do better in providing care to those with long-term needs even in times of fiscal restraint through creative planning and use of best practices. Gerontological nurse

BOX 6.4   A Swedish Example of Long-Term Care

Roger is an 87-year-old widowed man who lives alone in the home he has owned for more than 40 years. He fell and broke his hip and received care in the hospital in his local municipality in Sweden. All of his care in the hospital, including rehabilitation, was covered by the government. When he was ready for discharge, a care plan meeting with Roger, his family and significant others, the district nurse in his municipality, a social worker, and therapists was held to evaluate how much care he will need following discharge. He will not be discharged until the plan is decided. If Roger is able to return home safely, he will receive personal care up to several times a day (getting up, dressing, grooming, toileting, meals, going to bed) at no charge to him. Services are supported through taxes and administered through the local municipalities.

If his family wants to provide some of this care, they can receive a stipend equivalent to the salary of the paid caregivers. Care plan meetings are held with the team to determine the type of services Roger needs, and the frequency; however, he can receive home assistance until his function improves and he is able to live safely at home. If he continues to need extensive care at home (24 hours a day) that is more expensive than nursing home care, he will be evaluated for nursing home care.

If he needs to move to a nursing home, he must go to a home in his area. Individuals with the greatest need have priority, and sometimes there is a waiting period before admission. He may pay a small fee for the nursing home depending on his income level but probably not more than $150 to $200 per month. The remaining costs are covered through the government benefits. The district nurse will continue to coordinate his care and evaluate his status while he is in the nursing home.

From in-person communication with Gabriella Engstrom, RN, PhD, February 2016.

educators, researchers, and providers must be knowledgeable about the full spectrum of LTPAC so that they can assist individuals and their caregivers to obtain the most appropriate care to enhance health and well-being. Nurses also must advocate for improved financing and delivery of LTSS so that quality, equitable, seamless, and affordable person-centered care is available for all in need of such services.

FORMAL LONG-TERM CARE SERVICE PROVIDERS

This section describes some of the types of facilities and programs that provide LTC services in the United States. Services available and characteristics of the individuals served are discussed. Most people would prefer to stay in their own home (age in place), but many factors can affect decision making about where to live as one ages (Chapter 21). Some older adults, by choice or by need, move from one type of residence to another. A number of options exist, especially for those with the financial resources that allow them to have a choice. Residential options range along a continuum from remaining in one's private house or apartment to senior retirement communities; shared housing with family members, friends, or others; residential care communities such as assisted living settings; and nursing facilities for those with the most needs.

It is important for nurses in all practice settings to be knowledgeable about the range of options so they can assist older adults and their families who may need to make decisions about relocation. Most nurses work in one setting and are not familiar

with the requirements of other settings or the needs of individuals in these settings. As a result, there are often significant misunderstandings and criticisms of care in different settings across the continuum. We can no longer work in our individual "silos" and not be concerned with what happens after the patient is out of our particular institution.

Community Care

Programs of All-Inclusive Care for the Elderly (PACE)

PACE is a Medicaid and Medicare program that provides community services to individuals who would otherwise need a nursing home level of care. Participants must meet the criteria for nursing home admission, prefer to remain in the community, and be eligible for Medicare or Medicaid. It is a full-service model that covers the cost of primary care, hospitalization, emergency department visits, approved specialty services, rehabilitation, home care, medication and treatment, and social and recreational services in a community center environment. PACE has been the only Medicare program that has required and paid for interdisciplinary team care using a capitated payment. Nursing has been central to the PACE care model since its inception. Outcomes of PACE include increased use of ambulatory services, lower rates of nursing home use and in-patient hospitalization, lower rates of functional decline, and better reported health status than among a comparison population (Cortes & Sullivan-Marx, 2016).

PACE is recognized as a permanent provider under Medicare and a state option under Medicaid. Currently there are 123 PACE programs operating 250 PACE centers in 31 states serving more than 45,000 participants. PACE has been approved by the US Department of Health and Human Services (USDHHS) Substance Abuse and Mental Health Services Administration (SAMHSA) as an evidence-based model of care. Models such as PACE are innovative care delivery models, and continued development of such models is important as the US population ages (National PACE Association, 2019).

Adult Day Services (ADS)

Adult day services (ADS) are community-based group programs designed to provide social and some health services to adults who need supervised care in a safe setting during the day. They also offer caregivers respite from the responsibilities of caregiving, and most provide educational programs, support groups, and individual counseling for caregivers. ADS are serving populations with higher levels of physical disability and chronic disease. Increasingly, ADS are being used to provide community-based care for conditions like Alzheimer's disease and for transitional care and short-term rehabilitation following hospitalization. Nearly half of all ADS participants have some level of dementia. Staff ratios in ADS are one direct care worker to six clients. Almost 80% of centers have professional nursing staff, 50% have a social worker, and 60% offer case management services. Most also offer transportation services.

Some ADS are private pay, and others are funded through Medicaid home and community-based waiver programs, state and local funding, and the US Department of Veterans Affairs (see Table 6.1). ADS hold the potential to meet the need for cost-efficient and high-quality LTC services, and continued expansion and funding are expected. ADS are an important part of the LTPAC continuum and a cost-effective alternative or supplement to home care or institutional care. Although further research is needed on patient and caregiver outcomes of ADS, findings suggest that they improve health-related quality of life for participants and improve caregiver well-being. Local Area Agencies on Aging are good sources of information about ADS and other community-based options.

Continuing Care Retirement Communities (CCRCs)

Life care communities, also known as CCRCs, provide the full range of residential options, from single-family homes to skilled nursing facilities, all in one location. Most of these communities provide access to these levels of care for a community member's entire remaining lifetime, and for the right price, the range of services may be guaranteed. Having all levels of care in one location allows community members to make the transition between levels without life-disrupting moves. For married couples where one spouse needs more care than the other, life care communities allow them to live nearby in a different part of the same community.

Most CCRCs are managed by not-for-profit organizations. Entrance fees can range from as low as $20,000 for a nonpurchase (rental) agreement to buy-in fees among the most expensive CCRCs of up to $500,000 or more depending on the size and location of the unit and the community. Monthly costs can be as low as $500 at some communities and as high as $3000 or more depending on type of contract and service plan. Costs of CCRCs are paid out-of-pocket and not covered by Medicare or Medicaid. Medicare would cover the cost of skilled care services for a resident of a CCRC.

Residential Care/Assisted Living (RC/AL)

Residential care/assisted living (RC/AL) facilities are nonmedical facilities that provide room, meals, housekeeping, supervision and distribution of medication, and personal care assistance with basic activities like hygiene, dressing, eating, bathing, and transferring. This level of care is for individuals who are unable to live by themselves but who do not need 24-hour nursing care. RC/AL facilities are known by more than 30 different names across the country, including adult congregate facilities, foster care homes, personal care homes, domiciliary care homes, board and care homes, rest homes, family care homes, retirement homes, and assisted living facilities.

RC/AL facilities are viewed as more cost-effective than nursing homes while providing more privacy and a homelike environment. Medicare does not cover the cost of care in these types of facilities. The majority of individuals in RC/AL pay for their care from their personal resources. Forty-seven percent of facilities accept Medicaid, although the number of residents with Medicaid is low at approximately 20%. Private and LTC insurance also may cover some costs. RC/AL services predominantly serve private pay and White residents. The rates charged and the services that those rates include vary considerably, as do regulations and licensing. States are responsible for regulating RC/AL facilities, and there are no federal quality standards or mandatory reporting on quality similar to the requirements for skilled

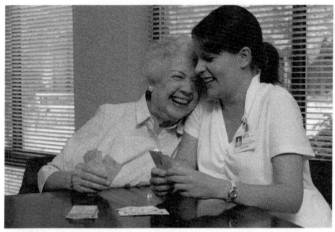

Providing nursing services in assisted living facilities promotes physical and psychosocial health. (From Potter PA: *Basic nursing: essentials for practice,* ed. 7, St. Louis, 2010, Mosby.)

nursing facilities. Less than half of these facilities have any type of RN or licensed practical nurse (LPN), and most states require only minimal training or certification or licensure for direct care workers (Siegel et al., 2021).

Assisted living. A popular type of RC/AL is the assisted living facility (ALF), also called *board and care homes* or *adult congregate living facilities.* ALF settings may be a shared room or a single-occupancy unit with a private bath, kitchenette, and communal meals. They all provide some support services, but if care needs increase, there is usually a charge for services. There are 28,900 assisted living and other residential care communities serving 811,500 residents in the United States (Zuraw & Rodriguez, 2021).

Assisted living is more expensive than independent living and less costly than skilled nursing home care, but it is not inexpensive (see Table 6.1). Costs vary by geographical region, size of the unit, and relative luxury. Forty-two percent of ALFs are small, with 4 to 10 beds, and 33% have between 26 and 100 beds. Most ALFs offer two or three meals per day, light weekly housekeeping, laundry services, and optional social activities. Each added service increases the cost of the setting but also allows for individuals with resources to remain in the setting longer, as functional abilities decline. Consumers are advised to inquire as to exactly what services will be provided and by whom if an ALF resident becomes more frail and needs more intensive care.

Many older adults and their families prefer ALFs to nursing homes because they cost less, are more homelike, and offer more opportunities for control, independence, and privacy. However, many residents of ALFs have chronic care needs and over time may require more care than the facility is able to provide. Services (e.g., home health, hospice, homemakers) can be brought into the facility, but some question whether this adequately substitutes for 24-hour supervision by RNs. Residential care facilities (RCFs) are not required to provide licensed nursing on a 24-hour basis, even though there is evidence that many residents in some facilities are frail, with many chronic illnesses, impaired self-care needs and cognition, and unmet care needs (Harrington et al., 2017) (Box 6.5).

- 32% are 75 to 84 years old; 51% are over 85 years old
- Female (72%)
- 38% need help with 3 to 5 activities of daily living; 61% need help with bathing; 45% need help with dressing; 37% need help with toileting; 18% need help with eating; 25% need help with bed transfer
- About 52% are cognitively impaired
- The median length of stay is about 22 months
- 59% move to a nursing facility
- 33% die while a resident of an assisted living facility

Data from National Center for Assisted Living: *Assisted living* (website), n.d. https://www.ahcancal.org/ncal/Pages/index.aspx. Accessed March 2018.

In an ALF there is no organized team of providers (i.e., nurses, social workers, therapists, pharmacists, dietitians) such as that found in skilled care facilities. The combination of congregate settings and residents who are frail meant that assisted living communities were particularly vulnerable to COVID-19. Little attention was paid by states and the federal government to COVID-19 preparations and precautions in this setting, and the exact number of individuals in assisted living communities who died from the virus is unknown since accurate reporting from these settings were not conducted.

With the growing numbers of older adults with dementia residing in ALFs, many of these facilities are establishing dementia-specific units. With the lack of regulatory requirements and inadequate staffing, the provision of high-quality care for individuals with dementia is questionable. It is important to investigate the services available and staff training when making decisions about the most appropriate placement for older adults with dementia. Continued research is needed on best care practices and outcomes of care for people with dementia in both ALFs and nursing homes. The Alzheimer's Association has issued a set of dementia care practices for ALFs and nursing homes (Alzheimer's Association, 2009) (Box 6.6).

The nonmedical nature of ALFs is a primary factor in keeping costs more reasonable than those in nursing facilities, but costs are still high for those without adequate funds. Appropriate standards of care must be developed, and care outcomes must be monitored to ensure that residents are receiving quality care in this setting, which is almost devoid of professional nursing. Available data about staff-to-resident ratios raise questions about care quality (Harrington et al., 2017). "The absence of oversight and regulations requires families to do extra due diligence before choosing a facility" (Gleckman, 2018). Further research is needed on care outcomes of residents in ALFs and the roles of unlicensed assistive personnel and RNs in these facilities.

Advanced practice gerontological nurses are well suited to the role of primary care provider in ALFs, and many have assumed this role. The American Assisted Living Nurses Association has established a certification mechanism for nurses working in these facilities and also has developed a *Scope and Standards of Assisted Living Nursing Practice for Registered Nurses*. The Assisted Living Federation of America and the National Center

Alzheimer's Association: Dementia Care Practice Recommendations for Assisted Living Residences and Nursing Homes. https://www.alz.org/media/documents/dementia-care-practice-recommend-assist-living-1-2-b.pdf.

American Assisted Living Nurses Association: Certification, scope, and standards of practice. https://alnursing.org/.

American Health Care Association/National Center for Assisted Living: Information, educational resources, guide to choosing an assisted living facility (ALF) and skilled nursing facility. https://www.ahcancal.org/Assisted-Living/Pages/default.aspx.

Argentum (formerly the Assisted Living Federation of America): Information, educational resources, guide to choosing an ALF. https://www.argentum.org/.

Centers for Medicare and Medicaid Services: Guide to choosing a nursing home; Nursing Home Compare; Nursing Home Quality Care Collaborative (NHQCC) learning; Partnership to Improve Dementia Care in Nursing Homes; Quality Assurance and Performance Improvement (QAPI). https://www.medicare.gov.

Eden Alternative: Nursing facility exemplifying culture change. https://www.edenalt.org/.

National Adult Day Services Association: https://www.nadsa.org/.

National Nursing Home Quality Improvement Campaign: Evidence-based and model-practice resources to support quality improvement. https://nursinghomehelp.org/educational/advancing-excellence/.

National Programs of All-Inclusive Care for the Elderly (PACE) Association: https://www.npaonline.org/pace-you.

Pioneer Network: Culture change information and toolkit. https://www.pioneernetwork.net/.

The Green House Project: Innovative long-term care model. https://thegreenhouseproject.org/.

The National Consumer Voice for Quality Long-Term Care: National voice representing consumers in issues related to long-term care; information and resources to help ensure quality care; Guide to Choosing a Nursing Home. https://theconsumervoice.org/.

for Assisted Living provide a consumer guide for choosing an assisted living residence (see Box 6.6).

Certified Nursing Facilities (Nursing Homes)

Certified nursing facilities offer 24-hour supervision and nursing care for those needing specialized care that cannot be provided elsewhere. Nursing homes are a complex health care setting that is a mix of hospital, rehabilitation facility, hospice, and dementia-specific units, and they are a final home for many older adults. When used appropriately, nursing homes fill an important need for families and older adults.

The settings called *nursing homes* or *nursing facilities* most often include up to two levels of care: a *skilled nursing care* (also called *subacute care*) facility is required to have licensed professionals with a focus on the management of complex medical needs, and a *chronic care* (also called *long-term* or *custodial*) facility is required to have 24-hour personal assistance that is supervised and augmented by professional and licensed nurses. Often, both kinds of services are provided in one facility.

There are approximately 15,600 certified nursing homes in the United States caring for 1.35 million residents

(Zuraw & Rodriguez, 2021). The majority of nursing homes (70%) are for-profit organizations, and 58% are operated by corporate chains. Private equity firms own about 11% of nursing facilities (Harrington et al., 2021). The number of nursing home beds is decreasing in the United States as a result of the increased use of RC/AL and more reimbursement by Medicaid programs for community-based care alternatives. However, in most areas of the country the supply and use of nursing homes is still greater than those of other LTC service options. Although the percentage of older adults living in nursing homes at any given time is low (4% to 5%), those who live to age 85 will have a 1 in 2 chance of spending some time in a nursing facility for subacute care, ongoing LTC, or end-of-life care.

Subacute Care (Short Term)

Subacute care is more intensive than traditional nursing home care and several times more costly, but far less costly than care in a hospital. Skilled nursing facilities are the most frequent site of postacute care (PAC) in the United States. More than a quarter of Medicare patients admitted to the hospital are discharged to PAC facilities, many with acute health conditions (Horney et al., 2017). In addition to skilled nursing care, rehabilitation services are an essential component of subacute units. The expectation is that the patient will be discharged home or to a less intensive setting. Length of stay is usually less than 1 month and is largely reimbursed by Medicare. Patients in subacute units are usually younger and less likely to be cognitively impaired than those in chronic care (long-term or custodial). Generally, higher levels of professional staffing are found in the subacute setting than in the chronic setting because of the acuity of the patient's condition.

Chronic Care (Long Term)

Chronic care (long-term) facilities care for patients who may not need the intense care provided in subacute units but still need ongoing 24-hour care. These individuals represent the most frail of all older adults. Their need for 24-hour care could not be met in the home or residential care setting or may have exceeded what the family was able to provide. These patients may include individuals with severe strokes, dementia, or Parkinson's disease, and those receiving hospice care. Residents of long-term chronic care facilities are predominantly women, 80 years or older, widowed, and dependent in ADLs and IADLs. About 50% of these residents are cognitively impaired, and these types of facilities are increasingly caring for people at the end of life. Twenty-three percent of Americans die in nursing homes, and this figure is expected to increase to 40% by 2040 (Stanford School of Medicine, 2019; Teno et al., 2013).

Interprofessional Team Model in Subacute and Long-Term Care

An interprofessional team, working with the resident and family, assesses, plans, and implements care in nursing facilities (Box 6.7). Rehabilitation and restorative care are increasingly important in light of shortened hospital stays that may occur before conditions are stabilized and the older adult is ready to

---

BOX 6.7   Interprofessional Teams in Nursing Homes

Patient
Family and significant others
Nurse
Primary care provider: physician, nurse practitioner
Physical, occupational, and speech therapists
Social worker
Dietitian
Discharge planner or case manager
Psychologist
Prosthetist and orthotist
Audiologist

---

function independently. The opportunity to work collaboratively with a team is one of the most exciting aspects of practice in LTC facilities.

Professional Nursing in Long-Term Care

There are a wide range of opportunities for professional nursing in skilled nursing facilities and projections of an increase in the need in the coming years. The setting provides opportunities for learning and practice in areas that are core to 21st-century nursing: managing chronic illness and palliative care in ways that are patient centered and evidence based, working with families, interprofessional teams, and developing systems for quality improvement. LTC should be marketed to young nurses as a bright future career that requires excellent technical and critical thinking skills and is more autonomous than other areas of nursing (Sherman & Touhy, 2017). Roles for professional nursing in LTC settings are discussed in Chapter 1.

Nursing homes are often blamed for all of the societal problems associated with the aging of our population. Daily, millions of dedicated caregivers in nursing homes are providing competent and compassionate care to very sick older adults against great odds, such as a lack of support, inadequate salaries and staff, inadequate funding, and a lack of respect. It is time for their stories to be told, and it is time to recognize their needs for adequate and well-trained staff to do this very important work. Although there are continued challenges and opportunities to improve care in nursing homes (and care in all settings for older adults) and in the fabric of the LTC system, many nursing homes provide an environment that truly represents the best of caring and quality of life. "The many positive aspects of nursing in LTC facilities are often overshadowed by an uncomplimentary image of care in this setting, influenced by a history laden with scandals and the media's readiness to highlight the abuses and substandard conditions demonstrated by a small minority. This negative image is compounded by reimbursement policies that significantly limit the ability to provide high-quality care" (Eliopoulos, 2010, p. 365).

Since the 1990s, more than 150 research studies have examined the effect of nurse staffing levels and improved quality outcomes in states with higher minimum staffing levels, particularly RN staffing, on care outcomes, with most finding positive effects with higher staffing levels and improved quality outcomes.

BOX 6.8   Expert Panel Recommendations: Professional Nursing in Nursing Homes

Bachelor of science in nursing (BSN) degree for directors of nursing

Increased staffing ratios for registered nurses (RNs), licensed practical nurses (LPNs), and nursing assistants

Most nursing homes should have a full-time clinical nurse specialist (CNS) or gerontological nurse practitioner (GNP) on staff

From Harrington C, Kovner C, Mezey M, et al.: Experts recommend minimum staffing standards for nursing facilities in the United States. *Gerontologist* 40(1):5–16, 2000.

Benefits of higher staffing levels, especially RN staffing, include lower mortality rates; improved physical functioning; less antibiotic use; fewer pressure ulcers, catheterized residents, and urinary tract infections; lower hospitalization rates; and less weight loss and dehydration. In addition to staffing levels, nursing staff training and competency have been identified as critical factors in ensuring high-quality care (Harrington et al., 2020). Yet despite the evidence of improved outcomes associated with professional nurse presence in nursing homes, federal rules require only one RN in the nursing facility for 8 hours a day, a figure quite shocking considering the ratio of RNs to patients in acute care, even in the face of shortages in this setting.

Many groups dealing with issues of the aging, as well as the American Nurses Association (ANA), have supported the critical need for adequate staffing in nursing homes. An expert panel on nursing homes provided comprehensive recommendations for improved RN staffing and increased gerontological nursing education requirements for all staff (Harrington et al., 2000) (Box 6.8). Federal regulations require adequate staffing to meet the needs of the residents, but research suggests that the majority of US nursing homes do not provide sufficient staffing to meet the basic quality standards. Over half of US nursing homes had lower RN, certified nursing assistant (CNA), and total nurse staffing levels than those recommended by experts, and one-quarter had very low staffing (Harrington et al., 2020). However, the federal government has not acted to mandate increases in minimum RN staffing requirements. Continued research on new models of care delivery and the appropriate mix of all levels of nursing staff in subacute and long-term units is needed to improve outcomes.

Nursing Assistants

Although it is important to promote professional nursing care for all older adults, nursing assistants provide the majority of direct care in nursing homes and significantly contribute to the quality of life for residents. Research results support the deep commitment and passion that nursing assistants bring to their jobs. The significance and importance of close personal relationships between nursing assistants and residents, often described as "like family," is emerging as a central dimension of quality of care and positive outcomes. The commitment and dedication of nursing home staff must be honored and supported. They have much to teach us about aging, nursing, and caring. Box 6.9 presents descriptions of caring themes expressed by nursing home caregivers in a research study examining caring practices.

BOX 6.9   How We Care: Voices of Nursing Home Staff

Responding to What Matters

Taking time to do the little things, competence, cleanliness, meeting basic needs, safe administration of medications, kindness and consideration

Caring as a Way of Expressing Spiritual Commitment

Spiritual beliefs lead staff to long-term care and continue to motivate and guide the special care they give to residents; they reflect a spiritual commitment to caring for residents as expressed in the golden rule: "Do unto others as you would like done to you."

Devotion Inspired by Love for Others

Deep connection between staff and residents described as being like family, caring for residents as you would for your own mother or father, sharing of good and bad times, going out on a limb to be an advocate, listening, and staying with residents when others had given up

Commitment to Creating a Home Environment

Nursing home is the resident's home, staff are guests in the home; the importance of cleanliness, privacy, good food, and feeling part of a family

Coming to Know and Respect Person as Person

Treating residents, families, and one another with respect and dignity, being recognized for the person you are, intimate knowing of likes and dislikes, individualized care

Adapted from Touhy T, Strews W, Brown C: Expressions of caring as lived by nursing home staff, residents, and families, *Int J Human Caring* 9:31, 2005.

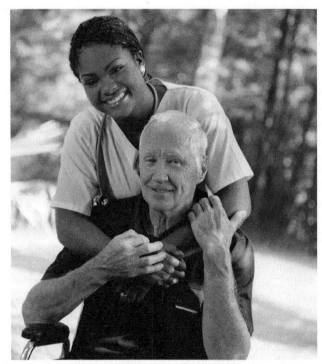

Caring relationships between staff and residents in long-term care enhance quality of care. (©iStock.com/Pamela Moore)

More than 15 million nursing assistants are employed in nursing homes, most of whom are under 55 years old and female, have a high school education or less, and have an income of $30,000 or less annually. The annual growth rate for nursing

RESEARCH HIGHLIGHTS

Care Aides' Relational Practices and Caring Contributions

Purpose

To explore the complexities of care; work environments; and knowledge, skills, and efforts of care aides who work in nursing homes.

Method

Qualitative focused ethnography was used. Twenty female and two male care aides from one privately funded and four publicly funded nursing homes in a western Canadian province were interviewed. Swanson's Middle Range Theory of Caring was used as a framework for the study. Descriptive analysis was used to identify the aides' perceptions and experiences and the fit between their perceptions and experiences, context of care, and Swanson's Middle Range Theory of Caring.

Results

The following four themes were identified: (1) desiring the ideal relationship; (2) establishing relationships with residents and their families; (3) maintaining

relationships with residents and their families; and (4) the reality of care aide work. Forming and maintaining relationships was viewed as a foundational and significant component of care aide work. The work occurs within a helping and caring framework and is not "just completing tasks." Care aides are the central and most accessible service providers in nursing homes, and the caring between the care aides and the residents and families is to be valued and nurtured.

Conclusions

Care aides are the central and most accessible service providers in nursing homes, and the caring between the care aides and the residents and families is to be valued and nurtured. The authors state: "The complexities of care and working environments are not well understood, and the knowledge, skills, and efforts of those who have chosen careers in residential care remain obscure and undervalued" (p. 24). Further research is needed to more fully explore the nature and expression of caring in nursing homes and its potential to improve both outcomes and quality of life.

Adapted from Andersen EA, Spiers J: Care aides' relational practices and caring contributions, *J Gerontol Nurs* 42(11):24–30, 2016.

assistants over the next decade is projected to be 9%, which is faster than average. Critical shortages of nursing assistants exist now in RCFs, skilled care, and home care, and these shortages will worsen in the future. Recruitment, retention, and high turnover rates are a problem in nursing homes. Low wages and inadequate benefits contribute to understaffing, particularly in for-profit facilities. Several recent studies have investigated the relationship of factors such as turnover, work satisfaction, staffing, and power relations to quality of care and positive outcomes in nursing homes. Results support the importance of developing a culture of respect in which the work of nursing assistants is understood and valued at all levels of the organization.

An important nursing role in LTC is the supervision and education of nursing assistants to enable them to competently perform in their role as an essential member of the care team. One of the most important components of the culture change movement (discussed later) is the creation of models of care that value and honor the important work of nursing assistants. Culture change must be equally concerned about the needs of residents and the well-being of staff (Thomas & Johansson, 2003). "An organization that learns to give love, respect, dignity, tenderness, and tolerance to all members of the staff will soon find these same virtues being practiced by the staff" (Thomas & Johansson, 2003, p. 3).

Until health care professionals and our society make a real commitment to providing adequate wages, individual supports (e.g., health insurance, education, career ladders), and an appreciation of their significant contribution to quality of nursing home care, these neglected workers cannot be expected to have the energy or incentive to extend themselves to the older adults in their care. Care of older adults who are frail and seriously ill persons is labor intensive and costly and requires specialized knowledge. Reasonable workloads, enhanced education and training, and adequate reimbursement are essential. The meaning and value of the work of nursing assistants must be supported by professional nurses and communicated to nursing

home owners, managers, legislators, and other health care professionals (Andersen & Spiers, 2016).

Resident Bill of Rights

Regulations have been created to protect the rights of the residents of nursing homes. Residents in LTC facilities have rights under both federal and state laws. The staff of the facility must inform residents of these rights and protect and promote their rights. The rights to which the residents are entitled should be conspicuously posted in the facility (Box 6.10). Also, the Long-Term Care Ombudsman Program is a nationwide effort

---

BOX 6.10   Bill of Rights for Long-Term Care Residents

- The right to voice grievances and have them remedied
- The right to information about health conditions and treatments and to participate in one's own care to the greatest extent possible
- The right to choose one's own health care providers and to speak privately with one's health care providers
- The right to consent to or refuse all aspects of care and treatments
- The right to manage one's own finances, if capable, or to choose one's own financial advisor
- The right to be transferred or discharged only for appropriate reasons
- The right to be free from all forms of abuse
- The right to be free from all forms of restraint to the extent compatible with safety
- The right to privacy and confidentiality concerning one's person, personal information, and medical information
- The right to be treated with dignity, consideration, and respect in keeping with one's individuality
- The right to immediate visitation and access at any time for family, health care providers, and legal advisors; the right to reasonable visitation and access for others

Note: This list of rights is a sampling of federal and several states' lists of rights of residents or participants in long-term care. Nurses should check the rules of their own state for specific rights in law for that state.

to support the rights of both the residents and the facilities. In most states, the program provides trained volunteers to investigate rights and quality complaints or conflicts. All reporting is anonymous. Each facility is required to post the name and contact information of the ombudsman assigned to the facility.

QUALITY OF CARE IN SKILLED NURSING FACILITIES

Nursing homes are one of the most highly regulated industries in the United States. The Omnibus Budget Reconciliation Act (OBRA) of 1987 and the frequent revisions and updates are designed to improve the quality of resident care and have had a positive impact. Some of the requirements of OBRA and subsequent legislation include the following: comprehensive resident assessments (Minimum Data Set [MDS]; Chapter 9), increased training requirements for nursing assistants, elimination of the use of medications and restraints for the purpose of discipline or convenience, higher staffing requirements for nursing and social work staff, standards for nursing home administrators, and quality assurance activities.

The Quality Assurance and Performance Improvement (QAPI) requires all nursing homes participating in Medicare or Medicaid programs to implement a QAPI program to assess quality of care provided to residents and to improve outcomes. The National Nursing Home Quality Improvement Campaign provides free, easy access to evidence-based and model-practice resources to support continuous quality improvement (see Box 6.6). The Skilled Nursing Facility Value-Based Purchasing (SNF VBF) Program, which began in 2019, rewards skilled nursing facilities with incentive payments for the quality of care they give to individuals with Medicare.

Nursing homes undergo regular unannounced surveys every 9 to 15 months, and surveys are also conducted in response to complaints. Detailed inspection data and penalties for violations for individual nursing homes are reported on the Centers for Medicare and Medicaid Services (CMS) Nursing Home Compare website (http://www.medicare.gov/NHCompare). Nursing homes were the first to publish online quality information, which is now available for hospitals and other health care organizations. Nursing homes also receive an overall quality rating using CMS's Five-Star Rating System based on annual inspection and complaint investigation data provided by state agencies, facility-reported nurse staffing hours per resident day, and quality measures based on MDS resident data.

Most nursing home quality measures have improved over time. Between 2011 and 2016, the use of physical restraints and antipsychotic medications, the number of pressure ulcers among high-risk residents, the percentage of residents experiencing pain and urinary tract infections, and the proportion of residents with ADL impairments that got worse declined. In 2014, 23.9% of long-stay nursing home residents were receiving an antipsychotic medication; since then, there has been a decrease of 35.4% to a national prevalence of 15.4% (CMS, 2019). The prevalence rate of antipsychotic use declined in nursing homes as a result of several proactive measures, but rates of antipsychotic use among individuals with dementia living in the community are rising.

Recommendations are to expand the efforts to curb the use of these drugs beyond nursing homes (Carter, 2018) (Chapter 26).

Disparities in care quality are associated with resident race or ethnicity, for-profit or nonprofit status (higher quality is associated with nonprofit status), and staffing levels. In spite of the benefits of using report cards, a recent study found that most hospital patients do not receive data about nursing home quality and receive only lists of nursing homes. Nurses involved in discharge planning are encouraged to use the CMS report cards so that patients' choices are based on quality data (Harrington et al., 2017). Box 6.11 presents CMS quality measures.

Choosing a Quality Nursing Home

Although the national rating system for nursing homes is helpful for evaluating quality, CMS advises consumers to use additional sources of information because the rating system provides only a "snapshot" of the care in individual nursing homes following one inspection and should not substitute for visiting nursing homes. The most appropriate method of choosing a nursing home is to personally visit the facility, meet with the director of nursing, observe care routines, discuss the potential resident's needs, and use a format such as the one presented in Box 6.12 to ask questions to evaluate the facility. CMS provides a nursing home checklist on its website, and the National Consumer

---

BOX 6.11 Quality Measures for Long-Term Care Facilities

Percentage of Short-Stay Residents With:
- Moderate to severe pain
- Pressure ulcers that are new or worsened
- Seasonal influenza vaccine
- Pneumococcal vaccine
- Antipsychotic medication
- Improvements in function
- Any cause hospital readmission
- Community discharge for 100 days without readmission
- Outpatient emergency department visit

Percentage of Long-Term Residents With:
- One or more falls with a major injury
- Urinary tract infections
- Moderate to severe pain
- Pressure ulcers that are new or worsened
- Loss of bowel and bladder control
- Use of a bladder catheter
- Physical restraints
- A need for increased help with daily activities
- Weight loss
- Depressive symptoms
- Antipsychotic medication
- Seasonal influenza vaccine
- Pneumococcal vaccine
- Ability to move independently worsened
- Antianxiety or hypnotic medication

From Centers for Medicare & Medicaid Services: *Quality measures* (website), 2020. https://www.cms.gov/Medicare/Quality-Initiatives-Patient-Assessment-Instruments/NursingHomeQualityInits/NHQIQuality Measures. Accessed January 2021.

BOX 6.12   Selecting a Nursing Home

Central Focus
- Residents and families are the central focus of the facility.

Interaction
- Staff members are attentive and caring.
- Staff members listen to what residents say.
- Staff members and residents smile at one another.
- There is a prompt response to resident and family needs.
- Meaningful activities are provided on all shifts to meet individual preferences.
- Residents engage in activities with enjoyment.
- Staff members talk to residents with cognitive impairments; residents with cognitive impairments are involved in activities designed to meet their needs.
- Staff members do not talk down to residents, talk as if they are not present, or ignore yelling or calling out.
- Families are involved in care decisions and daily life in the facility.

Milieu
- Calm, active, friendly
- Presence of community, volunteers, children, plants, animals

Environment
- No odor, clean, and well maintained
- Rooms personalized
- Private areas

- Protected outside areas
- Equipment in good repair

Individualized Care
- Restorative programs for ambulation, ADLs
- Residents well dressed and groomed
- Resident and family councils
- Pleasant mealtimes, good food, residents have choices
- Adequate staff to serve meals and assist residents
- Flexible meal schedules, food available 24 hours per day
- Ethnic food preferences available

Staff
- Well trained, high level of professional skill
- Professional in appearance and demeanor
- RNs involved in care decisions and care delivery
- Active staff development programs
- Physicians and advanced practice nurses involved in care planning and staff training
- Adequate staff (more than the minimum required) on each shift
- Low staff turnover

Safety
- Safe walking areas indoors and outdoors
- Monitoring of residents at risk for injury
- Restraint-appropriate care, adequate safety equipment and training on its use

ADLs, activities of daily living; *RNs,* registered nurses.
Adapted from Rantz MJ, Mehr DR, Popejoy L, et al.: Nursing home care quality: a multidimensional theoretical model, *J Nurs Care Qual* 12:30–46, 1998.

Voice for Quality Long-Term Care also provides resources for choosing a nursing home and understanding quality measures (see Box 6.6).

Nurses play an important role in helping individuals and their family and significant others to understand the discharge process and their posthospital needs, particularly if discharge to a skilled nursing facility is planned. CMS recommends that an evaluation of discharge be performed at least 48 hours before discharge, but ideally discharge planning should begin on admission. Patient and family education should include the role of skilled nursing facilities in rehabilitation, role of members of the interprofessional team, interpretation of five-star ratings, and other information on how to choose a facility.

The Culture Change Movement

Across the United States, and internationally, the movement to transform nursing homes from the typical medical model into "homes" that nurture quality of life for older adults and support and empower frontline caregivers is changing the face of LTC. Begun by the Pioneer Network, a national not-for-profit organization that serves the culture change movement, many facilities are changing from a rigid institutional approach to one that is person centered. CMS has endorsed culture change in the federal nursing home regulations and also has released a self-study tool for nursing homes to assess their own progress toward culture change.

Culture change is the "process of moving from a traditional nursing home model—characterized as a system unintentionally

designed to foster dependence by keeping residents, as one observer put it, 'well cared for, safe, and powerless'—to a regenerative model that increases residents' autonomy and sense of control" (Brawley, 2007, p. 9). The ultimate vision of culture change is to improve the lives of residents and staff by centering facility's philosophies, organizational structures, environmental designs, and care around practices that support residents' needs and preferences.

Older adults in need of LTC want to live in a homelike setting that does not look and function like a hospital. They want a setting that allows them to make decisions they are used to making for themselves, such as when to get up, take a bath, eat, or go to bed. They want caregivers who know them and understand and respect their individuality and their preferences. Box 6.13 presents some of the differences between an institution-centered culture and a person-centered culture.

While further research is needed, some results suggest that person-centered care is associated with improved organizational performance, including higher resident and staff satisfaction, better workforce performance, and higher occupancy rates (Duan et al., 2020). Examples of philosophies and programs of culture change are the Eden Alternative (companion animals, indoor plants, frequent visits by children, involvement with the community), the Green House Project (small homes designed for 10 to 12 residents), and the Wellspring Model. The Eden Alternative is best known for the addition of animals, plants, and visits from children to nursing homes. However, cats and dogs are not the heart of culture change. Truly transforming a nursing home starts at the top and requires the involvement of all levels of staff and changes in values, attitudes, structures, and management practices. The principles central to culture change are presented in Box 6.14. Strategic and cost-efficient methods of assisting nursing homes to implement culture change are needed and will require strong nursing leadership.

USING CLINICAL JUDGMENT TO PROMOTE HEALTHY AGING: EXCELLENCE IN LONG-TERM CARE

Nurses play a key role in improving quality of care in LTC through evidence-based practice and leadership in quality improvement initiatives. Nursing research has contributed significantly to the evidence-based interventions to improve quality of care in the nursing home. Further research needs to be directed to other LTPAC settings. For many, nursing in LTC offers the opportunity to practice the full scope of nursing, establish long-term relationships with patients and families, and make a significant difference in patient outcomes. Although medical management is important, the need for expert nursing is the most essential service provided. More and more nursing graduates will practice in LTPAC settings, and education must prepare them for these roles. Nurses are increasingly recognized as important to improved health outcomes for the individual with LTC needs.

KEY CONCEPTS

- Nurses need to develop the clinical judgment skills to identify and evaluate solutions and nursing actions to promote excellence in care outcomes for older adults in LTC.
- LTC describes a variety of services, including medical and nonmedical care (assistance with ADLs and IADLs), provided on an ongoing basis to people of all ages who have a chronic illness or physical, cognitive, or developmental disabilities.
- LTC can be provided informally or formally in a range of environments, from an individual's home to the home of a friend or relative, an adult day health center, independent and ALFs, CCRCs, skilled nursing facilities, long-term chronic care facilities, and hospice.
- The total spectrum of health care in the United States has been expanded to include LTPAC services, which include nursing homes, ALFs, home care, and hospice.

- The bulk of LTC throughout the developed world is informal unpaid care provided by family members. Without family caregivers, the present level of LTC could not be sustained.
- The number of older adults needing LTSS is dramatically increasing year after year, and the challenge of ensuring the quality and financial stability of care provision is one faced by governments in both the developed and the developing world.
- LTC coverage in the United States is expensive, fragmented, overly reliant on institutional care, and primarily financed by individuals themselves or their caregivers or by Medicaid.
- Nursing homes are the settings for the delivery of around-the-clock care for those needing specialized care that cannot be provided elsewhere. Nursing homes are a complex health care setting that is a mix of hospital, rehabilitation facility, hospice, and dementia-specific units, and they are a final home for many older adults.

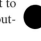

- Quality of care in nursing homes is improving. In skilled nursing facilities nationwide, the average performance has improved. Professional nurse staffing results in improved outcomes.

- Culture change in nursing homes is a growing movement to develop models of person-centered care and improve outcomes and quality of life.

NEXT-GENERATION NCLEX® (NGN) EXAMINATION–STYLE QUESTIONS

Mrs. Adams is an 87-year-old widowed female. She is being admitted to a rural long-term care (LTC) facility following hospitalization for uncontrolled hypertension. Prior to hospitalization, she had been living alone and it was determined that she had not been taking her medications for hypertension, osteoporosis, depression, and coronary artery disease. The nurse completing her admission interview concludes by asking Mrs. Adams what time she usually eats, stating that the facility serves food cafeteria-style between 0600 and 0800 hours for breakfast, 1100 and 1300 hours for lunch, and 1700 and 1900 hours for dinner. Residents are assisted to bed by 2200 hours. Her bath days will be Tuesday, Thursday, and Saturday mornings. The nurse gives Mrs. Adams an activity schedule with the daily offerings and states that if she does not like any of them, the staff would try to find something else she enjoys.

Highlight the statements above that correspond to a patient-centered culture.

NURSING STUDY

Transitions Across the Continuum

Ray is 85 years old and was recently admitted to the hospital from his own home following a fall with resultant fracture of the right hip. He was brought to the hospital by paramedics after a neighbor checked on him because they had not heard any sounds from his apartment. He had been lying on the floor for 8 hours, unable to call for help. He lives alone in a one-bedroom condominium. His wife of 50 years died 4 years ago. His three adult children and their families live out of state but keep in close contact with their father and visit several times a year. The last time they saw their father was 4 months before his hospitalization.

Before the hip fracture, Ray was fairly capable of taking care of himself, but since the death of his wife, his memory and mood have declined. He is hard of hearing in both ears but often refuses to wear his hearing aids, claiming that they distort all sounds and are a bother. He only occasionally left his apartment and had lost a great deal of weight. His neighbors reported that he was falling frequently and there were repeated calls to 911 for assistance. He had several "fender-benders" and had limited his driving to shopping and church. His

children were becoming increasingly worried about him living alone. He refused to consider moving to live nearer or with his children or to an assisted living facility. He did not want to be a bother to his children. His home is full of family pictures, pictures from his worldwide travels with his wife, memorabilia from his days as a police officer, and antique furniture. He has a little dog who gives him great enjoyment.

Following a surgical repair of his fractured hip, Ray experienced delirium and his mental status declined. He received physical therapy but had difficulty following the orders for partial weight bearing on the affected leg. He became incontinent and required an adult brief. He also developed a necrotic pressure ulcer on his right heel. The hospital case manager recommended to the family that Ray be transferred to a skilled nursing facility for further rehabilitation, treatment of the pressure ulcer, and possible long-term care placement. It was felt that he could not return safely to his home because of his mental status and functional decline. His finances were limited, so a home that accepts both Medicare and Medicaid was recommended.

CLINICAL JUDGMENT QUESTIONS AND ACTIVITIES

1. If you were in the role of a hospital case manager, how might you have helped the family in the nursing study with the discharge decision?
2. Would Ray, the gentleman in the nursing study, be appropriate for an ALF upon discharge from the hospital? Why or why not? What services would need to be in place for him to be discharged to an ALF? How would he pay for these services?
3. Would Ray, the gentleman in the nursing study, be appropriate for discharge home following hospitalization? What would home health provide under Medicare? What other services might he need? How would he pay for these services?
4. What are some of the obstacles that families of older adults face when their loved one needs a great deal of care? Do you

think that families should provide the care rather than place loved ones with 24-hour care needs in nursing homes? If this was your family, what challenges might be present in providing 24-hour care for a loved one?

5. Would you be willing to pay more taxes or be required to purchase LTC insurance to pay for LTC? Do you think individuals should be responsible for paying for their own LTC needs?
6. Would you consider nursing practice in LTC? Why or why not? What can education programs do to more adequately prepare students for practice in LTC and encourage them to consider working in these settings?

RESEARCH QUESTIONS

1. What are the experiences of older adults seeking care assistance to remain in their own homes?
2. What are the differences in the characteristics of residents of ALFs and nursing homes?
3. How do outcomes of care differ for older adults living in ALFs and nursing homes?
4. What are the best practice approaches to the provision of LTC for older adults?
5. How do younger adults and older adults in different countries feel about increased taxes for government support of LTC?
6. Are younger people preparing for their future LTC needs?
7. What is the relationship between a culture change model and care outcomes in nursing homes?
8. How does the role of the professional nurse differ between acute and long-term care?

REFERENCES

Alzheimer's Association: *Dementia care practice: recommendations for assisted living residences and nursing homes* (website), 2009. https://www.alz.org/national/documents/brochure_DCPRphases1n2.pdf. Accessed March 2018.

Andersen EA, Spiers J: Care aides' relational practices and caring contributions, *J Gerontol Nurs* 42(11):24–30, 2016.

Bailey M, Dubnow S: *Covid cases plummet 83% among nursing home staffers despite vaccine hesitancy* (website), 2021. https://khn.org/news/article/covid-cases-plummet-among-nursing-home-staffers-despite-vaccine-hesitancy/#:~:text=Covid%20Cases%20Plummet%2083%25%20Among%20Nursing%20Home%20Staffers%20Despite%20Vaccine%20Hesitancy,-By%20Melissa%20Bailey&text=New%20covid%2D19%20infections%20among,Johns%20Hopkins%20University%20data%20shows. Accessed March 2021.

Brawley E: What culture change is and why an aging nation cares, *Aging Today* 28:9–10, 2007.

Carter EA: *Off-label antipsychotic use in older adults with dementia: not just a nursing home problem* (website), 2018. https://www.aarp.org/ppi/info-2018/off-label-antipsychotic-use-in-older-adults-with-dementia.html. Accessed June 2021.

Centers for Disease Control and Prevention (2021). Nursing home care. https://www.cdc.gov/nchs/fastats/nursing-home-care.htm. Accessed December 2021.

Centers for Medicare and Medicaid Services (CMS): *National partnership to improve dementia care in nursing homes: antipsychotic medication use data report* (website), 2019. https://www.nhqualitycampaign.org/files/AP_package_20180131.pdf. Accessed March 2018.

Cortes TA, Sullivan-Marx EM: A case exemplar for national policy leadership: expanding Program of All-Inclusive Care for the Elderly (PACE), *J Gerontol Nurs* 42(3):9–14, 2016.

Cubanski J, Koma W, Damico A, et al.: *How much do Medicare beneficiaries spend out of pocket on health care?* (website), 2019. https://www.kff.org/report-section/how-much-do-medicare-beneficiaries-spend-out-of-pocket-on-health-care-appendix-table/.

Duan Y, Mueller C, Yu F, Talley K: The effects of nursing home culture change on resident quality of life in U.S. nursing homes: an integrative review, *Res Gerontol Nurs,* 13(4), 2020. https://journals.healio.com/doi/abs/10.3928/19404921-20200115-02. Accessed December 2021.

Eliopoulos C: *Gerontological nursing,* Philadelphia, 2010, Wolters Kluwer/Lippincott Williams & Wilkins.

Fulmer T, Koller C, Rowe J: *Reimagining nursing homes in the wake of COVID-19* (website), 2020. https://nam.edu/reimagining-nursing-homes-in-the-wake-of-covid-19/. Accessed March 2021.

Genworth: *Cost of care survey* (website), 2020. https://www.genworth.com/aging-and-you/finances/cost-of-care.html.

The Gerontological Society of America: *Pandemic-driven disruptions in oral health* (website), 2021. https://www.geron.org/images/gsa/documents/Pandemic-Driven_Disruptions_in_Oral_Health.pdf. Accessed April 2021.

Gleckman H: *What we don't know—but should—about assisted living facilities* (website), 2018. https://www.forbes.com/sites/howardgleckman/2018/02/05/what-we-dont-know-but-should-about-assisted-living-facilities/?sh=fdb03a2e0438. Accessed June 2021.

Golden R, Shier G: What does "care transitions" really mean? *Generations* 36(4):6–12, 2012–2013.

Gorges R, Konetzka R: Factors associated with racial differences in deaths among nursing home residents with COVID-19 infection in the US, *AMA Netw Open,* 2021 4(2):e2037431, 2021. doi:10.1001/jamanetworkopen.2020.37431.

Harrington C, Kovner C, Mezey M, et al.: Experts recommend minimum staffing standards for nursing facilities in the United States, *Gerontologist* 40(1):5–16, 2000.

Harrington C, Montgomery A, King T, et al.: These administrative actions would improve nursing home ownership and financial transparency in the post COVID-19 period. In *Health Affairs,* 2021. doi:10.1377/hblog202110208.597573 Accessed February 11, 2021.

Harrington C, Ross L, Chapman S, et al.: Nurse staffing and coronavirus infections in California nursing homes, *Policy Polit Nurs Pract* 21(3):174–186, 2020.

Harrington C, Wiener J, Ross L, et al.: *Key issues in long-term services and supports quality* (website), 2017. https://www.kff.org/report-section/key-issues-in-long-term-services-and-supports-quality-appendix/. Accessed June 2021.

Horney C, Capp R, Boxer R, et al.: Factors associated with early readmission among patients discharged to post-acute care facilities, *JAGS* 65(6):1109–1205, 2017.

Lynn J: The "fierce urgency of now": geriatrics professionals speaking up for older adult care in the United States, *JAGS* 67(10):2001–2003, 2019.

National PACE Association: *What is PACE?* (website), 2019. https://www.npaonline.org/. Accessed March 2019.

Nguyen V: *Fact sheet long-term support and services* (website), 2017. https://www.aarp.org/content/dam/aarp/ppi/2017-01/Fact%20Sheet%20Long-Term%20Support%20and%20Services.pdf. Accessed June 2021.

Ouslander J, Grabowski D: COVID-19 in nursing homes: calming the perfect storm, *JAGS* 68(10):2153–2162, 2020.

Reinhard S, Accius J, Houser A, et al.: *Picking up the pace of change: a state scorecard on long-term services and supports for older adults, people with physical disabilities, and family caregivers,* 2017, AARP, Commonwealth Fund, SCAN Foundation. http://www.long-termscorecard.org. Accessed June 2021.

Roy A: *Nursing home deaths from COVID-19: U.S. historical data* (website), 2020. https://freopp.org/nursing-home-deaths-from-covid-19-u-s-historical-data-b4ad44cfc48e. Accessed June 2021.

Shen K, Loomer L, Abrams H, et al.: Estimates of Covid-19 cases and deaths among nursing home residents not reported in federal data, *Jama Network Open,* 2021 4(9):e21222885.

Sherman R, Touhy T: An exploratory descriptive study to evaluate Florida nurse leader challenges and opportunities in nursing home setting, *SAGE Open Nurs* 3:1–7, 2017.

Siegel E, Bowers B, Carder P, et al.: Assisted living: optimal person-environment fit, *Res Gerontol Nurs* 14(1):5–10, 2021.

Stanford School of Medicine: *Palliative care* (website), 2019. https://palliative.stanford.edu/home-hospice-home-care-of-the-dying-patient/where-do-americans-die/. Accessed June 2021.

Teno J, Gozalo P, Bynum J, et al.: Change in end-of-life care for Medicare beneficiaries, *JAMA* 309(5):470–477, 2013.

Thomas W, Johansson C: Elderhood in Eden, *Top Geriatr Rehabil* 19:282–290, 2003.

Touhy T, Strews W, Brown C: Expressions of caring as lived by nursing home staff residents, and families, *Int J Hum Caring* 9:31–37, 2005.

Zuraw L, Rodriguez CH: *Caring for an aging nation* (website), 2021. https://khn.org/news/article/caring-for-an-aging-nation/. Accessed June 2021.

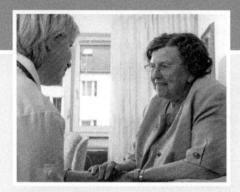

CHAPTER 7

Therapeutic Communication With Older Adults

Theris A. Touhy

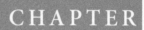

http://evolve.elsevier.com/Touhy/TwdHlthAging

A STUDENT SPEAKS

When they told us we were going to a senior center to interview an older person about their life, I was really nervous. My grandparents are no longer living, and I really wasn't close to them when they were alive. I have little contact with older people, and to tell you the truth, I find them a little boring. Seems to me they are always complaining and criticizing and talking about the good old days. I am just not sure what I am going to learn from this assignment. I plan to go into pediatrics, so it isn't very relevant to me.

James, age 22

AN OLDER ADULT SPEAKS

I love living in my retirement community, but I tell you, I miss being around younger people. My grandchildren live far away, and I don't see them often. I would enjoy being around the young folks more. They really bring a new perspective on things and have a lot of enthusiasm and energy. It's good to keep up on the new things they are involved in. I think older people and younger people could learn a lot from each other.

Frances, age 82

LEARNING OBJECTIVES

On completion of this chapter, the reader will be able to:

1. Describe the importance of communication in the lives of older adults.
2. Discuss how ageist attitudes affect communication.
3. Understand the significance of the life story in coming to know older adults.
4. Discuss the modalities of reminiscence and life review.
5. Use clinical judgment to generate solutions and nursing actions and to evaluate outcomes to facilitate therapeutic communication with older adults individually and in groups.

Communication is the single most important capacity of human beings. Few things are more dehumanizing than the inability to communicate effectively and engage in social interaction with others. The need to communicate, to be listened to, and to be heard does not change with age or impairment. Meaningful communication and active engagement with society contributes to healthy aging and improves an older adult's chances of living longer, responding better to health care interventions, and maintaining optimal function.

For some individuals, opportunities for social interaction may be more limited because of loss of family and friends, illnesses, and sensory and cognitive losses. The ageist attitudes of the public, and of health professionals, also present barriers to communicating effectively with older adults (Fick & Lundebjerg, 2017; Saliba, 2017). Good communication skills are the basis for accurate assessment, care planning, and the development of caring relationships between the nurse and the older adult.

This chapter discusses the effect of health professionals' attitudes toward aging on their communication with older adults and communication skills essential to therapeutic interaction. The significance of the life story, reminiscence, life review, and communication with groups of older adults are also included in this chapter. Communication with individuals with hearing and vision loss is discussed in Chapters 12 and 13, and communication with individuals with cognitive impairment is discussed in Chapter 26.

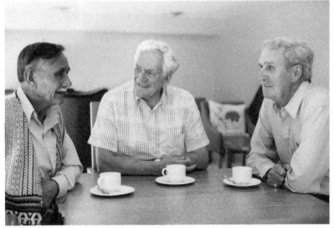

Group of older men talking over coffee. (©iStock.com/Squared-pixels.)

AGEISM AND COMMUNICATION

Beliefs in myths and stereotypes about aging and ageist attitudes on the part of health professionals, society, and older adults themselves can interfere with the ability to communicate effectively. For example, if a nurse believes that all older adults have memory problems or are unable to learn or process information, that nurse will be less likely to engage in conversation, provide appropriate health information, or treat the individual with respect and dignity. If an older individual believes that illness is inevitable with increased age, that individual may fail to report changes in health or adopt health promotion strategies. Although ageism is found cross-culturally, it is more prevalent in the United States, where aging is often viewed with sadness, fear, and anxiety. Some research indicates that individuals in many non-Western cultures are more tolerant of older adults, perceive older adults as significantly more important to their society, and engage in less avoiding behaviors toward older adults.

Robert Butler (1969), the first director of the National Institute on Aging, defined ageism as the systematic stereotyping of and discrimination against people because they are old, in the way that racism and sexism discriminate against color and gender. Ageism is the only form of discrimination and prejudice that we will all encounter if we live long enough. The Frame-Works Institute (2017) (https://www.frameworksinstitute.org/issues/aging/) proposes a current definition that includes both interpersonal and societal effects of ageism. "Ageism is discrimination based on prejudices about age. When ageism is directed at older adults, it often involves the assumptions that older adults are less competent, less attractive, and less vigorous than younger people. Ageism has a huge negative impact on older adults throughout all areas of life" (Sweetland et al., 2017, p. 22) (Box 7.1). Age biases have been associated with poor cognitive, functional, and mental health outcomes and are a risk factor for abuse (National Center of Elder Abuse, 2021).

We saw the effect of ageism during the COVID-19 pandemic in underresourced nursing homes and a lack of attention to the

BOX 7.1   Public Perceptions of Aging

- **Someone else's problem**—"What are we going to do with those older people?"
- **Undesirable and an inescapable decline**—almost exclusively associated with decline and deterioration
- **Isolated**—aging perceived as a personal or family problem, not a challenge that society shares
- **Fatalistic**—tied to fears of decline, depression, and dependence. Fears make aging viewed with dread and impedes policies and solutions that address both the challenges and opportunities
- **Out of sight and out of mind**—fears and misperceptions lead to a lack of attention to older adults and does little to enhance the experience of aging

From Fick D, Lundebjerg N: When it comes to older adults, language matters, *J Geron Nurs*, 43(9):2–4, 2017.

provision of adequate protective equipment and assistance in managing the pandemic. The World Health Organization repeatedly had to address public opinion that COVID-19 was not a serious concern because of initial public beliefs that it affected only older people (Fraser et al., 2020; Kendall-Taylor et al., 2021). Ageism will continue to have long-term negative impacts, including elder abuse, depression, and early mortality, that discriminate against older adults and eventually affect all of us (Kendall-Taylor et al., 2021).

Ageism also affects health professionals, and with few exceptions, studies of attitudes of students in the health professions toward aging reflect negative views. Examples of the effect of ageism include the small number of students who choose to work in the field of aging and the lack of education of health professionals in the care of older adults, even though the majority of their patients are older (Kydd et al., 2014). Other effects include spending less time with older patients, taking a more authoritarian role, having less patience, providing less information, and neglecting to address important psychosocial and preventive factors. It is important for nurses who care for older adults to be aware of their own attitudes and beliefs about aging and the effect of these attitudes on communication and care provision. Enhancing one's interpersonal communication skills and examining personal and societal attitudes toward aging are the foundation for therapeutic interactions with older adults. Educators play an important part in shaping attitudes of students in the health professions toward older adults (Kydd et al., 2014; Chapter 1).

Elderspeak

Elderspeak is a form of patronizing speech, similar to "baby talk," which is often used to talk to very young children (Box 7.2). Elderspeak is most likely a cognitive component of ageism. It is especially common in communication between health care professionals and older adults in hospitals and nursing homes but also occurs in non–health care settings (Corwin, 2017). Recent research reported that at least one example of elderspeak was identified in 84% of video recording transcripts of interactions between residents and staff during daily care activities. Collective pronoun substitution (e.g., "We are going to take a bath") and inappropriate terms of endearment, such as honey, hon, sweetheart, and sweetie, were used most commonly (Williams, Shaw, et al., 2017).

BOX 7.2   Characteristics of Elderspeak

- Using a singsong voice, changing pitch and tone, and exaggerating words
- Using short and simple sentences
- Speaking more slowly
- Using limited vocabulary
- Repeating or paraphrasing what has just been said
- Using pet names (diminutives) such as "honey" or "sweetie" or "grandma"
- Using collective pronouns such as "we"—for instance, "Would we like to take a bath now?"
- Using statements that sound like questions

Elderspeak is most often used without maliciousness or conscious awareness, and nurses may view it as an effective way to communicate with older adults, especially those with cognitive impairment. However, research has shown that use of this form of speech conveys messages of dependence, incompetence, and control. A majority of older adults interpret elderspeak as disrespectful or patronizing. Elderspeak is associated with lower rates of communication ability, social isolation, increased dependence, and cognitive decline. Use of elderspeak doubles the rates of challenging behaviors of individuals with dementia (Shaw et al., 2020; Chapter 26). Other examples of communication that conveys ageist attitudes are ignoring the older adult and talking to family and friends as if the person were not present and limiting interaction to task-focused communication only.

THERAPEUTIC COMMUNICATION WITH OLDER ADULTS

Basic communication strategies that apply to all situations in nursing, such as attentive listening, authentic presence, nonjudgmental attitude, clarifying, giving information, seeking validation of understanding, keeping focus, and using open-ended questions, are all applicable in communicating with older adults. Basically, older adults may need more time to give information or answer questions simply because they have a larger life experience from which to draw information. Sorting thoughts requires intervals of silence, and therefore listening carefully without rushing the older adult is important. Word retrieval may be slower, particularly for nouns and names (Chapter 8).

Open-ended questions are useful but also can be difficult. Those who wish to please, especially when feeling vulnerable or somewhat dependent, may wonder what it is you want to hear rather than what it is they would like to say. The most productive communication will focus initially on the issue of major concern to the individual, regardless of the priority of the nursing evaluation. When using closed questioning to obtain specific information, be aware that the individual may feel on the spot, and thus the appropriate information may not be immediately forthcoming. This is especially true when asking questions to determine mental status. The older adult may develop a mental block because of anxiety or feel threatened if questions are asked in a quizzing or demeaning manner. Older adults also may be reluctant to disclose information for fear of the consequences. For example, if they are having problems remembering things or are experiencing frequent falls, sharing this information may mean that they might have to relinquish desired activities or even leave their home and move to a more protective setting.

When communicating with individuals in a bed or wheelchair, position yourself at their level rather than talking over a side rail or standing above them. Pay attention to their gaze, gestures, body language, and the pitch, volume, and tone of their voice to help you understand what they are trying to communicate. Thoughts unstated are often as important as those that are verbalized. You may ask, "What are you thinking about right now?" Clarification is essential to ensure that you and the individual have the same framework of understanding. Many generational, cultural, and regional differences in speech patterns and idioms exist. Frequently seek validation of what you hear. If you tend to speak quickly, particularly if your accent is different from that of the patient, try to speak more slowly and give the person time to process what you are saying.

THE LIFE STORY

As we age, we accumulate complex stories from long years of living. Storytelling is a complementary and alternative therapy that nurses can use to enhance communication with older adults (Westerhof & Bohlmeijer, 2014). The life story can tell us a great deal about the person and is an important part of the assessment process. Stories provide important information about etiology, diagnosis, treatment, prognosis, and experience of living with an illness from the individual's point of view. Listening to stories is also a way of demonstrating cultural competence (Chapter 4). The nurse can learn much about an individual's history, communication style, relationships, coping mechanisms, strengths, fears, affect, and adaptive capacity by listening thoughtfully as the life story is constructed.

Listening to memories and life stories requires time and patience and a belief that the story and the person are valuable and meaningful. A memory is an incredible gift given to the nurse, a sharing of a part of oneself when one may have little else to give. The more personal memories are saved for persons who will patiently wait for their unveiling and who will treasure them. Stories are important. "The people who come to see us bring us their stories. They hope they tell them well enough so that we understand the truth in their lives. They hope we know how to interpret their stories correctly" (Coles, 1989, p. 7).

The life story as constructed through reminiscing, journaling, life review, or guided autobiography has held great fascination for gerontologists in the past 30 years. The universal appeal of the life story as a vehicle of culture, a demonstration of caring and generational continuity, and an easily stimulated activity has held allure for many professionals. The most exciting aspect of working with older adults is being a part of the emergence of the life story: the shifting and blending patterns.

Reminiscing

Reminiscing is an umbrella term that can include any recall of the past. Reminiscing occurs from childhood onward, particularly at life's junctures and transitions. Robert Butler (2003) emphasized that in the past, reminiscing was considered a sign of cognitive decline or what we now call Alzheimer's disease. Older adults who talked about the past and told the same stories again and again were said to be boring and living in the past. However, reminiscing is now considered a key developmental skill across the entire life span but an especially important psychological task of older adults. The focus of reminiscing changes as we age, and older adults reminisce more frequently for death preparation and to teach and inform others.

For the nurse, reminiscing is a therapeutic intervention important in coming to know and understand the older adult. The work of several gerontological nursing leaders, including Irene Burnside, Priscilla Ebersole, and Barbara Haight, has contributed to the body of knowledge about reminiscence and its importance in nursing. The International Center for Life Story Innovations and Practice (ICLIP), formerly the International Institute of Reminiscence and Life Review (IIRLR), is located at the University of Connecticut. This interdisciplinary organization focuses on the study of reminiscence and life review and is a valuable resource for nurses and members of other disciplines involved in research or practice. The *International Journal of Reminiscence and Life Review* is published by the ICLIP. An online certificate program for reminiscence and life story work is also available (Box 7.3).

Reminiscence can have many goals. It not only provides a pleasurable experience that improves quality of life but also increases socialization and connectedness with others, provides cognitive stimulation, improves communication, facilitates personal growth, and can decrease depression scores (Chapter 30). The process of reminiscence can occur in individual conversations with older adults, can be structured as in a nursing history, or can occur in a group where each person shares memories and listens to others sharing their memories. Digital storytelling is another medium that can be used with older adults to record their stories and memories across a variety of platforms, including tablets and smartphones in a format that can be shared with others (see Box 7.3).

Virtual reality (VR) is also being used to stimulate reminiscence and provide pleasurable experiences such as revisiting childhood neighborhoods, travel, nature, and other experiences that trigger positive memories. VR technology is also being used to allow health care staff to experience dementia, hearing loss, and other conditions (Bleiberg, 2018). Studies are ongoing to evaluate whether using VR might reduce feelings of isolation from the outside world (such as the isolation we all faced during the COVID-19 pandemic) (Spencer, 2021).

Intergenerational reminiscence activities could have benefits for both older and younger individuals. In several studies, benefits include increased engagement, enthusiasm, appreciation, respect, and empathy for the older adult (Yamashita et al., 2018). Reminiscence can be used by family caregivers to enhance communication and strengthen relationships with family members who are experiencing cognitive impairment (Karlsson et al., 2017). Nurses in long-term care facilities who engaged in reminiscence activities reported knowing older adults better, thereby enhancing their personhood (see the Research Highlights box). Boxes 7.4 and 7.5 provide some suggestions for encouraging reminiscence, and group work is discussed later in the chapter.

RESEARCH HIGHLIGHTS

Functions and Value of Reminiscence for Nursing Home Staff

Purpose

To understand the extent to which reminiscence is used by nursing home staff with cognitively impaired individuals, the reasons why nursing home staff engage in reminiscence activities, and the value they attribute to these activities. The degree to which engagement in reminiscence activities by nursing staff contributed to knowledge about residents also was explored.

Method

Participants included 23 licensed nursing staff and 20 certified nursing assistants (CNAs) in three suburban nursing homes in Connecticut. Homes ranged in size from 107 to 353 beds. Instruments included a survey that used key elements and ideas from previously validated reminiscence surveys and a modified version of the Reminiscence Functions Scale–Brief Version.

Results

Most of the participants (86%) found reminiscence to be enjoyable and valuable in their personal and professional lives. However, fewer than half reported engaging in these activities frequently or very frequently. The authors stated that there may be many reasons for this (lack of time, belief that it is not valuable, or the view that engaging in reminiscence activities or sharing personal experiences with residents is unprofessional). The most frequently used functions of reminiscence were to calm anxiety, help residents to see meaning in life, and reorient confused residents.

Conclusion

Those who engaged in reminiscence activities more often reported knowing residents better—a hallmark of high-quality care. The impediments to reminiscing in this setting and strategies to increase this practice require further study. A key finding from previous research indicates that residents would prefer to reminisce with staff more frequently and that the intervention of reminiscence enhances nurse-patient relationships.

Data from Kris A, Henkel L, Krauss K, et al: Functions and value of reminiscence for nursing home staff, *J Gerontol Nurs* 43(6):35–44, 2017.

BOX 7.3 Resources for Best Practice

Center for Digital Storytelling: Training and resources to assist people in using digital media to tell meaningful stories from their lives. https://elmcip.net/organization/center-digital-storytelling.

Gerontological Society of America: Communicating with older adults: an evidence-based review of what really works. https://secure.geron.org/cvweb/cgi-bin/msascartdll.dll/ProductInfo?productcd=1947_Comm-Adults.

International Center for Life Story Innovations and Practice (ICLIP), formerly the International Institute of Reminiscence and Life Review (IIRLR): Resources for reminiscence and life review. https://iclip.nursing.uconn.edu/message-from-the-director/.

StoryCenter: Resources for digital storytelling. https://www.storycenter.org/about.

The Old Women's Project: Making visible how old women are directly affected by issues of social justice and ageism. http://www.oldwomensproject.org/.

TimeSlips: Examples of storytelling with individuals with dementia, training, and certification. http://www.timeslips.org/.

BOX 7.4   Suggestions for Encouraging Reminiscence

- Listen actively without correction or criticism. Older adults are presenting their version of their reality; our version belongs to another generation.
- Encourage older adults to discuss various ages and stages of their lives. Use questions such as "What was it like growing up on that farm?", "What did teenagers do for fun when you were young?", and "What was World War II like for you?"
- Be patient with repetition and do not interrupt. Sometimes people need to tell the same story often to come to terms with the experience, especially if it was meaningful to them. If they have a memory loss, it may be the only story they can remember, and it is important for them to be able to share it with others.
- Be attuned to signs of depression in conversation (dwelling on sad topics) or changes in physical status or behavior and provide appropriate assessment and intervention.
- If a topic that the person does not want to discuss arises, change to another topic.
- If individuals are reluctant to share because they do not feel their life was interesting, reassure them that everyone's life is valuable and interesting and tell them how important their memories are to you and others.
- Keep in mind that reminiscing is not an orderly process. One memory triggers another in a way that may not seem related; it is not important to keep things in order or to verify accuracy.
- Keep the conversation focused on the person reminiscing, but do not hesitate to share some of your own memories that relate to the situation being discussed. Participate as equals and enjoy each other's contributions.
- Respond positively and give feedback by making caring, appropriate comments that encourage the person to continue.
- Use props and triggers such as photographs and memorabilia (e.g., a childhood toy or antique, short stories or poems about the past, favorite foods, YouTube videos, old songs).
- Use open-ended questions to encourage reminiscing. If working with a group, you can prepare questions ahead of time, or you can ask the group members to pick a topic that interests them. One question or topic may be enough for an entire group session.

BOX 7.5   Sample Questions to Encourage Reminiscence

- How did your parents meet?
- What do you remember most about your mother? Father? Grandmother? Grandfather?
- What are some of your favorite memories from childhood?
- What was the first house you remember?
- What were your favorite foods as a child?
- Did you have a pet as a child?
- What do you remember about your first job?
- How did you celebrate birthdays or other holidays?
- If you were married, what are your memories of your wedding day?
What was the greatest accomplishment or joy in your life?

Reminiscing and Storytelling With Individuals Experiencing Cognitive Impairment

Cognitive impairment does not necessarily preclude older adults from participating in reminiscence or storytelling groups. Opportunities for telling the life story, enjoying memories, and achieving ego integrity should not be denied to individuals based on their cognitive status. Modifications must be made according to the cognitive abilities of the person, and although individual life review from a psychotherapeutic approach is not an appropriate modality, individuals with mild to moderate memory impairment can enjoy and benefit from group work focused on reminiscence and storytelling.

Emerging evidence suggests that reminiscence is an important nonpharmacological intervention for individuals with dementia. Reminiscence and storytelling provide a structure and mechanism for communication and engaging in interaction and can enhance quality of life and improve mood (Testad et al., 2014). Results of a study examining the use of reminiscence with people with dementia living in long-term care (Cooney et al., 2014) reported positive outcomes for the residents, staff, and family members. Outcomes for the resident included increased opportunities to socialize and interact, increased enjoyment, and potential changes in behavior (e.g., being more talkative and engaging with residents and staff more). For the staff, increased knowledge about the resident and engaging in relationships were associated with job satisfaction. Family members felt that their relative was better known and cared about (as opposed to cared for). For family caregivers, communication skills training that involves reminiscence and life review activities between the caregiver and family member with dementia can increase the quantity and quality of communication between care recipients and caregivers, lower caregiver stress and burden, and reduce behavioral problems.

When the nurse is working with a group of persons who are experiencing cognitive impairment, the emphasis in reminiscence groups is on sharing memories, however they may be expressed, rather than on specific recall of events. There should be no pressure to answer questions such as "Where were you born?" or "What was your first job?" Rather, discussions may center on jobs people had and places they have lived. Using additional props, such as music, pictures, and familiar objects (e.g., an American flag, an old coffee grinder) and doing familiar activities that trigger memories (e.g., having a tea party, folding linens) can prompt many recollections and sharing. The leader of a group with participants who have memory problems must assume a more active approach.

The TimeSlips program (Basting, 2003, 2006, 2013) is an evidence-based innovation, cited by the Agency for Healthcare Research and Quality (AHRQ, 2014), that uses storytelling to enhance the lives of people with cognitive impairment. Positive outcomes associated with the program include enhanced verbal skills and provider reports of positive behavioral changes, increased communication, increased sociability, and less confusion. TimeSlips is a beneficial and cost-effective therapeutic intervention that can be used in many settings. See http://www.timeslips.org/ for more information and examples and online training and certification (see Box 7.3).

Using the TimeSlips format, group members looking at a picture are encouraged to create a story about the picture. The pictures can be fantastical and funny, such as from greeting cards, or more nostalgic, such as Norman Rockwell paintings. All contributions are encouraged and welcomed, there are no right or wrong answers, and everything that the individuals say is included in the story and written down by the scribe. Stories are read back to the participants during the session, using their names to identify their contributions. At the beginning of each session, the story from the last session is read to the participants. Care is taken to compliment each member for his or her contribution to the wonderful story. The stories that emerge are full of humor and creativity and often include discussions of memories and reminiscing.

One of the authors of this text (T. Touhy) has used the TimeSlips storytelling modality extensively with mildly to moderately impaired older adults with great success as part of a research study on the effect of therapeutic activities for persons with memory loss. Qualitative responses from group participants and families indicated their enjoyment with the process. At the end of the 16-week group, the stories were bound into a book and given to the participants with a picture of the group and each member's name listed. Many of the participants and their families have commented on the pride they feel about their "book" and have even shared them with grandchildren and great-grandchildren.

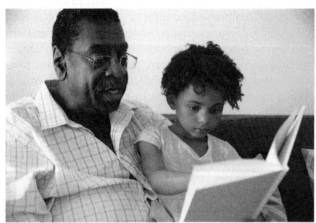

A grandfather sharing stories with his granddaughter. (©iStock. com/monkeybusinessimages.)

Life Review

Robert Butler (1963) first noted and brought to public attention the review process that normally occurs in the older person as the realization of approaching death creates a resurgence of unresolved conflicts. Butler called this process *life review*. Life review occurs quite naturally for many persons during periods of crisis and transition. However, Butler (2003) noted that in old age, the process of putting one's life in order increases in intensity and emphasis. Life review occurs most frequently as an internal review of memories, an intensely private and soul-searching activity.

Life review is a more formal therapy technique than reminiscence and takes a person through his or her life in a structured and chronological order. Life review therapy, guided autobiography, and structured life review are psychotherapeutic techniques based on the concept of life review. Gerontological nurses participate with older adults in both reminiscence and

life review, and it is important to acquire the skills to be effective in achieving the purposes of both of these techniques.

Life review may be especially important for older adults experiencing depressive symptoms and those facing death (Kris et al., 2017). However, life review should occur not only when we are old or facing death but also frequently throughout our lives. This process can assist us to examine where we are in life and change our course or set new goals. Butler (2003) commented that ongoing life review by an individual may help avoid the overwhelming feelings of despair that may surface for some individuals at the end of life when there may not be time to make changes.

COMMUNICATING WITH GROUPS OF OLDER ADULTS

Group work with older adults has been used extensively in institutional settings to meet myriad needs in an economical manner. Nurses have led groups of older adults for a variety of therapeutic reasons. Expert gerontological nurses, such as Irene Burnside and Priscilla Ebersole, have extensively discussed advantages of group work both for older adults and for group leaders and have provided in-depth guidelines for conducting groups. Box 7.6 presents some of the benefits of group work.

Many groups can be managed effectively by staff with clear goals and guidance and training. Volunteers, nursing assistants, students, and recreational staff can be taught to conduct many types of groups, but groups with a psychotherapy focus require a trained and skilled leader. With training and supervision, nursing students co-leading groups can enhance leadership and communication skills. Older adults in the group thoroughly enjoy spending time with younger

---

BOX 7.6   Benefits of Group Work With Older Adults

- Group experiences provide older adults with an opportunity to try new roles—those of teacher, expert, storyteller, or even clown.
- Groups may improve communication skills for lonely, shy, or withdrawn older people and those with communication disorders or memory impairment.
- Groups provide peer support and opportunities to share common experiences, and they may foster the development of warm friendships that endure long after the group has ended.
- The group may be of interest to other residents, staff, and relatives and may improve satisfaction and morale. Staff, in particular, may come to see their patients in a different light—not just as persons needing care but as persons.
- Active listening and interest in what older people have to say may improve self-esteem and help older adults feel like worthwhile persons whose wisdom is valued.
- Group work offers the opportunity for leaders to be creative and use many modalities, such as music, art, dance, poetry, exercise, and current events.
- Groups provide an opportunity for the leader to assess the person's mood, cognitive abilities, and functional level on a weekly basis.

Adapted from Burnside IM: Group work with older persons, *J Gerontol Nurs* 20:43, 1994.

BOX 7.7 Special Considerations in Group Work With Older Adults

- The leader must pay special attention to sensory losses and compensate for vision and hearing loss.
- Pacing is different, and group leaders must slow down in both physical and psychological actions depending on the group's abilities.
- Group members often need assistance or transportation to the group, and adequate time must be allowed for assembling the members and assisting them to return to their homes or rooms.
- Time of day that a group is scheduled is important. Meeting time should not conflict with bathing and eating schedules, and evening groups may not be good for older people, who may be tired by then. For community-based older people, transportation logistics may become complicated in the evening.
- Groups generally should include people with similar levels of cognitive ability. Mixing cognitively intact older adults with those who have memory and communication impairments requires special skills. In groups of people with varying abilities, alert persons tend to ask, "Will I become like them?" whereas those with memory and communication impairments may become anxious when they are aware that they cannot perform as well as the other members.
- Many older people likely to be in need of groups may be depressed or have experienced a number of losses (health, friends, spouse). Discussion of losses and sad feelings can be difficult for group leaders. A leader prone to depression would not be appropriate.
- Remind members of the termination date for the group so that they can prepare and not experience another loss.
- Leaders must be prepared for some members to become ill, deteriorate, and die. Plans for recognition of missing members will need to be clear.
- Leaders are continually confronted with their own aging and attitudes toward it. Co-leaders are ideal and can support each other. If leading the group alone, locate someone with expertise in group work with older adults who can discuss the group experiences with you and provide support and direction. Students generally should work in pairs and will need supervision.
- Evaluate each group session and the total group experience. Involve the group members in the evaluation.

Data from Burnside IM: Group work with older persons, *J Gerontol Nurs* 20:43, 1994; Stinson C: Structured group reminiscence: an intervention for older adults, *J Contin Educ Nurs* 40(11):521–528, 2009.

BOX 7.8 Group Work: The Wisdom of Older Adults

While the chapter author was conducting a weekly reminiscence group with older adults who were cognitively impaired, we were told by the supervisor that one of our members had died. One of the group members had been a priest, so we asked him to say a prayer for our deceased group member. He did so beautifully, and the group was grateful. The next week, to our surprise, the supposedly deceased member showed up for the group (she had been in the hospital). We didn't know how to handle the situation, but the other members came to our rescue by saying, "Father's prayers really worked this time." Older people's wisdom and humor can teach us a lot.

---

individuals, and they have much wisdom to share. Some basic considerations for group work are presented in this chapter, but nurses interested in working with groups of older adults should consult a text on group work for more in-depth information.

Groups can be implemented in many settings, including adult day health programs, retirement communities, assisted living facilities, nutrition sites, and nursing homes. Examples of groups include reminiscence groups, psychoeducational groups, caregiver support groups, and groups for people with memory impairment or other conditions such as Parkinson's disease or stroke. Groups can be organized to meet any level of human need; some meet multiple needs.

Group Structure and Special Considerations

Implementing a group intervention follows a thorough assessment of environment, needs, and the potential for various group strategies. Major decisions regarding goals will influence the strategy selected. For instance, individuals with diabetes in an acute care setting may need health care teaching on diabetes. The nurse sees the major goal as education and restoring order (or control) in each individual's lifestyle. The strategy best suited for that would be motivational or educational. A group of people experiencing mild neurocognitive impairment may benefit from a support group to express feelings or a group that teaches memory-enhancing strategies. Successful group work depends on organization; attention to details; agency support; evaluation and consideration of the older person's needs and status; and caring, sensitive, and skillful leadership.

Group work with older adults is different from that with younger age groups, and there are some unique aspects that require special skills and training and an extraordinary commitment on the part of the leader. Irene Burnside's (1994) pioneering work in this area remains a model for group work with older adults. Although these unique aspects may not apply to all types of groups of older adults, some strategies are presented in Box 7.7. Box 7.8 shares a story about the wisdom and humor of older adults.

USING CLINICAL JUDGMENT TO PROMOTE HEALTHY AGING: THERAPEUTIC COMMUNICATION

Throughout this chapter we have tried to convey the potential for honest and hopeful communication with individuals as they age. Communicating with older adults requires special skills, patience, and respect. We must break through the barriers and continue to reach toward the humanity of the individual with the belief that communication is the most vital service we offer. This is the heart of nursing. Skilled, sensitive, and caring individual and group communication strategies with older adults are essential to meeting needs and are the basis for therapeutic nursing relationships. Just as all people have the need to communicate and have their basic needs met, they also have the right to experiences that are meaningful and fulfilling. Age, language impairment, or mental status does not change these needs. Communication with individuals with cognitive impairment is discussed in Chapter 25.

KEY CONCEPTS

- Communication is a basic need regardless of age or impairment.
- It is important for nurses who care for older adults to be aware of their own attitudes and beliefs about aging and the effect of these attitudes on communication, care provision, and health and well-being.
- The life history of an individual is a story to be developed and treasured. This is particularly important toward the end of life.

- Storytelling is a complementary and alternative therapy that nurses can use to come to know older adults and enhance communication.
- In a rapidly changing society, the shared life histories of older adults provide a sense of continuity among the generations.
- Group work can meet many needs and is satisfying and rewarding for both the older adult and the group leader.

NEXT-GENERATION NCLEX® (NGN) EXAMINATION–STYLE QUESTIONS

A nursing unit is focusing closely on patient satisfaction, which originates with appropriate and professional interactions between patients and nurses. One of the nurse leaders is providing feedback to all staff nurses about ways to enhance therapeutic communication with older adults. When accompanying a staff nurse on the unit who is caring for an 88-year-old female patient named Alma who is hospitalized for generalized weakness and intermittent changes in mental status, the nurse leader observes this interaction:

Interaction observed between staff nurse and patient	Staff RN: "Hi, Alma honey, I'm Pat and I am going to be your nurse today. Today, the first thing we are going to do this morning is work together to get you ready for breakfast. Are you hungry, sweetie?" Alma: "Yes, I'm hungry." Staff RN: "Great. I saw your breakfast tray, and it has eggs, toast, and a fruit cup. Does all of that sound good to you?" Alma: "Yes, I eat all of those things." Staff RN: "Good. Other than being hungry, how are you feeling this morning?" Alma: (no response) Staff RN: "Are you feeling better than yesterday?" Alma: "Well…I am kind of feeling…" (searching for words) Staff RN (very quickly): "I think you look much better than yesterday." Alma: "I think my son is coming to see me today. Did I tell you about when he was a little boy and had to be hospitalized too?" Staff RN: "I'm glad he is coming by. I don't think you have told me that story about his hospitalization." Alma: "He was about 10 years old and was riding a bike when a car nearly hit him. He fell off into a ditch and broke a leg and an arm, and he also hit his head very hard. I was scared that I was going to lose him. I'm so glad he eventually got better." Staff RN: "That had to be really scary for you as well as for your son. I'm so glad that he recovered and is able to come visit you today. Perhaps you both can share other stories about his childhood that make you both happy."

Click to highlight statements by the staff nurse that require the nurse leader to provide feedback to improve the staff nurse's therapeutic communication abilities.

CLINICAL JUDGMENT QUESTIONS AND ACTIVITIES

1. Observe communication styles of people talking to older adults (e.g., in restaurants, stores, and the health care setting). Do you see examples of elderspeak?
2. Watch some commercials on television that feature older adults. What image do they portray?
3. Ask an older adult whom you know to tell you his or her life story. Reflect on whether you learned anything surprising.

4. If you were going to create a digital life story of your own life, what kinds of music, pictures, and artifacts would you include to help people know about your life?
5. Sit with another student and share your life stories. Reflect on what this exercise meant to you and to the other person.

RESEARCH QUESTIONS

1. Are there particular care settings and activities in which elderspeak is more prevalent?
2. What benefits do older adults experience in sharing their life stories?
3. Can digital storytelling be used to promote more positive attitudes toward older adults among nursing students?
4. Does the use of reminiscence and storytelling lead to a more holistic approach to care of older adults?

REFERENCES

Agency for Healthcare Research and Quality: Weekly group storytelling enhances verbal skills, encourages positive behavior change, and reduces confusion in patients with Alzheimer's and related dementias (website), 2014. https://innovations.ahrq.gov/profiles/weekly-group-storytelling-enhances-verbal-skills-encourages-positive-behavior-change-and/. Accessed February 2021.

Basting AD: Reading the story behind the story: context and content in stories by people with dementia, *Generations* 27:25–29, 2003.

Basting AD: Arts in dementia care: "This is not the end . . . it's the end of this chapter, *Generations* 30:16–20, 2006.

Basting AD: Time Slips: creativity for people with dementia, *Age Action* 28(4):1–5, 2013.

Bleiberg L: Virtual reality opens the door to new worlds, *AARP*, 2018. Oct. 15. https://www.aarp.org/caregiving/home-care/info-2018/virtual-reality-triggers-memory.html#quest1 Accessed February 2022.

Burnside IM: Group work with older persons, *J Gerontol Nurs* 20:43, 1994.

Butler R: The life review: an interpretation of reminiscence in the aged, *Psychiatry* 26:65–76, 1963.

Butler R: Age-ism: another form of bigotry, *Gerontologist* 9:243–246, 1969.

Butler R: Age, death and life review. In Doka K, editor: *Living with grief: loss in later life*, Washington, DC, 2003, Hospice Foundation.

Coles R: The call of stories, Boston, 1989, Houghton Mifflin.

Cooney A, Hunter A, Murphy K, et al.: Seeing me through my memories": a grounded theory study on using reminiscence with people with dementia living in long-term care, *J Clin Nurs* 23:3564–3574, 2014.

Corwin AI: Overcoming elderspeak: a qualitative study of three alternatives, *Gerontologist* 58:724–729, 2017.

Fick DM, Lundebjerg NE: When it comes to older adults, language matters, *J Gerontol Nurs* 43(9):2–4, 2017.

FrameWorks Institute: *Framing strategies to advance aging and address ageism as policy issues* (website), 2017. https://frameworksinstitute.org/toolkits/aging/elements/items/aging_frame_brief.pdf. Accessed February 2021.

Fraser S, Lagace M, Bongue B, et al.: Ageism and COVID-19: what does our society's response say about us? *Age Ageing* 49:682–695, 2020.

Karlsson E, Zingmark K, Axelsson K, et al.: Aspects of self and identify in narrations about recent events: communication with individuals with Alzheimer's disease enabled by a digital photograph diary, *J Gerontol Nurs* 43(6):25–31, 2017.

Kendall-Taylor N, Neumann A, Schoen J: Advocating for age in an age of uncertainty (website), 2021. https://ssir.org/articles/entry/advocating_for_age_in_an_age_of_uncertainty#. Accessed February 2021.

Kris AE, Henkel LA, Krauss KM, et al.: Functions and value of reminiscence for nursing home staff, *J Gerontol Nurs* 43(6):35–44, 2017.

Kydd A, Touhy T, Newman D, et al.: Attitudes toward caring for older adults in Scotland, Sweden and the United States, *Nurs Older People* 26(2):33–40, 2014.

National Center on Elder Abuse: Ageism (website), 2021. https://ncea.acl.gov/NCEA/media/Publication/NCEA_RB_Ageism.pdf. Accessed May 2021.

Saliba D: Looking at our words as if seeing them for the first time, *J Gerontol Nurs* 43(9):47–48, 2017.

Shaw C, Gordon J, Williams K: Understanding elderspeak: an evolutionary concept analysis, *Innov Aging* 4(Suppl 1):451, 2020.

Spencer T: *Can virtual reality help seniors? Stanford study hopes to find out* (website), 2021. https://www.mercurynews.com/2021/06/08/can-virtual-reality-help-seniors-study-hopes-to-find-out/.

Sweetland J, Volmert A, O'Neill M: *Finding the frame: an empirical approach to reframing aging and ageism* (website), 2017. http://frameworksinstitute.org/assets/files/aging_elder_abuse/aging_research_report_final_2017.pdf. Accessed February 2021.

Testad I, Corbett A, Aarsland D, et al.: The value of personalized psychosocial interventions to address behavioral and psychological symptoms in people with dementia living in care home settings: a systematic review, *Int Psychogeriatr* 26:1083–1098, 2014.

Westerhof GJ, Bohlmeijer ET: Celebrating fifty years of research and applications in reminiscence and life review: state of the art and new directions, *J Aging Stud* 29:107–114, 2014.

Williams K, Shaw C, Lee A, et al.: Voicing ageism in nursing home dementia care, *J Gerontol Nurs* 43(9):16–20, 2017.

Yamashita T, Hahn S, Kinney J, et al.: Impact of life stories on college students' positive and negative attitudes toward older adults, *Gerontol Geriatr Educ* 39(3):326–340, 2018.

Cognitive Health and Learning

Theris A. Touhy

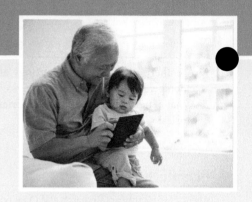

http://evolve.elsevier.com/Touhy/TwdHlthAging

A STUDENT SPEAKS

I was shocked the other day when I got a message on my Facebook page from my grandmother. I had no idea that older adults even knew about Facebook, but my Gram says she has 30 friends and has reconnected with some of her classmates from high school. She's been pretty lonely since Grandpa died, and I wouldn't be surprised if she finds her old boyfriend next. Older adults can be pretty cool.

Kate, age 19

AN OLDER ADULT SPEAKS

Imagine, they tell us now that our brain continues to develop even though we are older. I thought it was all downhill to dementia when I turned 70. My nurse practitioner advised me to get involved in some activities for stimulating my brain and improving my memory. I found a free class at the high school where I could learn French, something I have always wanted to do. I am having such fun and am already looking at brochures for river cruises through France.

Marie, age 74

LEARNING OBJECTIVES

On completion of this chapter, the reader will be able to:

1. Explain cognitive changes with increasing age and nursing actions to enhance cognitive health throughout life.
2. Discuss factors influencing learning in late life and appropriate teaching and learning strategies.
3. Use clinical judgment to identify and evaluate solutions and nursing actions to enhance cognitive health and learning in later life.

The processes of normal cognition and learning in late life, nursing actions to enhance cognitive health, and effective teaching and learning are discussed in this chapter. Evaluation of cognition is discussed in Chapter 9 and 25, and care of older adults with mild and major neurocognitive disorders is discussed in Chapter 26.

ADULT COGNITION

Cognition is the process of acquiring, storing, sharing, and using information. Components of cognitive function include language, thought, memory, executive function (planning, organizing, remembering, paying attention, solving problems), judgment, attention, and perception. The determination of intellectual capacity and performance has been the focus of a major portion of gerontological research. Emerging research suggests that cognitive function and intellectual capacity is a complex interplay of age-related changes in the brain and nervous system and many other factors such as education, environment, nutrition, life experiences, physical function, emotions, biomedical and physiological factors, and genetics (Agency for Healthcare Research and Quality [AHRQ], 2017).

Before the development of sophisticated neuroimaging techniques, conclusions about brain function as we age were based on autopsy results (often on diseased brains) or on results of cross-sectional studies conducted with older adults who were institutionalized or had coexisting illnesses. Changes seen were considered unavoidable and the result of the biological aging process rather than disease. As a result, the bulk of research has focused on the inevitable cognitive declines rather than on cognitive capacities. There are many old myths about aging and the brain that may be believed by both health professionals and older adults. It is important to understand cognition and memory in late life and dispel the myths that can have a negative effect on wellness and may, in fact, contribute to unnecessary cognitive decline (Box 8.1).

Changes in the aging nervous system (Box 8.2) cause a general slowing of many neural processes, but they are not consistent with deteriorating mental function, nor do they interfere with daily routines. Age-related changes in brain structure, function, and cognition are also not uniform across the whole brain or across individuals. Research suggests that the reason older brains respond more slowly is because they take longer to process constantly increasing amounts of information.

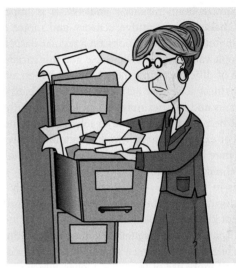

Alex Comfort, an early gerontologist, described the slowed response time of an older adult: By the time you are 80 years old, you have a lot of files in the file cabinet. Your secretary is 80 years old, so it also takes her a lot longer to locate the files, go through them, find the one you want, and bring it to you.

Cognitive functions may remain stable or decline with increasing age. The cognitive functions that remain stable include attention span, language skills, communication skills, comprehension and discourse, and visual perception. The cognitive skills that decline are verbal fluency, logical analysis, selective attention, object naming, and complex visuospatial skills. Overall cognitive abilities remain intact, and it is important to remember that if brain function becomes impaired in old age, it is the result of disease, not aging (Crowley, 1996).

Neuroplasticity

It is very important to know that the aging brain maintains resiliency or the ability to compensate for age-related changes. Developing knowledge refutes the myth that the adult brain is less plastic than the child's brain and less able to strengthen and increase neuronal connections. We now know that the brain has the capacity for neuronal replacement. The old adage "use it or lose it" applies to cognitive and physical health. Stimulating the brain increases brain tissue formation, enhances synaptic regulation of messages, and improves the development of cognitive reserve (CR).

CR is based on the concept of neuroplasticity and refers to the strength and complexity of neuronal dendrite connections from which information is transmitted and cognition and mentation emerges. The greater the strength and complexity of these connections, the more the brain can absorb damage before cognitive functioning is compromised. "CR can be increased or decreased due to two complex, overarching processes—positive or negative neuroplasticity. Positive

---

BOX 8.1   Myths About Aging and the Brain

MYTH: People lose brain cells every day and eventually just run out.
FACT: Most areas of the brain do not lose brain cells. Although you may lose some nerve connections, it can be part of the reshaping of the brain that comes with experience.
MYTH: You cannot change your brain.
FACT: The brain is constantly changing in response to experiences and learning, and it retains this "plasticity" well into aging. Changing our way of thinking causes corresponding changes in the brain systems involved; that is, your brain believes what you tell it.
MYTH: The brain does not make new brain cells.
FACT: Certain areas of the brain, including the hippocampus (where new memories are created) and the olfactory bulb (scent-processing center), regularly generate new brain cells.
MYTH: Memory decline is inevitable as we age.
FACT: Many people reach old age and have no memory problems. Participation in physical exercise, stimulating mental activity, socialization, healthy diet, and stress management helps maintain brain health. The incidence of dementia does increase with age, but when there are changes in memory, older adults need to be evaluated for possible causes and receive treatment.
MYTH: There is no point in trying to teach older adults anything because "you can't teach an old dog new tricks."
FACT: Basic intelligence remains unchanged with age, and older adults should be provided with opportunities for continued learning. Minimizing barriers to learning such as hearing and vision loss and applying principles of geragogy enhance learning ability.

Modified from American Association of Retired Persons: *Myths about aging and the brain* (website), 2006. https://www.aarp.org/health/brain-health/info-2017/common-myths-aging-brains-fd.html. Accessed February 2019.

BOX 8.2   Changes in the Central Nervous System

Neurons
- Shrinkage in neuron size and gradual decrease in neuron numbers
- Structural changes in dendrites
- Deposit of lipofuscin granules, neuritic plaque, and neurofibrillary bodies within the cytoplasm and neurons
- Loss of myelin and decreased conduction in some nerves, especially peripheral nerves

Neurotransmitters
- Changes in the precursors necessary for neurotransmitter synthesis
- Changes in receptor sites
- Alteration in the enzymes that synthesize and degrade neurotransmitters
- Significant decreases in neurotransmitters, including acetylcholine, glutamate, serotonin, dopamine, and gamma-aminobutyric acid

neuroplasticity is the brain's ability to make more and stronger connections between neurons in response to novel situations. Negative neuroplasticity refers to the atrophy of such connections in response to low stimulation or physiological insults" (Vance, 2012, p. 28).

To maximize brain plasticity and CR, it is important to engage in challenging cognitive, sensory, and motor activities and meaningful social interactions on a regular basis throughout life. People vary in the CR they have, and this variability may be because of differences in genetics, overall health, education, occupation, lifestyle, leisure activities, or other life experiences. Brain diseases and injuries may be less apparent in those with greater CR because they are able to tolerate lost neurons and synapses. For example, people who have attained more years of education may have high levels of Alzheimer's pathology, but few if any clinical symptoms.

Changes in the brain with aging, once seen only as compensation for declining skills, are now thought to indicate the development of new capacities. These changes include using both hemispheres more equally than younger adults, thus enhancing bilateral communication potential, greater density of synapses, and more use of the frontal lobes, which are thought to be important in abstract reasoning, problem solving, and concept formation (Davis et al., 2017). The scaffolding theory of aging and cognition suggests that the increased frontal lobe activation with age is a marker of an adaptive brain that engages in compensatory scaffolding in response to the challenges of declining neural structures and function. The scaffolding can be considered a form of positive neuroplasticity that accompanies aging (Reuter-Lorenz & Park, 2014).

Later adulthood is no longer seen as a period when growth has ceased and cognitive development has halted; rather, it is seen as a life stage programmed for plasticity and the development of unique capacities. The renewed emphasis on the development of cognitive capabilities that can develop with age provides a view of aging that reflects the history of many cultures and provides a much more hopeful view of both aging and human development. While "some areas experience decline (e.g., memory and processing speed), improvements are noted in areas such as wisdom, knowledge, and resilience" (Fick, 2016, p. 6) (Chapter 35).

Fluid and Crystallized Intelligence

Fluid intelligence and crystallized intelligence are factors of general intelligence that can be measured in standardized IQ tests. Fluid intelligence (often called *native intelligence*) consists of skills that are biologically determined, independent of experience or learning. It involves the capacity to think logically and solve problems in novel situations, independent of acquired knowledge. Fluid intelligence can be likened to "street smarts." Crystallized intelligence is composed of knowledge and abilities that the person acquires through education and life ("book smarts") and is demonstrated largely through one's vocabulary and general knowledge. Crystallized intelligence is long-lasting and improves with experience.

Older adults perform more poorly on performance scales (fluid intelligence), but scores on verbal scales (crystallized intelligence) remain stable. This has been known as the classic aging pattern. The tendency to do poorly on performance tasks was attributed to changes in sensory and perceptual abilities and psychomotor skills. However, research by Ramscar et al. (2014) questions this and postulates that older adults need more time to process the knowledge they have gained from their experiences. "In other words, you get slower when you're older because you're smarter" (Hill, 2017). Testing methods also may contribute to differences.

Memory

Memory is defined as the ability to retain or store information and retrieve it when needed. Memory is a complex set of processes and storage systems. Biological, functional, environmental, and psychosocial influences affect memory development throughout adulthood. Recall of newly encountered information seems to decrease with age, and memory declines are noted in connection with complex tasks and strategies. Even though some older adults show decrements in the ability to process information, reaction time, perception, and capacity for attentional tasks, the majority of functioning remains intact and sufficient. Tips for improving memory are presented in Table 8.1.

Familiarity, previous learning, and life experience compensate for the minor loss of efficiency in the basic neurological processes. In unfamiliar, stressful, or demanding situations, however, these changes may be more marked (e.g., hospitalization). Healthy older adults may complain of memory problems, but their symptoms do not meet the criteria for mild or major neurocognitive impairment (Chapter 25). The term *age-related cognitive decline (ARCD)* has been used to describe memory loss that is considered normal given a person's age and educational level. This may include a general slowness in processing, storing, and recalling new information and difficulty remembering names and words. However, these concerns can cause great anxiety in older adults who may fear dementia (Box 8.3). Many medical or psychiatric difficulties (delirium, depression) also influence memory abilities, and it is important for older adults with memory complaints to have a comprehensive evaluation (Chapters 9, 25, and 26). Healthy People 2030 includes an objective addressing evaluation of cognitive symptoms.

♥ HEALTHY PEOPLE 2030

- Increase the proportion of adults with a subjective cognitive decline who have discussed their symptoms with a provider

Data from US Department of Health and Human Services: *Healthy People 2030* (website), 2020. https://health.gov/healthypeople.

Cognitive Health

Healthy cognitive aging (healthy brain aging) is comprehensive and proactive; it implies that cognitive health is much more than simply a lack of decline with aging. A healthy brain is "one that can perform all mental processes that are collectively known as cognition, including the ability to learn new things, intuition, judgment, language, and remembering" (Centers for Disease

TABLE 8.1 Tips for Improving Your Memory

Technique	Example
Pay attention to the task at hand; minimize distractions, avoid multitasking.	When listening to someone giving you directions while you are driving, do not keep the radio on.
Involve your senses.	To help remember the names of people you are meeting, look them in the eye, shake their hand, and repeat their name. Use auditory cues such as timers, alarm clocks, cell phone reminders.
Use repetition.	Say what you are trying to remember several times. Say things aloud ("I am putting my car keys on the hall table"). Review new learning at the end of the day.
Chunk it and organize it.	When trying to remember a telephone number, chunk it into 3 pieces of information (area code, 3-digit prefix, and a 4-digit number). Write things down, organize routine tasks, try to prepare things in advance when you have time to concentrate.
Use mnemonic devices (clues to help you remember; visual images, acronyms, rhymes, and alliterations).	Use the word HOMES to remember the names of the Great Lakes: Huron, Ontario, Michigan, Erie, and Superior. Remember the months of the year with 30 days using the rhyme "Thirty days has September…" Search the alphabet when trying to remember something. Do an internet search for what you are trying to remember.
Relate information to what you already know.	Remember a new address by thinking of someone you know who lives on the same street.
Get adequate sleep, use stress-relieving techniques, and engage in physical activity.	Sleep is necessary for memory consolidation, and the key memory-enhancing activity occurs during the deepest stages of sleep. Cognitive training and memory training exercises may improve sleep. Mindfulness meditation encourages more connections between brain cells and increases mental acuity and memory ability. Exercise increases oxygen to the brain, reduces the risk of illness, enhances helpful brain chemicals, and protects brain cells.

Adapted from Grobol J: *8 tips for improving your memory* (website), 2010. http://psychcentral.com/blog/archives/2010/09/03/8-tips-for-improving-your-memory. Accessed February 17, 2014; Smith M, Robinson L: *How to improve your memory* (website), n.d. http://www.helpguide.org/articles/memory/how-to-improve-your-memory.htm. Accessed February 17, 2014.

BOX 8.3 Memory and Thinking: What's Normal and What's Not?

Normal Aging/ARCD
Making a bad decision once in a while
Missing a monthly payment
Forgetting which day it is and remembering it later
Sometimes forgetting names or what word to use
Losing things from time to time

Dementia
Making poor judgments and decisions a lot of the time
Problems taking care of monthly bills/managing finances
Losing track of the date, year, or time of year
Trouble having a conversation
Misplacing things often and being unable to find them

ARCD, Age-related cognitive decline.
From National Institute on Aging: *Memory and thinking: what's normal and what's not?* (website), n.d. https://www.nia.nih.gov/health/memory-and-thinking-whats-normal-and-whats-not. Accessed February 2019.

USING CLINICAL JUDGMENT TO PROMOTE HEALTHY AGING: COGNITIVE HEALTH

Solutions, Nursing Actions, and Outcomes

Nurses need to educate people of all ages about effective strategies to enhance cognitive health and vitality and to promote cognitive reserve and brain plasticity. Fig 8.2 presents a checklist to promote healthy brain aging that can be used by clinicians. Blood pressure management (particularly in midlife), physical activity (Chapter 19), adherence to a Mediterranean diet (MetDiet) or a combined MetDiet and Dietary Approaches to Stop Hypertension (DASH) diet plan (Chapter 15), social engagement, and cognitive stimulation may reduce the risk of cognitive decline (McEvoy et al., 2017). The CDC and the National Institute on Aging have large-scale programs focused on healthy brain aging and provide resources that nurses can use in health-promotion education (Box 8.5). Education provided about cognitive health should be tailored to specific communities and cultural subgroups because there are differences in perceptions about cognitive health among these groups. More research is needed to understand adaptations of interventions for specific communities and cultural subgroups (Chapter 4).

There is no strong evidence that cognitive stimulation activities have a lasting, beneficial effect on cognition. Additional research is needed, but remaining intellectually engaged throughout life is important. There is some evidence that such activities may protect the brain by establishing cognitive reserve. They may help the brain become more adaptable in some mental functions so it can compensate for age-related brain changes and health conditions that affect the brain (National Institute on Aging, 2020). Game playing (Scrabble, Trivial Pursuit, cards), puzzles, learning a new language, developing a new hobby, taking a class, volunteering, reading, and engaging in interesting conversations are all ways to stimulate the brain. Among the various types of cognitive stimulating activities, games such as cards or puzzles seem to be particularly useful.

Control and Prevention [CDC], 2017). Attention to cognitive health, beginning at conception and continuing throughout life, is just as important as attention to physical and emotional health. Many of the behaviors influencing physical and emotional health also promote cognitive health (Fig. 8.1). Box 8.4 presents four steps to a beautiful mind.

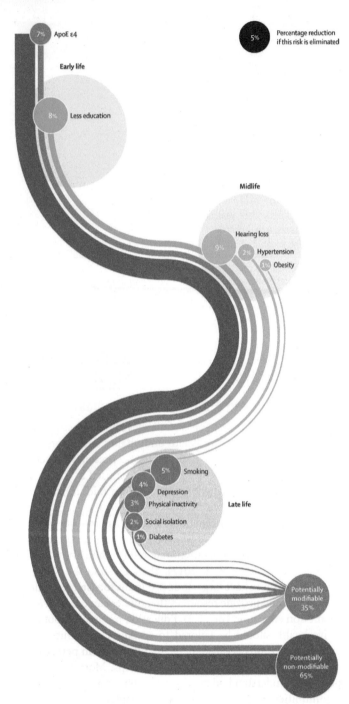

Fig. 8.1 Risk factors for dementia. From The Lancet Commission's new life-course model, showing potentially modifiable—and nonmodifiable—risk factors for dementia. *ApoE,* Apolipoprotein E. (Reprinted from Livingston G, Sommerlad A, Orgeta V, et al.: Dementia prevention, intervention, and care, *Lancet* 390[10113]:2673–2674, 2017. Copyright 2017, with permission from Elsevier.)

The brain exercising activity chosen should meet the following criteria: (1) it is new, unfamiliar, and out of your comfort zone; (2) it is challenging and takes some mental effort; and (3) it is fun and stimulates your interest and enjoyment. At present, there is no evidence that long-term cognitive effects are obtained with commercial computer-based "brain training" applications

> ### BOX 8.4   **Four Steps to a Beautiful Mind**
>
> **The Nourished Mind:** A diet low in saturated fats and cholesterol, rich in good fats like polyunsaturated fats and omega-3 fatty acids, and packed with protective nutrients such as vitamin E and lutein may protect brain cells and promote brain health.
>
> **The Mentally Engaged Mind:** Brain cells, like muscle cells, can grow bigger and stronger with cognitive challenges and stimulation. Continued learning and new activities, skills, and interests help build connections in the brain and enhance function.
>
> **The Socially Connected Mind:** Social connectedness is vital to health, wellness, and longevity. A rich social network supports brain health and provides individuals with better resources and stimulation.
>
> **The Physically Active Mind:** Physical activity is important and is associated with improved cognitive skills or reduced cognitive decline.

Data from National Center for Creative Aging: *Four steps to a beautiful mind,* Washington, D.C., 2014.

and no evidence that cognitive training can delay dementia (AHRQ, 2017; National Institute on Aging, 2020). Tips for best practice to promote cognitive health are presented in Box 8.6.

LEARNING IN LATER LIFE

Basic intelligence remains unchanged with increasing years, and older adults should be provided with opportunities for continued learning. Adapting communication and teaching to enhance understanding requires knowledge of learning in late life and effective teaching and learning strategies with older adults. *Geragogy* is the application of the principles of adult learning theory to the design of teaching situations with older adults. The older adult demands that teaching situations be relevant; new learning must relate to what the person already knows and should emphasize concrete and practical information. Aging may present barriers to learning, such as hearing and vision losses and cognitive impairment. Pain and discomfort also can interfere with learning. Moreover, the process of aging may accentuate other challenges that had already been factors in a person's life, such as cultural and cohort variations (Chapter 4) and education.

Some older adults may have special learning needs based on educational deprivation in their early years and consequent anxiety about formalized learning. Attention to literacy level and cultural variations is important to enhance learning and the usefulness of what is learned. Mood is extremely important in terms of what individuals (both young and old) will recall. In other words, when we attempt to measure recall of events that may have occurred in a crisis situation or an anxiety state, recall will be impaired. This is significant for health care professionals who give information to older adults who are ill or upset, particularly in times of crisis such as hospital discharge.

Learning Opportunities

Opportunities for older adults to learn are available in many formal and informal modes: self-teaching, college attendance, participation in seminars and conferences, public television programs, CDs, internet courses, and countless others. In most

1. Counseled regarding smoking cessation
   Comments:

2. Advised to follow guidelines proposed jointly by the American Heart Association and the American ☐ College of Sports Medicine regarding daily physical activity
   Comments:

3. Counseled regarding healthy nutrition (e.g., Mediterranean diet, DASH [Dietary Approaches to ☐ Stop Hypertension] diet)
   Comments:

4. Counseled regarding the importance of intellectually challenging and creative leisure activities ☐
   Comments:

5. Counseled regarding strategies to promote emotional resilience and reduce psychological distress ☐ and depression (e.g., relaxation exercises, mindfulness-meditation practices)
   Comments:

6. Advised to maintain an active, socially integrated lifestyle ☐
   Comments:

7. Discussed strategies to achieve and maintain optimal daily sleep ☐
   Comments:

8. Provided education about strategies to reduce risk of serious head injury (e.g., wearing seat belts, ☐ wearing helmets during contact sports, bicycling, skiing, skateboarding)
   Comments:

9. Provided education about strategies to reduce exposure to hazardous substances (e.g., wearing ☐ protective clothing during the administration of pesticides, fumigants, fertilizers, and defoliants)
   Comments:

10. Provided education and counseling regarding negative health effects of alcohol consumption ☐ more than recommended as safe by the National Institute of Alcoholism and Alcohol Abuse
    Comments:

11. Provided education about importance of achieving and maintaining healthy weight to promote ☐ overall health
    Comments:

12. Discussed and implemented strategies to achieve optimal blood pressure control ☐
    Comments:

13. Discussed and implemented strategies to achieve optimal control of dyslipidemia (e.g., high ☐ cholesterol)
    Comments:

14. Discussed and implemented strategies to achieve optimal control of blood sugar/diabetes ☐
    Comments:

15. Discussed risks and benefits of medications, supplements, herbal remedies, and vitamins to ☐ promote brain health
    Comments:

16. Discussed and implemented secondary prevention of stroke strategies (e.g., daily baby aspirin) ☐
    Comments:

Fig. 8.2 Checklist for Promoting Healthy Brain Aging. (Courtesy Center for Healthy Brain Aging, Saint Louis University School of Medicine, St. Louis, MO. From Desai A, Grossberg G, Chibnall J: Healthy brain aging: a road map, *Clin Geriatr Med* 26:1–16, 2010.)

BOX 8.5 Resources for Best Practice

Cognitive Health

- **National Institutes of Health:** Cognitive and Emotional Health Project: The Healthy Brain. https://trans.nih.gov/cehp/.
- **Centers for Disease Control and Prevention:** Healthy Brain Initiative: State and Local Public Health Partnerships to Address Dementia: The 2018–2023 Road Map. https://www.cdc.gov/aging/pdf/2018-2023-Road-Map-508.pdf.
- **National Institute on Aging:** Memory, Forgetfulness, and Aging: What's Normal and What's Not. https://www.nia.nih.gov/health/memory-forgetfulness-and-aging-whats-normal-and-whats-not.

colleges and universities, older adults are taking classes of all types. Fees are usually lower for individuals older than 60 years of age, and older adults may choose to work toward a degree or audit classes for enrichment and enjoyment. Senior centers and local school districts often provide a wide array of adult education courses as well. Road Scholar (formerly Elderhostel) is an example of a program designed for older adults that combines continued learning with travel. The program offers trips to all 50 states and 150 countries. Road Scholar offers intergenerational programs for grandparents and grandchildren ages 4 and older (https://www.roadscholar.org/). "Skip gen" travel (travel with

BOX 8.6   Tips for Best Practice

Cognitive Health

- Dispel myths about brain aging and teach about cognition and aging.
- Educate people of all ages about factors that influence cognitive health.
- Be aware of cultural differences in perceptions of cognitive health and adapt education accordingly.
- Advise older adults to have a comprehensive assessment if they are experiencing cognitive decline.
- Encourage socialization and participation in intellectually stimulating activities, exercise, and healthy diets (e.g., Mediterranean diet, Dietary Approaches to Stop Hypertension [DASH] diet).
- Teach chronic illness prevention strategies and ensure good management of chronic illnesses.
- Share resources for cognitive training (memory enhancing techniques, computer games, puzzles, card games).

grandchildren alone) is experienced by a third of grandparents (Ianzito, 2019).

Information Technology and Older Adults

Older adults comprise the fastest growing population using computers and the internet. Forty-six percent of older adults use Facebook and 38% use YouTube. More than half of internet users ages 65 and older use Facebook (Gramlich, 2019). More than any other age group, older adults perceive the internet as a valuable resource to help them more easily obtain information and connect to loved ones. This could range from using a cell phone to set medication reminders to using Skype and FaceTime to interact with long-distance grandchildren. Many individuals are also using email to communicate with their health care providers. Organizations such as Cyber-Seniors and AARP provide basic computer and internet training for older adults.

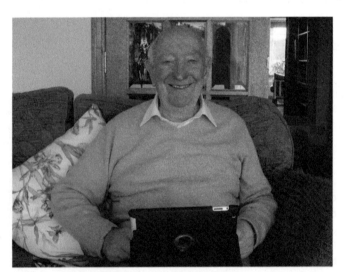

This is what 90 looks like.

With the aging of the baby boomers and the young tech-savvy adults, the future of technology in care and service for older adults can only be imagined. Traditional ways of providing health information and services are changing, and both public and private institutions are increasingly using the internet and other technologies. However, not all older adults share the benefits that technology offers. Results of a recent study reported the presence of a deep digital divide within the older population. Individuals who were older, less educated, poorer, and/or members of an ethnic minority group (Black, Afro-Caribbean, or Hispanic American) were up to five times less likely to have access to digital health information than those who were younger and more highly educated, had a higher income, or were European American (see Research Highlights box). The effects of the COVID-19 pandemic have highlighted how essential access to the internet and to digital health information is in all communities. Lack of access to digital health information significantly contributes to health disparities and poor outcomes (Tappen et al., 2021).

RESEARCH HIGHLIGHTS

Digital Health Information Disparities in Older Adults: A Mixed Methods Study

Purpose

To describe the extent of computer ownership, internet access, and digital information use among older African Americans, Afro-Caribbeans, Hispanic Americans, and European Americans and to explore the differences found.

Methods

A mixed methods approach in which quantitative data was obtained from 562 participants over the age of 60 years as part of a larger study. Participants included 100 Blacks, 113 Afro-Caribbeans, 129 Hispanic Americans, and 220 White, non-Hispanic European Americans.

Qualitative data was obtained from 49 older adults who participated in focus groups: 28 were low-income Blacks and Afro-Caribbeans, 12 were low- to middle-income Hispanic Americans, and 9 were middle- to high-income European Americans.

Results

A deep digital divide was evident in both the community sample and the focus groups. Individuals who were older, less educated, poorer, and/or members of an ethnic minority group were up to five times less likely to have access to digital health information than those who were younger and more highly educated, had a higher income, or were European American. Among the focus group participants, only 2 of the 28 low-income Blacks and Afro-Caribbean participants had an internet-enabled device or convenient internet access source.

Conclusion

The barriers identified may be underappreciated by developers of health-related information. At the policy level, national connectivity plans are needed and greater effort to provide universal internet access needs to be made. Digital information needs to be more customized and culturally sensitive as well as available in patients' primary language. Until internet access is universal, health information must include printed materials, telephone calls, in-person groups, family assistance, individual meetings, and mailings for disadvantaged and minority older adults who remain affected by this disparity.

Data from Tappen R, Cooley M, Luckmann R, et al.: Digital information disparities in older adults: a mixed methods study, *J Racial Ethn Health Disparities* Jan 7:1–11, 2021.

USING CLINICAL JUDGMENT TO PROMOTE HEALTHY AGING: LEARNING AND INFORMATION TECHNOLOGY

Solutions, Nursing Actions, and Outcomes

Nurses need to use a person-centered approach in using technology. This includes involving older adults in development, testing, and evaluation of technology; considering individual needs, preferences, and characteristics; and customizing the approach for each individual's identified goals (Hill, 2017). Nurses can share resources available for older adults who want to learn computer skills and adaptations that can make connections as user-friendly as possible (e.g., touch screens, voice systems) for those who may have limitations.

Nurses and other health professionals need to develop skills in the understanding and use of consumer health information and teach clients how to evaluate the reliability and validity of health information on the internet. Using social media as a platform for health promotion and health education presents exciting possibilities. Continued attention to access to technology, especially among disadvantaged groups, and also efforts to enhance culturally and linguistically appropriate materials are essential. Chapter 21 further discusses technology in practice. Healthy People 2030 addresses information technology.

♥ HEALTHY PEOPLE 2030

- Increase the proportion of adults with broadband internet
- Increase the proportion of adults offered online access to their medical record
- Increase the proportion of persons who use electronic personal health management tools
- Increase the proportion of persons who use the internet to communicate with their health care provider
- Increase the proportion of quality health-related websites
- Increase the proportion of health-related websites that meet three or more evaluation criteria for disclosing information that can be used to assess information reliability

Data from US Department of Health and Human Services: *Healthy People 2030* (website), 2020. https://health.gov/healthypeople.

HEALTH LITERACY

Health literacy is defined as the degree to which individuals have the capacity to obtain, process, and understand basic health information and services needed to make appropriate health decisions (CDC, 2017). Limited health literacy has been linked to increased health disparities, poor health outcomes, inadequate preventive care, increased use of health care services, higher health care costs, higher risk of mortality for older adults, and several health care safety issues, including medical and medication errors (Cutilli et al., 2018).

Some older adults may be disproportionally affected by inadequate health literacy. Older adults have lower health literacy scores than all other age groups, and more than half of individuals over 65 years of age are at the below-basic level (MacLeod et al., 2017). Older adults are a heterogeneous group in their characteristics and literacy skills, so strategies to enhance understanding of health information need to be individualized. However, as the major consumers of health care in this country, many older adults are at risk for poor outcomes related to understanding of health care information and navigating the health care system.

Health literacy plays a major role in improving health and health care quality for all Americans. In the past, health literacy was viewed in terms of individual patient deficits (lack of knowledge regarding health issues) but is now recognized as a complex issue that involves the patient, the health care professional, and the health care system. Nearly 9 in 10 adults do not have the level of proficiency in health literacy skills necessary to successfully navigate the health care system. Income and education are the strongest predictors of health literacy. However, anyone can have low health literacy, including people with good literacy skills. Most people will have trouble understanding health information at some point in their lives.

In today's complex health care system, health literacy also includes the ability to obtain and apply relevant information, understand visual information, operate a computer, search the internet and evaluate websites, calculate or reason numerically, and interact with health professionals. Healthy People 2030 presents objectives for health literacy. The overall goal is to use health communication strategies and health information technology to improve population health outcomes and health care quality, and to achieve health equity.

♥ HEALTHY PEOPLE 2030

Health Literacy

- Increase the proportion of adults whose health care provider checked their understanding
- Decrease the proportion of adults who report poor communication with their health care provider
- Increase the proportion of adults whose health care providers involved them in decisions as much as they wanted
- Increase the proportion of persons who report that their health care provider always gave them easy-to-understand instructions about what to do to take care of their illness or health condition
- Increase the proportion of adults with limited English proficiency who say their providers explain things clearly

Data from US Department of Health and Human Services: *Healthy People 2030* (website), 2020. https://health.gov/healthypeople.

USING CLINICAL JUDGMENT TO PROMOTE HEALTHY AGING: HEALTH LITERACY

Solutions, Nursing Actions, and Outcomes

An integral part of the nursing role across the continuum is provision of health information. Older adults are the major users of health care, so nurses will have many opportunities to provide health education to this age group. Knowledge of health literacy and its relationship to health status in older adults is a growing area of concern. In addition to poorer health literacy skills, some older adults also may have multiple risk factors that affect their ability to understand and use health information (sensory changes, cognitive

---

BOX 8.7   **Resources for Best Practice**

Health Literacy

- Centers for Disease Control and Prevention: The Healthy Brain Initiative: A National Public Health Road Map to Maintaining Cognitive Health. https://www.cdc.gov/aging/pdf/thehealthybraininitiative.pdf.
- Agency for Healthcare Research and Quality (AHRQ): Health Literacy Universal Precaution Toolkit. https://www.ahrq.gov/sites/default/files/publications/files/healthlittoolkit2_3.pdf.

---

changes, complex medical regimens). Knowledge of the principles of geragogy, an understanding of health literacy, excellent communication skills, creativity, cultural competence, and knowledge of what matters most to the person are essential.

There are many widely available resources (Box 8.7) that nurses can use to evaluate health literacy and design effective teaching programs (brochures, one-to-one or group teaching, web resources). Identifying high-risk older adults (non-English speakers, less than high school education) can assist in targeting interventions (Chapter 4). Several validated easy-to-administer health literacy screening tools are readily available (Wide Range Achievement Test–Revised [WRAT-R], Rapid Estimate of Adult Literacy in Medicine, Test of Functional Health Literacy in Adults, and Newest Vital Sign assessment).

Health literacy screening in clinical care settings would be beneficial for older adults. The *Health Literacy Universal Precautions Toolkit* (AHRQ, 2013) (Box 8.7) was developed to help structure the delivery of care as if every patient had limited health literacy. This strategy may benefit everyone, regardless of health literacy levels, because it improves understanding.

Patient education materials should use plain language and provide information at no higher than a sixth-grade level in the person's language (may vary depending on person's abilities), be culturally appropriate, and use varying methods to communicate information (pictures, videos). Written material is clear and effective when it meets the following criteria: (1) attracts the intended reader's attention; (2) holds the reader's attention; (3) makes the reader feel respected and understood; (4) helps the reader understand the messages in the material; and (5) moves the reader to take action. Translation of materials should be done by certified medical interpreters or a native speaker of the target language rather than by the literal translation of English to another language because many concepts cannot be translated.

Individuals should be able to both understand and use the information presented. Using the "teach-back" (also known as "show-me" or "closing the loop") method involves having people explain back to you or demonstrate what you have told them. For example, you might say, "I want to be sure you understand your

medication correctly. Can you tell me how you are going to take this medicine?" Because medication management is a high-risk activity for older adults, attention to improving older adults' ability to understand their medications and take them correctly is essential. In addition to effective teaching, simplified drug regimens, and use of assistive medication management devices, pharmaceutical companies should be encouraged to develop educational materials at lower literacy levels to ensure comprehension. Box 8.8 presents strategies to improve health literacy in older adults.

There are relatively few studies specifically examining health literacy in older adults and strategies to improve health literacy. Nurses should be advocates for continued development and research on the most effective age-specific, culturally appropriate health literacy materials and interventions. Interventions for diverse populations are particularly important.

BOX 8.8   **Tips for Best Practice**

Strategies to Improve Health Literacy in Older Adult Learners

Manage the Teaching Environment
- Schedule appointment for when the individual is rested
- Ensure comfort (appropriate seating, room temperature, pain medication if needed)
- Limit session to 10 to 15 minutes
- Observe for signs of fatigue, discomfort during session

Improve Oral Communication
- Pay attention to vision and hearing deficits (face individual, speak slowly, keep pitch of voice low, eliminate background noise)
- Adapt materials for culture, language, health literacy
- Limit content to three to five points and repeat key points frequently
- Be specific and concrete; use plain language
- Connect new learning to past experiences
- Conclude with brief summary of essential points

Modify Written Communication
- Use 16- to 18-point Arial font for written material with both uppercase and lowercase letters
- Use high contrast on printed materials (dark colors for text and lighter for background, black print on white)
- Use gestures, demonstrations, and pictures in addition to printed material
- Bold key points
- Avoid charts with rows and columns
- Use a lot of white space

Evaluate Comprehension
- Use "teach-back" methods to ensure understanding
- Have the individual paraphrase instructions
- Have the individual demonstrate and provide feedback
- Encourage the individual to teach family or caregivers in your presence

---

KEY CONCEPTS

- Although there are changes in the aging brain, cognitive function, in the absence of disease, remains adequate. Any changes in cognitive function require appropriate evaluation.
- The aging brain maintains resiliency or the ability to compensate for age-related changes and can strengthen and increase neuronal connections.

- Late adulthood is no longer seen as a period when growth has ceased and cognitive development has halted; rather, it is seen as a life stage programmed for plasticity and the development of unique capacities.
- Attention to brain health throughout life is just as important as attention to physical health.

- Learning in late life can be enhanced by using principles of geragogy and adapting teaching strategies to minimize barriers such as hearing and vision impairment and low literacy.
- Older adults are disproportionally affected by inadequate health literacy, and nurses must ensure that health information is provided in an appropriate manner to ensure understanding.
- Older adults who are less educated, poorer, and/or members of an ethnic minority group (Black, Afro-Caribbean, or Hispanic American) have been found to be up to five times less likely to have access to digital health information than those who were younger and more highly educated, had a higher income, or were European American.
- Lack of access to digital health information significantly contributes to health disparities and poor outcomes.

NEXT-GENERATION NCLEX® (NGN) EXAMINATION–STYLE QUESTIONS

Mr. Stanton, an 88-year-old widower, is preparing for discharge following hospitalization for community-acquired pneumonia. He has a history of hypertension and osteoarthritis but is otherwise healthy. He lives by himself in a split-level home, in an established neighborhood. He has two grown children who live in neighboring cities. He worked most of his life as a laborer, having dropped out of school in the eighth grade to help provide for his family. Mr. Stanton states that he never did well in school and was happy to leave the classroom to work in the fields to help his parents put food on the table. He wears bifocal glasses and a hearing aid on the right ear. He admits to not wearing the hearing aid all the time, as his arthritis makes it difficult to adjust the device. His blood pressure is 138/86 mm Hg, respirations are 18 breaths per minute, heart rate is 92 beats per minute, and temperature is 98.4°F. His oxygen saturation is 94% on room air. He becomes short of breath and begins to cough, bringing up thick sputum, with exertion. The nurse comes to Mr. Stanton's room to go over his discharge instructions, prepares his room to facilitate teaching, and reviews the teaching materials with him. His discharge medications include:

Levofloxacin 750 mg daily

Prednisone taper:
- Day 1: 10 mg PO (by mouth) before breakfast, 5 mg after lunch and after dinner, and 10 mg at bedtime
- Day 2: 5 mg PO before breakfast, after lunch, and after dinner and 10 mg at bedtime
- Day 3: 5 mg PO before breakfast, after lunch, after dinner, and at bedtime
- Day 4: 5 mg PO before breakfast, after lunch, and at bedtime
- Day 5: 5 mg PO before breakfast and at bedtime
- Day 6: 5 mg PO before breakfast

Lisinopril/hydrochlorothiazide 20 mg/25 mg daily

Acetaminophen 500 mg every 4 hours as needed for pain

Multivitamin daily

Which strategies should the nurse take to improve health literacy for the client? *(Select all that apply.)*

1. Schedule discharge teaching for a time when the client is rested and ready to learn.
2. Ensure that the client is wearing glasses and hearing aids.
3. Use proper medical terminology.
4. Limit the teaching session to 15 minutes.
5. Use bright colored paper for handouts to gain the client's attention.
6. Use charts to organize content on printed materials.
7. Use 12-point Times New Roman font.
8. Ensure that the teaching environment is free from background noise.

CLINICAL JUDGMENT QUESTIONS AND ACTIVITIES

1. Review the myths about aging and the brain (see Box 8.1). Were any of the facts surprising to you?
2. Partner with another student and use the checklist of promoting cognitive health (see Fig. 8.2). Discuss what areas may need improvement to enhance cognitive health in aging.
3. What types of health teaching would you provide to a young adult to enhance their cognitive health in aging?
4. Work with another student and design a brochure for a group of culturally diverse older adults about interventions to enhance cognitive health. What adaptations would you incorporate to ensure understanding and cultural appropriateness?

RESEARCH QUESTIONS

1. What do older adults of different cultures believe about aging and brain function?
2. What types of cognitive stimulating activities do older adults report engaging in on a daily basis?
3. What strategies to improve the understanding of health information are most effective for older adults?
4. What are the learning needs of older adults related to the use of computers?
5. What do older adults perceive as the benefits of participation in social networking sites such as Facebook?

REFERENCES

Agency for Healthcare Research and Quality (AHRQ): *Health Literacy Universal Precautions Toolkit* (website), 2013. www.ahrq.gov/professionals/quality-patient-safety/quality-resources/tools/literacy-toolkit/index.html. Accessed February 2021.

Agency for Healthcare Research and Quality (AHRQ): Interventions to prevent age-related cognitive decline, mild cognitive impairment, and clinical Alzheimer's-type dementia, *Comp Eff Rev,* 188, 2017. https://effectivehealthcare.ahrq.gov/topics/cognitive-decline/research-2017/ Accessed February 2021.

Centers for Disease Control and Prevention (CDC): *What is a healthy brain? New research explores perceptions of cognitive health among diverse older adults* (website), 2017. https://www.cdc.gov/aging/pdf/Perceptions_of_Cog_Hlth_factsheet.pdf. Accessed February 2021.

Crowley S: Aging brain's staying power, *AARP Bulletin,* 37(1)1996.

Cutilli C, Simko L, Colbert A, et al.: Health literacy, health disparities, and sources of health information in U.S. older adults, *Orthop Nurs* 37(1):54–65, 2018.

Davis S, Luber B, Murphy D, et al.: Frequency-specific neuromodulation of local and distant connectivity in aging and episodic memory function, *Hum Brain Mapp* 38(12):5987–6004, 2017.

Fick D: Promoting cognitive health, *J Gerontol Nurs* 42(7):4–6, 2016.

Gramlich J: *10 facts about Americans and Facebook use* (website), 2019. https://www.pewresearch.org/fact-tank/2019/05/16/facts-about-americans-and-facebook/. Accessed February 2021.

Hill N: Person-centered technology for older adults, *J Gerontol Nurs* 43(4):3–4, 2017.

Ianzito C: *New trend: grandparents vacationing with grandchildren* (website), 2019. https://www.aarp.org/travel/vacation-ideas/family/info-2019/skip-generation-travel.html. Accessed June 2021.

MacLeod S, Musich S, Gulyas S, et al.: The impact of inadequate health literacy on patient satisfaction, healthcare utilization, and expenditures among older adults, *Geriatr Nurs* 38(4):334–341, 2017.

McEvoy C, Guyer H, Langa K, et al.: Neuroprotective diets are associated with better cognitive function: the Health and Retirement Study, *J Am Geriatr Soc* 65:1857–1862, 2017.

National Institute on Aging: *Cognitive health and older adults* (website), 2020. https://www.nia.nih.gov/health/cognitive-health-and-older-adults. Accessed June 2021.

Ramscar M, Hendrix P, Shaoul C, et al.: The myth of cognitive decline: non-linear dynamics of lifelong learning, *Top Cogn Sci* 6(1):5–42, 2014.

Reuter-Lorenz PA, Park DC: How does it STAC Up? Revisiting the scaffolding theory of aging and cognition, *Neuropsychol Rev* 24(3):366–370, 2014.

Tappen R, Cooley M, Luckmann R, et al.: Digital Health information disparities in older adults: a mixed methods study, *J Racial Ethn Health Disparities* Jan 7:1–11, 2021. doi:10.1007/s40615-020-00931-3.

Vance DE: Potential factors that may promote successful cognitive aging, *Nursing (Auckl)* 2:27–32, 2012.

CHAPTER 9

Recognizing and Analyzing Cues to Maximize Outcomes

Kathleen Jett

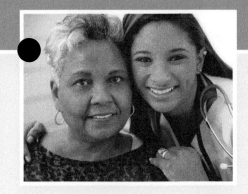

A STUDENT SPEAKS

It takes so long to get a health history from older adults—they have so many stories. Most of them have had their health problems for longer than I have been alive! I have learned to listen carefully, to determine the priorities for their nursing care.

Michelle, age 19

AN OLDER ADULT SPEAKS

Whenever I go to one of my doctors, I feel like they are rushing through and never really give me a good examination. Then I had an appointment with a nurse practitioner who specializes in us older folks. I couldn't believe the difference. I not only felt listened to but also felt like I got the best exam I have had in a long time. I am sure she will help me get better!

Henry, age 76

LEARNING OBJECTIVES

On completion of this chapter, the reader will be able to:

1. List the essential components of a comprehensive health assessment of an older adult.
2. Recognize cues from the physical assessment of older adults that differ in meaning from those for younger adults.
3. Discuss the advantages and disadvantages of the use of standardized assessment instruments.
4. Describe the purpose of the functional assessment when caring for an older adult.

In the promotion of healthy aging, gerontological nurses conduct skilled and comprehensive assessments of, and with, the persons who entrust themselves to their care. That is, the nurse recognizes and analyzes the cues needed for clinical judgment. The process is more complex than that used with younger adults, even when it is limited to a single problem. Recognizing cues with older adults takes more time than it does with younger adults because of the increased complexities associated with simply having lived longer. There is often an atypical presentation of a health problem in older adults, increasing the difficulty of analysis in a timely manner (Table 9.1). An interprofessional team may be needed to assess the physical health, functional and cognitive abilities, and mood of an older adult who is frail. When it is necessary to use a medical interpreter, simply collecting data will double the amount of time that will be needed (Chapter 4).

Assessment of the older adult requires the gerontological nurse to listen patiently, allow for pauses, ask questions that are not often asked, observe for very subtle cues, obtain data from all available sources, and analyze them quickly to be able to differentiate normal age-related changes from those that threaten health outcomes. The quality and speed of both observation and analysis are born of experience.

The analysis of the cues provides information critical to hypothesis development and prioritization leading to the development of an action plan that enhances healthy aging, decreases the potential for complications related to chronic conditions, and increases older adults' self-efficacy and self-care empowerment. The initial analysis serves as a baseline, a snapshot of the person's health status at that point in time. Subsequent visits or encounters allow the opportunity for evaluation of outcomes of previous interventions and treatments. These ongoing contacts also provide new opportunities for continued analysis that may affect the action plan as the person moves along the wellness trajectory.

Health assessment, the process of recognizing and analyzing cues, is a complex process that entire textbooks address in detail; often the books have short sections relative to the older adult. In this chapter we provide an overview of the recognition and analysis of cues leading to the critical prioritization of

TABLE 9.1	**Examples of Atypical Cues Related to Emerging Health Problems in Older Adults**	
Cues in Older Adult	**Cues in Younger Adult**	**Possible Implications**
Incontinence, falls, confusion, fatigue, dizziness	Dysuria, frequency, urgency	Urinary tract infection
Fall, weakness, confusion, hypotension, tachypnea	Chest pain, diaphoresis, nausea, dyspnea	Myocardial infarction
Tachypnea, hypoxia, slight cough, confusion, weakness, fatigue	Productive cough, chills, fever, elevated white blood count	Pneumonia
Memory and concentration decline, cognitive and behavioral changes, increased sleeping	Depressed mood, crying, withdrawal, weight loss, insomnia	Depression

hypotheses when working with older adults within the context of the complex changes during aging. The geriatric assessment leads to the generation of solutions and evaluation of outcomes related to common conditions in the lives of older adults. Subsequent chapters in this text specific to common issues, such as falls, continence, caregiver burden, and safety, include information about the augmented assessments needed when worrisome cues are identified.

THE HEALTH HISTORY

The health history marks the beginning of the nurse-patient relationship in the assessment process. The health history in an older adult will take longer due to multiple factors, including the high number of concurrent illnesses (Box 9.1). The collection of health data may begin when the older adult completes a form in advance of the health care contact, through a face-to-face interview, or most often through a combination of the two. The minimum information needed for the health history includes demographic information, past medical history, immunizations, allergies, current medications, dietary supplements (prescribed, over the counter, "home remedies," and herbals), functional status, and social status. Other aspects as time permits include family history, past or present occupation, and recreation and leisure activities. Too often an incomplete aspect of the health history is the presence or absence of advance directives (Chapters 31 and 34). Copies of these and other related documents should be obtained and entered into the electronic medical record (EMR).

A discussion of functional status may be one of the more difficult parts of the health history because it deals with the degree of a person's ability to manage independently. It includes a history of falls or injuries and the ability to manage everyday activities, such as cooking and shopping, and driving. These must be discussed with the utmost tact to avoid embarrassing the person who has developed limitations, such as the inability to hold

BOX 9.1 Factors Affecting the Collection of Information for the Health History

Visual and auditory acuity
Manual dexterity
Language and health fluency
Adequacy of translation of materials
Availability of a trained interpreter as needed
Cognitive ability and reading level

a spoon without spilling its contents because of tremors. Most often, the history of functional status is in the form of a screening tool, several of which are discussed later in this chapter.

The social component of the health history includes living environment and resources and support available. Such inquiries can be made during the functional assessment. Several of the instruments discussed later in this chapter address the collection of these data. Assessment includes recognition and analysis of cues related to social networks and specifically who would be available if support, physical care, or transportation were needed. It is very important to include information about those who are involved in health care decision making, such as health care surrogates (Chapter 31). The gerontological nurse must be cognizant of the fact that persons in their 90s and 100s may have limited social networks, having outlived children and perhaps all other relatives.

Review of Systems

The review of systems (ROS) is the person's subjective report of symptoms (or lack of them) in each body system, that is, what cues to aging changes and potential health problems are perceived by the individual. In a younger adult the ROS is likely to be quick, with most systems asymptomatic. However, as one ages and collects health problems, this review becomes more complex and time consuming because of the extent that the systems are inter related (Box 9.2). A conventional approach may not reveal the data needed to complete the analysis of the potential effect any one problem has on a person's overall function and health status. Cues are more often nonspecific, vague, or attributed incorrectly to normal aging (Box 9.3). Due to the extended time needed for a ROS with an older adult, the systems reviewed begins with those associated with the subjective reported symptoms (i.e., the person's own prioritized concern). The nurse must be able to quickly determine which other systems are most relevant to the assessment. At times only the most urgent issues can be addressed, and the mnemonic OLD CART can provide a guide for this (Table 9.2). When no symptoms are mentioned by the patient, the ROS begins with the systems associated with the person's chronic conditions or the problems that are most urgent in the country at the time (e.g., COVID-19), age of the patient, or social determinants of health (Box 9.4).

It is ideal to obtain the history from the person directly. All assistive sensory devices must be available and in working order (e.g., functioning hearing aids, clean glasses) (Table 9.3). Still, it may be necessary to speak with a proxy, that is, someone who knows the person well and has permission to speak

BOX 9.2   Tips for Best Practice

Areas of Emphasis in Subjective Review of Systems With Older Adults

Constitutional
- Perception of health status
- Changes in the level of energy?
- Still driving?
- Change in living situation?
- Significant life events?

Senses
- Changes in vision? Sudden or slowly and what type?
- Changes in hearing acuity? In certain situations or noted by others?
- Recent check for cerumen impaction? Recent hearing aid "checkup"?
- Increase in dental caries, changes in taste, bleeding gums, or level of current dental care?
- Changes in smell?
- Changes in sensation? Less or more? Pain?

Respiratory
- Cough, changes?
- Shortness of breath and, if so, under what circumstances?
- Need to sleep in chair or elevated on pillows?
- If taking "inhalers/puffers," are more doses required to achieve the same result?

Cardiac
- Chest, shoulder, or jaw pain and under what circumstances?
- Sense of heart palpitations?
- Weight changes?

Vascular
- Cramping or pain in extremities?
- Edema, what time of the day and how much (can still wear usual shoes)?
- Change of color of the skin and, if so, what color and where?

Urinary
- Changes in urine stream or difficulty starting stream?

- Incontinence and, if this is new, under what circumstances and amount?

Sexual
- Change in usual arousal, desire, or ability to participate in physical sexual activity?
- Changes with aging that may affect sexual activity (e.g., vaginal dryness, erectile dysfunction)?

Musculoskeletal
- Falls or near falls since last seen?
- Pain in joints, back, or muscles?
- Changes in gait?
- If stiffness is present, when is it the worst and is it relieved by activity?
- If limited mobility or movement, effect on day-to-day life? Independence?

Neurological
- Changes in sensation, especially in extremities?
- Changes in memory or mood?
- Ability to perform usual cognitive activities? Change in memory?
- Changes in sense of balance, proprioception, or episodes of dizziness?

Gastrointestinal
- Change in level of continence?
- Change in bowel function: diarrhea, constipation, bloating?
- Dyspepsia or reflux?
- Change in appetite, weight changes?
- Abdominal pain?

Integument
- Frequency of injury, speed of healing?
- Itching and dryness?
- New lesions? Changes in skin lesion?
- Unusual bruising?

BOX 9.3   Am I Just Getting Older or Is This a Problem?

Mrs. Brown arrives in the medical office for a follow-up of her hypertension and arthritis. She is 89 years old and lives alone in her home of 50 years. She reports that she seems to have lost a little energy and has noted that her memory is not as good as it once was. She recently stopped driving and is dependent on neighbors for trips to the grocery and other errands. She feels that these changes are not significant and that they just may be because she had a birthday last week.

BOX 9.4   Aging and Social Determinants of Health

Food security
Stable income/employment
Accessible and safe housing and neighborhoods
Reliable and affordable transportation
Availability of social network and activities

From Pooler J, Srinivasan M: *Social determinants of health and the aging population* (website), 2018. https://impaqint.com/sites/default/files/issue-briefs/Issue%20Brief_SDOHandAgingPopulation_0.pdf.

TABLE 9.2   Problem-Oriented Assessment Mnemonic

O	Onset of problem
L	Location of problem
D	Duration of problem
C	Characteristics (e.g., signs, symptoms)
A	Aggravating factors (what makes it worse)
R	Relieving factors (What makes it better)
T	Treatments already tried

on the person's behalf. In some cases, the person with a cognitive impairment can still be part of the process when simple language is used, such as "Are you having any pain today?" or "Where are you hurting?"

Kleinman's explanatory model provides questions to supplement the usual data collected in the health history (Kleinman, 1980). It enables the nurse to better understand the older adult and plan effective strategies for individualized outcomes (see Chapter 4, Box 4.12).

TABLE 9.3   Factors Interfering With the Quality of the Health History and Potential Actions

Factor	Nursing Actions
Visual deficit	Directed lighting, offer to clean glasses.
Hearing deficit	Confirm person's ability to understand speaker, speak clearly while facing patient with no obstruction of the view of speaker's mouth, reduce or eliminate background noise.
Reduced energy	If possible, conduct assessment when the patient is most energetic. Provide for comfortable seating, prioritize data collection from most to least relevant. Be alert for signs of fatigue.

PHYSICAL HEALTH

The ROS accompanies or is followed by the physical examination to recognize the cues needed to perform clinical judgment. It is also used to support or refute the subjective report and further prioritize hypotheses. When this is done depends on the setting and the stamina of the older adult. The order in which it is done depends on the nurse-patient relationship. Although a "head-to-toe" approach is often taught, in a new relationship or with someone more fearful of the encounter, an "out-to-in" approach may be more acceptable. In this approach, the nurse begins with an assessment of "noncontact activities," such as weight and height; moves to examination of the extremities; and eventually examines the heart and lungs or genitalia. An observational functional exam can flow from the gross neurological exam of muscle strength and balance. While it may be customary for a patient to disrobe, working around the clothing of an older adult may be preferable when the low room temperatures in care settings are combined with age-related decreases in cold tolerance. Auscultating the heart through one thin layer of a smoothed cotton fabric (no synthetics) may be adequate for experienced nurses. In a symptomatic person or a person who has any positive findings, skin-to-stethoscope contact is necessary.

It is ideal to be able to auscultate all four areas (aortic, pulmonic, tricuspid, and mitral) of the heart, with the length of time spent in each area dependent on what is heard. For example, if a murmur or irregular rhythm is detected in the aortic area, then 60 seconds would be a reasonable time to auscultate; if the nurse auscultates for less time, the irregularity may be missed. The first three areas are often easier to auscultate in an older woman than in a younger woman because of the age-related increased laxity of the breast tissue.

When a comprehensive assessment is needed, this is often done over the course of multiple appointments or days, depending on the level of complexity of the current health problems and functional status of the individual.

The manual techniques of the physical exam, such as the use of the otoscope, do not differ from those used with younger adults; however, it is always necessary to consider the normal changes with aging and their effect on both the exam and the

cues recognized (Box 9.5). When either physical or cognitive limitations are present, it is not always possible to perform the physical exam as thoroughly as would be ideal (Box 9.6). For example, in the outpatient setting, observing objective abdominal cues may not be possible if the person cannot assume a lying position because of arthritis, kyphosis, or other skeletal deformity. Instead, the best that can be done is for the person to lean as far back in the chair as possible and then for the examiner to observe, auscultate, percuss, and palpate as usual. This is documented as a "limited abdominal exam."

It is always best that the assessment begins with the most obvious cues or critical systems, that is, those that have the most potential to put the person at risk, such as cues that support the geriatric syndromes (Box 9.7). In many cases, the aspects of the exam that require special attention are determined by the setting and purpose of the assessment. It is always necessary to be aware of cultural rules of etiquette that influence the physical examination (Box 9.8).

Using a Mnemonic for the Collection of Cues in Physical Assessment

Novice nurses should neither be expected to nor expect themselves to conduct a comprehensive assessment of older adults quickly but should expect to see their skills and efficiency increase over time. Nurses of all levels of experience must be mindful to conduct thorough assessments in order to provide the safest quality care possible.

The use of a mnemonic specifically applicable to the aging adult can guide the nurse in the recognition of essential cues, so that "nothing is missed." Two mnemonics that gerontological nurses use to organize, recognize, and prioritize hypotheses in the assessment of older adults are *SPICES* and *FANCAPES*. Once recognized, analysis of cues helps the nurse to differentiate normal aging changes from concerns requiring nursing actions and prioritizing the outcomes. If the analysis indicates that more detailed assessments are needed, the nurse will be able to do this as discussed in subsequent chapters.

FANCAPES

The mnemonic *FANCAPES* stands for Fluids, Aeration, Nutrition, Communication, Activity, Pain, Elimination, and Socialization. Developed by Barbara Bent (2005) in her work as a geriatric resource nurse at Missouri Hospital in Ashville, North Carolina, it can be used in any setting.

F: Fluids. Observation and analysis of cues indicative of a person's state of hydration. These include physiological, situational, functional, and psychological factors that contribute to the maintenance of adequate fluid intake. Information critical to the nurse's ability to prioritize needs of an older adult includes the ability of the person to obtain adequate fluids (functional data), to recognize or express thirst (situational and psychological data), and to swallow effectively (physiological data). Medications are reviewed to identify those with the potential to affect intake or output. Recognition and analysis of each of these cues are especially important when working with older adults who are frail, impaired in any way, or in situations where they are not

BOX 9.5   Tips for Best Practice

Special Considerations When Conducting a Physical Assessment With an Older Adult

Height and Weight
- Height loss associated with age-related changes and progressive osteoporosis.
- Weight gain: especially important if the person has any heart disease; be alert for early signs of heart failure.
- Weight loss: be alert for indications of malnutrition from dental problems, depression, or cancer. Check for mouth lesions from ill-fitting dentures. There is an increased rate of mortality for rapid weight loss in persons with dementia.

Temperature
- Change from baseline: Even a low-grade fever could be an indication of a serious illness. Temperatures as low as 100°F may indicate developing sepsis.

Blood Pressure
- Bilateral readings required. Best information from ambulatory monitoring. Positional blood pressure readings should be obtained because of the high occurrence of orthostatic hypotension (drop of 20/10 mm Hg or more when changing from sitting to standing).

Skin
- Check for skin cancer, especially in those with solar damage. Due to thinning, "tenting" is not a good indicator of hydration status.

Ears
- Increased hair in the canals may make visualization of the tympanic membrane difficult.
- It may not be possible to straighten out the canal completely. Begin by pulling back gently with otoscope in canal until tympanic membrane is visible.
- Cerumen dries, and impactions are common. Common cause of reversible hearing loss. These must be removed before hearing or tympanic membrane can be assessed adequately.

Hearing
- Cerumen impactions common cause of reversible hearing loss.
- High-frequency hearing loss (presbycusis) is age-related and common.
- Evaluate functional hearing by determining the volume needed by nurse for consistent understanding of conversation and directions.

Eyes
- Small pupils common (miosis). Normal if equal bilaterally. Minimal pupillary reflex.
- Gray ring around the iris (arcus senilis) normal. Sagging of upper lids may interfere with vision.
- Watch for entropion and ectropion.

Vision
- If Snellen chart is not available, a newspaper can be used for test of visual acuity.
- Changes may not be reported.
- Increased glare sensitivity, decreased contrast sensitivity, and need for more light to see and read can be expected but also may indicate cataracts.
- Decreased color discrimination may affect ability to self-administer medications safely.

Mouth
- Excessive dryness common and exacerbated by many medications. Periodontal disease common. Decreased sense of taste and thirst. Tooth surface abraded.

- If dentures warn, observe for irritation to mucosa and fit.

Neck
- Because of loss of subcutaneous adipose tissue, it may appear that carotid arteries are enlarged when they are not.

Chest/Pulmonary
- Any kyphosis will alter the location of the lobes, making careful assessment more important. Crackles in lower lobes may clear with cough.
- Risk for aspiration pneumonia increased and therefore increased importance of the lateral exam and measurement of accurate oxygen saturation.

Heart
- Listen carefully for murmurs and third and fourth heart sounds. Fourth heart sounds are somewhat common. A third heart sound is suggestive of heart failure.
- Presence of edema, especially lower extremities.

Extremities
- Dorsalis pedis and posterior tibial pulses difficult to palpate. Must look for other indications of vascular integrity. Mild edema common.

Abdomen/Gastrointestinal
- Because of deposition of fat in the abdomen, auscultation of bowel tones may be difficult.
- If concerned about incontinence or constipation, gentle rectal exam may be needed, hemorrhoids common. Occult blood test can be done at same time.

Musculoskeletal
- Osteoarthritis very common and pain often undertreated. Ask about pain and function in joints. Conduct very gentle passive range-of-motion (ROM) exercises if active ROM exercises are not possible. Do not push past comfort level. Observe for gait disorders. Observe the person get in and out of chair to assess independent function and fall risk.
- Although there is a gradual decrease in muscle strength, it should remain equal bilaterally.
- Observe for Heberden's and Bouchard's nodes.
- Observe gait.
- Assess painful areas and joints last.

Neurological
- Greatly diminished or absent ankle jerk (Achilles) tendon reflex is common and normal. Decreased or absent vibratory sense of the lower extremities are common. Slowed reflexes are normal but should be equal. Verbal fluency should be intact; assess quality of conversation. Slight, insignificant memory loss common.

Genitourinary: Male
- Pendulous scrotum with less rugae; smaller penis; thin and graying pubic hair.

Genitourinary: Female
- Small to nonpalpable ovaries; short, dryer vagina; decreased size of labia and clitoris; sparse pubic hair. Use utmost care with exam to avoid trauma to the tissues.

able to independently access fluids. A reduced sense of thirst is a common age-related change, with the potential of detrimental effect on health outcomes (Chapter 16).

A: Aeration and circulation. Aeration includes both inhalation of oxygen and exhalation of waste products. Circulation is a means to distribute oxygenated blood and nutrients throughout

BOX 9.6 An Abbreviated Exam

Alice has severe dementia. She spends most of her time walking around the unit where she lives. When she gets tired, she lays down on the floor or in whatever bed she is near, occupied or not. When an exam in the outpatient clinic was needed, the only way we could examine her was to very quietly and gently "follow her around" as she wandered. An aide was with her and knew exactly how to redirect her back to the clinic hallway.

BOX 9.7 Geriatric Syndromes[a]

Falls and gait abnormalities
Frailty
Delirium
Urinary incontinence
Sleep disorders
Pressure injury

[a]Note that there is considerable discussion about the exact "conditions" that are considered "geriatric syndromes." There is agreement that a syndrome is something that does not neatly fit into another disease category.

BOX 9.8 Tips for Best Practice

Key Points to Consider in Observing Cultural Rules and Etiquette

- Be aware of past experiences in the health care setting.
- Ask if there are persons (e.g., males in the family) who need to be present or involved in some way with the exam.
- Respect the communication style used in the health care setting.
- Do not intrude into personal space without permission.
- Determine general health orientation related to time (past, present, future).
- Inquire as to appropriate wording reference to the person; presume use of last name unless otherwise welcomed (e.g., Mrs. Jones).
- Inquire as to acceptability of touch during appropriate parts of the exam.
- Inquire as to the acceptability of the gender of the health care provider.

BOX 9.9 Cues Suggestive of Compromised Respiratory Function

Cyanosis of face, lips, nails, fingers, or toes
Shortness of breath, respiration with effort
Bradypnea or tachypnea
Restlessness
Chest pain or tightness

BOX 9.10 Factors Decreasing the Accuracy of a Pulse Oximetry Reading

Darkly pigmented skin and nail bed
Baseline poor peripheral circulation
Thick fingertip skin
Cool body temperature
Current tobacco use
Fingernail polish
Hand raised above heart level
Movement during measurement
Poor-quality oximeter

the body. Because of the close relationship between these two systems, they should be assessed simultaneously.

Careful pulmonary auscultation in the older adult should include the apices and lateral aspects of the lower lobes. Assessment of the respiratory rate and depth at rest and with activity should always be conducted due to the high rate of cardiopulmonary disease in late life and the potential for rapid decompensation. Not all older adults will present signs of decompensation, and the nurse must be alert to other potential cues that indicate respiratory compromise (Box 9.9). Assessment of the cardiovascular system is addressed in detail in Chapter 23.

The measurement of the oxygen saturation rate is an assessment regarding blood oxygen levels. It is easily estimated in any setting with a small, inexpensive fingertip device. It should be a model approved by the US Food and Drug Administration (FDA). Many people with heart disease or a recent COVID-19 infection already have these at home and can provide the nurse with very useful historical information or alert the person to the need for urgent care. However, there is always a risk for inaccuracies, and it is the nurse's responsibility to make sure that persons

and the people closest to them are aware of this (Box 9.10) (see also Pulse Oximeter Accuracy and Limitations, https://www.fda.gov/medical-devices/safety-communications/pulse-oximeter-accuracy-and-limitations-fda-safety-communication).

Careful attention to symptoms of fluid overload must be done anytime a person is receiving intravenous fluids. These symptoms include crackling lung sounds, shortness of breath, elevations in blood pressure, edema, and changes in mental status (delirium). Analysis of these cues is a priority in caring for older adults due to the speed with which heart failure can develop in older adults.

N: Nutrition. Protein-calorie malnutrition is common among individuals who are frail and those who live alone, are socially isolated, or are poor. Nutritional assessment is a complex process but especially important in frail older adults or those with dementia. A frail older adult who is losing weight even with an adequate intake or is malnourished for any reason has an increased risk for premature death from all causes (Söderström et al., 2017). Assessment of nutritional status and potential actions to improve outcomes are addressed in Chapter 15.

C: Communication. Communication that is impaired to some extent becomes more common with aging and may be misdiagnosed as delirium or dementia. Instead of making any assumptions before links between communication and cognition abilities can be analyzed, the nurse observes carefully for cues indicating hearing or vision loss. Communication is further at risk when the person suffers from any psychiatric or cardiovascular condition. Solutions to improve outcomes are discussed in Chapters 12 and 13.

A: Activity. The ability to move independently and the capacity to participate in enjoyable physical activities are important parts of healthy living. This does not change with aging. However, an activity assessment varies greatly because of the range of abilities among those referred to as "older adults." It is often tempting to provide movement assistance to any older adult, but this prevents the observation of important cues that may indicate an activity concern. Observation of the movement needed for activity occurs throughout all nursing contact, from when the person enters an examination room to when the person lies in a hospital bed. This information also can be used when the nurse considers teaching needs regarding home safety, fall risk, the need for assistive devices, and the degree to which the person can participate in exercises (Chapters 19, 20, and 21). Assessment of activity and mobility are often accomplished by the combined efforts of nurses, nursing assistants, occupational and physical therapists, and home caregivers (as appropriate) (Chapters 20 and 21). Any sudden change indicates the need for prompt analysis and determination of urgency of response (e.g., signs of a stroke; Chapter 23).

P: Pain. The assessment of pain includes that which is physical, psychological, and spiritual. One rarely occurs in isolation. Many nurses hear their patients implore, "What did I do to deserve this [pain]?" Because of the increasing amount of discomfort common with each decade of life (e.g., progression of arthritis or number of losses), assessment of pain requires particular attention by gerontological nurses and is addressed in detail in Chapter 29.

E: Elimination. Although difficulties with bowel and bladder functioning are not normal parts of aging, they are more common in older adults than they are in younger adults and can be triggered by such things as immobility attributable to physical limitations (e.g., post-stroke) or medications (e.g., diuretics). Incontinence can result from cognitive changes that affect the ability to identify the sensations indicating a need to void or defecate. The nurse observes for cues indicating dependence on others for assistance to maintain continence (e.g., getting to the toilet in time). The nurse may observe soiled underwear, the upper edge of an incontinence brief, or perigenital skin irritation indicating the use of personal protective pads.

Constipation and urinary retention may or may not be reported but are suggested by the routine use of laxatives or medications prescribed for the treatment of benign prostatic hyperplasia (BPH). Although the nurse may identify other more urgent findings, the patient may personally prioritize elimination needs. The nurse should then include these needs within the plan of care.

Discussing elimination function may be difficult for the older adult. The assessment begins by providing a safe and nonjudgmental avenue of communication, and finding mutually acceptable, understandable, and culturally appropriate language are ways to approach this difficult topic (Chapter 17).

S: Social skills. Socialization and social skills include the individual's ability to navigate in society, to give and receive love and friendship, and to feel self-worth. The nurse will assess whether the person seems able to ask for things from friends, family, and strangers. Other pertinent nursing assessment questions include "Who are the caregivers and how long are they available?", "Does the person belong to any social network or group, such as a church, synagogue, ashram, or temple that serves as a source of support?", and "Is the monthly income adequate to meet needs (e.g., medication and food)?"

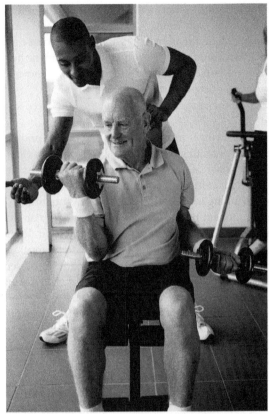
©iStock.com/Dean Mitchell.

SPICES

As with FANCAPES, the mnemonic *SPICES* helps the nurse remember elements that must be assessed when caring for an older adult (Fulmer & Wallace, 2012; Montgomery et al., 2008). *SPICES* refers to six common areas that have been identified as highly related to risk for hospitalization and very serious geriatric syndromes (Yeager, 2019). Recognition of cues related to potential *S*leep disorders, *P*roblems with eating, *I*ncontinence, *C*onfusion, *E*vidence of falls, and *S*kin breakdown is required in care of the older person, particularly someone who has one or more unstable medical conditions or is at high risk for physical or functional decline. As with FANCAPES, any abnormal cue must be rapidly analyzed to determine how quickly intervention needs to take place to avoid any reversible problems. All SPICES cues have the potential of significantly affecting a person's health, self-esteem, and well-being (Box 9.11).

BOX 9.11   Resources for Best Practice

- The website of the Hartford Institute for Geriatric Nursing (https://hign.org/consultgeri-resources/try-this-series) provides a free compilation of many evidence-based tools for individual use. In many cases, videos demonstrating their administration are included.

FUNCTIONAL ABILITY

Whereas FANCAPES and SPICES address primarily physical cues, functional assessments have been designed to predict and monitor an individual's ability to perform the activities or tasks needed for daily living. Other aspects of the functional assessment include the individual's ability to negotiate physical and social environments. The functional assessment helps the gerontological nurse work with the individual to move toward healthy aging by accomplishing the following:

- Recognize the specific areas in which help is needed or not needed
- Recognize changes in abilities from one time to another
- Recognize potential risks to safety in a living situation

The functional assessment is composed of elements that are considered mutually exclusive and scored arbitrarily. For example, drinking is observed in totality; it is not broken down into its component parts, such as picking up a cup or swallowing water. The nurse analyzes if the person (1) can do the task alone, (2) needs assistance, or (3) is not able to perform the task at all. This type of scoring has not been found to be sensitive enough to evaluate small changes in outcomes. The scoring may be done by self-report, proxy, or observation. It should be noted that some research has found that self-reports overestimate functional ability and differ from that of proxy reports (Griffiths et al., 2020; Li et al., 2015). While universal human needs have been identified, the way in which they are met are socially and culturally determined.

The instruments are beneficial in that they provide caregivers with a common cue nomenclature and metric for analysis and therefore have the potential to increase the consistency of care. When analysis suggests a hypothesis of functional deficit, a more detailed assessment is expected of the gerontological nurse or care team (see specialized chapters).

Although loss of some function is often considered a "normal change of aging," as in other aspects of the assessment, when sudden changes are found, further analysis is urgent. Reversible causes must always be sought, and appropriate actions to address these must be implemented promptly. Worsening of functional status associated with chronic conditions is an important indicator of movement toward death and reduced quality of life (Volpato and & Guralnik, 2018; Yeager, 2019).

Activities of Daily Living

Basic functions related to personal needs are referred to as *activities of daily living* (ADLs) (Box 9.12). Two of these, dressing (including grooming) and bathing, require higher cognitive function than the others. The ability to feed oneself, in at least some rudimentary manner, remains intact until late in dementia, assuming other health problems (e.g., dominant-side stroke) do not interfere.

Katz Index

ADLs were first classified as such by Sidney Katz and colleagues in 1963 (Katz et al., 1963). The Katz Index has served as a basic framework for most of the subsequent screening tools. The ADLs are considered only in dichotomous terms: the ability to complete the task independently (one point) or the complete inability to do so (zero points). With equal weight on all activities, this index cannot be used to identify specific areas of need, cannot show change in any one task, and cannot evaluate specific outcome of actions. Over the years this instrument has been refined to afford more sensitivity to the nuances of analyses indicating functional status (Nikula et al., 2003).

Barthel Index (BI)

The Barthel Index (BI) (Mahoney & Barthel, 1965) is a quick and reliable instrument for the recognition of cues related to ability to perform ADLs as well as mobility. It can be completed in 2 to 3 minutes using self-report or in about 20 minutes when direct observational recognition is necessary. The activities are scored in various ways. The BI has been found to be sensitive enough for both the early identification of needs and the evaluation of outcomes, especially following a stroke (Quinn et al., 2011).

Functional Independence Measure

The Functional Independence Measure (FIM) is also especially useful when working with those who have had strokes or spinal cord injuries. The FIM guides the collection of comprehensive cues relative to the ability to perform ADLs, as well as mobility, cognition, and social functioning. Analysis provides for the hypotheses of needs during an inpatient stay and the development of outcome goals associated with discharge planning (Cournan, 2011; Rayegani et al., 2016). The activities are scored using a seven-point scale from totally independent to totally dependent. In some studies, the reliability of the BI and FIM were found to be comparable (Sangha et al., 2005). In others, the FIM was deemed preferable. It is a required tool in the rehabilitation setting in US Department of Veterans Affairs (VA) hospitals and rehabilitation centers in the United States (Shulkin, 2017). Information about this tool is easily found on the internet.

Functional Assessment Staging Tool

The Functional Assessment Staging Tool (FAST) is unique in that it identifies the cues specific to functional change in persons with a progressive dementia such as Alzheimer's disease (Table 9.4). It was designed by geriatrician Barry Reisberg (1988) to assist clinicians to quantify the level or stage of dis/ability and, in doing so, help the family know what to expect and how to prepare for the changes ahead. It uses an ordinal scale from stage 1 (no functional impairment, associated with any cognitive impairment) to 7 (unable to perform any ADLs, associated with very severe [late stage] cognitive impairment). The FAST has been found to be reliable and valid (Boltz, 2021; Sclan & Reisberg, 1992).

Instrumental Activities of Daily Living

Those activities considered necessary for independent living are referred to as *instrumental activities of daily living or IADLs* (Box 9.13). This does not mean that the person performs the tasks,

---

BOX 9.12	Activities of Daily Living
• Bathing	• Transferring
• Dressing	• Continence
• Toileting	• Eating

TABLE 9.4 Functional Assessment Staging Tool (FAST)

Stage 1—Normal adult	Shows no functional decline.
Stage 2—Normal older adult	Shows personal awareness of some functional decline.
Stage 3—Early Alzheimer's disease	Demonstrates noticeable deficits in demanding job situations.
Stage 4—Mild Alzheimer's disease	Requires assistance in complicated tasks such as handling finances or planning parties.
Stage 5—Moderate Alzheimer's disease	Requires assistance in choosing proper attire.
Stage 6—Moderately severe Alzheimer's disease	Requires assistance dressing, bathing, and toileting. Experiences urinary and fecal incontinence.
Stage 7—Severe Alzheimer's disease	Speech ability declines to about a half-dozen intelligible words.
	Demonstrates progressive loss of abilities to walk, sit up, smile, and hold up head.

From Reisberg B: Functional Assessment Staging (FAST), *Psychopharmacol Bull* 24:653–659, 1998. Copyright ©1984 by Barry Reisberg, MD. Reproduced with permission.

BOX 9.13 Instrumental Activities of Daily Living

- Ability to use telephone
- Abilities related to travel
- Shopping
- Self-medication administration
- Food preparation
- Handling finances
- Housekeeping
- Laundry

BOX 9.14 Evelyn: Moving From Dependence to Independence

When I first met Evelyn, she was 65 years old and recently widowed. She had married young, moving from her parents' home into that of her husband. During their entire marriage she had never driven, pumped gas, shopped alone, or taken care of anything but personal and child care, cooking, and house cleaning. She knew nothing about their finances. She had significant instrumental activities of daily living (IADLs) deficits but had no choice but to learn how to take care of herself independently after her husband died. She never did learn how to drive very well!

just that the person could perform them if called upon to do so (Box 9.14). It is generally agreed that the ability to perform IADLs requires higher cognitive and physical functioning than do the ADLs.

The Lawton IADL Scale

The original Lawton IADL Scale assigned scores from zero (lowest functioning) to eight (highest functioning) for each activity (Lawton & Brody, 1969). The level of functioning is determined by a summary score. It may be useful as a screening tool to establish an overall baseline of general functioning but, like the Katz Index, it is not sensitive to changes in any one area. The original tool and the subsequent iterations take about 15 minutes to administer using self-report, proxy report, or clinician-observed

cues. Persons with dementia will progressively lose the ability to perform IADLs beginning with those associated with the highest neuropsychological functioning, such as handling finances and shopping. Unfortunately, this scale may be biased by age and culture (Cress, 2017; LaPlante, 2010).

COGNITION

A cognitive assessment is usually referred to as a "mental status exam." The cues analyzed include level of consciousness, general appearance and interactional behavior, orientation, attention and concentration, memory, judgment and insight, executive function/planning, speech, and language (Boltz, 2021). Another common cue is mathematical ability or calculation. Multiple instruments have been developed and tested, with descriptions of several that are frequently used appearing below. When the analysis suggests potential problems, the need for a more in-depth assessment is indicated before any hypotheses are possible, especially to determine if there are any potentially reversible conditions present.

A mental status exam of any kind may be particularly stressful to the person and significant others. An environment and relationship of trust leads to the most accurate analysis possible with the least amount of embarrassment. The assessment may be described as similar to auscultation of the heart, to "see how the brain is doing." Like most other assessments, these are best administered when the person is comfortable, rested, and free of pain (Boltz, 2021). Gerontological nursing requires the sensitivity to note subtle changes that may indicate a reversible health problem or new or evolving conditions.

Short Portable Mental Status Questionnaire

The Short Portable Mental Status Questionnaire (SPMSQ), created in 1975 by Dr. Eric Pheiffer, is a 10-item instrument used as a screen for cognitive impairment from any cause. It is easy to administer and widely available, including in a downloadable and fillable PDF version (https://geriatrics.stanford.edu/culturemed/overview/assessment/assessment_toolkit/spmsq.html) (Table 9.5). Nurses have used it to assess altered cognition, but it cannot predict self-care or progression of dementia. It is similar in content, sensitivity, and specificity to the Mental Status Questionnaire (MSQ) (McDougall, 1990).

Mini-Mental State Examination

The Mini-Mental State Examination (MMSE) has been the gold standard used in more detailed screening (recognition of cues) and assessment (analysis) of cognitive status (Folstein et al., 1975; Mitchell, 2009). Completion requires functional vision, hearing, and manual dexterity. With training and practice the MMSE takes 7 to 10 minutes to administer (Patnode et al., 2020). The score must be adjusted for those with low education levels and disability (Commonwealth of Australia, 2014). Using the original 30-item instrument, a score of 24 to 30 is considered "normal," 18 to 23 is suggestive of mild cognitive impairment, and 0 to 17 is suggestive of severe cognitive impairment. Although the MMSE is still widely available, it is no longer in the public domain and permission for its use must be requested (http://www.parinc.com).

TABLE 9.5   Short Portable Mental Status Questionnaire

Question	Correct	Incorrect
What is the date, month, year?		
What is the day of the week?		
What is the name of this place?		
What is your phone number?		
How old are you?		
Where were you born?		
Who is the current president?		
Who was the president before him[/her]?		
What is your mother's maiden name?		
Please count backwards from 20 by 3's.		

Scoring number of incorrect responses: 0–2 normal, 3–4 mild impairment, 5–7 moderate impairment, 8+ severe impairment.

From Pfeiffer E: A short portable mental status questionnaire for the assessment of organic brain deficit in elderly patients, *J Am Geriatr Soc* 23:433–441, 1975.

Montreal Cognitive Assessment

The Montreal Cognitive Assessment (MoCA) may be more sensitive than the MMSE and has been tested in several countries (Fujiwara et al., 2010; Memória et al., 2013). Due to the complexity of the tasks within each component, the preprinted tool is necessary for administration and analysis. Training and certification in use of this tool are now required. Past math abilities, vision adequate to see printed figures, functional hearing, and ability to use a pencil or pen are necessary. A video demonstrating the use of the instrument and further instructions are available at http://www.mocatest.org.

Clock Drawing Test

In use since 1992, the Clock Drawing Test is quick and easy to administer and score. The results have been highly correlated with the MMSE across the world (Aprahamian et al., 2010;

Ehreke et al., 2010). It is not appropriate for use with those who are blind or who have limiting conditions such as tremors or a stroke that affects the dominant hand. While reading fluency is not necessary, completion requires number fluency, the ability to hear and see, manual dexterity adequate to use a writing implement, and experience with analog clocks (Fig. 9.1). Scoring is based on the analysis of the position of both the numbers and the hands. This tool cannot be used as the sole measure of dementia, but it does test for constructional apraxia as an early indicator and has been found by some to be useful for indicating that dementia is *unlikely* (Janssen et al., 2017; Nair et al., 2010). The clock test is an evidence-based instrument that has been found to be useful across cultures and languages and is not influenced by educational level (Borson et al., 1999).

Mini-Cog

The Mini-Cog builds on the Clock Drawing Test (Boltz, 2021; Borson et al., 2000). It has been found to be as accurate and reliable as the MMSE but less biased, easier to administer and score, and possibly more sensitive to dementia (Mitchell & Malladi, 2010). The Mini-Cog combines the assessment of short-term memory with those of executive function from the clock test (Boxes 9.15 and 9.16). It is equally reliable with non–English-speaking as with English-speaking individuals and is minimally affected by education, gender, and ethnicity (Boltz, 2021). It takes 3 to 5 minutes to administer and, like the other screening tools discussed in this chapter, only serves as a means of recognizing and analyzing cues that have been found to be pertinent to dementia. Like the clock test, it requires number fluency and the ability to hear and see, hold a pencil, and have experience with analog clocks.

MOOD

Evidence-based instruments that have been developed and tested can help the nurse to recognize cues related to mood,

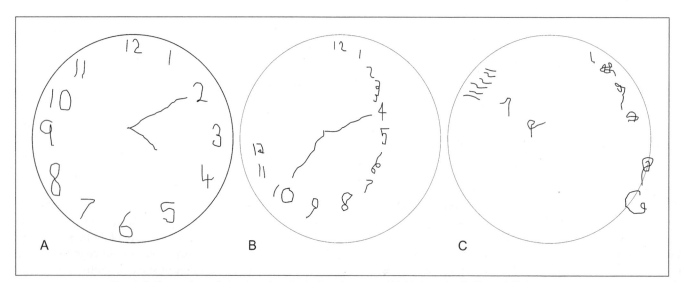

Fig. 9.1 Examples of results of a clock drawing test. (A) Unimpaired. (B and C) Impaired. (From Stern TA, Rosenbaum JF, Fava M, et al: *Massachusetts General Hospital comprehensive clinical psychiatry,* St Louis, 2008, Mosby.)

BOX 9.15 Instructions for the Administration of the Mini-Cog and Clock Drawing Tests

1. State three unrelated words, such as "chair," "coin," "tree"; state each word clearly and slowly, about 1 second for each.
2. Ask the person to repeat these words; if the person is unable to do so, you may repeat the words up to three times to give the person three attempts to immediately say them back to you correctly.
3. The person is asked to draw a clock as in the Clock Drawing Test.
   a. Provide the person with a piece of plain white paper with a circle drawn on it.
   b. Ask the person to draw numbers in the circle so that it looks like a clock, and then to put the hands in the circle to read "10 after 4."
4. The person is asked to recall the three words from step 1.

TABLE 9.6 Geriatric Depression Scale (Short Form)

Are you basically satisfied with your life?	Yes	No*
Do you often get bored?	Yes*	No
Do you often feel helpless?	Yes*	No
Do you prefer to stay at home, rather than going out and doing new things?	Yes*	No
Do you feel pretty worthless about the way you are now?	Yes*	No

*Each answer indicated by an asterisk counts as 1 point. Two points suggests depression in older adults.
From Heidenblut S, Zank S: Screening for depression in old age with very short instruments: the DIA-S4 compared to the GDS5 and GDS4, *Gerontol Geria Med* 6:1–9, 2020.

BOX 9.16 Scoring of the Mini-Cog and Clock Drawing Tests

Scoring

Points are awarded for recalled words first. The following scoring system is used: none remembered, dementia likely; all three words remembered, dementia unlikely; recall of either one or two words, then results of the clock drawing must be taken into consideration: normal (all numbers and hands correct) or abnormal (any errors).

There are several suggestions by psychologists about how the clocks are scored. All consider (1) the symmetry of the numbers (able to plan ahead): if all numbers are included, repeated, or missed; whether they are inside or outside of the circle; if they appear as numbers; and (2) the hands of the clock: whether the numbers appear at all and if they are in the correct place relative to the numbers (abstract thinking).

coherency, logic, thought content, and perception (such as presence or absence of delusions or hallucinations). Assessment of mood is especially important in gerontological nursing due to the potential for adverse effects of medications and of the number of illnesses, such as stroke and Parkinson's disease, frequently associated with depression and anxiety. Older adults with unrecognized depression may appear to have signs suggestive of dementia, and many persons with dementia are also depressed (Bowker et al., 2012; Yeager, 2019). The interconnection between the mental status and mood calls for skill and sensitivity on the part of the nurse to ensure that cues in older adults are recognized and analyzed promptly and accurately.

The Geriatric Depression Scale and the Cornell Scale for Depression in Dementia are tools frequently used to assess depression in older adults. Tools useful for assessing persons who are demonstrating cues related to possible anxiety are discussed in Chapter 30.

Geriatric Depression Scale

The Geriatric Depression Scale (GDS) was developed as a 30-item tool specifically for screening older adults (Brink et al., 1982; Yesavage et al., 1983). Shortened 15-item and 5-item versions have been developed and validated (Valpato & Guralik, 2018). The 5-item GDS takes about 1 minute to administer and has an accuracy of as much as 90% (in predicting depression) (Heidenblut & Zank, 2020; Hoyl et al., 1999) (Table 9.6). A score

of 2 or more is an indicator for late life depression. It has been suggested that the short version can be used by some who are aphasic but are able to use a point-board. It also has been found to be useful in persons with some dementia with a score of 15 or above on the MMSE.

The GDS has been extremely successful in identifying depression because it deemphasizes patient reports of physical symptoms, decreased libido, and changes in appetite (Lach et al., 2010). It has been tested extensively with translations in multiple languages (Ortiz & Romero, 2008). The ConsultGeri resource of the Hartford Institute for Geriatric Nursing offers a free training video on the administration of the GDS 15-item version (https://hign.org/consultgeri/try-this-series/geriatric-depression-scale-gds). Free scoring calculators are also available from a number of websites.

Cornell Scale for Depression in Dementia

Persons with cognitive impairments tend to underreport symptoms, and therefore the GDS is less accurate when used by those who score below 15 on the MMSE (Burke et al., 2019). The Cornell Scale for Depression in Dementia (CSDD) was designed to identify depression in persons who have moderate to severe cognitive impairments (Alexopoulos et al., 1988; Lim et al., 2012; Sheehan, 2012). With 19 items, it takes approximately 20 minutes to administer; behaviors are ranked as 0 = absent, 1 = mild or intermittent, and 3 = severe. A score of 5 or lower indicates absence of clinically significant depression, effective treatment, or remission (Maust et al., 2012). A caregiver is asked if any of the behaviors have been observed in the *week* before the interview. This is followed briefly by an interview with the person with dementia, to the extent possible. The CSDD can be downloaded for free.

COMPREHENSIVE GERIATRIC ASSESSMENT

In some cases, an integrated assessment approach is needed rather than an individual instrument or collection of separate instruments, that is, an approach that combines physical, functional, and psychosocial components. The most well-known comprehensive tools are the Resident Assessment Instrument (RAI) and the Outcome and Assessment Information Set (OASIS). The RAI is required for persons in skilled nursing facilities, and the OASIS is required for persons receiving skilled care from a home health agency. Although they are lengthy and labor intensive, once completed they can be invaluable in setting and evaluating health outcomes. An early tool still in use is the OARS Multidimensional Functional Assessment Questionnaire (OMFAQ). Once completed it includes data related to social functioning as well.

Resident Assessment Instrument (RAI)

In 1986, what was then referred to as the Institute of Medicine (IOM) completed a study indicating that although considerable variation existed, residents in skilled nursing facilities in the United States were receiving an unacceptably low quality of care (IOM, 1986). As a result, nursing home reform was legislated as part of the Omnibus Budget Reconciliation Act (OBRA) of 1987. The creators of OBRA recognized the challenging work of caring for increasingly ill persons discharged from acute care settings to nursing homes and, along with this, the need for complex clinical judgment performed by an interprofessional team regarding the care or action that is needed, planned, implemented, and evaluated.

In 1990, the Resident Assessment Instrument (RAI) was created and mandated for use in all skilled nursing facilities that receive compensation from either Medicare or Medicaid (see Chapter 5). The RAI is a collection of comprehensive assessment items profiling physical and cognitive health, mood, social status, and functional ability of a person upon admission to a skilled nursing facility and at designated times thereafter (Centers for Medicare and Medicaid Services [CMS], 2021a). Many evidence-based instruments are included in the RAI, with the largest being the Minimum Data Set (MDS). As the cues are recognized and analyzed, specific areas of need are hypothesized that guide the development of actions. The initial assessment serves as the framework for the baseline goals and outcomes for the individual. The nurse and other members of the care team can track the patient's progress and amend the

action plan as appropriate. Quality Measures provide information to the public regarding specific factors indicative of the care that is provided in a facility and give the facility information about specific areas in need of improvement. The Quality Measures are divided into "short stay" (<100 days) and "long stay" (Box 9.17). These have been updated and revised and now are considered in terms of "Meaningful Measures" or those indicators that have been found to have the most impact on outcomes (CMS, 2020).

As outcomes are achieved and resources are made available, the RAI/MDS leads to discharge to a lower level of care, such as returning home or moving to an assisted living facility. For a person whose condition is one of progressive decline, the RAI leads to actions focused on comfort.

Use of the RAI is dynamic and outcome oriented. It is used to gather definitive information and promote healthy aging in a specific care setting and in a comprehensive manner. It is coordinated by nurses and requires their signature attesting to its accuracy. The Quality Measures, along with the RAI, are used in several countries outside the United States, including provinces in Canada.

Outcome and Assessment Information Set (OASIS-D)

The skilled care provided in the home is based on and documented in the Outcome and Assessment Information Set (OASIS). While the fifth version is now in use (in 2021), the sixth revision, OASIS-E, will be required for use 1 year following the end of the COVID-19 pandemic (CMS, 2021b). The data collected are very comprehensive, focus on patient outcomes, and are designed to address the prioritized needs, prevent unnecessary rehospitalization, and ensure safety in the home setting (Box 9.18). Completion is required for all care that is compensated by Medicare or Medicaid and forms the basis for the level of reimbursement. As with other instruments used in care settings, the OASIS is completed at the time the care is begun and at intervals thereafter. Nurses provide additional information

---

> BOX 9.17 **Examples of Quality Measures Highly Relevant to Persons Receiving Care in Skilled Nursing Facilities**
>
> | Short Stay Residents | Long-Term Stay Residents |
> |---|---|
> | Self-report of moderate to severe pain | Number of hospitalizations per 1,000 resident days |
> | Pressure injury: new or worsened | Emergency room visits per 1,000 resident days |
> | One or more falls with major injury | Percentage of residents: |
> | Assessed for/given seasonal influenza vaccination | Experienced one or more falls with a major injury |
> | Assessed for/given pneumococcal vaccine | High-risk residents with pressure-ulcers |
> | Newly received antipsychotic medication | Developed a urinary tract infection |
> | Re-hospitalized 30 days after an admission. | Developed bowel or bladder incontinence |
> | Had an emergency room visit | Has/had catheter inserted into bladder |
> | Successful return home | Is physically restrained |
> | Functional abilities assessed and goals part of treatment plan | Has increased need for assistance with ADLs |
> | Medicare spending per patient | Ability to move independently worsened |
> | | Has/had excessive weight loss |
> | | Shows depressive symptoms |
> | | Received an antipsychotic, antianxiety or hypnotic medication |
> | | Needs and got flu or pneumonia vaccine |
>
> From Centers for Medicare and Medicaid Services (CMS): *Quality measures* (website), 2020. https://www.cms.gov/Medicare/Quality-Initiatives-Patient-Assessment-Instruments/QualityMeasures.

BOX 9.18 Risk for Hospitalization From the OASIS Assessment

- History of falls (2 or more falls—or any fall with an injury—in the past 12 months)
- Unintentional weight loss of a total of 10 pounds or more in the past 12 months
- Multiple hospitalizations (2 or more) in the past 6 months
- Multiple emergency department visits (2 or more) in the past 6 months
- Decline in mental, emotional, or behavioral status in the past 3 months
- Reported or observed history of difficulty complying with any medical instructions (e.g., medications, diet, exercise) in the past 3 months
- Currently taking 5 or more medications
- Currently reports exhaustion
- Other risk(s) not listed in 1–8
- None of the above

OASIS, Outcome and Assessment Information Set.

necessary to generate solutions within the context of the existing environmental and personal factors. Clinical judgment at this level is exceedingly complex. Training is required for the accurate use of the OASIS instrument.

The OARS Multidimensional Functional Assessment Questionnaire

The classic Older Americans Resources and Services (OARS) was developed at the Center for the Study of Aging and Human Development at Duke University and later updated as the OARS Multidimensional Functional Assessment Questionnaire (OMFAQ) (Duke University Center for the Study of Aging and Human Development, 2021). The updated instrument serves to help determine (1) the ability, disability, and capacity level at which the person can function; and (2) the extent and intensity of the use of available resources. In the first section, the assessment is divided into five subscales that may be used separately or alone. The person's functional capacity in each area is rated on a scale of 1 (excellent functioning) to 6 (totally impaired functioning). A cumulative impairment score (CIS) is calculated ranging from the most capable (6) to total disability (30). It takes approximately 45 minutes to administer and requires training. The OMFAQ and training materials can be purchased for a nominal fee from the Center

for the Study of Aging and Human Development at Duke University (http://www.sites.duke.edu/centerforaging/?s=OMFAQ&submit=).

CLINICAL JUDGMENT TO PROMOTE HEALTHY AGING

Many evidence-based instruments are available to facilitate the recognition of cues that result in a score. The nurse can then use those data to assist in determining a hypothesis. In some cases, the instruments used to gather a baseline initial assessment can be repeated to evaluate outcomes. When the nurse knows how and when to use an instrument or tool, quicker assessment and prioritization of care can take place. Each tool has strengths and weaknesses, as does each completed assessment. The use of a mnemonic or an assessment instrument serves to assist the nurse in performing this role.

Whether the nurse is working with a standardized instrument or creating a new one, the goal is always to recognize the cues needed for the careful analyses leading to the prioritization of hypotheses; the development of coordinated, integrated, safe, and individualized solutions and actions; and the evaluation of outcomes regardless of the care setting or health status. Urgent solutions are developed for prioritized problems and long-term solutions to promote wellness.

The nurse is expected to collect data accurately and to do so in the most efficient yet caring manner possible. Many factors affect the recognition of cues in the older adult: differentiating the effects of aging from those originating from disease, determining the presence of comorbidities, underreporting of symptoms by older adults, manifesting atypical presentations or nonspecific presentations of illnesses, and increasing numbers of iatrogenic illnesses.

Careful clinical judgment is necessary when assessing and prioritizing problems in older adults, especially those with multiple chronic conditions. Symptoms may be ascribed to normal aging rather than to a disease process that may be developing, necessitating careful and often problem-oriented assessments. The symptoms also may be thought to be indications of a pathological process when they are normal changes with aging. Cues suggestive of one hypothesis can exacerbate or mask those of another. The gerontological nurse is challenged to provide the highest level of excellence in the assessment of the older adult without burdening the person in the process.

KEY CONCEPTS

- Recognition and analyses of cues relative to physical, psychological, and functional status are essential to identifying specific needs that will lead to the development of prioritized hypotheses.
- Once hypotheses are determined, the nurse generates solutions and implements interventions needed to achieve healthy aging outcomes.
- The quality of cues is affected by the source of collection, that is, whether by self-report, report by proxy, or through nurse observation.
- Evidence-based mnemonics and instruments are available for most aspects of the assessment of the older adult.
- Knowledge of and sometimes training in the use of an assessment instrument may be necessary for the nurse to use it reliably and accurately.
- Multiple factors can affect assessment when working with older adults.

NEXT-GENERATION NCLEX® (NGN) EXAMINATION–STYLE QUESTIONS

The nurse is conducting the first home visit for Mr. Ortiz, an 86-year-old Hispanic male, following his discharge from the hospital for community-acquired pneumonia. His medical history includes diabetes, chronic obstructive pulmonary disease (COPD), and arthritis. He lives alone with his wife, who suffers from dementia.

Assessment findings include blood pressure of 90/60 mm Hg, heart rate of 90 beats per minute, respirations 20 breaths per minute, temperature 97.3°F, and oxygen 89% on room air. His heart has a regular rate and rhythm; rhonchi in the left lower lobe are auscultated; abdomen has normoactive bowel sounds, soft and nontender; no peripheral edema; skin is dry, warm, and pale. He reports feeling very fatigued but believes that it from his long-standing COPD. Able to sleep if he uses several pillows. Does not feel that he sleeps soundly, as he feels he must stay alert in case his wife needs him. He has pain in his back and ribs with coughing; he denies shortness of breath. Mr. Ortiz states that his appetite has not yet returned; he is trying to eat but feels full quickly. States that his last bowel movement was yesterday; it was soft.

Considering FANCAPES, underline priority cues that require further analysis. Which type of information is still needed for the initial assessment?

Vital signs indicate at the least that his heart is beating faster to compensate for low blood pressure. Low blood pressure, rapid pulse, dry skin, and fatigue all indicate possible dehydration. Poor eating and sleep disruption could contribute to his fatigue. He is at **high risk for falling and rapid decompensation**. Need more information about nutrition, pain, and social support, especially help with caretaking.

CLINICAL JUDGMENT QUESTIONS AND ACTIVITIES

1. Of the assessment tools that are available to you, which are the most reasonable to perform within the limitations of an acute care setting? Give your rationale for the choices.
2. How would any of your answers to the preceding question change in a skilled nursing facility? In an assisted living facility? In the home setting? What is your rationale?
3. If you cannot do a complete head-to-toe examination and detailed history, list the parts that are essential when assessing an older adult, in order of priority.
4. Review the literature and present to your class two instruments that are applicable for use in cultures or languages other than the ones for which they were created.
5. Select the instrument or the portion of an instrument you are the least comfortable with and role-play with a classmate in conducting the assessment until you become comfortable.

RESEARCH QUESTIONS

1. What is the importance of measuring ADLs and IADLs in older adults?
2. What makes an assessment tool effective?

REFERENCES

Alexopoulos GS, Abrams RC, Young RC, et al.: Cornell Scale for Depression in Dementia, *Biol Psychiatry* 23:271–284, 1988.

Aprahamian I, Martinelli JE, Neri AL, et al.: The accuracy of the Clock Drawing Test compared to that of standard screening tests for Alzheimer's disease: results from a study of Brazilian elderly with heterogeneous educational backgrounds, *Int Psychogeriatr* 22:64–71, 2010.

Bent B: FANCAPES assessment increases in longevity lead to need for expertise in geriatric care, *Adv Healthcare Netw Nurs* 7(14):10, 2005.

Boltz M: Dementia: assessment and care [Ex Ed.]. In Boltz M, editor: *Evidence-based geriatric nursing protocols for best practices*, 3, New York, 2021, Springer, pp 333–352.

Borson S, Brush M, Gil E, et al.: The Clock Drawing Test: utility for dementia detection in multiethnic elders, *J Gerontol A Biol Sci Med Sci* 54(11):M534–M540, 1999.

Borson S, Scanlan J, Brush M, et al.: The Mini-Cog: a cognitive "vital signs" measure for dementia screening in multi-lingual elderly, *Int J Geriatr Psychiatry* 15(11):1021–1207, 2000.

Bowker LK, Price JD, Smith SC, editors: *Oxford handbook of geriatric medicine*, 2, 2012, OxfordOxford University Press.

Brink TL, Yesavage JA, Lum O, et al.: Screening tests for geriatric depression, *Clin Gerontol* 1:37–43, 1982.

Burke AD, Goldfarb D, Bollam B, et al.: Diagnosing and treating depression in patients with Alzheimer's disease, *Neurol Ther* 8(2):325–350, 2019.

Centers for Medicare and Medicaid Services (CMS): *Quality measures* (website), 2020. https://www.cms.gov/Medicare/Quality-Initiatives-Patient-Assessment-Instruments/QualityMeasures.

Centers for Medicare and Medicaid Services (CMS): *Minimum Data Set (MDS) 3.0 Resident Assessment Instrument (RAI) manual* (website), 2021a. https://www.cms.gov/Medicare/Quality-Initiatives-Patient-Assessment-Instruments/NursingHomeQualityInits/MDS30RAIManual.

Centers for Medicare and Medicaid Services (CMS): *OASIS Data Sets* (website), 2021b. https://www.cms.gov/Medicare/Quality-Initiatives-Patient-Assessment-Instruments/HomeHealthQualityInits/OASIS-Data-Sets.

Cournan M: Use of the Functional Independence Measure for outcomes measurement in acute inpatient rehabilitation, *Rehabil Nurs* 36(3):111–117, 2011.

Cress CJ: *Handbook of geriatric care management*, 4, Burlington, MA, 2017, Jones and Bartlett.

Duke University Center for the Study of Aging and Human Development: *Older Americans resources and services* (website), 2021. https://sites.duke.edu/centerforaging/services/older-americans-resources-and-services/.

Ehreke L, Luppa M, König HH, et al.: The Clock Drawing Test a screening tool for the diagnosis of mild cognitive impairment? A systematic review, *Int Psychogeriatr* 22:56–63, 2010.

Folstein MF, Folstein SE, McHugh PR: Mini-Mental State: a practical method for grading the cognitive state of patients for the clinician, *J Psychiatr Res* 12:189–198, 1975.

Fujiwara Y, Suzuki H, Yasunaga M, et al.: Brief screen tool for mild cognitive impairment in older Japanese: validation of the Japanese version of the Montreal Cognitive Assessment, *Geriatr Gerontol Int* 10(3):225–232, 2010.

Fulmer T, Wallace M: *Fulmer SPICES: an overall assessment tool for older adults*, New York, 2012, Hartford Institute for Geriatric Nursing https://hign.org/sites/default/files/2020-06/Try_This_General_Assessment_1.pdf.

Griffiths AW, Smith SJ, Martin A, et al.: Exploring self-report and proxy-report quality-of-life measures for people living with dementia in care homes, *Qual Life Res* 29(2):463–472, 2020.

Heidenblut S, Zank S: Screening for depression in old age with very short instruments: the DIA-S4 compared to the GDS5 and GDS4, *Gerontol Geria Med* 6:1–9, 2020.

Hoyl MT, Alessi CA, Harker JO, et al.: Development and testing of a five-item version of the Geriatric Depression Scale, *J Am Geriatr Soc* 47(7):873–878, 1999.

Institute of Medicine (IOM): *Improving the quality of care in nursing homes*, Washington, DC, 1986, The National Academies Press https://www.nap.edu/catalog/646/improving-the-quality-of-care-in-nursing-homes.

Janssen J, Koekkoek PS, Moll van Charante EP, et al.: How to choose the most appropriate cognitive test to evaluate cognitive complaints in primary care, *BMC Fam Pract*, 2017 18(101).

Katz S, Ford AB, Moskowitz RW, et al.: Studies of illness in the aged: the index of ADL: a standardized measure of biological and psychosocial function, *JAMA* 185:914–919, 1963.

Kleinman A: *Patient and healers in the context of culture: an exploration of the borderland between anthropology, medicine, and psychiatry*, Berkeley, CA, 1980, University of California Press.

Lach HW, Chang YP, Edwards D: Can older adults accurately report depression using brief forms?, *J Gerontol Nurs* 36:30–37, 2010.

LaPlante MP: The classic measure of disability of activities of daily living is biased by age but an expanded IADL/ADL measure is not, *J Gerontol B Psychol Sci Soc Sci* 65(6):720–732, 2010.

Lawton MP, Brody EM: Assessment of older people: self-maintaining and instrumental activities of daily living, *Gerontologist* 9:179–186, 1969.

Li M, Harris I, Lu ZK: Differences in proxy-reported and patient-reported outcomes: assessing health and functional status among Medicare beneficiaries, *BMC Med Res Methodol*, 2015 15.

Lim HK, Hong SC, Won WY, et al.: Reliability and validity of the Korean versions of the Cornell Scale for Depression in Dementia, *Psychiatry Invest* 9(4):332–338, 2012.

Mahoney FI, Barthel DW: Functional evaluation: the Barthel Index, *Md State Med J* 14:61–65, 1965.

Maust D, Cristancho M, Gray L, et al.: Psychiatric rating scales. In Aminoff MJ, Boller F, Swaab DF, editors: Psychiatric rating scales, *Handbook of clinical neurology* 106:227–237, 2012.

McDougall GJ: A review of screening instruments for assessing cognition and mental status in older adults, *Nurse Pract* 15(11):18–28, 1990.

Memória CM, Yassuda MS, Nakano EY, et al.: Brief screen for mild cognitive impairment: validation of the Brazilian version of the Montreal cognitive assessment, *Int J Geriatr Psychiatry* 28(1):34–40, 2013.

Mitchell AJ: A meta-analysis of the accuracy of the Mini-Mental Status Examination in the detection of dementia and mild cognitive impairment, *J Psychiatr Res* 43:411–431, 2009.

Mitchell AJ, Malladi S: Screening and case finding tools for the detection of dementia. Part 1. Evidence-based meta-analysis of multidomain tests, *Am J Geriatr Psychiatry* 18:759–782, 2010.

Montgomery J, Mitty E, Flores S: Resident condition change: should I call 911?, *Geriatr Nurs* 29:15–26, 2008.

Nair AK, Gavett BE, Damman M, et al.: Clock Drawing Test ratings by dementia specialists: interrater reliability and diagnostic accuracy, *J Neuropsychiatry Clin Neurosci* 22(1):85–92, 2010.

Nikula S, Jylhä M, Bardage C, et al.: Are ADLs comparable across countries? Sociodemographic associates of harmonized IADL measures, *Aging Clin Exp Res* 15(6):451–459, 2003.

Ortiz I, Romero L: Cultural implications for assessment and treatment of depression in Hispanic elderly individuals, *Ann Longterm Care*, 2008 16(45).

Patnode CD, Perdue LA, Rossom RC, et al.: Screening for cognitive impairment in older adults: updated evidence report and systematic review for the US Prevention Services Task Force, *JAMA* 323(8):764–785, 2020.

Quinn TJ, Langhorne P, Stott DJ: Barthel Index for stroke trials: development, properties and application, *Stroke* 42:1146–1151, 2011.

Rayegani SM, Raeissadat SA, Alikhani E, et al.: Evaluation of complete functional status of patients with stroke by Functional Independence Scale on admission, discharge, and six months post-stroke, *Iran J Neurol* 15(4):202–208, 2016.

Reisberg B: Functional Assessment Staging (FAST), *Psychopharmacol Bull*, 1988 24(653).

Sangha H, Lipson D, Foley N, et al.: A comparison of the Barthel Index and the Functional Independence Measure as outcome measures in stroke rehabilitation: patterns of disability scale usage in clinical trials, *Int J Rehabil Res* 28:135–139, 2005.

Sclan SG, Reisberg B: Functional Assessment Staging (FAST) in Alzheimer's disease: reliability, validity, and ordinality, *Int Psychogeriatr* 4:55–69, 1992.

Sheehan B: Assessment scales in dementia, *Ther Adv Neurol Disord* 5(6):349–358, 2012.

Shulkin DJ: *Physical medicine and rehabilitation outcomes for inpatient rehabilitation units, VHA Directive 1225*, Washington, DC, 2017, Department of Veterans Affairs https://www.va.gov/vhapublications/ViewPublication.asp?pub_ID=5328.

Söderström L, Rosenblad A, Adolfsson ET, et al.: Malnutrition is associated with increased mortality in older adults regardless of the cause of death, *Br J Nutr* 117(4):532–540, 2017.

Volpato S, Guralnick JM: The different domains of the comprehensive geriatric assessment. In Pilotto A, Martin FC, editors: *Comprehensive geriatric assessment*, Cham, Switzerland, 2013, Springer International, pp 11–27.

Yeager JJ: Assessment of the older adult. In Meiner SE, Yeager JJ: *Gerontological nursing*, 6, St Louis, 2019, Elsevier, pp 54–75.

Yesavage JA, Brink TL, Rose TL, et al.: Development and validation of a geriatric depression screening scale: a preliminary report, *J Psychiatr Res* 17:37–49, 1983.

10 CHAPTER

Using Laboratory Data in Clinical Judgment

Kathleen Jett

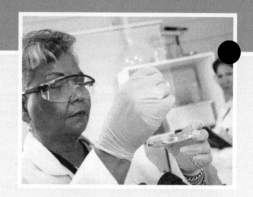

http://evolve.elsevier.com/Touhy/TwdHlthAging

A STUDENT SPEAKS

I always thought that as people got older, their blood sugars went up a little and that was okay. Now I realize that an elevation in fasting glucose means a potential problem regardless of one's age.

Susan, age 20

AN OLDER ADULT SPEAKS

Every time I turn around, somebody wants my blood. They say that they need to "watch me closely," but I am not sure what that has to do with my blood. What if they take too much and it causes me to get sick?

Sung Ye, age 92

LEARNING OBJECTIVES

On completion of this chapter, the reader will be able to:

1. Recognize the key laboratory tests used to monitor common health problems in later life.
2. Analyze the meaning of deviations in key laboratory values that are the most important to the older adult.
3. Recognize the precautions the nurse should take when interpreting laboratory values in older adults.

Since ancient times, the diagnosis of medical problems was based in part on the results of laboratory tests. The results were thought to be quantitative measures of health or illness. "Standards" or "reference ranges" were statistically determined based on the results drawn from adults with no known health problems.

However, a comparable "reference range" for older adults has not been established (Lapin & Mueller, 2017). First, the older one is, the more likely one is to have acquired at least one or more chronic diseases (multimorbidity), any of which *could* influence laboratory findings. Second, it has been well established that aging is a continuous and progressive decline in physiological function, which has the *potential* to affect the findings (Chapter 3). Finally, age-related reference ranges cannot account for the high degree of *individual variability* that occurs during senescence. Factors to consider include physical endurance, nutritional status, mobility, cognitive status, genetic makeup, and predominant diseases (Lapin & Mueller, 2017).

Unfortunately, structural factors also influence laboratory results that are particularly relevant to frail older adults. For example, Laboratory A performs phlebotomy services for Nursing Home A. One day the phlebotomist is late, arriving after breakfast, but "fasting" tests are drawn nonetheless, and the discrepancy may or may not make it to the attention of the medical or nursing provider. On most days Nursing Home A is the first of several stops for Laboratory A, and specimens are chronically late getting to the analytical laboratory. If any abnormalities are found, are they reflections of health or disease or aging or structural problems? As the availability of "point-of-care tests" (POCTs) increases, some of these problems will be resolved.

The nurse's analysis of laboratory values assumes special meaning when working with older adults. In this chapter the most common laboratory data collected from older adults are reviewed.

HEMATOLOGICAL TESTING

Hematological testing refers to that associated with the blood and lymph and their component parts: red blood cells (RBCs), white blood cells (WBCs), and cell fragments called *platelets*. Together the cells float in a fluid matrix called *plasma*. A basic complete blood count (CBC) provides the number of RBCs, WBCs, platelets, and the hematocrit and hemoglobin indices. A CBC with a "differential" refers to the inclusion of the subtypes of the WBCs: granulocytes (neutrophils, basophils, and eosinophils) and agranulocytes (lymphocytes and monocytes).

Hematological laboratory tests are often used to diagnose infection, anemia, or to check for the presence of potential side effects of treatment such as chemotherapeutic agents. They also are used to assist in determining a hypothesis related to reported fatigue, weakness, shortness of breath, or headache and the cues of increased heart rate, low blood pressure, or pallor. Several conditions more common in older adults affect the results, especially dehydration, malnutrition, infection, and inflammation.

Red Blood Cell Count

The primary function of the RBCs (erythrocytes) is to transport molecules of hemoglobin. They are produced primarily by the bone marrow of the long bones. If the person is dehydrated, the RBC will be artificially high and the cues to anemia cannot be recognized. Once the person is hydrated, anemia may be found. As it is normal for the sense of thirst to decrease with age, hydration status must be considered before completing any analysis of these data. With an average life span of 120 days, the RBCs are constantly being replenished in younger adults. In older adults red blood cells are still replaced as needed, but more slowly due to declines in hematopoietic reserves. This becomes a potential problem with a loss of blood, such as after repeated phlebotomy or with frank bleeding. Recovery from the loss takes much longer, increasing the risk of falling, delirium, and other geriatric syndromes (Chapter 22).

A low RBC count for whatever reason is referred to as anemia and becomes more common with increasing frailty or an accumulation of chronic diseases. An overproduction of RBCs, or polycythemia, may be the result of heart failure or chronic pulmonary disease as the body fights the associated hypoxia.

Hemoglobin and Hematocrit

Hemoglobin (Hgb), a conjugated protein, is the main component of the RBC. It contains iron and the red pigment porphyrin. The iron is part of protein synthesis in the mitochondria, essential for generating cellular energy and transporting oxygen from the lungs to the tissues and carbon dioxide from the tissues to the lungs.

> ## ⚡ SAFETY TIP
>
> A hemoglobin level equal to or less than 5 g/dL, or more than 20 g/dL, is considered a "critical value" regardless of age and may require urgent intervention. Older adults may begin to exhibit cues of the physiological distress with a reduced RBC well before a critical value is reached.

The lower the Hgb, the more often the nurse will recognize impaired mobility and cognition, frailty, and falls in older adults (Reuben et al., 2020). If there is a sudden drop, it may be the result of trauma, such as a subdural hematoma following a fall, and is always a medical emergency. If the Hgb drops slowly (a "slow bleed"), an older adult may complain of fatigue, confusion, shortness of breath, or difficulty with ambulation. A common cause is unrecognized gastrointestinal (GI) bleeding, especially associated with the use of nonsteroidal antiinflammatory drugs (NSAIDs). For those nearing the end of life, the invasive testing needed to determine the exact etiology may not be appropriate, and the cause may remain undetermined.

The term *hematocrit* means "to separate blood." It is the *relative percentage* of packed RBCs to the plasma in blood after the two have been separated (often referred to as "spun down"). Although they measure different aspects of the RBCs, the hematocrit and hemoglobin values are comparative numbers, with the Hgb level approximately one-third of the hematocrit value. For example, a person with a Hgb level of 12 g/dL will have a hematocrit of approximately 36%. A sudden increase in the hematocrit is a cue to possible dehydration, whereas a decrease signals the nurse to look for signs of malnutrition or bleeding.

> ## ⚡ SAFETY TIP
>
> **Caution With the Interpretation of Hematocrit and Hemoglobin Levels**
> Elevations in hematocrit and hemoglobin levels may be the result of a pathological process but are more often an early sign of hypovolemia from malnutrition, dehydration, or severe diarrhea. The volume depletion must be corrected before an accurate analysis can be done.

Iron. The primary source of iron is the consumption of iron-containing foods such as dark-green leafy vegetables and red meats. Adequate iron is necessary for cellular protein synthesis and energy. Iron is transported into bone marrow by the plasma protein *transferrin* for storage and later use. The serum concentration of iron is determined by a combination of its absorption and storage and the breakdown and synthesis of Hgb. Iron studies include measurements of serum iron, total iron binding capacity (TIBC), ferritin, and transferrin levels.

> ## EVIDENCE-BASED PRACTICE
>
> A serum ferritin level is the most useful test to differentiate iron deficiency anemia from that associated with long-term chronic disease (now referred to as "chronic inflammation").

The TIBC is a measure of the combination of the amount of iron already in the blood and the amount of transferrin available in the blood serum. Ferritin is a complex molecule made up of ferric hydroxide and a protein; its measurement reflects body iron stores. If the person has adequate iron, the body can respond quickly to the demand for increased oxygen and energy and to replenish iron lost through bleeding.

Anemia. Anemia is diagnosed any time a man's Hgb drops to <13 g/dL or a woman's drops to <12 g/dL (Box 10.1). Although not a normal part of aging, there is an increasing prevalence of anemia with age. Vitamin deficiency associated with protein and energy malnutrition, more common in aging, increases the risk. Between 10% and 24% of those living in the community and at least 65 years of age have diagnosed anemia, as do between 48% and 54% of those residing in nursing homes. The incidence is highest among Blacks compared with Whites and Hispanics (Ershler, 2017).

BOX 10.1 Common Reasons for Anemia in Older Adults

Iron deficiency
Vitamin B$_{12}$/folate deficiency
As a result of renal insufficiency
Chronic inflammation, especially due to chronic illness
Unexplained

BOX 10.2 Potential Cues That May Indicate Anemia in Older Adults

Fatigue
Decreased mobility
Decreased cognitive function or confusion
Increased frailty
Falls
Shortness of breath or dyspnea at rest or with exertion
Tachycardia

Screening for anemia is rarely done in the younger, healthy population. In geriatrics it is more common, especially if cues indicate that a potential problem is present (Box 10.2). Diagnostic testing for anemia includes a CBC with differential, iron studies, and the measurement of several vitamins, especially folic acid and vitamin B12. The gerontological nurse also should carefully consider an assessment of diet any time anemia is suspected or found to be present (Chapter 15).

Anemia that is progressive and untreated or not responsive to treatment will result in the person's death. The gerontological nurse must be able to recognize that it is the potential causative factor for several vague problems and geriatric syndromes (Chapter 22).

White Blood Cells

WBCs (or leukocytes) are the cells of the lymphatic system and tissues that function primarily to protect the body from infection and other foreign invaders such as allergens. They are produced by the bone marrow and thymus and are stored in the lymph nodes, spleen, and tonsils, then travel to the site of invasion. The healthy adult has 5000 to 10,000 WBCs/mm³. The number and type are regulated largely by the endocrine system and by the body's need for a particular type of cell at a point in time. Each cell has a life span of 13 to 20 days, after which it is destroyed in the lymphatic system and excreted in feces. An excess is referred to as *leukocytosis,* and a deficiency as *leukopenia.* Both conditions are more common in the older adult because of adverse side effects of commonly used medications and increased incidence of infection. Medications that can cause leukopenia include some antibiotics, anticonvulsants, antihistamines, analgesics, sulfonamides, and diuretics. On the other hand, leukocytosis may be a side effect of other drugs, including allopurinol, aspirin, heparin, or steroids (Dugdale, 2020).

Granulocytes

Neutrophils. Neutrophils are produced in the bone marrow every 7 to 14 days and are in circulation for about 6 hours. They fight illness by phagocytizing bacteria and other products perceived to be foreign. *Neutrophilia,* or increased numbers of neutrophils, is a nonspecific finding. It may be an indicator of several conditions more common in late life, including connective tissue diseases, such as rheumatoid arthritis; a side effect of medications, such as corticosteroids; or a result of trauma, such as a fall with or without physical injury.

Eosinophils and basophils. Eosinophils ingest antigen-antibody complexes induced by immunoglobulin-E–mediated reactions to attack allergens and parasites. High eosinophil counts are found in people with type I allergies such as hay fever and asthma. Eosinophils are known to diminish in late life due to age-related reductions in immune function (Chapter 27). Basophils transport histamine, a factor in immune and antiinflammatory responses. Like eosinophils, they play a role in allergic reactions but are not involved in bacterial or viral infections.

Agranulocytes

Lymphocytes. Lymphocytes play key roles in the immune system (Lin et al., 2016). Among the types are T and B cells. T cells are produced by the thymus and are active in cell-mediated immunity; B cells are produced in the bone marrow and are involved in the production of antibodies (humoral immunity). While T-cell activity is especially important in late life, due in part to age-related immunosenescence, T-cell responses and T-cell–macrophage activity are slowed (Chapter 3). Measurement of the number of T cells is included in the monitoring of the health status and treatment response of persons who are immunocompromised, such as those who are receiving chemotherapeutic agents or are infected with the human immunodeficiency virus (HIV).

Monocytes. Monocytes are the largest of the leukocytes. When matured, they become macrophages and help defend the body against foreign substances or, more importantly, what the body perceives are foreign substances. The macrophages migrate to a site in the body where they can remove microorganisms, dead RBCs, and foreign debris through the physiological process of phagocytosis. There may be a decline in monocyte function in later life, which leads to a reduced physiological capacity to fight infection. This value must be watched carefully, especially in ill or frail older adults.

Infection

Due to age-related decreases or delayed responses in the immune system, an infection in an older adult is particularly dangerous. A mild rhinovirus (e.g., cold) can quickly become bacterial bronchitis or even life-threatening pneumonia. Older adults are significantly more likely than younger adults to die from infections such as influenza and COVID-19.

Theoretically, one way to determine the intensity of an infection is through the measurement of the WBCs. This is ordered as a "CBC with differential." A WBC count greater than 10,000/mm³ alone is indicative of a potential infection, especially in an older adult. However, up to 50% of those with pneumonia initially will have WBCs that are within normal limits. Up to 95% will have a *left shift*—an abnormally high number of immature neutrophils

BOX 10.3   Atypical Cues of Potential Infection in Older Adults

Decreased functional status
Decreased cognition or confusion
Anorexia and reduced intake
Incontinence
Falls
Fatigue
Exacerbation of a chronic disease, especially diabetes or heart failure
Reduced level of consciousness

(Reuben et al., 2020). Unfortunately, with aging it becomes more and more difficult to detect early indicators of infection. WBC elevation is delayed, and the person may be afebrile early in the infection. Similarly, signs of pneumonia on a chest x-ray may be initially absent. These changes require the gerontological nurse to be knowledgeable and vigilant to atypical cues to infection in older adults that can be easily misinterpreted until too late (Box 10.3).

⚡ SAFETY TIP

Waiting for the "usual signs" of infection in an older adult may result in the person's death. Instead, the nurse must be alert for more subtle signs of illness and respond to these earlier rather than later.

Platelets

Platelets are small, irregular particles known as thrombocytes, an essential ingredient in clotting. They are formed in the bone marrow, lungs, and spleen and released when a blood vessel is injured. As they arrive at the site of injury, they become "sticky," forming a plug at the site to stop the bleeding and to help trigger what is known as the *clotting cascade*. Although the platelet count does not change with aging, there is an increase in the concentrations of coagulation enzymes (factors VII and VIII and fibrinogen). This and other developments indicate a greater possibility of a pathological hypercoagulability. At the same time, older adults are more likely to have blood diatheses (unusual susceptibility to bleeding), resulting in unexplained bruising, nosebleeds, or excessive bleeding with surgery. If any of these signs are present, a platelet count and coagulation studies may be done. Counts of 150,000 to 400,000/mm³ are considered normal. Counts of less than 100,000/mm³ are considered *thrombocytopenia*.

⚡ SAFETY TIP

Spontaneous hemorrhage may occur when the platelet count falls below 20,000/mm³. There is a significantly exacerbated risk of excessive bleeding when anticoagulants (e.g., warfarin, apixaban [Eliquis]) are used in the presence of thrombocytopenia.

When the platelet count is elevated, it is referred to as *thrombocythemia*. It can occur at any age but is more common in those 50 to 70 years old. While the cause is unknown, both abnormal bleeding and clotting can still occur when the count is greater than 1 million/mm³ (National Heart, Lung, and Blood Institute [NHLBI], n.d.). The gerontological nurse caring for older adults, especially those who are frail or who have vague symptoms, is expected to monitor patients at risk for bleeding. A basic understanding of the meaning of the patient's hematological laboratory findings is expected. For frail older adults, such as those in long-term care facilities, thrombocytopenia can quickly lead to death should bleeding occur, such as from NSAID-related gastric bleeding or from an unrecognized subdural hematoma following a fall.

MEASURES OF INFLAMMATION

Erythrocyte Sedimentation Rate

The *erythrocyte sedimentation rate* (ESR), also referred to as the "sed rate," is a proxy measure for the degree of inflammation, infection, necrosis, infarction, or advanced neoplasm that is present. It is slightly elevated in many older adults, most likely attributable to the prevalence of long-standing chronic disease and consequential inflammation (Ferri, 2015). An ESR greater than 100 mm/h is strongly associated with a serious illness; however, when there is no obvious reason for the elevation, the test should be repeated before further testing is done. The ESR may be useful for monitoring several inflammatory diseases and their treatments, such as polymyalgia rheumatica, temporal arteritis, or rheumatoid arthritis (Chapter 28). An ESR that becomes elevated due to a sudden event such as heart failure will stay elevated for weeks (Litao & Kamat, 2014). However, the ESR is a nonspecific test, and this always must be recognized when considering the results.

VITAMINS

Vitamin deficiencies are common in later life and should be considered any time the person complains of vague symptoms (especially fatigue), cognitive impairment develops, wound healing is delayed, or anemia is suspected. Those at highest risk are persons with protein-calorie malnutrition. Vitamin B deficiencies are more likely in those who have been undernourished for long periods of time, such as many of those living in low-income countries, who have been neglected, or who have end-stage dementia (Mathew & Jacobs, 2014). Vitamin D deficiencies are now being found in both apparently healthy and ill adults.

B Vitamins

The two B vitamins that are especially important in aging are folic acid (folate) and B_{12}.

Folate (B_9)

Folate is formed by bacteria in the intestines; it is necessary for the normal functioning of both RBCs and WBCs and for DNA synthesis (Huether et al., 2019). It is stored in the liver and can be found in eggs, milk, green leafy vegetables, yeast, liver, and fruit. Decreases in folate may indicate protein-energy malnutrition, several types of anemia, and liver and renal disease. It is common among persons with chronic alcohol abuse and persons who take any one of several medications, including phenytoin, trimethoprim-sulfamethoxazole, and methotrexate. Prolonged deficiencies can result in cognitive impairment and depression; vitamin B_9 and vitamin B_6 (pyridoxine) levels should be done prior to the diagnoses of either of these conditions.

Due to the number of foods that are enriched with folic acid, the deficiencies and associated anemias are much less common than they were in the past. Nonetheless, the nurse must be alert for potential folate deficiencies when the person has significant nutritional deficits, such as in those who are very frail or abuse alcohol. Folic acid is the manufactured version of folate available as a supplement and added to foods.

Vitamin B_{12}

Vitamin B_{12} (manufactured as synthetic cyanocobalamin) is a water-soluble vitamin required for the normal development of RBCs, for several neurological functions, and for DNA synthesis. Symptoms suggestive of low B_{12} are fatigue, weakness, and memory loss; it can lead to anemia, neuropathy, and cognitive impairments. It cannot be synthesized in the human body and thus must be provided by the diet or supplementation. B_{12} deficiency is common in older adults because of the high prevalence of atrophic gastritis associated with malabsorption (Wong, 2015). Conditions that lead to folate and B_{12} deficiency can result in megaloblastic anemia (large RBCs that do not function properly). Tests of B_{12} and folate levels are now part of the standard workup for dementia or unexplained neurological or functional decline (Sink & Yaffe, 2021).

Vitamin B_{12} is found in the proteins of foods such as eggs, fish, shellfish, and especially meat, but typically only half of the B_{12} is absorbed when ingested by healthy adults with normal gastric function. It is primarily extracted from proteins in the stomach in the presence of gastric acid and other compounds, including intrinsic factor (IF). Pernicious anemia is a type of anemia characterized by lowered IF production by gastric cells. The age-related decrease in the production of gastric acid and IF significantly increases the risk for vitamin B_{12} deficiency. In addition, those who do not eat, cannot afford to eat, or limit their eating of meat should always take supplemental B_{12}.

Vitamin D

Vitamin D is produced in the skin when exposed to ultraviolet light (UV) through the conversion of 7-dehydrocholesterol to vitamin D_3 (cholecalciferol). Levels are measured in the blood considering vitamin D_2 and D_3, and total levels are affected by multiple personal, atmospheric, geographic, and climactic factors. Although there has been no clear consensus on what level indicates a deficiency, a total of less than 50 nmol/L is often used (Neville et al., 2021). Vitamin D deficiencies have been found to be common among all ages but especially in older adults. Vitamin D is a key component in maintaining bone and muscle strength. As of this writing there is a growing consensus regarding the relationship between vitamin D deficiency and poor

prognosis for older adults hospitalized with severe COVID-19 infections. There have been many suggestions that those who enter hospitals with preexisting deficiencies had higher mortality rates, but supplementation did not appear to help (Ali, 2020; Pereira et al., 2020). There is no support that supplementation without deficiency provides benefit (Bennouar et al., 2021).

Those with decreased exposure to UV light, such as many who live in institutional settings or at the extremes of the hemispheres (e.g., Inuit living near the Arctic Circle), are at higher than usual risk for vitamin D deficiencies. The age-related decreases in the ability to synthesize vitamin D in the aging skin exacerbate the risk considerably, even more so in persons with darkly pigmented skin (Webb et al., 2018). Ensuring adequate intake is essential for healthy aging through food, sun exposure, and dietary supplements. Four hundred to 1000 units daily has been recommended as a minimum dose for supplementation for older adults (over-the-counter vitamin D_3) (Ramasamy, 2020).

BLOOD CHEMISTRY STUDIES

Blood chemistry studies include an assortment of laboratory tests used to identify and measure circulating elements and particles in the plasma and blood, including thyroxin-stimulating hormone, glucose, proteins, amino acids, nutritive materials, excretion products, hormones, enzymes, vitamins, minerals, and electrolytes. Due to the number of medications taken and common chronic diseases in older adults, typical tests include lipids (cholesterol and triglycerides), vitamins D and B_{12} (discussed earlier), and thyroid-stimulating hormone. Some of these tests are used for screening and others for monitoring specific health problems or treatments. All tests are individually selected and must be justified by a current diagnosis for reimbursement (Table 10.1). Nurses must become familiar with the names and test components used by the laboratory that provides services to their patients. The advanced practice nurse is expected to know when urgent and disease-monitoring blood chemistry studies are needed and what to do with the results.

Basic and Comprehensive Metabolic Panels

A basic metabolic panel involves seven or eight different measures (Chem 7 or BMP [8 tests]). They measure renal function (creatinine and blood urea nitrogen [BUN]), blood glucose, electrolyte balance, and acid-base balance. The comprehensive

TABLE 10.1 Examples of Laboratory Testing and Associated Diagnoses	
Diagnosis	**Examples of Justified Laboratory Test**
Hypertension	Basic metabolic panel (monitoring renal function and electrolytes related to treatment)
Altered mental status	Complete blood count, comprehensive metabolic panel, vitamin D, vitamin B_{12}, thyroid-stimulating panel, urine analysis (culture and sensitivity if positive)
Dyslipidemia	Lipid panel, liver function (usually part of the comprehensive metabolic panel)

metabolic panel (CMP) includes all the measures found in the BMP plus measures of nutritional status (albumin) and basic liver function.

Electrolytes are inorganic substances that help maintain cellular homeostasis. They regulate hydration and acid-base balance (blood pH) and are critical for nerve and muscle function. An imbalance could be related to a number of things, including overhydration or dehydration. If there is an imbalance of calcium, sodium, or potassium levels, muscle weakness or contractions may occur. Because older adults are more sensitive to electrolyte imbalances, these should be checked any time there is a sudden change in mental status, an adjustment or addition of a medication (e.g., diuretic), a change in fluid intake, or a transfer of the patient from one setting to another (e.g., home to hospital, nursing home to hospital, general unit to intensive care unit). Excessive diuresis, medication interactions, dehydration, and diarrhea are probably the most common causes of electrolyte imbalances in older adults.

A normal age-related change is decreased renal function. Since all electrolytes are excreted by the kidneys, older adults are more at risk for imbalances. Those at the highest risk are acutely ill, frail, reside in long-term care facilities, or take multiple medications (Chapter 11). Imbalances can occur quickly and be life-threatening in older adults. While all electrolyte abnormalities are important, the ones most often seen by gerontological nurses are associated with sodium and potassium.

⚡ SAFETY TIP

A minor electrolyte imbalance may have little effect in younger adults but may have significantly deleterious effects in older adults, especially those who are medically or cognitively fragile. In the older adult, the symptoms to an imbalance of any kind include weakness, fatigue, immobility, falling, or delirium (altered mental status).

Sodium

Serum sodium (Na+) is necessary for the maintenance of blood pressure, the transmission of nerve impulses, and the regulation of body fluids. The serum sodium level is a measurement of the balance between ingested and excreted sodium relative to body fluid (Table 10.2). Sodium is always accompanied by chloride (Cl−) as sodium chloride.

TABLE 10.2 Signs and Symptoms of Disturbances in Sodium Levels

	Hyponatremia	Hypernatremia
Signs	Plasma Na+ ≤130 mmol/L (approximately)	Plasma Na+ ≥150 mmol/L (approximately)
	Drop in blood pressure	Poor skin turgor
	Tachycardia	Dry mucous membranes
Symptoms	Mental status changes	Mental status changes

Hyponatremia. The causes of hyponatremia can be divided into three types: increased extracellular fluid (ECF) volume, impaired water excretion (e.g., renal insufficiency), and, least often in late life, the syndrome of inappropriate antidiuretic hormone (SIADH) secretion. In most cases the cause of hyponatremia is multifactorial in older adults. Several medications place a person at higher risk, including thiazide diuretics and several antidepressants, including mirtazapine (Remeron). Those with poor diets (i.e., low salt and protein accompanied by *increased* intake of water) are also at risk (Filippatos et al., 2017).

Hyponatremia is usually asymptomatic until the plasma sodium concentration drops below 130 mEq/L. Malaise, confusion, headache, and nausea may be recognizable symptoms with levels of 125 to 130 mEq/L or less. With further loss, seizures and coma secondary to cerebral edema may develop quickly, and cues suggestive of these conditions must be recognized and analyzed promptly to prioritize care. Hypovolemic hyponatremia is always accompanied by a significant drop in postural blood pressure and tachycardia as the body attempts to compensate. In the most severe cases, hyponatremia can result in a high mortality rate. Hyponatremia is one of the more common causes of delirium in older adults. *Slow replacement is necessary.*

Hypernatremia. An elevation of plasma sodium concentration (>145 mEq/L) indicates a deficit in total body water relative to total body sodium (i.e., less water intake than output). It is usually caused by either reduced or impaired thirst (normal part of aging), prolonged nausea and vomiting, or limited access to water. It is common among older adults, especially those who are taking diuretics or who are frail, hospitalized, or living in long-term care facilities where they are dependent on others for assistance obtaining fluids. Symptoms of hypernatremia include confusion, thirst, weakness, nausea, and muscle twitching (Lewis, 2021a). The mortality rate in the older adult is considerable unless nursing interventions are prioritized promptly (Shah et al., 2014).

Potassium

Potassium (K+) is an electrolyte found primarily within the cells. It is essential in maintaining cell osmolality, ensuring muscle functioning, and transmitting nerve impulses. It is a key component in the maintenance of the acid-base balance. Serum potassium levels should remain within an expected range but will decrease as age-related lean body mass decreases. When the person is taking any K+-sparing or wasting medications, as is common in later life, potassium level must be closely monitored.

Hypokalemia. Excess renal (e.g., diuresis) or GI tract (e.g., diarrhea) loss are the most common causes of hypokalemia (K+ <3.5 mEq/L). Mild hypokalemia is asymptomatic (i.e., no cues may be initially recognized), but muscle weakness and polyuria develop as the loss increases. Through polyuria body fluid is reduced and the relative serum potassium increases. Potassium levels less than 3.0 mEq/L are critical, and signs include cramping, confusion, fatigue, paralytic ileus, electrocardiogram (ECG) changes and tachycardia, fibrillation, and sudden death (Lewis, 2021b). Chronic low levels of potassium may lead to significant renal tubular dysfunction.

Hyperkalemia. Hyperkalemia (K+ >5.5 mEq/L) most often results when potassium is not adequately excreted via the

BOX 10.4 Signs and Symptoms of Disturbances in Potassium Levels

Hypokalemia	Hyperkalemia
Generalized muscle weakness	Impaired muscle activity
Fatigue	Weakness
Muscle cramps	Muscle pain or cramps
Constipation	Increased GI motility
Ileus	Bradycardia
Flaccid paralysis	Cardiac arrest
Hyporeflexia	ECG changes:
Hypercapnia	P wave flattened
Tetany	T wave large, peaked
ECG changes:	QRS broad
Q-T interval prolonged	Biphasic QRS-T complex
T wave flattened or depressed	
ST segment depressed	

ECG, Electrocardiogram; *GI*, gastrointestinal.

TABLE 10.3 Cues to Hypoglycemia and Hyperglycemia in Older Adults

Hypoglycemia	Hyperglycemia
Confusion	No cues may be present
Fatigue	Fatigue
Tachycardia	Dehydration
Tremors	Obtunded or coma
Headache	
Reduced level of consciousness	
Obtunded or coma	

kidneys. However, it is also found in those with acidosis, inadequate monitoring of potassium-sparing medications such as angiotensin-converting enzyme (ACE) inhibitors, or excessive potassium supplementation, all highly relevant to older adults. The signs and symptoms of a disturbance in potassium levels may not be evident until cardiac toxicity occurs (Box 10.4) (Malkina & Hadley, 2021).

⚡ SAFETY TIP

If a person is prescribed a potassium-sparing medication such as an angiotensin-converting enzyme (ACE) inhibitor at the same time as a potassium supplement is given, hyperkalemia should be expected in most circumstances. When taking a potassium-wasting medication like furosemide without a potassium supplement (e.g., K-Dur), hypokalemia is likely. Both are life-threatening.

Glucose

Glucose is a complex sugar produced by the pancreas. Glucose and fat circulate in the blood as sources of physiological energy. A consistent supply always must be available to the brain. When not in use, it is stored in skeletal muscle and the liver as glycogen. The level of fasting glucose in the body is between about 70 and 99 mg/dL. Although the required levels do not change with aging, confusion and depressed central nervous system activity are possible with even slight hypoglycemia. Fasting blood glucose levels are in the high normal range, and it takes longer to return to normal levels after eating. These changes appear to be most likely related to a decrease in the insulin sensitivity of the tissues (Chapter 27). Elevations are well tolerated, and due to a blunted reaction to hyperglycemia it may not be evident until the person is in a hyperosmolar hyperglycemic state (HHS) or coma (Table 10.3). Analysis and prioritization of hypotheses are done within the context of time since the person has eaten.

Glycosylated hemoglobin A_{1C}. Laboratory testing of blood glucose and plasma glucose levels provide "snapshot" information at any one time. About 6.5% of the hemoglobin in the RBCs can combine with glucose through the process of glycosylation. The glucose attachment is not easily reversible and therefore stays for the life of the RBC, approximately 120 days, and provides a good estimate of the average blood glucose and measured through a glycosylated hemoglobin A_{1C} (Hgb A_{1C}) blood test. An A_{1C} of 8% correlates with an estimated average glucose of about 200 mg/dL. In nondiabetics, less than 5.7% is the normal range regardless of one's age; however, the A_{1C} goal for diabetes is now individually determined. Strict glycemic control and a consequential low A_{1C} is an independent risk factor for frailty (Yanase et al., 2018).

However, the "normal" A_{1C} is based on a White, healthy adult population. Several studies have found that there are significant differences in "average" Hgb A_{1C} results among Blacks, Asians, and Latinx in the United States when it is compared to that of Whites. In all cases the levels were higher (American Diabetes Association, 2020; Cavagnolli et al., 2017). The results can be further skewed in persons with conditions that alter the life span of the RBC, such as those taking erythropoietin to stimulate RBC growth.

Albumin

Albumin is a protein that makes up about 60% of the blood protein and has been part of a nutritional assessment and an indicator of liver and kidney function. More recent research indicates that a low level reflects chronic inflammation rather than protein stores or weight (Alves et al., 2018). As inflammation is now considered a part of the aging process (Chapter 3), it is not surprising that albumin levels drop with aging. The concentration of serum albumin also depends on many factors such as body losses, hepatic synthesis, rate and extent of protein breakdown, malnutrition, malabsorption, and immobility.

Although serum protein measurements are commonly ordered, they are neither sensitive nor specific for nutritional health and are often in the low range of normal in older adults. Dehydration will show a deceptive increase in albumin levels at the same time albumin levels appear to decrease with overhydration, liver and renal disease, malabsorption, and changes from an upright position to a supine position during the blood draw (Connor, 2020). The half-life of albumin is about 3 weeks, so changes are not quickly apparent except in sudden and acutely severe conditions. However, albumin levels are most useful as an indicator of the severity of illness and the risk of mortality. Prealbumin (transthyretin) has a half-life of only 2 to 3 days and is therefore a more sensitive marker for change. A low prealbumin level can confirm poor nutritional status and serve to monitor for active treatment.

URIC ACID

Uric acid is a naturally occurring end product of purine metabolism. It is usually measured in specific serum chemistry studies but is also found in the urine. Two-thirds of the amount normally produced is excreted by the kidneys and therefore can be used as a measure of renal function. Elevations in uric acid levels (>7 mg/dL) are found when there is either *overproduction* or *underexcretion*. It is used in but not a requirement for diagnosing gout. Warfarin, frequently taken by older adults, represses the uric acid level, complicating the analysis of laboratory data (Ferri, 2015). While all persons with gout have an elevated uric acid level (>13 mg/dL), others with elevated uric acid levels do not have cues suggestive of gout. Several conditions and situations can result in increased uric acid levels, such as hypothyroidism; binge alcohol drinking; some medications, especially thiazide diuretics, aspirin, and those given for Parkinson's disease, surgery, or an acute medical illness. The use of thiazide diuretics in the person with preexisting elevations in uric acid levels may trigger an acute episode or an exacerbation of chronic gout (Chapter 27). The levels increase slightly with age.

PROSTATE-SPECIFIC ANTIGEN

A blood test to measure the prostate-specific antigen (PSA) had been the primary screening tool for prostate cancer. After detailed examination of the science it was concluded that while there was a slight benefit to this testing, there were significant potential harms. The harms all relate to the large number of false positives; an elevated PSA also may result from enlargement, inflammation, or stimulation of the prostate during a rectal exam prior to the laboratory test. The false positives led to aggressive additional testing or treatment when cancer was not actually present. Common harms of treating the "cancer" included impotence, incontinence (bowel and bladder), or death from unnecessary surgery. In 2018, the US Preventive Services Task Force (USPSTF) recommended that PSA no longer be used for screening except in certain circumstances (Box 10.5). The PSA continues to be used as a gross measure of men's responsiveness to *treatment* of prostate cancer. When appropriate, screening for prostate cancer using the PSA usually begins at the age of 55. It is recommended that screening is stopped at the age of 70 (USPSTF, 2018).

LABORATORY TESTING FOR CARDIAC HEALTH

Heart disease remains the primary cause of noninfectious deaths worldwide. As a result, the gerontological nurse must be knowledgeable about the most common laboratory testing related to cardiac function. These include measures performed after acute cardiac events and those used in the determination of cardiac health and health risk.

BOX 10.5 Prostate Screening With the PSA

The most recent U.S. Prevention Services Task Force guidelines recommend against screening for men over 70 years of age. Screening for others is to be considered. African American men more often develop more aggressive forms of prostate cancer and at a younger age than their white counterparts. While there is still inadequate research relating to African American men, screening may be somewhat helpful. There also may be some benefit for screening men with a strong family history of prostate cancer. Those with two to three close relatives may be at risk for a genetic type of the cancer. The evidence to support routine screening is not conclusive.

From US Preventive Services Task Force: *Prostate cancer: screening* (website), 2018. https://www.uspreventiveservicestaskforce.org/uspstf/document/RecommendationStatementFinal/prostate-cancer-screening.

Acute Cardiac Events

Older adults who appear to have acute and unexpected changes may be having, or recently had, an acute ischemic event and need immediate transportation to an emergency department for evaluation unless otherwise indicated in their advance directive confirmed at the time of event. Initial testing for an acute myocardial infarction (AMI) will include at least an ECG and measurement of cardiac enzymes or tissue markers (creatinine kinase and troponin). Measurement of inflammation with the high-sensitivity C-reactive protein (hs-CRP) and ESR are often used in combination.

Creatinine Kinase

The enzyme creatinine kinase (CK) is present in various parts of the body and in several forms (called isoenzymes). An elevation in CK may occur in rhabdomyolysis and cerebrovascular accidents, both of which are common among older adults (Ferri, 2015). An elevation in the isoenzyme CK-MB is associated with cardiac tissue injury and in the diagnosis of an AMI and several conditions. The CK-MB level rises in the first 3 to 6 hours after the onset of AMI symptoms, peaks at 12 to 24 hours (unless the ischemia continues), and returns to normal in 12 to 48 hours; therefore it is not a useful measure after that period. A number of medications used to manage chronic diseases can cause false CK-MB testing results (Box 10.6). For the best diagnosis, CK-MB is used as a comparative measure with troponin (Reuben et al., 2020).

Troponin

A troponin is a skeleton and cardiac muscle protein not normally found in the blood. Either transient or persistent troponin I and troponin T elevations can be caused by both acute cardiac

---

BOX 10.6 Medications That Can Cause False CK-MB Results

Anticoagulants	Alcohol
Aspirin	Lovastatin
Dexamethasone	Lidocaine
Furosemide	Propranolol
Captopril	Morphine
Colchicine	

CK, Creatinine kinase.

and noncardiac events or conditions. Of the multiple causes, the most relevant to the older adult and therefore most important to the gerontological nurse are hypertension, acute congestive heart failure, sepsis, rhabdomyolysis, and acute central nervous events (Reuben et al., 2020). A troponin T of 0.50 ng/mL or more indicates a strong probability of an AMI. This sensitive marker is seen within the first 48 hours after the AMI and remains elevated for 5 to 7 days. The cardiac troponin I can be seen in the first 3 to 4 hours, peaking at 24 hours and persisting for up to 7 days. The higher the troponin I, the higher the risk of death (Ferri, 2015).

Due to the asymptomatic ("silent") nature of the AMI in many older adults, the troponins may be measured incidentally to another acute health problem. An elevated troponin with a normal CK-MB can be used to identify reinfarction both in the first week after an AMI and in the ensuing 5 years (Reuben et al., 2020).

Monitoring Cardiovascular Risk and Health

Increasing attention has been given to three biochemical markers that are believed to have value in the detection of heart disease, in the assessment for risk of cardiovascular disease, or for decreasing the risk of future cardiac events. These are hs-CRP, homocysteine, and brain natriuretic peptide. Detection and monitoring of dyslipidemia and elevated triglyceride levels are important for determining both health and health risk (Takata et al., 2014).

hs-CRP

C-reactive protein (CRP) is produced by the liver and increases whenever there is inflammation somewhere in the body. It is recommended that persons with at least one risk factor for coronary artery disease have at least one measurement of serum CRP to establish a baseline for later comparison (Reuben et al., 2020).

Although originally used to determine solely cardiac events, CRP has been found to be a useful indicator for other forms of inflammation, such as after an injury, following surgery, or in the presence of infection. The CRP can also be used as a marker for cardiac risk, such as identifying those with "silent" atherosclerosis prior to a cardiac event (Ferri, 2015). Tests of both CRP and ESR are used at the time of an acute event for the determination of tissue damage associated with an AMI. It normalizes in 3 to 7 days. The high-sensitivity assay hs-CRP has increased the accuracy of the measurement even at low levels.

Homocysteine

Serum homocysteine is a naturally occurring amino acid produced during the metabolism of proteins such as meat. The range considered normal increases with age (>59 years old: 5.8–11.9 μmol/L). Elevations are associated with and increase the risk for dementia, atherosclerosis, strokes, AMI, and peripheral vascular disease. Elevations are also present in B6, B12, and folic acid deficiencies (Ferri, 2015).

B-type Natriuretic Peptide

B-type natriuretic peptide (BNP) and the N-terminal pro-B-type natriuretic peptide (NT-proBNP) are produced by the heart and released when it is stretched. The values increase with age and are higher in women (Zhang et al., 2019). Elevations are found in several cardiac conditions but most often in acute heart failure. An elevated BNP is a predictor of mortality from sudden death in those with cardiovascular disease (Zhang et al., 2015). BNP and NT-proBNP levels are also used to monitor the effectiveness of treatment of heart disease.

Lipid Panels

Elevated cholesterol and triglycerides have been found to be health risks regardless of age. When uncontrolled, they are major predictors of coronary heart disease. Laboratory testing is usually done as a lipid panel. This provides a total cholesterol, a low-density lipoprotein (LDL), a high-density lipoprotein (HDL), and a triglyceride level. It is done both as a routine health screen and as a means of monitoring the response to treatment. Fasting for 12 to 15 hours before the test is required for accuracy.

Cholesterol. Cholesterol is a sterol compound used by the body to stabilize cell membranes. It is metabolized in the liver, where it is combined with LDL, HDL, and very-low-density lipoprotein (VLDL). There continues to be considerable discussion regarding the necessity of treating hypercholesterolemia in persons over the age of 75 (Spencer-Bonilla et al., 2021).

High-density lipoprotein (HDL). Referred to as "good cholesterol," HDL transports cholesterol to the liver for degradation. In general, the HDL should be greater than 60 mg/dL, but the HDL-LDL ratio is probably more important.

Low-density lipoprotein. Referred to as "bad cholesterol," LDL transports cholesterol from the liver into the body.

For many years there had been widespread belief in a direct relationship between high cholesterol and the development of heart disease at any age. Goals for specific levels of each component of the lipid panel were predetermined. The most recent guidelines of the American Heart Association suggest that there is no longer a "one size fits all." It is now recommended that multiple factors be considered when the "numbers" are reviewed and a 10-year risk for an acute myocardial infarction is calculated (https://static.heart.org/riskcalc/app/index.html#!/baseline-risk). Persons of South Asian descent have the highest risk (Grundy et al., 2019). Nonetheless, a total cholesterol level of 200 mg/dL or more has also been suggested to increase neuropsychiatric symptoms in Alzheimer's disease, especially in men (Hall et al., 2014). A total cholesterol level *less than 160 mg/dL* in a frail older adult is a risk factor for increased mortality. In one study hypolipidemia was associated with increased severity of COVID-19 infected individuals (Wei et al., 2021)

Triglycerides. Triglycerides are produced in the liver and circulated in the blood. Most of the serum triglycerides combine with the VLDL. Excess blood levels are deposited into fatty tissue for later energy use. Reasons for elevated levels include chronic renal failure, poorly controlled diabetes, and genetic predisposition. Severely elevated triglyceride levels (>2000 mg/dL) are a strong risk factor for pancreatitis (Mathew & Jacobs, 2014).

LABORATORY TESTS OF RENAL HEALTH

Renal function decreases substantially with age, but in most cases the body can adequately compensate for this, and laboratory findings stay "within normal limits." However, laboratory findings may be *unreliable* in those with reduced lean body mass (a normal change with aging), excessive dietary intake of protein, alterations in metabolism, and strenuous physical activity before measurement. Because of the frequency of health problems and medications that affect renal health, measuring and monitoring renal functioning are particularly important to the older adult and the gerontological nurse. Laboratory indices particularly diagnostic of renal disease are elevated BUN and creatinine levels. These are included in metabolic panels.

Blood Urea Nitrogen

Urea nitrogen is the end product of protein metabolism. The blood urea nitrogen (BUN) is used as a gross measurement for renal functioning and level of hydration. Blood levels are often in the high-normal range because of the age-related changes to the liver and kidney. Changes over time in the BUN level may be more important than any one laboratory result, especially in the assessment of dehydration, renal insufficiency, or renal failure. *Azotemia* is an elevation of BUN level. Prerenal azotemia refers to elevations before blood reaches the kidneys; causes include shock, severe dehydration, congestive heart failure, and excessive protein catabolism such as in starvation.

Creatinine

Creatinine is a waste product resulting from the breakdown of muscle that is normally produced in energy metabolism; its level is highly dependent on muscle mass. If muscle mass remains the same, the serum creatinine level should be constant. The reduced lean muscle mass of normal aging will result in a decreased creatinine level. The BUN creatinine ratio is usually considered together in the evaluation of renal function.

The glomerular filtration rate (GFR) is a measure of the flow of filtered fluid through the kidneys and derived from blood creatinine levels. As the GFR normally decreases with aging, the nurse must take this into consideration any time a nephrotoxic medication is administered or prescribed. The GFR is an estimated number and is usually calculated by the laboratory.

The calculation of the creatinine clearance (CrCl) is an alternate means of the measurement of renal function. The age, race, sex, weight, and serum creatinine are required. Multiple calculators are available online, for example, at http://nephron.com/cgi-bin/CGSI.cgi (Chapter 11).

MONITORING FOR THERAPEUTIC BLOOD LEVELS

The monitoring of blood levels of certain medications is especially important at any time but more so in later life as medications requiring blood level monitoring are prescribed more often and inappropriate dosing can more easily be life-threatening.

Anticoagulants

Anticoagulation therapy has become the mainstay of stroke prevention for persons with atrial fibrillation and artificial heart valves and in the treatment or prevention of deep vein thrombosis (Chapter 23). When the blood is excessively anticoagulated, the person is at risk for life-threatening bleeding. When the levels of anticoagulants in the blood are too low, the protective qualities are lost.

Traditional anticoagulants (warfarin, heparin, and low-molecular-weight heparin) must be monitored closely to ensure that the correct dose is being administered. The newer anticoagulants with a direct mechanism of action (DOACs) (e.g., Xarelto, Pradaxa) do not require laboratory monitoring. Concentrations of the latter can be measured by a combination of liquid chromatography and mass spectrometry, but there is wide variability and associated therapeutic dosages have not yet been determined.

The activated partial thromboplastin time (APTT), the activated clotting time (ACT), and/or the anti–factor Xa level are used to monitor intravenous (IV) heparin infusions. Monitoring of low-molecular-weight heparin (Lovenox) is not required but can be accomplished with the anti–factor Xa in the presence of renal failure, at the extremes of body weight, or in any situation where there is an increased risk for bleeding.

In the past, precise monitoring of the anticoagulation effects of warfarin (Coumadin, Jantoven) was difficult because of the amount of variation in results between laboratories. To overcome these difficulties, an international normalized ratio (INR) is now used. The INR can be measured by a laboratory or at the point of care (POC), such as in a clinic or a care facility, using a device similar to a blood glucose monitor. Most of the time standard ranges are used: 2.0 to 3.0 for those treated for atrial fibrillation or flutter and 2.5 to 3.5 for persons with a mechanical heart valve, deep vein thrombosis, or pulmonary embolism. Some persons self-monitor, with their cardiologists receiving the results and adjusting the dose of the warfarin as needed. Specially trained pharmacists and registered nurses often perform the POC INR test.

Digoxin

Digoxin (Lanoxin) is a drug that is prescribed to control ventricular response to chronic atrial fibrillation and in persons with heart failure. It is no longer considered appropriate to use this as a first-line treatment because of side effects and interactions (AGS, 2019). If used, it is initiated slowly and carefully to prevent too rapid a reduction in heart rate.

> ⚡ **SAFETY TIP**
>
> The normal therapeutic range of digoxin is 0.9 to 2.0 ng/mL, with toxicity occurring at levels greater than 3.0 ng/mL. However, because of the normal changes with aging that affect pharmacokinetics, toxicity may be evident at levels well below 3.0 ng/mL.
> Observing for signs of toxicity, regardless of laboratory results, is probably more meaningful; this is especially important for an older adult who is receiving a dose higher than 0.125 mg/day (not recommended) (Box 10.7).

Once the patient's dose is stabilized, the nurse monitors the effect of the medication by measuring the heart rate before drug

BOX 10.7   Cues of Possible Digitalis ("dig") Toxicity

Lethargy	Visual disturbances
Confusion	Irregular or slowed pulse
Anorexia	Sense of palpitations
Nausea and/or vomiting	Syncope
Diarrhea	

Note: The same cues may be recognized with the ingestion of foxglove, oleander, or lily of the valley.

administration, by observing for cues indicating possible side effects or adverse drug events, and by assuring that blood levels are obtained at any time there are changes dose or in the person's health.

Thyroid Panels

A thyroid panel is used to both diagnose thyroid disorders and monitor their treatment. The panel includes measurement of the level of thyroid-stimulating hormone (TSH), free triiodothyronine (T_3), and free thyroxin (T_4). Each of these is considered relative to the others and used to make a diagnosis (Chapter 27). A thyroid panel is always done to "rule out" a disorder prior to a diagnosis for depression or dementia is made. In most cases, treatment can be monitored based on TSH levels alone. Testing is repeated initially at 6- to 8-week intervals until a euthyroid state is reached and confirmed. After that, only annual reevaluations are necessary unless there is a change in the person's health status. The nurse is in a key position to monitor the thyroid function of the patient by ensuring timely and appropriate laboratory testing of TSH level.

URINE STUDIES

Urine is the end product of metabolism and should only contain products that have exceeded the body's threshold of usefulness. If the kidneys are working well and the urine level of a compound is elevated, there should be a corresponding elevation in the blood. However, if the kidney is diseased, urine levels may be deceptively low. The most common urine test in the everyday care of older adults is a urinalysis.

A macroscopic urinalysis ("urine dip") may be performed in any setting but is often done microscopically in a diagnostic laboratory. In healthy aging, the findings do not differ by age, but abnormalities are frequently found because of the high rate of diabetes, renal insufficiency, subclinical bacteriuria, and proteinuria.

A urine specimen is collected either by using the clean-catch method or via catheterization. In the outpatient setting, it is best that the specimen be collected at the laboratory or sent to the lab immediately. If necessary, it may be collected and refrigerated. Any specimen that has not been properly stored or tested promptly must be disposed of and a new one obtained. The cleaner and fresher the specimen, the more accurate the laboratory analysis. It may be impossible to obtain a clean-catch specimen from someone who cannot understand directions or has urinary or fecal incontinence. If so, the nurse must depend on

more gross signs of health or illness based on color and odor of the urine and changes in amount of incontinence or mental status and behavior. There is a long history of conflicting evidence of the accuracy and reliability of urine testing using the "dipstick" method in the outpatient setting even when it is automated with a POC device. Both laboratory and outpatient office analyses will yield results for urine specific gravity, pH, and the presence of urine protein, glucose, ketones, blood, bilirubin, nitrates, leukocytes, and blood.

> ⚡ **SAFETY TIP**
>
> A finding of hematuria, even in outpatient macroscopy, always requires further evaluation.

The specific gravity is a measure of the adequacy of the renal concentrative mechanism and measures hydration and therefore is a useful measure when caring for frail older adults. Specific gravity in the adult is normally between 1.005 and 1.030. These values decrease with aging because of the 33% to 50% decline in the number of nephrons, which impairs the ability of the kidney to concentrate urine. The urine pH indicates its acid-base balance. An alkaline pH (higher pH) is usually caused by bacteria (which may indicate a urinary tract infection), a diet high in citrus fruits and vegetables, or the intake of sodium bicarbonates. Acidic urine (lower pH) occurs with starvation, dehydration, and diets high in meats and cranberries. A urine albumin level of almost 30 mg/dL translates into a considerably high rate of proteinuria and always indicates a need for further evaluation of renal function. Ascorbic acid and aspirin can cause false-negative results for glucose. Ketones may be positive in high-protein diets, "crash" diets, or starvation.

Nitrates and/or leukocytes usually are found only in the presence of infection. With additional data indicating the presence of more than 100,000 bacteria, a culture is usually indicated and a subsequent testing of sensitivity of the bacteria to select antibiotics is done. This is often ordered as a "U/A, C & S as indicated" (urine analysis, culture and sensitivity if UA is positive). However, due to the potential lethality of any infection in frail and ill older adults, medical treatment may be based on the results of the initial urinalysis and nonlaboratory cues while waiting for the 3 or 4 days needed to obtain culture results.

USING CLINICAL JUDGMENT TO PROMOTE HEALTHY AGING

All nurses caring for older adults are expected to have skills in basic laboratory interpretation, knowledge of the appropriate timing of the testing, and awareness of factors that could affect both the collection of specimens and the results. Advanced practice nurses are responsible for knowing when and what testing to order and to use the results for prescriptive and educational actions to promote healthy aging.

Laboratory findings are often reported in relationship to a range of normalized values or reference ranges referred to as

TABLE 10.4   Potential Age-Related Changes That Can Affect Laboratory Findings and Potential Nursing Actions

Age-Related Change	Potential Result	Reference Range
Delays in RBC production	Increased risk for anemia	Male: $4.3–5.9 \times 10^6/mm^3$ Female: $3.5–5 \times 10^6/mm^3$
↓ T-cell activity	Decreased response to treatment	Total T lymphocytes: $800–2200/mm^3$
↓ Eosinophils	Increased allergic reactions	1%–4% of lymphocytes
↓ Monocytes	Reduced ability to fight an infection	2%–8% of lymphocytes
↑ Coagulation enzymes	Increased risk for clot development	Varying for 7 different factors
↑ ESR	Delayed recognition of pathology	Male: 0–15 mm/h Female: 0–20 mm/h
↓ B_{12}	Fatigue, weakness, memory loss	160–950 pg/mL
↓ K+	Quicker hypokalemia	3.6–5.2 mEq/L
↑ Uric acid	Increased risk for gout	2–7 mg/dL
↑ Homocysteine	Increased risk for cardiovascular diseases, stroke, and dementia	<15 mcmol/L
↑ BNP	Increased risk of heart disease	<100 pg/mL
↓ Albumin	Increased concentrations of protein-bound medications	3.4–5.4 g/dL
↑ BUN	Increased risk for misinterpretation	7–20 mg/dL
↓ Creatinine level	Increased risk for misinterpretation	Male: 0.74–1.35 mg/dL Female: 0.59–1.04 mg/dL
↓ GFR	Increased risk of renal damage from nephrotoxic drugs Potential need for lower doses or dosage adjustment of renally excreted drugs	60 (little support for variation by race)
↓ Specific gravity	Increased risk for misinterpretation	1.0005–1.030

Note: The age-related change may place the person in the high or low range of the reference range, not outside of it.
BNP, B-type natriuretic peptide; *BUN*, blood urea nitrogen; *ESR*, erythrocyte sedimentation rate; *GFR*, glomerular filtration rate; *K+*, potassium; *RBC*, red blood cell.

"within normal limits" (WNL). Age-related changes have the potential to affect results; in health, they should remain within the reference range, increasing or decreasing to higher or lower normal limits (Table 10.4). Special diligence is needed to interpret the results within the context of the normal changes with aging, the person's overall health status, and the presence or absence of nonlaboratory cues.

Diagnostic laboratory tests and regular screening tests are commonly used when caring for a resident of a nursing home. The skill of basic interpretation of these is especially important in this setting where frail older adults are vulnerable to dramatic responses to subtle changes. The nurse must ensure that when abnormalities are recognized, the person is treated promptly and appropriately and care needs are prioritized. Protocols for establishing routine laboratory testing procedures for long-term care vary widely from one institution to the next and from one laboratory to the next. Gerontological nurses advocate good resident care by requesting laboratory tests and developing protocols to comply with recommended evidence-based standards for screening and monitoring for both long-term and short-term residents in all settings.

Laboratory values are helpful tools to augment the recognition of changes in health status and response to treatment, but they are not enough for treatment of the whole person. Abnormal laboratory results should trigger comprehensive patient assessments (Chapter 9). The nurse analyses the results to prioritize care and develop solutions and actions for promoting the healthiest outcomes possible.

KEY CONCEPTS

- The normal range of diagnostic laboratory results does not differ by age.
- Because of more limited reserves, the older adult is often more sensitive to slight variations in biological parameters.
- The nurse is often responsible for the initial interpretation of laboratory results. The nurse cannot depend entirely on laboratory values when considering the possibility of medication toxicity.
- The interactions between medications and chronic disorders complicate the interpretation of laboratory values in older adults.

NEXT-GENERATION NCLEX® (NGN) EXAMINATION–STYLE QUESTIONS

An 84-year-old male, Mr. Jones, is being admitted to the nursing home where you work. He has already had his morning medications. He has a history of heart disease, hypertension, diabetes, constipation, and anemia of chronic inflammation. He denies any fever, chest pain, numbness or tingling, leg swelling, or palpitations. His diabetes has been under good control while at home, but he has difficulty telling you how much insulin he has been taking. His skin is cool to the touch. He is lethargic, but you notice that he also has some muscle twitching. He has an order to have blood tests done today, including a complete blood count (CBC) and a complete metabolic panel. You request these tests and get the following results later in the evening. Medications include lisinopril, 20 mg/day; Lasix, 40 mg/day; potassium, 5 mEq/day; Lantus insulin, 12 units every morning; laxative as needed; multivitamin daily. Blood sugar before supper last night was 243. Vital signs now: pulse 100, blood pressure (BP) 110/50, respirations 10.

	Result	Reference Range
Sodium	135 mEq/L	136–48 mEq/L
Potassium	5.8 mEq/L	3.6–5.2 mEq/L
Chloride	96 mEq/L	96–106 mEq/L
Glucose	60 mg/dL	70-99 mg/dL fasting <140 mg/dL 2 hours after eating
BUN	25 mg/dL	7–20 mg/dL
Creatinine	1.8 mg/dL	0.74-1.35 mg/dL
Albumin	2.4 g/dL	3.4–5.4 g/dL
WBCs	7000/mm³	5000–10,000/mm³
RBCs	$4.0 \times 10^6/\mu L$	$4.3–5.9 \times 10^6/mm^3$

BUN, Blood urea nitrogen; *RBCs,* red blood cells; *WBCs,* white blood cells.

You note that Mr. Jones has several laboratory results that are not in the acceptable reference range. You know that there are no adjustments that must be made due to age, but there are several deviations that place him at higher risk than a younger person for further or rapid deterioration.

Match the cues recognized on your assessment that are supported by the abnormal laboratory results.

He has difficulty telling you how much insulin he has been taking.	
Skin is slightly cool to the touch.	
He is lethargic.	
Some muscle twitching.	
Taking a potassium-sparing medication at the same time as a potassium-wasting medication and a potassium supplement.	
Elevated pulse and BP and lowered respirations.	

Highlight the one item of laboratory data you will use to determine the highest priority in care at this time.

When you review the medications with the physician or nurse practitioner, which do you determine has the highest risk for causing harm?

CLINICAL JUDGMENT QUESTIONS AND ACTIVITIES

1. The next time you are working with an older adult, either as a nurse/nurse practitioner or as a student nurse, review the most recent laboratory report and determine which variations are more likely a reflection of the person's disease state rather than age.
2. In a classroom discussion, consider a 90-year-old with increasing dyspnea and fatigue. If you were ordering or requesting laboratory tests for this person, which ones would you choose in order of priority?
3. Summarize laboratory values that are considered the most "critical" in older adults and require some type of immediate response.

RESEARCH QUESTIONS

1. In what way do food and alcohol intake affect the accuracy of laboratory test results?
2. If someone has had several chronic diseases for an extended period of time and yet is active and "healthy," what laboratory findings may still be outside of the normal limits?

REFERENCES

Ali N: Role of vitamin D in preventing of COVID-19 infection, progression, and severity, *J Infec Public Health* 13(10):1373–1380, 2020.

Alves FC, Sun J, Qureshi AR, et al.: The higher mortality associated with low serum albumin is dependent on systemic inflammation in end-stage kidney disease, *PLoS One*, 2018 13(1):e0190410.

American Diabetes Association: Classification and diagnosis of diabetes: standards of medical care in diabetes—2020, *Diabetes Care* 43(Suppl 1):S14–S31, 2020.

American Geriatrics Society (AGS): American Geriatrics Society 2019 updated Beers Criteria for potential inappropriate medication use in older adults, *JAGS* 67(4): 674–694, 2019.

Bennouar S, Cherif AB, Kessira A, et al.: Vitamin D deficiency and low serum calcium as predictors of poor prognosis in patients with severe COVID-19, *J Am Coll Nutr* 40(2):104–110, 2021.

Cavagnolli G, Pimentel AL, Freitas P, et al.: Effect of ethnicity on HbA1c levels in individuals without diabetes: systematic review and metanalysis, *PLoS One*, 2017 12(2):e0171315.

Connor GJ: *Lab values interpretation: the ultimate laboratory tests manual of reference ranges and what they mean*, Berlin, 2020, GD Publishing Ltd.

Dugdale DC: *Blood differential* (website), 2020. https://medlineplus.gov/lab-tests/blood-differential/.

Ershler WB: Blood disorders in older adults. In Fillit HM, Rockwood K, Young JB, editors: *Brocklehurst's textbook of geriatric medicine and gerontology*, Philadelphia, 2017, Elsevier, pp 757–771.

Ferri FF: *Ferri's best test: a practical guide to clinical laboratory medicine and diagnostic imaging*, Philadelphia, 2015, Saunders.

Filippatos TD, Makri A, Elisaf MS, et al.: Hyponatremia in the elderly: challenges and solutions, *Clin Interv Aging* 12:1957–1965, 2017.

Grundy SM, Stone NJ, Bailey AL, et al.: 2018 AHA/ACC/AACVPR/AAPA/ABC/ACPM/ADA/AGS/APhA/ASPC/NLA/PCNA guideline on the management of blood cholesterol: executive summary: a report of the American College of Cardiology/American Heart Association Task Force on clinical practice guidelines, *J Am Coll Cardiol* 73(24):3168–3209, 2019.

Hall JR, Wiechmann AR, Johnson LA, et al.: Total cholesterol and neuropsychiatric symptoms in Alzheimer's disease: the impact of total cholesterol level and gender, *Dement Geriatr Cogn Disord* 38(5–6):300–309, 2014.

Huether SE, Rote NS, McCance KL: Structure and function of the hematologic system. In McCance KL, Huether SE, editors: *Pathophysiology: the biologic basis for disease in adults and children*, ed 8, St Louis, 2019, Elsevier, pp 945–981.

Lapin A, Mueller E: Laboratory diagnosis and geriatrics: more than just reference intervals for older adults. In Fillit HM, Rockwood K, Young JB, editors: *Brocklehurst's textbook of geriatric medicine and gerontology*, Philadelphia, 2017, Elsevier, pp 220–225.

Lewis JL: *Hypernatremia* (website), 2021a http://www.merckmanuals.com/professional/endocrine-and-metabolic-disorders/electrolyte-disorders/hypernatremia.

Lewis JL: *Hypokalemia* (website), 2021b. http://www.merckmanuals.com/professional/endocrine-and-metabolic-disorders/electrolyte-disorders/hypokalemia.

Lin Y, Kim J, Metter EJ, et al.: Changes in blood lymphocyte numbers with age in vivo and their association with the levels of cytokines/cytokine receptors, *Immun Ageing* 13:24, 2016.

Litao MK, Kamat D: Erythrocyte sedimentation rate and C-reactive protein: how best to use them in clinical practice, *Pediatr Ann* 43(10):417–420, 2014.

Malkina A, Hadley L: Fluid and electrolyte abnormalities. In Walter LC, Chang A, editors: *CURRENT diagnosis and treatment: geriatrics*, ed 3, New York, 2021, McGraw Hill, pp 402–409.

Mathew MK, Jacobs MS, et al.: Malnutrition and feeding problems. In Ham RJ, Sloane PD, Warshaw GA, et al, editors: *Ham's primary care geriatrics: a case-based approach*, ed 6, Philadelphia, 2014, Elsevier, pp 315–322.

National Heart, Lung, and Blood Institute (NHLBI): *Thrombocythemia and thrombocytosis* (website), n.d. https://www.nhlbi.nih.gov/health-topics/thrombocythemia-and-thrombocytosis.

Neville JJ, Palmiere T, Young AR: Physical determinants of vitamin D photosynthesis: a review, *JBMR Plus* 5(1):e10460, 2021.

Pereira M, Damascena AD, Azevedo LM, et al.: Vitamin D deficiency aggravates COVID-19: systematic review and meta-analysis, *Crit Rev Food Sci Nutr* 4:1–9, 2020. doi:10.1080/10408398.2020.1841090 Nov.

Ramasamy I: Vitamin D metabolism and guidelines for vitamin D supplementation, *Clin Biochem Rev* 41(3):103–126, 2020.

Reuben DB, Herr KA, Pacala JT, et al.: *Geriatrics at your fingertips*, ed 22, New York, 2020, American Geriatric Society.

Shah MK, Workeneh B, Taffet GE: Hypernatremia in the geriatric population, *Clin Interv Aging* 9:1987–1992, 2014.

Sink K, Yaffe K: Cognitive impairment and dementia. In Walter LC, Chang A, editors: *CURRENT diagnosis and treatment: geriatrics*, ed 3, New York, 2021, McGraw Hill, pp 57–68.

Spencer-Bonilla G, Chung S, Sarraju A, et al.: Statin use in older adults with stable atherosclerotic cardiovascular disease, *J Am Geriatr Soc* 69(4):979–985, 2021.

Takata Y, Ansai T, Soh I, et al.: Serum total cholesterol concentration and 10-year mortality in an 85-year-old population, *Clin Interv Aging* 9:293–300, 2014.

US Preventive Services Task Force (USPSTF): *Final recommendation statement: prostate cancer: screening* (website), 2018. https://www.uspreventiveservicestaskforce.org/Page/Document/RecommendationStatementFinal/prostate-cancer-screening1.

Webb AR, Kazantzidis A, Kift RC, et al.: Colour counts: sunlight and skin types as drivers of vitamin D deficiency at UK latitudes, *Nutrients* 10(4):457, 2018.

Wei X, Zeng W, Su J, et al.: Hypolipidemia is associated with the severity of COVID-19, *J Clin Lipidol* 14(3):297–304, 2021.

Wong CW: Vitamin B12 deficiency in the elderly: is it worth screening?, *Hong Kong Med J*, 2015 21(2):155064.

Yanase T, Yanagita I, Muta K, et al.: Frailty in elderly diabetes patients, *Endocr J* 65(1):1–11, 2018.

Zhang C, Huang D, Shen D, et al.: Brain natriuretic peptide as the long-term cause of mortality in patients with cardiovascular disease: a retrospective cohort study, *Int J Exp Med* 8(9):16364–16368, 2015.

Zhang J, Wang X, Xiao W, et al.: NT-proBNP is associated with age, gender and glomerular filtration rate in a community-dwelling population, *Int J Clin Exp Med* 12(10):12220–12227, 2019.

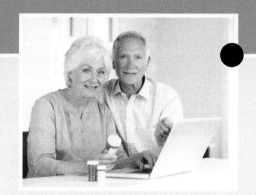

11 CHAPTER

Safe Medication Use

Kathleen Jett

http://evolve.elsevier.com/Touhy/TwdHlthAging

A STUDENT SPEAKS

Whenever I see patients in the clinic, I try to think very carefully about what can be stopped before adding any medications, but since most of them have so many illnesses at the same time, I sometimes wonder where I can start!

Helen, age 32, gerontological nurse practitioner student

AN OLDER ADULT SPEAKS

Every time I go to the clinic, I get another prescription. It just doesn't seem like I need to take so many medications, so sometimes I don't.

Annie, age 72

LEARNING OBJECTIVES

On completion of this chapter, the reader will be able to:

1. Describe the pharmacokinetic and pharmacodynamic changes that are normal changes with aging.
2. Describe potential problems associated with medication therapy in late life.
3. Recognize medications that are more commonly used in late life.
4. Recognize potentially inappropriate use of medication and explain how it affects healthy aging.
5. Recognize the early cues suggestive of adverse medication reactions and events and generate solutions to respond to these and prevent them.
6. Discuss barriers to medication adherence in older adults.
7. Develop nursing actions to promote safe medication practices and prevent medication toxicity.

In the United States, persons 65 years of age and older are prescribed more medications than any other age group. Although the exact statistics vary from study to study, all findings indicate that as one ages, the number of prescribed medications, dietary supplements, and herbal products taken increases (Hales et al., 2019).

When used appropriately, pharmacological interventions can enhance the quality of life and promote healthy aging. When used inappropriately, they can contribute to both morbidity and mortality at any age. Unfortunately, even when medications are prescribed, administered, and taken appropriately, adverse medication reactions and events can and do occur, especially in older adults. The reasons for this are many and include reduced organ function and physiological reserve and varying levels of skills of nurses and other health care professionals.

This chapter reviews the effect of aging on pharmacokinetics and pharmacodynamics (Box 11.1). Issues in medications are discussed, including polypharmacy, medication interactions, adverse medication reactions and events, and the uses of psychoactive agents relative to the aging adult.

PHARMACOKINETICS

Pharmacokinetics is the study of the movement and action of a medication in the body from the time it is administered to the time it is excreted. Pharmacokinetic processes determine the concentration of medications in the body, which in turn determines the effect. The concentration of the medication at different times depends on how the medication is absorbed, distributed, and metabolized, and excreted. Changes in renal

BOX 11.1 Age-Related Changes Affecting Pharmacokinetics and Pharmacodynamics

Absorption
Reduced saliva
Presbyphagia
Altered gastric pH
Delayed stomach emptying
Slowed intestinal motility

Distribution
Reduced cardiac output and reduced circulation
Reduced body water
Increased adipose tissue
Reduced serum albumin and other plasma proteins

Metabolism
Reduced liver mass
Reduced hepatic blood flow
Reduced enzyme activity

Excretion
Reduced glomerular filtration rate
Reduced renal tubular function

function and the increased permeability of the blood-brain barrier have the greatest impact on pharmacodynamics in older adults (Steinman & Holmes, 2021).

Absorption

There are several normal age-related changes that have the potential to affect absorption and therefore the amount of the medication available for both therapeutic and adverse effects. Most medications are administered orally. This is potentially problematic due to an age-related reduction in saliva; if this is severe (xerostomia) due to confounding factors, swallowing tablets and capsules can be difficult. A liquid formulation may be easier unless pathology-related dysphagia is present.

⚡ SAFETY TIP

Xerostomia

Medications associated with xerostomia include antihistamines, antidepressants, antipsychotics, clonidine, and diuretics. Chewing of sugar-free gum may increase salivation and comfort. There are also over-the-counter, quickly dissolving tablets, which increase oral moisture.

Age-related decreases in esophageal motility (presbyphagia) further contribute to swallowing difficulties and in extreme cases can cause tissue erosions (Shim et al., 2017). With sublingual administration, medication is absorbed directly into the systemic circulation through the mucous membrane, but a dry mouth will reduce or delay buccal absorption. Transdermal and rectal administration may be useful when a person cannot swallow or tolerate oral or sublingual medications, such as for those nearing the end of life.

Age-related changes in the gastrointestinal tract have several potential effects. Changes to the gastric mucosa may either increase or decrease initial absorption. Increases in gastric pH retard the action of acid-dependent medications. Delayed stomach emptying may diminish or negate the effectiveness of short-lived medications that could become inactivated before reaching the small intestine. Some enteric-coated formulations of medications, such as aspirin, which are specifically meant to bypass stomach acidity, may be delayed so long that their action begins in the stomach and may cause gastric irritation or nausea and bleeding. Once a medication has been administered orally (or enterally), it must be absorbed into the bloodstream. This usually begins in the stomach and continues through the large intestine. Slowed intestinal motility, although not a normal change of aging, is frequently encountered in late life. This additional time the medication has contact with the intestinal walls increases the risk for adverse reactions and unpredictable effects.

Nurses working with older adults are usually familiar with the transdermal drug delivery system (TDDS). Designed for the slow absorption of fat-soluble medications, it has been found to be extremely useful for those who require very small doses of a medication over a longer period. This route is more convenient, more acceptable, and potentially more reliable than other routes, especially for persons with cognitive disorders. Ideally the TDDS provides for a more constant rate of absorption and eliminates concern about variation in gastrointestinal absorption, gastrointestinal intolerance, and medication interaction. Placing patches on the skin requires manual dexterity, and self-administration is not always possible, especially for persons with orthopedic deformities such as osteoarthritis. Transdermal absorption is unreliable for the person who is underweight or overweight. The characteristic thin, dry older skin also may affect absorption of the intended dose at the intended time. TDDS fentanyl, the most commonly used patch in older adults, can be fatal if it is either intentionally or unintentionally ingested (Thornton & Darracq, 2020).

⚡ SAFETY TIP

Use of the TDDS

The previous TDDS patch must be removed at the time a new one is applied to maintain a consistent dose. A new place should be chosen to decrease the risk of skin irritation.

Distribution

A medication is transported through systemic circulation to receptors on the cells of the target organ where a therapeutic effect is initiated. The organs with high blood flow (e.g., brain, kidneys, lungs, liver) receive the highest concentrations rapidly. Distribution to organs of lower blood flow (e.g., skin, muscles, fat) occurs more slowly and results in lower concentrations of the medication in these tissues. Impaired peripheral circulation, common in late life, can negatively affect medication distribution.

Normal changes with aging include decreased total body water, increased body fat, and reduced lean tissue. By the age of 70, adipose tissue increases to 36% in healthy older men and 45% in healthy older women. Body water decreases by 17%, and extracellular volume decreases by 40% between the ages of 20 and 65 (Slattum et al., 2017). Lipophilic (fat-soluble) medications (such as diazepam) concentrate in adipose tissue more than in other tissues. If there is an excessive accumulation in the adipose tissue, more will be available, and this can result in a potentially fatal overdose. Hydrophilic (water-soluble) medications, such as digoxin, will have higher serum levels and can also cause adverse events even at the lowest doses.

Distribution also depends on the availability of plasma protein in the form of lipoproteins, globulins, and especially albumin (Box 11.2). Many medications are bound to plasma protein for distribution. In healthy adults of any age, a predictable percentage of an absorbed medication is inactivated as it is bound to the protein. The remaining free medication is available to provide a therapeutic effect.

Serum albumin levels decrease with age (Lapin & Mueller, 2017) (Fig. 11.1). This is further reduced in those with acute illness, a long-standing chronic condition, or frailty. This decrease in albumin-binding capacity unpredictably increases the amount of free medication. If two or more medications compete for the more limited protein (e.g., levothyroxine, digoxin) and binding is further reduced, higher plasma drug levels may result and cues that may indicate toxicity should be recognized quickly; this is especially dangerous in medications that both bind with albumin and have a narrow therapeutic window, such as warfarin.

Metabolism

Drug metabolism is the process wherein a pharmaceutical substance (substrate) is transformed into a metabolite that can be used and eliminated from the body more easily. Aging results in reduced liver mass and blood flow, so when medications make a "first pass" through the liver, fewer are metabolized (prepared for elimination) and therefore remain available for therapeutic action. Liver metabolism is facilitated by the isoenzymes in the cytochrome P450 enzyme system. The system is more affected by inherent genetics than aging, and the genetics show considerable racial variation (Gao et al., 2021) (Box 11.3). People may be poor (slow), intermediate, rapid, or ultra-rapid metabolizers of a medication, depending on their genetic variation in the number of active isoenzymes and subsequent plasma concentration of a particular drug (Boxes 11.4 and 11.5) (Horn, 2008). There are also many medications that either inhibit or induce (increase) the activity of a metabolic enzyme. Plasma concentrations of free drugs become more variable as we age. When there is an increased serum level, either less frequent or lower doses are needed to achieve the same effect (e.g., levothyroxine, digoxin). Due to the high number of medications typically taken by older adults, metabolism and therefore effect of medications are fraught with risk and unpredictability.

BOX 11.3   Potential Racial Differences (Phenotypic Disparities) in Metabolism Capacity

Warfarin is metabolized well by cytochrome CYP2C9, with at least two genetic variants. These variants can account for up to 22% of the total of CYP2C9 in Whites, resulting in slower metabolism. The same variants can account for only 1.5% of the total in Blacks, resulting in relatively rapid metabolism of warfarin.

Data from Gao S, Bell EC, Zhang Y, et al: Racial disparities in drug disposition in the digestive tract, *Int J Mol Sci* 22(3):e1038, 2021.

BOX 11.2   Medications That Bind Strongly to the Plasma Protein Albumin

Ceftriaxone	Valproic acid
Ibuprofen	Warfarin
Naproxen	

BOX 11.4   Fast and Slow Metabolizers

For many years I conducted a "Coumadin Clinic" where people taking coumadin had their INR checked and their coumadin dosage adjusted accordingly. Several required only about 7 mg a week to maintain a therapeutic level and were likely slow metabolizers. Several others required 50 to 60 mg a week and were likely to be rapid or ultra-rapid metabolizers. All would self-identify as White.

INR, International normalized ratio.
Data from Gao S, Bell EC, Zhang Y, et al: Racial disparities in drug disposition in the digestive tract, *Int J Mol Sci* 22(3):e1038, 2021.

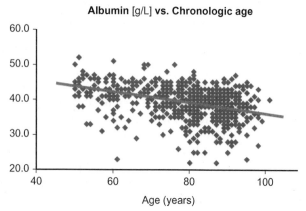

Albumin [g/L] vs. Chronologic age

Fig. 11.1 Correlation of albumin levels with age. (From Lapin A, Mueller E: Laboratory diagnosis and geriatrics: more than just reference intervals for older adults. In Fillit HM, Rockwood K, Young JB, editors: *Brocklehurst's textbook of geriatric medicine and gerontology,* ed 8, Philadelphia, 2017, Elsevier, pp 220–225.)

BOX 11.5   Metabolism and Pain Relief

Codeine is converted to morphine through the CYP2D6 metabolism in the liver. People who are genetically deficient in this would be "poor metabolizers" and are likely to feel little effect (pain relief) from codeine. A highly active CYP2D6 substrate leading to ultrarapid metabolism will lead to severe adverse effects due to a rapid rise in plasma concentration of morphine.

Data from Gao S, Bell EC, Zhang Y, et al: Racial disparities in drug disposition in the digestive tract, *Int J Mol Sci* 22(3):e1038, 2021.

Excretion

Medications are excreted either unchanged or as metabolites. A few are eliminated through the lungs, or in bile and feces. A small amount is eliminated through hair, sweat, saliva, tears, and semen. The renal system is the primary site of elimination as a medication or metabolite passes through the kidneys, into the bladder, and is excreted. The efficiency of excretion can be measured by the glomerular filtration rate (GFR).

Age-related changes in renal function (lost glomerular and tubular function) have a significant effect on medication and metabolite excretion (drug clearance). Most people lose 1% of their GFR per year starting at about 20 years of age (Slattum et al., 2017). This change reduces the body's ability to eliminate medications in a timely manner by prolonging their half-life, or the amount of time it takes to reduce a medication's therapeutic effect by one-half. This results in more opportunities for accumulation and can lead to potential toxicity or other adverse events.

The creatinine clearance (CrCl) is closely associated with an estimated GFR. There are a number of ways to calculate this; the most available means is with the Cockcroft-Gault Calculator. The plasma creatinine level and a person's weight, gender, and age are needed for the calculation. Many free automatic calculators are available online (e.g., http://nephron.com/cgi-bin/CGSI.cgi). The CrCl allows the nurse to determine which person needs medication dosage adjustment due to renal insufficiency and impairment. When there is uncertainty as to the accuracy of this calculation or a need for more certainty, a cystatin-C assay can done.

PHARMACODYNAMICS

Pharmacodynamics refers to the physiological interactions between a medication and the body, specifically the chemical compounds introduced into the body and the receptors on cell membranes. These receptors are cellular proteins with unique shapes and ionic charges that bind to a very specific medication, like a glove to a hand. When this binding occurs, a structural change in the receptor protein is initiated, which in turn leads to a biochemical cascade resulting in a therapeutic effect.

The older a person becomes, the more likely that person will have unreliable pharmacodynamics. Although it is not always possible to explain or predict all the alterations, several are well known. Those of special note for older adults are the side effects associated with sedating and anticholinergic medications. The side effects of these and other medications that depress the central nervous system can significantly increase the rate of delirium, confusion, agitation, functional decline, and the risk for accidental injury (Box 11.6) (Reuben et al., 2020; Steinman & Holmes, 2021). Age-related decreases in thirst sensation may lead to dehydration and subsequent alterations in drug metabolism. Decreased responsiveness of the alpha-adrenergic system results in decreased sensitivity to beta-agonist and beta-antagonist medications (e.g., beta blockers). Baroreceptor reflex responses decrease with age, causing increased susceptibility to orthostatic hypotension and the need to pay special attention to antihypertensive medications.

BOX 11.6 Medications With Strong Anticholinergic and Sedating Properties With Select Side Effects of Each

Examples of Medications	Select Potential Side Effects
Antihistamines	Constipation
Antimuscarinics (for urinary incontinence)	Dry mouth
	Blurred vision
Antispasmodics	Dizziness
Benzodiazepines	Confusion
Antipsychotics	Urinary retention
Antidepressants	Functional impairment
Opioids	Increased heart rate

ISSUES IN MEDICATION USE

Polypharmacy

A review of polypharmacy across the world found a prevalence between 10% and 90% (Khezrian et al., 2020). An estimated 39% of persons at least 65 years old living in the United States are taking at least five different medications (Steinman & Holmes, 2021). All studies reported increases over time and increases by age, and a linear relationship between the number of medications taken and subsequent drug-related problems (Khezrian et al., 2020). Although 5 medications are sometimes used as an arbitrary indicator of polypharmacy and 10 or more as excessive polypharmacy, there is no consensus as to the definition (Steinman & Holmes, 2021; Taghy et al., 2020). It may mean simply multiple medications used at the same time or multiple medications used for the same problem. Multimorbidity (multiple concurrent chronic conditions), demographic, socioeconomic status, and self-assessed health status have all been found to be major predictors of polypharmacy, but other determinants have been noted as well (Box 11.7). Polypharmacy occurred most often in persons treated for chronic obstructive pulmonary disease (COPD), diabetes, depression, heart disease, hypertension, and pain (Khezrian et al., 2020).

The focus is now on the consideration of risk and benefits and classified as either appropriate or problematic polypharmacy. When the doses of medications have been optimized, their choice is evidence-based, and the intent is to improve quality of life while minimizing harm, polypharmacy may be appropriate. When multiple medications have been prescribed

---

BOX 11.7 Determinants of Polypharmacy

Increased age	Systemic inflammation
Smoking: current or history of	Chronic pain
Gender: male	Urinary incontinence
Inactivity	Gastric disturbances
Higher socioeconomic status	Dependent ADLs
Poor self-assessed health	Multiple prescribers
Obesity	Cardiovascular disorders
Increased provider accessibility	

ADLs, Activities of daily living. From Khezrian M, McNeil CJ, Murray AD, et al: An overview of prevalence, determinants, and health outcomes of polypharmacy, *Ther Adv Drug Saf,* 11:1–10, 2020.

BOX 11.8 Consequences of Polypharmacy

Increased health care cost
Adverse drug reactions and events
Drug interactions (drug, supplement, disease)
Difficulty with compliance
Reduced functional status
Cognitive impairment
Falls with fractures
Urinary incontinence
Poor nutrition
Medication cascade
Frailty
Hospitalization
Death

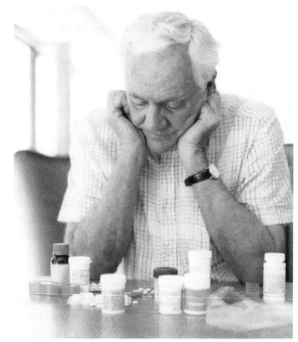

Polypharmacy. (From ©iStock.com/Squaredpixels.)

without consideration of the available evidence; the desired benefit has not been obtained; or there is an unfavorable risk-benefit balance, high potential for interactions, or unacceptable burden, the polypharmacy is considered problematic (Levy, 2017; Payne, 2016). It may occur unintentionally if an existing medication regimen is not considered when new prescriptions are given.

Polypharmacy is exacerbated by the combination of a high use of health care specialists and a reluctance of prescribers to discontinue potentially unnecessary medications that have been prescribed by someone else. This can lead to the continued use of medications that may no longer be necessary. When any number of the hundreds of over-the-counter (OTC) supplements such as vitamins and herbs are added to those medications prescribed, the polypharmacy becomes even riskier. When communication among patients, nurses, other health care providers, and caregivers becomes fragmented, the risk for duplicative medications, inappropriate medications, potentially unsafe dosages, and potentially preventable interactions is heightened. Polypharmacy is extremely common among older adults, with multiple potential consequences (Box 11.8). To address these concerns, there has been an effort to facilitate widespread use of "deprescribing" solutions as well as policy changes to reduce the use of potential inappropriate medications in long-term care facilities. The issues of polypharmacy are the increased risk for medication interactions and for adverse events. The more the medications, the greater the risk.

Drug Interactions

The more prescribed medications and any other substances a person takes (e.g., herbs, vitamins, dietary supplements, foods), the greater the possibility one or more will interact with another and that inappropriate prescribing or use will occur (Payne, 2016; Zwicker et al., 2021). At the same time, the more chronic conditions one has, the more likely it is that a medication for one condition will affect the body in such a way as to influence another condition. When two or more products of any kind are taken at the same time or closely together (including food), one may potentiate another (i.e., cause it to have stronger effects than when given alone) or antagonize the other (lower the potency or inactivate it), or cause adverse drug reactions and events. The nurse caring for frail elders is especially challenged because of

the physical and social vulnerability and medical complexity common in late life; medication interactions are more likely and adverse reactions more often lethal.

Drug-Herb/Supplement Interactions

As the popularity of medicinal herbs and other dietary supplements rises, so does the risk for interactions with prescribed medications. Although much remains unknown, new knowledge is added almost daily upon which gerontological nurses base their practice. For example, a number of herbs have a direct effect on coagulability. When these herbs are taken with warfarin, the risk of bleeding may increase significantly. If the herb influences the results of the international normalized ratio (INR) or other measure of coagulation, adjustments to the warfarin dose will lead to inappropriate and potentially dangerous consequences. The interactions presented in Table 11.1 represent only a small fraction of the many real and potential problems when prescribed medications are combined with an herb or a dietary supplement.

Drug-Food/Beverage Interactions

Many foods interact with medications, producing increased, decreased, or variable effects. For example, calcium in dairy products will bind to levothyroxine, tetracycline, and ciprofloxacin, greatly decreasing their absorption; lovastatin absorption is increased by a high-fat, low-fiber meal. Grapefruit juice contains substances that inhibit CYP3A4 isoenzyme 3A4–mediated metabolism in the gut wall and liver and increase the bioavailability of multiple medications (Table 11.2). The most common drug-food/beverage interaction of the type is between grapefruit juice and the statins to lower cholesterol.

Spironolactone, prescribed for end-stage heart failure, increases potassium (K^+) reabsorption by the renal tubule. If a

TABLE 11.1 Select Herb-Drug Interactions[a]

Herb	Medication	Complication	Nursing Action
Cinnamon	Antihyperglycemics	May increase effects	Avoid use, careful monitor of glucose
Coenzyme Q10	**Anticoagulants,** antihypertensives	Reduced anticoagulation effect, decreased antihypertensive effect	Use only with caution and under supervision and close monitoring.
Echinacea	**Any anticoagulant drug** such as warfarin sodium; digoxin	Risk of bleeding increases; therapeutic digoxin level may be altered	Advise person not to take without provider approval
Garlic	**Any anticoagulant or antiplatelet drug** such as warfarin sodium, streptokinase, aspirin, other NSAIDs	Risk of bleeding increases	Advise person not to take without provider approval; stop 7 days before surgery
	Antihypertensives	Increased hypotensive effect	Advise provider of use
	Antivirals, such as ritonavir	Altered drug effect	Advise against use
	Antimetabolites such as cyclosporine	Risk of less effective response	Advise against use
	Insulin or oral hypoglycemic agent such as pioglitazone or tolbutamide	Serum glucose control may improve; less antidiabetic drug needed	Monitor blood glucose levels
Ginkgo	Aspirin, other NSAIDs, heparin sodium, warfarin sodium, **any anticoagulant**	Increases risk for bleeding	Teach person not to take without approval of provider; stop 36 hours before surgery
	Antiplatelet drugs such as ticlopidine		
	Antidiabetic drugs: insulin, oral DMT2 drugs such as metformin	May alter blood glucose levels	Monitor blood glucose level closely
	Antidepressants, MAOIs, SSRIs	May cause abnormal response or decrease effectiveness	Advise not to take with these drugs
	Antihypertensives	May cause increased effect	Monitor blood pressure
	Antiseizure medications	Increased risk for seizure	Advise against use
Ginseng	Insulin and oral antidiabetic drugs	Blood glucose levels may be altered	Monitor blood glucose levels closely
	Anticoagulant and antiplatelet drugs	Increases risk for bleeding	Advise use with caution and provider oversight
	Aspirin and other NSAIDs		
	Antihypertensives, cardiac drugs such as calcium channel blockers	May alter effects of drug	Advise against use unless provider monitors closely
	Immunosuppressants	May interfere with action	Advise against use
	Stimulants	May cause additive effect	Advise against use
Green tea	**Warfarin,** statins, acetaminophen	May alter anticoagulant effects, increase risk of side effects	Advise against use
	Stimulants, caffeine	May cause additive effect	Advise to use with care
St. John's wort	Triptans such as sumatriptan, zolmitriptan	May increase risks of serotonergic adverse effects, serotonin syndrome, cerebral vasoconstriction	Advise against use
	Statins	May decrease plasma concentrations of these drugs	Monitor levels of lipids
	Digoxin	Decreases effects	Advise against use
	Alprazolam	May decrease effect of drug	Advise against use
	Ketoprofen	Photosensitivity	Advise sunblock use
	Tramadol and some SSRIs	Increased risk for serotonin syndrome	Advise against use
	Olanzapine	Increased risk for serotonin syndrome	Advise against use
	Paroxetine	Sedative-hypnotic intoxication	Advise against use
	Theophylline	Increases metabolism; decreases drug blood level	Monitor drug effects
	Albuterol		
	Warfarin	May decrease anticoagulant effect	Advise against use
	Amlodipine	Lowers efficacy of calcium channel	Advise against use
	Estrogen or progesterone	May decrease effect of hormones	Advise that this effect may occur
Saw palmetto	**Anticoagulants**	No longer recommended for BPH	Do not take

[a]The interactions listed represent only a few of the possible herb-drug interactions.
BPH, Benign prostatic hyperplasia; *DMT2,* diabetes mellitus type 2; *MAOIs,* monoamine oxidase inhibitors; *NSAIDs,* nonsteroidal antiinflammatory drugs; *SSRIs,* selective serotonin reuptake inhibitors.
Data from: Anderson, L. (2020). *18 herbal supplements with risky drug interactions.* https://www.drugs.com/slideshow/herb-drug-interactions-1069; Pruitt, R, Lemanski, A., & Carroll, A. (2018). Herbal supplements: Research findings and safety. *The Nurse Pract, 43*(5), 32–37.

TABLE 11.2 Common Drug-Food/Beverage Interactions With Nursing Teaching Points

Food	Drug	Potential Effect	Nursing Teaching
Fiber	Digoxin	Absorption of drug into fiber, reducing drug action	Take at different times of the day
Foods with vitamin K	Warfarin	Decreased effect of drug	Do not take or take regularly so that dosage of warfarin can be stabilized
Food	Many antibiotics	Reduced absorption rate of drug	Watch for association
Vitamin B$_6$ supplements	Levodopa-carbidopa	Inactivates antiparkinsonian effect	Avoid if possible
Grapefruit juice	Multiple medications[a]	Altered metabolism and elimination can increase concentration of drug	Avoid all grapefruit juice products
Citrus juice	Calcium channel blockers	Gastric reflux exacerbated	Avoid juice, do not take medications for reflux to treat instead of avoiding
Foods or beverages containing magnesium, calcium, iron, aluminum	Levothyroxine	Inactivates levothyroxine	Take at least 1 hour before taking anything else, same time daily

[a]See Food and Drug Administration: *Grapefruit juice and some drugs don't mix* (website), 2017. https://www.fda.gov/consumers/consumer-updates/grapefruit-juice-and-some-drugs-dont-mix.

BOX 11.9 Examples of Foods and Beverages to Avoid When Taking Warfarin

Kale	Broccoli
Spinach	Brussels sprouts
Collards	Asparagus
Swiss chard	Green tea
Mustard greens	Cranberry juice
Turnip greens	Alcohol
Parsley	

patient ingests a diet high in potassium (e.g., KCl salt substitute, molasses, oranges, bananas) along with a potassium-sparing medication (e.g., lisinopril), K$^+$ levels can rise significantly and quickly reach intoxication (see Chapter 10, Box 10.4). The vitamin K$^+$ in many foods antagonizes (decreases) the anticoagulant effects of warfarin and may significantly increase the coagulability of the blood (Reuben et al., 2020) (Box 11.9).

⚡ **SAFETY TIP**

Vitamin K and Warfarin

It is recommended that a patient taking an anticoagulant such as warfarin who choose to continue to eat foods high in vitamin K, such as greens, ingest a consistent amount to avoid variations in their international normalized ratio (INR) (Chapter 10).

Drug-Drug Interactions

The polypharmacy that may be a necessary part of disease management in later life significantly increases both the risk for and the frequency of drug-drug interactions. These may occur at any time from preparation to excretion. For example, persons who cannot swallow after a stroke may receive all feedings and medications enterally. To safely pass through a feeding tube, medications intended for oral administration must be converted to a soluble form to pass through it without clogging and yet also remain in their original form. When several medications are crushed, mixed, and then dissolved in water for administration, a new product is created, and drug-drug interactions may have already begun.

⚡ **SAFETY TIP**

Safe Administration of Medications Through Enteral Feeding Tubes

Persons who receive their medications via the enteral route are at high risk for medication errors. The possible outcomes of such errors include occluded tube, reduced medication effect, medication toxicity, patient harm, and patient death. The three most common errors are incompatible route, improper preparation, and improper administration. Most often this preparation occurs at the bedside, further increasing the risk for errors. Safe administration of enteral medications is a time-consuming process that requires detailed knowledge of the medications (and their formulation) and skill to prepare them appropriately.

Altered absorption can occur when one medication binds with another in the small intestine to form a nonabsorbable compound. For example, ciprofloxacin and iron compounds are both taken frequently by older adults. When taken at the same time they bind together, and both lose their therapeutic effect. Other medications may compete for the same receptor site, creating varied bioavailability of one or both drugs. Interference with enzyme activity may alter metabolism and cause deficiencies or toxicities. Antispasmodic medications slow gastric and intestinal motility even further than that present in normal aging. In some instances, this may be desired if the prolonged effect is beneficial (e.g., stool softener) but may prove harmful when it leads to an accumulation and potential medication intoxication.

Altered distribution is a common cause of adverse medication reactions in older adults and is an especially important issue in patients with lowered albumin levels. As discussed earlier, a reaction may be caused by displacement of one medication from its receptor site by another medication. Thus they are common among chronically ill, frail older adults, such as many of those residing in long-term care facilities (Slattum et al., 2017).

Age-related decreases in renal function alter excretion when one medication changes the urine pH such that another medication is either reabsorbed or excreted to a greater extent than is desired. For example, probenecid increases the active transport of uric acid out of the renal tubules but decreases the transport of penicillin, thereby prolonging its half-life while increasing its therapeutic effect and risk for adverse events.

Pharmacodynamic medication interactions can be especially dangerous for older adults, especially the additive pharmacological effects of two or more similar medications. Together they are more potent than they are separately (Slattum et al., 2017). The frequency of polypharmacy in later life and drug-drug interactions has significant implications for the prescribing, administration, and recognition of the cues of both the effects and the side effects of medications taken by older adults (Table 11.3).

Drug-Disease Interactions

In some instances, an underlying disease state or condition can make a person more susceptible to the unwanted effects of a medication and increase the risk for an adverse drug reaction or event (Table 11.4). For example, many oral decongestants containing pseudoephedrine may increase blood pressure as do nonsteroidal anti-inflamatories such as ibuprofen and Naprosyn.

These interactions are particularly relevant to older adults due the high frequency of combined polypharmacy and multimorbidity.

Adverse Drug Reactions and Events

Adverse drug reactions (ADRs) and *adverse drug events* (ADEs) occur when there is a noxious response or side effect to a medication. They can result either from the administration of a single medication or from the interaction between multiple medications, supplements, or foods/beverages as previously discussed. There are multiple potential causes of an increased rate of ADRs and ADEs in late life (Box 11.10). It is reasonable to assume that many ADRs in older adults go unrecognized because the cues are often atypical and unrecognized as such or are misinterpreted as changes associated with normal aging or one of the many chronic diseases common in later life (Box 11.11). The most troublesome are those medications with a long half-life or a narrow therapeutic window (Steinman & Holmes, 2021) (Box 11.12). The number of medications taken and medication overuse and underuse, rather than the age of the individual alone, increase the risk.

The effects of such reactions may range from a minor annoyance to death and are a common cause of hospitalization (Zwicker et al., 2021). The prevalence of potentially inappropriate medications among older adults have ranged from 34.1% to 57.7%, many of which were found to be associated with ADRs, ADEs, and hospitalizations (Fahmi et al., 2019; Thomas & Thomas, 2019). Four types of medications (warfarin, insulin,

---

TABLE 11.3   Very High-Risk Drug-Drug Interactions

Drug or Class	Interacting Drug or Class	Potential Effect
Angiotensin-renin inhibitors, potassium-sparing diuretics	Others of the same	Increased risk for hypokalemia
Opioids	Sedatives/hypnotics, especially benzodiazepines	Excess sedation, respiratory depression
Anticholinergics	Other anticholinergics or sedatives/hypnotics	Cognitive decline, urinary retention
CNS-active drugs	Use of three or more CNS-active drugs at the same time (SSRIs, SNRIs, antipsychotics, benzodiazepines, opioids)	Increased falls, fractures, cognitive decline
Steroids, oral or parenteral	NSAIDs	Peptic ulcer disease, GI bleeding
Warfarin	Amiodarone, ciprofloxacin, macrolides (excluding azithromycin), Septra, NSAIDs	High risk for bleeding, need to monitor INR frequently

CNS, Central nervous system; *GI,* gastrointestinal; *INR,* international normalized ratio; *NSAIDs,* nonsteroidal antiinflammatory drugs; *SNRIs,* serotonin–norepinephrine reuptake inhibitors; *SSRIs,* selective serotonin reuptake inhibitors.

TABLE 11.4   Potential Consequences of Health Condition and Medication Combination

Condition	Medication	Consequences
History of peptic ulcer	Aspirin	Gastric bleeding
Chronic obstructive pulmonary disease (COPD)	Oral corticosteroid	Steroid effect
Hypertension or heart failure	Nonsteroidal antiinflammatory drug (NSAID)	Worsening

---

BOX 11.10   Causes of Increased Prevalence of Adverse Drug Reactions and Adverse Drug Effects in Late Life

Alterations in pharmacokinetics
Suboptimal monitoring
Multiple health care providers
Atypical presentations
Increased age (especially >85 years old)
Cognitive decline
Polypharmacy
Iatrogenesis: inappropriate prescribing or dosing, treating symptom of side effect, self-medication
Poor medication adherence
Underreport or underrecognition of side effects
Increased societal use of herbal preparations and supplements

BOX 11.11   Atypical Cues of Potential Adverse Drug Reactions in Older Adults

Fatigue	Incontinence
Falls	Depression
Confusion	Agitation

BOX 11.12   High-Risk Medications Due to Narrow Therapeutic Windows

Anticoagulants	Some antibiotics
Antihyperglycemic agents	Antipsychotics
Sedatives	Chemotherapeutic agents
Narcotics	

oral antiplatelet drugs, and oral hypoglycemics) accounted for 67% of emergency hospitalizations (Rochon et al., 2021).

Sometimes an ADR can be predicted from the pharmacological action of the medication, such as bone marrow suppression from chemotherapeutic agents or bleeding from anticoagulants. At other times they are unpredictable, such as a new allergic reaction to an antibiotic. Allergic reactions become more common in older adults as the immune system decreases in function (Chapter 27).

When an ADR reaches the level of harm, it is referred to as an *adverse drug event* (ADE). Many of these must be reported to the US Food and Drug Administration (FDA) or other regulatory body. Although reporting previously was limited to prescribed substances, this has been expanded to include any other products (such as dietary supplements) *for which health-related claims are made* (FDA, 2015). Most reporting is voluntary. However, it is strongly encouraged because such information is an important part of protecting the public from harm.

Although ADRs and ADEs still occur, there has been considerable progress in the development of solutions to reduce their likelihood (Box 11.13), especially in the recognition of age-related pharmacokinetic and pharmacodynamic changes in later life. We now know of many medications that have been identified as potentially inappropriate for use by older adults or that should be prescribed in lower dosages due to their high risk. There also has been a recognition that the risk of ADEs for some medications is so high when taken with other medications that they are simply not recommended for use in any older adult. To minimize the likelihood of an ADR, the initial dose may be low and then slowly increased until a safe therapeutic level is reached. In the absence of an ADR or in fear of it, a medication may be underprescribed. A common adage related to medication dosing in older adults is "Start low, go slow, but go" when needed.

Box 11.13   Tips for Best Practice

Using Technology to Reduce Adverse Drug Effects (ADEs)

Computer-based drug-interaction programs and electronic medical records are important tools used to minimize the risk for ADEs.

PSYCHOACTIVE MEDICATIONS

Psychoactive medications are those that affect mental function, which in turn affect behavior and how the world is experienced. The gerontological nurse, especially one working in a long-term care setting, is likely to be responsible for older adults who are receiving psychoactive medications, especially those for the treatment of depression, anxiety, and bipolar disorder (Chapter 30). Medications with psychoactive properties have a higher than usual risk for adverse events, in part due to increased permeability of the blood-brain barrier. When they must be prescribed and administered, it must be with an acute awareness of how age-related changes affect their absorption, distribution, excretion, and hepatic function.

To control the burgeoning use of psychotropic medications in nursing homes, the Centers for Medicare and Medicaid Services (CMS) issued a clarification of instructions to guide those who were responsible for monitoring the overall quality of patient care in a facility (usually state surveyors) (CMS, 2021). This classification of medications may never be used as a "quick fix" and should be used only when a thorough assessment had been completed, nonpharmacological approaches have proven ineffective, and the patient would clearly benefit from their use (Steinman & Holmes, 2021).

One specific class of psychoactive medications, antipsychotics, is sometimes prescribed to persons with neurodegenerative disorders and behavior disturbances due to hallucinations and delusions that place the person and those around the person in danger. These should never be used unless all nonpharmacological means have been tried. Persons taking these medications must be monitored with special care.

Antipsychotics

Antipsychotic medications are used to treat major depressive disorders, bipolar disorders, and psychoses, including those associated with the dementias when antidepressants have failed. Their mechanism of action centers on blocking dopamine receptor pathways in the brain, and they also affect the hypothalamic and thermoregulatory pathways. They are often ranked in relation to their side effects, especially sedation, hypotension, and extrapyramidal (and anticholinergic) side effects (EPSEs). Other side effects of these medications include neuroleptic malignant syndrome (NMS) and movement disorders.

The first such medications to be produced (in the 1950s) are now referred to as "typical antipsychotics" (e.g., haloperidol, chlorpromazine), and the newer, second-generation medications (developed since the 1990s) are classified as "atypicals" (e.g., quetiapine [Seroquel]). The dangers associated with the use of any of these requires that their use be significantly justified and that a careful cost-benefit analysis be done.

⚡ SAFETY TIP

Permanent Adverse Effects

To prevent permanent adverse effects, first-generation typical antipsychotics can never be given to someone with known or suspected Lewy body dementia.

When used appropriately and cautiously, antipsychotics can provide a person with relief from frightening and incapacitating symptoms. Inappropriate use of antipsychotic medications may mask a reversible cause for the psychosis (such as delirium, infection, dehydration, fever, or electrolyte imbalance), an adverse medication effect, or a sudden change in the environment. Because of the seriousness, frequency, and number of side effects and associated complications, these medications are prescribed at the lowest dose possible and for the shortest time possible. When antipsychotic medications are prescribed, more caution than usual must be used, and the patient must be monitored closely.

> ⚡ **SAFETY TIP**
>
> Examples of side effects of antipsychotic medications include drowsiness, dizziness, weight gain, constipation, low blood pressure, tremors, restlessness, rigidity, and muscle spasms (National Institute of Mental Health, 2016).

Malignant Syndrome

Because antipsychotics affect the thermoregulatory pathway, patients taking them cannot tolerate excess environmental heat. Even mild elevations of core temperature can result in liver damage, resulting in *neuroleptic malignant syndrome* (NMS). Acute NMS is characterized by high fever, rigidity, altered mental status, and other symptoms of autonomic instability such as tachycardia and pallor. The nurse or caregiver therefore must protect the person from NMS by making sure the environment is cool at all times and the person is adequately hydrated. Direct sunlight should be avoided. Because the person may not share or be able to share discomfort about the heat, subjective reports of altered body temperature cannot alert the nurse to search for related signs or symptoms. Any circumstance resulting in dehydration greatly increases the risk of heat stroke, which in late life is associated with mortality.

Movement Disorders

NMS is not commonly seen in older adults taking antipsychotics. The more common adverse side effects are movement disorders, also referred to as *extrapyramidal syndrome* (EPS), and include acute dystonia, akathisia, parkinsonian symptoms, and tardive dyskinesia (TD). Although more common with the typical antipsychotics, they can occur with any of them. The prescribing provider should be notified immediately any time such cues are recognized. Many of them are potentially life-threatening, and in most cases the offending medication must be stopped immediately, with a potential need for hospitalization.

Acute Dystonia

An acute dystonic reaction is an abnormal involuntary movement consisting of a slow and continuous muscular contraction or spasm of the mouth, jaw, face, and neck. The jaw may lock (trismus), the tongue may roll back and block the airway, the neck may arch backward (opisthotonos), or the eyes may close. In an oculogyric crisis, the eyes are fixed in one position. Often this creates a feeling of needing to look up constantly without the ability to gaze downward. The cues may be recognized within hours or days after the initiation of a medication or after a dose increase and may continue from a few minutes to many hours.

Akathisia

Akathisia is a compulsion to be in motion, a sense of restlessness, being unable to be still, having an unrelenting desire to move, and feeling "like crawling out of my skin." Other signs include pacing, fidgeting, and marked restlessness. Akathisia is often mistaken for worsening psychosis instead of the adverse medication reaction that it is. The cues may be recognized at any time during therapy.

Parkinsonian Symptoms

Some of the side effects of antipsychotic medications may appear as if someone has Parkinson's disease. Signs include a tremor, bradykinesia, and rigidity that may progress to the inability to move. The tremor is bilateral compared to one that is unilateral in true Parkinson's disease. An inflexible facial expression and appearing bored and apathetic may be recognized and mistakenly thought to be suggestive of depression instead of an adverse side effect. While these symptoms are more common with the higher-potency antipsychotics, they may be recognized within weeks to months of initiation of antipsychotic therapy.

Tardive Dyskinesia

When antipsychotics have been used continuously for at least 3 to 6 months, patients are at risk for the development of the repetitive and irreversible movement disorder called tardive dyskinesia (TD). Those most at risk are older adults who have been treated for schizophrenia, schizoaffective disorder, or bipolar disorder. The indications of TD usually appear first as choreiform or wormlike movements of the tongue accompanied by other facial movements including grimacing, blinking, and frowning. Slow, maintained, involuntary twisting movements of the limbs, trunk, neck, face, and eyes (involuntary eye closure) also have been recognized (Cornett et al., 2017). Risk factors for the development of TD are increased age, female, dementia, African, or African American. No treatment completely reverses the effect of TD, but it can worsen over time. Therefore it is essential that the nurse be attentive for early recognition of cues so that the health care provider can make prompt changes to the psychotropic regimen. The scheduled and repeated use of a standardized monitoring instrument such as the Abnormal Involuntary Movement Scale (AIMS) is recommended. The instrument as well as a video demonstrating its use can be found at https://www.psychiatrictimes.com/view/aims-abnormal-involuntary-movement-scale.

USING CLINICAL JUDGMENT TO PROMOTE HEALTHY AGING

The gerontological nurse is the key professional involved in making sure that the medications prescribed to and taken by older adults are administered or taken correctly and safely, their effectiveness is monitored, and adjustments are made promptly when needed. Nurses know that one of the most common medication errors is incorrect administration (i.e., wrong time or wrong dose), and that errors frequently occur during transitions from one care setting to another. The nurse can take advantage of the transition as an opportunity to carefully and expertly reconcile all medications and supplements that are taken and note any special risks for drug-drug, drug-supplement, drug-food, or drug-disease interaction. Nurses should be aware of scientific advancements in pharmacogenetics.

In acute care hospitals and long-term care facilities, nurses are responsible for both administering medications and monitoring their effect, especially changes in level of frailty and fluid and dietary intake. Nurses ensure that appropriate laboratory testing is done as needed. They conduct ongoing assessments that determine hypothesis prioritization and actionable nursing interventions that promote safe medication use and self-administration whenever possible.

The promotion of safe medication use requires attention to the potential for ADRs and ADEs, as well as misuse, overuse, and underuse of medications (Box 11.14). Medication overuse (using a drug when not indicated), underuse (not using one when it would be beneficial), and misuse (using one drug when a better alternative is available, a drug that is contraindicated, or that of a neighbor's who had a similar problem) are common occurrences in the life, health, and death of older adults. For example, most older adults are prescribed a proton pump inhibitor for stress ulcer prophylaxis when they are admitted to a hospital. About half of these prescriptions continue after discharge for no known reason (Steinman & Holmes, 2021). Establishing safe usage includes a determination of the patient's self-medication management ability, monitoring the effect and interactions of current medications and other products (e.g., herbals), and evaluating effectiveness of any education provided. Ideally the nurse should know what resources are available, such as the clinical pharmacist and knowledgeable community pharmacists.

Recognizing and Analysing Cues

The initial step in ensuring that medication use is safe, effective, and appropriate is to conduct a comprehensive medication review. This process should be ongoing, but particular attention

---

BOX 11.14 Issues Related to Underuse of Appropriate Medications

Patient Issues
Excessive fear of adverse effects
Lack of agreement by person of the need for the medication
Inadequate resources: financial and inability to obtain
Changes in condition attributed to "old age"

Provider Issues
Distraction of other clinical issues
A sense of futility
Unrecognized ageism, racism, classism, and gender discrimination
Regimen not compatible with person's lifestyle
Undiagnosed condition or missed signs or symptoms of illness
Unrecognized cognitive or sensory limitations

---

is required at any time a new medication is prescribed, a new symptom is reported, or a new cue is observed that indicates a potential reaction or interaction, and during each transition from one care location to another.

⚡ SAFETY TIP

Maintain a High Level of Suspicion

Consideration of a possible adverse drug effect or interaction is imperative at any time a new cue of any kind is recognized.

Both actual and potential problems must be considered. The earlier a potential ADR or ADE is recognized, the less the risk of a cascading of ever-worsening effects, such as dizziness leading to a fall and a fall leading to a fracture and a fracture leading to a premature death. Risk can be reduced through the early recognition of a "prescribing cascade" where more medications are added to treat side effects, reactions, or interactions.

In health care institutions, clinical pharmacists may interview patients about their medication history, but more often this is done through the combined efforts of the licensed nurse and the prescribing care provider (e.g., physician, nurse practitioner). In an ambulatory care setting, the gerontological nurse should not reconcile medications by asking an older adult, "Has anything changed since your last visit?" Instead the "brown bag" approach is highly recommended (Steinman & Holmes, 2021; Zwicker et al., 2021). The person is asked to bring the bottles of all of the medications being taken, including prescription medications, OTCs, herbals, and other dietary supplements, to the hospital or office. To prevent possible misunderstandings or determine misuse, as each bottle is reviewed, the nurse asks what the person thinks each medication is for and how, when, and with what it is taken. The person is asked not to read the label if possible and will guide later patient teaching if needed. At times it may be necessary to compare the dates indicating when the prescriptions were last filled with the number of pills, capsules, or patches remaining or even to call a pharmacy to determine frequency of refills. At least half of all older adults do not take their medications as prescribed, making it extremely important to obtain this information to avoid overprescribing; therefore it is always necessary to ask how many doses are missed in a usual week (Steinman & Holmes, 2021). This may provide indications of level of adherence and compatibility of the prescribed drug regimen with the person's lifestyle and resources. Determination of adherence is particularly important when checking medications that are taken for chronic problems that are asymptomatic, such as hypertension. The sensitive nurse may be told: "I don't have hypertension, so I don't take it."

⚡ SAFETY TIP

Incidental Nonadherence

A person who is instructed to take a medication "three times a day with meals" cannot follow these directions if only two meals a day are eaten. It is unlikely that an older adult with a limited income will fill a prescription that is not covered under that person's prescription drug plan (Chapter 5) or that has a high copay.

BOX 11.15 Medication Review: A Search for Cues Related to Safe Medication Use

1. Is the medication working to improve the patient's symptoms?
   a. What are the desired therapeutic effects of the medication?
   b. What is the time frame for the therapeutic effects?
   c. Is the medication appropriate to the problem and the patient?
   d. Has the length of time been appropriate to determine efficacy?
2. Is the medication harming the patient?
   a. What physiological changes are occurring?
   b. What laboratory values are changing?
   c. What mental status changes are occurring?
   d. What functional changes are occurring?
   e. Is the patient experiencing side effects?
   f. Is the medication interacting with anything?
   g. Can cues of adverse drug events and reactions be recognized and by whom?
3. Does the patient understand the following?
   a. Why is the medication being taken?
   b. How and when is the medication supposed to be taken?
   c. The risks for interactions and adverse reactions?
   d. How to reduce or manage side effects and who to report these to?
   e. What limitations are imposed by taking the medication (e.g., avoiding alcohol, avoiding direct sun, avoiding becoming overheated)?

BOX 11.16 Tips for Best Practice

Review Points Particularly Important When Working With Older Adults

- Have nonpharmacological actions already been attempted?
- Is the dose the lowest possible while still effective?
- Is a prescribing cascade present?
- Is the medication affordable and obtainable?
- Can a less expensive medication be equally safe and effective?
- Has the person involved in decision making regarding medication use been involved in teaching?
- Are medications that have been obtained from others being used?
- Are recently discontinued medications or "leftover" prescriptions still in use? Any duplications (e.g., both atenolol and Tenormin)?
- Are effective reminder systems in place or available?
- Are needed medication blood levels current?
- Are there any indications of hepatic or renal insufficiencies?
- Can packaging and lids be removed?
- Is there manual dexterity adequate to self-administer all medications required?
- Is storage and disposal safe and available?
- Are there any cognitive limitations that will affect safe drug use?
- Are atypical cues to adverse reactions and events recognizable?

The review or assessment must be conducted with utmost tact and respect and in a nonjudgmental manner, otherwise it is likely that the needed information will not be forthcoming. By conducting the assessment in this manner, the nurse can discover discrepancies between the prescribed dosage and the dosage taken, potential interactions, and potential or actual ADRs. While the essentials of the comprehensive medication review are the same as those for younger adults (Box 11.15), additional information is needed to provide expert care to those in later life (Box 11.16).

The analysis of the review data should include the identification of unnecessary or potentially inappropriate medications (PIMs) as well as those medications that are potential prescribing omissions (PPOs). For example, all older adults taking opioids for any length of time also should be prescribed a routine stool softener and may need a routine laxative as well, but this may have been "missed." The appropriate use of medications in the older adult means that such products are used when needed but only as necessary and then at the minimum dose needed to achieve the desired effects, and in a way where the risks relative to benefits have been considered within the greater context of the person's life expectancy, health, lifestyle, and values. The use of PIMs has been found to be associated with confusion, falls, frailty, and unnecessary morbidity and mortality.

The Screening Tool of Older Person's Prescriptions/Screening Tool to Alert Doctors to Right Treatment (STOPP/START) and the Beers Criteria (American Geriatrics Society [AGS], 2019) are both evidence-based and recommended for use in the identification of potentially inappropriate prescribing (Thomas & Thomas, 2019). Both tools include lists of medications to avoid or use with caution and are widely used or mandated to address overuse or underuse and to maximize health outcomes (Zwicker et al., 2020). Based on the Beers Criteria, the AGS

offers alternatives to commonly prescribed medications that should be avoided (Health in Aging, 2019).

STOPP/START

The STOPP/START instrument is widely available and offers a ranking of medications under a stoplight system of red (avoid) and green (consider if appropriate). The instrument provides guidance in a medication review, to reach an agreement with the patient about treatment and to optimize the impact of medicines while minimizing medication-related problems. A person-centered approach is recommended while considering benefits versus risks, interlinked symptoms, comorbidities, and medication-related side effects and interactions. It is expected that discussions include risks and benefits of the treatment plan and their values and preferences, in order to help a patient make fully informed decisions regarding medication use that takes into account the patient's knowledge, beliefs, and cultural patterns (NHS, 2016).

Beers Criteria

The Beers Criteria are the result of an exhaustive review of medications considered to be frequently prescribed to older adults. The 2019 list includes (1) those medications that are "potentially inappropriate" for use with older adults, (2) those that are potentially inappropriate for older adults with certain conditions, (3) those that should avoided or have their dose changed for people with impaired renal function, and (4) a list of drug-drug interactions documented to be harmful to older adults (Box 11.17).

While the Beers Criteria have been incorporated into regulatory policy, the authors of the 2019 document emphasize the need to have it serve as a guide rather absolute direction. The Criteria are a part of the quality measures for the National Committee for Quality Assurance (NCQA) and the Healthcare

BOX 11.17 High-Risk and Potentially Inappropriate Medications for Older Adults

Oral anticoagulants
Sliding-scale insulin
Long-acting sulfonylureas
Digoxin
Opioids
Nonsteroidal antiinflammatory drugs (NSAIDs)
Anticholinergics
Antipsychotics (only as necessary for persons with dementia related psychosis)
Benzodiazepines
Proton pump inhibitors for longer than 8 weeks
H2-receptor antagonists
Demerol: *always contraindicated*

Data from American Geriatrics Society: American Geriatrics Society 2019 updated Beers Criteria for potentially inappropriate medication use in older adults, *J Am Geriatr Soc* 67(4):674–694, 2019; Hamilton H, Gallagher P, Ryan C, et al: Potentially inappropriate medications defined by STOPP criteria and the risk of adverse drug events in older hospitalized patients, *Arch Intern Med* 171(11):1013–1019, 2011.

TABLE 11.5 Examples of Changes With Aging That May Interfere With Medication Self-Administration

Change With Aging	Consequence
Sensory	
Decreased visual acuity	Greater difficulty in reading instructions
Decreased sensation	Greater difficulty in manipulating medications
Decreased salivation	Greater difficulty in swallowing
Mechanical	
Decreased fine motor coordination	Greater difficulty in manipulating medications and packaging
Stiffening of large joints	Greater difficulty in self-administering medications

BOX 11.18 Knowing Whom You Are Talking To

M. François came to the clinic as a new patient with uncontrolled hypertension. The nurse practitioner, through an interpreter, spent a lot of time with him explaining how to take his medications, what they were for, and so on. He and his presumed caregiver sat quietly and appeared to understand. When he returned a month later his blood pressure was still out of control. There was a different person with him who asked all the questions that were addressed at the first appointment. On further inquiry it was found that rather than miss an appointment, a neighbor had brought M. François to the clinic. His niece who "takes care of things" had been unavailable and was now present.

Effectiveness Data and Information Set (HEDIS) (NCQA, 2018). When a potentially inappropriate medication is prescribed in the long-term care setting without documentation of an overwhelming benefit of its use, it can be considered a form of medication misuse by the prescribing practitioner.

SOLUTIONS AND NURSING ACTIONS: SAFE MEDICATION USE

In all settings, a vital nursing function is to provide education leading to safe medication use and to ensure that the older adult is aware of potential side effects, how to minimize their risk, and what to do about them should they occur. Through education the nurse assists the patient and family in adapting the medication regimen to normal age-related changes, functional ability, lifestyle, and life patterns (Table 11.5). However, education can be particularly challenging when working with older adults. The following nursing actions may be helpful in promoting safe medication use.

Education

Identify key persons: Determine who, if anyone, manages the person's medications, helps the person, or assists with decision making; and with the person's permission, make sure that the helper is present when any teaching is done (Box 11.18).

Consider the teaching and learning environment: Minimize distraction and avoid competition with television, grandchildren, or others demanding the patient's attention; make sure the person is comfortable and is not hungry, thirsty, tired, too warm or too cold, in pain, or in need of the toilet.

Optimize timing: Provide the teaching during the best time of the day when the learners are most engaged and energetic. Keep the education sessions short and succinct.

Facilitate communication: Ensure that you are understood. Make sure the learner's glasses are clean and on and hearing aids are functioning and in place if they are needed. Use simple and direct language, avoid medical or nursing jargon (e.g., "intake"), yet always strive for clarity (Box 11.19). Speak clearly, facing the person at head level and with light on your face to facilitate the lip-reading used to augment hearing loss. Use formal language (e.g., Mr. Jones) unless you have permission to do otherwise. Do not touch the patient unless it is indicated to you that it is acceptable to do so (e.g., patient lays a hand on yours; Chapter 4). If the person is blind and reads braille, obtain instructions in this format whenever possible. If the person has limited language proficiency in the country in which care is delivered, a trained medical interpreter will be needed (Chapter 4).

Reinforce teaching: All education is supported by written or graphic materials that are understandable to the patient. They are provided in a font size that compensates for reduced visual acuity if needed. If the person or helper is literate, the materials must be provided at the appropriate educational level and in the language that can be understood. For those with limited literacy, symbols may be needed, such as sunrise, sunset, food, or bed. Most people have at least rudimentary number fluency.

BOX 11.19   A Potentially Lethal Misunderstanding

I visited Mrs. Helena to enroll her in a research study. As we reviewed her health and current medications, she shared that she had not been feeling well. She reported that in the past she had been told that the "little white pills" would make her feel better, and so she had taken five or more in the last couple of hours and did not understand why she was not improved. When I looked at her pill bottle, I saw that the "little white pill" was digoxin. I called an ambulance urgently and reported that she had accidentally taken a potentially toxic (and fatal) dose of a prescribed medication.

Kathleen Jett

Evaluate teaching: In the ambulatory care setting, teaching is evaluated as medications are reconciled at each encounter. Medications are reviewed with the same questions as in the previous encounter (e.g., why taken, when, how, misses). With further discussion the goal is to determine if any variation from expected knowledge and use are related to teaching or learning difficulty or a patient-centered issue. Using the LEARN model in the assessment process may be helpful in the evaluation of teaching (Chapter 4).

Medication Reminders

A safe, optimal, and feasible medication plan is one that the patient can adhere to. Due to the sheer volume of medications and supplements taken, some reminder mechanisms are frequently required. Although there is a wide array of these reminder tools available on the market today, most older adults continue to use the strategies they have developed over the years to remember to take their medications. These may be as simple as a using an egg carton as a storage box or turning a bottle upside down once the medication has been taken for the day, or as intense as having a family member or friend call the person at designated times. Encourage the person to use techniques that have worked in the past or to develop new strategies to ensure correct and timely medication use when needed (Lavan et al., 2016). A safe, optimal, and feasible medication regimen and reminder system is one that the patient can and is willing to adhere to.

Evaluating Outcomes

Lastly, it is necessary for the gerontological nurse to monitor and evaluate both nursing actions and prescribed treatments for use, side effects, and efficacy (Table 11.6). Monitoring and evaluating involves recognition of changes in physical and functional status (e.g., vital signs, performance of activities of daily living, sleeping, eating, hydrating, eliminating) and mental status (e.g., attention and level of alertness, memory, orientation, behavior, mood, emotional display and affect, content and characteristics of interactions). Monitoring means ensuring that blood levels are measured when they are needed—for example, regular thyroid-stimulating hormone (TSH) levels for all persons taking thyroid replacement therapy, INRs for all persons taking warfarin, or periodic hemoglobin A_{1C} levels for all persons with diabetes (Chapter 27). Accurate monitoring is dependent on the

TABLE 11.6   Medications Commonly Prescribed to Older Adults and Cues for Monitoring for Effectiveness

Class of Medication	Cues
Antibiotics and antivirals	Signs of infection: symptom reduction
Antihyperlipidemics	Lipids and triglycerides within normal limits for the person Liver function testing: no changes in function Blood glucose: no elevation
Cardiac medications	Heart rate and rhythm are within the desired parameters for the person
Anticoagulants	Presence or absence of bleeding, clotting times (international normalized ratio [INR], prothrombin time) within acceptable limits
Antihypertensives	Heart rate and rhythm are within the desired parameters for the person and without orthostatic hypotension No unexplained weight gain or loss
Antihyperglycemics	Hemoglobin A1C is maintained between 6.0 and 7.0 for all but frail patients (Chapter 27)
Antiparkinsonians	Improved functional status Less visible immobility
Analgesics	Improved symptoms of pain and inflammation

nurse possessing and understanding the relevant information about the treatments and medications that are prescribed and administered. Quality patient care requires nurses to promptly communicate their analyses and hypotheses to the patient's nurse practitioner or physician.

Deprescribing

With the recognition of the frequency of problematic polypharmacy, the concept of "deprescribing" has received considerable attention of late. Deprescribing is a process that includes the recognition of PIMs and the development of interventions that can lead to cessation of some medications or supplements or reducing the dosages as low as possible without losing their effectiveness. The Beers Criteria or the STOPP instrument can be used as a guide for recognition of PIMs.

Although the prescriber (e.g., nurse practitioner) holds a lead role in deprescribing, the bedside and office nurses are involved as well. This may involve making suggestions to the prescriber or becoming the key negotiator working with the patient or family member who resists recommended changes to the drug regimen. The nurse will hear, "I don't understand; I/mom/dad has always taken this" or "We/I tried that before and it did not work."

Medications occupy a central place in the lives of many older persons: cost, acceptability, interactions, adverse reactions and events, and the need to schedule medications appropriately all combine to create many difficulties. The nurse can promote healthy aging through knowledge of the effect of normal age-related changes on pharmacodynamics and pharmacokinetics and awareness of the key issues in medication use in older adults in all care settings.

All medications have indications, side effects, interactions, and individual patient reactions. The nurse must determine whether side effects are minimal and tolerable or serious (Table 11.7). Asking subjective questions and observing the patient's interactions, behavior, mood, emotional responses, and daily habits provide essential data.

The desired outcomes of evidence-based nursing actions related to safe medication use by older adults include minimizing problematic polypharmacy; avoiding adverse medication reactions, events, and interactions; and facilitating adherence to medication regimens that promote healthy aging or comfort while dying. For those who do not have a medical home or require additional support, older persons can be referred to the Medication Therapy Management program that may be available to them through their prescription drug plans (https://www.medicare.gov/drug-coverage-part-d/what-medicare-part-d-drug-plans-cover/medication-therapy-management-programs-for-complex-health-needs).

The nurse is well situated to coordinate care, identify the patient's goals, determine what the patient needs to learn in order to understand prescribed medications, and arrange for follow-up care to determine the outcome of medication teaching.

TABLE 11.7 Medications Commonly Prescribed to Older Adults and Cues of Toxicity

Medication	Cues
Benzodiazepines (e.g., Ativan)	Ataxia, restlessness, confusion, depression, anticholinergic effect
Cimetidine (Tagamet)	Confusion, depression
Digitalis (digoxin)	Confusion, headache, anorexia, vomiting, arrhythmias, blurred vision or visual changes (halos, frost on objects, color blindness), paresthesia
Furosemide (Lasix)	Electrolyte imbalance, hepatic changes, pancreatitis, leukopenia, thrombocytopenia
Levodopa (L-Dopa)	Muscle and eye twitching, disorientation, asterixis, hallucinations, dyskinetic movements, grimacing, depression, delirium, ataxia
Nonsteroidal antiinflammatory drugs (NSAIDs), such as Advil and Naprosyn	Photosensitivity, fluid retention, anemia, nephrotoxicity, visual changes, bleeding, blood pressure elevations
Ranitidine (Zantac)	Liver dysfunction, blood dyscrasias
Sulfonylureas: first generation (e.g., Diabinese)	Hypoglycemia, hepatic changes, heart failure, bone marrow depression, jaundice

KEY CONCEPTS

- The therapeutic goal of pharmacological intervention is to reduce the targeted symptoms and control disease conditions without undesirable side effects.
- One must always be alert for cues that require further analysis related to potential medication-medication, medication-herb/supplement, and medication-food/beverage interactions.
- Polypharmacy significantly increases the risk of medication interactions and adverse events. The risk for polypharmacy increases with each prescriber seen.
- Any time there is a change in a person, it is reasonable to first consider it a a potential cue of medication effect; this is of paramount importance when caring for older adults and those who are frail.
- Medication misuse may be triggered by prescriber practices, individual self-medication, physiological idiosyncrasies, altered biodegradability, nutritional and fluid states, and inadequate assessment before prescribing.

- Patients cannot comply with a prescription or treatment when it interferes with the practicalities of life or is distressful to the individual's well-being or when misunderstanding or disability prevents compliance.
- The side effects of psychotropic medications vary significantly; thus these medications must be selected with care and monitored closely when prescribed for the older adult.
- The cues indicating a positive response to psychotropic medications are reduced distress, clearer thinking, and enhanced safety for the person and those around that person.
- It is always expected that psychotropic pharmacological approaches augment rather than replace nonpharmacological approaches.
- Older adults are particularly vulnerable to develop movement disorders (extrapyramidal symptoms, parkinsonian symptoms, akathisia, dystonia) with the use of antipsychotics.

NEXT-GENERATION NCLEX® (NGN) EXAMINATION-STYLE QUESTIONS

Mrs. Rosa Donato is a 78-year-old widow who lives alone in a large city. She is very proud of her adult children and often tells others stories about when she and her husband immigrated to the United States from Italy when her children were small. She is a devout Catholic and attends mass each morning. Her treks to church, to the senior center, and to her various physicians (internist; orthopedic, cardiac, and ophthalmic specialists) constitute her social life. She had only a few years of primary education and has little written

Highlight the cues that will help determine if Mrs. Donato is at risk for adverse interactions and effects or medication misuse.
Underline the first and second priority hypotheses (i.e., those that put her at most immediate risk for a poor outcome).

English fluency. According to the staff at the senior center, she still clings to many of her "old country" ways. She speaks a mixture of English and Italian. She reports that her knees "give out" and that she has "sugar" and "water" problems. She admits that she has been increasingly short of breath of late and her knees have been aching more than usual. She has been diagnosed with arthritis, mild diabetes, and heart failure. One day the nurse at the senior center noticed her pulling a paper bag of medication bottles from her purse. She sat down to talk with Rosa about them and soon realized that she had only a vague idea of what most of them were for and tended to take them whenever she felt she needed them. When a student nurse arrived at the center she was asked to speak with Mrs. Donato. She is taking digoxin, Lasix, a potassium supplement, lisinopril, Zocor, and glyburide. She also takes ibuprofen, garlic, and ginseng. She takes Xanax for sleep.

Select from the following potential solutions. Which one would be most likely to be effective in your first approach to Mrs. Donato?

1. Call her children to learn if they have any concerns about their mother.
2. Ask one of her children to visit when you are scheduled to next be at the senior center so that the three of you can discuss Mrs. Donato's priorities.
3. Ask Mrs. Donato to describe her health problems and whether any of the medications she is taking addresses the problem.
4. Ask Mrs. Donato how she is supposed to take each of her medications.

CLINICAL JUDGMENT QUESTIONS AND ACTIVITIES

1. Mrs. J., a patient of yours in a long-term care setting, is calling out repeatedly for a nurse; other patients are complaining, and you simply cannot be available for long periods to quiet her. Considering the setting and the Beers Criteria, what would you do to manage the situation?
2. When you are given a prescription for medication, what do you ask about it?
3. Do you think most older adults seek adequate information about their medications before taking them?

RESEARCH QUESTIONS

1. Where would you obtain medication information for persons with limited English proficiency?
2. Why do older adults often self-treat with OTC and herbal medicines?
3. What are the nursing roles in preventing adverse medication events?
4. Among the following three teaching strategies, which works the best: computer-assisted medication teaching, telephone teaching, or in-person medication teaching? Why?

REFERENCES

American Geriatrics Society (AGS): American Geriatrics Society 2019 updated Beers Criteria for potentially inappropriate medication use in older adults, *J Am Geriatr Soc* 67(4):674–694, 2019.

Centers for Medicare and Medicaid Services (CMS): *National partnership to improve dementia care in nursing homes* (website), 2021. https://www.cms.gov/Medicare/Provider-Enrollment-and-Certification/SurveyCertificationGenInfo/National-Partnership-to-Improve-Dementia-Care-in-Nursing-Homes.

Cornett EM, Novitch M, Kaye AD, et al.: Medication-induced tardive dyskinesia: a review and update, *Ochsner J* 17(2):162–174, 2017.

Fahmi ML, Azmy MT, Noorizan EU, et al.: Inappropriate prescribing defined by STOPP and START criteria and its association with adverse drug event among hospitalized older patients: a multicentre prospective study, *PLoS ONE* 14(7):e219898, 2019.

Gao S, Bell EC, Zhang Y, et al.: Racial disparities in drug disposition in the digestive tract, *Int J Mol Sci* 22(3):e1038, 2021.

Hales CM, Servais J, Martin CB, et al: *Prescription drug use among adults aged 40–79 in the United States and Canada* (website), 2019. https://www.cdc.gov/nchs/products/databriefs/db347.htm.

Health in Aging: *Tip sheet: alternative for medications listed in the AGS Beers Criteria® for potentially inappropriate medication use in older adults* (website), 2019. https://www.healthinaging.org/tools-and-tips/tip-sheet-alternatives-medications-listed-ags-beers-criteriar-potentially.

Horn JR: (2008). *Get to know an enzyme: CYP2D6* (website), 2008. https://www.pharmacytimes.com/view/2008-07-8624.

Khezrian M, McNeil CJ, Murray AD, et al.: An overview of prevalence, determinants, and health outcomes of polypharmacy, *Ther Adv Drug Saf* 11:1–10, 2020.

Lapin A, Mueller E: Laboratory diagnosis and geriatrics: more than just reference intervals for older adults. In Fillit HM, Rockwood K, Young JB, editors: *Brocklehurst's textbook of geriatric medicine and gerontology*, ed 8, Philadelphia, 2017, Elsevier, pp 220–225.

Lavan AH, Gallagher PE, O'Mahony D: Methods to reduce prescribing errors in elderly patients with multimorbidity, *Clin Interv Aging* 11:857–866, 2016.

Levy HB: Polypharmacy reduction strategies: tips on incorporating American Geriatrics Society Beers and Screening Tool of Older People's Prescriptions Criteria, *Clin Geriatr Med* 33(2):177–187, 2017.

National Institute of Mental Health (NIMH): *Mental health medications (website)*, 2016, www.nimh.nih.gov/health/topics/mental-health-medications.

NHS: *STOPP START toolkit: supporting medication review in Cumbria (website)*, 2016. https://www.hqsc.govt.nz/assets/Medication-Safety/prescribing-toolkit/STOPPSTART-toolkit-Cumbria-2016.pdf.

Payne R: The epidemiology of polypharmacy, *Clin Med (Lond)* 16(5):465–469, 2016.

Reuben DB, Herr KA, Pacala JT, et al.: *Geriatrics at your fingertips*, ed 19, New York, 2020, American Geriatrics Society.

Rochon PA, Schmader KE, Givens J: *Drug prescribing for older adults* (website), 2021. https://www.uptodate.com/contents/drug-prescribing-for-older-adults.

Shim YK, Kim N, Park YH, et al.: Effects of age on esophageal motility: use of high-resolution esophageal impedance manometry, *J Neurogastroenterol Motil* 23(2):229–236, 2017.

Slattum PW, Ogbonna KC, Peron EP: The pharmacology of aging. In Fillit HM, Rockwood K, Young JB, editors: *Brocklehurst's textbook of geriatric medicine and gerontology*, ed 8, Philadelphia, 2017, Elsevier, pp 160–165.

Steinman MA, Holmes HM: Principles of prescribing and adherence. In Walter LC, Change A, editors: *CURRENT diagnosis and treatment: geriatrics*, ed 3, New York, 2021, McGraw Hill, pp 105–120.

Taghy N, Cambon L, Cohn J-M, et al.: Failure to reach a consensus in polypharmacy definition: an obstacle to measuring risks and impacts—results of a literature review, *Ther Clin Risk Manag* 16:57–73, 2020.

Thomas RE, Thomas BC: A systematic review of studies of the STOPP/START 2015 and the American Geriatric Society Beers 2015 Criteria in patients ≥65 years, *Curr Aging Sci* 12(2):121–154, 2019.

Thornton SL, Darracq MA: Patch problems? Characteristics of transdermal drug delivery system exposures reported to the national poison data system, *J Med Toxicology* 16(1):33–40, 2020.

US Food and Drug Administration (FDA): *FDA 101: Dietary supplements* (website), 2015. https://www.fda.gov/ForConsumers/ConsumerUpdates/ucm050803.htm .

Zwicker D, Carvajal C, Fulmer T: Reducing adverse drug events in the older adult. In Boltz M (Ed): *Evidence-based geriatric nursing protocols for best practice*, ed 3, New York, 2021, Springer, pp 408–438.

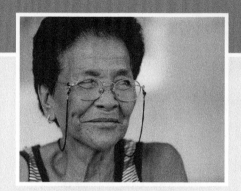

CHAPTER 12

Visual Health

Theris A. Touhy

http://evolve.elsevier.com/Touhy/TwdHlthAging

A STUDENT SPEAKS

I kind of understand the problems vision impairment can cause as one ages. I am pretty blind without my glasses. I can't even see the alarm clock numbers. I worry about what my vision will be when I am older. I took care of a woman in the assisted living facility with macular degeneration. I asked her how the disease affects her vision. The woman put her hand in front of my face and said, "I can see your hair, the color, and some of the space around you, but I cannot see your face or the color of your skin." She seems to cope pretty well and uses low-vision devices to help her manage her life. It frightened me a little but also gave me hope that even with this kind of vision loss she is able to function and stay in pretty good spirits. I am going to get some information about how to keep my eyes healthy. I hadn't thought about the things I could do now that might help as I age.

Debbie, age 27

AN OLDER ADULT SPEAKS

One of the great frustrations is the matter of eyesight. One can get used to large print and hope for black letters on white paper, but why do modern publishers seem to prefer the shiny, slick off-white paper and pale ink in minuscule print? Thank goodness for restaurants with lighted menus and my new iPhone with a bright light.

Lyn, age 85

LEARNING OBJECTIVES

On completion of this chapter, the reader will be able to:

1. Describe the impact of vision changes on quality of life and function.
2. Describe the importance of health education and screening for vision problems.
3. Identify effective communication strategies for older adults with vision impairment.
4. Use clinical judgment to recognize and analyze cues and identify and evaluate solutions and nursing actions to enhance visual health.
5. Gain awareness of assistive devices to enhance vision.

VISION IMPAIRMENT

Incidence and Prevalence

Vision loss is not an inevitable part of the aging process, but age-related changes contribute to decreased vision. Even older adults with good visual acuity (20/40 or better) and no significant eye disease show deficits in visual function and need accommodations to enhance vision and safety. With age, there is a higher risk of developing age-related eye diseases and other conditions (hypertension, diabetes) that can result in vision losses if left untreated.

Vision loss is a leading cause of age-related disability. More than two-thirds of those with visual impairment are older than

65 years of age, and adults older than 80 years account for 70% of the cases of severe visual impairment. The World Health Organization (WHO, 2020) defines visual impairment as visual acuity worse than 20/70 but better than 20/400 (legal blindness) in the better eye, even with corrective lenses.

Visual impairment worldwide has decreased since the 1990s because of increased availability of eye care services (particularly cataract surgery), promotion of eye care education, and improved treatment of infectious diseases. However, vision impairment is a major public health problem across the globe that is expected to increase substantially with the aging of the population. Rates of blindness and visual impairment in disadvantaged, minority populations, particularly African American and Latinx subpopulations who have an increased prevalence of diabetes and hypertension, are expected to increase even further. In the United States, the leading causes of visual impairment are cataracts, glaucoma, diabetic neuropathy, and age-related macular degeneration (AMD). Globally, uncorrected refractive errors (myopia, hyperopia, or astigmatism), glaucoma, and unoperated cataract are the leading causes of visual impairment.

CHANGES IN VISION WITH AGE

Changes in eye structure begin early, are progressive in nature, and are both functional and structural. The structures most affected are the cornea, anterior chamber, lens, ciliary muscles, and retina. All of the age-related changes affect visual acuity and accommodation. Although presbyopia (decreased near vision due to aging) is first seen between 45 and 55 years of age, 80% of those older than 65 years have fair to adequate far vision past 90 years of age. Nearly 95% of adults older than 65 years wear glasses for close vision.

Extraocular Changes

Like the skin elsewhere, the eyelids lose elasticity and drooping (senile ptosis) may result. In most cases, this is only a cosmetic concern. In some cases, it can interfere with vision if the lids sag far enough over the lower lid margin. Spasms of the orbicular muscle may cause the lower lid to turn inward. If it stays this way, it is called *entropion*. With the curling of the lid, the lower lashes also turn inward, causing irritation and scratching of the cornea. Surgery may be needed to prevent permanent injury. Decreases in orbicular muscle strength may result in *ectropion*, or an out-turning of the lower lid (Fig. 12.1). Without the integrity of the trough of the lower lid, tears run down the cheek instead of bathing the cornea. This, along with an inability to close the lid completely, leads to excessively dry eyes (xerophthalmia) and the need for use of artificial tears. The individual also may need to tape the eyes shut during sleep. A reduction of goblet cells in the conjunctiva is another cause for drying of the eyes in the older adult. Goblet cells produce mucin, which slows the evaporation of tear film and is essential for eye lubrication and movement.

Ocular Changes

The cornea is the avascular transparent outer surface of the eye globe that refracts (bends) light rays entering the eye through

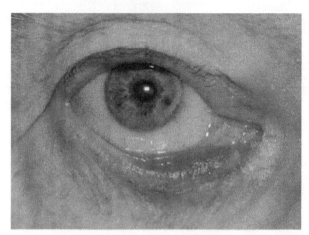

Fig. 12.1 Ectropion. (From Swartz MH: *Textbook of physical diagnosis: history and examination,* ed 6, Philadelphia, 2009, Saunders.)

the pupil. With aging, the cornea becomes flatter, less smooth, and thicker, with the changes noticeable by its lackluster appearance or loss of sparkling transparency. The result is the increased incidence of astigmatism. The anterior chamber is the space between the cornea and the lens. The edges of the chamber include the canals that control the volume and movement of aqueous fluid within the space. With aging, the chamber decreases slightly in size and volume capacity because of thickening of the lens. Resorption of the intraocular fluid becomes less efficient and may lead to eventual breakdown in the absorption process. If the change is greater, it can lead to increased intraocular pressure (IOP) and the development of glaucoma.

The iris is a ring of muscles inside the anterior chamber. The iris surrounds the opening into the eye (the pupil), gives the eye color, and regulates the amount of light that reaches the retina. With age the iris becomes paler in color as a result of pigment loss and increases in the density of collagen fibers. A normal age-related change in the iris is linked to other neurological changes—that is, slowed response to sensory stimuli, in this case, to light and dark. Slowness to dilate in dark environments creates moments when older adults may have difficulty seeing where they are going (e.g., moving from a well-lit area to a dark area such as in a movie theater).

Because of the slow ability of the pupils to accommodate to changes in light, glare can be a major problem. Glare is caused by not only sunlight but also reflection of light on any shiny object, such as headlights or polished floors. The use of sunglasses outdoors (and indoors if considerable glare exists) can be helpful. The effect of glare from headlights of oncoming vehicles increases safety risks with driving (night blindness). Persistent pupillary constriction is known as *senile miosis*. It may be noted during the physical exam but is considered a normal finding if it is bilateral. At the edges of the cornea and the iris is a small ring known as the *limbus*. In some older adults, a gray-white ring or partial ring, known as *arcus senilis*, forms 1 to 2 mm inside the limbus. It does not affect vision and is composed of deposits of calcium and cholesterol salts.

The lens, a small, flexible, biconvex, crystal-like structure just behind the iris, is responsible for visual acuity as it adjusts the light entering the pupil and focuses it on the retina. Age-related

TABLE 12.1 Changes in the Eye Caused by Aging

Structure	Change	Consequence
Cornea	Thicker and less curved	Increase in astigmatism
	Formation of a gray ring at the edge of cornea (arcus senilis)	Not detrimental to vision
Anterior chamber	Decrease in size and volume caused by thickening of lens	Occasionally exerts pressure on Schlemm canal and may lead to increased intraocular pressure and glaucoma
Lens	Increase in opacity	Decrease in refraction with increased light scattering and decreased color vision (green and blue); decreased dark adaptation; cataracts
	Loss of elasticity	Loss of accommodation (presbyopia: loss of focus for near objects)
Ciliary muscles	Reduction in pupil diameter, atrophy of radial dilation muscles	Persistent constriction (senile miosis); decrease in critical flicker frequencya
Retina	Reduction in number of rods at periphery, loss of rods and associated nerve cells	Increase in the minimum amount of light necessary to see an object
Macula	Atrophy (age-related macular degeneration)	Loss of vision
Vitreous	Liquefaction of vitreous and decrease in gel volume	Posterior vitreous detachment causing "floaters"; risk for retinal detachment

aThe rate at which consecutive visual stimuli can be presented and still be perceived as separate.
From McCance KL, Huether SE: *Pathophysiology*, ed 7, St Louis, 2014, Mosby.

changes in the lens are probably universal, but many of the changes are thought to result from exposure to ultraviolet light. The constant compression of lens fibers with age, the yellowing effect, and the inefficiency of the aqueous humor, which provides the lens with nutrition, all have a role in altered lens transparency. Lens cells continue to grow but at a slower rate than previously. The lens can no longer focus (refract) close objects effectively, described as decreased accommodation.

Changes to the suspensory ligaments, ciliary muscles, and parasympathetic nerves also contribute to the decreased accommodation. Finally, light scattering increases and color perception decreases. For the person who was myopic (near-sighted) earlier in life, this change actually may improve vision. Lens opacity (cataracts) begins to develop around the fifth decade of life. The origins are not fully understood, although ultraviolet light contributes, with cross-linkage of collagen creating a more rigid and thickened lens structure.

Intraocular Changes

The vitreous humor, which gives the eye globe its shape and support, loses some of its water and fibrous skeletal support with age. Opacities other than cataracts can be seen by the person as lines, webs, spots, or clusters of dots moving rapidly across the visual field with each movement of the eye. These opacities are called "floaters" and are bits of coalesced vitreous humor that have broken off from the peripheral or central part of the retina. Most are harmless but annoying until they dissipate or one gets used to them. However, if the person sees a shower of these and a flash of light, immediate medical attention is required, and this is always considered an ocular emergency (retinal detachment).

The retina, which lines the inside of the eye, has less distinct margins and is duller in appearance than in younger adults. Fidelity of color is less accurate with blues, violets, and greens of the spectrum; warm colors such as reds, oranges, and yellows are more easily seen. Color clarity diminishes by 25% in the sixth decade and by 59% in the eighth decade. Some of this difficulty is linked to the yellowing of the lens and the impaired transmission of light to the retina, and the fovea may not be as bright. The average 80-year-old needs more than twice as much light as a 20-year-old to see equally well (McCance & Huether et al., 2014).

Drusen (yellow-white) spots may appear in the area of the macula. As long as these changes are not accompanied by distortion of objects or a decrease in vision, they are not clinically significant. Finally, the number of rods and associated nerves at the periphery of the retina is reduced, resulting in peripheral vision that is not as discrete or is absent. Arteries in the back of the eye may show atherosclerosis and slight narrowing. Veins may show indentations (nicking) at the arteriovenous crossings if the person has a long history of hypertension. Table 12.1 summarizes changes in the eye with age.

Consequences of Visual Impairment

Visual problems have a negative impact on quality of life, equivalent to that of life-threatening conditions such as heart disease and cancer. Loss of vision affects an individual's quality of life and ability to function in most daily activities such as driving, reading, maneuvering safely, dressing, cooking, taking medications, and participating in social activities. Decreased vision also has been found to be a significant risk factor for falls and other accidents and is associated with cognitive decline and depression, increased risk of institutionalization, and death. Vision loss not only severely impairs one's ability to be independent and self-sufficient but also has a "snowball effect" on the health and well-being of older adults, families, caregivers, and society at large. This cumulative effect is severely underestimated.

Prevention of Visual Impairment

Many age-related eye diseases have no symptoms in the early stages but can be detected early through a comprehensive

BOX 12.1   Promoting Healthy Eyes

- Have a comprehensive eye dilated eye exam
- Know your family's eye health history
- Eat right to protect your sight (diet rich in green leafy vegetables, fruit, and fish)
- Maintain a healthy weight
- Wear protective eyewear
- Quit smoking or never start
- Be cool and wear your shades
- Give your eyes a rest when doing computer work or focusing on any one thing. Every 20 minutes look away 20 feet in front of you for 20 seconds. This will help reduce eyestrain
- Clean your hands and your contact lenses properly
- Practice workplace eye safety (protective eye wear if required)

From National Eye Institute: *Information for healthy vision* (website), 2021. https://nei.nih.gov/healthyeyes/eyehealthtips. Accessed March 2021.

BOX 12.2   Resources for Best Practice

Vision Impairment

Centers for Disease Control and Prevention (CDC): Educational materials, videos illustrating vision with age-related macular degeneration (AMD), glaucoma, diabetic retinopathy. https://www.cdc.gov/features/healthyvision/index.html.

EyeCare America: Online referral center for eye care resources. https://www.aao.org/eyecare-america.

National Eye Health Education Program (NEHEP) and National Eye Institute (NEI): Educational and professional resources, vision and aging program: *See Well for a Lifetime Toolkit,* vodcasts on common visual problems, videos on eye disease. https://www.nei.nih.gov/learn-about-eye-health/resources-for-health-educators.

National Federation of the Blind: Educational information, resources. https://www.nfb.org/.

VisionAware (American Foundation for the Blind): Resources for independent living with vision loss, getting started kit for people new to vision loss, how to walk with a guide. https://www.visionaware.org.

dilated eye exam. However, knowledge about eye disease and treatments remains inadequate among both laypersons and medical professionals. Socioeconomic position and educational position are important social determinants that may influence access to and use of effective and appropriate eye care, thus influencing disease identification and treatment.

At all ages, attention to eye health and protection of vision are important (Box 12.1). Prevention and treatment of eye disease are important priorities for nurses and other health professionals. The National Eye Health Education Program (NEHEP) of the National Eye Institute (NEI) provides a program for health professionals with evidence-based tools and resources that can be used in community settings to educate older adults about eye health and maintaining healthy vision. Educational materials and outreach activities targeted to populations at high risk for eye diseases, including African Americans, American Indians, Alaska Natives, Hispanics/Latinos, and individuals with diabetes and a family history of glaucoma, are available (NEI, 2021a) (Box 12.2).

Vision loss from eye disease is particularly a concern in the developing countries, where 90% of the world's blind individuals live. Cataracts are the leading cause of blindness in economically challenged countries, largely as a result of limited service and treatment (WHO, 2020). The proportion of vision impairment attributable to cataract is higher in low- and middle-income countries than in high-income countries, and diseases such as diabetic retinopathy, glaucoma, and AMD are more common. Estimates are that 80% of all visual impairment can be avoided or cured. *Healthy People 2030* addresses visual health.

HEALTHY PEOPLE 2030

Goals for Visual Health

- Increase the proportion of adults who have had a comprehensive eye exam in the last 2 years
- Reduce vision loss from diabetic retinopathy
- Reduce vision loss from glaucoma
- Reduce vision loss from cataract
- Reduce vision loss from macular degeneration
- Increase the use of vision rehabilitation services by people with vision loss
- Increase the use of assistive and adaptive devices by people with vision loss
- Reduce vision loss from refractive errors
- Understand factors that affect use of protective eyewear in occupational and recreational settings
- Increase the number of states and DC that track eye health and access to eye care

Data from US Department of Health and Human Services: *Healthy People 2030* (website), 2020. https://health.gov/healthypeople.

DISEASES AND DISORDERS OF THE EYE

Cataracts

A cataract is an opacification (cloudiness) in the eye's normally clear crystalline lens, causing the lens to lose transparency or scatter light. Cataracts can occur at any age (babies can be born with them), but they are most common later in life. In the United States, about 70% of people older than age 75 have cataracts. Cataracts are categorized according to their location within the lens: nuclear, cortical, or posterior subcapsular (in the rear of the lens capsule). Nuclear cataracts are the most common type, and their incidence increases with age and cigarette smoking. Cortical cataracts also are more common with age, and their development is related to a lifetime of exposure to ultraviolet light. Older adults with diabetes are 60% more likely to develop cataracts than individuals without diabetes. Cataracts are also more likely to occur after glaucoma surgery or other types of eye surgery.

Cataracts form painlessly over time. The most common symptom is cloudy or blurred vision. Everything becomes dimmer, as if seen through glasses that need cleaning. Other symptoms include glare, halos around lights, poor night vision, a perception that colors are faded or that objects are yellowish, and the need for brighter light when reading. The red reflex may be absent or may appear as a black area. Fig. 12.2A illustrates

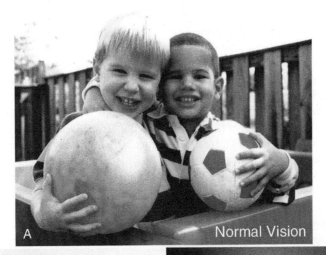

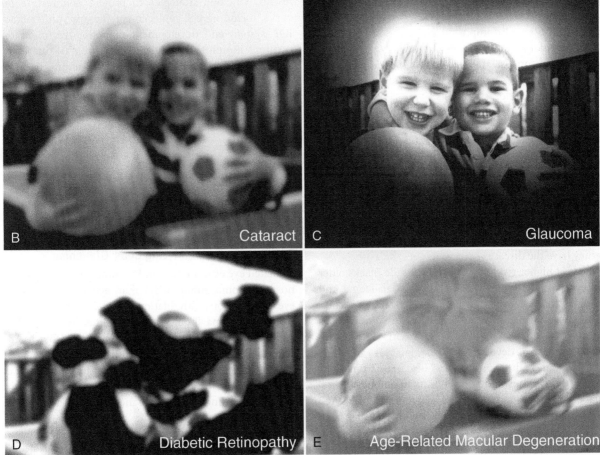

Fig. 12.2 (A) Normal vision. (B) Simulated vision with cataracts. (C) Simulated vision with glaucoma. (D) Simulated vision with diabetic retinopathy. (E) Simulated loss of vision with age-related macular degeneration. (From National Eye Institute, National Institutes of Health, 2010.)

normal vision; Fig 12.2B illustrates the effects of a cataract on vision. The NEI presents videos simulating eye disorders as well as information on eye health (Box 12.2).

Treatment of Cataracts

The treatment of cataracts is surgical, and cataract surgery is the most common surgical procedure performed in the United States. The surgery involves removal of the lens and placement of a plastic intraocular lens (IOL). Most often, cataract surgery involves only local anesthesia and is done on an outpatient basis. If the eye is normal except for the cataract, surgery will improve vision in 95% of cases. Significant postsurgical complications such as inflammation, infection, bleeding, retinal detachment, swelling, and glaucoma are rare. Individuals with medical problems such as diabetes and other eye diseases are most at risk for complications.

Solutions, Nursing Actions, and Outcomes: Cataract Surgery

Nursing actions when caring for the person experiencing cataract surgery include preparing the individual for significant changes in vision and adaptation to light and ensuring that the individual has received adequate counseling regarding realistic postsurgical expectations. Most people experience a small amount of discomfort after surgery. Some redness, scratchiness, or discharge from the eye may occur during the first day after surgery. There also may be a few black spots or shapes (floaters) drifting through the field of vision. Vision remains blurred for several days or weeks and then gradually improves as the eye heals.

If the person has bilateral cataracts, surgery is performed first on one eye, with the second surgery on the other eye a month or so later to ensure healing. Following surgery, the individual needs to avoid heavy lifting, straining, and bending at the waist. Eye drops may be prescribed to aid healing and prevent infection. Teaching fall prevention techniques and ensuring home safety modifications are also important because some research suggests that the risk for falls increases after surgery, particularly between first and second cataract surgeries. The vision imbalance that can occur if the person has one "good" eye and one "bad" eye contributes to the risk for falls.

Glaucoma

Glaucoma is a group of diseases that can damage the optic nerve. Glaucoma is the second leading cause of blindness in the United States. Glaucoma affects as many as 2.3 million Americans ages 40 years and older and 6% of those older than age 65. Because the most common form of the condition, primary open-angle glaucoma (POAG), affects side vision first, it may remain unnoticed for years. At least half of all persons with glaucoma are unaware they have the disease.

Individuals at higher risk for glaucoma include Blacks older than age 40 years; people with a family history of glaucoma; and everyone older than 60 years, especially Mexican Americans. The condition is four times more common in Latinx individuals and five times more common in Blacks than it is in Whites. Black Americans are at risk of developing glaucoma at an earlier age than other racial and ethnic groups, and blindness from glaucoma is four to five times more common than among Whites. Type 2 diabetes is associated with an 82% higher risk of POAG. Some genetic variants may be associated with elevated IOP; thus family history is an important risk factor. However, some people with one or more risk factors may never develop glaucoma, whereas others develop the disease and have no known risk factors. Other risk factors include trauma to the eye, severe myopia, or previous eye surgeries. Other high-risk groups are individuals with a history of corticosteroid use, trauma to the eye, myopia, or previous eye surgeries.

The damage to the optic nerve in glaucoma is irreversible, and regenerative attempts have been unsuccessful, so early diagnosis is essential. If detected early, glaucoma usually can be controlled and serious vision loss prevented. Signs of glaucoma can include headaches, poor vision in dim lighting, increased sensitivity to glare, "tired eyes," impaired peripheral vision, a fixed and dilated pupil, and frequent changes in prescriptions

for corrective lenses. Fig. 12.2C illustrates the effects of glaucoma on vision.

Angle-closure glaucoma is not as common as POAG and occurs when the angle of the iris causes obstruction of the aqueous humor through the trabecular network. Individuals with smaller eyes, Asians, and women are most susceptible. It may occur as a result of infection or trauma. IOP rises rapidly, accompanied by redness and pain in and around the eye, severe headaches, nausea and vomiting, and blurring of vision. It is a medical emergency, and blindness can occur in 2 days. Treatment is an iridectomy to ease pressure. Many drugs with anticholinergic properties, including antihistamines, stimulants, vasodilators, and sympathomimetics, are particularly dangerous for individuals predisposed to angle-closure glaucoma (NEI, 2021b).

The Glaucoma Research Foundation's goals for glaucoma research include strategies to protect and restore the optic nerve, including cell replacement therapy; understanding the IOP system and development of better treatment therapies; accurate monitoring of glaucoma's progression with emerging technologies to accurately track structural and functional changes; finding the genes responsible for glaucoma; and determining the risk factors for glaucoma (Glaucoma Research Foundation, 2021).

> **⚡ SAFETY TIPS**
>
> Redness and pain in and around the eye, severe headaches, nausea and vomiting, and blurring of vision occur with angle-closure glaucoma. It is a medical emergency, and blindness can occur in 2 days.

Recognizing and Analyzing Cues: Glaucoma

A dilated eye examination and tonometry are necessary to diagnose glaucoma. Adults older than age 65 should have annual eye examinations with dilation, and those with medication-controlled glaucoma should be examined at least every 6 months. Annual screening is also recommended for Black Americans and other individuals with a family history of glaucoma who are older than 40 years. Although standard Medicare does not cover routine eye care, it does cover 80% of the cost for dilated eye exams for individuals at higher risk for glaucoma and those with diabetes.

Management of glaucoma involves medications (oral or topical eye drops) to decrease IOP and/or laser trabeculoplasty and filtration surgery. Medications lower eye pressure either by decreasing the amount of aqueous fluid produced within the eye or by improving the flow through the drainage angle. Beta blockers are the first-line therapy for glaucoma, followed by prostaglandin analogues. Second-line agents include topical carbonic anhydrase inhibitors and alpha-2 agonists. The patient may need combinations of several types of eye drops.

In the hospital or long-term care setting, it is important to obtain a medical history to determine whether the person has glaucoma and to ensure that eye drops are given according to the prescribed treatment regimen. Without the eye drops, eye pressure can rise and cause an acute exacerbation of glaucoma.

Usually medications can control glaucoma, but laser surgery (trabeculoplasty) and filtration surgery may be recommended for some types of glaucoma. Surgery is usually recommended only if necessary to prevent damage to the optic nerve.

Diabetic Eye Disease

Diabetic eye disease includes diabetic retinopathy (DR) and diabetic macular edema (DME). Cataracts and glaucoma are also more prevalent in individuals with diabetes. All forms of diabetic eye disease have the potential to cause severe vision loss and blindness.

Diabetic Retinopathy

Diabetes has become an epidemic in the United States, and DR occurs in both type 1 and type 2 diabetes mellitus (Chapter 27). Risk increases the longer an individual has diabetes. Almost all people with type 1 diabetes eventually will develop retinopathy. Figure 12.2D illustrates the effects of DR on vision. People with type 2 diabetes are less likely to develop more advanced retinopathy than those with type 1. Chronically high blood sugar from diabetes is associated with damage to the tiny blood vessels in the retina, leading to DR. Blood and lipid leakage leads to macular edema and hard exudates (composed of lipids). In advanced disease, new fragile blood vessels form and hemorrhage easily. Because of the vascular and cellular changes accompanying diabetes, there is often also rapid worsening of other pathological vision conditions. DR progresses through four stages (Box 12.3).

Recognizing and Analyzing Cues: Retinopathy

Early detection and treatment of DR are essential. There are no symptoms in the early stages of DR. The disease often progresses unnoticed until it affects vision. Bleeding from abnormal retinal blood vessels can cause the appearance of "floating" spots that sometimes clear on their own. Without prompt treatment, bleeding often recurs, increasing the risk of permanent vision loss. Early signs are seen in the fundoscopic examination and include microaneurysms, flame-shaped hemorrhages,

cotton wool spots, hard exudates, and dilated capillaries. Constant, strict control of blood glucose levels, cholesterol levels, and blood pressure measurements and laser photocoagulation (LPC) treatments can halt progression of the disease.

Annual dilated fundoscopic examination of the eye is recommended beginning 5 years after diagnosis of type 1 diabetes and at the time of diagnosis of type 2 diabetes. Nurses need to provide education to diabetic patients about the risk of DR, the importance of early identification, and good control of diabetes. An increased likelihood of falls has been reported in individuals with mild to moderate nonproliferative DR. Fall prevention education should be provided to individuals with early-stage disease. Some experts are encouraging mass screening efforts. There is good treatment that can reverse vision loss and improve vision, but individuals must have access to screenings and eye examinations.

Diabetic Macular Edema

DME is the buildup of fluid (edema) in a region of the retina called the macula. DME is the most common cause of visual loss attributable to diabetes and the leading cause of legal blindness. The disease affects 1 in 25 adults ages 40 years and older with diabetes, and the incidence is higher in African Americans and Hispanics. About half of people with DR will develop DME. People with a history of high blood pressure and atherosclerosis are at a high risk of developing DME. Although it is more likely to occur as DR becomes worse, it can happen at any stage of the disease. Symptoms include blurred vision, loss of contrast, and patches of vision loss, which may appear as black dots or lines "floating" across the front of the eye (Genentech, 2021).

Treatment includes medications (often cortisone-type drugs), anti-VEGF (vascular endothelial growth factor) injection therapy, and laser therapy to cauterize leaky blood vessels and reduce accumulated fluid within the macula. Anti-VEGF therapy (Lucentis) is used alone or in conjunction with laser treatment to treat DR in individuals with DME. The treatment appears to be well tolerated but requires about 12 to 15 injections into the eye over 36 months (NEI, 2020).

Strict control of blood glucose, cholesterol, and blood pressure values; completion of annual dilated retinal examinations; and education about eye disease and diabetes are essential. However, in a recent study, only 44.7% of adults age 40 years and older with DME reported that they were told by a physician that diabetes had affected their eyes and 59.7% had received a dilated eye examination in the past year. Approximately 55% of individuals with DME are unaware they have the condition (Genentech, 2021). Advances in stem cell technology and tissue engineering in the past several years have opened the possibility of replacing lost retinal neurons that occur as a result of glaucoma, DR, and AMD.

Detached Retina

A retinal detachment can occur at any age but is more common after the age of 40 years. Emergency medical treatment is required, or permanent visual loss can result. There may be small areas of the retina that are torn (retinal tears or breaks) and will lead to retinal detachment. This condition can develop

---

BOX 12.3 Stages of Diabetic Retinopathy

1. **Mild nonproliferative retinopathy.** At this earliest stage, microaneurysms occur. They are small areas of balloon-like swelling in the retina's tiny blood vessels.
2. **Moderate nonproliferative retinopathy.** As the disease progresses, some blood vessels that nourish the retina are blocked.
3. **Severe nonproliferative retinopathy.** Many more blood vessels are blocked, depriving several areas of the retina with their blood supply. These areas of the retina send signals to the body to grow new blood vessels for nourishment.
4. **Proliferative retinopathy.** At this advanced stage, the signals sent by the retina for nourishment trigger the growth of new blood vessels. This condition is called proliferative retinopathy. These new blood vessels are abnormal and fragile. They grow along the retina and along the surface of the clear, vitreous gel that fills the inside of the eye. By themselves, these blood vessels do not cause symptoms or vision loss. However, they have thin, fragile walls. If they leak blood, severe vision loss and even blindness can result (NEI, 2017c).

in persons with cataracts or recent cataract surgery or trauma, or it can occur spontaneously. Symptoms include a gradual increase in the number of floaters and/or light flashes in the eye. It also manifests as a curtain coming down over the person's field of vision. Small holes or tears are treated with laser surgery or a freeze treatment called *cryopexy*. Retinal detachments are treated with surgery. More than 90% of individuals with a retinal detachment can be successfully treated, although sometimes a second treatment is needed. However, the visual outcome is not always predictable and may not be known for several months after surgery. Visual results are best if the detachment is repaired before the macula detaches, so immediate treatment of symptoms is essential (NEI, 2021c).

Age-Related Macular Degeneration

AMD is the most common cause of new visual impairment among people ages 50 years and older, although it is most likely to occur after age 60 (NEI, 2021d). The prevalence of AMD increases drastically with age, with more than 15% of White women older than age 80 years having the disease. Whites and Asian Americans are more likely to lose vision from AMD than are African Americans or Hispanics/Latinx. With the number of affected older adults projected to increase over the next 20 years, AMD has been called a growing global epidemic.

AMD is a degenerative eye disease that affects the macula, the central part of the eye responsible for clear central vision. The disease causes the progressive loss of central vision, leaving only peripheral vision intact. The early and intermediate stages usually start without symptoms, and only a comprehensive dilated eye exam can detect AMD. Objects may not appear to be as bright as they used to be, and individuals may attribute their vision problems to normal aging or cataracts. As AMD progresses, a blurred area near the center of vision is a common symptom. Over time, the blurred areas may grow larger and blank spots can develop in the central vision. AMD does not lead to complete blindness, but the loss of central vision interferes with everyday activities such as the ability to see faces, read, drive, or do close work, and can lead to impaired mobility, increased risk of falls, depression, and decreased quality of life. Fig. 12.2E illustrates the effects of AMD on vision.

AMD results from systemic changes in circulation, accumulation of cellular waste products, atrophy of tissue, and growth of abnormal blood vessels in the choroid layer beneath the retina. Fibrous scarring disrupts nourishment of photoreceptor cells, causing their death and loss of central vision. Risk factors include a family history of AMD, White race, and smoking. Smoking doubles the risk of AMD. At least 20 genes have been identified that affect the risk of developing AMD, and many more genetic risk factors are suspected (NEI, 2021d). Box 12.4 presents other ways to lower risk for AMD.

BOX 12.4   Lowering Risk for Age-Related Macular Degeneration

- Quit smoking—or don't start
- Get regular physical activity
- Maintain a healthy blood pressure and cholesterol levels
- Eat healthy foods, including green leafy vegetables and fish

---

BOX 12.5   Three Stages of Age-Related Macular Degeneration

There are three stages of age-related macular degeneration (AMD) defined in part by the size and number of drusen under the retina. It is possible to have AMD in one eye only or to have one eye with a later stage of AMD than the other.

- **Early AMD.** Medium-sized drusen deposits and no pigment changes, no loss of vision. Change can be detected only during a dilated eye exam.
- **Intermediate AMD.** Large drusen and/or pigment changes. There may be mild vision loss, but most people don't experience any problems. Changes can be detected only during a dilated eye exam.
- **Late-stage AMD.** Dry or wet macular degeneration that causes vision loss. It is possible to have both geographic atrophy and neovascular AMD in the same eye, and either condition can appear first.

There are three stages of AMD, defined in part by the size and number of drusen under the retina (Box 12.5). An individual can have AMD in one eye only or have one eye with a later stage of AMD than the other. Not everyone with early AMD will develop the later stage of the disease. In individuals with early AMD in one eye and no signs of AMD in the other eye, about 5% will develop advanced AMD after 10 years. For people who have early AMD in both eyes, about 14% will develop late AMD in at least one eye after 10 years. Having late AMD in one eye puts an individual at increased risk for late AMD in the other eye.

In late AMD, there is vision loss attributable to damage to the macula. There are two types of late AMD: geographic atrophy (dry AMD) and neovascular AMD (wet AMD). Neovascular AMD occurs when abnormal blood vessels behind the retina start to grow under the macula. These new blood vessels are fragile and often leak blood and fluid, which raise the macula from its normal place at the back of the eye. With wet AMD, the severe loss of central vision can be rapid, and many people will be legally blind within 2 years of diagnosis. Dry AMD progresses much more gradually than wet AMD and is also less likely to cause severe vision loss or other problems.

Recognizing and Analyzing Cues: Macular Degeneration

Early diagnosis is the key, and macular degeneration can be detected only with a dilated eye examination. There is no treatment for early AMD, but regular eye exams are necessary to monitor progression. An Amsler grid (Fig. 12.3) is used to determine clarity of vision. A perception of wavy lines is diagnostic of beginning macular degeneration. In the advanced forms of AMD, the person may see dark or empty spaces that block the center of vision. People with AMD are taught to test their eyes daily using an Amsler grid so that they will be aware of any changes.

Solutions, Nursing Actions, and Outcomes: Macular Degeneration

The NEI Age-Related Eye Disease Studies (AREDS/AREDS2) found that daily intake of certain high-dose vitamins and minerals can slow progression of the disease in individuals with intermediate AMD and those with late AMD in one eye. Supplementation with these formulations will not help people with early AMD and will not restore vision already lost. Individuals should discuss supplementation with AREDS formulations with their eye care professional (NEI, 2020).

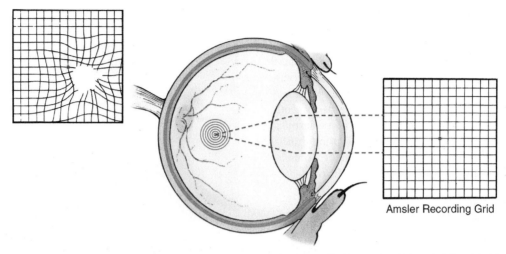

Fig. 12.3 Macular degeneration: distortion of center vision (*left*). Normal peripheral vision (*right*). (Illustration by Harriet R. Greenfield, Newton, MA.)

Treatment of wet AMD includes photodynamic therapy (PDT), LPC, and anti-VEGF therapy. Lucentis and Avastin (anti-VEGF therapy) are biological drugs that are the most common form of treatment in neovascular AMD. Abnormally high levels of a specific growth factor occur in eyes with wet AMD, which promote the growth of abnormal blood vessels. Anti-VEGF therapy blocks the effect of the growth factor. These drugs are injected into the eye as often as once a month and can help slow vision loss from AMD and, in some cases, improve sight. PDT with laser treatment is also used to manage AMD. There is also an implantable miniature telescope (IMT) approved by the US Food and Drug Administration (FDA) to help individuals 65 years of age and older with vision loss attributable to AMD (see Research Highlights A).

Dry Eye

Dry eye is not a disease of the eye but is a frequent complaint among older adults. Tear production normally diminishes as we age. The condition is termed *keratoconjunctivitis sicca*. It occurs most commonly in women after menopause. There may be age-related changes in the mucin-secreting cells necessary for surface wetting, in the lacrimal glands, or in the meibomian glands that secrete surface oil, and all of these may occur at the same time. The individual will describe a dry, scratchy feeling in mild cases (xerophthalmia). There may be marked discomfort and decreased mucus production in severe situations.

Medications can cause dry eye, especially anticholinergics, antihistamines, diuretics, beta blockers, and some hypnotics. Sjögren syndrome is a cell-mediated autoimmune disease whose

---

RESEARCH HIGHLIGHTS A

Understanding the Patient's Lived Experience of Neovascular Age-Related Macular Degeneration: A Qualitative Study

Purpose

The intent of this interpretive phenomenological study was to understand the individual's experience of neovascular age-related macular degeneration (AMD), including ongoing treatment with anti–vascular endothelial growth factor (anti-VEGF).

Method

The study took place in an Australian public hospital clinic. Thirteen female and 12 male participants between 67 and 90 years of age with a diagnosis of neovascular AMD in at least one eye who were receiving anti-VEGF therapy on a routine basis were interviewed. Thematic analysis identified two major themes: *Life negotiated by neovascular AMD* and *Uncertainty*.

Results

For most participants a diagnosis of AMD that required ongoing anti-VEGF injection was a life-changing event that evoked a range of feelings and fears from high anxiety to pragmatic acceptance. Participants expressed relief that the condition could be treated but they experienced apprehension at the thought of "having a needle into the eye." Positive experiences of the injection process helped with coping but anxiety increased if a new clinician was to give the injection or there were unexpected symptoms/complications (e.g., pain, intraocular bleeding). It was difficult for the participants to have to structure their lives around appointments and they described sadness at the loss of enjoyment of life that occurred as a result of the treatment and vision limitations.

Conclusion

A fear of blindness was pervasive. Many experienced a significant halt in disease progression and for some, improvement in vision. However, they struggled with the uncertainty about prognosis. The relationship between the health care facility staff and participants was critical in helping overcome anxieties. Reassurance, caring, communication, and feeling supported and known helped participants endure the rigors of the treatment and they were grateful for the treatment being available. Continuity of providers and treatment techniques and coming to know the patient and their unique experience are important.

From McCloud C, Lake S: Understanding the patient's lived experience of neovascular age-related macular degeneration: a qualitative study, *Eye (Lond)* 29(12):1561–1569, 2015.

manifestations include decreased lacrimal gland activity. The problem is diagnosed by an ophthalmologist using a Schirmer tear test, in which filter paper strips are placed under the lower eyelid to measure the rate of tear production. A common treatment is artificial tears or a saline gel, but dry eyes may be sensitive to them because of preservatives, which can be irritating. The ophthalmologist may close the tear duct channel either temporarily or permanently. Other management methods include keeping the house air moist with humidifiers, avoiding wind and hair dryers, and using artificial tear ointments at bedtime. Vitamin A deficiency can be a cause of dry eye, and vitamin A ointments are available for treatment.

Charles Bonnet Syndrome

Charles Bonnet syndrome (CBS) is a disease in which visual hallucinations occur as a result of vision loss. The cause of CBS is not well understood, but it is thought to be related to the brain continuing to interpret images, even in their absence. Individuals may see simple patterns of colors or shapes or detailed pictures of people, animals, buildings, or landscapes. Sometimes these images fit logically into a visual scene, but often they do not. Nurses are cautioned to understand the syndrome and not attribute symptoms to cognitive impairment or mental illness. The condition is similar to phantom limb syndrome, a condition in which individuals with a missing limb still feel their fingers or toes or experience itching. Similarly, when the brain loses input from the eye, it may fill the void by generating visual images on its own. The syndrome often goes away 1 year to 18 months after it begins. Interventions to lessen the symptoms include adequate lighting and encouraging the individual to blink, close the eyes, or focus on a real object for a few moments.

USING CLINICAL JUDGMENT TO PROMOTE HEALTHY AGING: VISUAL HEALTH

Vision impairment is common among older adults in connection with aging changes and eye diseases and can significantly affect communication, functional ability, safety, and quality of life. To promote healthy aging and quality of life, nurses who care for older adults in all settings can improve outcomes for visually impaired older adults by providing evaluation of vision changes, adapting the environment to enhance vision and safety, communicating appropriately, and providing appropriate health teaching and referrals for prevention, treatment, and assistive devices.

Solutions, Nursing Actions, and Outcomes: Visual Health

General principles in caring for persons with visual impairment include the following: use warm incandescent lighting; increase intensity of lighting; control glare by using shades and blinds; suggest yellow or amber lenses to decrease glare; suggest sunglasses that block all ultraviolet light; recommend reading materials that have large, dark, evenly spaced printing; and select colors with good contrast and intensity. Color contrasts are used to facilitate location of items. Sharply contrasting colors assist the partially sighted. For instance, a bright towel is much easier to locate than a white towel hanging on a beige wall. When choosing color, it is best to use primary colors at the top end of the spectrum rather than those at the bottom. If you think of the colors of the rainbow,

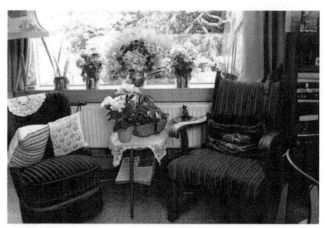

Fig. 12.4 Sitting Room (Højdevang Sogns Plejejem, Copenhagen, Denmark). (Photo courtesy Christine Williams, PhD, RN.)

it is more likely that people will see reds and oranges better than blues and greens. Fig. 12.4 beautifully illustrates the use of color in a nursing home in Copenhagen, Denmark.

Special Considerations in Long-Term Care Settings

Visual impairment among nursing home residents is higher than among adults of the same age living in the community. It is important to note the prevalence of older adults reporting both hearing and vision loss. An estimated 30% of those ages 80 years and older have dual sensory loss (DSL). Older adults with a single sensory deficit (either vision or hearing) can rely on the intact sensory function to compensate. Those with DSL lack this compensatory capability, and this increases challenges

---

RESEARCH HIGHLIGHTS B

Elderly People Need an Eye Examination Before Entering Nursing Homes

Purpose

To assess visual impairment and correct prescription and visual aids in a sample of 371 nursing home residents in 11 nursing homes.

Method

An eye examination by an optometrist and medical record review were conducted. Personnel were given a questionnaire concerning their assessment of the resident's visual abilities.

Results

Among those who received an assessment, a total of 22% were visually impaired, 13% socially blind, and 13% unable to cooperate; 32% had correct optics, 15% were recommended glasses, and 36% were referred for further diagnostics or checkup. The most common causes of impaired vision were cataract and age-related macular degeneration (AMD). Prior to assessment, many of the residents had no diagnosis of vision impairment, and in 1 in 4 cases, staff were unaware that the resident's vision was impaired.

Conclusion

Based on study results, the recommendation is made that every person referred to a nursing home receive an eye examination and relevant information be given to staff to allow them to assist the residents in the proper way due to vision-related issues

Data from Jensen H, Tubaek G: Elderly people need an eye examination before entering nursing homes, *Dan Med J* 64(2):A5825, 2017.

and poor outcomes. Research and public policies mainly address either hearing or vision loss. More attention must be paid to the design of nursing actions to assist individuals experiencing DSL (Ge et al., 2021). Nursing home residents with DSL are likely to experience cognitive impairment, functional disability, and communication difficulties. DSL also is associated with higher incidence of behavioral symptoms compared to nursing home residents with a single impairment (Petrovsky et al., 2019.

A study by Jensen and Tubaek (2017) found that cataracts and AMD were the most frequent causes of impaired vision among individuals in long-term care facilities. Information on eye diagnoses was often lacking in medical records, and staff were often unaware of the vision impairments of the individuals. Cognitive and hearing impairment often accompany visual impairment and can severely affect communication, safety, functional status, and quality of life (see Research Highlights B).

Ongoing evaluation of vision is important, and if function declines, a referral to an eye care professional is indicated. Information on needed visual aids that the individual uses (glasses, need for lighting, optical aids) is included in the plan of care. Treatments to improve visual acuity, such as cataract removal, if needed, should be accessible. Even in individuals with dementia who have clinically significant cataracts, surgery improves visual acuity, slows the rate of cognitive decline, decreases neuropsychiatric symptoms, and reduces caregiver stress.

Although it may sound like common sense, it is especially important that individuals who wear glasses are wearing them and that the glasses are cleaned regularly. Also important is asking the person or the person's family or significant other if the person routinely wears glasses and if the person is able to see well enough to function. There is limited research on visual impairment in nursing and assisted living facilities despite the scope of the concern and the need for improved interventions. Box 12.6 presents Tips for Best Practice in care for older adults with visual impairment.

Low-Vision Optical Devices

Technology advances in the past decade have produced some low-vision devices that may be used successfully in the care of

> ### BOX 12.6   Tips for Best Practice
> #### Communicating With Older Adults Who Have Visual Impairment
>
> - Perform ongoing evaluation of vision, including whether the individual is experiencing vision changes or might need evaluation or assistance.
> - Make sure you have the person's attention before speaking.
> - Clearly identify yourself and others with you. State when you are leaving to make sure the person is aware of your departure.
> - Position yourself at the person's level when speaking.
> - Ensure adequate lighting and eliminate glare.
> - When others are present, address the visually impaired person by prefacing remarks with the person's name or a light touch on the arm.
> - Select colors for paint, furniture, and pictures with rich intensity (e.g., red, orange).
> - Use large, dark, evenly spaced printing in a large font.
> - Use contrast in printed material (e.g., black marker on white paper).
> - Use a night light in bathroom and hallways and use illuminated switches.
> - Do not change room arrangement or the arrangement of personal items without explanations.
> - If in a hospital or nursing facility, use some means to identify individuals who are visually impaired and include visual impairment in the plan of care.
> - Use the analogy of a clock face to help locate objects (e.g., describe positions of food on a plate in relation to clock positions, such as meat at 3 o'clock, dessert at 6 o'clock).
> - Label eyeglasses and have a spare pair if possible; make sure glasses are worn and are clean.
> - Be aware of low-vision assistive devices such as talking watches, talking books, and magnifiers, and facilitate access to these resources.
> - If the person is blind, ask the person how you can help. If walking, do not try to push or pull. Let the person take your arm just above the elbow, and give directions with details (e.g., the bench is on your immediate right); when seating the person, place the person's hand on the back of the chair.

the visually impaired individual. These devices are grouped into devices for "near" activities (such as reading, sewing, and writing) and devices for "distance" activities (such as attending movies, reading street signs, and identifying numbers on buses and trains). Nurses can refer individuals with low vision or blindness to vision rehabilitation services, which may include assistance with communication skills, counseling, independent living and personal management skills; independent movement and travel skills; training with low-vision devices; and vocational rehabilitation. It is important to be familiar with agencies in your community that

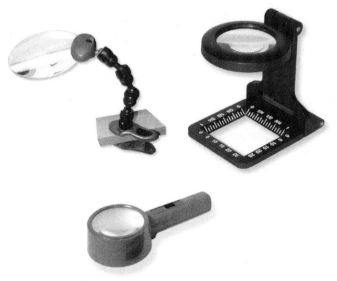

Magnifiers. (Reprinted with permission from Carson Optical.)

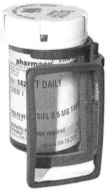

Prescription bottle magnifier. (Reprinted with permission from Carson Optical.)

offer these services. Persons with severe visual impairment may qualify for disability and financial and social services assistance through government and private programs, including vision rehabilitation programs.

Many low-vision assistive devices are available, including insulin delivery systems, talking clocks and watches, large-print books, magnifiers, telescopes (handheld or mounted on eyeglasses), electronic magnification through closed-circuit television or computer software, and software that converts text into artificial voice output. iPods have a setting for audio menus; Microsoft and Apple computer programs allow a person to change color schemes, select a high-contrast display, and magnify and enlarge print. Many websites also have an option for audio text. The e-Reader product from Kindle allows the user to increase font sizes up to 40 points in e-books and offers a Text-to-Speech feature. The iPad from Apple can enlarge text size up to 56 points and includes VoiceOver, a feature that reads everything displayed on the screen for you, making it fully usable for people with low to no vision. As individual needs are unique, it is recommended that before investing in vision aids, the individual consult with a low-vision center or low-vision specialist. Other vision resources are presented in Box 12.2.

KEY CONCEPTS

- Vision loss is a leading cause of age-related disability.
- The leading causes of visual impairment in the United States are diseases that are common in older adults: AMD, cataract, glaucoma, and DR.
- Many causes of visual impairment are preventable, so attention to keeping eyes healthy throughout life and early detection and treatment of eye disease are essential.
- Many eye diseases present with no symptoms, so regular eye examinations, including dilated examination, are important, particularly for at-risk groups.
- Visual impairment significantly affects quality of life and a person's ability to perform activities of daily living and function independently.

- An estimated 30% of those ages 80 years and older have DSL. Older adults with a single sensory deficit (either vision or hearing) can rely on the intact sensory function to compensate. Those with DSL lack this compensatory capability, and this increases challenges and poor outcomes. Research and public policies mainly address either hearing or vision loss. More attention must be paid to the design of nursing actions to assist individuals experiencing DSL.
- Nurses who care for visually impaired older adults in all settings can improve outcomes by assessing for vision changes, adapting the environment to enhance vision and safety, communicating appropriately, and providing appropriate health teaching and referrals for prevention, treatment, and assistive devices.

NEXT-GENERATION NCLEX® (NGN) EXAMINATION–STYLE QUESTIONS

Mrs. Hoang, 82 years old, was diagnosed with age-related macular degeneration (AMD) 15 years ago during a routine eye examination. She has developed progressively blurred central vision, making it difficult to read, watch TV, knit, and participate in other craft projects. She has an 80 pack-year history of smoking; she quit 15 years ago. She states that her mother had AMD. She is 5'6" and weighs 225 pounds (BMI 36.31 kg/m²). She has a history of hypertension and hypercholesterolemia. Mrs. Hoang's medications include a daily multivitamin containing lutein and omega-3 fatty acids, atenolol 50 mg twice a day, ezetimibe 10 mg daily, and acetaminophen occasionally for headaches. She tells the nurse she is frustrated at the continued loss of her vision and has stopped attending the senior center bingo night and arts and craft night because of her low vision. She scores 8 on the short-form Geriatric Depression Scale (GDS), indicating depression. Her blood pressure is 125/80 mm Hg, her heart rate is 78 beats per minute, her respirations are 16 breaths per minute, and her temperature is 97.2°F. The nurse discusses resources that are available from low-vision and rehabilitation services and answers Mrs. Hoang's questions. A 3-month follow-up appointment is scheduled.

For each client finding, use an X to indicate whether the teaching concerning low-vision and rehabilitation services was **Effective** (helped to meet expected outcomes), **Ineffective** (did not help to meet expected outcomes), or **Unrelated** (not related to the expected outcomes). Only one selection can be made for each client finding.

Client Finding	Effective	Ineffective	Unrelated
Score on GDS is 8			
Wears a talking watch			
Has magnifier but still does not attend bingo night			
Has electronic magnification for TV and computer			
Has access to audio books			

CLINICAL JUDGMENT QUESTIONS AND ACTIVITIES

1. How can nurses enhance awareness and education about vision disorders?
2. Have students attempt to ambulate, read, or take simulated medications while wearing sunglasses with lenses covered in Vaseline or with one lens covered.
3. What is the role of the nurse in the acute care setting or long-term setting in screening and evaluation of vision?
4. Develop a teaching plan for an individual with a new diagnosis of glaucoma.
5. What community resources are available in your area for individuals with vision impairment?

RESEARCH QUESTIONS

1. What do people think is helpful in enhancing communication with the visually impaired?
2. What content on visual impairment and nursing interventions is included in curricula of Bachelor of Science in Nursing (BSN) programs?
3. What factors influence the decisions of older adults to seek help for visual problems?
4. Which types of educational programs and outreach activities are most effective in educating older adults about prevention and treatment of eye diseases?
5. Are there differences in the views about visual health in aging among diverse groups of older adults?
6. What is the effect of visual rehabilitation services on performance of activities of daily living (ADLs) and instrumental activities of daily living (IADLs) and quality of life for visually impaired older adults?
7. Formulate a research question related to caring for visually impaired older adults in long-term care settings.

REFERENCES

Ge S, McConnell E, Wu B, et al.: Longitudinal association between hearing loss, vision loss, dual sensory loss, and cognitive decline, *J Am Geriatr Soc*, 69(3), 2021. doi:10.1111/jgs.16933.

Genentech: *Retinal diseases fact sheet (website)*, 2021. https://www.gene.com/stories/retinal-diseases-fact-sheethttps://www.gene.com/stories/retinal-diseases-fact-sheet. Accessed March 2021.

Glaucoma Research Foundation: *Research updates (website)*, 2021. https://www.glaucoma.org/?gclid=EAIaIQobChMI3Nm23pmP7wIV0MDACh2USgFVEAAYASAAEgIlg_D_BwE. Accessed March 2021.

Jensen H, Tubaek G: Elderly people need an eye examination before entering nursing homes, *Dan Med J* 64(2):A5825, 2017.

McCance KL, Huether SE: *Pathophysiology*, ed 7, St Louis, 2014, Mosby.

National Eye Institute (NEI): *National eye health education program (NEHEP) (website)*, 2021a. https://www.nei.nih.gov/learn-about-eye-health/outreach-campaigns-and-resources/national-eye-health-education-program. Accessed December 2021.

National Eye Institute (NEI): *Age-Related Eye Disease Studies (AREDS/AREDS2) (website)*, 2020. https://www.nei.nih.gov/research/clinical-trials/age-related-eye-disease-studies-aredsareds2. Accessed June 2021.

National Eye Institute (NEI): *What is glaucoma? (website)*, 2021b. https://www.nei.nih.gov/learn-about-eye-health/eye-conditions-and-diseases/glaucoma. Accessed March 2021.

National Eye Institute (NEI): *Facts about retinal detachment. (website)*, 2021c. https://www.nei.nih.gov/learn-about-eye-health/eye-conditions-and-diseases/retinal-detachment. Accessed March 2021.

National Eye Institute (NEI): *Facts about age-related macular degeneration (website)*, 2021d. https://nei.nih.gov/health/maculardegen/armd_facts. Accessed February 2021.

Petrovsky DV, Sefcik JS, Hanlon AL, et al.: Social engagement, cognition, depression, and comorbidity in nursing home residents with sensory impairments, *Res Gerontol Nurs* 12(5):217–226, 2019.

World Health Organization (WHO): *Blindness and vision impairment (website)*, 2020. https://www.who.int/news-room/fact-sheets/detail/blindness-and-visual-impairment. Accessed February 2021.

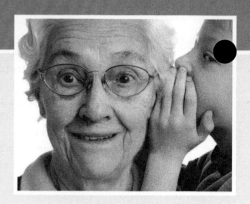

13 | CHAPTER

Auditory Health

Theris A. Touhy

http://evolve.elsevier.com/Touhy/TwdHlthAging

A STUDENT SPEAKS

My dad has had a hearing problem for a couple of years, and it has driven us all crazy. He won't admit he can't hear. It's always us mumbling or some other excuse. When you go in the house, the TV is so loud, no one can talk and visit. When I call him on his cell phone, he gets half of what I am saying. His responses are off the wall a lot of the time. I am sure there is something that would help him if he would accept it—it would sure help us!

Sophia, age 21

AN OLDER ADULT SPEAKS

A great annoyance of hearing loss is in the subtle aspects of living with a partner, who most probably has a hearing loss as well. You must often repeat what you say, and in lovemaking, whispering sweet words becomes a gesture for yourself alone.

Bob, age 80

LEARNING OBJECTIVES

On completion of this chapter, the reader will be able to:

1. Describe the impact of hearing changes on quality of life and function.
2. Identify the types of hearing loss and contributing factors.
3. Describe the importance of health education and screening to promote auditory health.
4. Identify effective communication strategies for older adults with hearing impairment.
5. Gain awareness of assistive devices to enhance auditory health.
6. Use clinical judgment to recognize and analyze cues and identify and evaluate solutions and nursing actions to enhance auditory health.

Although both vision and hearing impairment significantly affect all aspects of life, Oliver Sacks (1989), in his book *Seeing Voices,* presents a view that blindness may in fact be less serious than loss of hearing. Hearing loss interferes with communication with others and the interactional input that is so necessary to stimulate and validate. Helen Keller (1902) was most profound in her expression: "Never to see the face of a loved one nor to witness a summer sunset is indeed a handicap. But I can touch a face and feel the warmth of the sun. But to be deprived of hearing the song of the first spring robin and the laughter of children provides me with a long and dreadful sadness." Both hearing and vision impairment have a significant effect on the daily lives of older adults. Hearing impairment, in particular, is a burden on social life.

HEARING IMPAIRMENT

Hearing loss is the third most prevalent chronic condition and the foremost communicative disorder of older adults in the United States. Hearing loss is an underrecognized public health issue. Nearly two-thirds of adults ages 70 years and older have a hearing loss significant enough to impair daily communication. In all age groups, men are more likely than women to be hearing impaired, and Black Americans have a lower prevalence of hearing impairment than either White or Hispanic Americans (Lin & Whitson, 2017). Healthy People 2030 addresses objectives related to hearing impairment and older adults.

Age-related hearing loss (ARHL) is a complex disease caused by interactions between age-related changes (Table 13.1), genetics, lifestyle, and environmental factors. Factors associated with hearing loss include noise exposure, ear infections, smoking, and chronic disease (e.g., diabetes, chronic kidney disease, heart disease). Hearing loss may not be an inevitable part of aging, and increased attention is being given to the links between lifestyle factors (e.g., smoking, poor nutrition, hypertension) and hearing impairment (Box 13.1).

TABLE 13.1   Changes in Hearing Related to Aging

Changes in Structure	Changes in Function
Cochlear hair cell degeneration; loss of auditory neurons in spiral ganglia of organ of Corti	Inability to hear high-frequency sounds (presbycusis, sensorineural loss); interferes with understanding speech; hearing may be lost in both ears at different times
Degeneration of basilar (cochlear) conductive membrane of cochlea	Inability to hear at all frequencies, but more pronounced at higher frequencies (cochlear conductive loss)
Decreased vascularity of cochlea; loss of cortical auditory neurons	Equal loss of hearing at all frequencies (strial loss); inability to disseminate localization of sound

From McCance KL, Huether SE: *Pathophysiology*, ed 7, St Louis, 2014, Mosby.

BOX 13.1   Auditory Health

Avoid exposure to excessively loud noises.
Avoid cigarette smoking.
Maintain blood pressure and cholesterol levels within normal limits.
Eat a healthy diet.
Have hearing evaluated if there are any changes.
Avoid injury with cotton-tipped applicators and other cleaning materials.

Consequences of Hearing Impairment

The broad consequences of hearing loss have functional and clinical significance and should not be viewed as something a person accepts as part of aging. Hearing loss diminishes quality of life and is associated with multiple negative outcomes, including decreased function, miscommunication, depression, falls, loss of self-esteem, safety risks, poor cognitive function, and possible increased health service use secondary to unmet health care needs (Wallhagen & Strawbridge, 2017). Among older adults who are frail and have multiple comorbidities, hearing loss has been cited as a contributing factor in common geriatric syndromes. Failures in clinical communication are considered the leading cause of medical errors, and ARHL has a negative effect on clinical communication across both hospital and primary care clinical settings (Cudmore et al., 2017).

Hospitalized older adults with hearing impairment are vulnerable to adverse outcomes. These patients are at risk of being labeled confused and experiencing a loss of control, heightened fear and anxiety, and misunderstanding of the plan of care. Among older adults who are frail, hearing loss has been cited as a contributing factor in "common geriatric syndromes such as confusion, falls, social withdrawal, and failure to thrive" (Funk et al., 2018, p. 28). ARHL also has been linked to late life cognitive disorders, and correcting hearing loss may have a long-term protective effect against cognitive decline (Pabst et al., 2021). Hearing loss increases feelings of isolation and may cause older adults to become suspicious or distrustful or to display feelings of paranoia. All these consequences of hearing impairment further increase social isolation and decrease opportunities for meaningful interaction and stimulation. The two major forms of hearing loss are *conductive* and *sensorineural.*

Sensorineural Hearing Loss

Sensorineural hearing loss results from damage to any part of the inner ear or the neural pathways to the brain. Presbycusis (also called ARHL) is a form of sensorineural hearing loss that is related to aging and is the most common form of hearing loss. Presbycusis progressively worsens with age and is usually permanent. The cochlea appears to be the site of pathogenesis, but the precise cause of presbycusis is uncertain. Other causes of sensorineural hearing loss include hereditary or genetic factors, viral or bacterial infections, noise exposure, head trauma, and ototoxic medications (Meyer & Hickson, 2020).

Noise-induced hearing loss (NIHL) is the second most common cause of sensorineural hearing loss among older adults. Direct mechanical injury to the sensory hair cells of the cochlea causes NIHL, and continuous noise exposure contributes to damage more than intermittent exposure. NIHL is permanent but considered largely preventable. The rate of hearing impairment is expected to rise because of the growing number of older adults and also because of the increased number of military personnel who have been exposed to blast exposure in combat situations. NIHL may be reduced through the development of better ear-protection devices, education about exposure to loud noise, and emerging research into interventions that may protect or repair hair cells in the ear, which are key to the body's ability to hear (National Institute on Deafness and Other Communication Disorders [NIDCD], 2019).

Presbycusis

Presbycusis is a slow, progressive hearing loss that affects both ears equally. Because of its slow progression, many individuals ignore their hearing loss for years, considering it "just part of aging." It is common to hear older adults deny hearing impairment and accuse others of mumbling. Their spouses or significant others, however, often voice frustration over the hearing loss long before the individuals acknowledge it. Older adults initially may be unaware of hearing loss because of the gradual manner in which it develops and therefore may not report any problems. There is a low rate of hearing screening in primary care despite the high prevalence of hearing loss among older adults. Screening for hearing impairment and appropriate treatment are essential parts of primary care for older adults. Individuals residing in long-term care facilities should be screened for hearing impairment on admission and on an ongoing basis.

One of the first signs of presbycusis is difficulty hearing and understanding speech in noisy environments. A hallmark of presbycusis is difficulty separating the incoming speech signal from background noise. Presbycusis begins in the high frequencies and later affects the lower frequencies. High-frequency consonants are important to speech understanding. Changes related to presbycusis make it difficult to distinguish among some of the sibilant consonants such as *z, s, sh, f, p, k, t,* and *g*. People often raise their voices when speaking to a person with hearing impairment. When this happens, more consonants drop out of speech, making hearing even more difficult. Without consonants, the high-frequency–pitched language becomes disjointed and misunderstood. Older adults with presbycusis have difficulty filtering out background noise and often complain of difficulty understanding women's and children's speech (which is higher pitched) and conversations in large groups. Sensorineural hearing loss is treated with hearing aids and, in some cases, cochlear implants (see Box 13.3 for the Unfair Hearing Test, which simulates presbycusis).

Conductive Hearing Loss

Conductive hearing loss usually involves abnormalities of the external and middle ear that reduce the ability of sound to be transmitted to the middle ear. Otosclerosis, infection, perforated eardrum, fluid in the middle ear, tumors, or cerumen accumulations cause conductive hearing loss. Cerumen impaction is the most common and easily corrected of all interferences in the hearing of older adults (Fig. 13.1). When hearing loss is suspected or a person with existing hearing loss experiences increasing difficulty, it is important first to check for cerumen impaction as a possible cause. After accurate assessment, if cerumen removal is indicated, it may be removed through irrigation, cerumenolytic products, or manual extraction (Schwartz et al., 2017).

Cerumen interferes with the conduction of sound through air in the eardrum. The reduction in the number and activity of cerumen-producing glands results in a tendency toward cerumen impaction. Long-standing impactions become hard, dry, and dark brown. Individuals at particular risk of impaction are Blacks, individuals who wear hearing aids, and older

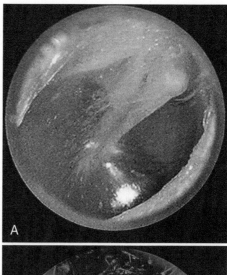

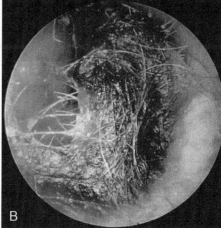

Fig. 13.1 **(A)** Normal eardrum. **(B)** Eardrum impacted with cerumen. (**A,** From Ball JW, Dains JE, Flynn FA, et al: *Seidel's guide to physical examination,* ed 8, St Louis, 2015, Mosby. **B,** From Swartz MH: *Textbook of physical diagnosis,* ed 7, Philadelphia, 2014, Saunders.)

men with large amounts of ear canal tragi (hairs in the ear) that tend to become entangled with the cerumen. One-third to two-thirds of nursing home residents and patients older than 65 years of age have cerumen impaction affecting hearing. It is very important to assess the ears for cerumen impaction in primary care evaluation and among long-term care residents. Protocols should be in place for safe removal of cerumen.

INTERVENTIONS TO ENHANCE HEARING

Hearing Aids

A hearing aid is a personal amplifying system that includes a microphone, an amplifier, and a loudspeaker. There are numerous types of hearing aids with either analog or digital circuitry. The size, appearance, and effectiveness of hearing aids have greatly improved (decreasing stigma), and many can be programmed to meet specific needs. Digital hearing aids are smaller and have better sound quality and noise reduction and less acoustic feedback; however, they are expensive. Completely-in-the-canal

(CIC) hearing aids fit entirely in the ear canal. These types of devices are among the most expensive and require good dexterity. Some models are invisible, placed deep in the ear canal, and replaced every 4 months. New hearing aids can be adjusted precisely for noisy environments and telephone usage through software built into smartphones.

Most individuals can obtain some hearing enhancement with a hearing aid, but among adults ages 70 years and older, fewer than 1 in 3 have ever used a hearing aid (Kimball et al., 2018). The kind of device chosen depends on the type of hearing impairment and the cost, but most users will experience hearing improvement with a basic to midlevel hearing aid. The investment in a good hearing aid is considerable, and a good fit is critical. Accessibility and affordability of hearing care are massive barriers for those with hearing impairment. Bilateral hearing aids cost an average of $4700 in the United States and require several visits to a hearing professional's office. The cost of hearing aids usually is not covered by health insurance or Medicare, another barrier to purchase.

For decades, the U.S. Food and Drug Administration (FDA) has regulated hearing aids as prescription medical devices – an arrangement that adds to the cost and effort individuals must expend to get them. In October 2021, the U.S. Food and Drug Administration issued a proposal intended to improve access to and reduce the cost of hearing aid technology for millions of Americans. The agency proposed a rule to establish a new category of over-the-counter (OTC) hearing aids. When finalized, the rule would allow hearing aids within this category to be sold directly to consumers in stores or online without a medical exam or a fitting by an audiologist. The proposed rule is designed to help increase competition in the market while also ensuring the safety and effectiveness of OTC and prescription hearing aids (U.S. Food and Drug Administration, 2021).

Adjustment to Hearing Aids

Nearly 50% of people who purchase hearing aids either never began wearing them or stop wearing them after a short period. Factors contributing to low hearing aid use after purchase include difficulty manipulating the device, annoying loud noises, being exposed to sensory overload, developing headaches, and perceiving stigma. Hearing aids amplify all sounds, making things sound different. ARHL is like any other physical impairment and requires counseling, rehabilitative training, patient education, environmental accommodations, and patience. The internet may be a valuable tool for aural rehabilitation and for improving adjustment to hearing aids and communication (teleaudiology) (Saunders, 2020). More research about factors that influence the decision to seek help for hearing loss is needed (Wallhagen & Strawbridge, 2017).

It is important for nurses who work with individuals wearing hearing aids to be knowledgeable about their care and maintenance. They can teach the individual, family, or formal caregiver proper use and care of hearing aids. Many older adults experience unnecessary communication problems when in the hospital or nursing home because their hearing aids are not inserted and working properly, need batteries, or are lost. In addition, individuals who wear hearing aids often come to the hospital in emergent situations without their hearing aids or do not bring them because they fear they will be lost or broken (Kimball et al., 2018).

Cochlear Implants

Cochlear implants are increasingly being used for older adults with sensorineural loss who are not able to gain effective speech recognition with hearing aids. Cochlear implants are safe and well tolerated and improve communication. Thorough evaluation of hearing and medical condition is necessary to determine if a cochlear implant may be indicated. A cochlear implant is a small, complex electronic device that consists of an external portion that sits behind the ear and a second portion that is surgically placed under the skin (Fig. 13.2). Unlike hearing aids that magnify sounds, the cochlear implant bypasses damaged portions of the ear and directly stimulates the auditory nerve.

Hearing through a cochlear implant is different from normal hearing and takes time to learn or relearn. Most insurance plans cover the cochlear implant procedure. The transplant carries some risk because the surgery destroys any residual hearing. Therefore cochlear implant users can never revert to using a hearing aid. Individuals with cochlear implants need to be advised to never have magnetic resonance imaging (MRI) because it may dislodge the implant or demagnetize its internal magnet.

Assistive Listening and Adaptive Devices

Assistive listening devices (also called personal listening systems) should be considered as an adjunct to hearing aids or used in place of hearing aids for people with hearing impairment. These devices are available commercially and can be used to enhance face-to-face communication and to better understand speech in large rooms such as theaters, to use the telephone, and to listen to television. Many movie theaters have both sound amplifiers and personal subtitle devices available. Hearing loop conduction systems are a newer technology and

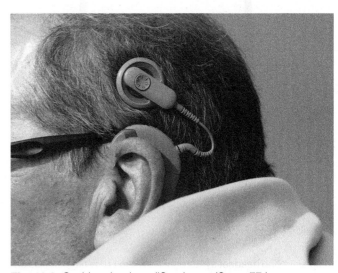

Fig. 13.2 Cochlear implant. (iStock.com/Garret77.)

consist of a copper wire that is installed around the periphery of a room or other venue to transmit the microphone or TV sound signal to hearing aids and cochlear implants that have "telecoil" receivers (built into most hearing aids and cochlear implants). Sound from the microphone or TV is received but background noises are not. This transforms the hearing aid into loudspeakers delivering sound for one's own hearing loss. These devices are widely used in Europe and becoming more available in the United States in places such as theaters, churches, subway information booths, taxi back seats, and home TV rooms.

Other examples of assistive listening and adaptive devices include smartphones and tablets with real-time speech-to-text transcription. Low-tech aids such as white boards or yellow pads can be useful. During the COVID-19 pandemic, the use of face masks brought barriers to hearing because they block lip movements and expressions and muffle the high-frequency portions of speech that are essential to speech and understanding. Face masks with clear windows are available but have been in short supply. Individuals with hearing impairment are fashioning their own clear masks (Chodosh et al., 2020). Alerting devices, such as vibrating alarm clocks that shake the bed or activate a flashing light, and sound lamps that respond with lights to sounds, such as doorbells and telephones, are also available. Special service dogs ("hearing dogs") are trained to alert people with a hearing impairment about sounds and intruders. Dogs are trained to respond to different sounds, such as the telephone, smoke alarms, alarm clock, doorbell or door knock, and name call, and lead the individual to the sound.

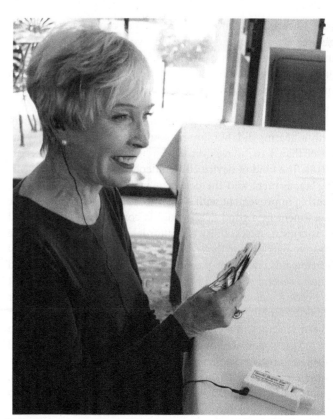

Pocket-sized amplifier. (With permission from Sonic Technology Products, Inc.)

The use of computers and e-mail also assists individuals with hearing impairment to communicate more easily. Programs such as Skype and FaceTime are also beneficial because they may allow the person to lip read and to adjust volume. Pocket-sized amplifiers (available at retail stores) are especially helpful in improving communication in health care settings, and nurses in a clinical setting should be able to obtain appropriate devices for use with individuals who are hearing impaired. These devices are safe and easy to use in inpatient settings, and both patients and nurses were very satisfied with their use (Kimball et al., 2018).

USING CLINICAL JUDGMENT TO PROMOTE HEALTHY AGING: AUDITORY HEALTH

Recognizing and Analyzing Cues: Hearing Impairment

Hearing impairment is underdiagnosed and undertreated in older adults. There is a low rate of hearing screening in primary care despite the high prevalence of hearing loss among older adults. Older adults initially may be unaware of hearing loss because of the gradual manner in which it develops and therefore may not report any problems. Screening for hearing impairment and appropriate treatment are essential parts of primary care for older adults (Wallhagen & Strawbridge, 2017). In hospitals and long-term care facilities, bedside screening for hearing impairment is important.

Nurses should note any nonverbal signs of a hearing deficit (e.g., cupping the ear, turning the head to one side when asked questions, misunderstanding questions). Ask the individual

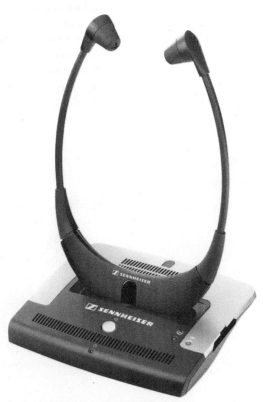

Voice-clarifying headset system for TV listening. (With permission from TV Ears, Inc.)

directly if there is a hearing impairment. Since many individuals are unaware of or deny hearing impairment, the screening should include a short discussion rather than yes-or-no questions. A suggested question is: "Can you tell me about any problems you have with hearing or misunderstanding questions?" It is important to identify barriers to hearing, such as background noise, unfamiliar accents, and call system speakers. The individual also should be asked the preferred method for enhancing hearing, such as writing or using personal sound amplifiers.

Obtaining information from the significant other about hearing problems also can be useful. Self-assessment instruments (Box 13.2) and the Hearing Handicap Inventory for the Elderly–Screening Version (HHIE-S) Box 13.3) also can be included. Box 13.3 presents information on resources for hearing impairment as well as simulation of presbycusis that may be helpful in understanding the condition. Question the person about prolonged noise exposure, past ear injuries, and use of potentially ototoxic medications.

Physical examination includes evaluation of the external ear to determine any evidence of infection and using an otoscope to visualize the inner ear, looking for any possible causes of conductive hearing loss, such as cerumen impaction or foreign objects. Inspect the tympanic membrane for integrity. Depending on findings, the patient may need to be referred for follow-up by a specialist. Results of a recent study reported that the finger rub test showed high sensitivity and requires little time and no special equipment, making it an effective screening tool in all settings. The test involves asking the individual to close the eyes; the clinician stands 6 to 10 inches in front of the individual with arms extended and rubs the thumb and middle finger together, first vigorously and then faintly, switching from side to side. Failure to hear the sound two out of three times is considered a positive test (Funk et al., 2018; Strawbridge & Wallhagen, 2017).

BOX 13.3 Resources for Best Practice
Hearing Impairment

American Tinnitus Association: Listen to the sounds of tinnitus; patient and professional information. https://www.ata.org/.

Experience hearing loss: Unfair hearing test. https://canadianadaptive.network/index.php/2019/04/26/we-challenge-you-to-an-unfair-hearing-test/.

Hartford Institute for Geriatric Nursing: Hearing Handicap Inventory for the Elderly–Screening Version (HHIE-S). https://hign.org/consultgeri/try-this-series/hearing-screening-older-adults.

National Institute on Aging: Hearing loss: a common problem for older adults (patient information). https://www.nia.nih.gov/health/hearing-loss-common-problem-older-adults#:~:text=Presbycusis%2C%20or%20age%2Drelated%20hearing,hear%20what%20others%20are%20saying.

National Institute on Deafness and Other Communication Disorders (NIDCD): Hearing loss and older adults patient information; interactive hearing test; "It's a noisy planet: protect their hearing"; resources for health professionals. https://www.nidcd.nih.gov/health/hearing-ear-infections-deafness.

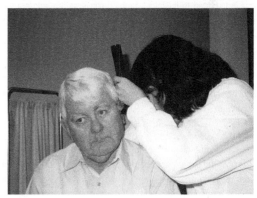

Proper technique for an otoscopic examination. (From Ignatavicius DD, Workman ML: *Medical-surgical nursing: patient-centered collaborative care*, ed 6, St Louis, 2014, Saunders.

Solutions, Nursing Actions, and Outcomes: Hearing Impairment

Nursing actions are based on history and examination findings and may include referral to an audiologist, education on hearing loss (including prevention and consequences), hearing aids, assistive listening devices, and communication techniques. Providing education to individuals and family members about hearing loss, how it affects one's communication, why it is important to address hearing loss early in the process, what hearing aids can and cannot do, and alternatives to the use of hearing aids is important and may enhance the effective use of hearing health care services (Wallhagen & Strawbridge, 2017) (see Research Highlights).

There are many evidence-based resources available that can be used to educate the patient and family and assist the nurse in designing educational materials (see Box 13.3). Using the information presented in this chapter, nurses can play an important role in providing older adults with the information they need to improve their hearing and avoid the negative consequences of untreated hearing loss. Effective communication strategies when working with individuals who are hearing impaired are presented in Box 13.4.

BOX 13.2 Do You Need a Hearing Test?

- Do you sometimes feel embarrassed when you meet new people because you struggle to hear?
- Do you feel frustrated when talking to members of your family because you have difficulty hearing them?
- Do you have difficulty hearing or understanding co-workers, clients, or customers?
  - Do you feel restricted or limited by a hearing problem?
  - Do you have difficulty hearing in the movies or in the theater?
  - Does a hearing problem cause you to argue with family members?
  - Do you have trouble hearing the TV or radio at levels that are loud enough for others?
  - Do you feel that any difficulty with your hearing limits your personal life or social life?
  - Do you have trouble hearing family or friends when you are together in a restaurant?

If you answered YES to 3 or more of these questions, you may want to see have a hearing evaluation.

From National Institute on Deafness and Other Communication Disorders: *Do you need a hearing test?* (website), 2019. https://www.nidcd.nih.gov/health/do-you-need-hearing-test. Accessed March 2021.

RESEARCH HIGHLIGHTS

Original Research: Understanding the Hospital Experience of Older Adults With Hearing Impairment

Purpose
To assess the hospital experience of older adults with hearing impairment and to use findings to formulate suggestions for improving nursing care.

Method
Participants were 5 men and 3 women, ranging in age from 70 to 95 years, who had a self-reported hearing loss and were hospitalized in a large 600-bed hospital in the Midwest United States. Interviews were conducted, and each interview began with an open-ended question asking participants to share their experiences as hospitalized patients with hearing loss. As each person's story unfolded, additional questions that arose naturally were asked. Interviews were recorded, and field notes were taken. Data were analyzed, and themes were compiled representing the patients' hospital experiences.

Results
All the participants discussed communication barriers in the hospital setting, including reluctance to share hearing problems with staff, frustration and embarrassment related to misunderstanding conversation, and not wanting to inconvenience staff. Barriers to understanding included speech and unfamiliar accents, staff speaking too loudly, and difficulty hearing telephone conversations and conversations through the call system speakers. Several disclosed that they only revealed hearing problems to staff who showed concern about and interest in helping with communication difficulties. Some participants had left their hearing aids at home out of concern about loss and replacement costs.

Conclusion
Based on findings, the following primary nursing actions were identified to improve the hospital experiences of older adults with hearing impairments:
1. **Assess:** Bedside screening for hearing impairment; ask individual if there is a hearing impairment and about circumstances that make hearing difficult (e.g., background noise, unfamiliar accents). Discuss patient's preferred method for reducing barriers (e.g., using personal sound amplifiers, communicating with paper and pen or written materials) and include methods in plan of care.
2. **Accommodate:** Give ample time to establish trust and rapport. Provide accommodations such as a quiet setting, minimizing noise, and speaking clearly and slowly. Document helpful actions and share information during hand-offs. Provide adequate supplies of personal sound amplifiers.
3. **Educate:** Educate patients and families on key communication strategies and provide a handout outlining strategies. Explain the importance of using hearing-assistive devices while in the hospital.
4. **Empower:** Encourage active participation in care. Tell patients it is important to inform nursing staff if they have trouble hearing and what will help them.
5. **Advocate:** Advocate for system-wide education on hearing impairment in older adults. Provide staff education to promote awareness of the consequence of hearing deficits on care outcomes, hearing screening techniques, and communication strategies.

Data from Funk A, Garcia C, Mullen T: Original research: understanding the hospital experience of older adults with hearing impairment, *Am J Nurs* 118(6):28–34, 2018.

BOX 13.4   Tips for Best Practice
Communication Strategies to Improve Hearing

- Never assume hearing loss is from age until other causes are ruled out (infection, cerumen buildup).
- Inappropriate responses, inattentiveness, and apathy may be symptoms of a hearing loss.
- Face the individual, and stand or sit on the same level; do not turn away while speaking (e.g., face a computer).
- Determine if hearing is better in one ear than another, and position yourself appropriately.
- If hearing aid is used, make sure it is in place and batteries are functioning.
- Lower your tone of voice, articulate clearly, and use a moderate rate of speech.
- Use nonverbal approaches: gestures, demonstrations, visual aids, and written materials.
- Reduce background noise (e.g., turn off television, close door).
- Utilize assistive listening devices such as pocket talker.
- Verify that the information being given has been clearly understood. Be aware that the person may agree to everything and appear to understand what you have said even when he or she did not hear you (listener bluffing).
- If the person is in a hospital or nursing facility, label the chart, note on the intercom button, and inform all caregivers that the patient has a hearing impairment.
- Share resources for the hearing-impaired and refer as appropriate.

From Adams-Wendling L, Pimple C: Evidence-based guideline: nursing management of hearing impairment in nursing facility residents, *J Gerontol Nurs* 34(11):9–16, 2008.

as buzzing, hissing, whistling, crickets chirping, bells, roaring, clicking, pulsating, humming, or swishing sounds. The sounds may be constant or intermittent and are more acute at night or in quiet surroundings. The most common type is high-pitched tinnitus with sensorineural loss; less common is low-pitched tinnitus with conduction loss, such as is seen in Ménière's disease. Tinnitus affects about 1 in 5 people.

Tinnitus is the number one service-related disability for US military personnel and veterans and is the leading cause of service-connected disability of veterans returning from Iraq or Afghanistan. Other high-risk groups include older adults; individuals employed in loud work environments; musicians and music lovers; motorsports and hunting enthusiasts; and individuals with depression, anxiety, and obsessive-compulsive disorder (American Tinnitus Association, 2019).

The exact physiological cause or causes of tinnitus are not known, but several likely factors are known to trigger or worsen tinnitus. Exposure to loud noises is the leading cause of tinnitus, and the exposure can damage and destroy cilia in the inner ear. Once damaged, the cilia cannot be renewed or replaced. Other possible causes of tinnitus include head and neck trauma, certain types of tumors, cerumen accumulation, jaw misalignment, cardiovascular disease, and ototoxicity from medications. More than 200 prescription and nonprescription medications list tinnitus as a potential side effect, aspirin being the most common.

There is some evidence that caffeine, alcohol, cigarettes, stress, and fatigue may exacerbate the problem, so lifestyle changes may be part of the plan of care. Tinnitus research

TINNITUS

Tinnitus is defined as the perception of sound in one or both ears or in the head when no external sound is present. It is often referred to as "ringing in the ears" but also may manifest goals center on (1) understanding the many forms of tinnitus; (2) understanding the mechanisms of tinnitus (area of brain where tinnitus signals arise at molecular, cellular, and systems levels); (3) studying the epidemiology of tinnitus; (4) developing methods to prevent tinnitus; (5) developing reliable diagnostic tools; (6) optimizing management therapy; and (7) discovering a definitive cure (American Tinnitus Society, 2019).

Solutions, Nursing Actions, and Outcomes: Tinnitus

Some persons with tinnitus will never find the cause; for others the problem may arbitrarily disappear. Hearing aids can be prescribed to amplify environmental sounds to obscure tinnitus, and there is a device that combines the features of a masker and a hearing aid, which emits a competitive but pleasant sound that distracts from head noise. Therapeutic modes of treating tinnitus include transtympanic electrical stimulation, iontophoresis, biofeedback, tinnitus masking with alternative sound production (white noise), cochlear implants, and hearing aids. Some have found hypnosis; cognitive behavioral therapy; acupuncture; and chiropractic, naturopathic, allergy, or drug treatment to be effective.

Nursing actions include discussions with the client regarding times when the noises are most irritating and having the person keep a diary to identify patterns. Assess medications for possibly contributing to the problem. Discuss lifestyle changes and alternative methods that some have found effective. Also refer clients to the American Tinnitus Association for research updates, education, and support groups (see Box 13.3).

KEY CONCEPTS

- Hearing impairment is the third most prevalent chronic condition among older Americans and the foremost communicative disorder.
- Age-related hearing loss (AHRL) is a complex disease caused by interactions among age-related changes, genetics, lifestyle, and environment.
- The two major forms of hearing loss are conductive and sensorineural.
- Presbycusis (also called ARHL) is a form of sensorineural hearing loss that is related to aging and is the most common form of hearing loss.
- Hearing aids and cochlear implants are used to improve hearing, and both require a period of adjustment and education.
- Hearing loss diminishes quality of life and is associated with multiple negative outcomes, including decreased function, increased likelihood of hospitalizations, miscommunication, medical errors, depression, falls, loss of self-esteem, safety risks, and cognitive decline.
- Screening for hearing loss is an essential component of assessment in older adults.
- Nurses need to provide education about hearing health, care of hearing aids, and assistive listening devices to enhance communication.

NEXT-GENERATION NCLEX® (NGN) EXAMINATION–STYLE QUESTIONS

The nurse is caring for a 68-year-old patient who was admitted for pneumonia. While interacting, the nurse notices that the patient frequently asks for questions or statements to be repeated and does not seem to hear if the nurse is not directly facing him. Further assessment reveals no remarkable external or internal structural auditory abnormalities. Later that evening, the patient's daughter arrives and confirms that the patient was diagnosed with presbycusis several months earlier, although he has not done anything about the diagnosis since then. When planning care, the nurse creates a list of interventions that can benefit the patient's ability to hear while hospitalized, upon discharge to outpatient care, and in the home environment.

For each setting, mark any potential nursing interventions that would be appropriate for the care of the patient from those listed in the table below. Each setting may support more than one potential nursing intervention. Each setting must have at least one response option selected.

Setting	Potential Nursing Interventions
Hospital	Stand beside the patient when speaking
	Articulate words clearly in a deeper voice
	Conduct discussions with the door to the room closed
	Perform cerumen removal to clear the ears
Outpatient care	Refer to an audiologist for auditory testing
	Teach that a cochlear implant will be required
	Request a prescription for ofloxacin
	Ask patient to repeat discharge instructions back
Home	Encourage routine cleaning of ear canals with cotton swabs
	Teach about smart devices with speech-to-text transcription
	Educate about ways to minimize background noises
	Refer to cognitive behavioral specialist to cope with ringing noise

NURSING STUDY

Hearing Impairment

Sonya is a 66-year-old high school nurse/consultant. She retired from the Army Nurse Corps with an officer's rank after serving for 20 years, much of it in the Korean conflict with heavy exposure to shelling in the early part of her career. She became aware of hearing loss at about age 45, and by age 55 it had become severe. While in the service she had considerable assistance from noncommissioned personnel and functioned well. When she entered civilian life, it became more difficult for her to manage, but she was unwilling to admit to others her major hearing deficit. During those years she simply attempted to cover it up as much as possible, and some of her coworkers thought she was rather obtuse; others suspected her deafness. When she took the position with the school district, she was involved with three high schools, numerous faculty members, and students, and interpersonal communication was a major aspect of her position. When she was evaluated at the end of the first year of her employment, it was pointed out that feedback indicated that she was inattentive. She admitted her hearing problem and was advised to get a hearing aid. She said, "I've known several people over the years who have hearing aids, and none of them were really satisfied with them. I guess that is why I have not gotten them before now." She complied but, after a few weeks, rarely wore her hearing aids. The personnel officer of the school board, after hearing several more complaints of inappropriate communication, told her she must wear the hearing aids if she wished to continue in her position. Sonya knew that hearing aids were essential, not only for communication but also for safety—she had almost been hit by a car while walking simply because she did not hear it coming. Yet she did not want to go back to the audiology clinic because they did not seem to know what they were doing, and each time she saw someone, the person gave her different information. She tried three different types of hearing aids that seemed of little help. She lost confidence in her ear, nose, and throat specialist because he had been unable to help her resolve the ringing in her ears. Now her school district has contracted with a health maintenance organization, and she is not even sure which health care provider she should see.

CLINICAL JUDGMENT QUESTIONS AND ACTIVITIES

Questions 1 and 2 refer to the Nursing Study.

1. What are some of the possible reasons Sonya suffered severe hearing loss at so young an age?
2. Discuss the reasons why Sonya may have discontinued wearing her hearing aids? What might you suggest that would help in adapting to a hearing aid?
3. Discuss the stigma of hearing loss and hearing aids.
4. Obtain a "hearing aid loaner" from your educator. Wear it for several hours and report your reactions in writing. List any difficulties experienced.
5. Listen to the Unfair Hearing Test (see Box 13.3).
6. Which of the various sensory or perceptual changes of aging would you find most difficult to handle?
7. Discuss the meanings and the thoughts triggered by the student's and older adult's viewpoints expressed at the beginning of the chapter. How do these vary from your own experience?

RESEARCH QUESTIONS

1. What do older adults think is helpful in enhancing communication with individuals who are experiencing hearing impairment?
2. What strategies are most effective in facilitating adaptation to hearing aids?
3. What are the challenges for older adults and their families and significant others in living with hearing loss?
4. What is the knowledge level of professional nurses related to hearing impairment and communication strategies to enhance communication?
5. What is the relationship between stigma and denial of hearing loss and wearing hearing aids?

REFERENCES

American Tinnitus Association: *Understanding the facts: tinnitus* (website), 2019. https://www.ata.org/understanding-facts. Accessed March 2021.

Chodosh J, Freedman M, Weinstein B, et al.: Face masks can be devastating for people with hearing loss, *BMJ* 370:m2683, 2020.

Cudmore V, Henn P, O'Tuathaigh CMP, et al.: Age-related hearing loss and communication breakdown in the clinical setting, *JAMA Otolaryngol Head Neck Surg* 143(10):105–1055, 2017.

Funk A, Garcia C, Mullen T: Original research: understanding the hospital experience of older adults with hearing impairment, *Am J Nurs* 118(6):28–34, 2018.

Keller H: *The story of my life*, Garden City, NY, 1902, Doubleday.

Kimball AR, Roscigno CI, Jenerette CM, et al.: Amplified hearing device use in acute care settings for patients with hearing loss: a feasibility study, *Geriatr Nurs* 39:279–284, 2018.

Lin FR, Whitson HE: The common sense of considering the senses in patient communication, *J Am Geriatr Soc* 65:1659–1660, 2017.

Meyer C, Hickson L: Nursing management of hearing impairment in nursing facility residents, *J Gerontol Nurs* 46(7):15–21, 2020.

National Institute on Deafness and Other Communication Disorders (NIDCD): *Noise-induced hearing loss* (website), 2019. https://www.nidcd.nih.gov/health/noise-induced-hearing-loss. Accessed March 2021.

Pabst A, Bar J, Rohr S, et al.: Do self-reported hearing and visual impairment predict longitudinal dementia in older adults?, *Jour Am Geriatr Soc* 69(6):1519–1528, 2021.

Sanders G: Evaluating evidence-based teleaudiology: Part 1 on hearing assessment. *In The Hearing Journal blog,* June 18, 2020 https://journals.lww.com/thehearingjournal/blog/OnlineFirst/pages/post.aspx?PostID=68.

Sacks O: *Seeing voices: a journey into the world of the deaf,* Berkeley, CA, 1989, University of California Press.

Schwartz S, Magit A, Rosenfeld R, et al.: Clinical practice guideline (update): earwax (cerumen impaction), *Otolaryngol Head Neck Surg* 156(1S):S1–S29, 2017.

Strawbridge WJ, Wallhagen MI: Simple tests compare well with a hand-held audiometer for hearing loss screening in primary care, *J Am Geriatr Soc* 65:2282–2284, 2017.

United States Food and Drug Administration: FDA issues landmark proposal to improve access to hearing aid technology for millions of Americans, *FDA News Release*, October 19, 2021. https://www.fda.gov/news-events/press-announcements/fda-issues-landmark-proposal-improve-access-hearing-aid-technology-millions-americans.

Wallhagen M, Strawbridge W: Hearing loss education for older adults in primary care clinics: benefits of a concise educational brochure, *Geriatr Nurs* 38(6):527–530, 2017.

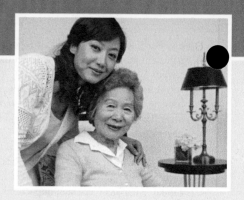

Healthy Skin

Theris A. Touhy

http://evolve.elsevier.com/Touhy/TwdHlthAging

A GRANDCHILD SPEAKS

An older woman and her little grandson, whose face was sprinkled with bright freckles, spent the day at the zoo. Many children were waiting in line to get their cheeks painted by a local artist who was decorating them with tiger paws.

"You've got so many freckles, there's no place to paint!" a girl in the line said to the little fellow. Embarrassed, the little boy dropped his head. His grandmother knelt down next to him.

"I love your freckles. When I was a little girl I always wanted freckles," she said, while tracing her finger across the child's cheek. "Freckles are beautiful."

The boy looked up. "Really?"

"Of course," said the grandmother. "Why, just name me one thing that's prettier than freckles?"

The little boy thought for a moment, peered intensely into his grandma's face, and softly whispered, "Wrinkles."

A STUDENT SPEAKS

My mother is always on me to take care of my skin so that it will look good when I am older. Stay out of the tanning salon and the sun, wear sunscreen all the time, use moisturizer. It's hard to think that 50 years from now I might not have this beautiful skin anymore unless I take better care of it now. Mom keeps pointing to a magnet on her refrigerator: "Wrinkled was not one of the things I wanted to be when I was older."

Janine, age 19

AN OLDER ADULT SPEAKS

I have that white Irish skin and have really had a lot of problems ever since I was 40 with precancerous lesions and even a basal cell skin cancer or two. Of course, we didn't know about sunscreen when I was growing up, and I remember lathering myself with baby oil and iodine to get a good tan (or a bad burn). I am pretty obsessive about going to the dermatologist every 3 months and staying out of the sun. A year ago, she saw an area on my back that looked suspicious, so a biopsy was done. Turned out it was a melanoma and was removed by a plastic surgeon, who told me that I was lucky it was found or I would have been dead in 6 months. The area was not unusual looking at all—no change, no irritation, no irregular borders, no elevation—looked like nothing. Best advice I can give is to make the skin checks regular. It may save your life.

Bob, age 77

LEARNING OBJECTIVES

On completion of this chapter, the reader will be able to:

1. Identify skin conditions commonly found in later life.
2. Identify preventive, maintenance, and restorative measures for healthy skin.
3. Identify risk factors for pressure injuries and describe nursing actions for prevention and treatment.
4. Use clinical judgment to recognize and analyze cues of skin problems in older adults and develop and evaluate solutions and nursing actions to promote healthy skin.

Gerontological nurses have an instrumental role in promoting the health of the skin of the persons who seek their care. The skin often may be overlooked when the focus is on management of disease or acute problems. However, skin problems can be challenging concerns, affecting health and compromising quality of life. Thorough evaluation and action based on age-related evidence-based protocols is important to healthy aging and best practice gerontological nursing.

SKIN

The skin is the largest organ of the body and accounts for 15% of body weight. The skin has at least seven physiological functions (Box 14.1). Exposure to heat, cold, water, trauma, friction, and pressure notwithstanding, the skin's function is to maintain

BOX 14.1   Physiological Functions of the Skin

- Protects underlying structures
- Regulates body temperature
- Serves as a vehicle for sensation
- Stores fat
- Is a component of the metabolism of salt and water
- Is a site for two-way gas exchange
- Is a site for the production of vitamin D when exposed to sunlight

a homeostatic environment. Healthy skin is durable, pliable, and strong enough to protect the body by absorbing, reflecting, cushioning, and restricting various substances and forces that might enter and alter its function, yet it is sensitive enough to relay subtle messages to the brain. When the integument malfunctions or is overwhelmed, discomfort, disfigurement, or death may ensue. However, the nurse can both promptly recognize and help to prevent many of the sources of danger to a person's skin in the promotion of the best possible health.

Age-Related Skin Changes

Many age-related changes in the skin are visible; similar changes in other organs of the body are not as readily observed. Although there are some changes related to the aging process, genetics and environmental factors (ultraviolet [UV] radiation, tobacco smoke, inflammatory responses, and gravity) contribute to these changes (McCance & Huether, 2014). Many skin problems are seen with aging, both in health and when compromised by illness or mobility limitations. Even though many worry about wrinkles and gray hair, the most common skin problems of aging are xerosis (dry skin), pruritus, seborrheic keratosis, herpes zoster (HZ), and cancer. Those who are immobilized or medically fragile are at risk for fungal infections and pressure injuries (PIs), both major threats to wellness. Table 14.1 provides an overview of skin changes related to aging.

TABLE 14.1   Changes in the Integument Related to Aging

Changes	Effects
Skin	
Epidermis	
Melanocytes decrease	Lightening of overall skin tone; decreased protection against ultraviolet radiation
Keratinocytes smaller; regeneration slower	Slowed wound healing
Noncancerous pigmented spots (freckles, nevi) enlarge	Mostly cosmetic
Increased lentigine ("age" or "liver" spots) and seborrheic keratosis common	Mostly cosmetic (see Fig. 14.2)
Dermatosis papulosa nigra, variant of keratosis in dark skin, increases	Clinically insignificant (see Fig. 14.3)
Dermis	
20% loss of thickness	Skin more transparent and fragile; skin tears and bruising occur easily
Dermal blood vessels decrease	Skin pallor and cooler skin temperature; increased susceptibility to skin cancer; diminished dermal clearance, absorption, and immunological response
Cross-linking increases; collagen synthesis decreases	Skin "gives less" under stress and tears easily
Elastin fibers thicken and fragment	Loss of stretch and elasticity; "sagging" appearance
Decreased sebum production	Skin becomes drier; risk for cracking and xerosis increases
Hypodermis	
Shifting of subcutaneous fat; loss of subcutaneous tissue	Skinfolds on the back of the hand diminish even with substantial weight gain; more risk for injury as cushioning decreases; wrinkling and sagging of skin
Reduced efficiency of eccrine glands	Temperature regulation compromised; risk for hyperthermia and hypothermia; moisture evaporates quickly; skin is drier
Fewer Meissner's and Pacinian corpuscles	Diminished tactile sensitivity; increased susceptibility to injury
Decreased Langerhans cells	Reduces skin's immune response
Hair	
Diminished melanocytes; loss of hair follicles	50% of population have gray or partly gray hair
Other changes	Men experience hair loss in vertex, frontal, and temporal areas; by 60 years of age, 80% of men are substantially bald; less pronounced in women. Race, gender, sex-linked genes, and hormonal balance influence maximum amount of hair one has and the changes that occur throughout life

TABLE 14.1	Changes in the Integument Related to Aging—cont'd
Changes	**Effects**
	Terminal hair can occur in face and chin area in women after menopause
	Amount of hair increases in ears, nose, eyebrows; axillary, extremity, and pubic hair diminishes or disappears
Nails	
Decreased circulation	Fingernails and toenails thicken and change in shape and color
	Nails become brittle, flat, or concave rather than convex; longitudinal striations; may appear yellow or grayish with poorly defined or absent lunulae; cuticle becomes thick and wide
	Onychogryphosis (thickening and distortion of nail plate) and fungal infection (onycholysis) common but not part of normal aging

COMMON SKIN PROBLEMS

Xerosis

Xerosis is extremely dry, cracked, and itchy skin. Xerosis is the most common skin problem experienced and may be linked to a dramatic age-associated decrease in the amount of epidermal filaggrin, a protein required for binding keratin filaments into macrofibrils. This leads to separation of dermal and epidermal surfaces, which compromises the nutrient transfer between the two layers of the skin. Xerosis occurs primarily in the extremities, especially the legs, but also can affect the face and the trunk. The thinner epidermis of older skin makes it less efficient, allowing more moisture to escape. Inadequate fluid intake worsens xerosis, as the body will pull moisture from the skin to combat systemic dehydration. Box 14.2 presents Tips for Best Practice in prevention and treatment of xerosis.

BOX 14.2 Tips for Best Practice

Prevention and Treatment of Xerosis

Assessment
- Evaluate for dehydration, nutritional deficiencies, systemic diseases (diabetes mellitus, hypothyroidism, renal disease), and open lesions
- Determine precipitating and alleviating factors
- Evaluate current treatment and effectiveness

Interventions
- Maintain environment of 60% humidity
- Promote adequate fluid intake; skin can be rehydrated only with water
- Creams, lubricants, emollients should be applied to towel patted–dry, damp skin immediately after a bath; water-laden emulsions without perfumes or alcohol should be used
- Mineral oil or Vaseline is effective and more economical than commercial lotions and oils
- Use only tepid water for bathing; avoid long-duration baths; daily baths and showers may not be needed; advise sponge bathing
- Use super-fatted soaps or skin cleansers (Cetaphil, Dove, Caress soaps; Neutrogena and Oil of Olay bath washes); avoid deodorant soaps except in places such as axilla and groin
- In cases of extreme dryness, petroleum jelly can be applied to affected area before bed (can use cotton gloves and socks to cover hands and feet)

Pruritus

One of the consequences of xerosis is *pruritus*, that is, itchy skin. It is a symptom, not a diagnosis or disease, and is a threat to skin integrity because of the attempts to relieve it by scratching. It is aggravated by perfumed detergents, fabric softeners, heat, sudden temperature changes, pressure, vibration, electrical stimuli, sweating, restrictive clothing, fatigue, exercise, and anxiety. Medication side effects are another common cause of pruritus. Pruritus also may accompany systemic disorders such as chronic renal failure and biliary or hepatic disease. Subacute to chronic generalized pruritus that awakens the individual is an indication to look for secondary causes (especially lymphoma or hematological conditions).

The gerontological nurse should always listen carefully to the patient's ideas of why the pruritus is occurring and to the patient's description of aggravating and relieving factors. If rehydration of the stratum corneum (outer layer of the skin) and other measures to prevent and treat xerosis are not sufficient to control itching, cool compresses or oatmeal or Epsom salt baths may be helpful. Failure to control the itching increases the risk for eczema, excoriations, cracks in the skin, inflammation, and infection arising from the usually linear excoriations resulting from scratching. The nurse should be alert to signs of infection.

Scabies

Scabies is a skin condition that causes intense itching, particularly at night. Scabies is caused by a tiny burrowing mite called *Sarcoptes scabiei*. Scabies is contagious and can be passed easily by an infested person to household members, caregivers, or sexual partners. Scabies can spread easily through close physical contact in a family, childcare group, or school class. Scabies outbreaks have occurred among patients, visitors, and staff in institutions such as nursing homes and hospitals. These types of outbreaks are frequently the result of delayed diagnosis and treatment of crusted (Norwegian) scabies. Individuals who are immunocompromised, disabled, or debilitated are at risk for this form of scabies.

Individuals with crusted scabies have thick crusts of skin that contain large numbers of scabies mites and eggs. In addition to spreading through skin-to-skin contact, crusted scabies can transmit indirectly through contamination of clothing, linen, and furniture. Because the characteristic itching and rash of scabies can be absent in crusted scabies, there may be misdiagnosis and delayed or inadequate treatment and continued transmission.

To diagnose scabies, a close skin examination is conducted to look for signs of mites, including their characteristic burrows. A scraping may be taken from an area of skin for microscopic examination to determine the presence of mites or their eggs.

Scabies treatment involves eliminating the infestation with prescribed lotions and creams. Two or more applications, about a week apart, may be necessary, especially for crusted scabies. Treatment usually is provided to family members and other close contacts even if they show no signs of scabies infestation. Medication kills the mites, but itching may not stop for several weeks. Oral medications may be prescribed for individuals with altered immune systems, for those with crusted scabies, or for those who do not respond to prescription lotions and creams. All clothes and linen used at least three times before treatment should be washed in hot, soapy water and dried with high heat. Rooms used by the person with crusted scabies should be thoroughly cleaned and vacuumed (Centers for Disease Control and Prevention [CDC], 2020a).

Purpura

Thinning of the dermis leads to increased fragility of the dermal capillaries and to easy rupture of blood vessels with minimal trauma. Extravasation of the blood into the surrounding tissue, commonly seen on the dorsal forearm and hands, is called *purpura*. Most cases are not related to a pathological condition. The incidence of purpura increases with age due to the normal changes in the skin. Persons who take blood thinners are especially prone to easily acquiring purpura. For those who find that they are prone to purpura, it is advisable to use protective garments such as long-sleeved pants and shirts. Health care personnel must be advised to be gentle while providing care to persons with sensitive or easily traumatized skin.

Skin Tears

Skin tears are painful, acute, accidental wounds, perhaps more prevalent than PIs, and are largely preventable. Although skin tears are frequently caused by trauma, they are slow to heal and may become chronic wounds. If not managed properly, they can be susceptible to secondary wound infections. Older adults who are dependent on others for total care are at greatest risk for skin tears, and independent ambulatory older adults are at second highest risk. Physiological changes in the skin such as dermal and subcutaneous tissue loss and xerosis contribute to risk factors for skin tears in older adults. The top causes of skin tears include equipment injury, patient transfers, falls, activities of daily living, and treatment and dressing or adhesive removal. The literature pertaining to the prevalence and incidence of skin tears and risk factors is very limited.

Skin tears should be classified using the International Skin Tear Advisory Panel (ISTAP) Classification System (Tiggelen et al., 2020) (Fig. 14.1). Prevention of skin tears is very important and needs attention by nurses in all settings. Comprehensive information on assessment and prevention can be found on the ISTAP website (see Box 14.7). Box 14.3 presents tips for skin tear prevention and treatment. Management of skin tears includes proper assessment of the skin tear category, control of bleeding, cleansing with nontoxic solutions (normal saline or nonionic surfactant cleaners), use of appropriate dressings that provide moist wound healing, protection of periwound skin, management of exudate, prevention of infection, implementation of prevention protocols, and education. Skin flaps, if present, should not be removed but instead rolled back over the open, cleaned area. Steri-Strips can be very useful; suturing is not recommended (Cheung, 2017; LeBlanc et al., 2016).

Keratoses

There are two types of keratosis: seborrheic and actinic. *Actinic keratosis* is a precancerous lesion, and *seborrheic keratosis* is a benign growth that appears mainly on the trunk, the face, the neck, and the scalp as single or multiple lesions. One or more lesions are present on nearly all adults older than 65 years and are more common in men. An individual may have dozens of these benign lesions. Seborrheic keratosis is a waxy, raised lesion, flesh colored or pigmented in various sizes. The lesions have a "stuck-on" appearance, as if they could be scraped off. Seborrheic keratoses may be removed by a dermatologist for cosmetic reasons (Fig. 14.2). A variant seen in

Type 1: No Skin Loss	Type 2: Partial Flap Loss	Type 3: Total flap loss

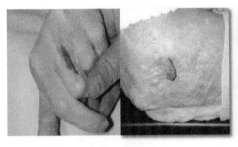 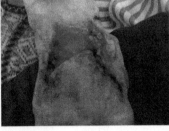 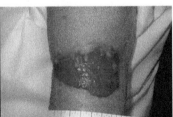

Linear or Flap Tear which can be repositioned to cover the wound bed	Partial Flap loss which cannot be repositioned to cover the wound bed	Total Flap loss exposing entire wound bed

Fig. 14.1 Skin tear classification. (From International Skin Tear Advisory Panel (ISTAP) Classification System: *Skin tear classification* [website], 2020. http://www.skintears.org/wp-content/uploads/2019/03/ISTAP-CLASSIFICATION.pdf. Accessed March 2021.)

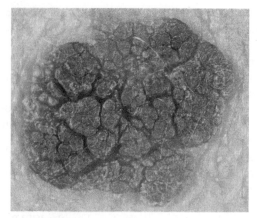

Fig. 14.2 Seborrheic keratosis in older adults. (From Habif TP: *Clinical dermatology: a color guide to diagnosis and therapy*, ed 5, St Louis, 2010, Mosby.)

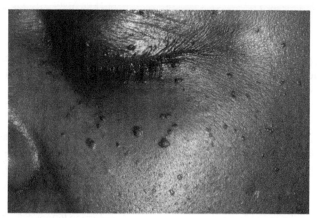

Fig. 14.3 Dermatosis papulosa nigra. (From Neville B, Damm DD, Allen CM, et al: *Oral and maxillofacial pathology*, ed 3, St Louis, 2009, Saunders.)

darkly pigmented persons occurs mostly on the face and appears as numerous small, dark, possibly tag-like lesions (Fig. 14.3).

Actinic keratosis is a precancerous lesion that is thought to be in the middle of the spectrum between photoaging changes and squamous cell carcinoma. Actinic keratosis is the most common precancer, affecting more than 58 million Americans (Skin Cancer Foundation, 2021). It is directly related to years of overexposure to UV light. Risk factors are older age and fair complexion. It is found on the face, the lips, and the hands and forearms—areas of chronic sun exposure in everyday life. Actinic keratosis is characterized by rough, scaly, sandpaper-like patches, pink to reddish-brown on an erythematous base (Fig. 14.4). Lesions may be single or multiple; they may be painless or mildly tender. The person with actinic keratoses should be monitored by a dermatologist every 6 to 12 months for any change in appearance of the lesions. Early recognition, treatment, and removal of these lesions are easy and important and may be combined with topical field therapy.

Herpes Zoster

HZ, or shingles, is a viral infection frequently seen in adults older than age 50, those who have medical conditions that compromise

BOX 14.3   Tips for Best Practice

Skin Tears: Prevention and Treatment

Prevention

- Identify high-risk individuals (extremes of age; fragile skin; history of skin tears or falls; impaired activity; dependent on other for care; decreased mobility, sensation, and cognition). Top causes of skin tears are equipment injury, patient transfers, activities of daily living, falls, and treatment and dressing removal.
- Have individual wear long sleeves or pants to protect extremities.
- Ensure adequate hydration and nutrition; provide a nutritional consultation.
- Lubricate skin with hypoallergenic moisturizer twice daily; apply to damp skin after bathing.
- Perform careful transfers; use a lift sheet to move and turn patients.
- Pad bed rails, wheelchair arms, leg supports, and furniture edges.
- Avoid use of adhesive products. Use nonadherent dressings and paper tape only as needed.
- Use gauze wrap, stockinettes, flexible netting, or other wraps to secure dressings.
- Use no-rinse, soapless bathing products and warm or tepid water for bathing.
- Caregivers need to keep nails short and not wear jewelry that can catch and contribute to skin tears.
- Implement fall prevention protocol.
- Educate patients, staff, and health care providers on prevention and management.

Treatment

- If skin tear occurs, assess and classify according to ISTAP classification system (see Fig. 14.1) and assess size.
- Gently cleanse skin with normal saline.
- Air dry or pat dry carefully.
- Approximate skin tear flap if present; consider Steri-Strips; do not suture.
- Use nonadherent dressings and skin sealants to protect surrounding skin.
- Draw an arrow on the dressing to indicate direction of skin tear to minimize further injury during dressing removal; consider doing a wound tracing.
  - Take time to remove dressings slowly ("low and slow").
  - Use adhesive removers when removing dressing to minimize trauma.

ISTAP, International Skin Tear Advisory Panel.
Data from LeBlanc K, Baranoski S: Skin tears: state of the science: consensus statements for the prevention, prediction, assessment and treatment of skin tears, *Adv Skin Wound Care* 24(Suppl 9):2, 2011.

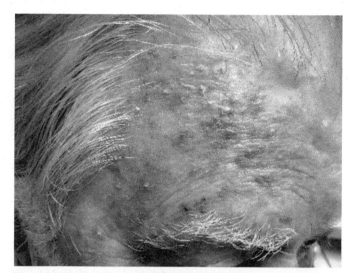

Fig. 14.4 Actinic keratosis. (Courtesy Dr. Robert Norman.)

the immune system, or people who receive immunosuppressive drugs. About 1 in 3 people in the United States will develop HZ in their lifetime. HZ is caused by reactivation of latent varicella-zoster virus (VZV) within the sensory neurons of the dorsal root ganglion decades after initial VZV infection is established. More than 90% of the world's population is infected with this virus, and about half of all cases occur in individuals ages 60 years or older (CDC, 2020b).

HZ always occurs along a nerve pathway, or *dermatome* (Fig. 14.5). The more dermatomes involved, the more serious the infection, especially if it involves the head. When the eye is affected, it is always a medical emergency. Most HZ occurs in the thoracic region, but it also can occur in the trigeminal area and cervical, lumbar, and sacral areas. HZ vesicles never cross the midline. In most cases, the severity of the infection increases with age.

It is important to differentiate HZ from herpes simplex. Herpes simplex does not occur in a dermatome pattern and is recurrent. The onset of HZ may be preceded by itching, tingling, or pain in the affected dermatome several days before the outbreak of the rash. During the healing process, clusters of papulovesicles develop along a nerve pathway. The lesions themselves eventually rupture, crust over, and resolve. Scarring may result, especially if scratching or poor hygiene leads to a secondary bacterial infection. HZ is infectious until it becomes crusty. HZ may be very painful and pruritic. Prompt treatment with the oral antiviral agents acyclovir, valacyclovir, and famciclovir may shorten the length and severity of the illness; however, to be effective, the medications must be started as soon as possible after the rash appears. Analgesics may help relieve pain. Wet compresses, calamine lotion, and colloidal oatmeal baths may help relieve itching.

Two shingles vaccines are licensed and recommended in the United States. Zoster vaccine live (ZVL, Zostavax) has been used since 2006, and recombinant zoster vaccine (RZV, Shingrix) has been used since 2017 and is recommended as the preferred shingles vaccine. It is recommended that individuals ages 50 years and older get the Shingrix vaccine even if they have had previous vaccination with Zostavax. Two doses of Shingrix are required, with the second dose given 2 to 6 months after the first dose. Shingrix should not be given within 2 months of receiving Zostavax.

Vaccination is recommended for all individuals ages 50 years and older who have no contraindications, including those who report a previous episode of HZ or who have chronic medical conditions (CDC, 2020b). Shingrix induces a strong and persistent immune response in older adults and is more than 90% effective at preventing shingles and long-term nerve pain (Bastidas et al., 2019). *Healthy People 2030* includes a goal of increasing the proportion of adults ages 19 years and older who receive recommended age-appropriate vaccines, with the overall goal of reducing or eliminating cases of vaccine-preventable diseases.

A common complication of HZ that is minimized for those who are immunized is postherpetic neuralgia (PHN), a chronic, often debilitating painful condition that can last months or even years. Older adults are more likely to have PHN and to have longer-lasting and more severe pain. Another complication of HZ is eye involvement, which occurs in 10% to 25% of zoster episodes and can result in prolonged or permanent pain, facial scarring, and loss of vision. The pain of PHN has been difficult to control and can significantly affect quality of life. Treatment should include medical, psychological, complementary, and alternative medicine options, as well as rehabilitation. The best evidence studies for medications indicate that the most effective are the tricyclic antidepressants, gabapentin and pregabalin, carbamazepine (for trigeminal neuralgia), opioids, tramadol, topical lidocaine patch, and duloxetine or venlafaxine. Other treatments include a high-concentration (8%) topical capsaicin patch, gastroretentive gabapentin, gabapentin enacarbil, and pregabalin in combination with lidocaine plaster, oxycodone, or transcutaneous electrical nerve stimulation (TENS) (Endo & Norman, 2014). Assessment and management of pain are discussed in Chapter 29.

Candidiasis (*Candida albicans*)

The fungus *Candida albicans* (referred to as "yeast") is present on the skin of healthy persons of any age. However, under certain circumstances and in the right environment, a fungal infection can develop. Persons who are obese or malnourished, are receiving antibiotic or steroid therapy, or have diabetes are at increased risk. *Candida* grows especially well in areas that are moist, warm, and dark, such as in skinfolds, in the axilla, in the groin area, and under pendulous breasts. It also can be found in the corners of the mouth associated with the chronic moisture of angular cheilitis. In the vagina it is also called a "yeast infection." If this is found in an older woman, it may mean that she has undiagnosed or poorly controlled diabetes.

Inside the mouth a *Candida* infection is referred to as "thrush" and is associated with poor hygiene and the immunocompromised individual, such as those who have long-term steroid use, who are receiving chemotherapy, or who test positive for or are infected with human immunodeficiency virus (HIV) or have acquired immunodeficiency syndrome (AIDS). In the mouth, candidiasis appears as irregular, white, flat to slightly raised patches on an erythematous base that cannot be removed by scraping. The infection can extend down into the throat and

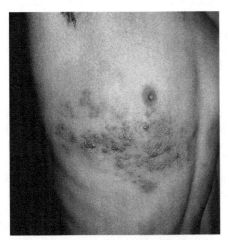

Fig. 14.5 Herpes zoster. (From Harding MM, Kwong J, Roberts D, et al: *Lewis's medicalsurgical nursing,* ed 11, St Louis, 2020, Mosby.)

cause swallowing to be painful. In severely immunocompromised persons the infection can extend down the entire gastrointestinal tract.

On the skin, *Candida* is usually maculopapular, glazed, and dark pink in persons with less pigmentation or grayish in persons with more pigmentation. If it is advanced, the central area may be completely red and/or dark and weeping, with characteristic bright red and/or dark satellite lesions (distinct lesions a short distance from the center). At this point the skin may be edematous, itching, and burning. The best approach to managing fungal infections is to prevent them, and the key to prevention is limiting the conditions that encourage fungal growth. Prevention is extremely important for persons who are obese, bedridden, incontinent, or diaphoretic (Box 14.4).

Photo Damage of the Skin

Although exposure to sunlight is necessary for the production of vitamin D, the sun is also the most common cause of skin damage and skin cancer. More than 90% of the visible changes commonly attributed to skin aging are caused by the sun (Skin Cancer Foundation, 2021). With aging, one accumulates years of sun exposure and the epidermis is thinner, significantly increasing the risk of skin cancer for older adults. The damage (photo or solar damage) comes from prolonged exposure to UV light from the environment or in tanning booths. Although the amount of sun-induced damage varies with skin type, genetics, and geographical location, much of the associated damage is preventable. People who use sunscreen with a sun protection factor (SPF) of 15 or higher show 24% less skin aging than those who do not use sunscreen daily. Ideally, preventive measures begin in childhood, but clinical evidence has shown that some improvement can be achieved at any time by limiting sun exposure and using sunscreens regularly regardless of skin tones.

SKIN CANCERS

Facts and Figures

More people are diagnosed with skin cancer each year in the United State than with all other cancers combined. At least 1 in 5 Americans will develop skin cancer by the age of 70. Skin cancer is a major public health problem, and skin cancers in the United States, unlike many other cancers, continue to rise (Skin Cancer Foundation, 2021). White populations generally have a much higher risk of getting nonmelanoma or melanoma skin cancers than dark-skinned populations, but individuals of all skin colors should minimize sun exposure. Individuals with pale or freckled skin, fair or red hair, and blue eyes belong to the highest risk group. About 90% of nonmelanoma skin cancers are associated with exposure to UV radiation from the sun.

Recent research suggests that individuals who have a nonmelanoma skin cancer before their mid-20s have a high risk of developing cancers of the bladder, brain, breast, lung, pancreas, and stomach. With age, the risk for developing cancer decreased but remained higher compared with individuals who did not have nonmelanoma skin cancer when young (Ong et al., 2014). The exact number of basal and squamous cell cancers is not known for certain because these cancers are not reported to cancer registries, but it is estimated that more than 2 million basal and squamous cell skin cancers are found each year. Most of these are basal cell cancers. Squamous cell cancer is less common, but rates are increasing. Most of these are curable; the type with the greatest potential to cause death is melanoma.

Basal Cell Carcinoma

Basal cell carcinoma is the most common malignant skin cancer. It occurs mainly in older age groups but is occurring more and more in younger persons. It is slow growing, and metastasis is rare. A basal cell lesion can be triggered by extensive sun exposure, especially burns, chronic irritation, and chronic ulceration of the skin. It is more prevalent in light-skinned persons. It usually begins as a pearly papule with prominent telangiectasias (blood vessels) or as a scar-like area with no history of trauma (Fig. 14.6). Basal cell carcinoma is also known to ulcerate. It may be indistinguishable from squamous cell carcinoma and is diagnosed by biopsy. Early detection and treatment are necessary to minimize disfigurement. Treatment is usually surgical with either simple excision or Mohs micrographic surgery.

Squamous Cell Carcinoma

Squamous cell carcinoma is the second most common skin cancer. This form of skin cancer is aggressive and has a high incidence of metastasis if not identified and treated promptly. Major risk factors include sun exposure, fair skin, and immunosuppression. Individuals in their mid-60s who have been or are chronically exposed to the sun (e.g., persons who work outdoors, athletes) are prime candidates for this type of cancer. Less common causes include chronic stasis ulcers, scars from injury, and exposure to chemical carcinogens, such as topical hydrocarbons, arsenic, and radiation (especially for individuals who received treatments for acne in the mid-20th century).

BOX 14.4   Tips for Best Practice

Candidiasis: Prevention and Treatment

- Identify high-risk individuals (e.g., obese, bedridden, incontinent, diaphoretic, immunocompromised) and limit conditions that encourage fungal growth.
- Provide adequate drying of target areas after bathing and prompt management of incontinent episodes. A hair dryer on the low setting can help dry hard-to-reach, vulnerable areas.
- A dry, folded washcloth or cotton sanitary pad can be placed under the breasts or between skinfolds to promote exposure to air and light.
- Use loose-fitting clothing and underwear; change clothing and bedding when damp.
- Avoid incontinence products that are tight or have plastic that touches the skin.
- Avoid use of cornstarch because it promotes growth of *Candida* organisms.
- Optimize nutrition and glycemic control.
- The goal of treatment is to eradicate the infection and may include the use of a prescribed antifungal medication for 7 to 14 days or until the infection is completely cleared. Antifungal preparations are available as powders, creams, and lotions. Powders are recommended because they trap moisture less than the other preparations do.

The lesion begins as a firm, irregular, fleshy, pink-colored nodule that becomes reddened and scaly, much like actinic keratosis, but it may increase rapidly in size. It also may be hard and wart-like with a gray top and horny texture, or it may be ulcerated and indurated with raised, defined borders (Fig. 14.7). Because it can appear so differently, it is often overlooked or thought to be insignificant. All persons, especially those who live in sunny climates, should be screened regularly by a dermatologist. Treatment depends on the size, histologic features, and patient preference and may include electrodesiccation and curettage, Mohs micrographic surgery, aggressive cryotherapy, or topical 5-fluorouracil. Once diagnosed with a squamous cell carcinoma, the person needs to be routinely followed because most recurrences occur within the first few years.

Melanoma

Melanoma, a neoplasm of the melanocytes, affects the skin or, less commonly, the retina. Melanoma has a classical multicolor, raised appearance with an asymmetrical, irregular border. It may appear to be of any size, but the surface diameter is not necessarily reflective of the size beneath the surface, similar in concept to an iceberg. It is treatable if diagnosed early, before it has a chance to invade surrounding tissue. Melanoma accounts for less than 2% of skin cancer cases, but it causes most skin cancer deaths. Eighty-six percent of melanomas can be attributed to exposure to UV radiation from the sun. Melanoma is highly curable if the cancer is detected in its earliest stages and treated promptly (Skin Cancer Foundation, 2021).

Incidence and Prevalence

In the past decade (2011–2021), the number of new invasive melanoma cases diagnosed annually increased by 44%. Overall, the lifetime risk of getting melanoma is about 1 in 50 for the White population, 1 in 1000 for the Black population, and 1 in 200 for the Hispanic population. Melanoma rates among middle-aged adults, especially women, have increased in the past 4 decades. Men have a higher rate of melanoma than women, and a person who has already had a melanoma has a higher risk of developing another one. Melanomas in Black individuals, Asians, and native Hawaiians most often occur on nonexposed skin with less pigment, with

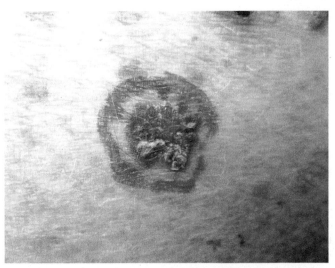

Fig. 14.7 Squamous cell carcinoma. (From Ham RJ, Sloane PD, Warshaw GA, et al: *Primary care geriatrics*, ed 6, Philadelphia, 2014, Saunders. Used with permission, University of Utah Department of Dermatology.)

up to 60% to 75% of tumors arising on the palms, plantar portion of the foot, mucous membranes, and nail regions.

Risk Factors

Risk factors for melanoma include a personal history of melanoma; the presence of atypical, large, or numerous (more than 50) moles; sun sensitivity; history of excessive sun exposure and severe sunburns; use of tanning booths; natural blond or red hair color; diseases or treatments that suppress the immune system; and a history of skin cancer. Only 20% to 30% of melanomas are found in existing moles, whereas 70% to 80% arise on apparently normal skin. The legs and backs of women and the backs of men are the most common sites of melanoma. Increasing age along with a history of sun exposure increases one's risk even further. An individual's risk for melanoma doubles if that person has had more than five sunburns, but just one blistering sunburn in childhood or adolescence more than doubles the chances of developing melanoma later in life. Blistering sunburns before the age of 18 years are thought to damage Langerhans cells, which affect the immune response of the skin and increase the risk for a later melanoma (Skin Cancer Foundation, 2021).

Indoor tanning. Although melanoma occurs more often in older adults, it is one of the most common cancers in people younger than 30 years. Exposure to indoor tanning, common in developed countries, is thought to be contributing to the increasing rates of melanoma and other skin cancers among younger individuals. Indoor tanning increases the risk of melanoma by 75% when use started before age 35 years. Indoor tanners are 2.5 times more likely to develop squamous cell cancer and 1.5 times more likely to develop basal cell cancer. Women who have ever tanned indoors are 6 times more likely to be diagnosed with melanoma in their 20s than those who have never tanned indoors.

Indoor tanning devices can emit UV radiation in amounts 10 to 15 times higher than the sun at its peak intensity. Worldwide, there are more skin cancer cases due to indoor tanning than there are

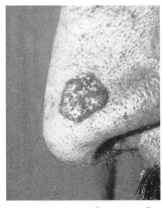

Fig. 14.6 Basal cell carcinoma. (Courtesy Gary Monheit, MD, University of Alabama at Birmingham School of Medicine.)

lung cancer cases due to smoking (Skin Cancer Foundation, 2021). This is considered a major public health issue, with many states limiting minors' access to tanning salons. Globally, many countries have banned indoor tanning altogether or banned it for individuals younger than 18 years. Tanning devices have been reclassified by the US Food and Drug Administration (FDA) to Class II (moderate-risk devices).

Solutions, Nursing Actions, and Outcomes: Promoting Healthy Skin

Age-related skin changes, such as thinning and diminished numbers of melanocytes, significantly increase the risk for solar damage and subsequent skin cancer. The nurse has an active role in the prevention and early recognition of skin cancers. This role may include working with community awareness and education programs and screening clinics and providing direct care. By far the most important preventive nursing action is to provide education on skin cancer risk factors and adequate lifelong protective measures (Box 14.5).

Careful skin inspection is essential, and the nurse is vigilant in observing skin for changes that require further evaluation. Patient education also includes teaching the individual how to examine the skin once a month to look for warning signs or any suspicious lesions. If the individual has a partner, partners can perform regular "checks" of each other's skin, watching for signs of change and the need to contact a primary care provider or dermatologist promptly. For the person with keratosis and multiple freckles (nevi), photographing the body parts may be a useful reference. The adage "when in doubt, get it checked" is an important one, and regular screenings should be a part of the health care of all older adults. The "ABCDE" approach to assessing such potential lesions is used (Box 14.6).

PRESSURE INJURIES (PIs)

Aging carries a high risk for the development of PIs; 70% of PIs occur in older adults. PIs are recognized as one of the geriatric

---

BOX 14.5	**Promoting Healthy Skin**

Sun Protection
- Seek the shade.
- Do not burn.
- Avoid indoor tanning booths and sunlamps.
- Wear hats with a brim wide enough to shade the face, ears, and neck, and clothing that adequately covers the arms, legs, and torso. Cover up with clothing, including a broad-brimmed hat and UV-blocking sunglasses.
- Use a broad-spectrum (UVA/UVB) sunscreen with an SPF of 30 or higher every day.
- Apply 1 ounce (2 tablespoons) of sunscreen to your entire body 30 minutes before going outdoors. Reapply every 2 hours or immediately after swimming or excessive sweating.
- Examine your skin head-to-toe every month.
- See your health care provider every year for a professional skin exam.

SPF, Sun protection factor; *UV,* ultraviolet; *UVA,* ultraviolet A; *UVB,* ultraviolet B.
Modified from Skin Cancer Foundation: *Prevention guidelines* (website), n.d. http://www.skincancer.org/prevention/sun-protection/prevention-guidelines. Accessed March 2019.

BOX 14.6	**Danger Signs: Remember ABCDE**

A Asymmetry of a mole (one that is not regularly round or oval)

B Border is irregular

C Color variation (areas of black, brown, tan, blue, red, white, or a combination)

D Diameter greater than the size of a pencil eraser (although early stages may be smaller)

E Elevation and enlargement[a]

[a]Lesions that change, itch, bleed, or do not heal are also alarm signals. From Skin Cancer Foundation: *Do you know your ABCDEs?* (website), 2018. https://www.skincancer.org/skin-cancer-information/melanoma/melanoma-warning-signs-and-images/do-you-know-your-abcdes. Accessed January 2018.

---

syndromes (Chapter 9), and *Healthy People 2030* has addressed this issue with a goal of reducing the rate of PI-related hospitalizations among older adults. Although prevention and treatment of PIs require an interprofessional approach, PIs are considered specifically a nurse-sensitive indicator by the US National Database of Nursing Quality Indicators (Al-Majid et al., 2017). Nurses play a key role in the prevention of PIs and selection of evidence-based treatment strategies.

Definition

A pressure injury is defined as localized damage to the skin and underlying soft tissue usually over a bony prominence or related to a medical or other device. The injury can present as intact skin or an open ulcer and may be painful. The injury occurs as a result of intense and/or prolonged pressure or pressure in combination with shear. The tolerance of soft tissue for pressure and shear also may be affected by microclimate, nutrition, perfusion, comorbidities, and condition of the soft tissue.

The National Pressure Injury Advisory Panel (NPIAP) and the European Pressure Ulcer Advisory Panel (EPUAP) constitute an international collaboration convened to develop evidence-based recommendations to be used throughout the world to prevent and treat pressure-related injuries. In 2016, the NPIAP began using the term *pressure injury* to replace *pressure ulcer* to more accurately describe PIs to both intact and ulcerated skin. The organization also changed its name from the National Pressure Ulcer Advisory Panel to the National Pressure Injury Advisory Panel. In addition to the change in terminology, Arabic numbers are now used in the names of the stages of PIs instead of Roman numerals. Stages have been more fully described, and two additional PI definitions have been added. In 2019, the third edition of the clinical guidelines was released (https://npiap.com/page/Guidelines) (Box 14.7).

Scope of the Problem

PIs cause pain, loss of function, extended length of hospitalization and long-term care stays, and increase in health care cost. Reported prevalence rates of HAPIs are as high as 38% in the acute care setting, 42% in critical care, 17% in home care, and 23% in long-term care. PIs are a major challenge worldwide and a major cause of morbidity, mortality, and health care burden

BOX 14.7 Resources for Best Practice
Pressure Ulcer Prevention and Treatment

Agency for Healthcare Research and Quality: Preventing pressure ulcers in hospitals: a toolkit for improving quality of care: (https://www.ahrq.gov/professionals/systems/hospital/pressureulcertoolkit/putool3a.html); Safety Program for Nursing Homes: On-Time Pressure Ulcer Prevention: https://www.ahrq.gov/professionals/systems/long-term-care/resources/ontime/pruprev/index.html.

Hartford Institute for Geriatric Nursing: Braden Scale and video demonstrating its use: https://hign.org/consultgeri/try-this-series/predicting-pressure-injury-risk.

International Skin Tear Advisory Panel (ISTAP): Skin Tears Tool Kit, best practice recommendations for holistic strategies to promote and maintain skin integrity, treatment of skin tears, classification system, educational materials: http://SkinTears.org.

National Pressure Injury Advisory Panel (NPIAP): International Pressure Ulcer Prevention Guidelines (available in 17 languages); PUSH Tool 3.0, Support Surface Standards Initiative; pressure ulcer photos; and other educational materials on prevention and treatment available online and via an application for iPhones, iPads, and Android devices: http://www.npiap.org.

VA Pressure Ulcer/Injury Resource (VA PUR) App: The app is available from the Apple App Store and Google Play Store.

Wound Source: Categories of wound-related devices and product information: http://www.woundsource.com.

BOX 14.8 Avoidable and Unavoidable Pressure Injuries

Avoidable: Development of a pressure injury while the facility did not do one or more of the following:
- evaluate the resident's clinical condition and pressure ulcer risk factors
- define and implement interventions that are consistent with resident needs, resident goals, and recognized standards of practice
- monitor and evaluate the impact of the interventions; or revise the interventions as appropriate

Unavoidable: Development of a pressure injury even though the facility:
- evaluated the resident's clinical condition and pressure ulcer risk factors
- defined and implemented interventions that are consistent with resident needs and goals
- recognized standards of practice
- monitored and evaluated the impact of the interventions
- revised the approaches as appropriate

From Centers for Medicare and Medicaid Services: *CMS manual system,* Publication No. 100-07 State Operations, Baltimore, 2004, Author.

globally (Ramundo et al., 2018). The epidemiology of PIs varies appreciably by clinical setting. Critically ill patients in the intensive care unit (ICU) are considered at the greatest risk for PI development as a result of high acuity and the multiple interventions and therapies they receive. Patients admitted to an ICU are twice as likely as other acute care patients to develop a HAPI. HAPI rates have decreased across the United States. However, despite growing resources invested into the development and implementation of evidence-based prevention protocols, the rates of facility-acquired PIs are still much higher in many clinical areas across the globe, especially in high-risk populations such as older adults and critically ill patients (Rondinelli et al., 2018).

Cost and Regulatory Requirements

Treatment of PIs is costly in terms of both health care expenditure and patient suffering. In 2008, the Centers for Medicare and Medicaid Services (CMS) included HAPIs as one of the preventable adverse events (health care–acquired conditions [HACs]). The development of a stage/category 3 or 4 PI is considered a "never event" (preventable serious medical error or adverse event that should never happen to a patient). Hospitals no longer receive additional reimbursement to care for a patient who has acquired PIs while in the hospital's care, and this has the potential to greatly increase the financial strain for facilities that fail to rise to this challenge. In long-term care facilities, when PIs develop after admission and are identified as avoidable, civil monetary penalties can be assessed (Box 14.8).

Characteristics

PIs can develop anywhere on the body but are seen most frequently on the posterior aspects, especially the sacrum, the heels, and the greater trochanters. Secondary areas of breakdown include the lateral condyles of the knees and the ankles. The pinna of the ears, occiput, elbows, and scapulae are other areas subject to breakdown. The heel is particularly prone to the development of PIs due to its anatomy. It consists of skin overlying a cup-like shell of connective tissue that essentially forms a sealed compartment, creating a compartment of fat with comparatively low vascularity that is prone to ischemia. The shell of connective tissue and sealed compartment structure inhibit distribution of external pressure. In addition, the small surface area of contact and little subcutaneous tissue lead to PI when pressure is exerted directly on bone (Ramundo et al., 2018).

⚡ SAFETY TIPS

Approximately 25% to 35% of pressure injuries are on heels. Those with peripheral vascular disease (PVD) are at high risk. Keep heels elevated off the bed with a pillow under the calf or use heel suspension boots. Prophylactic multilayer foam dressings, in conjunction with a pressure injury prevention program, are recommended for prevention of pressure injuries on the heel (Ramundo et al., 2018).

Classification

The EPUAP and NPIAP classification of PIs is presented in Box 14.9. The following two PI definitions also have been added:

Medical Device–Related Pressure Injury: Medical device–related pressure injuries (MDRPIs) result from the use of devices designed and applied for diagnostic or therapeutic purposes. The resultant PI generally conforms to the pattern or shape of the device. The injury should not be staged using the staging system.

Mucosal Membrane Pressure Injury: A mucosal membrane PI is found on mucous membranes with a history of a medical device in use at the location of the injury. Because of the anatomy of the tissue, these injuries cannot be staged.

PIs are always classified by the highest stage "achieved," and reverse staging is never used. This means that the wound is documented as the stage representing the maximal damage and

BOX 14.9 Pressure Injury Stages/Categories

Deep Tissue Pressure Injury (DTPI): Persistent Nonblanchable Deep Red, Maroon, or Purple Discoloration

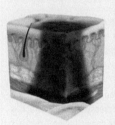
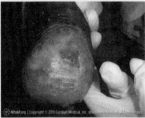

Heel, ethnic skin

Intact or nonintact skin with localized area of persistent nonblanchable deep red, maroon, or purple discoloration or epidermal separation revealing a dark wound bed or blood-filled blister. Pain and temperature change often precede skin color changes. Discoloration may appear differently in darkly pigmented skin. This injury results from intense and/or prolonged pressure and shear forces at the bone-muscle interface. The wound may evolve rapidly to reveal the actual extent of tissue injury or may resolve without tissue loss.

DTPI may evolve into a full thickness wound despite optimal care. If necrotic tissue, subcutaneous tissue, granulation tissue, fascia, muscle, or other underlying structures are visible, this indicates a full-thickness pressure injury (Unstageable, Stage 3, or Stage 4). Do not use DTPI to describe vascular, traumatic, neuropathic, or dermatological conditions. If PI is on a mucosal membrane, document, but do not stage.

Stage 1 Pressure Injury: Nonblanchable Erythema of Intact Skin

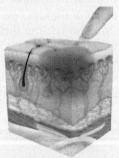
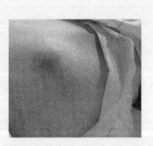

Intact skin with a localized area of nonblanchable erythema, which may appear differently in darkly pigmented skin. Presence of blanchable erythema or changes in sensation, temperature, or firmness may precede visual changes. Color changes do not include purple or maroon discoloration; these may indicate DTPI.

Stage 2 Pressure Injury: Partial-Thickness Skin Loss With Exposed Dermis

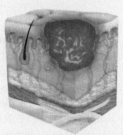
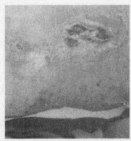

Partial-thickness loss of skin with exposed dermis. The wound bed is viable, pink or red, and moist, and may also present as an intact or ruptured serum-filled blister. Adipose (fat) is not visible and deeper tissues are not visible. Granula-

tion tissue, slough, and eschar are not present. These injuries commonly result from adverse microclimate and shear in the skin over the pelvis and shear in the heels. This stage should not be used to describe moisture-associated skin damage (MASD) including incontinence-associated dermatitis (IAD), intertriginous dermatitis (ITD), medical adhesive–related skin injury (MARS), or traumatic wounds (skin tears, burns, abrasions).

Stage 3 Pressure Injury: Full-Thickness Skin Loss

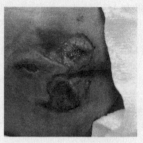
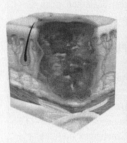

Full-thickness loss of skin, in which adipose (fat) is visible in the ulcer and granulation tissue and epibole (rolled wound edges) are often present. Slough and/or eschar may be visible. Undermining and tunneling may occur. Fascia, muscle, tendon, ligament, cartilage, and/or bone are not exposed. If slough or eschar obscures the extent of tissue loss this is an Unstageable Pressure Injury.

Stage 4 Pressure Injury: Full-Thickness Skin and Tissue Loss

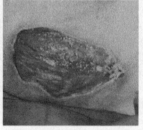
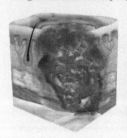

Full-thickness skin and tissue loss with exposed or directly palpable fascia, muscle, tendon, ligament, cartilage, or bone in the ulcer. Slough and/or eschar may be visible. Epibole (rolled edges), undermining, and/or tunneling often occur. Depth varies by anatomical location. If slough or eschar obscures the extent of tissue loss, this is an Unstageable Pressure Injury.

Unstageable Pressure Injury: Obscured Full-Thickness Skin and Tissue Loss

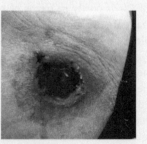
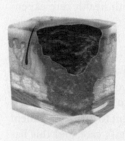

Full-thickness skin and tissue loss in which the extent of tissue damage within the ulcer cannot be confirmed because it is obscured by slough or eschar. If slough or eschar is removed, a Stage 3 or Stage 4 pressure ulcer will be revealed. Stable eschar (e.g., dry, adherent, intact without erythema or fluctuance) on an ischemic limb or the heels should not be removed.

PI, Pressure injury.
From National Pressure Ulcer Advisory Panel: *National Pressure Ulcer Advisory Panel (NPUAP) announces a change in terminology from pressure ulcer to pressure injury and updates the stages of pressure injury,* 2016. Reprinted with permission of the NPUAP, 2016; From National Pressure Ulcer Advisory Panel: *NPUAP position statement on staging—2017 clarifications,* 2017. Reprinted with permission of the NPUAP, 2017; DTPI photo: From NPUAP; Stages 1–4 photos: From Cameron MH, Monroe L: *Physical rehabilitation for the physical therapist assistant,* St Louis, 2011, Saunders; Unstageable photo: From Ham RJ, Sloane PD, Warshaw GA, et al: *Primary care geriatrics,* ed 6, Philadelphia, 2014, Elsevier.

depth that has occurred. As the wound heals, it fills with granulation tissue composed of endothelial cells, fibroblasts, collagen, and an extracellular matrix. Muscle, subcutaneous fat, and dermis are not replaced. A stage 4 PI that is healing does not revert to stage 3 and then to stage 2. It remains defined as a healing stage 4 PI.

Risk Factors

Many factors increase the risk of PIs, including changes in the skin, comorbid illnesses, nutritional status, frailty, surgical procedures (especially orthopedic and cardiac), cognitive deficits, incontinence, and reduced mobility (Box 14.10). A major risk factor is the combination of intensity and duration of pressure and tissue tolerance. Individuals confined to a bed or chair and who are unable to shift weight or reposition themselves at regular intervals are at high risk. Tissue tolerance, in addition to unrelieved pressure, contributes to the risk of a PI. Tissue tolerance is related to the ability of the tissue to distribute and compensate for pressure exerted over bony prominences. Factors that affect tissue tolerance include moisture, friction, shear force, nutritional status, age, sensory perception, and arterial pressure.

Prevention of Pressure Injuries

The importance of prevention of PIs has been frequently emphasized and is the key to treatment. Key elements of PI prevention are presented in Box 14.11. A comprehensive PI

BOX 14.11   Key Elements of a Pressure Injury Prevention Program

- Skin assessment for all patients looking for pressure injury
- Daily risk assessment
- Daily skin inspection
- Moisture management
- Optimizing nutrition and hydration
- Minimizing pressure (posture changes)
- Pressure injury nursing care education
- Establishment of a wound care team
- Interdisciplinary cooperation

From Jin Y, Jin T, Lee S: Automated pressure injury risk assessment system incorporated into an electronic record system, *Nurs Res* 66(6):462–472, 2017.

---

program that includes multiple interventions (care bundle) appears to be related to better outcomes. A care bundle is composed of a set of evidence-based practices that, when performed collectively and reliably, have been shown to improve patient outcomes. Involvement of the patient and family may enhance the effectiveness of care bundles. Core preventive actions include risk evaluation, evaluation of the skin, nutritional evaluation, repositioning, and appropriate support surfaces. Actions that address limited mobility, compromised skin integrity, and nutritional support have been associated with improvements in PI rates. Nurse practitioners assuming a leadership role as wound care consultants in acute care have been found to be instrumental in decreasing HAPI rates (Irvin et al., 2017).

Systematic prevention programs have been shown to decrease HAPIs. Use of the On-Time Pressure Ulcer Prevention program (Agency for Healthcare Research and Quality [AHRQ], 2014) has been shown to reduce the prevalence of PIs in long-term care. Tools to document PI healing and treatments and reports to monitor the healing process are available (see Box 14.7). Despite recognition of its importance, PI prevention strategies are not implemented consistently, and PIs continue to have a negative impact of patient outcomes and health care costs in a variety of care settings.

Education programs on PI, for both practicing nurses and student nurses, are essential and should be a part of institutional and educational curricula. Research conducted in the United States and internationally in other countries has demonstrated that nurses, both wound certified and not, have limited levels of PI knowledge (Ayello et al., 2017). Innovative approaches to education are important and may include "just in time" interactive educational methods, including mobile phone apps. The US Department of Veterans Affairs (VA) has developed an innovative mobile app for veterans and caregivers working to prevent and treat PIs—the VA Pressure Ulcer/Injury Resource app (VA PUR) (see Box 14.7). Continuing professional development for PI prevention and management needs to be interprofessional and include evidence-based educational material and strategies. Professional nursing checklists for competence and performance evaluations need to be implemented at all levels (novice to expert).

BOX 14.10   Pressure Injury Risk Factors

Prolonged Pressure/Immobilization

Lying in bed or sitting in a chair or wheelchair without changing position or relieving pressure over an extended period

Lying for hours on hard x-ray and operating tables

Neurological disorders (coma, spinal cord injuries, cognitive impairment, or cerebrovascular disease)

Fractures or contractures

Debilitation: older adult in hospitals and nursing homes

Pain

Sedation

Shearing forces (moving by dragging on coarse bed sheets)

Disease/Tissue Factors

Impaired perfusion; ischemia

Fecal or urinary incontinence; prolonged exposure to moisture

Malnutrition, dehydration

Chronic diseases accompanied by anemia, edema, renal failure, malnutrition, peripheral vascular disease, or sepsis

Previous history of pressure injuries

Additional Risk Factors for the Critically Ill

Norepinephrine infusion

Acute Physiology and Chronic Health Evaluation (APACHE II) score

Anemia

Age older than 40 years

Multiple organ system disease or comorbid complications

Length of hospital stay

From McCance KL, Huether SE: *Pathophysiology*, ed 7, St Louis, 2014, Elsevier.

Consequences of Pressure Injuries

PIs are costly to treat and prolong recovery and extend rehabilitation. Complications include the need for grafting or amputation, sepsis, or even death and may lead to legal action by the individual or a representative against the caregiver. The personal impact of a PI on health and quality of life is also significant and not well understood or researched. Findings from a study exploring patients' perceptions of the impact of a PI and its treatment on health and quality of life suggest that PIs cause suffering, pain, discomfort, and distress that are not always recognized or adequately treated by nursing staff. PIs have a profound impact on the patients' lives—physically, socially, emotionally, and mentally (Spilsbury et al., 2007).

Are Pressure Injuries Always Preventable?

PI development is a multicausal event. In the vast majority of cases, appropriate prevention and treatment interventions can prevent or minimize PI development. Some PIs are unavoidable despite provision of evidence-based care by the health care team. Both the NPIAP and the Wound, Ostomy, and Continence Nurses Society (WOCN Society) (Schmitt et al., 2017) have published statements on avoidable and unavoidable PIs. An unavoidable PI is an ulcer that forms because of an individual's clinical condition and risk factors, despite the proper application of standard preventative measures. The CMS has separated the skin changes associated with the dying process from PIs that may be avoidable versus unavoidable (Ayello et al., 2019). Clinical situations can severely impair efforts to prevent PIs. Some of these are preexisting deep tissue injury (DTI) (but no visible ulceration), immobility, hemodynamic instability, medical devices, compromised nutrition, and the patient who is nearing the end of life.

Skin Changes at the End of Life

Skin frailty is the suggested term for at-risk vulnerable skin. Skin frailty affects all ages from neonates to older adults and is multifactorial. Risk factors for skin frailty can be intrinsic, extrinsic, and modifiable or unmodifiable. If an individual's skin has enhanced vulnerability, the person is at increased risk of damage to the skin that can include skin tears, PIs, and skin changes at end of life. Skin changes at the end of life are related to skin frailty and are also known as skin failure. Skin failure is defined as "an event in which the skin and underlying tissue die due to the hypoperfusion that occurs concurrent with severe dysfunction or failure of other organ systems" (Beeckman et al., 2020, p 10).

The SCALE (Skin Changes at Life's End) Consensus Statement (Sibbald et al., 2009) states that the physiological changes of dying can cause unavoidable skin or soft tissue changes despite care interventions that meet or exceed the standard of care. Skin failure at the end of life is not the same as PIs. Preventing wound deterioration or healing may not be a realistic goal. The focus of wound management at the end of life is comfort and involves symptom control, stabilization of existing wounds, and prevention of additional wounds and infectious complications. If opportunity for wound healing is limited, maintenance of the wound in the present state may be the outcome. In some situations, palliative wounds may benefit from interventions such as surgical debridement or support surfaces even if the goal is not to heal the wound. The plan of care must be consistent with the patient and family goals and wishes.

In the last days or weeks prior to death, some individuals develop a condition known as Kennedy terminal ulcer (KTU), or the 3:30 syndrome, a subset of pressure ulceration. KTUs are unavoidable but may not be recognized by clinicians due to a lack of awareness of their existence. This can prevent accurate diagnosis and management of pain and discomfort.

KTUs present as small black spots due to hypoperfusion, appear very quickly, and grow in size, often in a few hours. Further research is needed to fully understand the development of unavoidable PI in situations of high risk such as at the end of life (Ayello et al., 2019; Beeckman et al., 2020). "There is a pressing need to define skin failure as a clinical syndrome and understand its pathophysiology because of its implications for both clinical care and health policy (Levine et al., 2022, p.1).

USING CLINICAL JUDGMENT TO PROMOTE HEALTHY AGING: PRESSURE INJURIES

Nursing staff, as direct caregivers, are key team members who perform evaluation of the skin, identify risk factors, and implement numerous preventive actions. The nurse alerts the health care provider of the need for prescribed treatments, recommends treatments, and administers and evaluates the changing status of the wounds and adequacy of treatments.

Recognizing and Analyzing Cues

An evaluation of the skin is performed on admission and whenever there is a change in the status of the patient (Box 14.12). In the long-term care facility, the Minimum Data Set (MDS) 3.0 provides an evidence-based assessment of skin integrity and PIs with accompanying care guidelines (Chapter 9). Evaluation begins with a history, detailed head-to-toe skin examination, nutritional evaluation, and analysis of laboratory findings. Laboratory values that have been correlated with risk for the development and poor healing of PIs include those that reflect anemia and poor nutritional status. Visual and tactile inspection of the entire skin surface with special attention to bony prominences is

---

BOX 14.12   Guidelines for Skin Assessment
Acute care: On admission, reassess at least every 24 hours or sooner if patient's condition changes
Long-term care: On admission, weekly for 4 weeks, then quarterly and whenever resident's condition changes
Home care: On admission and at every nurse visit

Data from National Pressure Ulcer Advisory Panel: *Pressure ulcer prevention points* (website), 2007. http://www.npuap.org/wp-content/uploads/2012/03/PU_Prev_Points.pdf. Accessed January 2018.

essential. The nurse looks for any interruption of skin integrity or other changes, including redness or *hyperemia.*

Special attention must be given to the assessment of dark skin because tissue injury will appear differently than in lighter skin. In darker-pigmented persons, redness and blanching may not be observed as early signs of skin damage. In dark skin, early signs of skin damage can manifest as a purplish color or appear like a bruise. It is important to observe for induration, darkening, change in color from surrounding skin, or a shadowed appearance of the skin. The affected skin area, when compared with adjacent tissues, may be firm, warmer, cooler, or painful. PIs present differently among ethnically or racially diverse nursing home residents, and it is important to recognize early cues and take action to prevent progression (Bates-Jensen et al., 2021) (see Research Highlights).

RESEARCH HIGHLIGHTS

Natural History of Pressure Injury (PI) Among Ethnically or Racially Diverse Nursing Home Residents: The Pressure Ulcer Detection Study

Data from Bates-Jensen G, Anber K, Chen M, et al: Natural history

Purpose

To describe resident and nursing home (NH) characteristics of Black, Asian, White, and Hispanic individuals with PIs; compare PI location, severity, characteristics, and progression among the groups; and examine use of PI prevention among racially or ethnically diverse nursing home residents.

Method

Descriptive data were gathered on 270 PIs among 142 racially or ethnically diverse nursing home residents over 16 weeks. Residents were recruited from 19 NHs in the Los Angeles area. Most NHs were for-profit facilities, and PI rates for long-stay residents were higher than national and state averages. NH data, reflecting quality and resources, were gathered from NursingHomeCompare and Cal/QualityCare.org websites. Data included Centers for Medicare and Medicaid Services (CMS) 5-star rating; bed number and occupancy rate; current year total number of survey inspections, deficiencies, and citations; staffing level; and percentage of short-stay and long-stay residents with PIs.

Medical and demographic information was obtained from medical records and Minimum Data Set (MDS) data. Repositioning, pressure reduction (beds and devices), and nutrition prevention interventions were obtained from medical records. The Braden Scale was used monthly, skin health was assessed weekly by research staff, and PI assessment was conducted.

Results

Most participants were at risk for PIs and totally dependent or required extensive assistance for bed mobility and transfers. Approximately one-half had a PI on more than one anatomic location. There was a range of quality among the NHs. More than half had one or two stars for CMS quality of care ratings; one-half reported licensed nursing home staff below the state average, and one-third reported high nurse aide levels. No differences were found on NH bed size, occupancy rate, and CMS ratings.

PI location did not vary across race or ethnicity groups, and no differences existed on PI severity, but Asian participants developed significantly more PIs than other groups. No differences in prevention interventions were observed across the groups. Only one-half of the participants used pressure reduction devices. Nutritional supplements were used for all participants. More Black and Asian participants had a diagnosis of peripheral vascular disease (PVD), which was associated with heel PIs in these groups.

Conclusion

Use of prevention was less than optimal for all racial or ethnic nursing home residents with PIs, and all groups would benefit from increased prevention interventions. Nutritional supplements for added protein and calories and increased use of heel boots and other pressure reduction devices are indicated for all residents with PIs. Black and Hispanic residents' PIs were generally more severe, and these individuals may need more vigorous prevention efforts early in the PI course. Increased attention to prevention and skin assessment in Asian individuals is indicated. Black and Hispanic residents were more likely to have PIs with no surrounding skin discoloration, and nurses may need to use techniques beyond visual observation to evaluate for PI deterioration—for example, use of palpation for edema or induration or use of biophysical measures to detect deep inflammatory changes at the wound site.

If pressure is present, it should be relieved and the area reassessed in 1 hour. Pressure areas and surrounding tissue should be palpated for changes in temperature and tissue resilience. Blisters or pimples with or without hyperemia and

of pressure injury among ethnically/racially diverse nursing home residents: the pressure ulcer detection study, *Jour Gerontol Nurs* 47(3):37–46, 2021.

scabs over weight-bearing areas in the absence of trauma should be considered suspect. Inspection is best accomplished in nonglare daylight or, if that is not possible, with focused lighting. Special attention should be directed to affected areas when an individual uses orthotic devices such as corsets, braces, prostheses, postural supports, splints, slings, or casts and to areas of skin around other devices such as endotracheal and tracheostomy tubes.

MDRPIs result from the use of devices designed and applied for diagnostic purposes. It is important to correctly position the equipment and select correct securement devices. Using thin hydrocolloids, film dressings, barrier products, or pressure-reducing dermal gel pads underneath the device will reduce friction and shear (Beeckman et al., 2020). There is little information available on the risks or frequency of device-related PIs.

Early identification of risk status is critical so that timely interventions can be designed to address specific risk factors. The Braden Scale for Predicting Pressure Sore Risk, developed by nurses Barbara Braden and Nancy Bergstrom, is widely used and clinically validated. The Braden Scale is available online and used in most health care institutions (see Box 14.7). This scale evaluates the risk of PIs based on a numerical scoring system of six risk factors: sensory perception, moisture, activity, mobility, nutrition, and friction or shear.

Because the Braden Scale does not include all the risk factors for PIs, it is recommended that it be used as an adjunct rather than in place of clinical judgment. A thorough patient history, to determine other risk factors such as age, medications, comorbidities (diabetes, peripheral vascular disease), and history of PIs, is important to fully address the risk of PI development so that appropriate preventive interventions can be developed. Some authors propose that the Braden Scale subscale scores, rather than the cumulative score, should be the focus of prevention efforts (Alderden et al., 2017).

Solutions, Nursing Actions, and Outcomes

The goal of prevention is to help maintain skin integrity against the various environmental, mechanical, and chemical assaults that are potential causes of breakdown. Nursing actions include (1) eliminating friction and irritation to the skin, such as from shearing; (2) reducing moisture so that tissues do not macerate; (3) managing incontinence; (4) enhancing mobility; and (5) displacing body weight from prominent areas to facilitate circulation to the skin. The nurse should be familiar with the types of supportive surfaces so that the most effective products are used. The Support Surface Algorithm (SSA) is an evidence-based tool that helps determine a strong protocol for addressing PIs (see Box 14.7). Use lifting devices to move the person rather than dragging the person during transfers and position changes. Use pillows or foam wedges so that skin surfaces do not touch and use devices that eliminate pressure on heels.

Repositioning is generally regarded as one of the most important and effective measures for preventing PIs, but there is no consensus on the frequency or type of repositioning most effective for individual patients. For some, 4-hour repositioning may be adequate, whereas for others even hourly repositioning would not prevent PI. Historically, 2-hour turning has been recommended regardless of the individual need. Hampton (2017) argues that this recommendation originated from Florence Nightingale, who recognized the importance of repositioning when caring for soldiers in the Crimean War. She did not stipulate the timing for repositioning, but it took 2 hours to work around the large ward. Hence the myth of turns every 2 hours was born.

Techniques for proper positioning are directed at offloading pressure and individualized for each person. These techniques include a change in body position, head of bed adjustment, microshifting, and use of the appropriate pillows, wedges, and sleep surfaces. Continuous bedside pressure mapping (CBPM) devices (Fig. 14.8) enable caregivers and patients to visualize, assess, and monitor pressure points between the patient and the support surface (beds or wheelchairs) and to undertake the necessary interventions to successfully offload pressure. The pressure sensing mat measures pressure from thousands of discrete points and converts pressure (measured in mmHg) into color, with red, orange, and yellow corresponding to higher pressures and blue and green corresponding to lower pressures. Based on systematic review and meta-analysis, the current literature demonstrates that PI-monitoring devices are associated with a strong reduction in the risk of developing PIs in acute and skilled nursing settings (Lucchini et al., 2020; Walia et al., 2016). These devices provide critical, real-time information to clinicians.

> ⚡ **SAFETY TIPS**
>
> Individuals placed on pressure redistribution mattresses continue to need turning and repositioning according to an individualized schedule.

Consultation with the nutritional team is important. Nutritional intake should be monitored, along with the serum albumin, hematocrit, and hemoglobin levels. Caloric, protein, vitamin, and/or mineral supplementation can be considered if there is evidence of deficiencies of these nutrients. It is recommended that individuals with PIs consume high-protein nutritional supplements in addition to dietary protein consumption of 1.25 to 1.5 g/kg/day. Use of multivitamins is also recommended, and multiple studies have shown increased healing with multivitamin use (Bates-Jensen et al., 2021). Routine use of higher than the recommended daily allowance of vitamin C and zinc for the prevention and/or treatment of PIs is not supported by evidence. The nurse promotes nutritional health by ensuring that the person receives adequate assistance with eating and that dining time is a pleasant experience for the person (Chapter 15). PI prevention education programs need to be provided to all levels of health care providers, patients, families, and caregivers.

Pressure Injury Evaluation

PIs are evaluated with each dressing change, and evaluations are repeated on a weekly, biweekly, and as-needed basis. The purpose is to specifically and carefully evaluate the effectiveness

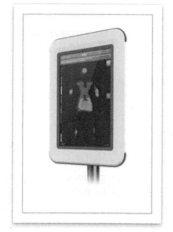
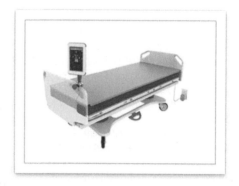

Fig. 14.8 Continuous bedside pressure mapping (CBPM) devices. (Used with permission from Wellsense, Inc.)

of treatment. Assessment of pain related to the PI (dressing changes, turning) is important so that appropriate treatment can be given to relieve pain (Chapter 29). The PUSH tool (Pressure Ulcer Scale for Healing) (Fig. 14.9) provides a detailed form that covers all aspects of evaluation but contains only three items and takes a short time to complete. Photographic documentation is highly recommended both at the onset of the problem and at intervals during treatment.

Pressure Ulcer Scale for Healing (PUSH)
PUSH Tool 3.0

NATIONAL PRESSURE ULCER ADVISORY PANEL

Patient Name_____ Patient ID# _____

Ulcer Location _____ Date _____

Directions:

Observe and measure the pressure ulcer. Categorize the ulcer with respect to surface area, exudate, and type of wound tissue. Record a sub-score for each of these ulcer characteristics. Add the sub-scores to obtain the total score. A comparison of total scores measured over time provides an indication of the improvement or deterioration in pressure ulcer healing.

LENGTH X WIDTH (in cm²)	**0** 0	**1** < 0.3	**2** 0.3 – 0.6	**3** 0.7 – 1.0	**4** 1.1 – 2.0	**5** 2.1 – 3.0	Sub-score
		6 3.1 – 4.0	**7** 4.1 – 8.0	**8** 8.1 – 12.0	**9** 12.1 – 24.0	**10** > 24.0	
EXUDATE AMOUNT	**0** None	**1** Light	**2** Moderate	**3** Heavy			Sub-score
TISSUE TYPE	**0** Closed	**1** Epithelial Tissue	**2** Granulation Tissue	**3** Slough	**4** Necrotic Tissue		Sub-score
							TOTAL SCORE

Length x Width: Measure the greatest length (head to toe) and the greatest width (side to side) using a centimeter ruler. Multiply these two measurements (length x width) to obtain an estimate of surface area in square centimeters (cm²). Caveat: Do not guess! Always use a centimeter ruler and always use the same method each time the ulcer is measured.

Exudate Amount: Estimate the amount of exudate (drainage) present after removal of the dressing and before applying any topical agent to the ulcer. Estimate the exudate (drainage) as none, light, moderate, or heavy.

Tissue Type: This refers to the types of tissue that are present in the wound (ulcer) bed. Score as a "4" if there is any necrotic tissue present. Score as a "3" if there is any amount of slough present and necrotic tissue is absent. Score as a "2" if the wound is clean and contains granulation tissue. A superficial wound that is reepithelializing is scored as a "1". When the wound is closed, score as a "0".

  4 – **Necrotic Tissue (Eschar):** black, brown, or tan tissue that adheres firmly to the wound bed or ulcer edges and may be either firmer or softer than surrounding skin.
  3 – **Slough:** yellow or white tissue that adheres to the ulcer bed in strings or thick clumps, or is mucinous.
  2 – **Granulation Tissue:** pink or beefy red tissue with a shiny, moist, granular appearance.
  1 – **Epithelial Tissue:** for superficial ulcers, new pink or shiny tissue (skin) that grows in from the edges or as islands on the ulcer surface.
  0 – **Closed/Resurfaced:** the wound is completely covered with epithelium (new skin).

www.npuap.org
11F

PUSH Tool Version 3.0: 9/15/98
©National Pressure Ulcer Advisory Panel

Fig. 14.9 Pressure Ulcer Scale for Healing (PUSH) tool. (Used with permission from National Pressure Injury Advisory Panel.)

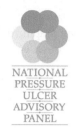

NATIONAL
PRESSURE
ULCER
ADVISORY
PANEL

Pressure Ulcer Healing Chart
To monitor trends in PUSH Scores over time
(Use a separate page for each pressure ulcer)

Patient Name_____ Patient ID# _____

Ulcer Location _____ Date _____

Directions:
Observe and measure pressure ulcers at regular intervals using the PUSH Tool.
Date and record PUSH Sub-scores and Total Scores on the Pressure Ulcer Healing Record below.

Pressure Ulcer Healing Record

Date												
Length x Width												
Exudate Amount												
Tissue Type												
PUSH Total Score												

Graph the PUSH Total Scores on the Pressure Ulcer Healing Graph below.

Pressure Ulcer Healing Graph

PUSH Total Score												
17												
16												
15												
14												
13												
12												
11												
10												
9												
8												
7												
6												
5												
4												
3												
2												
1												
Healed = 0												
Date												

www.npuap.org
11F

PUSH Tool Version 3.0: 9/15/98
©National Pressure Ulcer Advisory Panel

Fig. 14.9   cont'd

If there are no signs of healing from week to week or worsening of the wound is seen, then either the treatment is insufficient or the wound has become infected; in both cases, treatment must be changed. Determining the cause of the PI is important so that appropriate preventive measures can be implemented. The care team, in consultation with the individual and family, reviews the evaluation data and care plan and determines, if possible, whether the underlying cause is reversible so that appropriate treatment decisions can be made to ensure patient comfort. Consultation with a wound care specialist is advisable for wounds that are extensive or nonhealing. Specialized nurses such as enterostomal therapists or nurse practitioners, who may work with wound centers or surgeons, provide consultation in nursing homes, offices, or clinics.

Pressure Injury Dressings

The type of dressing selected is based on careful assessment of the condition of the PI; the presence of granulation, necrotic tissue, and slough; the amount of drainage; the microbial status; and the quality of the surrounding skin. If the wound has necrotic tissue, it must be debrided. Debridement methods include mechanical (whirlpool, wet-to-dry); sharp (scalpel, scissors); enzymatic (collagenase); and autolytic (hydrocolloid, hydrogel). Wound cleansing should be done with nontoxic preparations; normal saline is recommended. Other principles are presented in Box 14.13. Box 14.14 presents general guidelines for PI dressings.

There are many PI products and devices available but little research evidence regarding whether particular wound dressings or topical treatments and devices have a beneficial impact on wound healing, even compared with basic dressings (Westby et al., 2017). Quality research is needed on the effectiveness of the most widely used dressings and should include time to healing and whether healing occurs. Cost-effectiveness also should be considered. Although further research is needed, the use of prophylactic multilayer silicone foam dressings, particularly on the heel and sacrum, can help in the prevention of PIs and shear and friction injuries and improve the microclimate of the skin. Prophylactic dressings must be considered an adjunct treatment to be used alongside standard pressure-relieving measures (Ramundo et al., 2018).

Other general categories of wound care–related devices include compression therapy devices, off-weighting devices (offloading), adjunctive therapies such as electrical stimulation and ultrasound and hyperbaric oxygen therapy (HBOT), negative-pressure wound therapy (NPWT), and pressure redistribution surfaces (specialty beds, support surfaces). An evidence-based

---

BOX 14.13   Mnemonic for Pressure Injury Treatment: DIPAMOPI

D   Debride
I   Identify and treat infection
P   Pack dead space lightly
A   Absorb excess exudate
M   Maintain moist wound surface
O   Open or excise closed wound edges
P   Protect healing wound from infection and trauma
I   Insulate to maintain normal temperature

BOX 14.14   Factors to Consider in Selecting Pressure Injury Dressings

- Shallow, dry wounds with no or minimal exudate need hydrating dressings that add or trap moisture; very shallow wounds require cover dressing only (gels or transparent adhesive dressings, thin hydrocolloid, thin polyurethane foam, wound gel to add moisture).
- Shallow wounds with moderate to large exudate need dressings that absorb exudate, maintain moist surface, support autolysis if necrotic tissue is present, protect and insulate, and protect surrounding tissue (hydrocolloids, semipermeable polyurethane foam, calcium alginates, silicone-type foam). Cover with an absorptive cover dressing.
- Deep wounds with moderate to large exudate require filling of dead space, absorption of exudate, maintenance of moist environment, support of autolysis if necrotic tissue is present, protection, and insulation (copolymer starch, dextranomer beads, calcium alginates, foam cavity). Cover with gauze pad, abdominal dressing, transparent thin film, or polyurethane foam.

---

approach is recommended in the selection and prescription of equipment to prevent and manage wounds. Levine (2017) comments that NPWT is an expensive, cure-oriented treatment that is frequently overused in situations where treatment is hopeless. Health professionals need to consult reviews such as the Cochrane Review and clinical practice guidelines such as those from NPIAP when determining the most appropriate device or treatment. Specific product information can also be found at http://www.woundsource.com (see Box 14.7).

Provision of education to patients, families, and professional staff also must be included in any skin care program. Patient and family needs must be integrated into the plan of care. Teach the individual and the family about the normal healing process and keep them informed about progress (or lack of progress) toward healing, including signs and symptoms that should be brought to the health care professional's attention and education about any devices used.

KEY CONCEPTS

- The skin is the largest and most visible organ of the body; it has multiple roles in maintaining one's health.
- Maintaining adequate oral hydration and skin lubrication will reduce the incidence of xerosis and other skin problems.
- The best way to minimize the risk of skin cancer is to avoid prolonged sun exposure.
- The primary risk factors for PI development are immobility and reduced activity.
- Changes in the skin with age, comorbid illnesses, nutritional status, low body mass, shear, and friction also increase PI risk. Individuals at greatest risk include those who are confined to a bed or chair and unable to shift weight or reposition themselves.

- Structured protocols and prevention bundles should be present in all facilities and have been shown to reduce PI development.
- A PI is documented by stage, which reflects the greatest degree of tissue damage, and as it heals reverse staging is not appropriate.

- A PI covered in dead tissue (eschar or slough) cannot be staged until it is debrided.
- Darkly pigmented skin will not display the "typical" erythema of a stage 1 PI or early DTI; therefore early recognition and analysis of cues in dark-skinned individuals and closer vigilance is necessary.

NEXT-GENERATION NCLEX® (NGN) EXAMINATION–STYLE QUESTIONS

Ms. Patel, a 76-year-old female, is being admitted to skilled services following hospitalization for heart failure. She has a history of diabetes type 2, hypertension, osteoporosis, and peripheral vascular disease. She had a stroke 5 years ago and has left-sided hemiparesis. However, she can transfer herself from bed to wheelchair and propel herself around the facility. She is 5′6″ and laughs when she says she has shrunk a couple of inches over the past decade. Her weight is 225 pounds, and her body mass index (BMI) is 36.31 kg/m². Ms. Patel is oriented to person, place, and time. She denies any pain, although she says she takes acetaminophen at bedtime because her left side aches after a day of activity. Her blood pressure is 138/86 mm Hg, temperature 97.2°F, heart rate 96 beats per minute, respiratory rate 14 breaths per minute, and oxygen saturation 96% on room air. On examination there is a dark pink, maculopapular rash under her left breast; it has a scalloped border with a white rim. Her left lateral olecranon process has a half-moon–shaped wound with separation of the layers of skin with the edges rolled and the base of the wound red and moist. The sacrum has a shallow wound measuring 2.6 mm × 2 mm × 2 mm; the wound bed is viable, red, and moist. On her left ischial tuberosity, there is a wound measuring 5 mm × 4.5 mm × 4 mm. Slough covers 25% of the wound bed, and undermining that measures 3 mm is present from the 9 o'clock position to the 2 o'clock position. The wound has a moderate amount of serosanguineous drainage.

Ms. Patel's left lateral malleolus has an area the size of a dime that is nonblanchable and tender. On her left heel there is an intact, fluid-filled blister.

Choose the most likely options for the information missing from the statement below by selecting from the list of options provided.

The assessment findings indicate that the client has a _____ on her left lateral olecranon process, a _____ on her sacrum, a _____ on her left ischial tuberosity, a _____ on her left lateral malleolus, and a _____ on her left heel.

Options
Stage 1 pressure injury
Stage 2 pressure injury
Stage 3 pressure injury
Stage 4 pressure injury
Unstageable injury
Suspected deep tissue injury
Medical device–related injury
Skin tear
Maceration

CLINICAL JUDGMENT QUESTIONS AND ACTIVITIES

1. Describe the common skin conditions that an older adult is likely to experience.
2. What is the nurse's responsibility in health promotion related to skin integrity?
3. How would you counsel an older adult about getting the Shingrix vaccine even if they have had previous vaccination with Zostavax?
4. What are early cues to deep pressure tissue injury in dark-skinned individuals?
5. Which evidence-based protocols can the nurse use for prevention of pressure injuries?

RESEARCH QUESTIONS

1. What is the most effective strategy to inform younger people about the risk of skin cancer from sun and tanning bed exposure?
2. What is the knowledge level of older individuals about PI risk?
3. What are the major barriers identified by nursing staff to implementation of preventive interventions for PIs?
4. How effective are current patient education materials in enhancing knowledge of PI risk among racially and culturally diverse older individuals?

REFERENCES

Alderden J, Cowan L, Dimas J, et al.: Risk factors for hospital-acquired pressure injury in surgical critical care patients, *Am J Crit Care* 29(6):e128–e134, 2017.

Agency for Healthcare Research and Quality (AHQR) Safety Program for Nursing Homes: *On-time pressure ulcer prevention*, Rockville, MD, 2014, Agency for Healthcare Research and Quality Content last reviewed November.

Al-Majid S, Vuncanon B, Carlson N, et al.: The effect of offloading heels on sacral pressure, *AORN J* 106(3):194–200, 2017.

Ayello E, Zulkowski K, Capezuti E, et al.: Educating nurses in the United States about pressure injuries, *Adv Skin Wound Care* 30(2):83–94, 2017.

Ayello E, Levine J, Kennedy-Evans K, et al.: Reexamining the literature on terminal ulcers, SCALE, skin failure, and unavoidable pressure injuries, *Advances in Skin & Wound Care* 32(3):109–120, 2019.

Bastidas A, de la Sema J, El Idrissi M, et al.: Effect of recombinant zoster vaccine on incidence of herpes zoster after autologous stem cell transplantation: a randomized clinical trial, *JAMA* 322(2):123–133, 2019.

Bates-Jensen G, Anber K, Chen M, et al.: Natural history of pressure injury among ethnically/racially diverse nursing home residents: the pressure ulcer detection study, *J Gerontol Nurs* 47(3):37–46, 2021.

Beeckman E, Campbell K, LeBlanc K: *Best practice recommendation for holistic strategies to promote and maintain skin integrity* (website), 2020. http://www.skintears.org/wp-content/uploads/2020/05/best-practice-recommendations-holistic-strategies-promote-and-maintain-skin-integrity-ISTAP-2020.pdf. Accessed June 2021.

Centers for Disease Control and Prevention (CDC): *Scabies* (website), 2020a. https://www.cdc.gov/parasites/scabies/index.html.

Centers for Disease Control and Prevention (CDC): *Shingles (herpes zoster)* (website), 2020b. https://www.cdc.gov/shingles/index.html.

Cheung C: Older adults, falls, and skin integrity, *Adv Skin Wound Care* 30(1):40–46, 2017.

Endo J, Norman R, et al.: Skin problems. In Ham R, Sloane P, Warshaw G, et al, editors: *Ham's primary care geriatrics*, ed 6, Philadelphia, 2014, Elsevier Saunders, pp 573–587.

Hampton S. Could lateral tilt matresses be the answer to pressure ulcer prevention and management? Br Journal of Community Nursing 22 (Suppl 3): S6-12.

Irvin C, Sedlak E, Walton C, et al.: Hospital-acquired pressure injuries: the significance of the advanced practice registered nurse's role in a community hospital, *J Am Assoc Nurse Pract* 29(4):203–208, 2017.

LeBlanc K, Baronoski S, Christensen D, et al.: The art of dressing selection: a consensus statement on skin tears and best practice, *Adv Skin Wound Care* 29(1):32–46, 2016.

Levine JM: *Palliative wound care: a new frontier* (website), 2017. http://www.geripal.org/2017/09/palliative-wound-care-new-frontier.html. Accessed March 2020.

Levine JM, Delmore B, Cox J: Skin failure: concept review and proposed model, *Advances in Skin & Wound Care*:1–11, 2022 March file:///C:/Users/Terri/Downloads/Skin_Failure__Concept_Review_and_Proposed_Model.99883%20[2].pdfAccessed December 2021.

Lucchini A, Bambi S, Elli S, et al.: Continuous monitoring of contact pressures in a general ICU: a prospective observational study, *Assist Inferm Ric* 39(1):5–12, 2020.

McCance K, Heuther S: Structure, function, and disorders of the integument. In McCance KL, Huether SE, editors: *Pathophysiology*, ed 7, St Louis, 2014, Elsevier, pp 1616–1651.

Ong E, Goldacre R, Hoang U, et al.: Subsequent primary malignancies in patients with nonmelanoma skin cancer in England: a national record-linkage study, *Cancer Epidemiol Biomarkers Prev* 23:490–498, 2014.

Ramundo J, Pike C, Pittman J: Do prophylactic foam dressings reduce heel pressure injuries? *J Wound Ostomy Continence Nurs* 45(1):75–82, 2018.

Rondinelli J, Zuniga S, Kipnis P, et al.: Hospital-acquired pressure injury: risk-adjusted comparisons in an integrated healthcare delivery system, *Nurs Res* 67(1):16–25, 2018.

Schmitt S, Andries MK, Ashmore PM, et al.: WOCN Society position paper: Avoidable versus unavoidable pressure ulcers/injuries, *Jour of Wound Ostomy Continence Nursing* 44(5):458–468, 2017.

Sibbald R, Krasner D, Lutz J, et al.: SCALE: skin changes at life's end: final consensus statement, *Adv Skin Wound Care* 23(5):225–236, 2009.

Skin Cancer Foundation: *Skin cancer facts & statistics* (website), 2021. https://www.skincancer.org/. Accessed March 2021.

Spilsbury K, Nelson A, Cullum N, et al.: Pressure ulcers and their treatment and effects on quality of life: hospital inpatient perspectives, *J Adv Nurs* 57:494–504, 2007.

Tiggelen H, LeBlanc K, Campbell K, et al.: Standardizing the classification system of skin tears: validity and reliability of the International Skin Advisory Panel Classification system in 44 countries, *Br J Dermatol* 183(1):146–154, 2020.

Walia G, Wong A, Lo A, et al.: Efficacy of monitoring devices in support of prevention of pressure injuries: systematic review and meta-analysis, *Adv Skin Wound Care* 29:568–574, 2016.

Westby M, Dunville J, Soares M, et al. *Dressings and topical agents for treating pressure ulcers* (website), 2017. http://www.cochrane.org/CD011947/WOUNDS_which-dressings-or-topical-agents-are-most-effective-healing-pressure-ulcers. Accessed June 2021.

Nutritional Health

Theris A. Touhy

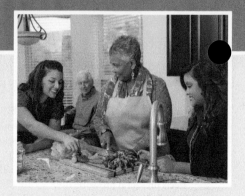

http://evolve.elsevier.com/Touhy/TwdHlthAging

A STUDENT SPEAKS

I work as a certified nursing assistant in a skilled nursing facility, and I am responsible for feeding 10 residents at the dinner meal. I try to get them to eat, but they eat very slowly, and we only have a limited amount of time. Sometimes I end up just mixing the food and getting them to take a few spoonfuls. The people with dementia need even more time, and I know that they are not getting enough to eat. It makes me feel terrible; we need so much more help to do a good job.

Marcia, age 21

AN OLDER ADULT SPEAKS

If I do reach the point where I can no longer feed myself, I hope that the hands holding my fork belong to someone who has a feeling for who I am. I hope my helper will remember what she learns about me and that her awareness of me will grow from one encounter to another. Why should this make a difference? Yet I am certain that my experience of needing to be fed will be altered if it occurs in the context of my being truly known . . . I will want to know about the lives of the people I rely on, especially the one who holds my fork for me. If she would talk to me, if we could laugh together, I might even forget the chagrin of my useless hands. We would have a conversation, rather than a feeding.

From Lustbader W: Thoughts on the meaning of frailty, Generations 13:21–22, 1999.

LEARNING OBJECTIVES

On completion of this chapter, the reader will be able to:

1. Discuss nutritional requirements and factors affecting nutrition for older adults.
2. Delineate risk factors for undernutrition and identify strategies for prevention and management.
3. Describe a nutritional screening and comprehensive evaluation.
4. Use clinical judgment to identify and evaluate solutions and nursing actions to promote adequate nutrition for older adults.
5. Use clinical judgment to recognize and analyze cues and identify and evaluate solutions and nursing actions for older adults with dysphagia.

NUTRITIONAL HEALTH

Adequate and affordable food supplies and improved nutrition are concerns worldwide, with some differences between developed and developing countries. Although issues vary among different areas of the globe, nutrition as a major contributor to health is a significant concern for all nations. The link between healthy eating patterns and healthy aging is well documented. The quality and quantity of diet are important factors in preventing, delaying the onset of, and managing chronic illnesses associated with aging. About half of all American adults have one or more preventable diet-related chronic diseases, including cardiovascular disease, type

2 diabetes, overweight and obesity, and certain cancers (National Center for Chronic Disease Prevention and Health Promotion, 2021) Adoption of healthful eating patterns and exercise has been shown to improve markers of age-associated diseases and reduce biological aging (Gerontological Society of America, 2021).

Proper nutrition means that all of the essential nutrients (i.e., carbohydrates, fat, protein, vitamins, minerals, and water) are adequately supplied and used to maintain optimal health and wellness. Although some age-related changes in the gastrointestinal (GI) system do occur (Box 15.1), these changes are rarely the primary factors in inadequate nutrition. Fulfillment of nutritional needs in older adults is more often affected by numerous other

BOX 15.1   Age-Related Changes Affecting Nutrition

Taste

Individuals have varied levels of taste sensitivity that seem predetermined by genetics, constitution, and age variations

The number of taste cells decreases, and the remaining cells atrophy as individuals age (beginning at age 40 to 60), but they can regenerate. Lag time in regeneration may contribute to diminished taste response

Mouth produces less saliva, which can affect sense of taste

Usually salty and sweet tastes lost first, followed by bitter and sour

Dentures, smoking, and medications can affect taste

Smell

Gradual decline in number of sensor cells that detect aromas, in nerves that carry signals to the brain, and in olfactory bulb that processes them; less mucus produced in nose

Increase in odor threshold and decline in odor identification

Many factors affect smell: nasal sinus disease, injury to olfactory receptors through viral infections, damage from industrial work before proper safety standards and equipment in place, smoking, medications, periodontal disease or dental problems

Changes in smell associated with Alzheimer's and Parkinson's diseases

Smelling food while it is cooking and participation in preparation can stimulate appetite

Digestive System

Changes do not significantly affect function; digestive system remains adequate throughout life

Decreased gastric motility and volume and reductions in secretion of bicarbonate and gastric mucus caused by age-related gastric atrophy, which results in hypochlorhydria (insufficient hydrochloric acid)

Decreased production of intrinsic factor can lead to pernicious anemia if stomach is not able to use ingested B12 vitamins

Protective alkaline viscous mucus of stomach lost because of increase in stomach pH, making stomach more susceptible to Helicobacter pylori infection and peptic ulcer disease, particularly with use of nonsteroidal antiinflammatory drugs (NSAIDs)

Presbyesophagus (decrease in intensity of propulsive waves) may occur, forcing the lower end to dilate, and may lead to digestive discomfort

Pathological processes seen with increasing frequency include gastroesophageal reflux disease (GERD) and hiatal hernia

Loss of smooth muscle in stomach delays emptying time, which may lead to anorexia or weight loss because of distention, meal-induced fullness, and premature satiety

Buccal Cavity

Teeth become worn, darker in color, prone to longitudinal cracks

Dentin becomes brittle and thick; pulp space decreases

Osteopenia of the facial bones and subtle changes to the connective tissues of the skin, sinuses, and oral cavity

Xerostomia (dry mouth) occurs in 30% of older individuals and can affect eating, swallowing, and speaking and lead to dental decay. More than 500 medications can affect salivary flow; artificial saliva preparations and adequate fluid intake can help

Regulation of Appetite

Appetite depends on physical activity, functional limitations, smell, taste, mood, socialization, comfort, medications, chronic illness, oral or dental problems

Individuals may be less hungry, fuller before meals, consume smaller meals, become more satiated following meal

Gastrointestinal hormones such as cholecystokinin (CCK) regulate satiety to varying degrees. With age, CCK is increased basally and following a meal and may have a more potent satiating effect. Disease states increase cytokine levels as a result of release by diseased tissues. Increase in CCK levels also occurs in malnutrition, which further decreases appetite

Endogenous opioid feeding and drinking drive may decline and contribute to decreased appetite and dehydration

Decreased stomach fundal compliance, decreased testosterone, and increased leptin and amylin also thought to contribute to decreased appetite

Ability to feed self or staff feeding techniques and mealtime ambience also affect appetite

Body Composition

Increase in body fat, including visceral fat stores

Decrease in muscle mass

Body weight usually peaks fifth or sixth decade of life and remains stable until age 65 or 70, after which there is a slow decrease in body weight for remainder of life

---

factors, including chronic disease, lifelong eating habits, ethnicity, socialization, income, transportation, housing, mood, food knowledge, functional impairments, health, and dentition.

This chapter discusses the dietary needs of older adults; the risk factors contributing to inadequate nutrition; and the effects of obesity, diseases, functional and cognitive impairments, and dysphagia on nutrition. Several conditions warrant further discussion because they are frequently encountered in older adults and are related to adequate diet and nutritional status. Dehydration and oral health are discussed in Chapter 16, and the effect of neurocognitive disorders on nutrition is discussed in Chapter 26. Readers are referred to a nutrition text for more comprehensive information on nutrition and aging and disease.

AGE-RELATED NUTRITIONAL REQUIREMENTS

United States Dietary Guidelines

The *Dietary Guidelines for Americans, 2020–2025*, published by the federal government, are designed to help individuals from infants to older adults and their families consume a healthy, nutritionally adequate diet. The Guidelines are used in developing federal food, nutrition, and health programs and policies. Eating patterns and their food and nutrient characteristics are a focus of the newest Guideline. Five overarching Guidelines are provided that encourage healthy eating patterns, recognize that individuals will need to make shifts in their food and beverage choices to achieve a healthy pattern, and acknowledge that all segments of our society have a role to play in supporting healthy choices.

The Guidelines provide an adaptable framework in which individuals can enjoy foods that meet their personal, cultural, and traditional preferences and fit within their budget (Box 15.2) (US Department of Agriculture & US Department of Health and Human Services, 2020). *Healthy People 2030* also provides goals and objectives for nutrition. The overall goal is to promote health and reduce chronic disease risk through the consumption of healthful diets and achievement and maintenance of healthy body weights (see Healthy People 2030).

HEALTHY PEOPLE 2030

Nutrition and Weight Status

- Reduce household food insecurity and hunger
- Reduce the proportion of adults with obesity
- Increase the proportion of adults who are at a healthy weight
- Increase the proportion of physician office visits made by adult patients who are obese that include counseling or education related to weight reduction, nutrition, or physical activity.
- Increase the proportion of primary care physicians who regularly measure the body mass index of their patients
- Reduce cholesterol in adults
- Increase the proportion of eligible people completing Centers for Disease Control and Prevention (CDC)–recognized type 2 diabetes prevention programs

Data from US Department of Health and Human Services: *Healthy people 2030* (website), 2020. https://health.gov/healthypeople.

MyPlate for Older Adults

Choose MyPlate is a visual depiction of daily food intake. The US Department of Agriculture (USDA) Human Nutrition Research Center on Aging at Tufts University provides a *MyPlate for Older Adults* emphasizing the nutritional needs of older adults in a framework based on the *Dietary Guidelines for Americans* (Fig. 15.1). The *MyPlate for Older Adults* depicts a colorful plate composed of approximately 50% fruits and vegetables; 25% grains, many of which are whole grains; and 25% protein-rich foods such as nuts, beans, fish, lean meat, poultry, and fat-free and low-fat dairy products such as milk, cheeses, and yogurts. Images of good sources of fluids, heart-healthy fats such as vegetable oils and soft margarines, and herbs and spices to be used in place of salt to lower sodium intake are also included.

Generally, older adults have lower energy requirements and need fewer calories because they may not be as active and metabolic rates decline. However, they still require the same or higher levels of nutrients for optimal health outcomes. The recommendations may need modification for individuals who have illnesses.

The Dietary Approaches to Stop Hypertension (DASH) eating plan is a recommended eating plan to assist with maintenance of optimal weight and management of hypertension (Fu et al., 2020). This plan consists of fruits, vegetables, whole grains, low-fat dairy products, poultry, fish, and restriction of salt intake. The Mediterranean diet (MedDiet) also has been

associated both with a lower incidence of chronic illness, weight gain, and impaired physical function and with improved cognition. This diet is characterized by a greater intake of fruits, vegetables, legumes, whole grains, and fish; a lower intake of red and processed meats; higher amounts of monosaturated fats, mostly provided by olive oil from Mediterranean countries; and lower amounts of saturated fats. The MIND (Mediterranean-DASH Intervention for Neurodegeneration Delay) combines the Med-Diet and the DASH diet. In a large representative sample of older adults, greater adherence to the MedDiet and the MIND diet was independently associated with better cognitive function and lower risk of cognitive impairment. Further research and clinical trials are needed to understand the role of dietary patterns in cognitive aging and brain disease (McEvoy et al., 2017).

Other Dietary Recommendations

Fats

Similar to other age groups, older adults should limit intake of saturated fat and trans fatty acids. High-fat diets cause obesity and increase the risk of heart disease and cancer. Less than 10% of calories per day should come from saturated fats.

Protein

The current protein reference nutrient intake (RNI) is 0.8 g protein/kg body weight in healthy adults of all ages. Many older adults fail to consume enough protein. An uneven or skewed protein intake pattern is also common in the United States, with adults typically ingesting the most protein at the evening meal and the least amount at breakfast. Inadequate protein intake along with skewed protein distribution among meals has been associated with reduced muscle protein synthesis, muscle mass, strength, and physical or functional performance.

Energy-protein deficiencies can cause a reduction in production of T cells and reduced innate and adaptive immunity, increasing the risk for infection (Bilder, 2016). In a recent study, older adults with higher protein intake had higher bone mineral density at the hip, whole body, and lumbar spine, and a lower risk of vertebral fracture (Weaver et al., 2021). A per-meal high-quality protein intake of 20 to 35 g has been suggested to improve protein syntheses needed for muscle protein repair and maintenance.

MyPlate for Older Adults

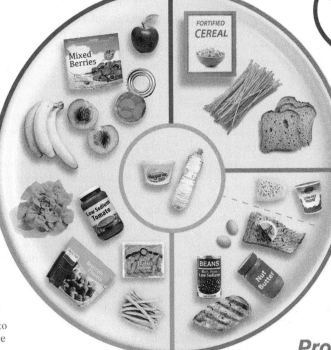

Fruits & Vegetables

Whole fruits and vegetables are rich in important nutrients and fiber. Choose fruits and vegetables with deeply colored flesh. Choose canned varieties that are packed in their own juices or low-sodium.

Healthy Oils

Liquid vegetable oils and soft margarines provide important fatty acids and some fat-soluble vitamins.

Herbs & Spices

Use a variety of herbs and spices to enhance flavor of foods and reduce the need to add salt.

Fluids

Drink plenty of fluids. Fluids can come from water, tea, coffee, soups, and fruits and vegetables.

Grains

Whole grain and fortified foods are good sources of fiber and B vitamins.

Dairy

Fat-free and low-fat milk, cheeses and yogurts provide protein, calcium and other important nutrients.

Protein

Protein rich foods provide many important nutrients. Choose a variety including nuts, beans, fish, lean meat and poultry.

Remember to Stay Active!

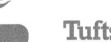

Fig. 15.1 MyPlate for Older Adults. (From Jean Mayer USDA Human Nutrition Research Center on Aging, Tufts University: *MyPlate for older adults*, Boston, 2020, Author. http://hnrca.tufts.edu/myplate/.

Intakes above the RNI of certain nutrients, such as protein, vitamin D, antioxidants, vitamin E, and selenium, are associated with beneficial effects on physical function and prevention of chronic diseases in older age. Older adults who are ill are the most likely segment of society to experience protein deficiency. Those with limitations affecting their ability to shop, cook, and consume food are also at risk for protein deficiency and malnutrition. In a study conducted by Gropper et al. (2020), protein intake differed among ethnic or racial groups, but all groups studied were below recommendations for protein intake (see Research Highlights).

Fiber

Fiber is an important dietary component that some older adults may not consume in sufficient quantities. Fiber is the indigestible material that gives plants their structure. It is abundant in raw fruits and vegetables and in unrefined grains and cereals. A daily intake of 25 g of fiber is recommended and must be combined with adequate amounts of fluid. Insufficient amounts of fiber in the diet, and insufficient fluids, contribute to constipation.

Vitamins and Minerals

Older adults who consume five servings of fruits and vegetables daily will obtain adequate intake of vitamins A, C, and E and potassium. However, Americans of all ages eat less than half of the recommended amounts of fruits and vegetables. Vitamin B_{12} plays a key role in antiaging, but 50% of adults over the age of 50 years are deficient. Vitamin B_{12} deficiency is a common and underrecognized condition. After age 50, the stomach produces less gastric acid, which makes vitamin B_{12} absorption less efficient. Older adults should increase their intake of the crystalline form of vitamin B_{12} from fortified foods such as whole-grain breakfast cereals. Other food sources include salmon, tuna,

⚡ RESEARCH HIGHLIGHTS

Increasing Protein Intake to Help Older Adults Increase Muscle Strength and Function: A Pilot, One-Arm Investigation Using Coaching and a Per-Meal Protein Prescription

Purpose

To evaluate the effects of nutrition education, diet coaching, and a protein prescription, and their association with muscle strength and function.

Method

Twenty White, non-Hispanic older adults received 10 weeks of telephone-based diet coaching, nutrition education, and a per-meal prescription on protein intake. Protein and energy intakes, weight, grip strength, 5-second chair rise, timed up and go (TUG) test, and 3-meter walk tests at baseline and 10 weeks.

Results

Participants had the lowest intake of protein at breakfast and the highest at dinner. The per-meal protein prescription and coaching helped participants identify protein-rich foods that could be consumed at breakfast and lunch to improve protein intake. Pre to 10-week post values significantly improved for protein intake/kg body weight, protein intake/meal, grip strength, and times for TUG, 3-meter walk, and chair rise test.

Conclusion

Given the positive findings of this pilot study, additional studies including a larger, more diverse group of participants and provision of a control group are needed to investigate the effectiveness of this approach and its effects on protein intake, muscle strength, and function.

Data from Gropper S, Exantus M, Jackson K, et al: Increasing protein intake to help older adults increase muscle strength and function: a pilot, single-arm investigation using coaching and a per-meal protein prescription, *J Aging Res & Lifestyle* 9:9–13, 2020.

grass-fed beef, sardines, eggs, and cottage cheese. Individuals who take proton pump inhibitors (e.g., Prilosec, Prevacid) show increased risk of vitamin B_{12} deficiency when these medications are taken for 2 years. Individuals consuming a vegetarian diet and those with some form of weight loss surgery are also more likely to be low in the vitamin.

OBESITY (OVERNUTRITION)

Most of the world's population live in countries where overweight and obesity kills more people than underweight. Every country, except for those in sub-Saharan Africa, faces alarming obesity rates that have risen 82% since 2000. More than two-thirds of individuals ages 65 and older are obese or overweight in the United States, with a higher prevalence in women than men (Balasubramanian et al., 2021). Since the 1990s, the prevalence of older adults who are obese has doubled. Overweight and obesity are associated with increased health care costs, functional impairments, disability, chronic disease, and nursing home admission. Obesity is a major risk factor for the most common disabling conditions: osteoarthritis, atherosclerosis, diabetes, and stroke (Batsis, 2019).

The World Health Organization (WHO, 2020) defines overweight and obesity as follows: overweight is a body mass index (BMI) greater than or equal to 25; obesity is a BMI greater than or equal to 30. However, there is no consensus about the best way to measure obesity in the older population. Normal changes in body composition may make BMI less accurate. Fat mass increases with age, and lean mass decreases; BMI underestimates total adiposity. In addition, most older adults also decline in height, resulting in overall overestimation of obesity.

Although there is strong evidence that obesity in younger people decreases life expectancy and has a negative effect on functionality and morbidity, less is known about the benefits and risks of obesity in older adults compared to children and adults. Older adults who are overweight or obese do not have the same risk of morbidity and mortality as younger individuals, particularly if obesity develops late in life. Maintaining a healthy weight throughout life can prevent many illnesses and functional limitations as a person grows older.

In what has been termed the *obesity paradox,* some research has found that for people who have survived to 70 years of age, mortality risk is lowest in those with a BMI classified as overweight (Kalish, 2016). Higher BMI is associated with an increased risk for osteoarthritis, diabetes, and disability, but when weight gain occurs in late life, there is less time to impose metabolic and cardiovascular health risks. Obesity may protect against bone density loss and hip fracture, and for older adults who are frail with severely decreased functional status, obesity may be regarded as a protective factor with regard to functionality and mortality.

Further research is needed to understand how long-term intentional weight loss and associated shifts in body composition affect the onset of chronic disease (Bowman et al., 2017). Weight loss recommendations for older adults should be carefully considered on an individualized basis with attention to the weight history and medical conditions. A critical goal is to maintain or increase quality of life and physical function. Since weight loss is accompanied by a decline in free fat mass, activities to maintain muscle strength, such as progressive resistance training, should be included in all weight loss plans for older adults.

MALNUTRITION (UNDERNUTRITION)

Malnutrition is a recognized geriatric syndrome. The most common definition of malnutrition is too little or too much energy, protein, and nutrients, which can cause adverse effects on a person's body and its function and clinical outcomes. Malnutrition happens when a person has an imbalance between the nutrients needed and those received, and can result from both overnutrition and undernutrition. The rising incidence of malnutrition among older adults has been documented in acute care, long-term care, and the community.

Malnutrition among hospitalized individuals is estimated to affect as many as 1 in 2 patients at admission, wheras many others develop malnutrition throughout hospitalization (Avelino-Silva & Jaluul, 2017). Up to 50% of older adult patients are malnourished when discharged from the hospital. Malnutrition is estimated to occur in up to 15% of community-dwelling older adults, 20% to 60% of hospitalized older adults,

BOX 15.4 Diagnostic Characteristics for Malnutrition

Two of the following characteristics must be present:
- Insufficient energy intake
- Weight loss
- Loss of muscle mass
- Loss of subcutaneous fat
- Localized or generalized fluid accumulation that may mask weight loss
- Diminished functional status as measured by handgrip strength

From Munoz N, Posthauer M, Cereda D, et al: The role of nutrition for pressure injury prevention and healing: The 2019 International Practice Guidelines Recommendations, *Adv Skin Wound Care* 33(3):123–136, 2020.

BOX 15.5 Risk Factors for Malnutrition

- Chronic diseases
- Acute illness or trauma
- Polypharmacy
- Overly restrictive diets
- Poor dentition
- Dysphagia
- Poor functional status; inability to prepare food
- Depression
- Altered mental status or dementia
- Social isolation and limited social supports
- Lack of transportation to purchase food
- Socioeconomic deprivation

and 30% to 85% of those living in nursing homes. These figures are expected to rise dramatically in the next 30 years with the aging of the population. Those at greatest risk are older women, minorities, and people who are poor or live in rural areas. Being 75 years of age and older is an independent risk factor for poor nutrition (Crogan, 2017; Tilly, 2017). Malnutrition among older adults is clearly a serious challenge for health professionals in all settings.

Characteristics

The understanding of malnutrition is evolving, and research is ongoing. No single marker has been identified to diagnose adult malnutrition of any etiology. Characteristics have been identified to determine malnutrition (Box 15.4). Malnutrition is a complex syndrome that can develop following two primary trajectories. It can occur when the individual does not consume sufficient amounts of micronutrients (i.e., vitamins, minerals, phytochemicals) and macronutrients (i.e., protein, carbohydrates, fat, water) required to maintain organ function and healthy tissues. This type of malnutrition can occur from prolonged undernutrition or overnutrition. In contrast, inflammation-related malnutrition develops because of injury, surgery, or disease states that trigger inflammatory mediators that contribute to increased metabolic rate and impaired nutrient use (Cederholm et al., 2019).

Inflammation is increasingly identified as an important underlying factor that increases risk for malnutrition and a contributing factor to suboptimal responses to nutritional intervention and increased risk for mortality. Weight loss frequently occurs in both trajectories, but weight alone is not an indicator of nutritional status. Individuals also experience malnutrition when they take in enough calories but miss important nutrients that affect their nutritional status (Tilly, 2017). Development of a consensus approach to identifying core attributes of malnutrition that consider ethnic or racial differences, and the presence of malnutrition among obese individuals, is important.

Consequences

Malnutrition is a precursor to frailty and has serious consequences, including infections, pressure injuries, anemia, hypotension, impaired cognition, sarcopenia (low muscle mass associated with aging) (Chapter 28), hip fractures, prolonged hospital stay, institutionalization, increased dependence, reduced quality of life, and increased morbidity and mortality (Tilly, 2017). Malnourished patients are twice as likely to develop pressure injuries and three times as likely to have infections. Almost half of the patients who fall during hospitalization are reported to be malnourished. There is an increased risk of nosocomial infections as a result of undernutrition, unintentional weight loss, and low serum albumin levels (Bilder, 2016). Finally, older adults who are admitted to the hospital with malnutrition are more likely to have longer hospital stays and die before discharge (Avelino-Silva & Jaluul, 2017). Many factors contribute to the occurrence of malnutrition in older adults (Box 15.5).

FACTORS AFFECTING FULFILLMENT OF NUTRITIONAL NEEDS

Lifelong Eating Habits

The nutritional state of a person reflects the individual's dietary history and present food practices. "Foodways are defined as the eating habits and culinary practices of a people, region, or historical period" (Furman, 2014, p. 80). This includes unique eating patterns of various cultural and religious groups. Foodways influence food preferences, meal expectation, and nutritional intake. Eating habits do not always coincide with fulfillment of nutritional needs and especially may affect the ability and desire to consume food that is not consistent with individual foodways. The meaning of food and mealtimes, often established in childhood, "become more poignant with age" (Furman, 2014, p. 83). It is important to understand cultural and religious beliefs and accustomed foodways (Box 15.6).

Lifelong habits of dieting or eating fad foods also echo through the later years. Individuals may fall prey to advertisements that claim specific foods can reverse aging or rid one of chronic conditions. Following the MyPlate for Older Adults (see Fig. 15.1) is best for an ideal diet, with changes based on particular problems, such as hypercholesteremia. Individuals should be counseled to base their dietary decisions on valid research and consultation with their primary care provider. For the healthy individual, essential nutrients should be obtained from food sources rather than relying on dietary supplements.

Socialization

The fundamentally social aspect of eating has to do with sharing and the feeling of belonging that it provides. All of us use food as a means of giving and receiving love, friendship, or belonging. The presence of others during meals is a significant predictor of caloric intake. The meaning and enjoyment of eating often can be challenged as one ages; requires hospitalization or nursing home residence; or experiences chronic illnesses, depression, isolation, and functional limitations. Disinterest in food also may result from the effects of medication or disease processes. Misuse and abuse of alcohol are prevalent among older adults and are growing public health concerns. Excessive drinking interferes with nutrition. Drinking alcohol depletes the body of necessary nutrients and often replaces meals, thus making an individual susceptible to malnutrition (Chapter 30).

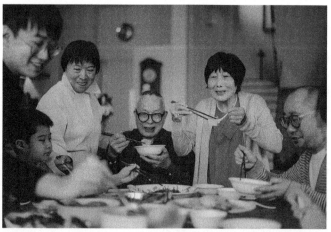

Enjoying a meal together. (© iStock.com/monkeybusinessimages.)

The elderly nutrition program, authorized under Title III of the Older Americans Act (OAA), is the largest national food and nutrition program specifically for older adults. Programs and services include congregate nutrition programs, home-delivered nutrition services (Meals on Wheels), and nutrition screening and education. The program is not means tested, and participants may make voluntary confidential contributions for meals. The OAA does require targeting services to those in greatest social and economic need. A large percentage of program participants are likely to be socioeconomically deprived, minorities, living alone, and individuals experiencing disability or poor health.

Facilitators of good nutrition in these types of programs include adherence to traditional (culturally appropriate) diet and peer networks. Home-delivered meals have been shown to be most effective in improving nutrition and other outcomes for older adults (Tilly, 2017). Increased attention should be given to providing meals that include traditional foods and evaluating the effectiveness of these kinds of programs on nutritional health. With the emphasis on community-based care rather than institutional care, expansion of nutrition services should be a priority (Chapter 6).

Socioeconomic Deprivation

There is a strong relationship between poor nutrition and socioeconomic deprivation. Older adults are the fastest-growing food-insecure population in the United States, which means they are not sure where or how they will get their next meal. In 2018, according to the most recent report issued in 2020, 7.3% of all senior households were food insecure (Feeding America, 2020). Older adults are likely to be food insecure if they live in a southern state, have a disability, are younger than 69 years, live with a grandchild, and/or are African American or Hispanic (National Council on Aging, 2018).

Individuals with low incomes may need to choose among fulfilling needs such as food, heat, telephone bills, medications, and health care visits. Some older people eat only once per day in an attempt to make their income last through the month. The COVID-19 pandemic has had a large effect on food insecurity for individuals of all ages.

The Supplemental Nutrition Assistance Program (SNAP), a program of the USDA, Food and Nutrition Services, offers nutrition assistance to eligible, socioeconomically deprived individuals and families, but older adults are less likely than any other age group to use food assistance programs. Three in five older adults who qualify for SNAP do not participate. Some individuals may not see the benefit, and others, especially those who lived through the Great Depression, are very reluctant to accept "welfare." Low participation rates are also a result of barriers related to mobility and technology.

To enhance outreach to older adults, SNAP works with state agencies, nutrition educators, and neighborhood and faith-based organizations to assist those eligible for nutrition assistance to make informed decisions about applying for the program and accessing benefits. The Seniors Farmers' Market Nutrition Program, federally funded by the Farm Bill, provides low-income seniors with access to locally grown fruits, vegetables, honey, and herbs. In addition, the program goals include increasing the domestic consumption of agricultural commodities through farmers' markets, roadside stands, and community-supported agricultural programs (National Council on Aging, 2021). The National Council on Aging's (NCOA) Benefits Checkup (see Box 15.3) is a free online service to screen seniors with limited incomes for benefits.

Transportation

Available and easily accessible transportation may be limited for older adults. Many small, long-standing neighborhood food stores have been closed in the wake of the expansion of larger supermarkets, which are located in areas that serve a greater segment of the population. Small convenience stores may not have a selection of healthy foods. It may become difficult to walk to the market, to reach it by public transportation, or to carry a bag of groceries while using a cane or walker. Fear is apparent in older adults' consideration of transportation. They may fear walking in the street and being mugged, not being able to cross the street in the time it takes the traffic light to change, or being knocked down or falling as they walk in crowded streets. Despite reduced senior citizen bus fares, many older adults remain very fearful of attack when using public transportation. Functional impairments also make the use of public transportation difficult for others.

Transportation by taxicab or other transportation services may be unrealistic for an individual on a limited income, but sharing a taxicab with others who also need to shop may enable the older adult to go where food prices are cheaper and to take advantage of sale items. Senior citizen organizations in many parts of the United States have been helpful in providing older adults with van service to shopping areas. In housing complexes, it may be possible to schedule group trips to the supermarket. Many urban communities have multiple sources of transportation available, but the individual may be unaware of them. Resources in rural areas are more limited. It is important for nurses to be knowledgeable about transportation resources in the community.

In addition, many older adults may have difficulty shopping and preparing meals. Often individuals have to rely on others to shop for them, and this may be a cause of concern depending on the availability of support and the reluctance to be dependent on someone else, particularly family. For those who own a computer, shopping over the internet and having groceries delivered offers advantages, although prices may be higher than those in the stores.

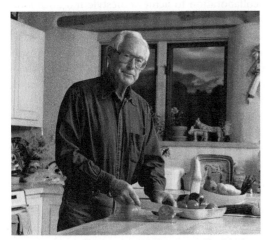

An older man preparing a meal. (Courtesy Corbis Images.)

Chronic Diseases and Conditions

Many chronic diseases and their sequelae pose nutritional challenges for older adults. Heart failure and chronic obstructive pulmonary disease (COPD) are associated with fatigue, increased energy expenditure, and decreased appetite. Dietary interventions for diabetes are essential but also may affect customary eating patterns and require lifestyle changes. Conditions of the teeth and dental problems also affect nutrition (Chapter 16). Functional and cognitive impairments associated with chronic disease interfere with the individual's ability to shop, cook, and eat independently. More detailed information on chronic illness can be found in Chapters 22–28.

The side effects of medications prescribed for chronic conditions may further impair nutritional status. There are clinically significant drug-nutrient interactions that result in nutrient loss, and evidence is accumulating that shows that the use of nutritional supplements may counteract these possible drug-induced nutrient depletions. A thorough medication review is an essential component of nutritional evaluation, and individuals should receive education about the effects of prescription medications, and herbals and supplements, on nutritional status (Chapter 11).

Gastrointestinal Conditions That Affect Nutrition

Although several physiological and functional changes in the gut are associated with aging, the majority of GI problems result from extrinsic factors. Polypharmacy; high-fat, high-volume meals; inactivity; and comorbid conditions are all aggravating factors. Some conditions that often affect nutritional intake—gastroesophageal reflux disease (GERD), diverticular disease, and dysphagia—are also discussed here.

Gastroesophageal reflux disease. GERD is a syndrome defined as mucosal damage from the movement of gastric contents backward from the stomach into the esophagus. It is the most common GI disorder affecting older adults. The majority of GERD is caused by abnormalities of the lower esophageal sphincter (LES). When this muscle relaxes and allows reflux or is generally weak, GERD may occur. Risk factors include hiatal hernia, obesity, pregnancy, cigarette smoking, or inhaling secondhand smoke. People of all ages can develop GERD, some for unknown reasons. GERD is diagnosed empirically based on history and response to treatment. When the symptoms do not resolve with standard treatment, an endoscopy is indicated (Iannetti, 2017).

Recognizing and analyzing cues: GERD. Although complaints of simple "heartburn" are often from dyspepsia, when other signs and symptoms are added it is a greater concern. The classic complaints indicative of GERD are heartburn plus regurgitation—a sensation of burning in the throat as partially digested food and stomach acid inappropriately return to the posterior oropharynx. Older adults more commonly have more atypical symptoms of persistent cough, exacerbations of asthma, laryngitis, and intermittent chest pain. Abdominal pain may occur within 1 hour of eating, and symptoms are worse when lying down with the added pressure of gravity on the LES.

Consumption of alcohol before or during eating exacerbates the reflux. Persistent symptoms of GERD may lead to esophagitis, peptic strictures, esophageal ulcers (with bleeding), and, most importantly, Barrett's esophagus, a precursor to cancer. The most serious complication is the development of pneumonia from the aspiration of stomach contents. Dental caries also may be caused by chronic exposure to gastric acids.

Solutions, nursing actions, and outcomes: GERD. The management of GERD combines lifestyle changes with pharmacological preparations, used in a stepwise fashion. Lifestyle modifications include eating smaller meals; stopping eating 3 to 4 hours before bed; avoiding high-fat foods, alcohol, caffeine, and nicotine; and sleeping with the head of the bed elevated. Weight reduction and smoking cessation are helpful. These strategies alone may control the majority of symptoms when complications are not present. Pharmacological preparations begin with over-the-counter antacids, such as Tums and Rolaids; progress to H2 blockers, such as ranitidine (Zantac); and then move to proton pump inhibitors, such as lansoprazole (Prevacid). In severe cases of GERD, surgical tightening of the LES may be necessary. The nurse works with the older adult to identify situations that aggravate GERD symptoms (e.g., overeating, consuming alcohol at mealtime) and develop strategies to best deal with them. The nurse also provides education regarding the alarm signs of GERD that should receive prompt evaluation by a health care provider (Box 15.7).

Diverticular disease. Diverticula are small herniations or saclike outpouchings of mucosa that extend through the muscle layers of the colon wall, almost exclusive of the sigmoid colon. They form at weak points in the colon wall, usually where arteries penetrate and provide nutrients to the mucosal layer. Usually less than 1 cm in diameter, diverticula have thin, compressible walls if empty or firm walls if full of fecal matter. Although the exact etiology of diverticular disease is unknown, it is thought to be related to a low-fiber diet, especially one accompanied by increased intraabdominal pressure and chronic constipation.

The prevalence of diverticular disease increases with age. Smoking and obesity have been linked to diverticulitis, and physical activity is associated with a decreased risk. The risk factors for diverticular disease can be found in Box 15.8. Diverticulitis is an acute inflammatory complication of diverticulosis.

Recognizing and analyzing cues: Diverticular disease. Most persons with diverticulosis are completely asymptomatic, and the condition is found only when a colonoscopy or computed tomography (CT) scan is performed for some other reason. Persons with uncomplicated diverticulitis complain of abdominal pain, especially in the left lower quadrant, and may have a fever

and elevated white blood cell count, although the latter symptoms may be delayed or absent in the older adult. The physical assessment may be completely negative. Rectal bleeding is typically acute in onset, is painless, and stops spontaneously.

The complications of diverticulitis are rupture, abscess, stricture, or fistula. With any perforation, peritonitis is likely. Individuals with these complications may have an elevated pulse rate or are hypotensive; however, in the older adult, unexplained lethargy or confusion may be seen also or instead. A mass in the left lower quadrant may be palpated. Complicated diverticulitis is always considered an emergency and requires hospitalization for treatment and possible surgical repair.

Solutions, nursing actions, and outcomes: Diverticular disease. For individuals with diverticulosis, the goal is prevention of diverticulitis. High-fiber diets (25 to 30 g/day) have been cited in American, European, and Asian studies as protective against diverticulosis. In addition, individuals should strive for intake of six to eight glasses of fluid per day, preferably with little caffeine. Acute diverticulitis can be quite painful. The nurse works with the individual to find effective and safe comfort strategies that include pain medication and creative nonpharmacological approaches such as massage, hot or cold packs, stretching exercises, relaxation, music, or meditation techniques. Uncomplicated diverticulitis is treated with antibiotics and a clear liquid diet and is usually managed in the outpatient setting.

In the promotion of healthy aging, the nurse works with the older adult to analyze diet, fluid intake, and activity level to ensure adequate motility and minimal pressure within the GI tract. If the person is overweight or obese, weight loss will decrease intraabdominal pressure and decrease the risk for the development of new diverticula. Additional nursing actions include collaboration to achieve lifestyle modifications, provision of education on the appropriate use of medications, warning signs of potential problems, and the best response to the signs or symptoms. When working with an older adult in a cross-cultural setting, it is especially important for the nurse to communicate effectively and incorporate cultural expectations and habits (e.g., diet) into the plan of nursing care.

Dysphagia. Dysphagia, or difficulty swallowing, is a prevalent and growing concern in the older adult population. Swallowing is a complex process, with some 50 pairs of muscles and many nerves working together to receive food into the mouth, prepare it, and move it from mouth to stomach. Normally, swallowing is a rapid and seamless act but involves several phases (Box 15.9). Dysphagia can occur secondary to deficits in any of the phases of swallowing. Any condition that weakens or damages the muscles and nerves used for swallowing may cause dysphagia. Examples of conditions that may cause dysphagia include diseases of the nervous system, such as amyotrophic lateral sclerosis (ALS) and Parkinson's disease.

Stroke or head injury may weaken or affect coordination of the swallowing muscles or limit sensation in the mouth and throat. Cerebrovascular accidents are the leading cause of neurological dysphagia and occurs in 20.7% to 46.3% with stroke (Khalil et al., 2020) (Chapter 23). In addition, cancer of the head, neck, or esophagus may cause swallowing problems. Memory loss and cognitive deficits also may make it difficult to chew or swallow (Box 15.10) (Chapters 25–26).

BOX 15.7 Warning Signs Suggesting Possible GERD Complication

- Anemia
- Anorexia
- Dysphagia
- Hematemesis
- Odynophagia
- Weight loss

GERD, Gastroesophageal reflux disease.

BOX 15.8 Risk Factors for Diverticular Disease

- Family history
- Personal history of gallbladder disease
- Low dietary intake of fiber
- Use of medications that slow fecal transit time
- Chronic constipation
- Obesity

BOX 15.9 Phases of Swallowing

1. Oral preparatory phase: food is chewed, mixed with saliva, and then formed into a softened mass (bolus) between the tongue and palate.
2. Oral transit phase: the bolus is sent posteriorly toward the base of the tongue.
3. Oropharyngeal phase: the bolus arrives at the base of the tongue and triggers the swallow reflex, which is automatic.
4. Pharyngeal phase: the bolus travels down from the base of the tongue past the closed and elevated larynx and to the entrance of the esophagus. This is a continuation of the automatic swallow reflex.
5. Esophageal phase: the esophageal muscle relaxes to allow the bolus into the upper esophagus, from where it is passed downward by waves of muscle contraction through the lower esophageal sphincter and into the stomach.

BOX 15.10 Risk Factors for Dysphagia

- Cerebrovascular accident
- Parkinson's disease
- Neuromuscular disorders (ALS, MS, myasthenia gravis)
- Dementia
- Head and neck cancer
- Traumatic brain injury
- Aspiration pneumonia
- Inadequate feeding technique
- Poor dentition

ALS, Amyotrophic lateral sclerosis; *MS,* multiple sclerosis.

The most common type of dysphagia is otopharyngeal dysphagia (OD). OD is a highly prevalent but largely unrecognized health issue. OD is considered a geriatric syndrome as it is highly prevalent among older adults, caused by multiple factors, is associated with several comorbidities and poor prognosis, and requires a multidimensional approach treatment (Engh & Speyer, 2021). Prevalence is highest in older adults with neurological conditions and increases with advancing age and frailty. Up to 47% of frail older adults hospitalized for acute illness suffer from OD, and it affects more than 50% of nursing home residents. Prevalence among independently living older adults 70 to 79 years old is 16% and in those over 80 years old is 33% Data suggest that there is a large population of community-living and nursing home residents with a certain level of dysphagia at baseline that is worsened with acute illness, hospitalization, and increasing frailty (Finucane, 2017).

Dysphagia is a serious problem and has negative consequences, including severe distress during meals, aspiration with the consequence of chronic bronchial inflammation and aspiration pneumonia, weight loss, reduced food and fluid intake with the consequence of malnutrition and dehydration, and increased risk of death. Aspiration is the most profound and dangerous problem for older adults with stroke who experience dysphagia. "Mortality rate is three times higher in patients who have aspirated than patients who do not aspirate, and there is a vicious cycle among dysphagia, malnutrition, aspiration, and aspiration pneumonia" (Khalil et al., 2020, p. 12).

Recognizing and analyzing cues: Dysphagia. Screening assessment is important and serves to identify those patients with the greatest risk of dysphagia. It is important to obtain a careful history of the older adult's response to dysphagia and to observe the person during mealtime. However, screening and swallowing evaluations are not routinely performed. In addition, nurse's knowledge of dysphagia has been shown to be limited (Artiles et al., 2020; Khalil et al., 2020). Early dysphagia screening and recognition by nurses are considered best practice for acute stroke patients to prevent complications.

Symptoms that alert the nurse to possible swallowing problems are presented in Box 15.11. If dysphagia is suspected, a comprehensive clinical assessment of swallowing and referral to a speech-language pathologist (SLP) are essential. A comprehensive exam includes a clinical swallowing evaluation, comprehensive medical history, physical exam of oral and motor function, and assessment of food intake. Instrumental assessment includes videofluoroscopy swallowing study (VFSS) and fiberoptic endoscopic evaluation of swallowing (FEES). Nothing-by-mouth (NPO) status should be maintained until the swallowing evaluation is completed.

Solutions, nursing actions, and outcomes: Dysphagia. After the swallowing evaluation, a decision must be made about the person's potential for functional improvement of the swallowing disorder and safety in swallowing liquid and solid food. The main goal of dysphagia therapy is to reduce morbidity and mortality associated with chest infections and poor nutritional status. Nurses work closely with speech therapy and the dietitian to implement interventions to prevent aspiration. Compensatory strategies include postural changes, such as chin tucks or head turns while swallowing, and modification of bolus volume, consistency, temperature, and rate of presentation. Diets may be modified in texture from pudding-like to nearly normal–textured

BOX 15.11 Symptoms of Dysphagia or Possible Aspiration

- Difficult, labored swallowing
- Drooling
- Copious oral secretions
- Coughing, choking at meals
- Holding or pocketing of food/medications in the mouth
- Difficulty moving food or liquid from mouth to throat
- Difficulty chewing
- Nasal voice or hoarseness
- Wet or gurgling voice
- Excessive throat clearing
- Food or liquid leaking from the nose
- Prolonged eating time
- Pain with swallowing
- Unusual head or neck posturing while swallowing
- Sensation of something stuck in the throat during swallowing; sensation of a lump in the throat
- Heartburn
- Chest pain
- Hiccups
- Weight loss
- Frequent respiratory tract infections, pneumonia

solids. Liquids may range from spoon-thick, to honey-like, to nectar-like, to thin. Commercial thickeners and thickened products are also available. The evidence is not strong that texture-modified food and thickened liquids reduce the impact of dysphagia. In addition, patients often do not prefer this kind of food, which may reduce nutritional intake.

Neuromuscular electrical stimulation has received clearance by the US Food and Drug Administration for treatment of dysphagia. This therapy involves the administration of small electrical impulses to the swallowing muscles in the throat and is used in combination with traditional swallowing exercises. Research on the appropriate management of swallowing disorders in older adults, particularly during acute illness and in long-term care facilities, is very limited, and additional study is essential.

The development of dysphagia screening tools that are valid in different settings (acute care, long-term care) is important. A protocol for preventing aspiration in older adults with dysphagia, and directions to access a video presentation of dysphagia, can be found in Box 15.3. Suggested nursing actions helpful in preventing aspiration during hand feeding are presented in Box 15.12.

A comprehensive assessment of swallowing problems and other factors that influence intake must be conducted before initiating severely restricted diet modifications or considering the use of feeding tubes, particularly in older adults with end-stage dementia or those at the end of life (Chapter 25). There is little evidence of a reduction in the risk of aspiration pneumonia with tube feeding in any group of adult patients, and in fact, enteral nutrition is generally cited as a risk factor for aspiration pneumonia (Finucane, 2017). However, there may be

---

BOX 15.12 Tips for Best Practice

Preventing Aspiration in Patients With Dysphagia: Hand Feeding

- Provide a 30-minute rest period before meal consumption; a rested person will likely have less difficulty swallowing.
- The person should sit at 90 degrees during all oral (PO) intake.
- Maintain 90-degree positioning for at least 1 hour after PO intake.
- Adjust rate of feeding and size of bites to the person's tolerance; avoid rushed or forced feeding.
- Alternate solid and liquid boluses.
- Have the person swallow twice before the next mouthful.
- Stroke under the chin downward to initiate swallowing.
- Follow the speech therapist's recommendation for safe swallowing techniques and modified food consistency (may need thickened liquids, pureed foods).
- If facial weakness is present, place food on the nonimpaired side of the mouth.
- Avoid sedatives and hypnotics that may impair cough reflex and swallowing ability.
- Keep suction equipment ready at all times.
- Supervise all meals.
- Monitor temperature.
- Observe color of phlegm.
- Visually check the mouth for pocketing of food in cheeks.
- Check for food under dentures.
- Provide mouth care every 4 hours and before and after meals, including denture cleaning.

---

certain circumstances when providing temporary short-term tube feeding may be appropriate (e.g., individuals with stroke and resulting dysphagia and other conditions when it may be possible to resume oral nutrition at some point) (Chapter 26).

USING CLINICAL JUDGMENT TO PROMOTE HEALTHY AGING: NUTRITIONAL HEALTH

The role of nursing in evaluation of nutrition and development of solutions and nursing actions should be comprehensive and include attention to the process of eating, the entire ritual of meals, and the assessment of nutritional status within the interprofessional team. Nurses are often the first to identify patients in need of nutrition intervention and are integral to encouraging nutritional intake from admission to discharge. Comprehensive nutritional screening and assessment are essential in identifying older adults at risk for nutrition problems or who are malnourished. Evaluation of nutritional health can be difficult in the absence of severe malnutrition, and older adults are less likely than younger people to show signs of malnutrition and nutrient malabsorption.

There is no historical, clinical, or laboratory parameter by itself that qualifies as a reliable and valid indicator of nutritional status, thus a comprehensive assessment is essential to reveal deficits. Screening and identification of concerns identified should be conducted within 24 hours of admission and periodically reassessed throughout the stay. Nutrition risk screening using a validated tool such as the Mini-Nutritional Assessment Short-Form (MNA-SF) should be performed routinely and can be incorporated into annual health checks for those ages 75 years and older.

Recognizing and Analyzing Cues

Nutritional screening is the first step in identifying individuals who are at risk for malnutrition or have undetected malnutrition, and it determines the need for a more comprehensive assessment and nutritional interventions. The screening is preliminary and is not to be viewed as a replacement for comprehensive evaluation of the individual. Nutrition screening performed by nurses in the first few hours of hospitalization or admission to a long-term care facility sets the stage for quality care.

There are several screening tools specific to older individuals, and screening can be completed in any setting. The Nutrition Screening Initiative Checklist (Fig. 15.2) can be self-administered or completed by a family member or any member of the health care team. The MNA-SF (Fig. 15.3) provides a simple, quick method of identifying older adults who are at risk of malnutrition. The Self-MNA is a simple tool designed to help older adults determine if they are getting the nutrition they need. The Self-MNA is available in English, Bulgarian, Danish, Finnish, German, Greek, Italian, Portuguese, Spanish, and Swedish (see Box 15.3).

The Minimum Data Set 3.0 (MDS 3.0) (Chapter 9), used in long-term care facilities, is also a useful screening tool for nutritional risk. The MDS does not establish malnutrition but rather is a tool to generate a care plan. The MDS includes information that can be used to identify potential nutritional problems, risk

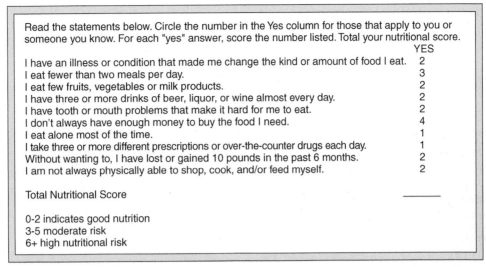

Read the statements below. Circle the number in the Yes column for those that apply to you or someone you know. For each "yes" answer, score the number listed. Total your nutritional score.

	YES
I have an illness or condition that made me change the kind or amount of food I eat.	2
I eat fewer than two meals per day.	3
I eat few fruits, vegetables or milk products.	2
I have three or more drinks of beer, liquor, or wine almost every day.	2
I have tooth or mouth problems that make it hard for me to eat.	2
I don't always have enough money to buy the food I need.	4
I eat alone most of the time.	1
I take three or more different prescriptions or over-the-counter drugs each day.	1
Without wanting to, I have lost or gained 10 pounds in the past 6 months.	2
I am not always physically able to shop, cook, and/or feed myself.	2
Total Nutritional Score	_____

0-2 indicates good nutrition
3-5 moderate risk
6+ high nutritional risk

Fig. 15.2 Nutrition Screening Initiative. (Courtesy The Nutrition Screening Initiative, Washington, DC.)

factors, and the potential for improved function. Triggers for more thorough investigation of problems include weight loss, alterations in taste, medical therapies, prescription medications, hunger, parenteral or intravenous feedings, mechanically altered or therapeutic diets, percentage of food left uneaten, pressure ulcers, and edema.

When risk for malnutrition is detected from screening, a comprehensive assessment is indicated and will provide the most conclusive data about a person's actual nutritional state. Interprofessional approaches are key to appropriate assessment and intervention and should involve medicine; nursing; dietary; physical, occupational, and speech therapy; and social work. The collective results provide the data needed to identify the immediate and the potential nutritional problems so that plans for supervision, assistance, and education in the attainment of adequate nutrition can be implemented. Components of a comprehensive evaluation include interview, history, physical examination, anthropometric data, laboratory data, food and nutrient intake, and functional assessment. A summary is presented in Box 15.13. Explanations of several components are discussed in the following sections.

Food and Nutrient Intake

Frequently, a 24-hour diet recall compared with the MyPlate for Older Adults (see Fig. 15.1) can provide an estimate of nutritional adequacy. When the individual cannot supply all of the requested information, it may be possible to obtain data from a family member or another source such as a shopping receipt. There will be times, however, when information will not be as complete as one would like or when the individual, too proud to admit to not eating, will furnish erroneous information. Even so, the nurse will be able to obtain additional data from the other three areas of the nutritional assessment.

Keeping a dietary record for 3 days is another tool. This can be completed by the individual, family, or caregivers. The diet recall includes what foods were eaten, when food was eaten, and the amounts eaten. Computer analysis of the dietary records provides information on energy and vitamin and mineral intake. Printouts can provide the individual and the health care provider with a visual graph of the intake. Accurate completion of 3-day dietary records in hospitals and long-term care facilities can be problematic, and intake may be either underestimated or overestimated. Standardized observational protocols to evaluate the process of eating meals should be developed to ensure accuracy of oral intake documentation and the adequacy and quality of feeding assistance during mealtimes. Nurses should ensure that direct caregivers are educated on the proper observation and documentation of intake and should closely monitor performance in this area.

Weight and Height Considerations

Weight change (from usual) offers the most useful information on nutritional status, and a detailed weight history should be obtained along with current weight. History should include a history of weight loss, if the weight loss was intentional or unintentional, and during what period it occurred. A history of anorexia is also important, and many older adults, especially women, have limited their weight throughout life. Debate continues in the quest to determine the appropriate weight charts for an older adult. Although weight alone does not indicate the adequacy of diet, unplanned fluctuations in weight are significant and should be evaluated.

Accurate weight patterns are sometimes difficult to obtain in long-term care settings. Procedures for weighing people should be established and followed consistently to obtain an accurate representation of weight changes. Weighing procedure should be supervised by licensed personnel, and changes should be reported immediately to the health care provider. One might meet correct weight values for height, but weight changes may be the result of fluid retention, edema, or ascites and merit investigation. A weight loss of 5% of usual body weight in 6 to 12 months is the most widely accepted definition for clinically important weight loss in older adults. In long-term care facilities, a loss of more than 5% of body weight in 1 month, more than

Mini Nutritional Assessment
MNA®

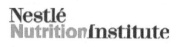

Last name: _____ First name: _____

| Sex: | Age: | Weight, kg: | Height, cm: | Date: |

Complete the screen by filling in the boxes with the appropriate numbers. Total the numbers for the final screening score.

Screening

A Has food intake declined over the past 3 months due to loss of appetite, digestive problems, chewing or swallowing difficulties?

0 = severe decrease in food intake
1 = moderate decrease in food intake
2 = no decrease in food intake ☐

B Weight loss during the last 3 months

0 = weight loss greater than 3 kg (6.6 lbs)
1 = does not know
2 = weight loss between 1 and 3 kg (2.2 and 6.6 lbs)
3 = no weight loss ☐

C Mobility

0 = bed or chair bound
1 = able to get out of bed / chair but does not go out
2 = goes out ☐

D Has suffered psychological stress or acute disease in the past 3 months?

0 = yes   2 = no ☐

E Neuropsychological problems

0 = severe dementia or depression
1 = mild dementia
2 = no psychological problems ☐

F1 Body Mass Index (BMI) (weight in kg) / (height in m)^2

0 = BMI less than 19
1 = BMI 19 to less than 21
2 = BMI 21 to less than 23
3 = BMI 23 or greater ☐

IF BMI IS NOT AVAILABLE, REPLACE QUESTION F1 WITH QUESTION F2.
DO NOT ANSWER QUESTION F2 IF QUESTION F1 IS ALREADY COMPLETED.

F2 Calf circumference (CC) in cm

0 = CC less than 31
3 = CC 31 or greater ☐

Screening score (max. 14 points)

12 - 14 points: Normal nutritional status
8 - 11 points: At risk of malnutrition
0 - 7 points: Malnourished ☐☐

References

1. Vellas B, Villars H, Abellan G, *et al.* Overview of the MNA® - Its History and Challenges. *J Nutr Health Aging.* 2006;**10**:456-465.
2. Rubenstein LZ, Harker JO, Salva A, Guigoz Y, Vellas B. Screening for Undernutrition in Geriatric Practice: Developing the Short-Form Mini Nutritional Assessment (MNA-SF). *J. Geront.* 2001; **56A**: M366-377
3. Guigoz Y. The Mini-Nutritional Assessment (MNA®) Review of the Literature - What does it tell us? *J Nutr Health Aging.* 2006; **10**:466-487.
4. Kaiser MJ, Bauer JM, Ramsch C, et al. Validation of the Mini Nutritional Assessment Short-Form (MNA®-SF): A practical tool for identification of nutritional status. *J Nutr Health Aging.* 2009; **13**:782-788.
® Société des Produits Nestlé, S.A., Vevey, Switzerland, Trademark Owners © Nestlé, 1994, Revision 2009. N67200 12/99 10M
For more information: <u>www.mna-elderly.com</u>

Fig. 15.3 Mini Nutritional Assessment (MNA). (From http://www.mna-elderly.com/forms/mini/mna_mini_english.pdf.)

BOX 15.13   Components of Nutritional Assessment

Dietary History and Current Intake
- Food preferences and habits; meaning and significance of food to the individual; do they eat alone?
- Cultural or religious food habits
- Ability to obtain and prepare food, including adequate finances to obtain nutritious food
- Social activities and normal patterns; meal frequency
- Control over food selection and choices
- Fluid intake
- Alcohol intake
- Special diet
- Vitamins, minerals, and supplement use
- Chewing or swallowing problems
- Functional limitations that impair independence in eating
- Cognitive changes affecting appetite or ability to feed self
- Depression screen if indicated

History and Physical
- Chief complaint, medical history, chronic conditions, presence or absence of inflammation (fever, hypothermia, signs of systemic inflammatory response), usual weight and any loss or gain, fluid retention, loss of muscle or fat, oral health and dentition, medication use

Anthropometric Measurements
- Body mass index
- Height
- Current weight and usual adult weight
- Recent weight changes
- Skinfold measurements

Biochemical Analysis
- Complete blood count
- Protein status
- Lipid profile
- Electrolytes
- Blood urea nitrogen (BUN)–creatinine ratio

Food and Nutrient Intake
- Periods of inadequate intake (nothing-by-mouth [NPO] status)
- 24-hour or 3-day diet record

Functional Assessment
- Hand-grip strength
- Standard functional assessment (Chapter 7)

Adapted from Mathew M, Jacobs M: Malnutrition and feeding problems. In Ham R, Sloane P, Warshaw G, et al, editors: *Primary care geriatrics: a case-based approach*, ed 6, Philadelphia, 2014, Elsevier Saunders, p 318.

7.5% in 3 months, or more than 10% in 6 months is considered a significant indicator of poor nutrition and an MDS trigger.

Height always should be measured and never estimated or given by self-report. If the person cannot stand, an alternative way of measuring standing height is knee-height using special calipers. An alternative to knee-height measurements is a demispan measurement, which is half the total arm span. Measurement of BMI in older adults can be unreliable and does not provide the same clues to health status in older adults as it does in younger

people. A BMI of less than 23 classifies an older adult (older than age 65) as underweight and may require nutrition intervention.

Biochemical Analysis and Measures of Visceral Protein

The relevance of laboratory tests of serum albumin, prealbumin, and transferrin, as indicators of malnutrition, is limited. These acute-phase proteins do not consistently or predictability change with weight loss, calorie restriction, or negative nitrogen balance. They appear to better reflect severity of inflammatory response rather than poor nutritional status. Further investigation of the significance of low protein levels is needed (Gropper et al., 2020; Weaver et al., 2021) (see Research Highlights).

Solutions, Nursing Actions, and Outcomes

Nurses hold a pivotal role in ensuring adequate nutrition to promote healthy aging. Inherent in the role is (1) observation of the individual for issues related to performance at mealtimes; (2) modification of the environment to be pleasurable for eating; (3) supervision of eating; (4) provision of guidance and support to staff on feeding techniques that enhance intake and preserve dignity and independence; and (5) evaluation of outcomes. Nurturing and nourishing have been described as the nurses' role in nutritional care (Jefferies et al., 2011). Collaboration with the interprofessional team (e.g., dietitian, pharmacist, social worker, occupational or speech therapist) is important in planning interventions.

For the community-dwelling older adult, nutrition education and problem solving with the older adult and family members or caregivers on how to best resolve the potential or actual nutritional deficit is important. Causes of poor nutrition are complex, and all of the factors emphasized in this chapter are important to assess when planning individualized interventions to ensure adequate nutrition for older adults. Box 15.3 presents resources to assist older adults in planning for good nutrition.

Older adults in hospitals and long-term care facilities are more likely to be admitted with malnutrition, be at high risk for malnutrition, and have disease conditions that contribute to malnutrition. Severely restricted diets, long periods of NPO status, and insufficient time and staff for feeding assistance also contribute to inadequate nutrition. Older adults with dementia are particularly at risk for weight loss and inadequate nutrition (Chapters 25-26). Prevention of undernutrition and malnutrition and the maintenance of dietary needs and food are also ethical responsibilities. No older adult should be hungry or thirsty because of the inability to shop, cook, buy and prepare food, or eat independently. Nor should any older adult have to suffer because of a lack of assistance with these activities in whatever setting the person may reside.

Feeding Assistance

The incidence of eating disability in long-term care is high, with estimates that 50% of all residents cannot eat independently. Inadequate staffing in long-term care facilities is associated with poor nutrition and hydration. Classic research by gerontological nurse expert Kayser-Jones (1997) and many subsequent studies have shown that it can be an impossible task to feed the number of people who need assistance. In response to concerns about the lack of adequate assistance during mealtime in long-term care facilities, the Centers for Medicare and Medicaid Services (CMS) implemented a rule that allows feeding assistants with 8 hours of approved training to help residents with eating. Feeding assistants must be supervised by a registered nurse (RN) or licensed practical/vocational nurse (LPN/LVN). Family members also may be willing and able to assist at mealtimes and provide a familiar social context for the patient. Assistance with meals in hospitals is also a concern, and some acute care facilities have volunteer programs to address the unique needs of hospitalized patients. Further research is needed on the effectiveness of feeding assistance programs in hospital settings (Box 15.14).

Approaches to Enhancing Intake in Long-Term Care

In addition to adequate staff, many innovative and evidence-based ideas can improve nutritional intake in nursing facilities. Many suggestions are found in the literature: home-like dining rooms; cafeteria-style service; refreshment stations with easy access to juices, water, and healthy snacks; kitchens on the nursing units; choice of mealtimes; finger foods; visually appealing pureed foods with texture and shape.

Attention to the environment in which meals are served is important. Feeding older adults who have difficulty eating is complex and requires patience, time, and skill. It can become mechanical and devoid of feeling. The feeding process becomes rapid, and if it bogs down and becomes too slow, the meal may be ended abruptly, depending on the time the caregiver has allotted for feeding the person. Any pleasure derived through socialization and eating and any dignity that could be maintained are often absent (see "An Older Adult Speaks" at the beginning of this chapter). Other suggestions can be found in Box 15.15, and suggestions to improve intake for individuals with dementia are presented in Chapter 26.

Restrictive Diets and Caloric Supplements

The use of restrictive therapeutic diets (low cholesterol, low salt, no concentrated sweets) for frail older adults in long-term care often reduces food intake without significantly helping the clinical status of the individual. Dispensing a small amount of calorically dense oral nutritional supplement (2 calories/mL) during the routine medication pass may have a greater effect on weight gain than a traditional supplement (1.06 calories/mL) with or between meals. Small volumes of nutrient-dense supplement may have less of an effect on appetite and will enhance food intake during meals and snacks. This delivery method allows

---

BOX 15.14 Tips for Best Practice
Improving Nutritional Intake in Hospitals

- Assess nutritional and oral health status, including ability to eat and amount of assistance needed.
- Ensure proper fit and cleanliness of dentures and denture use.
- Provide oral hygiene, and allow the person to wash his or her hands before meals.
- Ask yourself if you would want to eat the food in the environment in which it is presented.
- Ensure environment is conducive to eating (remove objects such as urinals and bed pans; clear bedside tables).
- Position patient for safe eating (head of bed elevated or sit in a chair if possible).
- Stop nonessential clinical activity during meals (e.g., procedures, rounds, medication administration).
- Ensure that all nursing staff are aware of the patients who need assistance with eating and that adequate help is provided.
- Ensure that all necessary items are on the tray; prepare all food on the tray if needed; butter bread, open containers, provide straws, provide adaptive equipment as needed.
- Consider volunteers or family members to assist with eating and train and supervise.
- Administer medication for pain or nausea on a schedule that provides comfort at mealtime.
- Determine food preferences; provide for choices in food; include foods appropriate to cultural and religious customs.
- Accurately assess dietary intake using a validated method.
- Make dietary changes/referrals readily.
- Limit periods of nothing-by-mouth NPO status and provide food as soon as patient is able to eat.
- Consider liberalizing therapeutic diet if intake is inadequate; offer diet options/alternatives as indicated, including flavor enhancement.

From Furman E: The theory of compromised eating behavior, *Res Gerontol Nurs* 7(2):78–86, 2014.

BOX 15.15 Tips for Best Practice
Improving Nutritional Intake in Long-Term Care

- Assess nutritional and oral health status.
- Assess ability to eat and amount of assistance needed.
- Serve meals with the person in a chair rather than in bed when possible.
- Sit while feeding the person who needs assistance, use touch, and carry on a social conversation.
- Provide analgesics and antiemetics on a schedule that provides comfort at mealtime.
- Determine food preferences; provide for choices in food; include foods appropriate to cultural and religious customs.
- Consider buffet-style dining, use of steam tables rather than meal delivery service from trays, café- or bistro-type dining.
- Make food available 24 hours/day—provide snacks between meals and at night.
- Do not interrupt meals to administer medication if possible.
- Encourage family members to share the mealtimes if possible, for a heightened social situation.
- If caloric supplements are used, offer them between meals or with the medication pass.
- Ensure proper fit of dentures and denture use.
- Provide oral hygiene and allow the person to wash the hands before meals.
- Provide soft music during the meal.
- Use small, round tables seating six to eight people. Consider using tablecloths and centerpieces.
- Seat people with like interests and abilities together in communal dining areas and encourage socialization.
- Involve in restorative dining programs.
- Make diets as liberal as possible depending on health status, especially for frail elders who are not consuming adequate amounts of food.
- Consider a referral to occupational therapist for individuals experiencing difficulties with eating.

nurses to observe and document consumption. A growing body of evidence suggests that this form of supplementation might improve outcomes of hospitalized patients, including length of stay, costs, and readmissions (Malafarina et al., 2021).

Further studies and randomized clinical trials are needed to evaluate the effectiveness of nutritional supplementation. The American Geriatrics Society (2014 a, b) recommends avoiding high-calorie supplements for treatment of anorexia in older adults. Instead, recommendations are to optimize social supports, provide feeding assistance, and clarify patient goals and expectations. Unintentional weight loss is a common problem for medically ill or frail older adults. Although high-calorie supplements increase weight in older adults, there is no evidence that they affect other important clinical outcomes, such as quality of life, mood, functional status, or survival.

Pharmacological Therapy

The American Geriatrics Society (2014 a, b) does not recommend drugs that stimulate appetite (orexigenic drugs) to treat anorexia or malnutrition in older people. Use of drugs, such as megestrol acetate, results in minimum improvement in appetite and weight gain, no improvement in quality of life or survival, and increased risk of thrombotic events, fluid retention, and death. Systematic reviews of cannabinoids, dietary polyunsaturated fatty acids (cocosahexaenoic acid [DHA] and eicosapentaenoic acid [EPA]), thalidomide, and anabolic steroids have not identified adequate evidence for the efficacy and safety of these agents for weight gain. Box 15.3 provides a resource for an evidence-based protocol on evaluation and management of mealtime difficulties.

Patient Education

Education should be provided on nutritional requirements for health, special diet modifications for chronic illness management, the effect of age-associated changes and medication on nutrition, effective feeding techniques, dysphagia recognition and screening, and community resources to assist in maintaining adequate nutrition. Medicare covers nutrition therapy for select diseases, such as diabetes and kidney disease.

KEY CONCEPTS

- Diet can affect longevity and, when combined with lifestyle changes, reduce disease risk.
- Clinical judgment begins with the recognition and analysis of cues through observation, physical data, and integration of the range of complex factors that may affect nutritional health, including lifelong eating habits, income, chronic illness, dentition, mood disorders, capacity for food preparation, and cognitive and functional limitations.
- An interprofessional approach to nutritional evaluation is the most effective in developing solutions and improving outcomes.
- Overweight and obesity are major public health concerns around the globe. The proportion of older adults who are obese has doubled in the past 30 years.
- A rising incidence of malnutrition among older adults has been documented in acute care, long-term care, and the community and is expected to rise dramatically in the coming years. It is important to remember that overweight or obese individuals are also at risk for malnutrition.
- Malnutrition is a precursor to frailty and has serious consequences, including infections, pressure ulcers, anemia, hypotension, impaired cognition, hip fractures, prolonged hospital stay, institutionalization, and increased morbidity and mortality.
- A comprehensive evaluation of nutritional status is an essential component of the assessment of older adults.
- The role of nursing in evaluation of nutritional status and design of nursing actions should be comprehensive and include attention to the process of eating and the entire ritual of meals within an interprofessional approach.
- Making mealtimes pleasant and attractive for the older adult who is unable to eat unassisted is a nursing challenge; mealtimes must be made enjoyable, and adequate assistance must be provided.
- Dysphagia is a serious problem and has negative consequences, including weight loss, malnutrition, dehydration, aspiration pneumonia, and even death. Early recognition of cues, identification of risk factors, observation for signs and symptoms, referral for evaluation, and collaboration with SLPs on actions to prevent aspiration are essential.

NEXT-GENERATION NCLEX® (NGN) EXAMINATION–STYLE QUESTIONS

The nurse is completing the monthly nursing assessment of Mr. Dawson. Mr. Dawson is a 92-year-old male. He has been at the long-term care facility for the past 5 years. His weight this month is 300 pounds (BMI 26.6 kg/m²). His blood pressure is 145/82 mm Hg, heart rate 90 beats per minute, respirations 18 breaths per minute, and temperature 97.4°F. He responds to questions appropriately. During the physical examination at 0900 hours, the nurse notes that Mr. Dawson is drooling and coughing intermittently. His upper dentures fall when he opens his mouth for evaluation. His lungs are clear on examination, and his heart has regular rhythm.

Choose the most likely options for the information missing from the statements below by selecting from the lists of options provided.

The nurse recognizes that _____, _____, and _____ put Mr. Dawson at increased risk of _____, and he should be _____ until the _____ is completed.

Options
Overnutrition
Swallowing evaluation
Depression
Coughing after eating
NPO
Dry mouth
Dysphagia
Copious secretions
Difficulty chewing
Occupational therapy

NURSING STUDY

Nutrition

Helen, 77 years old, had dieted all her life—or so it seemed. She often chided herself about it. "After all, at my age who cares if I'm too fat? I do. It depresses me when I gain weight and then I gain even more when I'm depressed." At 5 feet, 4 inches tall and 138 pounds, her weight was ideal for her height and age, but Helen, like so many women of her generation, had incorporated the image of women on TV who weigh 105 pounds as her ideal. She had achieved that weight for only a few weeks three or four times in her adult life. She had tried high-protein diets, celery and cottage cheese diets, fasting, commercially prepared diet foods, and numerous fad diets. She always discontinued the diets when she perceived any negative effects. She was invested in maintaining her general good health. Her most recent attempt at losing 30 pounds on an all-liquid diet had been unsuccessful and left her feeling constipated, weak, irritable, and mildly nauseated and experiencing heart palpitations. This really frightened her.

Her physician criticized her regarding the liquid diet but seemed rather amused while reinforcing that her weight was "just perfect" for her age. In the discussion, the physician pointed out how fortunate she was that she was able to drive to the market, had sufficient money for food, and was able to eat anything with no dietary restrictions. Helen left his office feeling silly. She was an independent, intelligent woman; she had been a successful manager of a large financial office. Before her retirement 7 years ago, her work had consumed most of her energy. There had been no time for family, romance, or hobbies. Lately, she had immersed herself in reading the Harvard Classics, as she had promised herself she would when she retired. Unfortunately, now that she had the time to read them, she was losing interest. She knew that she must begin to "pull herself together" and "be grateful for her blessings" just as the physician had said.

CLINICAL JUDGMENT QUESTIONS AND ACTIVITIES

Questions 1 to 5 refer to the Nursing Study above.

1. In the nursing study, discuss how you would counsel Helen regarding her weight.
2. If Helen insists on dieting, what diet would you recommend, considering her age and activity level?
3. What lifestyle changes would you suggest to Helen?
4. What are the specific health concerns that require attention in Helen's case?
5. What factors may be involved in Helen's preoccupation with her weight?
6. Choose one of the contributing factors to malnutrition and list nursing actions to reduce risk.
7. Assess your nutrition using the Nutrition Screening Initiative and discuss your score and risk.

RESEARCH QUESTIONS

1. What are the dietary patterns of older men living alone?
2. What percentage of women and men older than age 60 are satisfied with their weight?
3. What factors influence older adults to implement dietary changes suggested by nurses, dietitians, or primary care providers?
4. What nursing actions can enhance the nutritional intake of older adults who are frail and residing in nursing facilities?
5. What is the level of knowledge about dysphagia among acute care and long-term care nurses?

REFERENCES

American Geriatrics Society: *Choosing wisely: five things physicians and patients should question* (website), 2014a. http://www.choosingwisely.org/american-geriatrics-society-releases-second-choosing-wisely-list-identifies-5-more-tests-and-treatments-that-older-patients-and-providers-should-question/. Accessed January 2021.

American Geriatrics Society: Feeding tubes in advanced dementia position statement, *J Am Geriatr Soc* 62(8):1590–1593, 2014. https://www.ncbi.nlm.nih.gov/pubmed/25039796.linical_guidelines_recommendations. Accessed June 2021.

Artiles C, Regan J, Donnellan C: Dysphagia screening in residential care settings: a scoping review, *Int J Nurs Stud*, 2020. epub https://doi.org/10.1016/j.ijnurstu.2020.103813.

Avelino-Silva T, Jaluul O: Malnutrition in hospitalized older patients: management strategies to improve patient care and clinical outcomes, *Int J Geront* 11(2):56–61, 2017.

Balasubramanian P, Kiss T, Tarantini S, et al.: Obesity-induced cognitive impairment in older adults: a microvascular perspective, *Am J Physiol Heart Circ Physiol* 320(2):H740–H761, 2021. https://doi.org/10.1152/ajpheart.00736.2020.

Batsis J: Obesity in the older adult: special issue, *J Nutr Gerontol Geriatr* 38(1):1–5, 2019.

Bilder GE: *Human biological aging*, Hoboken, NJ, 2016, Wiley-Blackwell.

Bowman K, Delgado J, Henley WE, et al.: Obesity in older people with and without conditions associated with weight loss: follow-up of 955,000 primary care patients, *J Gerontol A Biol Sci Med Sci* 72(2):203–209, 2017.

Cederholm T, Jensen G, Gonzalez M, et al.: GLIM criteria for the diagnosis of malnutrition: a consensus report from the global clinical nutrition community, *J Cachexia Sarcopenia Muscle* 10(1):207–217, 2019.

Crogan N: Nutritional problems affecting older adults, *Nurs Clin North Am* 52:433–445, 2017.

Engh M, Speyer R: Management of dysphagia in nursing homes: a national survey, *Dysphagia*, 2021. doi:10.1007/s00455-021-10275-7.

Feeding America: *Senior food insecurity studies* (website), 2020. https://www.feedingamerica.org/research/senior-hunger-research/senior. Accessed June 2021.

Finucane T: Questioning feeding tubes to treat dysphagia, *JAMA Intern Med* 177(3):443, 2017.

Fu J, Liu Y, Zhang L, et al.: Nonpharmacological interventions for reducing blood pressure in adults with prehypertension to established hypertension, *JAHA*, 9(19), 2020. https://doi.org/10.1161/JAHA.120.016804.

Furman E: The theory of compromised eating behavior, *Res Gerontol Nurs* 7(2):78–86, 2014.

Gropper S, Exantus M, Jackson K, et al.: Increasing protein intake to help older adults increase muscle strength and function: a pilot, single-arm investigation using coaching and a per meal protein prescription, *J Aging Res & Lifestyle* 9:9–13, 2020.

Iannetti A: Updates on the management of GERD disease, *J Gastrointest Dig Syst* 7:523, 2017.

Jefferies D, Johnson M, Ravens I: Nurturing and nourishing: the nurses' role in nutritional care, *J Clin Nurs*(20):317–330, 2011.

Kalish V: Obesity in older adults, *Prim Care* 43(1):137–144, 2016.

Kayser-Jones J: Inadequate staffing at mealtime: implications for nursing and health policy, *J Gerontol Nurs* 23:14–21, 1997.

Khalil N, Esa R, Ismaeel M: Critical care nurses' knowledge and practices regarding dysphagia care of acute ischemic stroke patient, *World J Pharm Med* 6(3):12–18, 2020.

Malafarina V, Rexach J, Masanes F, et al.: Results of high-protein, high-calorie oral nutritional supplement in malnourished older people in nursing homes: an observational, multicenter, prospective, pragmatic study (PROT-e-GER), *Jour Am Med Dir Assoc* 22(9):1919–1926, 2021.

McEvoy C, Guyer H, Langa K, et al.: Neuroprotective diets are associated with better cognitive function: the Health and Retirement Study, *J Am Geriatr Soc* 65:1857–1862, 2017.

National Council on Aging: *SNAP and senior hunger facts*, 2018. https://www.ncoa.org/news/resources-for-reporters/get-the-facts/senior-hunger-facts/. Accessed December 2021.

National Council on Aging: *7 facts about older adults and SNAP* (website), 2021. https://www.ncoa.org/article/7-facts-about-older-adults-and-snap. Accessed April 2021.

National Center for Chronic Disease Prevention and Health: *How you can prevent chronic disease* (website), 2021. https://www.cdc.gov/chronicdisease/about/prevent/index.htm. Accessed June 2021.

The Gerontological Society of America, *What's hot: Cellular nutrition and its influence on age-associated cellular decline*, November, 2021. https://www.geron.org/images/gsa/documents/whatshotcellularnutrition.pdf. Accessed February 2022.

Tilly J: *White paper: opportunities to improve nutrition for older adults and reduce risk of poor health outcomes* (website), 2017. http://nutritionandaging.org/opportunities-to-improve-nutrition-for-older-adults-and-reduce-risk-of-poor-health-outcomes/. Accessed April 2021.

US Department of Agriculture & US Department of Health and Human Services: *Dietary guidelines for Americans, 2020–2025*, ed 9, Washington, DC, 2020, Authors https://www.dietaryguidelines.gov/sites/default/files/2020-12/Dietary_Guidelines_for_Americans_2020-2025.pdf. Accessed June 2021.

Weaver A, Tooze J, Cauley J, et al.: Effect of dietary protein intake on bone mineral density and fracture incidence in older adults in the Health, Aging, and Body Composition Study, *J Gerontol A Biol Sci Med Sci* 76(12):2213–2222, 2021 https://doi.oeg/10.1093/gerona/glab068.

World Health Organization (WHO): *Obesity* (website), 2020. https://www.who.int/health-topics/obesity#tab=tab_1. Accessed June 2021.

16 CHAPTER

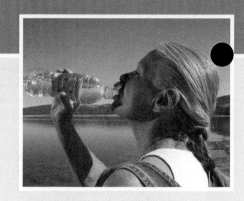

Hydration and Oral Health

Theris A. Touhy

http://evolve.elsevier.com/Touhy/TwdHlthAging

A STUDENT SPEAKS

I never thought that part of my nursing care was brushing someone's false teeth. I didn't even know my patient had false teeth until he asked me to help him take them out. Thank goodness he was able to tell me how to do it because I had no idea. He was really worried because he said the last time he was in the hospital, no one had taken them out for several days and he got a sore under them that was very painful. Together we got them out, cleaned, and back in with no problems. Made me realize how important the little things really are.

Jeff, age 22

AN OLDER ADULT SPEAKS

I know I don't drink enough water—coffee, yes; water, no. It's hard when you are in a wheelchair and only have one arm that works. This smart little student nurse really fixed me up. She gave me a plastic water bottle and attached it to my chair on my good side. Now wherever I go, the water goes.

Jack, age 84

LEARNING OBJECTIVES

On completion of this chapter, the reader will be able to:
1. Identify factors that influence hydration management in older adults.
2. Recognize and analyze early cues of dehydration and nursing actions for prevention and treatment.
3. Demonstrate understanding of the relationship between oral health and disease.
4. Discuss common oral problems that can occur with aging.
5. Use clinical judgment to identify and evaluate solutions and nursing actions to maintain hydration and oral health in a variety of settings.

HYDRATION MANAGEMENT

Hydration management is the promotion of an adequate fluid balance, which prevents complications resulting from abnormal or undesirable fluid levels. Water, an accessible and available commodity to almost all people, is often overlooked as an essential part of nutritional requirements. Water's function in the body includes thermoregulation, dilution of water-soluble medications, facilitation of renal and bowel function, and creation of requisite conditions for and maintenance of metabolic processes.

Daily needs for water usually can be met by functionally independent older adults through intake of fluids with meals and social drinks. However, a significant number of older adults (up to 85% of those 85 years of age and older) drink less than 1 liter of fluid per day. Older adults, except for those with fluid restrictions, should consume at least 1500 mL of fluid per day.

Maintenance of fluid balance (fluid intake equals fluid output) is essential to health, regardless of a person's age.

Age-related changes (Box 16.1; Fig. 16.1), medication use, functional impairments, and comorbid medical and emotional illnesses place some older adults at risk for changes in fluid balance, especially dehydration. Hydration habits, as described by Mentes (2012), also influence how and why individuals consume liquids. Each group has different hydration habits that can guide assessment and interventions. Providing targeted interventions to those at greatest risk may decrease the prevalence of dehydration (Box 16.2).

DEHYDRATION

Dehydration is considered a geriatric syndrome that is frequently associated with common diseases (e.g., diabetes, respiratory

BOX 16.1 Age-Related Changes Affecting Hydration Status

- Thirst sensation diminishes; thirst is not proportional to metabolic needs in response to dehydrating conditions
- Creatinine clearance declines, kidneys are less able to concentrate urine (particularly in individuals with illnesses affecting kidney function)
- Total body water decreases
- Loss of muscle mass and increase in proportion of fat cells; greater in women than men because they have a higher percentage of body fat and less muscle mass; fat cells contain less water than muscle cells

Adapted from Mentes JC: Managing oral hydration. In Boltz M, Capezuti E, Fulmer T, et al, editors: *Evidence-based geriatric nursing protocols for best practice*, ed 4, New York, 2012, Springer, pp 419–438.

illness, heart failure) and frailty. It is often an unappreciated comorbid condition that exacerbates an underlying condition such as a urinary tract infection, respiratory tract infection, or worsening depression. Dehydration is a significant risk factor for delirium, thromboembolic complications, infections, kidney stones, constipation and obstipation, falls, medication toxicity, renal failure, seizure, electrolyte imbalance, hyperthermia, and delayed wound healing. In community-dwelling older adults, physical performance and cognitive processing have been found to be affected even by mild dehydration (Mentes & Gaspar, 2020).

Dehydration takes various forms (Box 16.3). Water-loss dehydration (hypertonic, hyperosmotic, or intracellular dehydration) is common in older adults and results from deficient fluid intake (Hooper et al., 2016). Adults older than 65 years of age have the highest rates of acute care admissions for dehydration as a primary diagnosis. Although the prevalence of dehydration in older adults who are hospitalized has not been adequately studied, rates of 10% to 45% have been reported.

BOX 16.2 Typology of Hydration Problems

CAN DRINK: Capable of accessing and consuming fluids but may not know what adequate intake is or may forget to drink as a result of cognitive impairment. May need education about daily fluid needs and the importance of reporting any changes; verbal encouragement and prompting; easy access to fluids

CAN'T DRINK: Physically incapable of accessing or safely consuming fluids related to physical dependence or swallowing disorders. May need dysphagia prevention interventions; physical aids to assist with drinking (e.g., sports bottle, sippy cup); swallowing evaluation and safe swallowing techniques; oral care; foods rich in fluid (smoothies); adequate assistance

WON'T DRINK: Highest risk for dehydration. Capable of consuming fluids safely but do not because of fear of being incontinent; or have lower cognitive abilities and consume limited amounts of fluid at a time (sippers). Interventions may include offering frequent small amounts of fluid at each contact (preferred beverages); providing fluid with activities; implementing toileting programs; promoting education about maintaining fluid intake

END OF LIFE: Terminally ill individuals who may have hydration patterns described in other categories. Hydration will be dependent on resident and family preference, advance directives

From Mentes JC: A typology of oral hydration, *J Gerontol Nurs* 32(1):13–19, 2006.

Dehydration is estimated to be present in half of long-term care residents. In the long-term care setting, difficulties in communication, mobility, cognitive function, and eating difficulties prevent many from accessing fluid independently. Research results suggest that the majority of long-term care facility residents are not even consuming 1500 mL of fluids per day (Masot et al., 2018; Namasivayam-MacDonald et al., 2018). Adults ages 85 years and older, on average, drank the least amount of fluid at 850 cc/day (Mentes & Gaspar, 2020). A recent study reported

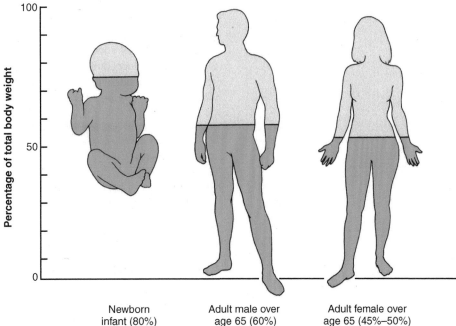

Proportion of Body Weight Represented by Water

Percentage of total body weight

Newborn infant (80%)   Adult male over age 65 (60%)   Adult female over age 65 (45%–50%)

Fig. 16.1 Changes in body water distribution with age. (From Thibodeau GA, Patton KT: *Structure & function of the body,* ed 13, St Louis, 2008, Mosby.)

BOX 16.3 Types of Dehydration

- **Water-loss dehydration (hypertonic, hyperosmotic, intracellular):** Results from insufficient fluid intake, which leads to an elevation of serum osmolarity and a drop in extracellular fluid volume.
- **Volume depletion (hypovolemia) (salt loss, extracellular dehydration):** Results from excess fluid loss as occurs in vomiting/diarrhea, excessive bleeding, loss of plasma. Serum is depleted of both fluid and electrolytes. Fluid loss occurs more abruptly than water-loss dehydration. Serum osmolarity may remain stable or decrease slightly.

From Hooper L, Bunn D, Aldelhamid A, et al: Water-loss (intracellular) dehydration assessed using urinary tests: how well do they work? Diagnostic accuracy in older adults, *Am J Clin Nutr* 104:121–131, 2016.

that hydration levels in an assisted care facility for individuals with memory impairment were lower than comparison groups of nursing home residents (Gaspar et al., 2019).

Risk Factors for Dehydration

The presence of physical or emotional illness, surgery, trauma, frailty, or conditions of higher physiological demands increases the risk of dehydration. Older adults are particularly at risk for dehydration, since their kidneys are less able to concentrate urine and some medications (diuretics) increase fluid excretion. However, the main reason for dehydration is reduced fluid intake (Namasivayam-MacDonald et al., 2018). Even simple disruptions in food and fluid intake (e.g., several missed meals) can precipitate an episode of dehydration (Mentes & Gaspar, 2020). When the fluid balance of older adults is at risk, the limited capacity of homeostatic mechanisms becomes significant (see Box 16.1; Fig. 16.1). Box 16.4 presents risk factors for dehydration.

BOX 16.4 Risk Factors for Dehydration

Age-related changes
Medications: diuretics, laxatives, angiotensin-converting enzyme (ACE) inhibitors, psychotropics
Use of four or more medications
Functional deficits
Communication and comprehension problems
Oral problems
Dysphagia
Delirium
Dementia
Hospitalization
Low body weight
Diagnostic procedures requiring fasting
Requiring physical assistance at meals
Being female
Inadequate assistance with fluid or food intake
Diarrhea
Fever
Vomiting
Infections
Bleeding
Draining wounds
Artificial ventilation
Fluid restrictions
High environmental temperatures
Multiple comorbidities

PROMOTING HEALTHY AGING: IMPLICATIONS FOR GERONTOLOGICAL NURSING: DEHYDRATION

Recognizing and Analyzing Cues

Prevention of dehydration is essential, but assessment is complex in older adults. Cues present differently than in younger individuals, and clinical signs may not appear until dehydration is advanced. Signs and symptoms may be nonspecific, making prevention and early identification of cues important. Skin turgor, assessed at the sternum and commonly included in the assessment of dehydration, is an unreliable marker in older adults because of the loss of subcutaneous tissue with aging. Dry mucous membranes in the mouth and nose, longitudinal furrows on the tongue, orthostasis, speech incoherence, rapid pulse rate, extremity weakness, dry axilla, and sunken eyes may indicate dehydration. Assessment of hydration status must be conducted on admission to the hospital, particularly for those who are frail, and must be monitored regularly throughout the individual's stay and at discharge (McCrow et al., 2016). In the long-term care setting, the Minimum Data Set (MDS) 3.0 (Chapter 9) assesses for dehydration and fluid maintenance.

The diagnosis of dehydration is biochemically proven. Serum osmolarity readings of 300 mOsmol/L or higher are indicative of dehydration in older adults (Hooper et al., 2016). Although most cases of dehydration have an elevated blood urea nitrogen (BUN) measurement, there are many other causes of an elevated BUN-creatinine ratio, so this test cannot be used alone to diagnose dehydration in older adults. Recent research reports that urinary measures reflecting hydration status in older adults (urine color, osmolarity, volume) should not be used because these measures are not sensitive or specific enough. However, urine patterns and color should be observed for changes.

Solutions, Nursing Actions, and Outcomes

Actions are derived from a comprehensive analysis of cues and consist of risk identification and hydration management (Box 16.5). Any older adult who has functional or cognitive impairments and is dependent on others for fluid intake is particularly at risk. Those who develop fever, diarrhea, vomiting, or a nonfebrile

BOX 16.5 Simple Screen for Dehydration

Drugs (e.g., diuretics)
End of life
High fever
Yellow urine turns dark
Dizziness (orthostasis)
Reduced oral intake
Axilla dry
Tachycardia
Incontinence (fear of)
Oral problems/sippers
Neurological impairment (confusion)
Sunken eyes

From Thomas D, Cote T, Lawhorne L, et al: Understanding clinical dehydration and its treatment, *J Am Med Dir Assoc* 9(5):292–301, 2008.

BOX 16.6 Tips for Best Practice

Ongoing Management of Oral Intake: Long-Term Care

1. Calculate a daily fluid goal.
   - All older adults should have an individualized fluid goal determined by a documented standard for daily fluid intake. At least 1500 mL of fluid/day should be provided.
2. Compare current intake to fluid goal to evaluate hydration status.
3. Provide fluids consistently throughout the day.
   - Provide 75% to 80% of fluids at mealtimes and the remainder during non-mealtimes, such as at medication times.
   - Offer a variety of fluids and fluids that the person prefers.
   - Standardize the amount of fluid that is offered with medication administration (e.g., at least 6 oz).
4. Plan for at-risk individuals.
   - Have fluid rounds midmorning and midafternoon.
   - Provide two 8-oz glasses of fluid in the morning and evening.
   - Offer a "happy hour" or "tea time," when residents can gather for additional fluids and socialization.
   - Provide modified fluid containers based on resident's abilities—for example, lighter cups and glasses, weighted cups and glasses, plastic water bottles with straws (attach to wheelchairs, deliver with meals).
   - Make fluids accessible at all times and be sure residents can access them—for example, filled water pitchers, fluid stations, or beverage carts in congregate areas.
   - Allow adequate time and staff for eating or feeding. Meals can provide two-thirds of daily fluids.
   - Encourage family members to participate in feeding and offering fluids.
5. Perform fluid regulation and documentation.
   - Document complete intake, including hydration habits.
   - Know volumes of fluid containers to accurately calculate fluid consumption.
   - In most settings, at least one accurate intake and output recording should be documented, including amount of fluid consumed and difficulties with consumption.
   - For individuals who are not continent, teach caregivers to observe incontinent pads or briefs for amount and frequency of urine, color changes, and odor, and report variations from individual's normal pattern.

Adapted from Mentes JC: Managing oral hydration. In Boltz M, Capezuti E, Fulmer T, et al, editors: *Evidence-based geriatric nursing protocols for best practice*, New York, 2012, Springer, pp 419–438.

BOX 16.7 Resources for Best Practice

Hartford Institute for Geriatric Nursing: Nursing Standard of Practice Protocols: hydration management; the Kayser-Jones Brief Oral Health Status Examination (BOHSE). https://consultgeri.org/trythis/general-assessment/issue-18.

Oral Cancer Foundation: Check Your Mouth—interactive website to assist individuals in self-screening for oral cancer or oral changes. http://www.checkyourmouth.org.

Rita Jablonski: Video: Providing Mouth Care for Persons with Dementia. https://www.youtube.com/watch?v=UIDL3YQPDNY.

Smiles for Life: National curriculum to help primary care clinicians integrate oral health care into care of patients. http://www.smilesforlifeoralhealth.org/buildcontent.aspx?tut=555&pagekey=62948&cbreceipt=0

---

infection should be monitored closely by implementing intake and output records and providing additional fluids. Acute situations such as vomiting, diarrhea, or febrile episodes should be identified quickly and treated. NPO (nothing by mouth) requirements for diagnostic tests and surgical procedures should be as short as possible for older adults, and adequate fluids should be given once tests and procedures are completed. A 2-hour suspension of fluid intake is recommended for many procedures. Education should be provided to older adults and their caregivers on the need for fluids and the signs and symptoms of dehydration.

Hydration management involves both acute and ongoing management of oral intake (Box 16.6). Oral rehydration therapy is the first treatment approach for dehydration. Individuals with mild to moderate dehydration who can drink and do not have significant mental or physical compromise due to fluid loss may be able to replenish fluids orally. Water is considered the best fluid to offer, but other clear fluids also may be useful depending on the person's preference.

Rehydration methods depend on the severity and the type of dehydration and may include intravenous or hypodermoclysis (HDC). A general rule is to replace 50% of the loss within the first 12 hours (or 1 L/day in afebrile individuals) or sufficient quantity to relieve tachycardia and hypotension. Further fluid replacement can be administered more slowly over a longer period of time. It is important to monitor for symptoms of overhydration (unexplained weight gain, pedal edema, neck vein distention, shortness of breath), especially in individuals with heart failure or renal disease. Individuals taking selective serotonin reuptake inhibitors (SSRIs) should have serum sodium levels and hydration status closely monitored due to risk for hyponatremia (Chapter 11). Increasing fluid intake may aggravate an evolving hyponatremia.

HDC (also known as clysis) is an infusion of isotonic fluids into the subcutaneous space. HDC is safe, easy to administer, and a useful alternative to intravenous administration for persons with mild to moderate dehydration, particularly those patients with altered mental status. HDC offers a wider range of infusion sites than traditional intravenous therapy and can be far less painful, especially when veins are difficult to find due to dehydration. HDC cannot be used in severe dehydration or for any situation requiring more than 3 L over 24 hours. Common sites of infusion are the lateral abdominal wall; the anterior or lateral aspects of the thighs; the infraclavicular region; and the back, usually the interscapular or subscapular regions with a fat fold at least 1 inch thick. Normal saline (0.9%), half-normal saline (0.45%), 5% glucose in water infusion (D5W), or Ringer's solution can be used. Other resources on hydration can be found in Box 16.7.

ORAL HEALTH

Orodental health is integral to general health. Orodental health is a basic need that is increasingly neglected with advanced age, debilitation, and limited mobility. Age-related changes in the oral cavity, medical conditions, poor dental hygiene, and lack of dental care contribute to poor oral health. Older adults who are dependent on caregivers for bodily care assistance exhibit worse oral hygiene than those who are self-sufficient. Poor oral health is recognized as a risk factor for dehydration, malnutrition, and a number of systemic diseases, including pneumonia, joint

---

BOX 16.8   Tips for Best Practice

Promoting Oral Health

Encourage annual dental exams, including for individuals with dentures.

Brush and floss twice daily; use a fluoride dentifrice and mouthwash.

Ensure that dentures fit well and are cleaned regularly.

Maintain adequate daily fluid intake (1500 mL).

Avoid tobacco.

Limit alcohol.

Eat a well-balanced diet.

Use an ultrasonic toothbrush (more effective in removing plaque).

Use a commercial floss handle for easier flossing.

Adapt toothbrush if manual dexterity is impaired. Use a child's toothbrush or enlarge the handle of an adult-size toothbrush by adding a foam grip or wrapping it with gauze or rubber bands to increase handle size.

If medications cause a dry mouth, ask the health care provider if other drugs can be substituted. If dry mouth cannot be avoided, drink plenty of water, chew sugarless gum, and avoid alcohol and tobacco.

---

infections, cardiovascular disease, and poor glycemic control in type 1 and type 2 diabetes. Certain oral and systemic conditions are related to one another (e.g., diabetes and periodontal disease, poor oral hygiene and aspiration pneumonia, dental pain and disruptive behaviors in invididuals with cognitive dysfunction or dementia). A connection between poor oral health and mortality has been identified in a cohort of older adults (Gerontological Society of America, 2021; Kohli et al., 2017).

Poor oral health is an important public health issue and a growing burden to countries worldwide. Health disparities are evident across and within regions and result from living conditions and availability of oral health services. Tips to promoting oral health are presented in Box 16.8. *Healthy People 2030* addresses oral health with the goal of improving oral health by increasing access to oral health care, including preventive services.

 HEALTHY PEOPLE 2030

Oral Conditions/Dental

- Reduce the proportion of older adults with untreated root surface decay
- Reduce the proportion of adults ages 45 years and older who have lost all their teeth
- Reduce the proportion of adults ages 45 years and older with moderate and severe periodontitis
- Increase the proportion of people with dental insurance
- Reduce the proportion of people who cannot get the dental care they need when they need it
- Increase the proportion of oral and pharyngeal cancers detected at the earliest stage
- Increase use of the oral health care system

Data from US Department of Health and Human Services: *Healthy People 2030* (website), 2020. https://health.gov/healthypeople.

Xerostomia (Mouth Dryness)

Xerostomia and hyposalivation are present in approximately 30% of older adults and can affect eating, swallowing, and speaking and contribute to dental caries and periodontal disease. Adequate saliva is necessary for the beginning stage of digestion, helping to break down starches and fats. It also functions to clear the mouth of food debris and prevent overgrowth of oral microbes. The flow of saliva does not decrease with age, but medical conditions and medications affect salivary flow. More than 400 medications, including antihypertensives, antidepressants, antihistamines, antipsychotics, diuretics, and antiparkinson agents, have a side effect of hyposalivation.

Treatment of Xerostomia

A review of all medications is important, and if medication side effects are contributing to dry mouth, medications may be changed or altered. Affected individuals should practice good oral hygiene practices and have regular dental care to screen for decay. Consumption of adequate water intake and avoidance of alcohol and caffeine are recommended. Over-the-counter saliva substitutes (Oral Balance Gel, Mouth Kote) and salivary stimulants such as Biotene, Xylitol gum, and sugarless candy can be helpful.

Oral Cancer

Oral cancers are more frequent with age. The median age at diagnosis is 61 years, and men are affected twice as often as women. Oral cancers are much more common in Hungary and France than in the United States and much less common in Mexico and Japan. The 5-year survival rate is 57% and has not improved significantly in decades. This is largely the result of late identification of the disease. Often oral cancers are discovered only when the cancer has metastasized to another location, most likely the lymph nodes of the neck. Oral cancer has a high risk of producing second primary tumors, and patients who survive a first encounter with the disease have up to 20 times higher risk for developing a second cancer.

There are several types of oral cancer, but around 90% are squamous cell carcinomas. Historically, the majority of individuals are over the age of 40 years at the time of discovery; however, the incidence is increasing in those younger than 40. Exact causes are becoming clearer and include the human papilloma virus 16 and the use of "smokeless" chewing or spit tobacco. In the younger age group, including those who have never used any tobacco products, human papilloma virus may be replacing tobacco as the primary causative agent. This virus is sexually transmitted between partners and is also responsible for more than 90% of all cervical cancers. Risk factors are listed in Box 16.9.

Early detection is essential, but more than 60% of oral cancers are not diagnosed until an advanced stage. Early signs and symptoms may be subtle and not recognized by the individual or health care provider. Common areas for oral cancer to develop are the tongue, tonsils and oropharynx, the gums, and the floor of the mouth. Oral examinations can assist in early identification

---

BOX 16.9   Risk Factors for Oral Cancer

Tobacco, including smokeless tobacco

Alcohol

Human papilloma virus 16

Genetic susceptibility

BOX 16.10 Signs and Symptoms of Oral and Throat Cancer

- Swelling or thickening, lumps or bumps, or rough spots or eroded areas on the lips, gums, or other areas inside the mouth
- Velvety white, red, or speckled patches in the mouth
- Persistent sores on the face, neck, or mouth that bleed easily
- Unexplained bleeding in the mouth
- Unexplained numbness, pain, or tenderness in any area of the face, mouth, neck, or tongue
- Soreness in the back of the throat; a persistent feeling that something is caught in the throat
- Difficulty chewing or swallowing, speaking, or moving the jaw or tongue
- Hoarseness, chronic sore throat, or changes in the voice
- Dramatic weight loss
- Lump or swelling in the neck
- Severe pain in one ear—with a normal eardrum
- Pain around the teeth; loosening of the teeth
- Swelling or pain in the jaw; difficulty moving the jaw

and treatment. All persons, especially those older than 50 years of age, with or without dentures, should have oral examinations on a regular basis. A new initiative from the Oral Cancer Foundation, *Check Your Mouth* (www.checkyourmouth.org), is built around an interactive website designed to help individuals learn to self-discover suspicious tissue changes in their own mouths. Box 16.10 presents common signs and symptoms of oral cancer. Once diagnosed, therapy options are based on diagnosis and staging and include surgery, radiation, and chemotherapy (Oral Cancer Foundation, 2021).

If detected early, these cancers can almost always be treated successfully. For those whose cancer is caught at a later stage, the results of surgical removal of the disease may require reconstruction of portions of the oral cavity or facial features. Adjunctive therapy may be required to assist in speech, chewing and swallowing, problems associated with lack of salivary function, as well as the fabrication of dental or facial prostheses. Individuals with treated oral cancer will need to have follow-up exams for the rest of their lives, since another cancer can develop later in the mouth, lung, throat, or other areas (Oral Cancer Foundation, 2021).

Oral Care

Nearly one-third of individuals older than age 65 have untreated tooth decay. Nearly 1 in 5 adults 65 years of age and older have lost all of their teeth (edentulous), primarily as a result of periodontitis. Periodontal disease increases with age; 70.1% of adults 65 years of age and older have periodontal disease. There has been a dramatic reduction in the prevalence of tooth loss as knowledge increases and more people use fluorides, improve nutrition, engage in new oral hygiene practices, and take advantage of improved dental health care. However, many individuals may not have had the advantages of new preventive treatment.

Older adults with the poorest of oral health tend to be those who are economically disadvantaged, lack insurance, and are members of racial and ethnic minorities. Being homebound, institutionalized, or experiencing functional and cognitive limitations that make performing oral hygiene difficult, contribute

to poor oral health (Centers for Disease Control and Prevention [CDC], 2021).

Access to dental care for older adults may be limited and cost prohibitive. In the existing health care system, dental care is a low priority. Medicare does not provide any coverage for oral health care services, and few Americans 75 years of age or older have private dental insurance. The cost of adding this basic and preventive Medicare benefit is estimated to be $29 per beneficiary per year, but it has not been added. Some Medicare Advantage plans offer reimbursement for routine procedures like teeth cleaning, with a fixed amount allotted yearly (Gerontological Society of America, 2021).

Medicaid coverage for dental varies from state to state, but funding has decreased and coverage can be limited. Older adults have fewer dentist visits than any other age group. Access to dentists in long-term care facilities is very limited, and many are unwilling to provide care in these facilities (Jablonski et al., 2017). If a long-term care resident needs dental care, this requires transportation to a dentist's office, which is not only costly but many times not possible because of the individual's condition. In many undeveloped countries, there is a shortage of trained dental professionals. Dental care is nonexistent except for that provided by groups such as medical and dental ministries from other countries.

USING CLINICAL JUDGMENT TO PROMOTE HEALTHY AGING: ORAL HEALTH

Recognizing and Analyzing Cues

Good oral hygiene and timely assessment of oral health are nursing responsibilities. Oral care is "oral infection control" (Jablonski-Jaudon et al., 2016, p 15). The relationship between poor oral health and systemic infections, such as pneumonia, is well documented (Jablonski et al., 2017). In addition, examination of the mouth can serve as an early warning system for some diseases and lead to early diagnosis and treatment. Assessment of the mouth, teeth, and oral cavity is an essential part of health assessment (Chapter 9) and especially important when an individual is hospitalized or in a long-term care facility. An oral exam should be included as part of a general medical exam in primary care. The MDS 3.0 requires information obtained from an oral assessment. Federal regulations mandate an annual examination for residents of long-term care facilities. Although the oral examination is best performed by a dentist, nurses in health care settings can provide oral health screenings using an instrument such as the Kayser-Jones Brief Oral Health Status Examination (BOHSE) (see Box 16.7).

Solutions, Nursing Actions, and Outcomes

Nurses may be involved in promoting oral health by teaching individuals or caregivers recommended interventions; screening for oral disease; making dental referrals; or providing, supervising, and evaluating oral care in hospitals and long-term care facilities. A recent report (Gerontological Society of America, 2021) suggested that responses instituted for provision of dental care during the COVID-19 pandemic could improve oral care

BOX 16.11 Tips for Best Practice

Providing Oral Care

1. Explain all actions to the individual; use gestures and demonstration as needed; cue and prompt to encourage as much self-care performance as possible.
2. If the individual is in bed, elevate the head by raising the bed or propping it with pillows and have the individual turn the head to face you. Place a clean towel across the chest and under the chin and place a basin under the chin.
3. If the individual is sitting in a stationary chair or wheelchair, stand behind the individual and stabilize the head by placing one hand under the chin and resting the head against your body. Place a towel across the chest and over the shoulders.
4. The basin can be kept handy in the individual's lap or on a table placed in front of or at the side of the patient. A wheelchair may be positioned in front of the sink.
5. If the individual's lips are dry or cracked, apply a light coating of petroleum jelly or use lip balm.
6. Inspect the oral cavity to identify teeth in ill repair, pain, lesions, or inflammation.
7. Brush and floss the individual's teeth (use an electric toothbrush if possible, with sulcular brushing). It may be helpful to retract the lips and cheek with a tongue blade or fingers to see the area that is being cleaned. Use a mouth prop as needed if the individual cannot hold the mouth open. If manual flossing is too difficult, use a floss holder or interproximal brush to clean the proximal surfaces between the teeth. Use a dentifrice containing fluoride. Brush the tongue.
8. Provide the conscious individual with fluoride rinses or other rinses as indicated by the dentist or hygienist.

BOX 16.12 Tips for Best Practice

Providing Denture Care

1. Remove dentures or ask individual to remove dentures. Observe ability to remove dentures.
2. Inspect oral cavity.
3. Rinse denture or dentures after each meal to remove soft debris. Do not use toothpaste on dentures because it abrades denture surfaces.
4. Once each day, preferably before retiring, remove denture and brush thoroughly.
   a. Although an ordinary soft toothbrush is adequate, a specially designed denture brush may clean more effectively. (**Caution:** Acrylic denture material is softer than natural teeth and may be damaged by being brushed with very firm bristles.)
   b. Brush denture over a sink lined with a facecloth and half-filled with water. This will prevent breakage if the denture is dropped.
   c. Hold the denture securely in one hand, but do not squeeze. Hold the brush in the other hand. It is not essential to use a denture paste, particularly if dentures are soaked before being brushed to soften debris. Never use a commercial tooth powder because it is abrasive and may damage the denture materials. Plain water, mild soap, or sodium bicarbonate may be used.
   d. When cleaning a removable partial denture, great care must be taken to remove plaque from the curved metal clasps that hook around the teeth. This can be done with a regular toothbrush or with a specially designed clasp brush.
5. After brushing, rinse denture thoroughly; then place it in a denture-cleaning solution and allow it to soak overnight or for at least a few hours. (**Note:** Acrylic denture material must be kept wet at all times to prevent cracking or warping.) In the morning, remove denture from the cleaning solution and rinse it thoroughly before inserting it into the mouth. Use denture paste if necessary to secure dentures.
6. Dentures should be worn constantly except at night (to allow relief of compression on the gums) and replaced in the mouth in the morning.

in long-term care facilities. Among those responses are mobile dentistry for people with dementia and teledentistry and teletriage to provide consultations and care. Box 16.11 presents information on providing oral hygiene.

Older adults and those who may care for them should be taught proper care of dentures and oral tissue to prevent odor, stain, plaque buildup, and oral infections. All nursing staff should be knowledgeable about care of dentures (Box 16.12). Dentures are very personal and expensive possessions, and the utmost care should be taken when handling, cleaning, and storing dentures, especially in hospitals and long-term care facilities. It is not uncommon to hear that dentures were lost, broken, or mixed up with those of others, or not removed and cleaned during a hospital or nursing home stay. Dentures should be marked, and many states require all newly made dentures to contain the client's identification. Denture marking kits are readily available and provide a simple, efficient, and permanent means of marking dentures.

Broken or damaged dentures and dentures that no longer fit because of weight loss or changes in the oral cavity are a common problem for older adults. Many older adults believe that there is no longer a need for oral care once they have dentures, but regular professional attention is important. Rebasing of dentures is a technique to improve the fit of dentures. Ill-fitting dentures or dentures that are not cleaned contribute to oral problems (lesions, stomatitis) and to poor nutrition and reduced enjoyment of food.

Oral Hygiene in Hospitals and Long-Term Care

Oral care is an often-neglected part of daily nursing care and should receive the same priority as other kinds of care. Illness, acute care situations, and functional and cognitive impairments make the provision of oral care difficult. Factors contributing to less than adequate oral care include inadequate knowledge of how to provide care, lack of appropriate supplies, inadequate training and staffing, and lack of oral care protocols. When the person is unable to carry out a dental or oral regimen, it is the responsibility of the caregiver to provide oral care. Most nursing curricula offer limited training and education in oral care practices, and graduates therefore may be unprepared to implement nursing actions to promote oral health (Red & O'Neal, 2020).

In the acute care setting, good oral care is crucial to the prevention of ventilator-associated pneumonia (VAP), one of the most common hospital-acquired infections and a leading cause of morbidity and mortality in intensive care units (ICUs). Attention to oral care is essential in all settings but often not consistently implemented. Mouth care may be perceived as a comfort measure rather than a critical component of infection control (see Research Highlights box). In an observational study of oral hygiene care interventions provided by nurses to older adults in postacute hospital settings, oral hygiene care was supported in just over one-third of encounters. Denture care was inconsistently performed; also, nurses did not encourage adequate self-care of natural teeth by patients and infrequently moisturized tissues (Coker et al., 2017).

The use of therapeutic rinses (e.g., chlorhexidine) that are broad-spectrum antimicrobial agents has been shown to help control plaque and reduce VAP by 40% (Erickson, 2016). These can be used in conjunction with brushing or instead of brushing in those unable to tolerate brushing. A correlation between tongue coating and aspiration pneumonia risk points to the benefit of including tongue cleaning as part of mouth care.

Individuals residing in long-term care facilities are particularly vulnerable to problems with oral care because of functional and cognitive impairments. A large number are dependent on staff for the provision of oral hygiene. Older adults with dementia often resist caregiving activities associated with mouth care. Care-resistant behavior (CRB) is one of the primary reasons for the omission of mouth care (Hoben et al., 2017; Jablonski-Jaudon et al., 2016). Long-term care residents with dementia who exhibit CRBs are three times more likely to have more tooth decay than those who allow mouth care.

RESEARCH HIGHLIGHTS

Observations of Oral Hygiene Care Interventions Provided by Nurses to Hospitalized Older Adults

Purpose
The purpose of the study was to report on the actual oral hygiene interventions that nurses were observed to provide to patients in postacute hospital settings during their evening rounds.

Method
Five hospital sites in southern Ontario were used. Twenty-five registered nurses and registered practical nurses were shadowed during their evening care. Observations were recorded and then categorized during data analysis. In addition to observation, nurses were engaged in conversation, and these conversations were audiotaped with consent.

Results
Practices observed were inconsistent with existing evidence in practice guidelines. The most notable exceptions related to the frequency and timing of oral hygiene care, caring for patients with dentures, cleaning the oral cavity, and keeping tissues moist. Little more than a third of patients were supported to complete their oral care. Rinsing with mouthwash was rarely done, and the hospital-supplied mouthwash was not antibacterial and would have been ineffective. Practice guideline recommendation for twice daily oral care was not met.

Conclusion
The study of adequate and feasible oral hygiene interventions is urgently needed.

Data from Coker SE, Ploeg J, Kaasalainen S, Carter N: Observations of oral hygiene care interventions provided by nurses to hospitalized older adults, *Geriatr Nurs* 38(1):17–21, 2017.

Nurse researcher Rita Jablonski has researched CRBs and developed the MOUTh intervention (*M*anaging *O*ral *H*ygiene *U*sing *Th*reat reduction strategies) to prevent and minimize CRBs to provide mouth care to older adults with dementia. Components include (1) an evidence-based mouth care protocol; (2) recognition of CRBs; and (3) strategies designed to lower the perception of mouth care as a threatening, scary, or assaultive activity. Strategies include approach, establishing rapport, avoiding elderspeak (Chapter 6), gestures or pantomime, cueing, and chaining (initiating the action with the expectation that the individual will take over). For a link to a video demonstrating techniques, see Box 16.7. Techniques may be applicable to other activities that trigger CRBs, such as bathing (Chapter 26) (Jablonski-Jaudon et al., 2016).

Many long-term care institutions have implemented programs, such as special training of nursing assistants for dental care teams, dental care champions, providing visits from mobile dentistry units on a routine basis, or using dental students to perform oral screening and cleaning of teeth (Kohli et al., 2017). An important nursing role in all health care settings is to assist in the development of oral care protocols, staff education, and monitoring of oral health care. Caregivers of older adults at home who require oral care also need education about the importance of oral care and techniques for providing oral care.

Other Considerations in Oral Hygiene Provision

Tube feeding is associated with significant pathological colonization of the mouth, greater than that observed in people who received oral feeding. Individuals with dysphagia (Chapter 15) often receive inadequate mouth care and experience poor oral health (Jablonski et al., 2017). Recommendations are that individuals receiving tube feeding should have their teeth brushed twice a day, but techniques and safety have not been determined (Huang et al., 2017). In hospitals, nurses routinely provide mouth care to patients unable to swallow using toothbrushes connected to wall suction. In a pilot study, Jablonski et al. (2017) examined the effectiveness of using soft toothbrushes dipped in alcohol-free mouthwash for individuals with dysphagia in long-term care settings without access to suction equipment. The protocol resulted in improved oral hygiene without aspiration. Research into the oral hygiene status of non–oral feeding patients and optimal and safe oral care interventions for individuals with dysphagia and tube feeding is needed, especially in long-term care and home settings (Ohno et al., 2017). Foam swabs are available to provide oral hygiene but do not remove plaque as well as toothbrushes. Foam swabs may be used to clean the oral mucosa of an edentulous older adult.

SAFETY TIPS

Lemon glycerin swabs should never be used for oral care. In combination with decreased salivary flow and xerostomia, they inhibit salivary production, causing dry mouth and promoting bacterial growth.

KEY CONCEPTS

- Age-related changes, medication use, functional impairments, and comorbid medical and emotional illnesses place some older adults at risk for changes in fluid balance, especially dehydration.
- Dehydration is considered a geriatric syndrome that is frequently associated with common diseases (e.g., diabetes, respiratory illness, heart failure) and declining stages of the older adult who is frail.
- In older adults, dehydration most often develops because of disease, age-related changes, and/or the effects of medication; dehydration is not primarily due to lack of access to water.
- Prevention of dehydration is essential, but assessment is complex in older adults. Cues present differently than in younger individuals, and clinical signs may not appear until dehydration is advanced. Signs and symptoms may be nonspecific, making prevention and early identification of cues important.
- Age-related changes in the oral cavity, medical conditions, poor dental hygiene, and lack of dental care contribute to poor oral health. Poor oral health is a risk factor for dehydration; malnutrition; and a number of systemic diseases, including pneumonia, joint infections, cardiovascular disease, and poor glycemic control in type 1 and type 2 diabetes.
- Good oral hygiene and timely assessment of oral health are essentials of nursing care.
- Nurses may be involved in promoting oral health by teaching individuals or caregivers recommended interventions; screening for oral disease and making dental referrals; or providing, supervising, and evaluating oral care in hospitals and long-term care facilities.

NEXT-GENERATION NCLEX® (NGN) EXAMINATION–STYLE QUESTIONS

The nurse is caring for a 77-year-old patient with a history of type 1 diabetes mellitus, hypertension, and chronic migraine headaches who has been admitted with nausea and vomiting, a dry cough, and mild shortness of breath. Assessment reveals temperature of 101.9°F (38.8°C), blood pressure of 90/62 mm Hg, respirations of 20 breaths/minute, dry mucous membranes, crackles in the lungs bilaterally, and intermittent confusion about where she is (yet she can provide her name and age). The chest x-ray shows bilateral infiltrates.

Laboratory results include the following:

Test	Results	Normal Range
Hemoglobin	18	Male 13.5–17.5 g/dL Female 12–16 g/dL
Hematocrit	55	Male 42%–52% Female 37%–47%
White blood cells	22,000	$4.5–10.5 \times 10^9$/L
Sodium	150	135–145 mEq/L
Potassium	6.2	3.5–5.3 mEq/L
Chloride	115	98–106 mEq/L
Magnesium	4	1.5–3.0 mEq/L

Select from the word choices listed below to complete the sentence.

The current conditions that place the patient at the highest risk for an adverse outcome include _____ and _____.

Word Choices
hypokalemia
infection
dehydration
xerostomia
hypernatremia
dental caries
ventilator-associated pneumonia

NURSING STUDY

Hydration Status

Violet Barnes is an 87-year-old woman who resides in a skilled nursing facility. Her diagnoses include dementia, hypertension, and diabetes. She is able to walk and feed herself with assistance. She knows her name and responds to conversation appropriately, although she is not oriented to time or place. Two days ago, she underwent a colonoscopy on an outpatient basis in the hospital for a suspected mass in the large intestine. She was maintained on nothing by mouth (NPO) for 12 hours before the procedure and returned to the skilled nursing facility after the procedure. Since she has returned, she has become very lethargic and is not able to respond to familiar caregivers. She is refusing any food or fluids offered. She has had four episodes of diarrhea, and her stool is being tested for *Clostridium difficile*.

CLINICAL JUDGMENT QUESTIONS AND ACTIVITIES

Questions 1 and 2 refer to the Nursing Study.

1. What risk factors for Violet's condition are present in the Nursing Study?
2. What preventive interventions by nursing would have been appropriate for Violet?

3. What are your suggestions for enhancing fluid intake for individuals with dementia residing in skilled nursing facilities?

RESEARCH QUESTIONS

1. What is the knowledge level of older adults about oral health practices?
2. What factors influence adequate dental care among older adults?
3. What strategies are most helpful in enhancing fluid intake of older adults in long-term care facilities?

4. What are the barriers to adequate oral care for older adults in hospitals and long-term care facilities?
5. What content related to oral health is included in your nursing education program?

REFERENCES

Centers for Disease Control and Prevention (CDC): *Facts about older adult oral health* (website), 2021. https://www.cdc.gov/oralhealth/basics/adult-oral-health/adult_older.htm. Accessed April 2021.

Coker E, Ploeg J, Kaasalaninen S, et al.: Observations of oral hygiene care interventions provided by nurses to hospitalized older people, *Geriatr Nurs* 38(1):17–21, 2017.

Erickson LE: The mouth-body connection, *Generations*, 2016 40(3).

Gaspar P, Scherb C, Rivera-Mariana F: Hydration status of assisted living memory care residents, *J Gerontol Nurs* 45(4):21–28, 2019.

Gerontological Society of America: *Pandemic-driven disruptions in oral health* (website), 2021. https://www.johnahartford.org/dissemination-center/view/gsa-report-pandemic-driven-disruptions-in-oral-health-10-transformative-trends-in-care-for-older-adults. Accessed April 2021.

Hoben M, Kent A, Kogagi N, et al.: Effective strategies to motivate nursing home residents in oral care and to prevent or reduce responsive barriers to oral care: a systematic review, *PLoS One*, 12(6):e0178913, 2017.

Hooper L, Bunn DK, Abdelhamid A, et al.: Water-loss (intracellular) dehydration assessed using urinary tests: how well do they work? Diagnostic accuracy in older people, *Am J Clin Nutr* 104:121–131, 2016.

Huang S, Chiou C, Liu H: Risk factors for aspiration pneumonia related to improper oral hygiene behavior in community dysphagia persons with nasogastric tube feeding, *J Dent Sci* 12(4):375–381, 2017.

Jablonski RA, Winstead V, Azuero A, et al.: Feasibility of providing safe mouth care and collecting oral and fecal microbiome samples from nursing home residents with dysphagia: proof of concept study, *J Gerontol Nurs* 43(9):9–15, 2017.

Jablonski-Jaudon RA, Kolanowski AM, Winstead V, et al.: Maturation of the MOUTh intervention: from reducing threat to relationship-centered care, *J Gerontol Nurs* 42(3):15–23, 2016.

Kohli R, Nelson S, Ulrich S, et al.: Dental care practices and oral health training for professional caregivers in long-term care facilities: an interdisciplinary approach to address oral health disparities, *Geriatr Nurs* 38(4):296–301, 2017.

Masot O, Lavedan A, Nuin C, et al.: Risk factors associated with dehydration in nursing homes: a scoping review, *Int J Nurs Stud* 82:90–98, 2018. doi:10.1016/j.ijnurstu.2018.03.020.

McCrow J, Morton M, Travers C, et al.: Associations between dehydration, cognitive impairment, and frailty in older hospitalized patients: an exploratory study, *J Gerontol Nurs* 42(5):19–27, 2016.

Mentes JC: Managing oral hydration. In Boltz M, Capezuti E, Fulmer T, editors: *Evidence-based geriatric nursing protocols for best practice*, ed 4, New York, NY, 2012, Springer, pp 419–438.

Mentes J, Gaspar P: Hydration management, *J Gerontol Nurs* 46(2):19–28, 2020.

Namasivayam-MacDonald A, Slaughter S, Morrison J, et al.: Inadequate fluid intake in long term care residents: prevalence and determinants, *Geriatr Nurs* 39:330–335, 2018.

Ohno T, Heshiki Y, Kogure M, et al.: Comparison of oral assessment results between non-oral and oral feeding patients: a preliminary study, *J Gerontol Nurs* 43(4):23–28, 2017.

Oral Cancer Foundation: *Oral cancer facts* (website), 2021. https://oralcancerfoundation.org/facts/. Accessed April 2021.

Red A, O'Neal P: Implementation of an evidence-based oral care protocol to improve the delivery of mouth care in nursing home residents, *J Gerontol Nurs* 46(5):33–38, 2020.

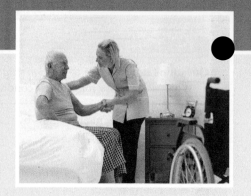

Elimination

Theris A. Touhy

http://evolve.elsevier.com/Touhy/TwdHlthAging

A STUDENT SPEAKS

My grandmother doesn't like to go out shopping with me anymore. She says she has to go to the bathroom all the time and can't walk fast enough to get to the bathrooms in the mall. She won't wear a protective garment or a pad because she says they smell. I hope I learn something in this class that will help her.

Molly, 20 years old

OLDER ADULTS SPEAK

"Being incontinent is like being a bad kid or a big baby."
"There's nothing that can be done. Well, I don't think there is anything else but a diaper."
"Sometimes I have to wet my bed before they get here, you know, and they are all busy and I have to wait for somebody."
"I do something that is very wrong. I try not to drink too much. How can you drink a lot, you would be soaked all the time?"

Comments from participants in a study of living with urinary incontinence in long-term care (MacDonald & Butler, 2007)

A NURSE SPEAKS

Urinary incontinence is a preventable and treatable condition and yet continence remains undervalued and UI remains underassessed. Even though UI is a basic nursing issue, nurses are not claiming it as one.

Comment from nurse in expert continence care (Mason et al., 2003, p. 3)

LEARNING OBJECTIVES

On completion of this chapter, the student will be able to:

1. Identify age-related changes and other contributing factors affecting bowel and bladder elimination.
2. Explain the types of urinary incontinence (UI) and their causes.
3. Identify risk factors for UI and accidental bowel leakage and describe appropriate nursing actions.
4. Use clinical judgment to recognize and analyze cues and identify and evaluate solutions and nursing actions to promote bowel and bladder health.

URINARY INCONTINENCE

Although some age-related changes (Box 17.1) in the renal and urological systems may contribute to UI (e.g. nocturia, frequent urination), UI should never be considered a normal part of aging and requires evaluation and treatment. Renal disease or urinary tract obstruction can amplify age-related declines. Nurses in all practice settings who care for older adults should be prepared to identify and analyze cues and use clinical judgment to implement nursing actions that promote continence.

UI is the involuntary loss of urine sufficient to be a problem. It is an important yet neglected geriatric syndrome. UI is a stigmatized, underreported, underdiagnosed, undertreated condition that is erroneously thought to be part of normal aging. Similar to other conditions experienced by older adults, many observed and reported cues of UI are ascribed to normal aging and accepted rather than being identified as indicators of the treatable condition.

BOX 17.1 Age-Related Changes in the Renal and Urological Systems

Kidneys

Decreased size and function begins in fourth decade; kidney is 20% to 30% smaller by end of eighth decade

Decrease in renal blood flow and glomerular filtration rate (GFR) (less pronounced in healthy individuals)

Diverticula of renal tubules in distal portion of nephron

Glucose reabsorption decreases (more glucose in the urine)

Decline in renal activation of vitamin D decreases intestinal absorption of calcium; more vitamin D is needed to counteract diminishing renal function

Ability to concentrate urine decreases; hyperkalemia more common; sudden large changes in pH or fluid load can quickly lead to hypervolemia or hypovolemia. These changes cause a high risk for adverse events if individual is exposed to changes in environment (high temperatures, renal-toxic medications) or to functional restrictions that limit ability to obtain adequate fluids

Ureters, Bladder, Urethra

Less tone and elasticity

Loss of bladder holding capacity

Total bladder capacity decreases to 300 mL from 600 mL

Urge to void occurs at lower bladder volume (160 to 300 mL)

Weakened contractions during emptying, which can lead to postvoid residual and increased risk for bladder infection

More urine produced at night; may be due to changes in circadian rhythm, output, or medications, or be indicator of sleep apnea

Increased collagen content, changes in gap junctions, increased space between myocytes, and changes in sensitivity of sensory afferents, all of which may contribute to involuntary bladder contractions and overactive bladder symptoms

Data from Gibson W, Wagg A: New horizons: urinary incontinence in older adults, *Age Ageing* 43:167–163, 2014; McCance K, Huether S: *Pathophysiology*, ed 7, St Louis, 2014, Elsevier.

BOX 17.2 Promotion of a Healthy Bladder

- Drink 8 to 10 glasses of water a day before 8 p.m.
- Eliminate or reduce the use of coffee, tea, brown cola, and alcohol, particularly before bedtime.
- Empty bladder completely before and after meals and at bedtime.
- Urinate whenever the urge arises; never ignore it.
- Limit the use of sleeping pills, sedatives, and alcohol because they decrease sensation to urinate.
- Make sure toilet is nearby with a clear path to it and good lighting, especially at night. Consider a grab bar or a raised toilet seat if there is difficulty getting on and off the toilet.
- Maintain ideal body weight.
- Get regular physical exercise.
- Avoid smoking.
- Seek professional treatment for complaints of burning, urgency, pain, blood in urine, or difficulties maintaining continence.

Without an adequate knowledge base of continence care and use of evidence-based practice protocols, nursing care will continue to consist of only containment strategies, such as the use of pads and briefs, to manage UI. Often, these are used out of convenience, nursing habit, patient preference, or lack of time (Colborne & Dahlke, 2017). Nurses are in a key position to generate solutions and take actions to enhance continence and improve function, independence, and quality of life. In addition, providing education about bladder health is an important nursing action for individuals of all ages (Box 17.2). There is a growing role for nurses in continence care, and advanced training and certification are available through specialty organizations such as the Society of Urologic Nurses and Associates and the Wound, Ostomy, and Continence Nurses Society.

Urinary Incontinence Facts and Figures

Because of the high prevalence and chronic but preventable nature of UI, it is most appropriately considered a public health problem. UI is more common in women than men by a ratio of 2 to 1. More than 50% of women and 25% of men ages 65 years and older, not residing in health care facilities or institutions, reported symptoms of UI of varying severities. The literature suggests that more than 70% of nursing home residents experience UI (McDaniel et al., 2020). UI is more prevalent than diabetes, Alzheimer's disease, and many other chronic conditions that have prompted more attention and treatment. The direct medical costs of UI are similar to those of coronary heart disease and higher than the costs of diabetes (Holtzer-Goor et al., 2015).

Risk Factors for Urinary Incontinence

UI is often the result of multiple risk factors (Box 17.3). "The maintenance of continence is complex and requires a functional lower urinary tract and pelvic floor, sufficient cognition to interpret the desire to void and locate a toilet, adequate mobility and dexterity to manipulate clothing and allow safe walking to the toilet, and an appropriate environment in which to allow this" (Gibson & Wagg, 2014, pp. 158–159). All of these factors need to be considered when recognizing and analyzing the range of cues contributing to UI symptoms.

Less than half of older adults with UI mention this problem to their health care provider. On average, women wait 6.5 years from the first time they experience symptoms until they obtain a diagnosis for their bladder control problems. Instead, they try to cope with the condition on their own, with variable success.

Individuals may not seek treatment for UI because they are embarrassed to talk about the problem or think that it is a normal part of aging. They may be unaware that successful treatments are available. Men may be unlikely to report UI to their primary care provider because they feel it is a woman's disease. Older individuals are less likely to receive evidence-based care for UI complaints than younger people (Hsu et al., 2016). Older adults want more information about bladder control, and nurses must take the lead in implementing approaches to continence promotion and public health education about UI.

Nurses are intimately involved in providing personal hygiene care and are often the ones to identify UI. However, studies have reported that nursing staff tend to view UI as an inconvenience rather than a condition requiring assessment and treatment. Negative attitudes toward the older adult population; lack of knowledge about UI; inadequate assessment, diagnosis, or proper documentation of the condition; and limited use of evidence-based protocols for UI contribute to inadequate assessment of UI.

BOX 17.3   Risk Factors for Urinary Incontinence

- Age
- Immobility, functional limitations
- Diminished cognitive capacity (dementia, delirium)
- Medications (those with anticholinergic properties, diuretics)
- Smoking
- High caffeine intake
- Low fluid intake
- Obesity
- Constipation, fecal impaction
- Pregnancy, vaginal delivery, episiotomy, forceps birth, large baby
- Environmental barriers
- High-impact physical exercise
- Diabetes, stroke, Parkinson's disease, multiple sclerosis, spinal cord injury
- Hysterectomy
- Pelvic muscle weakness, pelvic organ prolapse
- Childhood nocturnal enuresis
- Prostate surgery
- Estrogen deficiency
- Arthritis and/or back problems
- Malnutrition
- Depression
- Hearing or visual impairments
- Benign prostatic hyperplasia (BPH)

Older adults with dementia are at high risk of UI. Dementia does not cause UI but affects the ability of the individual to recognize the urge to void and to find a bathroom. Mobility problems and dependency in transfers are better predictors of continence status than dementia, suggesting that individuals with dementia may have the potential to remain continent as long as they are mobile and receive needed assistance to toilet. Drugs that increase urinary output and sedatives, tranquilizers, and hypnotics, which produce drowsiness, confusion, or limited mobility, promote incontinence by dulling the transmission of the desire to urinate.

Consequences of Urinary Incontinence

Elimination is a private matter, not publicized socially. In most cultures, children are taught early to deal with their own body waste. Deviations from this are socially unacceptable and can lead to chastisement, ostracism, and social withdrawal. UI affects quality of life and has physical, psychosocial, and economic consequences. UI is identified as a marker of frailty in community-dwelling older adults. UI affects self-esteem and increases the risk for depression, anxiety, loss of dignity and autonomy, social isolation, falls, skin breakdown, and avoidance of sexual activity (Ostaszkiewicz, 2017).

Older adults with UI experience a loss of independence and self-confidence and feelings of shame and embarrassment. In a survey of hospitalized older adults, 67% considered bladder and bowel incontinence to be a state the same as or worse than death. "Despite the value individuals place on being continent, many nurses do not consider incontinence to be a clinically important issue" (Ostaszkiewicz, 2017, p. 11). The psychosocial impact of UI affects the individual and family and professional caregivers. The provision of continence care to a dependent individual or an individual with cognitive impairment can be challenging and cause significant distress for both caregivers and care recipients. Continence care is frequently a trigger for agitation or aggression in individuals with cognitive impairment who may perceive intimate personal care interventions as frightening (Chapter 26).

Types of Urinary Incontinence

Incontinence is classified as either *transient* (acute) or *established* (chronic). *Transient* incontinence has a sudden onset, is present for 6 months or less, and is usually caused by treatable factors such as urinary tract infections (UTIs), delirium, constipation and stool impaction, and increased urine production caused by metabolic conditions such as hyperglycemia and hypercalcemia. Hospitalized older adults are at risk of developing transient UI and also may be at risk of being discharged without resolution of the condition. Use of medications such as diuretics, anticholinergic agents, antidepressants, sedatives, hypnotics, calcium channel blockers, and alpha-adrenergic agonists and blockers also can lead to transient UI. *Established* UI may have either a sudden or a gradual onset and is categorized into the following types: (1) stress, (2) urge, (3) overflow, (4) functional UI, and (5) mixed UI (Table 17.1).

TABLE 17.1   Types and Symptoms of Urinary Incontinence

Type	Symptoms
Stress	Loss of small amount of urine with activities that increase intraabdominal pressure (coughing, sneezing, exercising, lifting, bending) More common in women but can occur in men after prostate surgery or treatment Postvoid residual (PVR) low
Urge	Loss of moderate to large amount of urine before getting to toilet; inability to suppress need to urinate Frequency and nocturia may be present PVR low May be associated with overactive bladder (OAB) characterized by urinary frequency (>8 voids/24 h), nocturia, urgency, with or without urinary incontinence (UI). About half of individuals with OAB have urge UI
Overflow	Nearly constant urine loss (dribbling), hesitancy in starting urine, slow urine stream, passing small volumes of urine, feeling of incomplete bladder emptying; may be urge, stress, or mixed UI with high residuals PVR high
Functional	Lower urinary tract intact but individual unable to reach toilet due to environmental barriers, physical limitations, cognitive impairment, lack of assistance, difficulty managing belts, zippers, getting a dress up and undergarments down, or sitting on a toilet May occur with other types of UI; more common in individuals who are institutionalized
Mixed	Combination of more than one UI problem; usually stress and urge

USING CLINICAL JUDGMENT TO PROMOTE HEALTHY AGING: URINARY INCONTINENCE

Recognizing and Analyzing Cues

UI is more common and more severe in older adults and associated with sequelae not seen in younger people, such as increased risk for falls, fractures, hospitalization, and admission to long-term care. Cues to be examined will differ in older adults. A case-finding question about bladder and bowel problems (e.g., "Have you ever leaked urine/water?) is recommended as part of all interactions between older adults and clinicians (Shaw & Wagg, 2016). Health care personnel must begin to change their thinking about incontinence and acknowledge that it can be cured in about 80% of individuals (National Association for Continence, 2018). If it cannot be cured, it can be treated to minimize its detrimental effects. In older adults who are frail, interventions will improve UI in most cases, but complete continence may not be a realistic goal (Enberg & Li, 2017).

Recognizing and analyzing cues related to UI represent a multidimensional process targeted to identify continence patterns, alterations in continence, and contributing factors. If the individual is being admitted to a hospital, home care agency, or skilled nursing facility, it is important to document the presence or absence of UI, past continence patterns, the presence or absence of an indwelling urinary catheter, and the reasons for the catheter if present. Individuals in long-term care facilities should have an evaluation of continence on admission and whenever there is a change in cognition, physical ability, or urinary tract function. An environmental evaluation including the accessibility of bathrooms, the adequacy of room lighting, the availability of assistance, and the use of aids such as raised toilet seats or commodes is also important. The Minimum Data Set (MDS) 3.0 (Chapter 9) is used for continence assessment in the long-term care facility and provides an evidence-based overview of the important and relevant information to evaluate bladder continence based on the Medicare guidelines.

For individuals with UI, the nurse collaborates with the interprofessional team to (1) determine whether UI is transient or established (or both); (2) determine the type of UI; and (3) identify and document possible etiologies of the UI, including a review of risk factors (Spencer et al., 2017). Additional evaluation is presented in Box 17.4. Fig. 17.1 presents a bladder

---

BOX 17.4 Tips for Best Practice

Continence Assessment

Screening Questions
"Have you ever leaked urine/water? If yes, how much does it bother you?"
"Do you ever leak urine/water on the way to the bathroom?"
"Do you ever use pads, tissue, or cloth in your underwear to catch urine/water?"
"Do you dribble urine/water most of the time?"
"Do you have any burning, hesitancy, or pain with urination?"

Screening Instruments
Urogenital Distress Inventory–6
Incontinence Impact Questionnaire
Male Urogenital Distress Inventory
Bladder (Voiding) Diary (see Fig. 17.1)
    Kept for 3 to 7 days by the individual or caregiver
    Voiding record for even 1 day can be helpful

Patterns of Fluid Intake
Usual fluid intake over 24 hours
Types of fluids and time consumed
Decreased or increased urine output

Bowel Patterns
Frequency, consistency, straining
Use of laxatives

Exploration of Symptoms of Urinary Incontinence (UI)
When did UI start?
What have you done to manage the problem?
How often does it occur?
What things make it better or worse?
How severe is it?
Presence of voiding symptoms: hesitancy, straining, slow stream, intermittency, spraying
RED FLAGS: Hematuria, pain on urination

Focused History (Medical, Neurological, Gynecological, Genitourinary)
Review past health history: possible contributing factors to UI, pertinent diagnoses (heart failure, stroke, diabetes mellitus, multiple sclerosis, Parkinson's disease)

Medication Review
Review all medications, including over-the-counter (OTC), with focus on diuretics, anticholinergics, psychotropics, alpha-adrenergic blockers, alpha-adrenergic agonists, calcium channel blockers
Review use of alcohol

Focused Assessment
Screen for depression
Cognitive, functional

Observe Individual Using the Toilet
Ability to reach a toilet and use it, time it takes to reach the toilet, finger dexterity for clothing manipulation; character of the urine (color, odor, sediment); difficulty starting or stopping urinary stream

Physical Examination
Abdominal, rectal, genital: Assess for suprapubic distention indicative of urinary retention
Observe for signs of perineal irritation, itching, burning, lesions, discharge, tenderness, thin and pale genital tissues (atrophic vaginitis), dyspareunia, pelvic organ prolapse
Check for fecal impaction, tenderness

Other Tests That May Be Ordered
Urinalysis; culture and sensitivity if clinically significant systemic or urinary symptoms
If indicated, postvoid residual (PVR) (bladder sonography or catheterization) 16 minutes or less postvoid

Adapted from Shaw C, Wagg A: Urinary incontinence in older adults, *Med Older Adults* 45:1, 2016.

Bladder Diary ("Uro-Log")

Complete one form for each day for 4 days before your appointment with a health care provider. In order to keep the most accurate diary possible, you'll want to keep it with you at all times and write down the events as they happen. Take the completed forms with you to your appointment.

Your Name: _____

Date: _____

Time	Fluids		Foods		Did you urinate?		Accidents		
	What kind?	How much?	What kind?	How much?	How many times?	How much? (sm, med, lg)	Leakage How much? (sm, med, lg)	Did you feel an urge to urinate?	What were you doing at the time? Sneezing, exercising, etc.
Sample	Coffee	1 cup	Toast	1 slice	✓✓	med	sm	Yes (No)	Running
6-7 a.m.								Yes No	
7-8 a.m.								Yes No	
8-9 a.m.								Yes No	
9-10 a.m.								Yes No	
10-11 a.m.								Yes No	
11-12 noon								Yes No	
12-1 p.m.								Yes No	
1-2 p.m.								Yes No	
2-3 p.m.								Yes No	
3-4 p.m.								Yes No	
4-5 p.m.								Yes No	
5-6 p.m.								Yes No	
6-7 p.m.								Yes No	
7-8 p.m.								Yes No	
8-9 p.m.								Yes No	

Fig. 17.1 Bladder diary.

BOX 17.5 Resources for Best Practice

Assessing Continence: Video presentation of nurse conducting a continence assessment. https://www.youtube.com/watch?v=NHoZUFILEZs.

Catheter Out: Protocols, educational tools, toolkit. https://www.catheter-out.org.

Continence Product Advisor: Impartial advice for continence product users and health care professionals. https://www.continenceproductadvisor.org/.

International Continence Society: Educational materials, product guide, research, advocacy. https://www.ics.org/.

National Association for Continence (NAC): Comprehensive site for information on urinary and fecal incontinence for caregivers, professional clinicians, and individuals. Includes educational materials, management and treatment, resources, product guides. https://www.nafc.org/.

Safe Care Campaign: Preventing health care– and community-associated infections: urinary tract infections. https://www.safecarecampaign.org/.

Simon Foundation for Continence: Educational materials, resources, and products. Stool diary and Bristol Stool Form Scale. https://simonfoundation.org/.

diary useful in assessment of continence. Information on a video of a nurse conducting an evaluation for transient UI and other resources related to continence can be found in Box 17.5. More extensive examinations are considered after the initial findings are evaluated. Individuals who do not fit a simple pattern for UI should be referred promptly for urodynamic assessment.

Solutions, Nursing Actions, and Outcomes

Nursing actions focus primarily on the appropriate evaluation of continence, teaching about treatments, and implementation and evaluation of supportive and therapeutic modalities to promote and restore continence and to prevent incontinence-related complications, such as skin breakdown. The nurse should share appropriate resources and explain clinical information and differences in treatment choices. An important nursing role is to provide education to caregivers about UI and strategies to assist in practical and effective management (Box 17.6). Supportive and therapeutic modalities to promote and restore continence are discussed in the following section.

Lifestyle Modifications

Several lifestyle factors have been associated with either the development or the exacerbation of UI. These include increased fluid intake, smoking cessation, bowel management, avoiding caffeine and alcohol, physical activity, and weight reduction (if identified as contributing to UI) (See Research Highlights box). Women with stress UI who undergo a 5% to 10% weight loss experience a positive impact on UI symptoms. This is most likely due to the effects of reduced abdominal weight, intraabdominal pressure, and intravesicular pressure (Vasavada et al., 2021). The benefits of weight loss in older adults who are frail is more complex (Chapter 15). Good diabetic control to manage the hyperglycemic symptoms of osmotic diuresis and constipation management are also important.

BOX 17.6 Tips for Best Practice

Teaching About Urinary Incontinence (UI) Interventions

- Use therapeutic communication skills and a positive and supportive attitude to help individuals overcome any embarrassment about UI.
- Teach about the range of interventions available for management of UI.
- Share helpful resources for continence management.
- Share techniques found useful by others.
- Collaborate with the individual to help him or her choose the most appropriate and acceptable intervention based on needs.
- Assist individual to develop a detailed, realistic action plan and set goals.
- Determine an evaluation plan to assess the effectiveness of interventions.
- Review progress, identify any barriers to implementation, set alternative goals, or select alternate treatments if indicated.
- Reinforce effort and persistence.

From Wilde M, Bliss D, Booth J, et al: Self-management of urinary and fecal incontinence, *Am J Nurs* 114(2):38–45, 2014.

RESEARCH HIGHLIGHTS

Dancing to Treat Urinary Incontinence

Purpose

To evaluate the feasibility of using a combination of pelvic floor muscle exercises and virtual reality rehabilitation that involved dancing to treat mixed urinary incontinence (MUI) in older women.

Method

Participants were 24 women 65 years and older with at least 2 weekly episodes of MUI. Participants engaged in weekly treatment sessions and a home exercise program for 12 weeks. Evaluation was performed two times before and one time after the program. Effectiveness was evaluated through a bladder diary, pad test, symptom and quality of life questionnaire, and a satisfaction questionnaire.

Results

Results indicated that the frequency and quantity of urine leakage decreased and the patient-reported symptoms and quality of life improved significantly. About 91% of the participants were very satisfied with the treatment.

Conclusion

Further exploration of this type of combination therapy should be evaluated through further randomized controlled studies. The program was acceptable, efficient, and satisfying for the participants, encouraging exercise and social enjoyment while improving MUI.

Data from Elliott V, Bruin D, Dumoulin C: Virtual reality rehabilitation as a treatment approach for older women with mixed urinary incontinence: a feasibility study, *Neurourol Urodyn* 34(3):236–243, 2015.

Promotion of Continence-Friendly Environment

An evaluation of environmental, functional, and cognitive cues is important to determine factors that may affect the individual's ability to use the toilet in public settings, at home, and in the hospital and institutional settings. Observing the individual using the toilet should be included in any evaluation of UI. If the individual is in a hospital or institution, occupational therapists can be helpful in these assessments and provide suggestions and equipment for improved abilities (e.g., elevated toilet seat, grab bars).

Accessibility to toilets and the availability of toileting assistance in a timely manner are identified risk factors for UI, particularly for individuals in acute and long-term care facilities. Toileting aids such as grab bars, raised toilet seats, toilet visibility, signage, and images may be effective in older adults with cognitive impairment or visual-perceptual deficits. For those who are not able to go to the toilet independently, the availability of timely toileting assistance is critical to all other interventions for UI. In all settings, nurses play a key role in arranging the environment to facilitate toilet use and assisting the individual to maintain or return to continence.

Behavioral Techniques

Behavioral techniques, such as scheduled (timed) voiding, prompted voiding (PV), habit retraining, bladder retraining, and pelvic floor muscle exercises (PFMEs), are recommended as first-line treatment of UI. Because UI in older adults can have multiple precipitating factors, a single intervention may not be adequate, and more complex, multicomponent interventions may be required. Behavioral interventions have a good basis in research and can be implemented by nurses without extensive and expensive evaluation. Selection of a modality and interventions will depend on a comprehensive evaluation, the type of incontinence and its underlying cause, and whether the outcome is to cure or to minimize the extent and complications of the incontinence.

Scheduled (timed) voiding. Scheduled (timed) voiding is used to treat urge and functional UI in both older adults who are cognitively intact and those with cognitive impairment. The individual uses the toilet at fixed intervals, such as every 4 hours. The schedule or timing of voiding can be based on common voiding patterns (voiding on arising, before and after meals, midmorning, midafternoon, and bedtime).

Pelvic floor muscle exercises. PFMEs, also called Kegel exercises, involve repeated voluntary pelvic floor muscle contraction. The targeted muscle is the pubococcygeal muscle, which forms the support for the pelvis and surrounds the vagina, the urethra, and the rectum. The goal of the repetitive contractions is to strengthen the muscle and decrease UI episodes. PFMEs are recommended for stress, urge, and mixed UI in older women and have been shown to be helpful for men who have undergone prostatectomy. PFMEs also can be used to avoid an incontinence episode associated with urge UI.

Biofeedback may improve PFME teaching and outcomes, but further research is needed. Although biofeedback has long been used in medical offices, products are now accessible for people to use in the comfort of their own home, making effective training easier and more comfortable than ever. Medicare covers biofeedback for individuals who do not improve after 4 weeks of a trial of PFMEs. Reports of a study evaluating an app with instructions for PFMEs for treating stress UI suggest that it may be a feasible way to deliver high-quality care in a cost-effective manner to large groups of individuals (National Association for Continence, 2018; Sjöström et al., 2017). Box 17.7 presents a protocol for PFMEs.

Habit retraining. The individual's voiding pattern is identified, usually by means of a voiding diary (see Fig. 17.1). A schedule is then devised so that the individual uses the toilet to avoid UI episodes identified from the diary.

BOX 17.7   Pelvic Floor Muscle Training Exercises

Purpose
Prevent the involuntary loss of urine by strengthening the muscles under the uterus, bladder, and bowel.

Who Should Perform These Exercises?
Men and women who have problems with urine leakage or bowel control.

Identifying Pelvic Floor Muscles
When urinating, start to go and then stop. Feel the muscles in your vagina, bladder, or anus get tight and move up. These are the pelvic floor muscles. If you feel them tighten, you have done the exercise right.

   If you are still not sure you are tightening the right muscle, keep in mind that all the muscles of the pelvic floor relax and contract at the same time. Because these muscles control the bladder, rectum, and vagina, the following tips may help:

   Women: Insert a finger into your vagina. Tighten the muscles as if you are holding your urine; then let go. You should feel the muscles tighten and move up or down. These are the same muscles you would tighten if you were trying to prevent yourself from passing gas.

   Men: Insert a finger into your rectum. Tighten the muscles as if you were holding your urine; then let go. You should feel the muscles tighten and move up and down. These are the same muscles you would tighten if you were trying to prevent yourself from passing gas.

   Note: Nurses can teach correct muscle identification when performing a rectal or vaginal examination.

Pelvic Floor Muscle Exercises (PFME) Routine
1. Begin by emptying your bladder.
2. You can lie down, stand up, or sit in a chair.
3. Tighten the pelvic floor muscles and hold for a count of 10.
4. Relax the muscles completely for a count of 10.
5. Do 10 repetitions, 3 to 5 times a day.
6. Breathe deeply and relax your body when doing the exercises.
7. It is very important to keep the abdomen, buttocks, and thigh muscles relaxed when doing PFME.
8. After 4 to 6 weeks, most people see some improvement but it may take as long as 3 months. The regimen should be continued for 12 weeks.
9. After a few weeks, you can also try doing a single PFME contraction at times when you are likely to leak.

From US National Library of Medicine, NIH National Institutes of Health: *Pelvic floor muscle training exercises* (website), 2018. http://www.nlm.nih.gov/medlineplus/ency/article/003975.htm.

Bladder retraining. Bladder retraining aims to increase the time interval between the urge to void and voiding. This method is appropriate for individuals with urge UI who are cognitively intact and independent in toileting or after removal of an indwelling catheter. Bladder retraining involves frequent voluntary voiding to keep bladder volume low and suppression of the urge to void using PFMEs, distraction, or relaxation techniques. When the individual feels the urge to urinate, the urge control techniques are used. After the urge subsides, the individual walks at a normal pace to the toilet. The initial toileting frequency is every 2 hours and is progressively lengthened to 4 hours over the course of days or weeks, depending on tolerance.

Prompted voiding (PV). PV is a technique that combines scheduled voiding with monitoring, prompting, and verbal

BOX 17.8   Prompted Voiding Protocol: Long-Term Care

1. Contact resident every 2 hours from 8 a.m. to 9 p.m. (or the resident's usual bedtime).
2. Focus attention on voiding by asking if the resident is wet or dry.
3. Ask a second time if the resident does not respond.
4. Check clothes and bedding to determine if wet or dry. Give feedback on whether response was correct or incorrect.
5. Whether wet or dry, ask if the resident would like to use toilet or urinal.
If the resident says **YES**:
   Offer assistance.
   Record results on bladder record.
   Praise for appropriate toileting.
If the resident says **NO**:
   Repeat the question once or twice.
   If wet and declines to use the toilet, change him or her.
   Inform the resident you will be back in 2 hours and request that the resident try to delay voiding until then.
   If there has been no attempt to void in the past 2 to 3 hours, repeat the request to use the toilet at least twice more before leaving.
1. Offer fluids.
2. For nighttime management, use modified prompted voiding schedule, toilet when awake, or padding, depending on individual's sleep pattern and preferences.
3. If the individual who has been responding well has an increase in incontinence frequency despite adequate staff implementation of the protocol, further evaluation for reversible factors is indicated.

From Joseph Ouslander, MD, in-person communication, February 2016.

reinforcement (Box 17.8). The objective of PV is to increase self-initiated voiding and decrease the number of episodes of UI. The person is assisted to the toilet at predetermined times during waking hours if they request it and receives positive feedback for voiding successfully. PV is associated with modest short-term improvement in daytime UI in individuals residing in long-term care settings (Lai & Wan, 2017).

   Continence programs in long-term care facilities are required by Centers for Medicare and Medicaid Services (CMS) regulations. Monitoring and documentation of continence status in relation to implemented continence care is a quality-of-care indicator in this setting (Chapter 6). Individuals newly admitted to long-term care facilities who are incontinent (and able to use the toilet) should receive a 3- to 5-day trial of PV or other toileting programs. The trial can be helpful in demonstrating responsiveness to toileting and determining patterns of and symptoms associated with the incontinence. PV is also combined with functional intervention training in which direct caregivers incorporate strengthening exercises into toileting routines (Shaw & Wagg, 2016). Successful implementation of continence programs in long-term care requires a systems-based approach with consideration of individual-, group-, organizational-, and environmental-level factors.

Other Urinary Incontinence Management Techniques
Absorbent Products
Some individuals prefer to use absorbent products in addition to toileting interventions to maintain "social continence," and

a wide variety of products are available. Disposable types are available in several sizes, determined by hip and waist measurements, or as one size made to fit all. Many of these undergarments now look like regular underwear, and you even see them in stylish television commercials. Nurses should avoid the use of the word "diaper," since it is infantilizing and demeaning to older adults—the word "brief" is preferred. It is important that individuals are counseled to purchase proper continence products that will wick moisture away from the skin. These products are costly, but they protect skin integrity. Women may tend to use menstrual pads, but these do not absorb significant amounts of fluid. The National Association for Continence (see Box 17.5) provides comprehensive information on continence products.

Use of Intermittent Catheterization, Indwelling Catheters, and External Catheters

Intermittent catheterization is a technique used to manage involuntary loss of urine in individuals with urinary retention related to a weak detrusor muscle (e.g., diabetic neuropathy), those with a blockage of the urethra (e.g., benign prostatic hyperplasia [BPH]), or those with reflux incontinence related to a spinal cord injury. The goal is to maintain 300 mL or less of urine in the bladder. Most of the research on intermittent catheterization has been conducted with children or young adults with spinal cord injuries, but it may be useful for older adults who are able to self-catheterize. It provides an important alternative to indwelling catheterization.

Indwelling catheter use is not appropriate in any setting for long-term management of UI (more than 30 days), and there are specific criteria for acceptable reasons for an indwelling catheter (Box 17.9). Hospitalized older adults are more likely to have urinary catheters placed without indication, of which 50% have been shown to have been improperly used. Those with more care needs, cognitive impairment, and pressure injuries are at higher risk of catheter placement (Hu et al., 2017). Reasons for this include (1) convenience to manage UI; (2) lack of knowledge of risks associated with use and alternative

---

BOX 17.9 Appropriate Use of Indwelling Catheters

- Patient has acute urinary retention or bladder outlet obstruction
- Need for accurate measurement of urinary output in critically ill patients
- Perioperative use for selected surgical procedures: Urologic surgery or contiguous structures of the GU tract; anticipated prolonged duration of surgery (should be removed in PACU); patients anticipated to receive large-volume infusions or diuretics during surgery; need for intraoperative monitory of urinary output
- Assist in healing of open sacral or perineal wounds in incontinent patients
- Patient requires prolonged immobilization (potentially unstable thoracic or lumbar spine, multiple traumatic injuries such as pelvic fractures)
- To improve comfort for end of life care if needed

GU, Genitourinary; *PACU,* postanesthesia care unit.
From National Healthcare Safety Network: *Urinary tract infections catheter-associated urinary tract infection (CAUTI) and non-catheter-associated urinary tract infection (UTI) events* (website), 2021. https://www.cdc.gov/nhsn/pdfs/pscmanual/7psccauticurrent.pdf. Accessed April 2021.

---

treatments; (3) providers not tracking continued use; and (4) lack of valid continence assessment tools for older adults. Misuse of catheterization should be considered a medical error.

External catheters (condom catheters) are sometimes used in males who are incontinent and cannot use the toilet. Long-term use of external catheters can lead to fungal skin infections, penile skin maceration, edema, fissures, contact burns from urea, UTIs, and septicemia. The catheter should be removed and replaced daily and the penis cleaned, dried, and aired to prevent irritation, maceration, and the development of skin breakdown. If the catheter is not sized appropriately and not applied and monitored correctly, strangulation of the penile shaft can occur.

There is also an external female urinary collection device that is a feasible alternative to an indwelling urinary catheter or intervention for urinary incontinence and minimizes the risk for skin injury and infection. The collection device conforms to the perineal area between the labia and the urethra. The device is connected to low continuous suction providing a sump mechanism to collect and measure urine output. In addition, there is a continuous air flow promoting a microclimate environment to the perineum region (Beeson & Davis, 2018).

Pharmacological Approaches

Medications are not considered first-line treatment for UI but can be considered in combination with behavioral strategies in some cases. Behavioral therapy, alone or in combination with other interventions, is generally more effective than pharmacological treatments and should be the primary intervention (Balk et al., 2019). There are no pharmaceutical medications approved by the Food and Drug Administration (FDA) to treat stress UI. Low-dose estrogen administered vaginally to gently lubricate the tissues of the vagina also may be used to improve UI (National Association for Continence, 2018).

Pharmacological treatment (anticholinergic, antimuscarinic agents) may be indicated for urge UI and overactive bladder (OAB). Medication includes oxybutynin (Oxytrol, Ditropan, Ditropan XL), tolterodine (Detrol, Detrol LA), trospium chloride (Sanctura), darifenacin (Enablex), fesoterodine (Toviaz), and solifenacin (VESIcare) (National Association for Continence, 2018). All of these medications have similar efficacy in reducing urge UI frequency, and the choice of medication depends on avoidance of adverse drug effects, drug-drug and drug-disease interactions, dosing frequency, titration range, and cost. Beta-3 agonists (mirabegron) are a new class of medications for urge UI and OAB. They should not be used in individuals with severe uncontrolled hypertension, hepatic insufficiency, or bladder obstruction from BPH or in those taking antimuscarinic agents. These medications also can raise digoxin levels (Chapter 11).

Dosages of medications for urge UI and OAB should be started low and titrated with careful attention to side effects and drug interactions. A trial of 4 to 8 weeks is adequate and recommended. If one medication is not effective, another may be tried. Undesirable side effects of anticholinergic medications such as dry mouth and eyes, constipation, and cognitive impairment are problematic. People with narrow-angle glaucoma cannot use these medications, and they should not be combined with cholinesterase inhibitors. These medications can be especially problematic for those with cognitive impairment. None of these medications have been evaluated in older adults who are frail and should be considered only after all potentially remediable comorbid conditions and factors are evaluated and addressed and there has been an appropriate trial of behavioral and life-style interventions. With cautious use, there may be some benefit in pharmacological management of symptom control. Drug treatment generally should be avoided in individuals who make no attempt to use the toilet when assisted, become agitated when toileted, or are so cognitively and functionally impaired that there is no prospect for meaningful benefit (Enberg & Li, 2017).

Surgical Treatment and Nonsurgical Devices

Numerous surgical treatments for urge and stress UI are available for individuals when they are referred to a specialist. These include in-office urethral bulking agents, surgical placements of urethral slings and bladder neck suspensions for stress UI, and intradetrusor botulinum toxin injection. Nonsurgical injection of "bulking" material into the tissues around the urethra is a technique used to treat many UI issues such as OAB and male and female stress UI. The idea behind the injection therapy is to provide closure of the sphincter without obstructing it and therefore increasing the resistance to the outflow of urine. Multiple research studies have shown that in carefully selected patients, up to 80% of women become dry or improved after three treatment sessions. This is not a permanent solution, and repeated injections are necessary because the body absorbs the fluid over time (National Association for Continence, 2018).

For individuals with urge UI associated with OAB who have not responded to conservative or pharmacological therapies, sacral neuromodulation (SNM) may be recommended. SNM stimulates the sacral nerve root to control urination and can be an office-based 12-week treatment or a surgical implantation of a sacral neuromodulator system. Surgical SNM includes implantation of the Medtronic InterStim Therapy device, which is FDA-approved for bladder dysfunction, including UI and fecal incontinence, and has shown efficacy for decreasing symptoms of UI (El-Azab & Siegel, 2019). There is limited evidence on surgical treatments for UI in older adults who are frail; however, age alone is not a contraindication to surgical treatment (Enberg & Li, 2017; Searcy, 2017).

Nonsurgical Devices

There are a variety of intravaginal or intraurethral devices to relieve stress UI. These include intravaginal support devices, pessaries, external occlusive devices, and urethral plugs for women. For men, there are foam penile clamps. The pessary, used primarily to prevent uterine prolapse, is a device that is fitted into the vagina and exerts pressure to elevate the urethro-vesical junction of the pelvic floor. The individual is taught to insert and remove the pessary, much like inserting and removing a diaphragm used for contraception. The pessary is removed weekly or monthly for cleaning with soap and water and then reinserted. Adverse effects include vaginal infection, low back pain, and vaginal mucosal erosion. Another concern is the danger of forgetting to remove the pessary. An evaluation of the stress UI by the health care provider should be conducted to determine whether these devices would be helpful and the individual will be able to manage insertion and removal.

URINARY TRACT INFECTIONS (UTIs)

UTIs are the most common cause of bacterial sepsis in older adults and are 10 times more common in women than in men. The clinical spectrum of UTIs ranges from asymptomatic and recurrent UTIs to sepsis associated with UTI requiring hospitalization. There is significant disagreement in clinical practice as to what constitutes a UTI, and overdiagnosis of UTI is a significant problem in the older adult population. Recognizing and analyzing cues to UTIs in older adults is complex because signs and symptoms present differently, particularly in nursing home residents.

Cognitively impaired individuals may not be able to report symptoms, and nurses often rely on nonspecific signs and symptoms (lack of appetite, change in behavior) as indicators of UTI. It is widely believed that UTI in older adults can manifest atypically, but there is little evidence that nonspecific symptoms, when present in isolation, are reliable indicators of UTI (Johnson et al., 2021). The presence of nonspecific signs and symptoms in the absence of fever or urinary tract symptoms should trigger consideration of noninfectious conditions rather than a UTI.

Asymptomatic bacteriuria is transient and considered benign in older women. Significant bacteriuria and urinary symptoms are common, often occur together, and generally resolve spontaneously in noncatheterized, medically stable adults without structural or functional urinary tract abnormalities. Neither is linked strongly to serious urinary tract disease or to a likelihood of benefit from antibiotic treatment (Finucane, 2017). The American Geriatrics Society recommends that antimicrobials should not be used to treat bacteriuria in older adults unless specific urinary tract symptoms are present (American Geriatrics Society Choosing Wisely Workgroup, 2014). However, antibiotic treatment is common even though more than half of the antibiotics initiated for suspected UTIs are unnecessary or inappropriate (Crnich et al., 2017).

Urinalysis and screening urine cultures also should not be performed in individuals who are asymptomatic. As many as half of all positive urine cultures should be considered false positives for the presence of a UTI (Kistler et al., 2017; Johnson et al., 2021). The diagnosis of symptomatic UTI is made when the patient has both clinical features (painful urination, lower abdominal pain or tenderness, blood in urine, new or worsening urinary urgency or frequency, incontinence, and fever) and laboratory evidence of a UTI. Treatment is with antibiotics selected by identifying the pathogen, knowing local resistance rates, and considering adverse effects.

Catheter-Associated Urinary Tract Infections

Catheter-associated urinary tract infections (CAUTIs) are UTIs that occur in a patient with an indwelling catheter or within 48 hours of catheter removal. CAUTIs are one of the most common health care–associated infections (HAIs) in hospitals (Centers for Disease Control and Prevention [CDC], 2019). CAUTIs are the leading cause of secondary bloodstream infections and were among the first hospital-acquired conditions (HACs) targeted for nonpayment by Medicare in 2008. One of the goals of *Healthy People 2030* is to prevent, reduce, and ultimately eliminate HAIs, with an objective to reduce the rate of hospital admissions for UTIs among older adults.

Too often, catheters are inserted inappropriately and not removed in a timely manner. Continence evaluation and interventions are often lacking in acute care settings. Approximately 12% to 16% of hospital inpatients will have an indwelling catheter at some point during their hospitalization, and each day the catheter remains, a patient has a 3% to 7% increased risk of acquiring a CAUTI (National Healthcare Safety Network, 2021). Guidelines for appropriate catheter use are presented in Box 17.9. Recommendations to improve practice and decrease CAUTIs include appropriate use of indwelling catheters; standardized catheter removal protocols; catheter reminders, stop orders, nurse-initiated removal protocols; use of evidence-based guidelines to prevent CAUTIs: education of staff, patients, and families about CAUTI; and use of a urinary catheter bundle (Mody et al., 2017; Quinn et al., 2020). Box 17.10 presents Tips for Best Practice for prevention of CAUTI.

⚡ SAFETY TIPS

Long-term catheter use increases the risk of recurrent urinary tract infections leading to urosepsis, urethral damage in men, urethritis, or fistula formation. Indwelling catheters should be inserted only for appropriate conditions and must be removed as soon as possible, and alternatives should be investigated (e.g., condom catheters, intermittent catheterization, toileting programs).

BOX 17.10 Tips for Best Practice
Prevention of CAUTI: ABCDE

A Adherence to general infection control principles (hand hygiene, surveillance, aseptic catheter insertion, proper maintenance of a sterile, closed, unobstructed drainage system, and education)

B Be sure to use protocol in place to avoid unnecessary catherizations

C Condom catheters or other alternatives to an indwelling catheter such as intermittent catheterization should be considered in appropriate patients

D Do not use the indwelling catheter unless you must. Do not use antimicrobial catheters. Do not irrigate catheters unless obstruction is anticipated (e.g., as might occur with bleeding after prostatic or bladder surgery). Do not clean the periurethral area with antiseptics (cleansing of the meatal surface during daily bathing or showering is appropriate)

E Early removal of the catheter using a reminder or nurse-initiated removal protocol

CAUTI, Catheter-associated urinary tract infection.
From Centers for Disease Control and Prevention: *Healthcare-associated infections (HAI) progress report* (website), 2016. http://www.cdc.gov/hai/progress-report/index.html.

BOWEL ELIMINATION

Bowel function of older adults, although normally only slightly altered by the physiological changes of age (Box 17.11), can be a source of concern and a potentially serious problem, especially for older adults who are functionally impaired. Normal elimination should be an easy passage of feces, without undue straining or a feeling of incomplete evacuation or defecation. The urge to defecate occurs when the distended walls of the sigmoid and the rectum, which are filled with feces, stimulate pressure receptors to relax the sphincters for the expulsion of feces through the anus. Evacuation of feces is accomplished by relaxation of the sphincters and contraction of the diaphragm and abdominal muscles, which raises the intraabdominal pressure.

Constipation

Constipation is defined as a reduction in the frequency of stool or difficulty in formation or passage of stool. The Rome Criteria outline the operational definitions of constipation and should be used as a guide to diagnosis as well as a tool for teaching individuals about constipation (Box 17.12). Constipation is one of the most common gastrointestinal complaints encountered in clinical practice in all settings. Many individuals, both the lay public and health care professionals, may view constipation as a minor problem or nuisance. However, it is associated with impaired quality of life, significant health care costs, and a large economic burden. Constipation also can have very serious consequences, including fecal impaction, bowel obstruction, cognitive dysfunction, delirium, falls, and increased morbidity and mortality. Individuals with chronic constipation are

---

BOX 17.11 Age-Related Changes in the Bowel

Small Intestine
Villi become broader, shorter, and less functional; blood flow decreases
Proteins, fats, minerals (including calcium), vitamins (especially vitamin B_{12}), and carbohydrates (especially lactose) are absorbed more slowly and in lesser amounts

Large Intestine
Slowed peristalsis, blunted response to rectal filling, increased collagen deposition leading to dysmotility, fibro-fatty degeneration, and increased thickness of the internal anal sphincter

---

BOX 17.12 Rome III Criteria for Defining Chronic Functional Constipation in Adults

Two or more of the following for at least 12 weeks in the preceding 12 months:
- Straining with defecation more than 25% of the time
- Lumpy or hard stools more than 25% of the time
- Sensation of incomplete emptying more than 25% of the time
- Manual maneuvers used to facilitate emptying in more than 25% of defecations (digital evacuation or support of the pelvic floor)
- Fewer than three bowel movements per week

From Lacy B, Mearin F, Chang L, et al: Bowel disorders, *Gastroenterology* 150:1393–1407, 2016.

also at greater risk of developing colorectal cancer and benign colorectal neoplasms.

Constipation is a symptom, not a disease. It is a reflection of poor habits, delayed response to the colonic reflex, and many chronic illnesses—both physical and psychological—and a common side effect of medication. Diet and activity level play a significant role in constipation. Constipation and other changes in bowel habits also can signal more serious underlying problems, such as colonic dysmotility or colon cancer. Thorough evaluation is important, and these complaints should not be blamed on age alone.

Fecal Impaction

Fecal impaction is a major complication of constipation. Unrecognized, unattended, or neglected constipation eventually leads to fecal impaction. It is especially common in older adults who are incapacitated and institutionalized and those who require narcotic medications (e.g., end-of-life care). Symptoms and early cues indicating possible fecal impaction include malaise, loss of appetite, abdominal bloating or pain, nausea, vomiting, urinary retention, elevated temperature, incontinence of bladder or bowel, leaking of stool, alterations in cognitive status, fissures, hemorrhoids, and intestinal obstruction. Digital rectal examination for impacted stool and abdominal x-rays will confirm the presence of impacted stool. Continued obstruction by a fecal mass eventually may impair sensation, leading to the need for larger stool volume to stimulate the urge to defecate, which contributes to megacolon.

Paradoxical diarrhea, caused by leakage of fecal material around the impacted mass, may occur. Reports of diarrhea in older adults must be thoroughly evaluated before the use of antidiarrheal medications, which further complicate the problem of fecal impaction. Stool analysis for *Clostridium difficile* toxin should be ordered in patients who develop new-onset diarrhea, especially for those who live in a communal setting or have been recently hospitalized.

Removal of a fecal impaction is at times worse than the misery of the condition. Management of fecal impaction requires the digital removal of the hard, compacted stool from the rectum with use of lubrication containing lidocaine jelly. In general, this is preceded by an oil-retention enema to soften the feces in preparation for manual removal. Use of suppositories is not effective because their action is blocked by the amount and size of the stool in the rectum.

Several sessions or days may be necessary to cleanse the sigmoid colon and rectum totally of impacted feces. Once this is achieved, attention should be directed to planning a regimen that includes adequate fluid intake, increased dietary fiber, administration of medications if needed, and many of the suggestions presented later in the chapter for prevention of constipation. Protocols and policies for removal of a fecal impaction should be in place in all facilities.

For patients who are hospitalized or residing in long-term care settings, accurate bowel records are essential; unfortunately, they are often overlooked or inaccurately completed. Many older adults experience fecal impaction unnecessarily related to inadequate observation and monitoring of bowel function. Education about the importance of bowel function and the accurate reporting of size, consistency, and frequency of bowel movements should be provided to all direct care providers as well as to families caring for older adults in the home. This is especially important for individuals who are frail or experiencing cognitive impairment to prevent fecal impaction, a serious and often dangerous condition.

USING CLINICAL JUDGMENT TO PROMOTE HEALTHY AGING: BOWEL FUNCTION

Recognizing and Analyzing Cues

Identification of cues to altered bowel function and implementing nursing actions to promote bowel health represent an important nursing responsibility. Recognizing constipation can be a challenge because there may be a significant disconnect between the individual's definition of constipation and those of clinicians. Constipation has different meanings to different people. The recognition and analysis of cues begin with clarification of what the person means by constipation and discussion of the criteria for the diagnosis. It is important to note that alterations in cognitive status, incontinence, increased temperature, poor appetite, or unexplained falls may be the only clinical symptoms and early cues of constipation in individuals who are cognitively impaired or frail.

The precipitants and causes of constipation must be included in the evaluation of bowel function. A review of these factors also will determine whether the individual is at risk of altered bowel function and if any of the known risks are modifiable. It is important to obtain a bowel history, including usual patterns, frequency of bowel movements, size, consistency, any changes, and occurrence of straining and hard stools. However, recall of bowel frequency has been shown to be unreliable in establishing the presence of constipation. Having the individual keep a stool diary (Fig. 17.2) and monitoring stool consistency (described at the bottom of Fig. 17.2) will be more accurate. The Bristol Stool Form Scale (Lewis & Heaton, 1997) provides a visual description of stool appearance. Other important data to be obtained are presented in Box 17.13.

Solutions, Nursing Actions, and Outcomes
Nonpharmacological Treatment

The first action in evaluating constipation is to examine the medications the person is taking and to eliminate those that can cause constipation, preferably changing to medications that do not carry that side effect. Medications are the leading cause of constipation, and almost any drug can cause constipation. Nonpharmacological interventions for constipation that have been implemented and evaluated are as follows: (1) fluid and diet related, (2) physical activity, (3) environmental manipulation, (4) toileting regimen, and (5) a combination of these. Fluid intake of at least 1.5 L per day, unless contraindicated, is the cornerstone of constipation therapy, with fluids coming mainly from water.

A gradual increase in fiber intake, either as supplements or incorporated into the diet, is generally recommended. Fiber helps stools become bulkier and softer and move through the body more quickly. This will produce easier and more regular

STOOL DIARY

Complete this form for a week before your appointment with a healthcare provider. Use as many pages as needed. In order to keep the most accurate diary possible, you'll want to keep this with you at all times and write down the events as they happen. Take the completed forms with you to your appointment.

| NAME: |
| DATE: |

Date	Time	Incontinence Yes/No	Stool Seepage or Straining Yes/No	Stool Consistency 1-7 (See Below)	Urgency (unable to wait 15+ mins) Yes/No	Use of Pads Yes/No	Medications	Comments

STOOL CONSISTENCY Type 1: Separate hard lumps. Type 2: Sausage shaped but lumpy. Type 3: Like a sausage but with cracks on its surface. Type 4: Like a sausage or snake, smooth and soft. Type 5: Soft blobs with clear-cut edges (passed easily). Type 6: Fluffy pieces with ragged edges, a mushy stool. Type 7: Watery.

Provided by the National Association For Continence;
visit www.nafc.org for more information, locate a special special, and find support.

Fig. 17.2 Stool diary. (Available at https://static1.squarespace.com/static/597f302ed1758e9e17ad 4099/t/5aa656a3ec212d885d0665f1/1520850599951/Stool%2BDiary.pdf.)

BOX 17.13   Tips for Best Practice
Recognition and Analysis of Cues: Constipation

Sample Questions
- What is your usual bowel pattern?
- How many minutes did you sit on the bedpan or toilet before you had your bowel movement?
- How much did you have to strain before you had your bowel movement?
- Do you think you are constipated? If yes, why do you think so?
- Have you had any abdominal pain, nausea, vomiting, weight loss, blood in your bowel movement, or rectal pain?
- Have you had any bowel or rectal surgery?
- What type of physical activity do you engage in and how often?

Review of Food and Fluid Intake
Medication Review
- Include over-the-counter (OTC), herbal preparations, supplements

Psychosocial History
- With attention to depression, anxiety, and stress management

Review of Concurrent Medical Conditions
Other Measures
- Bowel diary
- Bristol Stool Form Survey

Focused Physical Examination
- Abdominal exam to detect masses, distention, tenderness, high-pitched or absent bowel sounds
- If these abnormalities are present, primary care provider should be contacted
- Rectal exam, following institutional policy, to identify painful anal disorders such as hemorrhoids or fissures, rectal prolapse, stool presence in the vault, strictures, masses, anal reflex

Other Tests as Indicated
- Complete blood count, fasting glucose, chemistry panel, thyroid studies
- Flexible sigmoidoscopy, colonoscopy, computed tomography scan, abdominal x-ray

From McKay S, Fravel M, Scanlon C: Management of constipation, *J Gerontol Nurs* 38(7):9–16, 2014.

bowel movements. High fiber intake is not recommended for individuals who are immobile or do not consume at least 1.5 L of fluid per day.

Physical activity. Physical activity is important as an intervention to stimulate colon motility and bowel evacuation. Daily walking for 20 to 30 minutes, if tolerated, is helpful, especially after a meal. Pelvic tilt exercises and range-of-motion (passive or active) exercises are beneficial for those who are less mobile or who are bedridden. Exercise and physical activity are discussed in Chapter 19.

Positioning. The squatting or sitting position, if the individual is able to assume it, facilitates bowel function. A similar position may be obtained by leaning forward and applying firm pressure to the lower abdomen or by placing the feet on a stool. Rocking back and forth while sitting solidly on the toilet may facilitate stool movement. Massaging the abdomen or rectum also may help stimulate the bowel.

Toileting regimen. Establishing a routine for toileting promotes or normalizes bowel function (bowel retraining). The gastrocolic reflex occurs after breakfast or supper and may be enhanced by a warm drink. Given privacy and ample time (a minimum of 10 minutes), many will have a daily bowel movement. However, any urge to defecate should be followed by a trip to the bathroom. Older adults dependent on others to meet toileting needs should be assisted to maintain normal routines and provided opportunities for routine toilet use. Box 17.14 presents a bowel training program.

Pharmacological Treatment

When changes in diet and lifestyle are not effective, the use of laxatives is considered. Use of these medications, both prescribed and OTC, is high. The extensive use of laxatives among older adults in the United States can be considered a cultural habit. In the past, weekly doses of rhubarb, cascara, castor oil, and other types of laxatives were consumed and believed by many to promote health. The belief that cleaning out the colon and having a daily bowel movement is paramount to maintaining good health persists in some groups. Providing information about normal bowel function, definition of constipation, and lifestyle modifications can assist in promoting healthy bowel habits without the use of laxatives.

If a laxative is indicated, there are several types with different actions and careful choice is important for older adults and needs to be based on symptoms and clinical status (Table 17.2). Older adults receiving opiates need to have a constipation prevention program in place because these drugs delay gastric emptying and decrease peristalsis. Correction of constipation associated with opiate use requires senna or an osmotic laxative to overcome the strong opioid effect. Stool softeners and bulking agents alone are inadequate.

Enemas. Enemas of any type should be reserved for situations in which other methods produce no response or when it is known that there is an impaction. Enemas should not be used on a regular basis. A normal saline or tap water enema (500 to 1000 mL) at a temperature of 105°F is the best choice. Sodium citrate enemas are another safe choice. Soapsuds and phosphate enemas irritate the rectal mucosa and should not be used. Oil

---

BOX 17.14 Tips for Best Practice
Bowel Training Program

1. Obtain a bowel history and establish a schedule for the bowel training program that is normal and comfortable for the patient and conforms to the patient's lifestyle.
2. Ensure adequate fiber and fluid intake (normalize stool consistency).
   a. Fiber
      i. Add high-fiber foods to diet (dried fruit, dried beans, vegetables, and wheat products).
      ii. Suggest adding 1 to 3 tablespoons of bran or Metamucil to the diet once or twice each day. (Titrate dosage based on response.)
   b. Fluid
      i. Consume 2 to 3 L daily (unless contraindicated).
      ii. Four ounces of prune, fig, or pear juice (or a warm fluid) may be given daily as a stimulus (e.g., 30 to 60 minutes before the established time for defecation).
3. Encourage an exercise program.
   a. Pelvic tilt, modified sit-ups for abdominal strength
   b. Walking for general muscle tone and cardiovascular system
   c. More vigorous program if appropriate
4. Establish a regular time for the bowel movement.
   a. Established time depends on the patient's schedule.
   b. Best times are 20 to 40 minutes after regularly scheduled meals, when the gastrocolic reflex is active.
   c. Attempts at evacuation should be made daily within 15 minutes of the established time and whenever the patient senses rectal distention.
   d. Instruct the patient about normal posture for defecation. (The patient normally sits on the toilet or bedside commode; for the patient who is unable to get out of bed, the left side–lying position is best.)
   e. Instruct the patient to contract the abdominal muscles and "bear down."
   f. Have the patient lean forward to increase the intraabdominal pressure by use of compression against the thighs.
   g. Stimulate the anorectal reflex and rectal emptying if necessary.
5. Insert a rectal suppository or mini-enema into the rectum 15 to 30 minutes before the scheduled bowel movement, placing the suppository against the bowel wall; or insert a gloved, lubricated finger into the anal canal and gently dilate the anal sphincter.

---

retention enemas are used for refractory constipation and in the treatment of fecal impaction.

 SAFETY TIPS

Sodium phosphate enemas (e.g., Fleets) should not be used in older adults because they may lead to severe metabolic disorders associated with high mortality and morbidity.

Alternative Treatments

Combinations of natural fiber, fruit juices, and natural laxative mixtures are often recommended in clinical practice, and some studies have found an increase in bowel frequency and a decrease in laxative use when these mixtures are used (Box 17.15). Although research is still limited, many modalities of complementary and alternative medicine, such as probiotic bacteria, traditional herbal medicines, biofeedback, and massage, are also used to treat constipation.

TABLE 17.2 Types of Laxatives: Actions, Use, Side Effects

Types of Laxatives	Actions, Use, Side Effects
Bulk-forming (e.g., psyllium, methylcellulose)	Usually first-line agents due to low cost and few adverse effects Do not use in presence of obstruction or compromised peristaltic activity Use with caution in older adults who are frail or bedbound and those with swallowing problems Must be taken with adequate fluid intake to avoid obstruction in esophagus, stomach, intestines Can cause abdominal distention and flatulence
Emollients and lubricants (e.g., docusate sodium, mineral oil)	Increase moisture content of stool Insufficient evidence to recommend docusate for prevention or treatment of constipation; may alleviate straining in selected patients who undergo rectal surgery or had myocardial infarction. Use with caution in older adults who are frail and may not have the strength to "push" when having a bowel movement since soft stool can accumulate in rectal vault The emollient laxative mineral oil should be avoided because of the risk of lipoid aspiration pneumonia
Osmotic laxatives (e.g., milk of magnesia [MOM], lactulose, sorbitol, polyethylene glycol [PEG], MiraLAX)	Cause water retention in the colon Avoid MOM in individuals with renal insufficiency since use can lead to hypermagnesemia or hyperphosphatemia Lactulose and sorbitol can cause diarrhea, abdominal cramping, and flatulence MiraLAX associated with less bloating and flatulence These medications can be added if bulk laxatives are ineffective
Stimulant laxatives (e.g., senna, bisacodyl)	Stimulate colorectal motor activity May cause cramping and electrolyte or fluid losses but when used appropriately, they are a safe and effective option, especially in those with opioid-induced constipation
Chloride channel stimulating (lubiprostone [Amitiza])	Stimulate ileal secretion and increase fecal water Generally safe, well tolerated, and effective in older adults with chronic constipation Side effects include nausea, diarrhea, headaches Expense of these medications may limit use except in individuals for whom other medications have failed or who have demonstrated intolerance to other agents

Data from McKay S, Fravel M, Scanlon C: Management of constipation, *J Gerontol Nurs* 38(7):9–16, 2014; Schuster B, Kosar L, Kamrul R: Constipation in older adults, *Can Fam Physician* 6(12):152–158, 2015.

BOX 17.15 Natural Laxative Recipe

Power Pudding

Ingredients
1 cup wheat bran
1 cup applesauce
1 cup prune juice

Directions
Mix and store in refrigerator. Start with administration of 1 tablespoon/day. Increase slowly until desired effect is achieved and no disagreeable symptoms occur.

ACCIDENTAL BOWEL LEAKAGE OR FECAL INCONTINENCE

Fecal incontinence (FI) is the involuntary passing of bowel movements, including solid stools, liquid stools, or mucus from the anus. There are two types of FI: urge incontinence and passive incontinence. With urge incontinence (the most common type), individuals feel a strong urge to have a bowel movement but cannot stop it before reaching a toilet. With passive incontinence, leakage of stool occurs without the individual being aware of it. The body may not sense when the rectum is full. FI can be transient (episodes of diarrhea, acute illness, fecal impaction) or persistent.

FI affects about 1 in 3 people who see a primary health care provider. Prevalence of FI varies with the study population: 2% to 17% in community-dwelling older adults; 50% to 65% in older adults in nursing homes; and 33% in hospitalized older adults. Age increases the prevalence of FI, but younger individuals also experience FI. Higher prevalence rates are found among patients with diabetes, irritable bowel syndrome, stroke (new onset, 30%; 16% at 3 years poststroke), multiple sclerosis, and spinal cord injury. Accurate estimates or prevalence are difficult to obtain because many people are reluctant to discuss this disorder and many primary care providers do not ask about it (National Institute of Diabetes and Digestive and Kidney Diseases, 2021).

Often FI is associated with UI, and up to 50% to 70% of patients with UI also carry the diagnosis of FI. UI and FI share similar contributing factors, including damage to the pelvic floor as a result of surgery or trauma, neurological disorders, functional impairment, immobility, and dementia. Bowel continence and defecation depend on coordination of sensory and motor innervation of the rectum and anal sphincters. Impairment of the anorectal unit, such as weakness from prolonged straining secondary to constipation, or overt anal tears seen after vaginal delivery in women (35%) are common causes of FI. Injury from obstetrical trauma is often delayed in onset, and many women do not manifest symptoms until after the age of 50 years. Fecal incontinence, like urinary incontinence, has devastating social ramifications for the individuals and families who experience it.

USING CLINICAL JUDGMENT TO PROMOTE HEALTHY AGING: ACCIDENTAL BOWEL LEAKAGE (FECAL INCONTINENCE)

Recognizing and Analyzing Cues

There is a great deal of stigma associated with FI, and individuals may feel ashamed and try to hide the problem. Using therapeutic communication and a positive and supportive attitude to help individuals overcome any embarrassment is important. An important point in assessment is the term chosen to describe FI. Although fecal incontinence is the most common terminology used, results of a large study of female patients showed that the term *accidental bowel leakage* was preferred over FI (Paquette et al., 2015).

Recognition and analysis of cues begin with a complete client history as in UI and investigation into stool consistency and frequency, use of laxatives or enemas, surgical and obstetrical history, medications, effect of bowel leakage on quality of life, focused physical examination with attention to the gastrointestinal system, and a bowel record. A digital rectal examination should be performed to identify any presence of a mass, impaction, or occult blood.

Solutions, Nursing Actions, and Outcomes

Nursing actions are aimed at assisting the individual in managing or restoring bowel continence. Dietary and medical management are recommended as first-line treatment options. Therapies similar to those used to treat UI, such as environmental manipulation (access to toilet), dietary alterations, habit training schedules, PFMEs, improving transfer and ambulation ability, sphincter training exercises, biofeedback, medications, and surgery to correct underlying defects, are effective. Simple treatments such as diet changes, medicines, bowel training, and exercises to strengthen pelvic floor muscles can improve symptoms by about 60%. These treatments can stop fecal incontinence in 1 in 5 people (National Institute of Diabetes and Digestive and Kidney Diseases, 2021). Providing resources and educational information is important and will help in

> ### BOX 17.16   Tips for Best Practice
> #### Nursing Actions for Accidental Bowel Leakage
>
> - Emphasize the importance of thorough evaluation.
> - Teach about the range of interventions available for management.
> - Share helpful resources for continence management.
> - Have individual keep a bowel diary and identify triggers. For example, if eating a meal or drinking a cup of coffee stimulates defecation, use the toilet at a given time after the trigger event. Have a regular toileting routine.
> - Encourage being prepared. Schedule outings, appointments, exercise routines around anticipated bowel patterns; suggest keeping a change of underwear, disposable underwear, clothing, and toileting supplies when out; use an absorbent pad and have bags to dispose of pad if soiled; fecal deodorants (over-the-counter pills that reduce the smell of stool and gas); wear darker clothing when away from home so that if soiling occurs, it will be less noticeable; when out, scan environment for toilet locations.
> - Keep a food diary to identify what foods and drinks affect FI. Avoid greasy and flatus-producing foods, dairy products, fruits with edible seeds, acidic citrus fruits, nuts, spicy foods, and other foods that trigger leakage. Bake or broil foods instead of frying; eat meals at regular times; eat after public events to reduce likelihood of leakage.

From National Institute of Diabetes and Digestive and Kidney Diseases: Fecal incontinence (website), 2017. https://www.niddk.nih.gov/search?s=all&q=fecal+incontinence. Accessed April 2021.

self-management (see Box 17.6). Other actions are presented in Box 17.16.

Pharmacological interventions may include the use of antidiarrheal medications and fiber therapy. Biofeedback also may be recommended, and some surgical options can be considered if conservative interventions are not successful. SNM also may be considered as a first-line surgical option and has been shown to reduce the frequency of episodes. Injection of bulking agents into the anal canal has been reported to reduce accidental bowel leakage, but guidelines suggest a weak recommendation for this treatment based on moderate-quality evidence (Paquette et al., 2015).

Further study is needed on these types of treatments. The effectiveness of interventions in FI will be self-evident but will take time. As in the treatment of UI, goals must be realistic. It cannot be stated too often or too strongly that nurses must always provide immaculate skin care to persons with incontinence because self-esteem and skin integrity depend on it.

KEY CONCEPTS

- Urinary incontinence is not a part of normal aging. UI is a symptom of an underlying problem and requires thorough recognition and analysis of cues to design nursing actions to promote bladder health.
- Urinary incontinence can be minimized or cured, and many therapeutic modalities that nurses can implement are available for treatment of UI. Behavioral and lifestyle approaches are first-line interventions.
- Health promotion teaching, identification of risk factors, comprehensive evaluation of UI, education of informal and formal caregivers, and use of evidence-based interventions are basic continence competencies for nurses.

- Nonpharmacological treatments (PFMEs, PV, bladder training, timed voiding, lifestyle modifications) are first-line treatments for UI.
- Asymptomatic bacteriuria is common in older women and does not need treatment.
- Indwelling catheter use is not appropriate in any setting for long-term management (>30 days) of UI except in certain clinical conditions. Proper insertion, care, and timely removal of indwelling catheters can reduce the number of CAUTIs.
- Evaluation and management of bowel function are important nursing responsibilities. The precipitants and causes of constipation must be included in the evaluation of bowel

function. Increased fluid intake, changes in diet, physical activity, bowel training programs, and review of medications with constipation side effects are important nonpharmacological interventions.

- A number of interventions for urinary incontinence are applicable to the management of fecal incontinence.

NEXT-GENERATION NCLEX® (NGN) EXAMINATION–STYLE QUESTIONS

Case Study 1

The assistive personnel report that Ms. Miller, an 87-year-old resident, has a change in her response level. Ms. Miller has late-stage Alzheimer's disease, hypertension, and osteoporosis. On regular days, she will attempt to speak to the staff even though her speech is garbled. She enjoys sitting up in bed or in a chair next to someone and listening to music. Upon assessment, Ms. Miller opens her eyes when her name is called but otherwise does not respond to verbal stimuli. Her blood pressure is 140/60 mm Hg, heart rate is 74 beats/minute, rhythm is regular, respiratory rate is even with 18 breaths/minute, temperature 98.9°F, with oxygen saturation of 95% on room air. Lungs sounds are clear to auscultation throughout lung fields, bowel sounds are hypoactive, abdomen is slightly distended, and Ms. Miller grunts with abdominal palpation. Ms. Miller has no peripheral edema, and her skin is warm, dry, and intact. Intake and output records from yesterday show a small bowel movement with each void and 50% meal intake. Laboratory results include:

- Blood urea nitrogen (BUN)/creatinine is 22 mg/dL and 1.6 mg/dL.
- Sodium (Na)/chloride (Cl) is 145 mmol/L and 105 mmol/L.
- Glucose is 105 mg/dL.
- Urine is amber and clear, pH 5.0, nitrite negative and leukocyte esterase trace, blood negative, white blood cells (WBCs) 2/high power field (hpf), and bacteria occasional.

Highlight the assessment data that require follow-up by the nurse.

Case Study 2

Ms. Franklin, 68 years old, is seen in the clinic for urinary incontinence. Her history includes hypertension, type 2 diabetes, and osteoarthritis, treated with lisinopril/hydrochlorothiazide 20 mg/25 mg daily, glipizide/metformin 2.5 mg/500 mg twice a day, and celecoxib 200 mg daily. She states that she delayed seeking care because she felt uncomfortable talking to her health care provider about the issue and thought all women experienced incontinence. The problem has worsened; she leaks through her incontinence liner pads at times. Two of her daughters convinced her to come to the clinic for treatment. Upon further questioning by the nurse, it is revealed that Ms. Franklin has reduced her caffeine intake to one cup of coffee per day but has also decreased her overall fluid intake to reduce her incontinence. When asked to describe her incontinence, she states that she loses urine before she can make it to the bathroom, and she needs to urinate frequently. She also gets up to use the bathroom several times each night. She states that her last bowel movement was this morning after breakfast; she normally has a soft bowel movement each day. Ms. Franklin's vital signs are blood pressure 125/82 mm Hg, heart rate 88 beats/minute, respirations 14 breaths/minute, temperature 97.9°F. She is 5′4″ and weighs 200 pounds. Her laboratory results include:

- BUN/creatinine is 22 mg/dL and 1.6 mg/dL.
- Na/Cl is 145 mmol/L and 105 mmol/L.
- Glucose is 115 mg/dL.
- Urine is amber and clear, pH 5.0, nitrite negative and leukocyte esterase negative, red blood cells (RBCs) 2/hpf, WBC 2/hpf, and bacteria negative.

Use an X to indicate which actions listed in the left column of the chart that follows would be included in the plan of care.

Actions	Plan of Care
Ask client to complete a 3-day bladder diary.	
Teach client to progressively lengthen toileting frequency to every 4 hours.	
Use a 3-day trial of prompted voiding combined with the use of absorbent products.	
Teach client pelvic floor muscle exercises.	
Encourage intake of 2 L of fluid per day.	
Reduce weight by 10%.	
Encourage client to use over-the-counter laxatives to maintain routine bowel movements.	

NURSING STUDY

Continence

Helen is an 80-year-old woman who lives in her own apartment in an assisted living residence. Helen is the mother of four adult children, whom she sees often, and enjoys family activities. She is independent in all activities of daily living and walks with a cane. She has osteoarthritis of the knees, and although she walks slowly, she is able to get around without any difficulty. Helen is 5 feet, 2 inches tall and weighs 150 pounds. She takes an antihypertensive medication and a diuretic. She has come to see the nurse practitioner in the on-site clinic for an annual physical examination. While the nurse practitioner is obtaining Helen's health history, he asks Helen if she has any problems with control of her urine, such as leaking or not getting to the bathroom before she loses urine. Helen replies: "Sometimes I do have some leaking of urine because I can't get to the bathroom quickly enough, so I wear a pad. It also sometimes happens when I cough or sneeze, but I don't think at my age there is much that can be done about that."

CLINICAL JUDGMENT QUESTIONS AND ACTIVITIES

Questions apply to Nursing Study: Continence.

1. What are the risk factors for UI in this situation?
2. What should be included in a more comprehensive assessment of Helen's stated problems with urine control?
3. What type of UI do you think Helen is experiencing?
4. What type of behavioral interventions might be helpful for Helen so that she has better urine control?
5. What health teaching would you provide to Helen related to urinary problems of older women?
6. What resources would you suggest for Helen to help her be more informed about her urine control concerns and how to manage them?

NURSING STUDY

Constipation

Stella, at age 78, has never had problems with her bowel movements. They have been regular—each morning about an hour after breakfast. In fact, she hardly thought about them because they had been so regular. While hospitalized for podiatric surgery last year, she never regained her usual pattern of bowel function. She was greatly distressed by this because it had been a symbol to her of her good health. Admittedly, she did not move about as much after the surgery, or as well, and had begun to use a cane. And she had heard that pain medications sometimes make one constipated, so she tried to use them sparingly despite the pain. She tried to reestablish her pattern of having a bowel movement every morning after breakfast but with little success. She then began to worry about constipation and to use laxatives. She thought, "This constipation really upsets me. I just don't feel like myself if I don't have a bowel movement every day."

CLINICAL JUDGMENT QUESTIONS AND ACTIVITIES

Questions apply to Nursing Study: Constipation.

1. What information will you need to obtain from Stella to help her determine the causes of her constipation?
2. What advice will you give Stella regarding the use of laxatives?
3. What dietary changes will you suggest to her, and how will you do this to encourage modifications?
4. What information regarding the relationships of medications to constipation will be useful to Stella?

RESEARCH QUESTIONS

1. Do childhood toilet training experiences and beliefs about elimination affect one's elimination functions later in life? How do these experiences vary across different cultures?
2. What is the knowledge level of graduating nursing students and practicing nurses in UI care?
3. What factors are associated with effective implementation and maintenance of PV programs in long-term care?
4. What are some of the reasons individuals do not seek professional help for incontinence concerns?
5. What types of techniques do individuals use to manage their incontinence problems and what is their level of satisfaction with the techniques?
6. How are decisions made by community-living individuals about the types of incontinence products to buy?
7. What are the specific concerns of older adults related to constipation?
8. What is the knowledge level of young, middle-aged, and older individuals about normal bowel function?

REFERENCES

American Geriatrics Society Choosing Wisely Workgroup: American Geriatrics Society identifies another five things that healthcare providers and patients should question, *J Am Geriatr Soc* 62(5):950–960, 2014.

Balk E, Rofeberg V, Adam G, et al. Pharmacological and nonpharmacological treatments for urinary incontinence in women: a systematic review and network meta-analysis of clinical outcomes, *Ann Intern Med* 170(7):465–479, 2019.

Beeson T, Davis C: Urinary management with an external female collection device, *J Wound Ostomy Continence Nurs* 45(2):187–189, 2018.

Centers for Disease Control and Prevention (CDC): *National and state healthcare-associated infections (HAI) progress report* (website), 2019. https://www.cdc.gov/hai/data/portal/progress-report.html. Accessed June 2021.

Colborne M, Dahlke S: Nurses' perceptions and management of urinary incontinence in hospitalized older adults, *J Gerontol Nurs* 43(10):46–55, 2017.

Crnich CJ, Jump RL, Nace DA: Improving management of urinary tract infections in older adults: a paradigm shift or therapeutic nihilism? *J Am Geriatr Soc* 65:1661–1663, 2017.

El-Azab AS, Siegel SW: Sacral neuromodulation for female pelvic floor disorders, *Arab J Urol* 17(1):14–22, 2019.

Enberg S, Li H: Urinary incontinence in frail older adults, *Urologic Nurs* 37(3):119–124, 2017.

Finucane TE: Urinary tract infection—requiem for a heavyweight, *J Am Geriatr Soc* 65:1650–1655, 2017.

Gibson W, Wagg A: New horizons: urinary incontinence in older adults, *Age Ageing* 43:157–163, 2014.

Holtzer-Goor KM, Gaultney JG, van Houten P, et al.: Cost-effectiveness of including a nurse specialist in the treatment of urinary incontinence in primary care in the Netherlands, *PLoS One*, 2015 10(10):e0138225.

Hsu A, Suskind A, Huang AJ: Urinary incontinence among older adults editor. In Lindquist L, editor: *New directions in geriatric medicine*, New York, 2016, Springer, pp 49–69.

Hu F, Chuan-Hsiu T, Huey-Shyan L, et al.: Inappropriate urinary catheter reinsertion in hospitalized older patients, *Am J Infect Control* 45(1):8–12, 2017.

Johnson M, Kleinpell R, Hulgan T, et al.: Evaluation of the management of UTIs in cognitively impaired older women in LTC, *Ann Longterm Care* 29(1):11–17, 2021.

Kistler CE, Zimmerman S, Scales K, et al.: The antibiotic prescribing pathway for presumed urinary tract infections in nursing home residents, *J Am Geriatr Soc* 65:1719–1725, 2017.

Lai CKY, Wan X: Using prompted voiding to manage urinary incontinence in nursing homes: can it be sustained? *J Am Med Dir Assoc* 18(6):509–514, 2017.

Lewis SJ, Heaton KW: Stool form scale as a useful guide to intestinal transit time, *Scand J Gastroenterol* 32:920–924, 1997.

Mason DJ, Newman DK, Palmer MH: Changing UI practice, *Am J Nurs* 103:129, 2003.

McDaniel C, Ratnani I, Fatima S, et al.: Urinary incontinence in older adults takes collaborative nursing efforts to improve, *Cureus* 12(7):e9161, 2020. doi:10.7759/cureus.9161.

MacDonald C, Butler L: Silent no more: elderly women's stories of living with urinary incontinence in long-term care, *J Gerontol Nurs* 33:14–20, 2007.

Mody L, Greene MT, Meddings J, et al.: A national implementation program to prevent catheter-associated urinary tract infection in nursing home residents, *JAMA Intern Med* 177(8):1154–1162, 2017.

National Association for Continence: *Urinary incontinence overview, facts and statistics* (website), 2018. https://www.nafc.org/urinary-incontinence/. Accessed April 2021.

National Healthcare Safety Network: *Urinary tract infections (catheter-associated urinary tract infection [CAUTI] and non-catheter-associated urinary tract infection [UTI] events)* (website), 2021. https://www.cdc.gov/nhsn/pdfs/pscmanual/7psccauticurrent.pdf. Accessed April 2021.

National Institute of Diabetes and Digestive and Kidney Diseases: Fecal incontinence (website), n.d. https://www.niddk.nih.gov/search?s=all&q=fecal+incontinence. Accessed April 2021.

Ostaszkiewicz J: A conceptual model of the risk of elder abuse posed by incontinence and care dependence, *Int J Older People Nurs* 13(2):e12182, 2017.

Paquette IM, Varma MG, Kaiser AM, et al.: The American Society of Colon and Rectal Surgeons clinical practice guideline for the treatment of fecal incontinence, *Dis Colon Rectum* 58:623–636, 2015.

Quinn M, Ameling JM, Forman J, et al.: Persistent barriers to timely catheter removal identified from clinical observation and interviews, *Jt Comm J Qual Patient Saf* 46(2):99–108, 2020.

Searcy JAR: Geriatric urinary incontinence, *Nurs Clin North Am* 52:447–455, 2017.

Shaw C, Wagg A: Urinary incontinence in older adults, *Med Older Adults*, 2016 45(1).

Sjöström M, Lindholm L, Samuelsson E: Mobile app for treatment of stress urinary incontinence: a cost-effectiveness analysis, *J Med Internet Res* 19(5):e154, 2017.

Spencer M, McManus K, Sabourin J: Incontinence in older adults: the role of the geriatric multidisciplinary team, *BC Med J* 59(2):99–105, 2017.

Vasavada S, Kim D, Carmel M, et al: *What is the role of weight loss in urinary incontinence treatment?* (website), 2021. https://www.medscape.com/answers/452289-172486/what-is-the-role-of-weight-loss-in-urinary-incontinence-treatment. Accessed June 2021.

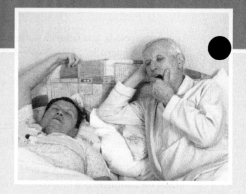

Sleep

Lenny Chiang-Hanisko, Theris A. Touhy

http://evolve.elsevier.com/Touhy/TwdHlthAging

A STUDENT SPEAKS

I am so stressed and tired all the time in this nursing program. The workload is so intense there is never enough time to sleep. When I have any time, I would go to bed at 7 p.m. and sleep until 11 in the morning if I could. When will I ever feel rested and not tired?

Marybeth, 22 years old

AN OLDER ADULT SPEAKS

The years have changed my sleep patterns. Bedtime rituals take longer. Nature wakens me two or three times a night for trips to the bathroom. Sleep returns at once unless my mind turns on and it gets launched on a needless project. The earlier remedies are called on to slow down the activities, or the next day is a disaster. My 90-year-old aunt, who slept very little and lightly and lay awake many nights, said she went to the bathroom several times just for something to do instead of just lying there.

Ricarda, 80 years old

LEARNING OBJECTIVES

Upon completion of this chapter, the reader will be able to:

1. Identify factors that affect sleep as we age.
2. Describe the signs, symptoms, treatment, and nursing actions for sleep disorders: insomnia, obstructive sleep apnea, restless legs syndrome/Willis-Ekbom disease, rapid eye movement sleep behavior disorder, circadian rhythm sleep disorder.
3. Use clinical judgment to identify and evaluate solutions and nursing actions for promotion of healthy sleep.
4. Educate individuals, families, and health care staff about sleep disorders and sleep hygiene measures.

Sleep is a basic need. Sleep occupies one-third of our lives and is a vital function that affects cognition and performance. Sleep is also a barometer of health, and attention to sleep and actions to address sleep concerns should receive as much attention as other vital signs. Research into the physiology of sleep suggests that the restorative function of sleep may be a consequence of the enhanced removal of potentially neurotoxic waste products that accumulate in the awake central nervous system.

Short sleep duration (6 hours or less per 24-hour period) and long sleep duration (≥9 to 10 hours per 24-hour period) are both associated with adverse health outcomes. At a population level, the optimal sleep duration in adults for good health is 7 to 9 hours, although individual variability exists. Gender differences exist in sleep disturbances, and sleep disturbances may be more common in women (World Association of Sleep Medicine, 2021). Sleep disturbance and deficiency have been linked with dementia and all-cause mortality. Poor sleep quality, difficulty maintaining alertness, and routine napping also contributed to risk of all-cause mortality. A recent study reported that sleeping fewer than 5 hours a night was associated with a twofold greater risk for incident dementia and that routinely taking 30 minutes or longer to fall asleep was associated with a 45% greater risk for incident dementia (Robbins et al., 2021).

Sleep problems constitute a global epidemic that threatens health and quality of life for up to 45% of the world's population. Because of the public health burden of chronic sleep loss and sleep disorders and the low awareness of poor sleep health, *Healthy People 2030* includes sleep health as a special topic area. The goal is to improve health, productivity, well-being, quality of life, and safety by helping people get enough sleep. Additional objectives are outlined in the Healthy People 2030 box.

❤ HEALTHY PEOPLE 2030

Sleep Health

Increase the proportion of adults with sleep apnea symptoms who get evaluated by a health care provider.
Increase the proportion of adults who get enough sleep.
Reduce the rate of motor vehicle crashes due to drowsy driving.

Data from US Department of Health and Human Services: *Healthy People 2030* (website), 2020. https://health.gov/healthypeople.

BIORHYTHM AND SLEEP

Our lives proceed in a series of rhythms that influence and regulate physiological function, chemical concentrations, performance, behavioral responses, moods, and the ability to adapt. It is clear that body temperature, pulse rate, blood pressure, and hormonal levels change significantly and predictably in a circadian rhythm. Circadian rhythms are linked to the 24-hour day by time cues (zeitgebers), the most important of which is the light-dark cycle. Biorhythms vary between individuals, and age-related changes in biorhythms (circadian rhythms) are relevant to health and the process of aging. With aging, there is a reduction in the amplitude of all circadian endogenous responses (e.g., body temperature, pulse rate, blood pressure, hormonal levels). Disruption of the circadian system is also associated with diseases like diabetes, cancer, and Alzheimer's.

The most important biorhythm is the circadian sleep-wake rhythm. As people age, the natural circadian rhythm may become less responsive to external stimuli, such as changes in light during the course of the day. The brain's ability to clear a protein (beta-amyloid) closely linked with Alzheimer's disease (Chapter 25) is tied to the circadian cycle. Recent research findings suggest that healthy sleep habits may prevent the protein from building up in the brain and open a path to potential Alzheimer's therapies. Taking care of our sleep or circadian rhythms by practicing good sleep hygiene (e.g., no bright lights at night, no TVs on while you sleep) may contribute to reducing the amyloid buildup over the lifespan, reducing the symptoms of Alzheimer's or delaying onset or progression of the disease (Clark et al., 2022). Actions to improve sleep hygiene are discussed later in the chapter.

SLEEP AND AGING

The predictable pattern of normal sleep is called sleep architecture. The body progresses through stages of sleep consisting of rapid eye movement (REM) sleep and non-rapid eye movement (NREM) sleep. Most of the changes in sleep architecture in healthy adults begin between the ages of 40 and 60 years. The age-related changes include less time spent in N3 sleep (formerly called stages 3 and 4) (slow wave sleep) and more time spent awake or in N1 sleep (formerly called stage 1). The changes contribute to fragmented sleep and early awakening (Suzuki et al., 2017). Declines in N3 sleep begin between 20 and 30 years of

BOX 18.1 The Stages of Sleep

Non-Rapid Eye Movement (NREM)
- 75% of night
- As we begin to fall asleep, we enter NREM sleep which is composed of N1-N3 (formerly Stages 1-4)

N1
- Between being awake and falling asleep
- Light sleep

N2
- Onset of sleep
- Becoming disengaged from surroundings
- Breathing and heart rate are regular
- Body temperature drops (so sleeping in a cool room is helpful)

N3
- Deepest and most restorative sleep
- Blood pressure drops
- Breathing becomes slower
- Muscles are relaxed
- Blood supply to muscles increases
- Tissue growth and repair occurs
- Energy is restored
- Hormones are released, such as growth hormone, essential for growth and development, including muscle development

Rapid Eye Movement (REM)
- 25% of night
- First occurs about 90 minutes after falling asleep and recurs about every 90 minutes, getting longer later in the night
- Provides energy to brain and body
- Supports daytime performance
- Brain is active and dreams occur
- Eyes dart back and forth
- Body becomes immobile and relaxed, as muscles are turned off

Adapted from National Sleep Foundation: *What happens when you sleep?* (website), n.d. https://sleepfoundation.org/how-sleep-works/what-happens-when-you-sleep. Accessed May 20, 2018.

age and are nearly complete by the age of 50 to 60 years. In adults older than 90 years of age, N3 sleep may disappear completely (Xiong & Hategan, 2019) (Box 18.1). Time spent in REM sleep also declines with age, and transitions between N1 and N2 (stages 1 and 2) are more common. REM sleep is viewed as important for older adults, since it is a time for the brain to replenish neurotransmitters essential for remembering, learning, and problem solving.

Research suggests that the deterioration of a cluster of neurons associated with regulating sleep patterns, the ventrolateral preoptic nucleus, may be responsible for sleep decline in aging. The more neurons that are lost, the more difficult it is for the person to sleep. For individuals with dementia, the link between the loss of neurons is greater and causes more problems with sleep (Petrovsky et al., 2018). The changes that occur in sleep with aging are summarized in Box 18.2.

Disruption of sleep occurs in up to 50% of individuals 65 years of age and older with chronic health conditions. The increase in sleep problems in older adults is associated with age-related changes in sleep; an increasing prevalence of multimorbidity (having at least two concurrent diseases); polypharmacy; psychosocial factors affecting sleep; physical, cognitive and functional impairment; and certain primary sleep disorders (e.g., obstructive sleep apnea, restless legs syndrome). This means that sleep disorders might arise from multiple different domains in older adults.

Sleep disturbance in older adults should be considered a geriatric syndrome, requiring consideration of multiple risk factors and a comprehensive treatment approach. Older adults in long-term care facilities show more prevalent sleep disturbances and disrupted sleep-wake patterns compared to community-dwelling older adults. About 72% report poor sleep quality. Older adults in long-term care facilities are more likely to have chronic conditions that contribute to sleep disturbances and to have poorer sleep hygiene than the general population of older adults (Kim & Yoon, 2020; see Research Highlights box).

SLEEP DISORDERS

Insomnia

Insomnia is the most common sleep disorder worldwide. The American Academy of Sleep Medicine defines insomnia as the subjective perception of difficulty with sleep initiation, duration, consolidation, or quality that results in some form of daytime impairment (Dopheide, 2020). Diagnostic criteria for insomnia include difficulty getting to sleep resulting in daytime dysfunction in an individual who has an adequate opportunity to sleep. Insomnia is a complex interaction of psychological cognitive arousal and altered circadian and homeostatic mechanisms.

Decreased function of the sleep-wake switch with age also may contribute to insomnia. Multiple brain centers work in concert to promote sleep and wakefulness.

Insomnia is classified as short-term, chronic, or other. It is short-term if symptoms occur for less than 3 months and chronic if symptoms occur three or more times a week for 3 months or longer. Insomnia can occur as a primary sleep disorder or as a symptom of another sleep disorder (e.g., sleep apnea, restless legs syndrome). The estimated prevalence of short-term insomnia is 9.5%, but about 1 in 5 cases of short-term insomnia transition to chronic insomnia, which can persist for years. The full clinical syndrome of chronic insomnia disorder occurs in about 10% of individuals (Dopheide, 2020). There are many influencing factors for insomnia, including physiological, psychological, and environmental (Box 18.3). Prescription and nonprescription medications and alcohol create sleep disturbances (Box 18.4). The times of day that medications are given also can contribute to sleep problems—for example, a diuretic given before bedtime or a sedating medication given in the morning.

BOX 18.3 Risk Factors for Sleep Disturbances in Older Adults

Physical Health
- Age-related changes in sleep architecture
- Comorbidities (cardiovascular disease, diabetes, pulmonary disease, musculoskeletal disorders); CNS disorders (Parkinson's disease, seizure disorder, dementia); GI disorders (hiatal hernia, GERD, PUD); urinary disorders (incontinence, BPH)
- Pain
- Polypharmacy
- Alcohol and substance abuse
- Lack of exercise
- Excessive napping; spending too much time in bed
- Sleep disorders (apnea, restless legs syndrome, periodic leg movement, rapid eye movement behavior disorder)
- Smoking

Psychological Health
- Depression, anxiety, delirium, psychosis
- Life stressors or response to stress
- Sleep-related beliefs
- Sleep habits (daily sleep-activity cycle, napping)
- Loneliness
- Loss of partner
- Being a worrier
- Family history of poor sleep
- Poor sleep hygiene

Physical Environment
- Environmental noises, institutional routines
- Caregiving for a dependent older adult
- Limited exposure to sunlight
- New environment

BPH, Benign prostatic hyperplasia; *CNS,* central nervous system; *GERD,* gastroesophageal reflux disease; *GI,* gastrointestinal; *PUD,* peptic ulcer disease.
Adapted from Teodorescu M: Sleep disruptions and insomnia in older adults, *Consultant* 54(3):166–173, 2014.

BOX 18.4 Medications Affecting Sleep

- Selective serotonin reuptake inhibitors (SSRIs)
- Antihypertensives (clonidine, beta blockers, reserpine, methyldopa)
- Anticholinergics
- Sympathomimetic amines
- Diuretics
- Opiates
- Cough and cold medications
- Thyroid preparations
- Phenytoin
- Cortisone
- Levodopa

Insomnia and Neurocognitive Disorders

Sleep disruption affects approximately 60% to 70% of older adults with neurocognitive disorders (NCDs) and varies by dementia subtype. Individuals with Lewy body dementia and Parkinson's dementia have the highest prevalence of sleep disruption (90%). Sleep disruptions or abnormal circadian rhythms are estimated to affect 25% to 60% of individuals with NCDs. Multiple factors contribute to sleep disruption in dementia, including degenerative changes in the suprachiasmatic nucleus (SCN) of the hypothalamus, which is related to circadian rhythm control (Scales et al., 2018).

Other factors that may affect quality of sleep in individuals with dementia include discomfort from musculoskeletal pain, respiratory distress, gastrointestinal discomfort, and urinary retention. Because the individual may not be able to report these sources of discomfort, careful observation and evaluation of pain and other sources of discomfort affecting sleep is important in improving sleep quality in individuals with NCDs (Evans & Kovach, 2020). In individuals with NCDs, sleep disruption is associated with increased neuropsychiatric symptoms and functional decline and is a major predictor of caregiver burden. Caregivers of individuals with NCDs also experience poor sleep quality, and this influences caregiver stress and health problems (Leggett et al., 2018; Petrovsky et al., 2018).

USING CLINICAL JUDGMENT TO PROMOTE HEALTHY AGING: SLEEP DISORDERS

Recognizing and Analyzing Cues

Sleep habits should be reviewed with older adults in all settings. Many people do not seek treatment for insomnia and may blame poor sleep on the aging process. Comprehensive assessment of sleep disturbances is important. For individuals in hospitals or nursing facilities, evaluation of sleep disturbances and awareness of contributing factors to poor sleep (pain, chronic illness, medications, alcohol use, depression, anxiety) are important. When assessing sleep, nurses should learn how well the person sleeps in the home setting, how many times the person is awakened at night, what time the person retires, level of physical activity during the day, and which rituals occur at bedtime.

Chronic insomnia is diagnosed by clinical evaluation. Polysomnography is not necessary for the diagnosis but may be indicated if sleep apnea or sleep-related movement disorders are suspected, the initial diagnosis is uncertain, behavioral or pharmacological treatment fails, or sudden arousals occur with violent behavior (American Adademy of Sleep Medicine, 2021). A sleep diary or log is also an important part of evaluation (Box 18.5). This information will provide an accurate account of the person's sleep problem and help identify the sleep disturbance.

BOX 18. 5 Sleep Diary

Instructions: Record the following for 2 to 4 weeks. Should be completed by the person or the caregiver if the person is unable. Record when you:
- Go to bed
- Go to sleep
- Wake up
- Get out of bed
- Take naps
- Exercise
- Consume alcohol
- Consume caffeinated beverages

BOX 18.6   Resources for Best Practice

- **Hartford Institute for Geriatric Nursing:** Epworth Sleepiness Scale: (https://hign.org/consultgeri/try-this-series/epworth-sleepiness-scale-ess) and Pittsburgh Sleep Quality Index (http://hbtinstitute.com/files/PSQIa.pdf).
- **National Heart, Lung, and Blood Institute:** Sleep apnea: https://www.nhlbi.nih.gov/health-topics/sleep-apnea.
- **Restless Legs Syndrome (RLS) Foundation:** Provider and patient teaching materials, RLS symptom diary: https://www.rls.org/file/symptom-diary.pdf.

A period of 2 to 4 weeks is needed to obtain a clear picture of the sleep problem. A self-rating scale, the Pittsburgh Sleep Quality Index (PSQI), can be used to measure the quality and patterns of sleep in the older adult, and daytime sleepiness can be evaluated with the Epworth Sleepiness Scale (Box 18.6). The Epworth Sleepiness Scale helps distinguish between the average amount of sleep and problems with sleep deprivation that require intervention. The Insomnia Severity Index is another tool to measure insomnia severity. Chronic insomnia is diagnosed by clinical evaluation.

Solutions, Nursing Actions, and Outcomes

Nonpharmacological Treatment

Treatment actions begin after a thorough sleep history has been recorded and, if possible, a sleep log obtained. Cognitive behavioral therapy for insomnia (CBTI) is recommended as first-line treatment of chronic insomnia. CBTI has a more durable benefit and fewer adverse effects than drug therapy and has demonstrated efficacy for insomnia in individuals with coexisting medical and psychiatric conditions, particularly depression, and in older adults. CBTI is a multidimensional approach combining psychological and behavioral therapies that include healthy sleep habits, relaxation techniques, circadian rhythm interventions, and cognitive therapy (Dolheide, 2020). Box 18.7 presents a guide to assessing sleep.

Despite recommendations for CBTI as first-line treatment, few individuals receive this treatment due to a lack of trained clinicians. Other approaches include computerized CBTI programs; telehealth approaches; and digital CBTI (dCBTI) products such as personal sleep monitoring devices (e.g., Fitbit) and applications that focus on relaxation, mindfulness, and meditation. Personal sleep monitoring devices are becoming increasingly popular and can be used as self-management tools in older adults with sleep disturbances to gain insight into their sleep and tailor individual interventions (Torossian et al., 2021).

Conventional exercise and tai chi have been found to be modestly effective in improving sleep with the beneficial effects sustained for 24 months (Su et al., 2021). In a systematic review and meta-analysis of randomized controlled trials, listening to music (calming-type music) is a potentially successful nonpharmacological intervention for improving sleep quality in adults. Further research is needed on effective interventions to improve sleep, but nurses can use the principles presented in Box 18.8 when caring for individuals with sleep concerns.

BOX 18.7   Tips for Best Practice

Recognizing and Analyzing Cues: Sleep Disturbances

Basic Sleep History Questions

- Where do you sleep at night (bed, couch, recliner chair)?
- Do you have any difficulty falling asleep?
- What do you do at night before you go to bed?
- Are you having any difficulty sleeping until morning?
- Are you having difficulty sleeping throughout the night?
- How often do you awaken and how long are you awake? What prevents you from falling back to sleep?
- Have you or someone else ever noticed that you snore loudly or stop breathing in your sleep?
- Do you find yourself falling asleep during the day when you do not want to?

Follow-Up Questions

- What time do you usually go to bed? Fall asleep?
- What prevents you from falling asleep?
- Do your legs kick or jump around while you sleep?
- Are you outside in natural light most days?
- Do you have any pain, discomfort, or shortness of breath during the night?
- What type of exercise do you get during the day?

Additional Assessment

- Individual's bed partner, family member, or caregiver also can be asked to provide information
- Obtain a medication and substance use history, including prescribed medications, over-the-counter drugs, dietary supplements, caffeine intake
- Review risk factors (obesity, arthritis, poorly controlled illnesses)
- Review depressive symptoms: weight loss, sadness, or recent losses
- Review involvement in social activities
- Review functional status, activities of daily living (ADL), and instrumental activities of daily living (IADL) performance

Objective Measures

- Sleep diary (keep for 24 hours daily for 2 to 4 weeks)
- Self-rating of sleep scales—Pittsburgh Sleep Quality Index; Epworth Sleepiness Scale; Insomnia Severity Scale
- On a scale of 1 to 10 (10 being the highest), how would you rate your sleep?

Adapted from Dean GE et al.: Protocol: excessive sleepiness. In Boltz M et al., editors: *Evidence-based geriatric nursing protocols for best practice*, New York, 2016, Springer, pp 431–441.

Sleep in hospitals and nursing homes. Sleep disturbances in individuals in hospitals and long-term care facilities is high, and promotion of a good sleep environment is important (Elliott et al., 2021). In hospitals and nursing facilities, nurses are in an excellent position to evaluate sleep and suggest actions to improve the quality of the sleep. "No other group of health care providers watch more people sleep than nurses" (Dean et al., 2016, p 438). Nurse-led sleep programs have been found to improve sleep quality and reduce depressive symptomatology in cognitively intact individuals in nursing facilities (Dolu & Nahcivan, 2018).

A multidisciplinary approach to identify sources of noise and light, such as equipment and staff interactions, could result in modification without compromising safety and quality of patient care. Decreasing nighttime noise is important, as sleep deprivation because of noise can potentially exacerbate

BOX 18.8   Solutions and Actions to Enhance Sleep

Healthy Sleep Habits

- Keep a consistent sleep schedule. Get up at the same time every day, even on weekends or during vacations.
- Set a bedtime that is early enough to get at least 7 hours of sleep.
- Don't go to bed unless sleepy.
- If you don't fall asleep after 20 minutes, get out of bed.
- Establish a relaxing bedtime routine.
- Use bed only for sleep and sex.
- Make bedroom quiet and relaxing. Keep the room at a comfortable, cool temperature.
- Limit exposure to bright light in the evenings.
- Turn off electronic devices at least 30 minutes before bedtime.
- Don't eat a large meal before bedtime. If hungry at night, eat a light, healthy snack.
- Exercise regularly and maintain a healthy diet.
- Avoid caffeine, alcohol, and tobacco in the late afternoon or evening.
- Reduce fluid intake before bedtime.
- Limit or avoid daytime napping.

Relaxation Techniques

- Diaphragmatic breathing
- Progressive relaxation
- White noise or music
- Guided imagery
- Stretching
- Yoga or tai chi

Circadian Rhythm Interventions

- Cue circadian rhythm by connecting with environmental signals (light exposure, meals, activity, medications).
- Maintain stable daytime routines with meals, activity, and medications.
- Increase duration and intensity of bright light or sunlight exposure during the day.
- Melatonin 1 to 2 hours before bedtime may be helpful.

Adapted from American Academy of Sleep Medicine: *Healthy sleep habits* (website), 2017. http://sleepeducation.org/essentials-in-sleep/healthy-sleep-habits. Accessed May 2021.

BOX 18.9   Tips for Best Practice

Suggestions to Promote Sleep When Hospitalized or in a Nursing Facility

- Allow individual to stay out of bed and out of the room for as long as possible before bed.
- Provide 30 minutes or more of sunlight exposure in a comfortable outdoor location.
- Provide low-level physical activity three times a day.
- Provide meaningful activities (individualized and group) during the daytime.
- Keep noise level at a minimum, speak in hushed tones, do no use overhead paging, reduce light in hallways and resident rooms.
- Institute a sleep improvement protocol—"do not disturb" times, soft music, relaxation, massage, aromatherapy, sleep masks, headphones, allowing patients to shut doors. Consider having a kit with music and aromatherapy that can be taken to bedside.
- Perform necessary care (e.g., turning, changing) when the individual is awake rather than awakening the individual between the hours of 10:00 p.m. and 6:00 a.m.
- Limit intake of caffeine and other fluids in excess before bedtime.
- Provide a light snack or warm beverage before bedtime.
- Discontinue invasive treatments when possible (Foley catheters, percutaneous gastrostomy tubes, intravenous lines).
- Encourage and assist to the bathroom before bed and as needed.
- Give pain medication before bedtime for patients with pain.
- Maintain comfortable temperature in room; provide blankets as needed.

delirium. Nursing staff should ensure that patients complete a full sleep cycle of 90 minutes before being awakened for nonemergency reasons such as checking for incontinence or doing routine tasks. Other actions are presented in Box 18.9.

Individuals with NCDs often have severe dysfunctions of their sleep-wake and rest-activity patterns (sundowning, excessive daytime sleepiness, nocturnal wandering, agitation, irritability, day-night reversal, decreased cognitive functioning). Daytime light exposure is a major synchronizer of circadian rhythms. When individuals with NCDs are in controlled environments (hospitals, long-term care facilities), daytime light exposure may be limited, exacerbating their symptoms. Tailored light interventions designed to maximally affect the circadian system have been reported to improve sleep in individuals with moderate to late-stage NCD (Figueiro et al., 2019).

Pharmacological Treatment

National guidelines emphasize that medications for chronic insomnia should be considered only in patients who are unable to participate in CBTI, patients who still have symptoms after this therapy, or those who require a temporary adjunct to CBTI (Edinger et al., 2021). A thorough assessment of sleep concerns is necessary before pharmacological treatment is initiated. The American Geriatrics Society (AGS, 2015) Beers Criteria strongly suggest avoiding any type of benzodiazepine for the treatment of insomnia in older adults because these medications are associated with adverse outcomes, including motor vehicle accidents, impaired cognition, and falls. Yet the use of prescription sedative and hypnotic medications, as well as over-the-counter (OTC) sleep aids, is increasing in the United States. Individuals over the age of 60 years receive 33% of all hypnotic prescriptions, although they constitute only 14% of the population. Use of narcotic pain medications and sedatives, and the use of alcohol in combination with these medications and other prescribed medications, is a growing concern (Chapter 30).

OTC drugs such as diphenhydramine, found in many OTC sleep products such as Tylenol PM, are often thought to be relatively harmless but should be avoided because of antihistaminic and anticholinergic side effects. Other OTC sleep aid preparations contain ingredients such as kava kava, valerian root, melatonin, chamomile, and tryptophan. Because these ingredients are not regulated, information and outcomes of efficacy may not be known. Endogenous nocturnal melatonin, a major loop for circadian rhythm, may have decreased levels in older adults. Melatonin, taken 1 to 2 hours before bedtime, may replicate the natural secretion pattern of melatonin and lead to improvements in the circadian regulation of the sleep-wake cycle.

The individual should report use of all OTC drugs to the health care provider since these drugs may interact with other medications. Routine use of OTC medications for sleep may

BOX 18.10   Tips for Best Practice

Use of Sleeping Medications

Provide health education on:

1. Normal changes in sleep patterns with age
2. Importance of appropriate assessment of sleep problems before any medications are used
3. Nonpharmacological treatment of sleeping problems as first-line treatment (cognitive behavioral therapy for insomnia, sleep hygiene, stimulus control, sleep restriction, relaxation techniques)
4. Avoiding over-the-counter (OTC) medications that contain diphenhydramine, which can have side effects of confusion, blurred vision, constipation, falls
5. Adverse effects of sleep medications, even OTC medications; include problems with daily function, changes in mental status, possibility of motor vehicle accidents, increase in daytime drowsiness, and increased risk for falls with only minimal improvement in sleep
6. Avoiding benzodiazepines (flurazepam, triazolam, temazepam) for sleep due to long-acting sedation effects
7. If sleeping medications are prescribed, the benzodiazepine receptor agonists (zolpidem, eszopiclone, zaleplon) or ramelteon are preferred; given at the lowest possible dose for short-term use only (2 to 3 weeks, never longer than 90 days); medications for sleep should be taken immediately before bedtime
8. Avoiding the use of alcohol, narcotic pain-relieving medications, and antianxiety medications if taking sleeping medications
9. Reviewing all medications, including OTC, with health care provider for interactions with sleeping medications
10. Using caution the day after taking sleeping medications, particularly with driving and activities that require full alertness; accidents are common

BOX 18.11   Risk Factors for Obstructive Sleep Apnea

- Increasing age
- Increased neck circumference (not as significant in older adults)
- Male gender
- Anatomical abnormalities of the upper airway
- Upper airway resistance and/or obstruction
- Family history
- Excess weight
- Use of alcohol, sedatives, or tranquilizers
- Smoking
- Hypertension

delay appropriate evaluation and treatment of contributing medical or psychological conditions, identification of sleep disorders, and appropriate counseling and treatment. An important nursing action is to educate individuals on the proper use of medications, their side effects, and their interactions with alcohol and other prescription drugs (Box 18.10).

Benzodiazepine receptor agonists, such as zolpidem (Ambien), eszopiclone (Lunesta), and zaleplon (Sonata), are considered benzodiazepine-like in their action because they induce sleep easily. Prolonged use of these drugs can lead to tolerance, dependence, rebound insomnia, residual daytime sedation, motor incoordination, increased risk of motor vehicle accidents, cognitive impairment, and increased risk for falls, with only minimal improvement in sleep latency and duration. In 2019 the US Food and Drug Administration (FDA) added a black box warning on patient medication guides and prescription information for insomnia drugs such as zolpidem, zaleplon, and eszopiclone, calling attention to side effects that can lead to serious injury or death. Rare but serious incidents have occurred when users of these medications experienced complex

⚡ SAFETY TIP

Thorough evaluation of sleep problems should be conducted before medication use. Nonpharmacological interventions are first-line treatment. If sleeping medications are used, they should be taken immediately before bedtime because of their rapid action. Short-term use (2 to 3 weeks, never more than 90 days) is recommended.

sleep behaviors: sleepwalking, sleep driving, and engaging in other activities when not fully awake.

Sleep Disordered Breathing and Sleep Apnea

Sleep disordered breathing (SDB) affects approximately 25% of older individuals (more men than women), and the most common form is obstructive sleep apnea (OSA). Untreated OSA is related to heart failure, atrial fibrillation, stroke, type 2 diabetes, cognitive decline, osteoporosis, and even death. OSA is characterized by complete or partial airway closure during sleep. Age-related decline in the activity of the upper airway muscles, resulting in compromised pharyngeal patency, predispose older adults to OSA.

A high body mass index (BMI) and large neck circumference have been identified as risk factors for OSA. Losing weight is recommended in obese individuals with OSA, as it improves overall health and reduces the severity of OSA. Weight loss improves OSA by several mechanisms, including reduction in fatty tissue in the throat (i.e., parapharyngeal fat and the tongue). Loss of abdominal fat increases mediastinal traction on the upper airway, making it less likely to collapse during sleep (Wang et al., 2020). Other risk factors for OSA are presented in Box 18.11.

Recognizing and Analyzing Cues

Symptoms of sleep apnea include loud periodic snoring, gasping and choking upon awakening, unusual nighttime activity such as sitting upright in bed or falling out of bed, morning headache, unexplained daytime sleepiness, complaints of insomnia, poor memory and intellectual functioning, and irritability and personality change. Symptoms of OSA and information from the sleeping partner, if present, are obtained. If the person has a sleeping partner, it is often the partner who reports the nighttime symptoms. If there is a sleeping partner, the partner may move to another room to sleep because of the disturbance to his or her own rest.

Recognition of OSA in older adults may be more difficult because there may not be a sleeping partner to report symptoms. If presenting symptoms suggest the disorder, a tape recorder can be placed at the bedside to record snoring and breathing sounds during the night. A medication review is always indicated when investigating sleep complaints. The upper airway, including the nasal and pharyngeal airways, should be examined for anatomical obstruction, tumors, or cysts. Comorbid conditions such as heart failure and diabetes should be evaluated and managed appropriately.

Solutions, Nursing Actions, and Outcomes

If OSA is suspected, a referral for a sleep study should be conducted. A sleep study or polysomnogram is a multiple-component test that electronically transmits and records specific physical activities during a full night of sleep. Sleep studies can be done in a special center or at home with a portable diagnostic device. Removable sensors are placed on the scalp, face, eyelids, chest, limbs, and a finger. The sensors record brain waves, heart rate, breathing effort and rate, oxygen levels, and muscle movements before, during, and after sleep. Mild, moderate, or severe sleep apnea can be diagnosed based on the number of sleep apnea events that occur in an hour during the sleep study (National Heart, Lung, and Blood Institute, 2018).

Therapy will depend on the severity and type of sleep apnea and the presence of comorbid illnesses. Treatment of sleep apnea may involve avoidance of alcohol and sedative-hypnotic medications, cessation of smoking, avoidance of supine sleep positions, increased physical activity, development of healthy sleep habits, and weight loss. There should be risk counseling about impaired judgment from sleeplessness and the possibility of accidents when driving.

Continuous positive airway pressure (CPAP) is the most commonly recommended treatment for OSA and generally can reverse this condition quickly with the appropriate titration of devices (Downey et al., 2018). The CPAP device delivers pressurized air through tubing to a nasal mask or nasal pillows, which are fitted around the head. The pressurized air acts as an airway splint and gently opens the individual's throat and breathing passages, allowing the individual to breathe normally, but only through the nose (Fig. 18.1). Teaching should be provided about the effects of untreated OSA with the need for treatment emphasized. Recent research findings suggest that treating OSA through CPAP may reduce the risk of developing Alzheimer's disease and other dementias in older adults (Dunietz et al., 2021).

A stepwise approach during the initiation of therapy and continued monitoring can foster better use of CPAP or prevent discontinuation of therapy. CPAP nonadherence is a major challenge, with estimates indicating that about half of individuals either discontinue the therapy or are not adherent (use for less than 4 hours per night) (Nadal et al., 2018). If the individual who requires CPAP needs surgery or pain management, precautions should be taken to make sure the airway stays open during surgery or when selecting pain medications.

Mandibular repositioning mouthpieces are devices that cover the lower and upper teeth and hold the jaw in a position that prevents it from blocking the upper airway. These devices may be recommended as an alternative treatment for individuals who prefer this type of device, experience adverse effects with CPAP, and have mild sleep apnea that occurs only while lying on their back. These devices are custom fit by a dentist who specializes in correcting tooth or jaw problems. The devices

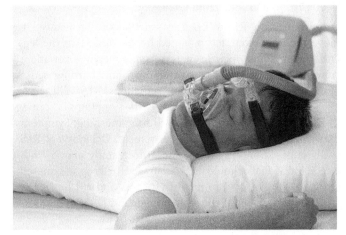

Fig. 18.1 Continuous positive airway pressure (CPAP) device. (© iStock.com/cherrybeans.)

require a stable dentition and may be problematic for individuals with dentures or extensive tooth loss. Implants that are surgically implanted can benefit some people with sleep apnea. The device senses breathing patterns and delivers mild stimulation to certain muscles that open the airways during sleep. The FDA has approved one implant as a treatment for sleep apnea. Further research is needed to determine how effective the implant is in treating sleep apnea.

Restless Legs Syndrome/Willis-Ekbom Disease (RLS/WED)

Restless legs syndrome/Willis-Ekbom disease (RLS/WED) is a neurological movement disorder of the limbs that is often associated with a sleep complaint. An estimated 7% to 10% of adults in North America and Europe have the disease. The disorder is familial in about 50% of individuals, and several predisposing genes have been identified through genome-wide association studies (Suzuki et al., 2017). RLS/WED is less common in Asian populations. Incidence is about twice as high in women, and although the disease may begin at any age (including childhood), many individuals who are severely affected are middle-aged or older. Symptoms become more frequent and last longer with age. RLS/WED may be a contributing factor to nighttime agitation in persons with Alzheimer's disease (Richards et al., 2020).

In most cases, RLS/WED is a primary idiopathic disorder, but it also can be associated with underlying medical disorders, including iron deficiency, end-stage renal disease (especially in individuals requiring dialysis), diabetes, and pregnancy. Other contributing factors being studied include iron metabolism and neurotransmitter dysfunctions involving dopamine and glutamate. Antidepressants, antihypertensives, and neuroleptic medications can aggravate RLS/WED symptoms. Increased BMI, caffeine use, alcohol or tobacco use, sleep deprivation, and sedentary lifestyle may also be contributing factors. Regular exercisers are 3.3 times less likely to have RLS than nonexercisers, and regular exercise has been found to reduce the severity of RLS/WED symptoms by an average of 40% (Restless Legs Syndrome Foundation, 2021).

Recognizing and Analyzing Cues

Individuals with RLS/WED have an uncontrollable need to move the legs, often accompanied by discomfort in the legs. Other symptoms include paresthesia; creeping sensations; crawling sensations; tingling, cramping, and burning sensations; pain; or even indescribable sensations. RLS/WED has a circadian rhythm, with the intensity of the symptoms becoming worse at night and improving toward the morning. Symptoms may be relieved temporarily by movement. Diagnosis of RLS/WED is based on symptoms, and a sleep study may be indicated. Individuals should be encouraged to keep a symptom diary for 7 to 14 days to identify triggers and aid in diagnosis. The Restless Legs Syndrome Foundation (2021) provides a symptom diary on their website (see Box 18.6).

Solutions, Nursing Actions, and Outcomes

Possible contributing conditions should be evaluated, and all individuals with symptoms should be tested for iron deficiency with a complete iron panel. If iron stores are low, iron replacement is needed. Medication treatment should start only when symptoms have a significant impact on quality of life in terms of frequency and severity; intermittent treatment might be considered in intermediate cases. The FDA has approved four drugs for treating RLS: ropinirole (Requip), pramipexole (Mirapex), gabapentin enacarbil (Horizant), and rotigotine (Neupro) (Restless Legs Syndrome Foundation, 2021).

Drugs such as methadone, codeine, hydrocodone, or oxycodone are sometimes prescribed to treat individuals with more severe symptoms of RLS who did not respond well to other medications. Side effects include constipation, dizziness, nausea, exacerbation of sleep apnea, and the risk of addiction; however, very low doses are often effective in controlling symptoms of RLS (National Institute of Neurological Disorders and Stroke, 2021). Nonpharmacological therapy includes stretching of the lower extremities; mild to moderate physical activity; hot baths; massage; acupressure; relaxation techniques; and avoidance of caffeine, alcohol, and tobacco.

Rapid Eye Movement Sleep Behavior Disorder (RBD)

REM sleep behavior disorder (RBD) is characterized by loss of voluntary muscle atonia during REM sleep associated with complex behavior while dreaming. Individuals report elaborate enactment of their dreams, often with violent content, during sleep. This may include violent behaviors, such as punching and kicking, with the potential for injury of both the individual and the bed partner. The mean age at emergence of RBD is 60 years, and it is more common in males (National Sleep Foundation, 2021).

The acute form of the disorder can be caused by toxic-metabolic abnormalities, drug or alcohol withdrawal, and medications (tricyclic antidepressants, monoamine oxidase inhibitors, cholinergic agents, selective serotonin reuptake inhibitors [SSRIs]). The chronic form is usually idiopathic and is identified as a potential prodrome of certain neurodegenerative diseases. Between 70% and 91% of individuals with

RBD go on to develop Parkinson's disease, Lewy body dementia, or multiple system atrophy. The prevalence of RBD in individuals with Parkinson's disease is estimated between 50% and 60%. Symptoms of RBD may precede the onset of classic symptoms of neurodegenerative diseases by 5 to 15 years. Diagnosis of RBD is based on history, symptoms, and a sleep study to test for the key features of the disorder.

Solutions, Nursing Actions, and Outcomes

Medications, including melatonin and clonazepam, may be used to suppress symptoms of dream enactment. A safe environment in the bedroom should be provided, and caregivers should receive support for ways to manage the disorder. Individuals with RBD and their caregivers may benefit from understanding that RBD behaviors of an angry or aggressive nature are not reflecting hidden relationship conflicts, nor will they resolve by scolding the patient (Edinger et al., 2021).

Circadian Rhythm Sleep Disorders

In circadian rhythm sleep disorders (CRSDs), relatively normal sleep occurs at abnormal times. Two clinical presentations are seen: advanced sleep phase disorder (ASPD) and irregular sleep-wake disorder (ISWD). The acute form of the disorder can be caused by toxic-metabolic abnormalities, drug or alcohol withdrawal, and medications (tricyclic antidepressants, monoamine oxidase inhibitors, cholinergic agents, selective serotonin reuptake inhibitors [SSRIs]). In ASPD, the individual begins and ends sleep at unusually early times (e.g., going to bed as early as 6 or 7 p.m. and waking up between 2 and 5 a.m.). Not all individuals with an advanced sleep phase have ASPD. If the sleep patterns do not bother the individual and there is no functional impairment, the individual may just be considered a "morning" person. In ISWD, sleep is dispersed across the 24-hour day in bouts of irregular length. Factors contributing to these disorders are age-related changes in sleep and circadian rhythm regulation combined with decreased levels of light exposure and activity.

A combination of good sleep hygiene practices and methods to delay the timing of sleep and wake times is recommended as treatment for ASPD. Bright light therapy is designed to promote the synchronization of circadian rhythms with environmental light-dark cycles through stimulation of the SCN area of the brain in the hypothalamus responsible for controlling circadian rhythms (Scales et al., 2018) (see Box 18.8). Bright light therapy is a reasonably low-cost treatment that, unlike medication usage, generally does not result in residual effects and tolerance. It should be noted that older adults may be less sensitive to light because of age-related changes, and this may influence the effectiveness of light therapy (Kim & Duffy, 2018).

In ISWD, the individual may obtain enough sleep over the 24-hour period, but time asleep is broken into at least three different periods of variable length. Erratic napping occurs during the day, and nighttime sleep is severely fragmented and shortened. Chronic insomnia and/or daytime sleepiness are present. ISWD is most commonly encountered in individuals with NCDs, particularly those who are institutionalized.

KEY CONCEPTS

- Sleep is a barometer of health and can be considered one of the vital signs.
- Sleep problems constitute a global epidemic affecting up to 50% of the world's population.
- In addition to age-related changes in sleep architecture, many chronic conditions interfere with quality and quantity of sleep in older adults. Complaints of sleep difficulties should be thoroughly investigated and not attributed to age.
- An important nursing role is recognition and analysis of cues suggesting sleep disturbances and identification and evaluation of nursing actions to improve sleep health.
- Nonpharmacological interventions are first-line treatments for sleep problems. CBTI is recommended for treatment of chronic insomnia.

- Benzodiazepines or other sedative-hypnotics should not be used in older adults as a first choice of treatment for insomnia.
- All sleeping medications, including OTC, have adverse effects that include daytime drowsiness, changes in mental status, and increased likelihood of falls.
- If sleeping medications are prescribed, benzodiazepine receptor agonists are preferred and should be given at the lowest possible dose and used only short term (2 to 3 weeks, never more than 90 days).
- SDB affects approximately 25% of older individuals (more men than women), and the most common form is OSA.
- Untreated OSA is related to heart failure, cardiac dysrhythmias, stroke, type 2 diabetes, and even death.

NEXT-GENERATION NCLEX® (NGN) EXAMINATION–STYLE QUESTIONS

A 59-year-old male patient seen last month for insomnia comes to the primary health care provider for a follow-up appointment. Upon assessment a month earlier, the patient reported difficulty sleeping after undergoing a recent stressful job loss and was prescribed zolpidem 10 mg before bedtime. The patient's partner says that although it seems easier for the patient to fall asleep at night since starting zolpidem, there is concern about the sleeping pattern. The patient says, "Sometimes I wake myself up and gasp for air; I guess it's because I snore so loud." The partner says, "It scares me because sometimes I look over and it looks like he isn't even breathing. Other times, I've found him in the kitchen making a sandwich but he doesn't remember doing it the next day. Last night I heard him, and when I got up to see what was happening, he had the car keys in his hand and said he was going for a drive at 3:00 a.m." The patient interrupts, stating, "That's not true—I didn't get up last night at all." Assessment today reveals a weight of 240 pounds (108.9 kg), height of 71 inches (180.3 cm), temperature of 97.9°F (36.6°C), blood pressure of 180/80 mm Hg, pulse of 90 beats/minute, respirations of 22 breaths/minute, clear oral cavity, 4+ tonsils, and negative cervical adenopathy. After the health care provider performs an examination, an order is placed for the patient to have a sleep study to determine if sleep apnea is a concern.

For each finding listed in the table below, indicate whether findings from this patient's assessment are more likely to be associated with obstructive sleep apnea or a medication-induced side effect of zolpidem.

Assessment Finding	Obstructive Sleep Apnea	Medication-Induced Side Effect
Reports waking self up and gasping for air		
Loud snoring		
Periodic episodes of "not breathing"		
Makes sandwiches at night and has no recollection the following day		
Tonsils assessed at 4+ size		
Takes car keys while reporting the intention to drive		

NURSING STUDY

Sleep

Gerald, 80 years old, had a sleeping disorder and was tired for most of the day and lonely at night. His wife of 45 years had recently moved into her sewing room, where she slept on the couch at night because she could no longer cope with Gerald's loud snoring. He sometimes even seemed to stop breathing, which kept her awake watching his abdomen rise and fall, or not. Sometimes he would awaken suddenly, gasping for air. However, Gerald had tolerated it because he thought nothing could be done for it. Because it had become a threat to his marriage, he became motivated to investigate possible solutions. Gerald said to his nurse clinician, "This isn't anything, but it upsets my wife." Although he did not admit it, he was also worried because he was beginning to feel rather weak and listless during the day. When he had consulted the clinic nurse, Gerald was diagnosed with obstructive sleep apnea. He found that some very practical means of dealing with this problem of sleep apnea were available, and if these were not effective, the nurse had reassured him that additional medical interventions could be helpful.

CLINICAL JUDGMENT QUESTIONS AND ACTIVITIES

Questions 1 to 3 refer to the Nursing Study.

1. What lifestyle factors may be increasing Gerald's episodes of sleep apnea?
2. Compose a list of 10 questions you would ask Gerald to obtain a clear picture of factors contributing to his sleep apnea. Discuss the rationale behind each question.
3. List some of the common methods for dealing with this problem that Gerald's nurse may have given to him.
4. In what circumstances is sleep apnea particularly dangerous to health?

RESEARCH QUESTIONS

1. Does better management of chronic disease improve sleep quality?
2. Does improving sleep quality have a favorable effect on the course of chronic illness?
3. What is the average time of the total sleep cycle as experienced by a healthy individual older than 70 years?
4. What type of exercise is effective for improved sleep?
5. Which nonpharmacological interventions are most effective for sleep and for what type of individual?
6. What are the concerns of caregivers of persons with dementia as they relate to sleep?
7. How do nurses in hospitals and nursing homes evaluate sleep quality for their patients or residents?

REFERENCES

American Academy of Sleep Medicine: Five things physicians and patients should question, *Choosing Wisely*, 2021 December 21.

American Geriatrics Society: 2015 Beers Criteria Update Expert Panel: American Geriatrics Society 2015 updated Beers Criteria for potentially inappropriate medication use in older adults, *J Am Geriatr Soc* 63(11):2227–2246, 2015.

Clark G et al.: Circadian control of heparin sulfate levels times phagocytosis of amyloid beta aggregates, PLOS Genetics 18(2):e1009994, 2022. doi:10.1371/journal.pgen.1009994.

Dean G et al.: Excessive sleepiness. In Boltz M et al., editors. *Evidence-based geriatric nursing protocols for best practice*, 5, New York, 2016, Springer, pp 431–441.

Dolu I & Nahcivan N: Impact of a nurse-led sleep programme on the sleep quality and depressive symptomatology among older adults in nursing homes: a randomized controlled study, *Int J Older People Nurs* 14(1):e12215, 2018. doi:10.1111/opn.12215.

Dopheide J: Insomnia overview: epidemiology, pathophysiology, diagnosis and monitoring, and nonpharmacological therapy, *Am J Managed Care* 26(4 Suppl):576–584, 2020.

Downey R et al.: *Obstructive sleep apnea (OSA) treatment and management* (website), 2018. https://emedicine.medscape.com/article/295807-treatment.

Dunietz G et al.: Obstructive sleep apnea treatment and dementia risk in older adults, *Sleep* 44(9):zsab076, 2021. doi:10.1093/sleep/zsab076 2021.

Edinger J et al.: Behavioral and psychological treatments for chronic insomnia disorder in adults: an American Academy of Sleep Medicine clinical practice guideline, *Jour of Clinical Sleep Medicine* 17(2):162–255, 2021.

Elliott Z et al.: Short-term physical health effects of sleep disruptions attributed to the acute hospital environment: a systematic review, *J Sleep Health* 7(4):508–518, 2021. doi:10.1016/j.sleh.2021.03.001.

Evans C & Kovach C: The association between physiological sources of pain and sleep quality in older adults with and without dementia, *Res Gerontol Nurs* 13(6):297–306, 2020.

Figueiro M et al.: Effects of a tailored lighting intervention on sleep quality, rest-activity, mood, and behavior in older adults with Alzheimer disease and related dementias: a randomized clinical trial, *J Clin Sleep Med* 15(12):1757–1767, 2019.

Kim D & Yoon J: Factors that influence sleep among residents in long-term care facilities, *Int J Environ Res Public Health*, 2020 17(6) 1889.

Kim JH & Duffy JF: Circadian rhythm sleep-wake disorders in older adults, *Sleep Med Clin* 13(1):39–50, 2018. doi:10.1016/j.jsmc.2017.09.004.

Leggett A et al.: What hath night to do with sleep?" The caregiving context and dementia caregivers' nighttime awakenings, *Clin Gerontol* 41(2):158–166, 2018.

Nadal N et al.: Predictors of CPAP compliance in different clinical settings: primary care versus sleep unit, *Sleep & Breath* 22(1):157–163, 2018.

National Heart, Lung, and Blood Institute: *Sleep apnea (website)*, 2018 https://www.nhlbi.nih.gov/health-topics/sleep-apnea Accessed June 2021.

National Institute of Neurological Disorders and Stroke: *Restless legs syndrome fact sheet (website)*, 2021 https://www.ninds.nih.gov/disorders/patient-caregiver-education/fact-sheets/restless-legs-syndrome-fact-sheet.

Petrovsky DV et al.: Sleep disruption and quality of life in persons with dementia: a state-of-the-art review, *Geriatr Nurs* 39(6):640–645, 2018.

Restless Legs Syndrome Foundation: *RLS symptom diary* (website), 2021. https://www.rls.org/understanding-rls/symptoms-diagnosis?

Richards K et al.: Nighttime agitation and restless leg syndrome in persons with Alzheimer's disease, *Res Gerontol Nurs* 13(6):280–288, 2020.

Robbins R et al.: Examining sleep deficiency and disturbance and their risk for incident dementia and all-cause mortality in older adults across 5 years in the United States, *Aging* 13(3):3254–3268, 2021.

Scales K et al.: Evidence-based nonpharmacological practice to address behavioral and psychological symptoms of dementia, *Gerontologist* 58(Suppl 1):S88–S102, 2018.

Sleep Foundation: *What is REM sleep behavior disorder?* (website), 2021 https://www.sleepfoundation.org/rem-sleep-behavior-disorder#:~:text=REM%20sleep%20behavior%20disorder%20is,describes%20abnormal%20behaviors%20during%20sleep.

Su P et al.: Effects of tai chi or exercise on sleep in older adults with insomnia: a randomized clinical trial, *JAMA Network Open*, 2021 4(2):e2037199. doi:10.1001/jamanetworkopen.2020.37199.

Suzuki K et al.: Sleep disorders in the elderly: diagnosis and management, *J Gen Fam Med* 18(2):61–71, 2017.

Torossian M et al.: Use of a personal sleep self-monitoring device for sleep self-management: a feasibility study, *J Gerontol Nurs* 47(1):28–34, 2021.

Wang S et al.: Effect of weight loss on upper airway anatomy and the apnea-hypopnea index: the importance of tongue fat, *Am J Respir Crit Care Med*, 2020 201(6) https://doi.org/10.1164/rccm.201903-0692OC.

World Association of Sleep Medicine: *World sleep day, toolkit* (website), 2021 https://worldsleepday.org/toolkit.

Xiong G & Hategan A: *Geriatric sleep disorder* (website), 2019. https://emedicine.medscape.com/article/292498-overview?pa=FoKIu4vX0dMcRVgVjSVTmYLaTejRnqVqku9xeP7q1BqUA5zw3fPxK-Tv30G3JQT0e8SIvl8zjYv73GUyW5rsbWA%3D%3D. Accessed December 2020.

Activity and Exercise

Theris A. Touhy

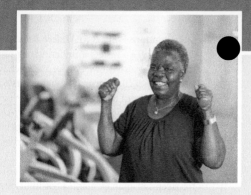

http://evolve.elsevier.com/Touhy/TwdHlthAging

A STUDENT SPEAKS

I work in a local gym on the weekends, and over the last several years, I have been amazed at the number of older adults who work out. We even have an older gentleman on staff who is a trainer. Some of them are really fit and look like they have been "gym rats" their whole lives. Others take it a bit easier, but they come a couple of times a week to lift weights or walk on the treadmill. The water aerobics classes are always full. There are also a few people recovering from knee replacements who do their exercises at the gym. I hope I can stay fit when I get old.

Jeff, age 20

AN OLDER ADULT SPEAKS

I am 82 years young. My girlfriends and I have had a walking club for 15 years. Coffee first and then our 1-mile walk down to the park. Now we are trying something new and are going to a yoga class at the local senior center. We've got our mats and our tights and are really enjoying ourselves. Of course, the lunch afterward is nice as well. My grandson thinks it's funny, but you should see the moves we are learning!

Peggy, age 74

LEARNING OBJECTIVES

On completion of this chapter, the reader will be able to:

1. Describe the relationship between physical activity and health.
2. Describe the guidelines for physical activity for older adults.
3. Identify components of assessment and screening to determine appropriate physical activity interventions and exercise programs.
4. Discuss adaptations of exercise for individuals with chronic illness, mobility limitations, and cognitive impairment.
5. Use clinical judgment to identify solutions and nursing actions to promote healthy activity and exercise patterns for older adults in all settings.

Physical activity is defined as any bodily movement produced by skeletal muscle that requires energy expenditure. This includes exercise and other activities such as playing, working, active transportation (walking, running, biking), household chores, and recreational activities. Exercise is a subcategory of physical fitness that is planned, structured, repetitive, and purposeful in the sense that improvement or maintenance of one or more components of physical fitness is the objective.

Few factors contribute as much to health in aging as being physically active. The adage "use it or lose it" certainly applies to muscles and physical fitness. Regular physical activity throughout life is essential for healthy aging. Physical activity enhances health and functional status while also decreasing the number of chronic illnesses and functional limitations often assumed to be a part of growing older (Box 19.1). The frail health and loss of function we often associate with aging are in large part due to physical inactivity. "Reduced physical mobility and immobility contribute to the development of geriatric syndromes (pressure injuries, urinary incontinence, falls, functional decline, and delirium)" (Gray-Miceli, 2017, p. 471).

PHYSICAL ACTIVITY AND AGING

Despite a large body of evidence about the benefits of physical activity to maintain and improve function, 28% of adults 50 years of age and older are physically inactive. The levels of

BOX 19.1 Health Benefits of Physical Activity

- Reduced risk of hypertension, coronary artery disease, heart attack, stroke, diabetes, colon and breast cancers, metabolic syndrome, depression
- Reduced adverse blood lipid profile
- Prevention of weight gain
- Improved cardiorespiratory and muscular fitness
- Enhanced neuronal function
- Reduced risk of falls and hip fracture
- Improved sleep quality
- Improved bone and functional health
- Enhanced neuronal function
- Decreased risk of early death (life expectancy increased even in persons who do not begin exercising regularly until age 75)
- Improved functional independence

BOX 19.2 Ways to Keep Fit During Aging

- After four unsuccessful attempts, Diana Nyad, 64 years old, became the first person to swim from Cuba to Florida without the use of a shark cage.
- Nellie, 83 years old, began swimming to ease the discomfort resulting both from a short left arm (the residual effect of poliomyelitis) and from a frozen left shoulder. She became an award-winning synchronized swimmer with 20 gold medals, 12 blue ribbons, and 13 trophies to her credit. Nellie continued to exercise this way despite the need to wear cataract goggles.
- James, 72 years old, was taking 40 mg of Lipitor daily for his high cholesterol level and lisinopril 40 mg for hypertension. He was a self-proclaimed couch potato. He joined Silver Sneakers, a program offered through his Medicare Advantage Plan, and started going to the gym. After a year of walking on the treadmill for 30 minutes three times a week and lifting weights, his cholesterol level and blood pressure value approached normal limits. His medications were reduced, and he was 10 pounds lighter. Even his 14-year-old grandson admired his biceps.
- Em, an 86-year-old nursing home resident, jogged every morning in place for about 5 minutes and then briskly walked around outside the facility. Although she had occasional lapses of memory, she was vital, erect, and interested in life around her.

physical activity among older adults have not improved over the past decade in the United States (Centers for Disease Control and Prevention [CDC], 2021; Du et al., 2019). Increasing physical activity for people of all ages is a global concern in both developed and developing countries. Physical inactivity is identified as a leading risk factor for global mortality (hypertension, smoking, high blood glucose level, physical inactivity, obesity). The Healthy People 2030 box outlines goals for physical activity.

♥ HEALTHY PEOPLE 2030

Physical Activity

- Reduce the proportion of adults who do no physical activity in their free time
- Increase the proportion of adults who do enough aerobic physical activity for substantial health benefits
- Increase the proportion of adults who do enough aerobic physical activity for extensive health benefits
- Increase the proportion of adults who do enough muscle-strengthening activity
- Increase the proportion of older adults with physical or cognitive health problems who get physical activity

Data from US Department of Health and Human Services: *Healthy People 2030* (website), 2020. https://health.gov/healthypeople.

Physical activity is important for all older adults, not just active healthy older adults. Reducing sedentary time, independent of physical activity, has cardiovascular, metabolic, and functional benefits. Older adults with chronic conditions should understand whether and how their conditions affect their ability to do regular physical activity safely. They should be as physically active as their abilities and conditions allow. Increasing physical activity improves health outcomes in individuals with chronic illnesses (regardless of severity) and in those with functional impairment and are especially important to older adults who are either frail or sarcopenic (Chapters 22 and 28). Improvements in insulin resistance, resting metabolic rate, glucose metabolism, blood pressure, body fat, and gastrointestinal transit time can

be obtained even through two 20-minute resistance-training sessions a week.

Exercise training also appears to improve brain health, lower the risk of dementia, and improve performance of activities of daily living (ADLs) in individuals with dementia, thus reducing caregiver burden (DiLorito et al., 2021; Ding et al., 2018; Marmeleira et al., 2018). Regardless of age or situation, the older adult can find some activity suitable for his or her condition. It is important to keep older adults moving in any way possible for as long as possible (Box 19.2).

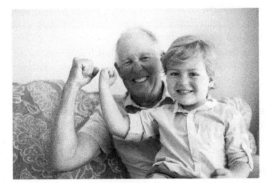

Physical activity is important for all older adults. (©iStock.com/ Squaredpixels.)

USING CLINICAL JUDGMENT TO PROMOTE HEALTHY AGING: ACTIVITY AND EXERCISE

Solutions, Nursing Actions, and Outcomes

Assessment of function and mobility are components of a health assessment for older adults (Chapters 9 and 20). Results from a recent study suggest that using a single question to assess physical activity in older women may be useful: "How would you describe your physical activity: not active, somewhat active, active, very active?" (Benton et al., 2020). For individuals 65 years of age and older, if they are relatively fit and have no limiting health conditions, initiation of a moderate-intensity exercise program is safe and does not require any type of cardiac screening (CDC, 2021). The consensus is that there is minimal cardiovascular risk to engaging in physical activity and a much greater risk in maintaining a sedentary lifestyle. Individuals with specific health conditions, such as cardiovascular disease and diabetes, may need to take extra precautions and seek medical advice before beginning an exercise program. Individuals who are frail will need more comprehensive assessment to adapt exercise recommendations to their abilities and ensure benefit without compromising safety.

Many older adults mistakenly believe that they are too old to begin a fitness program. Older adults are less likely to receive exercise counseling from their primary care providers than younger individuals. Research has noted that health care providers value the benefits of physical activity but have inadequate knowledge of specific recommendations. Nurses should be knowledgeable about recommended physical activity guidelines, educate individuals about the importance of exercise and physical activity, and provide exercise counseling on ways to incorporate exercise into daily routines. Giving an exercise prescription with specific advice about the type and frequency of exercise is important. Resources that nurses can use to assist older adults in beginning an exercise program are found in Box 19.3.

BOX 19.3   Resources for Best Practice

Physical Activity

Alzheimer's Society: Exercise and physical activity for individuals with dementia. https://www.alzheimers.org.uk/info/20029/daily_living/15/exercise_and_physical_activity/2.

Centers for Disease Control and Prevention (CDC): How much physical activity do older adults need? Comprehensive educational materials for individuals and professionals. https://www.cdc.gov/physicalactivity/basics/older_adults/index.htm.

Function-Focused Care: http://www.functionfocusedcare.org/.

Mobility Change Package and Toolkit: Guide to implementing a mobility program in hospitals. https://www.ahrq.gov/hai/tools/mvp/modules/technical/intro-early-mobility-fac-guide.html.3.

National Center on Health, Physical Activity and Disability: 14 weeks to a healthier you. http://www.ncpad.org/14weeks.

National Institute on Aging: Exercise and physical activity: your everyday guide: educational materials for individuals and professionals that can be used for teaching about exercise. Includes videos, stories, tracking tools, and tips for starting an exercise program. https://www.nia.nih.gov/health/how-older-adults-can-get-started-exercise.

US Department of Health and Human Services: Physical Activity Guidelines for Americans, ed 2. https://health.gov/sites/default/files/2019-09/Physical_Activity_Guidelines_2nd_edition.pdf.

YMCA: Online resources for chair exercises and chair yoga. https://www.youtube.com/watch?v=2luWm9wKqAk.

BOX 19.4   Exercise Guidelines

Older adults need at least:
- 2 hours and 30 minutes (150 minutes) of moderate-intensity aerobic activity every week (anything that gets your breathing harder and your heart beating faster) (e.g., brisk walking, swimming, bicycling, water aerobics, raking leaves or pushing a lawn mower)
- Muscle-strengthening activities that work all major muscle groups (hips, abdomen, chest, shoulders, and arms) at least 2 days a week
- Activities to improve balance (e.g., standing on one foot, yoga, tai chi) 2 to 3 times a week or incorporated in other exercises

Data from Centers for Disease Control and Prevention: *How much physical activity do older adults need?* (website), 2021. https://www.cdc.gov/physicalactivity/basics/adults/index.htm. Piercy K et al.: The physical activity guidelines for Americans, *JAMA* 320(19):2020–2028, 2018.

Physical Activity Guidelines

Guidelines for physical activity for adults 65 years of age and older who are generally fit and have no limiting health conditions are presented in Box 19.4. Types of recommended exercises are depicted in Fig. 19.1 and described more fully in Table 19.1. Multicomponent physical activity—combining more than one type of physical activity, such as aerobic activity, muscle strengthening activity, and balance training (e.g., dancing, yoga, water aerobics, gardening, sports)—has been shown to have more positive effects than a single exercise and may increase adherence (DiLorito et al., 2021). One does not have to perform exercises in 30-minute bouts; as little as 10 minutes of exercise has health benefits. Three 10-minute bouts of activity have the same fitness effects as one 30-minute bout. Individuals who are extremely frail may not be able to engage in aerobic activities and should begin with strength and balance training before participating in as little as 5 minutes of aerobic training.

Incorporating Physical Activity Into Lifestyle

One does not have to invest in expensive gym equipment or gym memberships to incorporate the recommended physical activity guidelines into one's daily routine. Hand weights (or using cans of food as weights), a chair, and an exercise mat can easily get the individual started. Individuals also may be able to integrate activity into daily life rather than doing a specific exercise. Examples include walking, golfing, tennis, biking, raking leaves, yard work or gardening, dancing, washing windows or

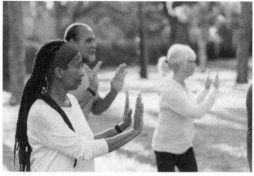

Tai chi can improve flexibility and balance and prevent falls. (©iStock.com/kali9.)

Be #Fit4Function with *Go4Life*®

Exercise and be active every day so you can keep doing what's most important to you.

Practice all 4 types of exercise fo the most benefits.

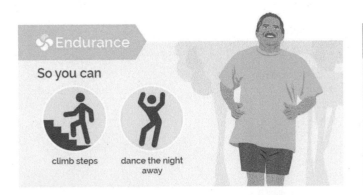

Endurance

So you can

climb steps | dance the night away

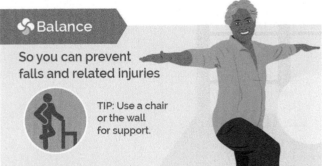

Balance

So you can prevent falls and related injuries

TIP: Use a chair or the wall for support.

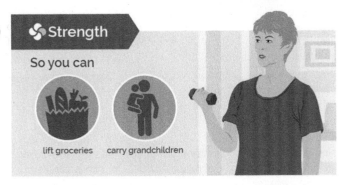

Strength

So you can

lift groceries | carry grandchildren

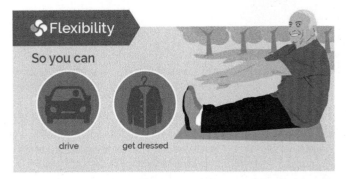

Flexibility

So you can

drive | get dressed

Visit go4life.nia.nih.gov and be #Fit4Function.

Get exercise ideas, motivational tips, and more from *Go4Life*®, an exercise and physical activity campaign for older adults from the National Institute on Aging at NIH.

Go4Life®

Fig. 19.1 Practice all 4 types of exercises for the most benefits. (Image courtesy the National Institute on Aging/National Institutes of Health.)

floors, washing and waxing the car, and swimming and water-based exercises. Exercise-based video games (e.g., Wii game system) offer other possibilities for exercise at all levels and have shown promising results (DiLorito et al., 2021). This technology is increasingly used by older adults in their own homes and in senior living facilities to encourage physical activity, improve balance, and provide enjoyable entertainment. Electronic tablets and smartphones are being evaluated for home-based exercise programs, and the use of personal fitness monitoring devices encourages exercise as well.

Many senior living communities and skilled nursing facilities (SNFs) provide gym equipment for residents. The Silver

TABLE 19.1   Guidelines for Teaching About Exercise

Exercise	Description	Benefits	Intensity	Frequency	Examples
Moderate-intensity aerobic activity	Continuous movement involving large muscle groups that is sustained for a minimum of 10 min; should make your heart beat faster	Improves cardiovascular functioning, strengthens heart muscle, decreases blood glucose and triglycerides, increases HDL, improves mood	On a 10-point scale, where sitting is 0 and working as hard as you can is 10, moderate-intensity aerobic activity is a 5 or 6. You will be able to talk but not sing the words to your favorite song	30 min, 5 days/wk Perform for at least 10 min at a time	Biking, swimming, and other water-based activities, dancing, brisk walking, lifestyle activities that incorporate large muscle groups (pushing a lawn mower, climbing stairs)
Muscle-strengthening activities	Activities that involve moving or lifting some type of resistance and work all major muscle groups (legs, hips, back, abdomen, chest, shoulders, arms)	Increases muscle strength, prevents sarcopenia, reduces fall risk, improves balance, modifies risk factors for cardiovascular disease and type 2 diabetes	To gain health benefits, muscle-strengthening activities need to be done to the point at which it is difficult to do another repetition without help. A repetition is one complete movement of an activity such as lifting a weight. An effort should be made to do 8–12 repetitions (one set) per activity or continue until it would be difficult to do another repetition without help	2 days/wk, but not consecutive days to allow muscles to recover between sessions	Lifting weights, calisthenics, working with resistance bands, Pilates, exercises that use the body's own weight for resistance (push-ups, sit-ups), heavy gardening (digging, shoveling), washing windows/floors
Stretching (flexibility)	A therapeutic maneuver designed to elongate shortened soft tissue structures and increase flexibility	Facilitates ROM around joints, prevents injury	Stretch muscle groups but not past the point of resistance or pain	At least 2 days/wk	Yoga, ROM exercises
Balance exercises	Movements that improve the ability to maintain control of the body over the base of support to avoid falling	Improves lower body strength, improves balance, helps prevent falls	Safety precautions are essential (holding on to a chair, working with another person)	Can be incorporated into regularly scheduled strength exercises. Older adults at risk of falling should do balance training for 3 or more days/wk	Tai chi, yoga, exercises such as standing on one foot, walking heel to toe or backward or sideways, leg raises, hip extensions (can be done holding on to a chair), standing up from a sitting position without using your hands

HDL, High-density lipoprotein; *ROM,* range of motion.
Data from Centers for Disease Control and Prevention: *How much physical activity do older adults need?* (website), 2015. https://www.cdc.gov/physicalactivity/basics/adults/index.htm. Accessed February 2018.

Sneakers program, the nation's leading exercise program for active community-dwelling older adults, is a membership benefit through some Medicare Advantage plans. Local community centers often provide exercise programs for older adults, and many gyms in the United States have reduced-cost memberships for individuals older than 65 years of age. Some have trainers on staff with expertise in exercises appropriate for older individuals. The nurse can share resources in the community,

and communities should be encouraged to provide accessible and affordable options for physical activity.

Maintaining motivation to adhere to a program of physical activity can present challenges for older adults. Making exercise programming enjoyable is recommended as a strategy to improve commitment and adherence to exercise activities. The benefits of group exercise in terms of social and emotional health have been reported, particularly among individuals

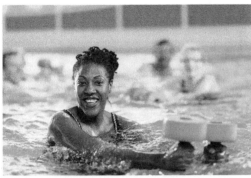

Aquatic programs are beneficial for older adults with mobility and joint problems. They improve circulation, muscle strength, and endurance and provide socialization and relaxation. (©iStock.com/FatCamera.)

who are at risk of social isolation (DiLorito et al., 2021). In a meta-analysis of exercise interventions for older adults, the most effective interventions were resistance training, meditative movement interventions, and exercise-based active video games. Resistance exercise programs have higher rates of adherence than aerobic exercise programs among older adults. The high prevalence of joint diseases, such as osteoarthritis (OA), may hamper successful performance of aerobic exercises that cause joint impact. Swimming is a low-risk activity that provides aerobic benefit, and water-based exercises are particularly beneficial for individuals with arthritis or other mobility limitations.

Chair-based exercises such as chair yoga, a gentle form of yoga practiced sitting in a chair or standing while holding on to the chair for support, is well suited to older adults with OA who cannot participate in traditional yoga or standing exercises, as well as to individuals with dementia (McCaffrey et al., 2017; Park et al., 2017, 2020). Results of chair yoga interventions with older adults with moderate to severe dementia reported an increase in quality-of-life score, including physical condition, mood, functional abilities, interpersonal relationships, and ability to participate in meaningful activities (Park et al., 2020). Research is needed on the types of physical exercise that are most effective for older adults, the use of assistive technologies to promote and monitor exercise, the benefits of group interventions, and the impact of significant others (e.g., caregivers) on encouraging

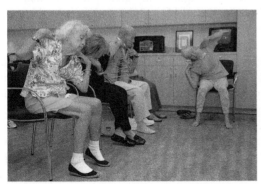

Age is not a barrier to fitness and exercise. Vera Paley, 95 years old, leads a yoga class. (Courtesy the Louis and Anne Green Memory and Wellness Center of the Christine E. Lynn College of Nursing at Florida Atlantic University.)

BOX 19.5   Tips for Best Practice
Physical Activity and Exercise Participation

- Provide appropriate screening before beginning an exercise program.
- Assess functional abilities and discuss how exercise can enhance function.
- Provide information about the benefits of exercise, emphasizing short-term benefits such as sleeping better, improved walking ability, decreasing fall risk.
- Clarify the misconceptions associated with exercise (fatigue, injury).
- Assess barriers to exercise and provide tips on how to overcome them.
- Provide an "exercise prescription" that specifies what exercises should be done and how often the person should exercise.
- Collaborate with the individual to set short- and long-term goals that are specific and achievable and match perceived needs, health, cognitive abilities, culture, gender, and interests.
- Encourage individual to keep a journal or diary to reflect experience and progress.
- Provide choices about types of exercises and design the program so that the person can do it at home or elsewhere.
- Begin with low-intensity physical activity for sedentary individuals.
- Initiate low-intensity activities in short sessions (<10 minutes) and include warmup and cooldown components with active stretching.
- Gradually progress from low to moderate intensity to obtain maximal benefits.
- Encourage use of proper, well-fitted footwear.
- Refer to community resources for physical fitness (e.g., YMCA, mall walking).
- Group-based programs and exercising with a buddy may be more successful.
- Try to make the program fun and entertaining (walking with favorite music, socializing with friends).
- Discuss potential exercise side effects and any symptoms that should be reported.
- Provide safety tips and situations that may require medical attention (Box 19.6).
- Share stories about the benefits of your own personal exercise program and those of older adults.
- Provide ongoing support and follow up on progress; support from experts and family and peers is a significant factor in encouraging continued participation.

exercise participation (DiLorito et al., 2021) Box 19.5 provides helpful tips nurses can use to encourage individuals to adopt physical activity. Box 19.6 presents safety precautions.

Special Considerations

The benefits of physical activity extend to individuals who are more physically impaired, those who are nonambulatory or experience cognitive impairment, and those residing in assisted living facilities or SNFs. In fact, these individuals may benefit most from an exercise program in terms of function and quality of life but often are not included in physical activity programs (Box 19.7). Residents of nursing facilities should be involved in an exercise program two to three times per week (Morley, 2016). There are many creative and enjoyable ideas for enhancing physical activity, such as using lower extremity cycling equipment, marching in place, tossing a ball, stretching, and using resistive bands.

Individuals with cognitive impairment often are not included in physical activity programs. Results of research suggest that

BOX 19.6 Tips for Best Practice
Exercise Safety

- Always wear comfortable, loose-fitting clothing and appropriate shoes for your activity.
- Warm up: Perform a low- to moderate-intensity warm up for 5 to 10 minutes.
- Drink water before, during, and after your exercise session.
- When exercising outdoors, evaluate your surroundings for safety: traffic, pavement condition, weather, and strangers.
- Wear clothes made of fabrics that absorb sweat and remove it from your skin.
- Never wear rubber or plastic suits. These could hold the sweat on your skin and make your body overheat.
- Wear sunscreen when you exercise outdoors.

Stop Exercising Right Away If You
- Have pain or pressure in your chest, neck, shoulder, or arm.
- Feel dizzy or sick.
- Break out in a cold sweat.
- Have muscle cramps.
- Feel acute (not just achy) pain in your joints, feet, ankles, or legs.
- Have trouble breathing. Slow down; you should be able to talk while exercising without gasping for breath.

Times Exercise Should Not Be Done
- Avoid hard exercise for 2 hours after a big meal. (A leisurely walk around the block is fine.)
- Do not exercise when you have a fever and/or viral infection accompanied by muscle aches.
- Do not exercise if your systolic blood pressure is greater than 200 mm Hg and your diastolic blood pressure is greater than 100 mm Hg.
- Do not exercise if your resting heart rate is greater than 120 beats/minute.
- Do not exercise if you have a joint that you are using to exercise (such as a knee or an ankle) that is red and warm and painful.
- If you have osteoporosis, always avoid stretches that flex your spine or cause you to bend at the waist and avoid making jerky, rapid movements.
- Stop exercising if you experience severe pain or swelling in a joint. Discomfort that persists should always be evaluated.
- Do not exercise if you have a new symptom that has not been evaluated by your health care provider, such as pain in your chest, abdomen, or a joint; swelling in an arm, leg, or joint; difficulty catching your breath at rest; or a fluttering feeling in your chest.

---

older adults with cognitive impairment who participate in exercise programs may improve strength and endurance, mood and behavior, cognitive function, and ability to perform ADLs. Elements of successful exercise interventions with individuals with dementia include individualized approaches, caregiver involvement, strength-training interventions, one-component exercises, and enjoyable activities (Rodriguez-Larrad et al., 2017). Although further research is needed to understand the level and intensity of exercise that is beneficial for each type of dementia, exercise should be a component of the plan of care (Li et al., 2020) (see Box 19.2).

Wheelchairs are a necessary adjunct at some level of immobility and for some individuals, but they are overused in nursing homes, with up to 80% of residents spending time sitting in a wheelchair every day. Often the individual is not assessed for

BOX 19.7 Positive Effects of Exercise in Long-Term Care

- Reduce frailty
- Enhance walking speed
- Improve function
- Decrease hospitalization
- Improve mobility
- Decrease falls
- Enhance cognition
- Decrease agitation
- Decrease dysphoria
- Enhance sleep
- Decrease sleep apnea
- Enhance quality of life

From Morley J: High-quality exercise programs are an essential component of nursing home care, *JAMDA* 17:373–375, 2016.

therapeutic treatment and restorative ambulation programs to improve mobility and function. Improperly maintained or ill-fitting wheelchairs can cause pressure ulcers, skin tears, bruises and abrasions, and nerve impingement and contribute to falls in nursing homes. If an individual is unable to ambulate without assistance, the person should be seated in a comfortable chair with frequent repositioning, and wheelchairs should be used for transport only. It is important that a professional evaluate the wheelchair for proper fit, provide training on proper use, and evaluate the resident for more appropriate mobility and seating devices and ambulation programs. There are many new assistive devices that could replace wheelchairs, such as small walkers with wheels and seats.

Maintaining Function Across Care Settings

Even though the focus in hospitals is on acute illness management, there is growing awareness of the need to also focus on functional status, especially in older adults. Hospitalization is associated with significantly greater loss of total, lean, and fat mass strength in older adults. Individuals older than age 85 experience the most functional decline with hospitalization. However, 34% of Medicare patients who were hospitalized experienced functional decline resulting in readmission (AARP, 2021). The onset of functional decline can occur in a matter of days and may start preadmission and continue after discharge, depending on the individual's condition and comorbid problems.

Functional decline leads to adverse events for older patients that are expensive to the health care system and cause stress for patients and families (Gray-Miceli, 2017; Swoboda et al., 2020). Bed rest, restricted activity or low mobility, and the tendency for staff to perform ADL care rather than encourage self-care all contribute to functional decline. Generally, older medical patients spend at least 83% of their acute care stay in bed and engage in only 2.4 minutes/day of moderate-level activity (Resnick et al., 2016a). Evidence demonstrates that nurses insufficiently promote mobility in older adults admitted to medical inpatient hospital units. Nurses need increased knowledge and awareness of older hospitalized adults' mobility needs, and older adults also need increased knowledge of the significance of mobility during hospitalization (Dermody & Kovach, 2017). Recommendations for reducing functional decline during hospitalization include structured exercise, progressive resistance strength training, and walking programs, with interdisciplinary approaches being most effective. Outcomes of early mobility to prevent functional decline include lower hospital costs, fewer delirium days, and improved functional independence (Lach, 2021). The American Geriatrics Society's (2019) CoCare: HELP program (formerly Hospital Elder Life Program) (Chapter 1) offers a free mobility change package and toolkit to guide organizations in implementing mobility programs (see Box 19.2).

Function-Focused Care

Function-focused care (FFC) is a "philosophy of care that involves teaching direct care workers to evaluate older adults' underlying capability with regard to function and physical activity and optimize their participation in all activities" (Resnick et al., 2021, p. 1) (Box 19.8). Examples include modeling behavior (e.g., during oral care, bathing), providing verbal cues during dressing, walking the individual to the dining room instead of transporting in a wheelchair, and doing resistance exercises with patients. Nurse researcher Barbara Resnick and her colleagues have conducted numerous studies evaluating the use of FFC care in improving function and physical activity, improving mood, and decreasing behavioral symptoms associated with dementia in older adults in hospitals, assisted living residences, and SNFs (Gray-Miceli, 2017; Lee et al., 2019; Resnick et al., 2016a, 2016b, 2021).

Nurses understand the importance of functional care yet often are not able to carry out functional care interventions.

Lack of organizational support, staff shortages, and lack of time and equipment have been identified as barriers to implementation. Suggestions to enhance the ability to provide this needed care include providing increased resources for the care of older adults; involving interdisciplinary teams, patients, and families in FFC; and creating environments in which FFC is a nursing expectation and functional decline is identified as a safety risk (Swoboda et al., 2020).

A family-centered, FFC intervention (Fam-FCC) incorporates an educational empowerment model for family caregivers that focuses on improving function during and after an acute care hospitalization. Outcomes of Fam-FCC include fewer 30-day hospital readmissions, less delirium severity, improved ADL performance, less decrease in walking ability, and an increase in preparedness for caregiving and less anxiety among family caregivers (Boltz et al., 2015). Box 19.2 includes information on FCC.

BOX 19.8   Tips for Best Practice
Function-Focused Care in Acute Care

- Ask or encourage the individual to move in bed and give the person time to move rather than moving the person yourself.
- Give step-by-step cues on how to move in bed (e.g., "Put your right hand on the rail and pull yourself over onto your left side.").
- Ask or encourage the individual to transfer and wait for the individual to move rather than transferring the individual yourself or automatically using lift equipment (use of assistive equipment depends on mobility and cognitive status).
- Give step-by-step cues and use gestures or demonstration on how to transfer safely (e.g., "Plant feet firmly on the floor and slide to the edge of the chair.").
- Ask or encourage the individual to walk or independently propel wheelchair and give the person time and step-by-step cues to perform the activity rather than doing it yourself.
- Encourage use of assistive devices; provide instruction on use and ensure that device is available and appropriate.

KEY CONCEPTS

- Few factors contribute as much to health in aging as being physically active.
- Physical activity enhances health and functional status while also decreasing the number of chronic illnesses and functional limitations often assumed to be a part of growing older.
- Despite a large body of evidence about the benefits of physical activity to maintain and improve function, physical activity levels of older adults remain low and have not improved over the past decade.
- Components of a health assessment for older adults should include assessment of function and mobility. Exercise counseling should be provided as a part of that assessment.

- The benefits of physical activity extend to older adults who are more physically frail, those who are nonambulatory or experience cognitive impairment, and those residing in assisted living facilities or SNFs. In fact, these individuals may benefit most from an exercise program in terms of function and quality of life.
- Nursing actions to assist older adults to improve physical activity include evaluation of functional ability, mobility, level of activity, education, and exercise counseling.

NEXT-GENERATION NCLEX® (NGN) EXAMINATION–STYLE QUESTIONS

A 65-year-old male patient who was hospitalized 3 weeks prior for general-ized weakness after an episode of dehydration has come to the health care provider's office today for a follow-up appointment. The patient, who ar-rived using a walker, reports adhering to discharge teaching and says, "I feel better than I did when I was in this hospital. I still don't feel great, but I think I'm on the right track." When asked to describe his daily activity routine, the patient says, "After breakfast, I sit in my chair and do some stretching of my arms and legs. I've been going outside a little bit each day. When I first went home from the hospital, I could only walk a few minutes before I was tired, even with my walker. Now I can walk twice a day for 10 minutes each, and I still use my walker so I won't fall. Next week I'm going to try to do three little walks with my walker. My wife also got me some of these little hand weights so when I sit down to watch TV, I do about 10 repetitions of lifting them up." The patient's wife says, "I am checking on him all day long and I always bring him a cup of water to drink every time I see him so that he stays hydrated." Assessment reveals a well-dressed and appropriately groomed older adult, temperature 98.9°F (37.2°C), blood pressure 122/70 mm Hg, respirations 18 breaths/minute, and moist mucous membranes.

Indicate whether today's assessment findings suggest that each item of posthospitalization dis-charge teaching by the nurse listed in the table below was effective or ineffective.

Discharge Teaching	Effective	Ineffective
Use a walker at all times to avoid falls		
Perform muscle-strengthening activities at least twice weekly		
Perform flexibility exercises at least twice weekly		
Work your way up to doing 10 minutes of activity three times daily		
Drink water before, during, and after activity		

NURSING STUDY

Exercise and Activity

Tom, 75 years old, had lost his wife, Ella, a year ago and had been feeling down and tired for much of each day. He had retired at age 70 from his job as a hous-ing contractor and had spent much of his time since then with Ella. They had been married for 50 years. He now sometimes seemed to sit in front of the television for most of the day without actually remembering what it was that he had viewed. Many of the couple's friends had moved away or relocated to retire-ment settings, and other than his daughter, who lived about 45 minutes from his house, Tom rarely saw anyone anymore. He had lived like this for nearly a year, and it had become his daily pattern of life. After a suggestion from his daughter, Tom took the initiative to go to the local senior center. He had lunch there nearly every day. At one point he was asked if he would allow a nursing student to spend time with him during her semester in a gerontology course. He agreed. In the course of her assessment, she (and he) found that his activity level was nearly completely sedentary. She gave Tom information about the ramifications of such a sedentary life. She pointed out that the center had an exercise class every day between 10.00 a.m. and 12 noon. Because he came to the center every day (except Saturday and Sunday) for lunch, it seemed a good thing to do. Tom said to the nursing student, "This isn't anything I am really interested in doing, but I will give it a try." Though he did not admit it, he was worried because he usually felt weak and listless during the day after lunch. When he did attend the first class, he found that there were both basic exercises and more advanced ones for older adults who had participated regularly for 6 months. He found that after a few weeks he was enjoying the social aspect of the exercise, if not the exercise itself. After nearly a year of fairly regular participation, Tom began play-ing golf with some of the men from the center. Once, he even attended a dance.

CLINICAL JUDGMENT QUESTIONS AND ACTIVITIES

Questions refer to the Nursing Study.

1. What lifestyle factors developed by Tom after his wife's death had become dangerous to his health?
2. Compose a list of 10 questions you would ask Tom to obtain a clear picture of factors contributing to his activity level. Discuss the rationale behind each question.

3. List some of the common methods for motivating Tom that his nursing student may have used.
4. Describe the level of activity that should be Tom's starting point and discuss symptoms he might expect as he increases his activity level.

RESEARCH QUESTIONS

1. What activities and exercises are most useful in maintaining mobility in older adults?
2. What factors increase adherence to an exercise program among community-dwelling older adults?
3. What are the benefits of group exercise programs?
4. What factors in the institutional environment induce immobility?

5. What are some creative ways to implement exercise in the long-term care setting?
6. How does the design of an exercise program differ for indi-viduals with cognitive impairment?

REFERENCES

AARP: Explaining post-hospital syndrome, AARP *Bulletin,* April 7, 2021, p 32.

American Geriatrics Society: *CoCare: HELP* (website), 2019. https://help.agscocare.org/About_AGS_CoCare_program_help.

Benton M et al.: Validity of a single activity question for clinical assessment of older women, *J Gerontol Nurs* 46(12):15–20, 2020.

Boltz M et al.: Testing family-centered, function-focused care in hospitalized persons with dementia, *Neurodegener Dis Manag* 5(3):203–215, 2015.

Centers for Disease Control and Prevention (CDC): *How much physical activity do adults need?* (website), 2021. https://www.cdc.gov/physicalactivity/basics/adults/index.htm.

Dermody G & Kovach C: Nurses' experience with and perception of barriers to promoting mobility in hospitalized older adults: a descriptive study, *J Gerontol Nurs* 43(11):22–29, 2017.

DiLorito C, et al.: Exercise interventions for older adults: a systematic review of meta-analyses, *J Sport Health Sci* 10(1):29–47, 2021.

Ding K et al.: Cardiorespiratory fitness and white matter neuronal fiber integrity in mild cognitive impairment, *J Alzheimers Dis* 61(2):729–739, 2018.

Du Y et al.: Trends in adherence to the physical activity guidelines for Americans for aerobic activity and time spent on sedentary behavior among US adults, 2007–2016, *JAMA Network Open* 2(7):e197597, 2019.

Gray-Miceli D: Impaired mobility and functional decline in older adults: evidence to facilitate a practice change, *Nurs Clin North Am* 52:469–487, 2017.

Lach H: Home sweet home: resources for promoting mobility for aging in place across settings, *J Gerontol Nurs* 47(5):3–6, 2021.

Lee S et al.: The effectiveness of function-focused care interventions in nursing homes: a systematic review, *J Nurs Res* 27(1):1–13, 2019.

Li B et al.: An integrative review of exercise interventions among community-dwelling adults with Alzheimer's disease, *Int J Older People Nurs* 15(1):e12287, 2020 https://doi.org/10.1111/opn.12287.

Marmeleira J et al.: Exercise merging physical and cognitive stimulation improves physical fitness and cognitive functioning in older nursing home residents: a pilot study, *Geriatr Nurs* 39:303–309, 2018.

McCaffrey R et al.: Chair yoga: feasibility and sustainability study with older community-dwelling adults with osteoarthritis, *Holist Nurs Pract* 31(3):148–157, 2017.

Morley JE: High-quality exercise programs are an essential component of nursing home care, *J Am Med Dir Assoc* 17:373–375, 2016.

Park J et al.: A pilot randomized controlled trial of the effects of chair yoga on pain and physical function among community-dwelling older adults with lower extremity osteoarthritis, *J Am Geriatr Soc* 65:592–597, 2017.

Park J et al.: Feasibility of conducting nonpharmacological interventions to manage dementia symptoms in community-dwelling older adults: a cluster randomized controlled trial, *Am J Alzheimers Dis Other Demen* 35:1533317519872635, 2020.

Resnick B et al.: Dissemination and implementation of function focused care for assisted living, *Health Educ Behav* 43(3):296–304, 2016.

Resnick B et al.: Feasibility and efficacy of function-focused care for orthopedic trauma patients, *J Trauma Nurs* 23(3):144–155, 2016.

Resnick B et al.: Testing the implementation of function-focused care in assisted living settings, *JAMDA* 22(8):1706–1713, 2021. doi:10.1016/j.jamda.2020.09.026.

Rodriguez-Larrad A et al.: Effectiveness of a multicomponent exercise program in the attenuation of frailty in long-term nursing home residents: study protocol for a randomized clinical controlled trial, *BMC Geriatr* 17:60, 2017.

Swoboda N, et al.: Nurses' perceptions of their role in functional focused care in hospitalized older people: an integrated review, *Int J Older People Nurs* 15: e12337, 2020.

Falls and Fall Risk Reduction

Theris A. Touhy

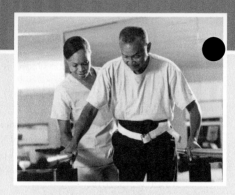

http://evolve.elsevier.com/Touhy/TwdHlthAging

A STUDENT SPEAKS

The thought of needing someone to help me shower and dress and transfer me from a chair to bed requires more acceptance than I have ever had to muster. I'm very good at making the best out of a bad situation, but somehow adapting to something like never walking again cannot be equated with a "bad situation." It is permanent, and it is the sacrifice of my precious independence. I was born on Independence Day! Thinking about these things overwhelms me with sadness.

Holiday, age 22

AN OLDER ADULT SPEAKS

I hate to have the family see me like this. You know, I was a military man. I took pride in the way I marched . . . or just stood at attention. I never imagined a time when I wouldn't be able to walk without assistance.

Jerry, age 78

LEARNING OBJECTIVES

On completion of this chapter, the reader will be able to:

1. Discuss the effects of impaired mobility on general function and quality of life.
2. Identify risk factors for impaired mobility and nursing actions to maintain and enhance mobility.
3. Recognize and analyze the cues that indicate fall risk.
4. Describe the effects of physical restraints and identify alternative safety interventions.
5. Use clinical judgment to identify and evaluate solutions and nursing actions to reduce falls and injury.

This chapter focuses on the importance of maintaining maximal mobility; assessing gait, mobility, and fall risk factors; implementing fall risk–reduction interventions; providing restraint-free care; and using clinical judgment to identify and evaluate solutions and nursing actions to maintain or enhance mobility and prevent falls.

MOBILITY AND AGING

Mobility is the capacity one has for movement within the personally available microcosm and macrocosm. This includes abilities such as moving oneself by turning over in bed, transferring from lying to sitting and from sitting to standing, walking, using assistive devices, or accessing transportation within the community environment. In infancy, moving about is the major mode of learning and interacting with the environment. Throughout life, movement remains a significant means of personal contact, sensation, exploration, pleasure, and control. Retaining pride and maintaining dignity, self-care, independence, social contacts, and activity are all needs identified as important to older adults, and all are facilitated by mobility.

Mobility and comparative degrees of agility are based on muscle strength, flexibility, postural stability, vibratory sensation, cognition, and perceptions of stability. Aging produces changes in muscles and joints (Chapter 28). Individuals who maintain regular physical activity and good health habits throughout life may have fewer of these changes (Chapter 19). Prenatal and postnatal development of muscle fibers and muscle growth during puberty also may have critical effects on musculoskeletal aging. Mobility is intimately linked to health status, quality of life, and healthy aging.

Gait and mobility impairments are not an inevitable consequence of aging but may occur as a result of chronic diseases or past or recent trauma. Mobility and gait impairments are caused by diseases and impairments across many organ systems. For some older adults, osteoporosis, Parkinson's disease, strokes, and arthritic conditions markedly affect movement and functional capacities. Mobility may be limited by paresthesias; hemiplegia; neuromotor disturbances; fractures; foot, knee, and hip problems; and respiratory diseases and other illnesses that deplete one's energy. All these conditions are likely to occur more frequently and have more devastating effects as one ages. Many older adults have some of these impairments, with women significantly outnumbering men in this respect (Chapter 22).

Difficulties in mobility are often the first sign of functional decline and may indicate that an individual could benefit from preventive actions. Impairment of mobility is an early predictor of physical disability and is associated with poor outcomes such as falling, loss of independence, depression, decreased quality of life, institutionalization, and death (Bergland et al., 2017). Maintenance of mobility and function is an essential component of best practice gerontological nursing and is effective in preventing falls, unnecessary decline, and loss of independence.

FALLS

Falls are defined as any sudden drop from one surface to a lower surface with or without injury. Falls are one of the most important geriatric syndromes and the leading cause of morbidity and mortality for older adults. Falls are the most common adverse event in health care facilities and the leading cause of injury-related emergency department (ED) visits and injury-related deaths in older adults. Of particular concern, rates of fall-related ED visits and hospitalizations are increasing (de Vries et al., 2018). Each year, about one-third of adults ages 65 years and older and half of those ages 80 years and older will fall. More than half of those will fall more than once (Pirker & Katzenschlager, 2017). Nearly half of all falls result in injury, of which 10% are serious.

About 3% to 20% of hospital inpatients fall at least once during their hospitalization (Quigley et al., 2016). Between 50% and 75% of nursing home residents fall annually, twice the rate of community-dwelling older adults, and these falls result in more serious complications than other falls (Centers for Disease Control and Prevention [CDC], 2021). Nearly 50% of hospital admissions and most nursing home placements are a direct result of fall-related injuries such as hip fractures, upper limb injuries, and traumatic brain injuries (Taylor-Piliae et al., 2017). Estimates are that up to two-thirds of falls may be preventable (Gray-Miceli et al., 2016). Falls are a significant public health problem. Various national studies from across the globe have demonstrated increasing fall-related incidence of injury, and this can be expected to increase substantially with the aging of the population (Fig. 20.1). Worldwide, falls are the second leading cause of accidental or unintentional injury deaths. *Healthy People 2030* includes several goals related to falls (see Healthy People 2030).

Healthy People 2030

Falls, Fall Prevention, and Injury

- Reduce fall-related deaths among older adults.
- Reduce the rate of emergency department visits due to falls among older adults.
- Reduce hip fractures among older adults.
- Increase the proportion of adults with dizziness or balance problems who have been referred to a specialist.
- Reduce fatal and nonfatal traumatic brain injuries.

Data from US Department of Health and Human Services: *Healthy People 2030* (website), 2020. https://health.gov/healthypeople.

⚡ SAFETY TIPS

The Quality and Safety Education for Nurses (QSEN) project has developed quality and safety measures for nursing and proposed targets for the knowledge, skills, and attitudes to be developed in nursing prelicensure and graduate programs. Education on falls and fall risk reduction is an important consideration in the QSEN safety competency, which addresses the need to minimize risk of harm to patients and providers through both system effectiveness and individual performance. Safe and effective transfer techniques are an important component of safety measures.

Consequences of Falls

Hip Fractures

More than 95% of hip fractures among older adults are caused by falling, usually by falling sideways. Hip fractures are associated with considerable morbidity and mortality. The likelihood of recovery to prefracture level of function is less than 50%, regardless of the individual's previous level of function.

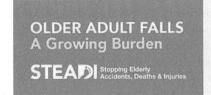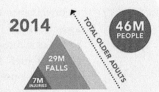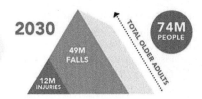

Fig. 20.1 Older adults falls: a growing burden. (From Centers for Disease Control and Prevention: STEADI Stopping Elderly Accidents, Deaths & Injuries, 2018.)

Returning to a high level of function is particularly low in individuals older than 85 years, with multiple comorbid conditions, or with dementia. Mattia et al. (2019) reported that the mortality rate in the first year after hip fractures surgery is high, ranging between 15% and 36%, and mortality rates a year after hip fracture were three to four times higher than expected in the general population. This excess mortality persists for 10 years after the fracture and is higher in men. White women have significantly higher hip fracture rates than Black women due to a higher incidence of osteoporotic changes.

The Fracture Risk Assessment Tool (FRAX), which assesses a person's 10-year risk of having an osteoporotic-related fracture, is commonly used for the prediction of fractures on the basis of clinical risk factors, with or without the use of femoral neck bone mineral density (US Preventive Services Task Force, 2018; Xu et al., 2020). The FRAX might be included in fall risk assessment measures for at-risk groups and can be completed online (Box 20.1). Osteoporosis is discussed in Chapter 28.

Traumatic Brain Injury

Older adults (75 years of age and older) have the highest rates of traumatic brain injury (TBI)–related hospitalization and death. Falls are the leading cause of TBI in this age group (CDC, 2020). Advancing age negatively affects the outcome after TBI, even with relatively minor head injuries. Factors that place the older adult at greater risk for TBI include the presence of comorbid conditions, use of antiplatelet and anticoagulant medications,

and changes in the brain with age. Preinjury use of antiplatelet and anticoagulant medications is especially problematic with head trauma and increases the risk of traumatic intracranial hemorrhage and premature disability and death.

Brain changes with age, although clinically insignificant, do increase the risk of TBIs and especially subdural hematomas, which are much more common in older adults. There is a decreased adherence of the dura mater to the skull, increased fragility of bridging cerebral veins, and increases in the subarachnoid space and atrophy of the brain, which create more space within the cranial vault for blood to accumulate before symptoms appear.

Although falls are the leading cause of TBI, older adults may experience TBI with seemingly more minor incidents (e.g., sharp turns or jarring movement of the head). Some individuals may not even remember the incident. In cases of moderate to severe TBI, there will be cognitive and physical sequelae obvious at the time of injury or shortly afterward that will require emergency treatment. However, older adults who experience a minor incident with seemingly lesser trauma to the head often present with more insidious and delayed symptom onset. Because of changes in the aging brain, there is an increased risk for slowly expanding subdural hematomas.

TBIs have been associated with an earlier age of dementia onset and a factor in increasing the risk of Parkinson's disease (Gardner et al., 2018; Schaffert et al., 2018). Results of a recent study suggested that sustaining just one head injury may increase the chance of developing dementia decades later by 25%. Women are more likely than men to develop dementia following head injury, and White individuals are at greater risk than Black individuals (Schneider et al., 2021).

TBIs are often missed or misdiagnosed among older adults. If clinicians do not have information on the usual cognitive status of the older adult, manifestations of TBI are often misinterpreted as signs of dementia, which can lead to inaccurate prognoses and limit implementation of appropriate treatment. Health professionals should have a high suspicion of TBI in an older adult who falls and strikes the head or experiences even a more minor event, such as sudden twisting of the head. For older adults who are receiving warfarin and experience minor head injury with a negative computed tomography (CT) scan, a protocol of 24-hour observation followed by a second CT scan is recommended. Box 20.2 presents signs and symptoms of TBI.

FALL RISK FACTORS

Falls are a symptom of a problem and are rarely benign in older adults. The etiology of falls is multifactorial and the result of a convergence of risk factors across biological and behavioral aspects of the individual and factors in the environment. Episodes of acute illness or exacerbations of chronic illness are times of high fall risk and falls may indicate impending illness. New-onset delirium is a common cause of falls (Morley, 2017). Nurse researcher Deanna Gray-Miceli et al. (2010, 2016) developed seven types of fall classifications based on research in nursing homes (Box 20.3).

BOX 20.1   Resources for Best Practice
Fall Prevention and Restraint Alternatives

- Agency for Healthcare Research and Quality (AHRQ): Preventing falls in hospitals: a toolkit for improving quality of care. https://www.ahrq.gov/professionals/systems/hospital/fallpxtoolkit/index.html.
- American Geriatrics Society: CoCare: HELP (formerly Hospital Elder Life Program). https://help.agscocare.org/About_AGS_CoCare_program_help.
- Centers for Disease Control and Prevention (CDC): STEADI (Stopping Elderly Accidents, Deaths and Injuries): educational materials for patients and providers; check for safety: a home fall prevention checklist for older adults; safe patient handling for schools of nursing (curricular materials). https://www.cdc.gov/steadi/materials.html.
- FRAX Tool: Evaluation of fracture risk. https://www.sheffield.ac.uk/FRAX/tool.aspx?country=9.
- Gericareonline: Story of Your Falls. http://www.gericareonline.net/tools/eng/falls/index.html.
- Hartford Institute for Geriatric Nursing (consultgeri.org): Hendrich II Fall Risk Model. http://www.wsha.org/wp-content/uploads/Hendrich-II-Fall-Risk.pdf; https://www.youtube.com/watch?v=jUwqXQU1Bmg; Avoiding restraints in hospitalized older adults with dementia. https://hign.org/consultgeri/try-this-series/avoiding-restraints-patients-dementia.
- National Council on Aging: National Falls Prevention Resource Center. https://www.ncoa.org/professionals/health/center-for-healthy-aging/national-falls-prevention-resource-center.
- The Joint Commission: Targeted Solutions Tool for Preventing Falls (TST): Provides in-depth support to help hospitals in fall prevention efforts. https://www.centerfortransforminghealthcare.org/tst_pfi.aspx.
- Veterans Affairs (VA) National Center for Patient Safety: Falls Toolkit. https://www.patientsafety.va.gov/professionals/onthejob/falls.asp.

BOX 20.2   Signs and Symptoms of Traumatic Brain Injury (TBI) in Older Adults[a]

Symptoms of Mild TBI

- Low-grade headache that will not dissipate
- Slowness in thinking, speaking, acting, or reading
- Getting lost or easily confused
- Feeling tired all the time, lack of energy or motivation
- Change in sleep pattern
- Loss of balance, feeling lightheaded or dizzy
- Increased sensitivity to sounds, lights, or distractions
- Blurred vision or eyes that tire easily
- Loss of sense of taste or smell
- Ringing in the ears
- Change in sex drive
- Mood changes

Symptoms of Moderate to Severe TBI

- Severe headache that gets worse or does not disappear
- Repeated vomiting or nausea
- Seizures
- Inability to wake from sleep
- Dilation of one or both pupils
- Slurred speech
- Weakness or numbness in the arms or legs
- Loss of coordination
- Increased confusion, restlessness, or agitation

[a]Older adults taking blood thinners should be seen immediately by a health care provider if they have a bump or blow to the head, even if they do not have any of the symptoms listed here.

BOX 20.3   Fall Classifications

- Falls due to acute events such as orthostatic hypotension, loss of balance, syncope
- Falls due to chronic events such as chronic dizziness or lower extremity weakness
- Falls due to medications
- Falls due to environmental mishaps
- Falls due to equipment malfunction
- Falls due to poor safety awareness
- Falls due to poor patient judgment

From Gray-Miceli D, deCordova P, Crane G, et al: Nursing home registered nurses' and licensed practical nurses' knowledge of causes of falls, *J Nurs Care Qual* 31(2):153–160, 2016.

⚡ SAFETY TIPS

A history of falls is a significant risk factor, and individuals who have fallen have three times the risk of falling again and being injured compared with persons who did not fall in the past year. Recurrent falls are often the result of the same underlying cause but also can be an indication of disease progression (e.g., heart failure, Parkinson's disease) or a new acute problem (e.g., infection, dehydration).

Individual risk factors can be categorized as either intrinsic or extrinsic. Intrinsic risk factors are unique to each individual and are associated with factors such as reduced vision and

hearing, unsteady gait, cognitive impairment, acute and chronic illnesses, effects of medications, and sleep disorders. Extrinsic risk factors are external to the individual and related to the physical environment and include lack of support equipment for bathtubs and toilets, height of beds, condition of floors, poor lighting, inappropriate footwear, and improper use of assistive devices. Falls in the young-old and the more healthy old occur more frequently because of external reasons; however, with increasing age and comorbid conditions, internal and locomotor reasons become increasingly prevalent as factors contributing to falls. The risk of falling increases as the number of risk factors increases. Most falls occur from a combination of intrinsic and extrinsic factors that combine at a certain point in time (Fig. 20.2).

Community-dwelling older adults may fall for different reasons than individuals living in long-term care. Environmental factors (indoors and outdoors) may bring a higher risk for falls when combined with current health conditions. Other factors also may influence risk for falls, including stressful life events such as illness; accidents; death of spouse, partner, close relatives, or friends; loss of pet; financial trouble; a move or change in residence; or giving up an important hobby. Falls in health care settings are more often related to the health status of the individual and the change in the person's environment. Inadequate staffing in health care settings is also a factor that may increase fall risk if patients attempt to get up for bathroom use or get out of bed because help is not readily available.

Fear of Falling (Fallophobia)

Even if a fall does not result in injury, falls contribute to a loss of confidence that leads to reduced physical activity, increased dependency, and social withdrawal. Fear of falling (fallophobia) may

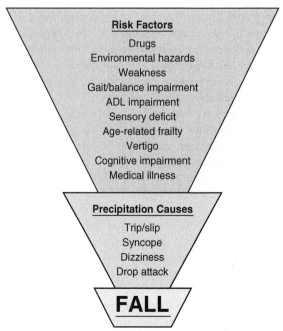

Fig. 20.2 Multifactorial nature of falls. *ADL,* Activities of daily living. (From Ham RJ, Sloane PD, Warshaw GA, et al: *Primary care geriatrics*, ed 6, Philadelphia, 2014, Elsevier Saunders.)

restrict an individual's life space (area in which an individual performs activities). Fear of falling is an important predictor of general functional decline and a risk factor for future falls. Fallophobia is a significant cue to identifying risk of falls and implementing nursing actions for prevention. Questions about fear of falling and effects on mobility always should be included in fall risk assessment.

Nursing staff also may contribute to fear of falling in their patients by telling them not to get up by themselves or by using restrictive devices to keep them from independently moving, further decreasing mobility, safety, and function and increasing fall risk. This often happens with older adults who are hospitalized for acute illness and is associated with poor outcomes, including loss of muscle mass and strength, long hospital stays, falls, and declines in activities of daily living (ADL) abilities post discharge (Chapter 19).

Gait Disturbances

More than 60% of community-dwelling individuals 80 years or older experience gait disorders. Gait deformities affect walking and balance and are associated with a threefold increase in fall risk. Marked gait disorders are not normally a consequence of aging alone but are more likely indicative of an underlying pathological condition. Arthritis of the knee may result in ligamentous weakness and instability, causing the legs to give way or collapse. Diabetes, dementia, Parkinson's disease, stroke, alcoholism, and vitamin B deficiencies may cause neurological damage and resultant gait problems (Pirker & Katzenschlager, 2017).

Foot Deformities

Foot deformities and ill-fitting footwear also contribute to gait problems and potential for falls. Frequent painful foot problems occur in about a quarter of older adults and have been shown to impair balance and foot function and more than double the risk of falling (Muchna et al., 2018). Care of the feet is an important aspect of mobility, comfort, and a stable gait and is often neglected. Little attention is given to one's feet until they interfere with walking and moving and ultimately the ability to remain independent. Foot problems are often unrecognized and untreated, leading to considerable dysfunction. Older adults may consider foot problems and foot pain to be part of aging rather than a treatable medical condition.

As we age, feet are subjected to a lifetime of stress and may not be able to continue to adapt, and inflammatory changes in bone and soft tissue can occur. Foot health and function may reflect systemic disease or give early clues to physical illness. Sudden or gradual changes in the condition of the nails or the skin of the feet or the appearance of recurring infections may be precursors of more serious health problems. Rheumatological disorders such as the various forms of arthritis also can affect the feet. Gout occurs most often in the joint of the great toe but is a systemic disease. Both diabetes and peripheral vascular disease (PVD) commonly cause problems in the lower extremities that can quickly become life-threatening.

Foot problems may include foot pain, nail fungus, dry skin, corns and calluses, bunions, and neuropathy (Fig. 20.3). Some older adults are unable to walk comfortably or at all because of neglect of corns, bunions, and overgrown nails. Other causes of

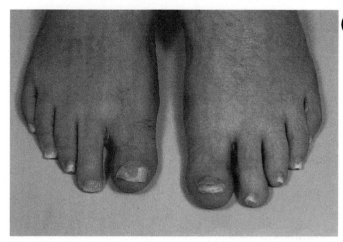

Fig. 20.3 Onycholysis, yellowing, crumbling, and thickening of the toenails. (From Bolognia J, Jorizzo JL, Rapini RP, editors: *Dermatology*, ed 2, St Louis, 2007, Mosby.)

problems may be traced to loss of fat cushioning and resilience with aging, diabetes, ill-fitting shoes, poor arch support, excessively repetitive weight-bearing activities, obesity, or uneven distribution of weight on the feet. Table 20.1 presents common foot problems.

Solutions, Nursing Actions, and Outcomes

Care of the foot takes a team approach, including the individual, the nurse, the podiatrist, and the primary health care provider. The feet should be assessed as part of a comprehensive examination of older adults. Nurses can identify potential and actual problems and make referral to or seek assistance as needed from the primary care provider or podiatrist for any changes in the feet (Box 20.4). Difficulty cutting toenails is common in older adults since it requires joint flexibility, manual dexterity, and visual acuity, and nurses often care for toenails. Appropriate cutting of toenails is important, and safety precautions are essential (Fig. 20.4).

Foot care for individuals with diabetes should be done only by a podiatrist or registered nurse with expertise. Individuals with diabetes or PVD should not have pedicures in commercial establishments. A comprehensive foot exam should be conducted annually for individuals with diabetes, including identification of risk factors for ulcers and amputations, testing for loss of sensation, and assessment of pedal pulses (Chapter 27). Individuals with foot concerns should be counselled about proper footwear.

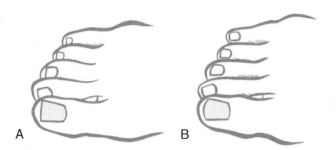

A   B

Fig 20.4 Cutting toenails. (A) Correct method. (B) Incorrect method.

TABLE 20.1   Common Foot Problems

Foot Problem	Prevention and Treatment
Corns and calluses: Growths of compacted skin that occur as a result of prolonged pressure, usually from ill-fitting, tight shoes. Corns are cone-shaped and develop on the top of toe joints or between opposing surfaces of the toes from prolonged squeezing. Once formed, corns will cause pain. Unless friction and pressure are relieved, will continue to enlarge and cause increasing pain	Over-the-counter preparations may remove temporarily but may burn surrounding tissue and should not be used by diabetics or those with neurological impairment or poor circulation. Foot care for individuals with diabetes or peripheral vascular disease should be performed by a nurse with expertise in foot care, a doctor, or a podiatrist **DO NOT** use razor blades, pocket knives, or scissors to remove corns and calluses Padding and protecting the area is the best practice (oval corn pads, gel pads, moleskin, lamb's wool, with a hole cut in the center for the corn) Daily lubrication of the feet; shoes with proper fit
Bunions: Bony deformities that develop over the medial aspect of the joint of the great toe or at the lateral aspect of the fifth metatarsal head (little toe) Occur from long-standing squeezing of first and second toes; may be a hereditary factor	May be treated with corticosteroid injections and antiinflammatory pain medications. Surgery is also an option Use custom-made shoes that provide forefront space (e.g., running shoes)
Hammer toes: A permanently flexed toe with a clawlike appearance resulting from muscle imbalance and pressure from big toe slanting toward second toe; the toe contracts, leaving a bulge on top of the joint. Result of ill-fitting shoes and often seen in conjunction with bunions	Professional orthotics or specially designed protective devices; properly fitting, nonconstricting shoes and/or surgical intervention
Fungal infections: May affect skin of feet *(tinea pedis)* and nails. Nail fungus *(onychomycosis)* is most common nail disorder. Nail plate degenerates, with color changes to yellow or brown and opaque, brittleness, and thickening of nail (see Fig. 20.3). Fine powdery collection of fungus forms under center of the nail, separating the layers and pushing it up, causing the sides of the nail to dig into the skin like an ingrown toenail	Wash hands after handling the feet. Culturing is the only way to diagnose; cure difficult to impossible due to limited circulation to the nails. Several oral medications available but expensive and of limited effectiveness; potentially toxic to liver and heart Photodynamic therapy (PDT) may be helpful Keep areas between the toes clean and dry and regularly exposed to sun and air. Topical antifungal powders are usual treatment. If diabetic, glycemic control is important

BOX 20.4   Tips for Best Practice

Recognizing and Analyzing Cues to Care of the Foot

Observation of Mobility
- Gait
- Use of assistive devices
- Footwear type and pattern of wear

Past Medical History
- Neuropathies
- Musculoskeletal limitations
- Peripheral vascular disease (PVD)
- Vision problems
- History of falls
- Pain affecting movement

Bilateral Assessment
- Color
- Circulation and warmth
- Pulses
- Structural deformities
- Skin lesions
- Lower-extremity edema
- Evidence of scratching
- Abrasions and other lesions
- Rash or excessive dryness
- Condition and color of toenails

Orthostatic and Postprandial Hypotension

Declines in depth perception, proprioception, and normotensive response to postural changes are important factors that contribute to falls. Estimates are that up to one-third of falls are related to syncope, and orthostatic hypotension (OH) and postprandial hypotension (PPH) contribute to syncope (Finucane et al., 2017; Morley, 2017). Clinically significant OH is a common clinical finding in older adults who are frail and has been reported to be present in up to 50% of older adults in nursing homes. OH is considered a decrease of 20 mm Hg (or more) in systolic pressure and/or a decrease of 10 mm Hg (or more) in diastolic pressure with position change from lying or sitting to standing. Assessment of OH in everyday nursing practice is often overlooked or assessed inaccurately and needs to be included as a competency in nursing education and practice. The detection of OH is of clinical importance to fall prevention because OH is treatable. However, there is considerable variability in the recommendations by clinical experts regarding the timing and position of blood pressure measurements, and further research is needed (Lipsitz, 2017) (Box 20.5).

PPH is associated with increased risk of syncope and falls. PPH occurs after ingestion of a carbohydrate meal and may be related to the release of a vasodilatory peptide, but research is needed on its epidemiology and pathophysiology. PPH is usually asymptomatic and may be overlooked. Patients with neurological disease and diabetes have a higher frequency of PPH.

BOX 20.5 Measuring Orthostatic Blood Pressure (BP)

- Orthostatic hypotension is more common in the morning, and therefore assessment should occur then.
- Have the individual lie down for 5 minutes.
- Measure the blood pressure and pulse rate in both arms. Use the arm with the higher blood pressure for measurements following position change.
- Have the individual stand (use safety precautions as needed). If unable to stand, measure blood pressure sitting with feet hanging.
- Take the blood pressure immediately after standing and ask about dizziness.
- Repeat blood pressure and pulse rate measurements after standing for 3 minutes and ask about dizziness.
- A drop in BP of ≥20 mm Hg or in diastolic BP of ≥10 mm Hg or experiencing light-headedness, dizziness, or loss of balance is considered abnormal.

From Momeyer M: Orthostatic hypotension in older adults with dementia, *J Gerontol Nurs* 40(6):22–29, 2014.

Lifestyle interventions such as increasing water intake before eating or eating smaller more frequent meals may be important, but further research is needed. Older individuals with risk factors should be cautioned against sudden rising from sitting or supine positions, particularly after eating. Measurement to detect OH should be conducted after any fall, particularly if related to a meal (Krbot Skorić et al., 2017).

Cognitive Impairment

Older adults with cognitive impairment are at double the risk of falling compared to age-matched individuals, with reports of 60% to 80% falling within a year of diagnosis of dementia. A twofold increased fall risk is present even in mild impairment (Peach et al., 2017). Cognition plays a crucial role in control of gait, and individuals with cognitive impairment may have an altered gait pattern. Other factors such as medications (neuroleptics), visual acuity, functional impairments, falls history, insight, memory, and behavior contribute to the complex mix of risk factors for falls in this population.

There is little research on fall prevention programs for individuals with cognitive impairment, but combined cognitive and physical interventions have been reported to improve balance, functional mobility, and gait speed in individuals with mild cognitive impairment (Chapter 19). Fall risk assessments should include more specific cognitive risk factors, and cognitive assessment measures need to be more frequently conducted with individuals at risk for falls. Research to evaluate the most effective fall risk–reduction programs for individuals at different stages of neurocognitive disorder is needed (Lach et al., 2017).

Vision and Hearing

Vision and hearing impairment have been associated with falls and should be assessed in older adults and corrected to the extent possible (Chapters 12 and 13). Poor visual acuity, reduced contrast sensitivity, decreased visual field, cataracts, and use of nonmiotic glaucoma medications all have been associated with falls. There is little research on interventions for either vision or hearing problems and falls and fractures.

Medications

Medications implicated in increasing fall risk include those causing potentially dangerous side effects, including drowsiness, mental confusion, problems with balance, loss of urinary control, and sudden drops in blood pressure with standing. These medications include antidepressants, antihypertensives, diuretics, some analgesics, sedative-hypnotics, and psychotropic medications. The association between psychotropic medications and falls is well established. The literature on cardiovascular medications as potential fall risk–increasing drugs is conflicting, and this needs further research.

In a systematic meta-analysis (de Vries et al., 2018), loop diuretics and digitalis were consistently associated with increased fall risk. In addition, the initiation of cardiovascular drugs showed an association with increased risk of falling. When cardiovascular drugs are prescribed, beginning with a smaller dose, increasing the dose slowly, monitoring response, and fall prevention teaching are important.

Medication review is an evidence-based strategy for reducing falls among older adults. Attention to medications should become a key focus of public health educational efforts and fall prevention in all settings. All medications, including over-the-counter (OTC) and herbal medications, should be reviewed and limited to those that are absolutely essential. The addition of any new medication should trigger a fall risk evaluation. Psychotropic prescribing should be considered carefully, initiated at low doses, and monitored closely. If these medications are being used, patient teaching should be provided related to fall risk; fall prevention interventions; appropriate dosing; use of other medications, such as benzodiazepines; and alcohol use (Chapter 30). Chapter 11 discusses safe medication use, and Chapter 26 discuss the use of these medications and alternative approaches for behavioral symptoms that may occur in individuals with dementia.

USING CLINICAL JUDGMENT TO PROMOTE HEALTHY AGING: FALLS AND FALL RISK REDUCTION

Recognizing and Analyzing Cues

The American Geriatrics Society/British Geriatrics Society (2010) *Clinical Practice Guideline: Prevention of Falls in Older Persons* recommends that fall risk assessment be an integral part of primary health care for the older adult. All older adults should be asked whether they have fallen in the past year and whether they experience difficulties with walking or balance. In addition, ask about falls that did not result in an injury, and the circumstances of a near-fall, mishap, or misstep, because this may provide important information for prevention of future falls.

Older adults may be reluctant to share information about falls due to fear of losing independence, so the nurse must use judgment and empathy in eliciting information about falls, assuring the individual that there are many modifiable factors to increase safety and help maintain independence. The intensity of the assessment will vary with the target population:

ASSESSMENT

Timed Up & Go (TUG)

Purpose: To assess mobility

Equipment: A stopwatch

Directions: Patients wear their regular footwear and can use a walking aid, if needed. Begin by having the patient sit back in a standard arm chair and identify a line 3 meters, or 10 feet away, on the floor.

① Instruct the patient:

NOTE: Always stay by the patient for safety.

When I say **"Go,"** I want you to:

1. Stand up from the chair.
2. Walk to the line on the floor at your normal pace.
3. Turn.
4. Walk back to the chair at your normal pace.
5. Sit down again.

② On the word "Go," begin timing.

③ Stop timing after patient sits back down.

④ Record time.

Time in Seconds: _____

An older adult who takes ≥12 seconds to complete the TUG is at risk for falling.

CDC's STEADI tools and resources can help you screen, assess, and intervene to reduce your patient's fall risk. For more information, visit www.cdc.gov/steadi

Patient	_____
Date	_____
Time	☐ AM ☐ PM

OBSERVATIONS

Observe the patient's **postural stability, gait, stride length, and sway.**

Check all that apply:

☐ Slow tentative pace
☐ Loss of balance
☐ Short strides
☐ Little or no arm swing
☐ Steadying self on walls
☐ Shuffling
☐ En bloc turning
☐ Not using assistive device properly

These changes may signify neurological problems that require further evaluation.

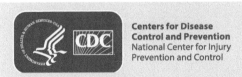

Centers for Disease Control and Prevention National Center for Injury Prevention and Control

2017

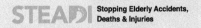 **Stopping Elderly Accidents, Deaths & Injuries**

Fig. 20.5 Timed Up & Go (TUG). (From Centers for Disease Control and Prevention: https://www.cdc.gov/steadi/pdf/TUG_Test-print.pdf. Accessed April 2019.)

ASSESSMENT

30-Second Chair Stand

Purpose: To test leg strength and endurance

Equipment: A chair with a straight back without arm rests (seat 17" high), and a stopwatch.

NOTE: Stand next to the patient for safety.

① **Instruct the patient:**

1. Sit in the middle of the chair.
2. Place your hands on the opposite shoulder crossed, at the wrists.
3. Keep your feet flat on the floor.
4. Keep your back straight, and keep your arms against your chest.
5. On **"Go,"** rise to a full standing position, then sit back down again.
6. Repeat this for 30 seconds.

② **On the word "Go," begin timing.**

If the patient must use his/her arms to stand, stop the test. Record "0" for the number and score.

③ **Count the number of times the patient comes to a full standing position in 30 seconds.**

If the patient is over halfway to a standing position when 30 seconds have elapsed, count it as a stand.

④ **Record the number of times the patient stands in 30 seconds.**

Number: _____   Score: _____

CDC's STEADI tools and resources can help you screen, assess, and intervene to reduce your patient's fall risk. For more information, visit www.cdc.gov/steadi

Patient _____

Date _____

Time _____   ☐ AM ☐ PM

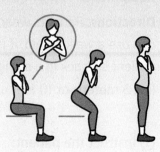

SCORING

**Chair Stand
Below Average Scores**

AGE	MEN	WOMEN
60-64	< 14	< 12
65-69	< 12	< 11
70-74	< 12	< 10
75-79	< 11	< 10
80-84	< 10	< 9
85-89	< 8	< 8
90-94	< 7	< 4

A below average score indicates a risk for falls.

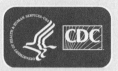

Centers for Disease Control and Prevention
National Center for Injury Prevention and Control

2017

2017

STEADI   Stopping Elderly Accidents, Deaths & Injuries

Fig. 20.6 30-Second Chair Stand. (From Centers for Disease Control and Prevention: https://www.cdc.gov/steadi/pdf/STEADI-Assessment-30Sec-508.pdf. Accessed April 2019.)

- Low-risk community-dwelling individuals should be asked at least once a year about fall occurrence and circumstances.
- Individuals who report a single fall should be evaluated for mobility impairment and unsteadiness using simple observational tests (Figs. 20.5 and 20.6), with those who demonstrate mobility problems or unsteadiness being referred for further assessment.
- High-risk populations (individuals who have had multiple falls in the past year, have abnormalities of gait and/or balance, have received medical attention related to a fall, or reside in a nursing facility) should undergo a more comprehensive and detailed assessment.

Comprehensive fall assessments include the following components: history of falls; medical history; complete physical examination (including vision and hearing); medication review (including alcohol and other drugs); functional assessment; cognitive assessment; gait, balance, and mobility; muscle strength; pain assessment; heart rate and rhythm; postural hypotension; feet and footwear; continence assessment; depression screening; cardiovascular assessment; skin assessment; sleep assessment; and nutrition assessment (Kruschke & Butcher, 2017) (Chapter 9).

Identifying Fall Risk

The following key questions can be asked during assessment and can alert clinicians to fall risk and the need for more follow-up: (1) Have you fallen in the past year? (2) Do you feel unsteady when standing or walking? (3) Are you worried about falling? Red flag risk factors such as osteoporosis, mobility problems, and anticoagulant therapy also alert the clinician of the need for further assessment. A patient self-assessment screening tool is available from the STEADI (*Stopping Elderly Accidents, Deaths, and Injuries*) program (CDC, 2021) (Box 20.1).

The National Center for Patient Safety recommends the Morse Fall Scale but not for use in long-term care. Other fall risk instruments include the Performance Oriented Mobility Assessment (Tinetti, 1986) and the Hendrich II Fall Risk Model (Hendrich et al., 2003), which also includes a modified Get Up and Go test. The Hendrich II Fall Risk Model has been validated with skilled nursing and rehabilitation populations and is also easy to use in the outpatient setting. In the skilled nursing facility, the Minimum Data Set (MDS 3.0) includes information about history of falls and hip fractures and an assessment of balance during transitions and walking (moving from seated to standing, walking, turning around, moving on and off toilet, and transfers between bed and chair or wheelchair) (Chapter 9).

Fall risk instruments are still commonly included in fall prevention programs, but instruments that are used need to be reliable and valid, and nurses need to use them judiciously. Often these instruments are completed in a routine manner, and risk factors are not identified or may not be known because of lack of assessment and knowledge of the individual's history. A fall risk score is not an adequate predictor of falls. To be able to prevent a fall, it is important to know why someone is at risk of falling, identification of the individual's actual fall and injury risk factors, factors that are modifiable and those that are not, treatment of modifiable factors, and helping patients compensate for those that are not modifiable. This information is obtained from comprehensive fall risk analysis. Additional research is needed to develop valid, reliable instruments to differentiate levels of fall risk in various settings.

Fall Screening and Assessment Guidelines in Hospitals and Nursing Facilities

Individuals admitted to acute or long-term care settings should have an initial fall assessment on admission, after any change in condition, and at regular intervals during their stay. Assessment is an ongoing process that includes multiple and continual types of assessment, reassessment, and evaluation following a fall or intervention to reduce the risk of a fall. An interprofessional team (physician or nurse practitioner, nurse, risk manager, physical and occupational therapists, and other designated staff) should be involved in planning care based on findings from an individualized assessment. Nurses bring expert knowledge of patient activities, abilities, and needs from a 24-hours-per-day, 7-days-per-week perspective to help the team implement the most appropriate interventions and evaluate outcomes.

Solutions, Nursing Actions, and Outcomes

Across settings of care, fall risk–reduction programs incorporating multifactorial and interprofessional approaches, aimed at multiple risk factors contributing to falls, are the most effective (Gray-Miceli et al., 2017; Isaranuwatchai et al., 2017). For fall prevention strategies to be most cost-effective, they should target those who are at highest risk for developing the outcome. The optimal bundle of interventions is not established, but suggested components are presented in Box 20.6.

BOX 20.6 Suggested Components of Fall Risk–Reduction Interventions

- Adaptation or modification of the home environment
- Withdrawal or minimization of psychoactive medications
- Withdrawal or minimization of other medications
- Detection and prevention of delirium
- Management of orthostatic hypotension
- Continence programs such as prompted voiding
- Management of foot problems and footwear
- Exercise, particularly balance, strength, and gait training
- Staff and patient education

From American Geriatrics Society/British Geriatrics Society: *2010 AGS/BGS clinical practice guideline: prevention of falls in older persons, summary of recommendations* (website), 2010. https://geriatricscare-online.org/application/content/products/CL014/html/CL014_BOOK001.html.

BOX 20.7 System-Level Actions for Fall Prevention in Acute Care

- Nurse champions
- Teach backs (all patients and families receive education about their fall and injury risks)
- Comfort care and safety rounds
- Safety huddle post fall
- Protective bundles: Patients with risk factors for serious injury, such as osteoporosis, anticoagulant use, and history of head injury or falls, are automatically placed on high fall risk precautions and interventions to reduce risk of serious injury
- Bundles may include interventions such as a bedside mat on the floor at the side of the bed, a height-adjustable bed, helmet use, hip protectors, and comfort and safety rounds

---

The focus of a fall risk–reduction program may differ according to the setting (community, hospital, home, long-term care), and further research is needed to determine the type, frequency, and timing of interventions best suited for specific populations. Choosing the most appropriate actions to reduce the risk of falls depends on appropriate evaluation at various intervals depending on the individual's changing condition and tailoring interventions to individual cognitive function, language, and health literacy.

A one-size-fits-all approach is not effective. In assessing fall risk and implementing the most appropriate interventions, listening to the story of the individual's experience related to falling and the personal impact the fall experience has had on the person's life is important. In collaboration with the older adult, the nurse can more effectively design individualized actions to enhance independence, mobility, and safety and to reduce fall risk (Gray-Miceli, 2017).

Fall Risk Reduction in Acute and Long-Term Care

Fall risk–reduction programs in hospitals and long-term care settings should be designed to meet organizational needs and to match patient population needs and the clinical realities of the staff. A systems-level quality improvement approach, including educational programs for staff, has been reported to reduce fall rates in hospitals and nursing facilities (Quigley et al., 2016). Systems-level actions for fall prevention in acute care are presented in Box 20.7. Some examples of effective programs in acute care settings include Acute Care of the Elderly (ACE) units, Nurses Improving Care for Healthsystem Elders (NICHE), the Geriatric Resource Nurse (GRN) model, and American Geriatrics Society CoCare: HELP (formerly Hospital Elder Life Program) (Chapter 1).

The Agency for Healthcare Research and Quality (2021) offers comprehensive guides for fall prevention programs in acute and long-term care (see Box 20.1). In addition to interventions presented in Box 20.7, other innovative programs in nursing facilities include the Visiting Angels and neighborhood watch teams. In the Visiting Angels program, alert residents

---

▸ RESEARCH HIGHLIGHTS

A Longitudinal Fall Prevention Study for Older Adults

Purpose

To implement and evaluate the effectiveness of a nurse practitioner–led comprehensive fall prevention program designed to improve gait and balance and reduce falls for older adults in a community setting. The fall prevention program ("Stay Standing") included exercise, medication review with suggested reductions in polypharmacy and potentially inappropriate medications (PIMs), patient education on medications, home modifications to improve safety, and referrals for vision and foot problems. The CDC's STEADI toolkit was used to design and evaluate the program.

Method

Participants included 18 older adults with a mean age of 75.45 years. A quantitative, repeated measures design was used for the study. The intervention group was enrolled in the fall prevention program, whereas the control group received usual care. Measurements of outcome variables (gait and balance scores, number of falls, increased knowledge about medications) were made at baseline and compared at 3, 6, 9, and 12 months for the intervention group; a comparison of falls between the intervention and control group was made at 12 months. The nurse practitioners conducted the initial baseline visit as well as the follow-up visits.

Results

The program was effective in improving lower extremity strength, decreasing falls, and increasing understanding of polypharmacy and PIMs. A program that focuses on multimodal assessment, treatment, and follow-up can be expected to reduce the number of falls and improve gait and balance.

Conclusion

Even though the research evidence shows that fall prevention programs are effective, the practice of recommending strategies to reduce falls by primary care providers is not consistent. The CDC's STEADI toolkit (see Box 20.1) provides guidance in designing and evaluating fall prevention programs. Nurse practitioners are particularly well suited to implementing and maintaining a fall prevention program in a primary care practice.

Data from Frith K, Hunter A, Coffey S: A longitudinal fall prevention study for older adults, *J Nurse Pract* 15(4):295–300, 2019.

---

visit and converse with residents who are cognitively impaired in the late afternoon and evening when fall risk starts to rise. Neighborhood watch teams involve the evening and night staff in morning reviews of any fall or incident that happened during the night.

Fall Risk Reduction in the Community

Group and home-based exercise programs, along with home safety interventions, reduce the rate of falls and risk of falling in community-dwelling older adults (Research Highlights). Vision screening, medication reduction, assessment of cardiovascular syncope and postural hypotension, using hip protectors and other assistive devices, and providing education on falls and fall prevention also have been associated with decreased fall risk. Impaired balance was the strongest predictor for falls in this population, followed by problems moving around in the home. Home-based tai chi chuan (TCC) has been shown to improve balance and physical performance and reduce falls among older adults in community settings more than conventional lower extremity exercise training (Nyman, 2020).

Recognizing and analyzing the cues to fall risk is important to implement nursing actions to tailor fall prevention programs in the home setting and during transitions of care (Zhao et al., 2017). Transitional care programs should include a fall

---

BOX 20.8 Evaluation Post Fall

Initiate emergency measures as indicated.

History
- Description of the fall from the individual or witness
- Individual's opinion of the cause of the fall
- Circumstances of the fall (trip or slip)
- Person's activity at the time of the fall
- Time of day and location of the fall
- Presence of comorbid conditions, such as a previous stroke, Parkinson's disease, osteoporosis, seizure disorder, sensory deficit, joint abnormalities, depression, cardiac disease
- Medication review
- Associated symptoms, such as chest pain, palpitations, light-headedness, vertigo, loss of balance, fainting, weakness, confusion, incontinence, or dyspnea
- Presence of acute illness

Physical Examination
- Vital signs: postural blood pressure changes, fever, or hypothermia
- Head and neck: visual impairment, hearing impairment, nystagmus, bruit
- Heart: arrhythmias or valvular dysfunction
- Neurological signs: altered mental status, focal deficits, peripheral neuropathy, muscle weakness, rigidity or tremor, impaired balance
- Musculoskeletal signs: arthritic changes, range of motion (ROM) changes, podiatric deformities or problems, swelling, redness or bruises, abrasions, pain on movement, shortening and external rotation of lower extremities

Functional Assessment
- Functional gait and balance: observe resident rising from chair, walking, turning, and sitting
- Balance test, mobility, use of assistive devices or personal assistance, extent of ambulation, restraint use, prosthetic equipment
- Activities of daily living: bathing, dressing, transferring, toileting

Environmental Assessment
- Staffing patterns, unsafe practice in transferring, delay in response to call light
- Faulty equipment
- Use of bed, chair alarm
- Call light within reach
- Wheelchair, bed locked
- Adequate supervision
- Clutter, walking paths not clear
- Dim lighting
- Glare
- Uneven flooring
- Wet, slippery floors
- Poorly fitted seating devices
- Inappropriate footwear
- Inappropriate eyewear

---

prevention component. In all settings, an important nursing action is to teach older adults and direct caregivers about fall prevention. The CDC's STEADI program provides excellent free materials on fall prevention.

Other Fall Risk–Reduction Actions

Postfall Assessments

Postfall assessment (PFA) is an integral component of fall prevention programs in institutional settings. It is important to identify underlying causes of falls and risk factors, and the PFA is a way of critically examining each fall. The purpose of the PFA is to identify the clinical status of the individual, verify and treat injuries, identify underlying causes of the fall when possible, and assist in implementing appropriate individualized risk reduction interventions. Incomplete analysis of the reasons for a fall can result in repeated incidents. If the patient cannot tell you about the circumstances of the fall, information should be obtained from staff or witnesses. Standard "incident report" forms do not provide adequate PFA information.

Conducting a postfall huddle (after action review) as soon as possible after a fall is recommended for PFA. Staff at all levels should be involved, as should be the patient, if able, to discuss the fall—what happened, how it happened, why it happened, how the outcome could be avoided the next time, and a follow-up plan (Buckner & Sherry, 2019). Other components to be addressed in PFA are presented in Box 20.8. The Department of Veterans Affairs National Center for Patient Safety provides comprehensive information about fall assessment, fall risk reduction, policies, and procedures and includes a postfall huddle guide. For falls that happen outside the hospital or skilled nursing facility, individuals can complete the "Story of Your Falls" to provide PFA information (Box 20.1).

Environmental Modifications

Among community-living older adults, falls are more likely to occur during ADLs but occur most frequently when the individual is transferring or changing physical positions (sitting to standing; using a bathtub, shower, or toilet; or walking downstairs). Environmental modifications alone have not been shown to reduce falls, but when included as part of a multifactorial program, they may be of benefit in risk reduction. A home safety assessment and home modification interventions are effective in reducing the rates of falls, especially for individuals at high risk of falling and those with visual impairments (Chapter 21).

In institutional settings, the patient care environment should be assessed routinely for extrinsic factors that may contribute to falls and corrective action taken. About 50% to 70% of falls in hospitals occur while transferring between bed and chair, and 10% to 20% occur in bathrooms (Quigley et al., 2016). Patients should be able to access the bathroom or be provided with a bedside commode, routine assistance to toilet, and programs such as prompted voiding (Chapter 17). Dual-stiffness flooring, which incorporates a layer of compressible material meant to cushion falls, can reduce fractures in nursing

BOX 20.9   Environmental Safety Check

- Outdoor grounds and indoor floor surfaces checked for spills, wet areas, and unevenness
- Hallways and doorways have clear paths free of clutter and equipment
- Proper illumination and functioning of lights, including night lights
- Tabletops, furniture, and beds are sturdy and in good repair
- Grab rails and nonskid appliques or mats are in place in the bathroom (toilet and shower)
- Appropriate footwear is available and used
- Adaptive aids are available, work properly, and are in good repair
- Bed rails do not collapse when used for transitioning or support
- Bed wheels lock
- Patient gowns and clothing do not cause tripping
- IV poles are sturdy if used during ambulation, and tubing does not cause tripping

BOX 20.10   Tips for Best Practice

Use of Assistive Devices

Cane Use
- Place your cane firmly on the ground before you take a step, and do not place it too far ahead of you. Put all of your weight on your unaffected leg, and then move the cane and your affected leg at a comfortable distance forward. With your weight supported on both the cane and your affected leg, step through with your unaffected leg.
- Wear low-heeled, nonskid shoes. It's best to have individuals wear the kind of shoes they are accustomed to wearing, and consideration should be given to properly fitted orthotic shoes as appropriate.
- Every assistive device must be adjusted to individual height; the top of the cane should align with the crease of the wrist.
- Choose a size and shape of cane handle that fits comfortably in the palm; like a tight shoe, it will be a constant irritant if it is not properly fitted.
- Cane tips are most secure when they are flat at the bottom and have a series of rings. Replace tips frequently because they wear out, and a worn tip is insecure.

Walker Use
- When using a walker, stand upright and lift or roll the walker with both hands a step's length ahead of you. Lean slightly forward and hold the arms of the walker for support. Step toward it with the affected leg and then bring the unaffected leg forward.

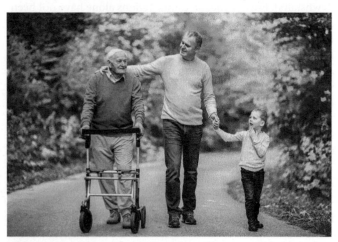

Maintaining ambulation and safety with appropriate assistive devices. (©iStock.com/Jovanmandic.)

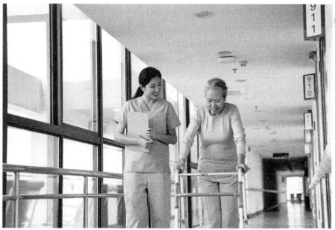

A physical therapist helping a client to ambulate. (©iStock.com/imtmphoto.)

homes (Morley, 2017). Important areas to check for safety are presented in Box 20.9.

Assistive Devices

Research on multifactorial interventions including the use of assistive devices has demonstrated benefits in fall risk reduction. Many devices are designed for specific conditions and limitations. Physical therapists provide training on use of assistive devices, and nurses can supervise correct use. Improper use of these devices can lead to increased fall risk (Box 20.10). For the community-dwelling individual, Medicare may cover up to 80% of the cost of assistive devices with a written prescription. New technologies such as "smart canes" that assess gait and fall risk or that "talk" and provide feedback to the user, sensors that detect when falls have occurred or when risk of falling is increasing, and other developing assistive technologies hold the potential to significantly improve functional ability, safety, and independence for older adults (Chapter 21) (Muchna et al., 2018).

Safe Patient Handling

Lifting, transferring, and repositioning patients are the most common tasks that lead to injury for health care staff and patients in hospital and nursing home environments. Handling and moving patients offer multiple challenges because of variations in size, physical abilities, cognitive function, level of cooperation, and changes in condition. Evidence-based practices for safe patient handling include: (1) use of patient-handling equipment and devices; (2) patient-care ergonomic assessment protocols; (3) no-lift policies; (4) training on proper use of patient handling equipment and devices; and (5) patient lift teams. Examples of helpful equipment are ceiling- and floor-based dependent lifts, sit-to-stand assists, ambulation aids, motorized hospital beds, powered shower chairs, and friction-reducing devices. Key aspects of patient assessment to improve safety for patients and staff are presented in Box 20.11.

Hip Protectors

The use of hip protectors for individuals who are at risk for hip fractures may be considered, and there is some evidence that they may be protective, but further research is needed to determine their effectiveness. Compliance has been a concern related to the ease of application and removing them quickly enough for toileting, but newer designs that are more attractive and practical may assist with compliance issues. In 2020, the Food and Drug Administration (FDA) approved hip protector garments for the prevention of hip fractures in older adults with known osteoporosis.

Alarms, Motion Sensors, and Staff Observation

Alarms, either personal or chair and bed, are often used in fall risk–reduction programs. Alarms were designed to be early warning systems, but there has been no research to support their effectiveness in preventing a fall. Use of alarms may increase patient agitation, especially in individuals who are cognitively impaired. Silent alarms, visual or auditory monitoring systems, motion detectors, and physical staff presence may be more effective. Continuous video monitoring has been noted as an effective intervention to significantly reduce the incidence of patient falls and the likelihood of injury if the patient does experience a fall. Motion sensors inside patient rooms may be another viable, cost-efficient, unobtrusive solution to prevent and detect falls (Potter et al., 2017). One of the most effective methods used in fall prevention is rounding every 1 to 2 hours to assess patient needs. The use of sitters is very costly, and evidence is scant that adding sitters to usual care reduces falls (Greeley et al., 2020).

RESTRAINTS AND SIDE RAILS

Definition and History

A physical restraint is defined as any manual method or physical or mechanical device, material, or equipment that immobilizes or reduces the ability of a patient to move the arms, legs, body, or head freely. A chemical restraint is when a drug or medication is used as a restriction to manage the individual's behavior or restrict freedom of movement. Historically, restraints and side rails have been used for the "protection" of the patient and for the security of the patient and staff. Originally, restraints were used to control the behavior of individuals with mental illness considered to be dangerous to themselves or others (Evans & Strumpf, 1989).

Research over the past 30 years by nurses such as Lois Evans, Neville Strumpf, and Elizabeth Capezuti has shown that the practice of physical restraint is ineffective and hazardous. The use of physical restraints in long-term care settings was effectively addressed more than 30 years ago through nursing home reform legislation, resulting in a major reduction of physical restraint use in these facilities. The Joint Commission and the Centers for Medicare and Medicaid Services (CMS) have focused on restraint reduction strategies in acute care over the past 15 to 20 years, but the use of restraints remains a concern, particularly in intensive care units (ICUs). Physical restraint use is part of public reporting for nursing homes through the CMS Nursing Home Compare website and a critical quality indicator (Chapter 6). Restraint use is considered a nurse-sensitive indicator.

Consequences of Restraints

Physical restraints, intended to prevent injury, do not protect patients from falling, wandering, or removing tubes and other medical devices. Physical restraints actually may exacerbate many of the problems for which they are used and can cause serious injury or death and emotional and physical problems. Physical restraints are associated with higher death rates, injurious falls, nosocomial infections, incontinence, contractures, pressure ulcers, agitation, and depression. Injuries occur as a result of the patient attempting to remove the restraint or attempting to get out of bed while restrained.

The use of restraints is a great source of physical and psychological distress to older adults and may intensify agitation and contribute to depression. Side rails may be seen as a barrier rather than a reminder of the need to request assistance with transfers. As well, for some older adults, especially those with a history of trauma (such as that induced by war, rape, or domestic violence), side rails may cause fear and agitation and a feeling of being jailed or caged (Box 20.12).

Side Rails

Side rails are no longer viewed as simply attachments to a patient's bed but are considered restraints with all the accompanying concerns just discussed. Side rails are now defined as restraints or restrictive devices when used to impede a person's ability to voluntarily get out of bed when the person cannot lower the rails by themselves. Restrictive side rail use is defined as two full-length or four half-length raised side rails. The proper use of side rails can be considered a means

---

BOX 20.12 Being Restrained

"I felt like a dog and cried all night. It hurt me to have to be tied up. I felt like I was nobody, that I was dirt. It makes me cry to talk about it. The hospital is worse than a jail."

"I don't remember misbehaving, but I may have been deranged from all the pills they gave me. Normally, I am spirited, but I am also good and obedient. Nevertheless, the nurse tied me down, like Jesus on the cross, by bandaging both wrists and ankles. . . . It felt awful, I hurt and I worried. Callers, including men friends, saw me like that and thought I lost something. I lost a little personal prestige. I was embarrassed, like a child placed in a corner for being bad. I had been important . . . and to be tied down in bed took a big toll. . . . I haven't forgotten the pain and the indignity of being tied."

BOX 20.14 Suggestions From Advanced Practice Nursing Consultation on Restraint-Free Fall Prevention Actions

- Compensating for memory loss (e.g., improving behavior, anticipating needs, providing visual and physical cues)
- Improving impaired mobility; reducing injury potential
- Evaluating nocturia and incontinence; reducing sleep disturbances
- Implementing restraint-free fall prevention interventions based on conducting careful individualized assessments; what works for one individual may not necessarily be effective for another
- Careful medication review
- Change emphasis from a focus on falls to a focus on safe mobility

---

BOX 20.13 Tips for Best Practice

Dealing With Tubes, Lines, and Other Medical Devices

- First question: "Is the device really necessary?" Remove it as soon as possible.
- Preoperative teaching about the device; use guided exploration and mirror to help the patient understand what devices are in place and why.
- Provide comfort care to the site—oral and nasal care, anchoring of tubing, topical anesthetic on site.
- Indwelling catheters should be used only if the patient needs intensive output monitoring or has an obstruction.
- Weigh risks and benefits of restraint versus therapy alternatives available (e.g., replace IV tubing with saline lock; deliver meds by intramuscular route, consider intermittent IV administration or hypodermoclysis).
- Use camoflauge: clothing or elastic sleeves, temporary air splint (occupational therapy can be helpful), skin sleeves to prevent IV tube dislodgment.
- Use mitts instead of wrist restraints; use roll belts instead of vest restraints.
- Use diversional activity aprons (zipping, unzipping, threading exercises, dials and knobs, busy box, therapeutic activity kit, twiddle [activity muff]).
- Hide lines by placing them in unobtrusive places; hang IV bags behind the patient's line of vision; have patient wear long sleeves or double surgical gowns with cuffs to prevent access.
- Enteral tubes: If essential, use percutaneous endoscopic gastrostomy (PEG) instead of nasogastric (NG); if NG is used, use smallest lumen possible to minimize irritation; consider taping with an occlusive dressing.
- For men with indwelling catheters, shave area just above pubis and tape catheter to pubis. Never secure catheter to leg (causes discomfort and can cause a fistula). Run tubing around back of leg and connect to a leg bag. Patients should wear underpants or pajama pants to camoflauge catheter.

---

of assisting in-bed movement and getting in and out of bed. If the patient uses a half- or quarter-length upper side rail to assist in getting in and out of bed, the side rail is not considered a restraint. Side rails manufactured for use on hospital beds have been redesigned and are no longer a threat to patient entrapment, but use of outmoded designs and incorrect assembly continue to be a concern. CMS requires nursing homes to conduct individualized assessments of residents, provide alternatives, or clearly document the need for restrictive side rails.

Restraint-Free Care

Restraint-free care is now the standard of practice and an indicator of quality care in all health care settings, although transition to that standard is still in progress, particularly in acute care settings. Physical restraint use in acute care is now predominantly in ICUs, particularly for patients with medical devices and those with delirium. Physical restraint is more likely to be used in ICUs because nurses fear tube dislodgement related to greater frequency of invasive lines and mechanical ventilation. However, physical restraints are not effective in preventing unplanned endotracheal extubation and increase its risk threefold (Hall et al., 2018). Daily evaluation of the necessity of medical devices (IV lines, nasogastric tubes, catheters, endotracheal tubes), and securing or camouflaging (hiding) the device, is important (Box 20.13). Both the American Geriatrics Society and the American Board of Internal Medicine recommend that physical restraints not be used to manage behavioral symptoms of hospitalized older adults with delirium (American Geriatrics Society, 2014). Further research is needed in ICU settings to determine the best strategies to manage delirium (Chapter 26).

Implementing best practice nursing in fall risk reduction and restraint-free care is a complex clinical decision-making process and calls for recognition and analysis of cues to physical and psychosocial concerns contributing to patient safety; knowledge of restraint alternatives; interdisciplinary teamwork; and institutional commitment. Nursing staff can benefit from educational programs focused on correcting misperceptions related to physical restraint application and the use of alternatives. The use of advanced practice nurse consultation in implementing alternatives to restraints has been most effective. Important areas of focus derived from research on advanced practice nurse consultations are presented in Box 20.14. Many of the suggestions on safety and fall risk reduction in this chapter can be used to promote a safe and restraint-free environment. Fall risk reduction and alternative strategies to restraints are presented in Box 20.15.

BOX 20.15 Tips for Best Practice

Fall Risk Reduction and Restraint Alternatives

Individual

- Work with the interdisciplinary team; nurses cannot manage these compli-cated challenges alone
- Perform fall risk screening; evaluate gait, balance, and mobility; and recognize the multifactorial nature of falls
- Refer to physical therapy for walking and/or strengthening programs as appropriate
- Check for postural hypotension
- Use a behavior log to track when the person in trying to get up and/or when the person seems agitated
- Recognize signs and symptoms of delirium
- Evaluate ability to see and hear adequately. If individual wears glasses, hear-ing aid, or dentures, ensure that devices are worn
- Ensure that pain is well managed
- Involve family and all staff in fall risk–reduction education and activities
- Identify individuals at risk for falls (ID bracelet, door sign, red socks)

Patient Room

- Evaluate ability to transfer in and out of bed and adjust height of bed for safety
- Use a concave mattress if trying to get out of bed
- Use bed boundary markers to mark the edges of the bed, such as mattress, rolled blanket, or "swimming noodles" under sheets
- Place a soft floor or a mattress by the bed to cushion any falls
- Use a water mattress to reduce movement to the edge of the bed
- Remove wheels from bed
- Clear the floor of debris or excess furniture; ensure that floors are nonskid

- Place call bell within reach and make sure individual can use it (attach to patient's garment or obtain adapted call device)
- Ensure that all personal items are within reach
- Ensure that ambulation devices are within reach and used properly
- Trapeze or patient assist handles to enhance mobility in bed
- Make every effort to keep the individual ambulatory
- Stay alert for falls, especially at change of shift
- Provide diversional activities (catalogs, puzzles, therapeutic activity kit)

Bathroom

- Evaluate continence and establish toileting plan, if appropriate
- Bedside commode available if needed
- Grab bars in bathroom and shower; shower chair
- Elevated toilet seat
- Clothing easy to pull down for toileting
- Make sure individual knows location of bathroom and can find it (keep door open, picture of toilet on the door, clear path, night lights, light inside toilet bowl, glow-in-the-dark footprints going from bed to toilet)

On the Unit

- Remove environmental hazards
- Keep individual in supervised area or room with view of nursing station
- Sit in reclining chair: chair with deep seat, bean bag chair, rocker
- Provide meaningful activities
- Provide hip protectors, helmets, arm pads for at-risk ambulatory individuals
- Provide a restraint management cart with alternative restraint products ar-ranged in order of restrictiveness

KEY CONCEPTS

- Mobility provides opportunities for exercise, exploration, and pleasure and is the crux of maintaining independence.
- As one ages, illnesses and changes in bones, muscles, and lig-aments affect balance and gait and increase instability. Gait and mobility impairments are not an inevitable consequence of aging but often a result of chronic diseases or remote or recent trauma.
- Impairment of mobility is an early predictor of physical dis-ability and associated with poor outcomes such as falling, loss of independence, depression, decreased quality of life, institutionalization, and death.
- Falls are one of the most important geriatric syndromes and the leading cause of morbidity and mortality for individuals older than 65 years of age.
- The risk of falling increases with the number of risk factors. Most falls occur from a combination of intrinsic and extrin-sic factors that unite at a certain point in time.

- Clinical judgment is required to recognize and analyze cues to fall risk and implement nursing actions to prevent falls. Evaluations must be ongoing and include analysis of any fall that occurs.
- Postfall assessments (PFAs) must be used to identify multi-factorial, complex fall and injury risk factors in those who have fallen.
- Physical restraints, intended to prevent injury, do not pro-tect patients from falling, wandering, or removing tubes and other medical devices. Physical restraints actually may exac-erbate many of the problems for which they are used and can cause serious injury or death and emotional and physical problems.
- Restraint-free care is the standard of practice in all settings, and knowledge of restraint alternatives and safety measures is essential for nurses.

NEXT-GENERATION NCLEX® (NGN) EXAMINATION–STYLE QUESTIONS

Ms. Parra, 68 years old, arrives in the emergency department via ambulance. The report from emergency services personnel indicates that she fell in her home, with loss of consciousness. The nurse obtains her history. The client states that she slipped in the bathroom while getting up to urinate during the night; the need to urinate was urgent and she feels she rushed more than usual. When she fell, she hit her head on the sink and passed out. She was wearing her medical alert watch; it notified emergency services that she had fallen. Ms. Parra's medical history includes hypertension and osteoarthritis in her knees. Her medications include atenolol 50 mg daily, meloxicam 7.5 mg daily, and acetaminophen as needed. Although she has never fallen before, her daughter bought her the medical alert watch when she noticed how stiff Ms. Parra became after short periods of inactivity. Vital signs include a blood pressure of 100/68 mm Hg, heart rate of 58 beats per minute, respirations of 16 breaths per minute, temperature of 99.5°F, and oxygen saturation of 98% on room air. Results of laboratory work include the following:

- White blood cell count: 12.5 × 103 cells/mm³
- Hemoglobin and hematocrit: 16 g/dL and 45%
- Platelet count: 100,000 cells/mm³
- Blood urea nitrogen and creatinine: 23 mg/dL and 1.2 mg/dL
- Sodium: 142 mEq/L
- Glucose: 100 mg/dL
- Urinalysis: Urine is amber and clear, pH 7.0, nitrite negative and leukocyte esterase positive, blood 5/high-power field (hpf), white blood cells (WBCs) 10/hpf, and bacteria 100,000 colony-forming units (CFUs)/mL.

Highlight the assessment data above that require follow-up by the nurse.

NURSING STUDY

Fall Risk Reduction

Jim is an 80-year-old World War II veteran who has resided in the skilled nursing facility for 2 years. His diagnoses include Alzheimer's disease, hypertension, and depression. Medications include an antihypertensive drug and an antidepressant. He is able to walk but has an unsteady gait and requires assistance. Due to his cognitive status, he often attempts to ambulate alone and today was found on the floor in the bathroom. No injuries were immediately apparent, and he says he is fine. His partner of 30 years is requesting that restraints be applied to prevent him from suffering injuries from falling.

CLINICAL JUDGMENT QUESTIONS AND ACTIVITIES

Questions pertain to the Nursing Study.
1. What risk factors for falls are present in the Nursing Study?
2. What interventions are appropriate to ensure safety for Jim?
3. How would you respond to the partner's request for the use of restraints?
4. In your clinical practice setting, what observations do you have related to the use of restraints?

RESEARCH QUESTIONS

1. What types of gait disorders trigger falls and in what situations?
2. How does cognitive impairment influence risk of falls?
3. What is the knowledge level of practicing nurses regarding nursing actions for fall risk reduction in hospitals?
4. What are the psychological reactions of older adults to the use of assistive devices for ambulation?
5. What factors among community-dwelling older adults are most hazardous for mobility?
6. What are the major reasons that individuals are restrained in ICUs, and what interventions are most effective in decreasing restraint use in this setting?

REFERENCES

Agency for Healthcare Research and Quality: *Falls prevention* (website), 2021. https://www.ahrq.gov/topics/falls-prevention.html. Accessed June 2021.

American Geriatrics Society: American Geriatrics Society identifies another five things that healthcare providers and patients should question, *J Am Geriatr Soc* 62(5):950–960, 2014.

American Geriatrics Society/British Geriatrics Society: *2010 AGS/BGS clinical practice guideline: prevention of falls in older persons, summary of recommendations* (website), 2010. https://geriatric-scareonline.org/ProductAbstract/updated-american-geriatrics-societybritish-geriatrics-society-clinical-practice-guideline-for-prevention-of-falls-in-older-persons-and-recommendations/CL014. Accessed May 2021.

Bergland A, Jorgensen L, Emaus N, et al.: Mobility as a predictor of all-cause mortality in older men and women: 11.8 year follow-up in the Tromso study, *BMC Health Serv Res* 17(1):22, 2017.

Buckner T, Sherry D: Improving falls in nursing homes: a post-fall huddle quality improvement project, *Int Jour Adv Nurs Studies* 8(2):33, 2019.

Centers for Disease Control and Prevention (CDC): *Traumatic brain injury and concussion* (website), 2020. https://www.cdc.gov/traumaticbraininjury/get_the_facts.html.

Centers for Disease Control and Prevention (CDC): *Older adult fall prevention* (website), 2021. https://www.cdc.gov/falls/index.html.

de Vries M, Seppala L, Daams J, et al.: Fall-risk-increasing drugs: a systematic review and meta-analysis: I. Cardiovascular drugs, *J Am Med Dir Assoc*, 2018 19(4) 371.e1–371.e9.

Evans L, Strumpf N: Tying down the elderly: a review of literature on physical restraint, *J Am Geriatr Soc* 37:65–74, 1989.

Finucane C, O'Connell M, Donoghue O, et al.: Impaired orthostatic blood pressure recovery is associated with unexplained and injurious falls, *J Am Geriatr Soc* 65:474–482, 2017 +.

Gardner R, Byers A, Barnes D, et al.: Mild TBI and risk of Parkinson disease: a chronic effects of neurotrauma consortium study, *Neurology* 90(20):e1771–e1779, 2018.

Gray-Miceli D: Impaired mobility and functional decline in older adults: evidence to facilitate a practice change, *Nurs Clin North Am* 52:469–487, 2017.

Gray-Miceli D, deCordova P, Crane G, et al.: Nursing home registered nurses' and licensed practical nurses' knowledge of causes of falls, *J Nurs Care Qual* 31(2):153–160, 2016.

Gray-Miceli D, Mazzia L, Crane G: Advanced practice nurse-led statewide collaborative to reduce falls in hospitals, *J Nurs Care Qual* 32(2):120–125, 2017.

Gray-Miceli D, Ratcliffe S, Johnson J: Use of a postfall assessment tool to prevent falls, *West J Nurs Res* 32(7):932–948, 2010.

Greeley A, Tanner E, Mak S, et al.: Sitters as a patient safety strategy to reduce hospital falls: a systematic review, *Ann Int Med* 172(5):317–324, 2020.

Hall D, Zimbro K, Maduro R, et al.: Impact of a restraint management bundle on restraint use in an intensive care unit, *J Nurs Care Qual* 33(2):143–148, 2018.

Hendrich AL, Bender PS, Nyhuis A: Validation of the Hendrich II Fall Risk Model: a large concurrent case/control study of hospitalized patients, *Applied Nursing Research* 16(1):9–21, 2003.

Isaranuwatchai W, Perdrizet J, Markle-Reid M, et al.: Cost-effectiveness analysis of a multifactorial fall prevention intervention in older home care clients at risk for falling, *BMC Geriatr* 17:199, 2017.

Krbot Skorić M, Crnosija M, Habek M, et al.: Postprandial hypotension in neurological disorders: systematic review and meta-analysis, *Clin Auton Res* 27(4):263–271, 2017.

Kruschke C, Butcher H: Evidence-based practice guideline: fall prevention for older adults, *J Gerontol Nurs* 43(11):15–21, 2017.

Lach H, Harrison B: Phongphanngam S: Falls and fall prevention in older adults with early-stage dementia: an integrative review, *Res Gerontol Nurs* 10(3):139–148, 2017.

Lipsitz LA: Orthostatic hypotension and falls, *J Am Geriatr Soc* 65:470–471, 2017.

Mattia M, Ambrosi E, Chiari P, et al.: One-year mortality after hip fracture surgery and prognostic factors: a prospective cohort study, *Sci Rep* 9(1):18718, 2019.

Morley JE: The future of long-term care, *J Am Med Dir Assoc* 18:1–7, 2017.

Muchna A, Najafi B, Wendel CS, et al.: Foot problems in older adults: associations with incident falls, frailty syndrome, and sensor-derived gait, balance, and physical activity measures, *J Am Podiatr Med Assoc* 108(2):126–139, 2018.

Nyman S: Tai chi for the prevention of falls among older adults: a critical analysis of the evidence, *J Aging Phys Act* 29(2):343–352, 2020.

Peach T, Pollock K, van der Wardt V, et al.: Attitudes of older people with mild dementia and mild cognitive impairment and their relatives about falls risk and prevention: a qualitative study, *PLoS One*, 2017 12(5):e0177530.

Pirker W, Katzenschlager R: Gait disorders in adults and the elderly: a clinical guide, *Wien Klin Wochenschr* 129(3–4):81–95, 2017.

Potter P, Allen K, Costantinou E, et al.: Evaluation of sensor technology to detect fall risk and prevent falls in acute care, *Jt Comm J Qual Patient Saf* 43(8):414–421, 2017.

Quigley P, Barnett S, Bulat T, et al.: Reducing falls and fall-related injuries in medical-surgical units: one-year multihospital falls collaborative, *J Nurs Care Qual* 31(2):139–145, 2016.

Schaffert J, LoBue C, White CL, et al.: Traumatic brain injury history is associated with an earlier age of dementia onset in autopsy-confirmed Alzheimer's disease, *Neuropsychology* 32(4):410–416, 2018.

Schneider A, Selvin E, Latour L, et al.: Head injury and 25-year risk of dementia, *Alzheimers Dement* 17(9):1432–1441, 2021.

Taylor-Piliae RE, Peterson R, Mohler MJ: Clinical and community strategies to prevent falls and fall-related injuries among community-dwelling older adults, *Nurs Clin North Am* 52:489–497, 2017.

Tinetti ME: Performance-oriented assessment of mobility problems in elderly patients, *J Am Geriatr Soc* 34(2):119–126, 1986.

US Preventive Services Task Force: Screening for osteoporosis to prevent fractures: US Preventive Services Task Force recommendation statement, *JAMA* 319(24):2521–2531, 2018.

Xu G, Yamamoto Y, Hayashi K, et al.: The accuracy of different FRAX tools in predicting fracture risk in Japan: a comparison study, *J Orthop Surg (Hong Kong)*, 2020 28(2) 2309499020917276.

Zhao JG, Zeng XT, Wang J, et al.: Association between calcium or vitamin D supplementation and fracture incidence in community-dwelling older adults: a systematic review and meta-analysis, *JAMA* 318(24):2466–2482, 2017.

21 CHAPTER

Safe and Secure Environments

Theris A. Touhy

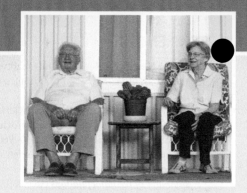

A STUDENT SPEAKS

During the community nursing experience my client decided to stay in her own home in spite of being barely able to shuffle around. A community program provided a homemaker for a few hours daily. She had to rely on the goodwill of neighbors when the budget for those services was discontinued. She wants so much to remain in her own home. I worry about her but don't know what I should do.

Jennifer, age 24

AN OLDER ADULT SPEAKS

I have been in my home for 50 years and widowed for 25 of those 50. The upkeep on my home is expensive and my resources are limited. I'm hoping I can manage to remain here, but I need some modifications to make it safe and I really don't know how to go about getting assistance to make the necessary changes.

Esther, age 79

LEARNING OBJECTIVES

On completion of this chapter, the reader will be able to:

1. Recognize and analyze cues to the effects of declining health, reduced mobility, isolation, and unpredictable life situations on older adults' perception of security.
2. Explain the underlying vulnerability of older adults to natural and human-generated or human-made disasters and the effects of extreme temperatures.
3. Identify resources for disaster preparedness.
4. Use clinical judgment to identify and evaluate nursing actions to maintain a safe environment for older adults.
5. Consider the impact of available transportation and driving in relation to independence and safety.
6. Discuss the use of assistive technologies to promote self-care, safety, and independence.
7. Identify the components of an elder-friendly community to enhance the ability to age in place.

ENVIRONMENTAL SAFETY

A safe environment is one in which one is capable, with reasonable caution, of carrying out activities of daily living (ADLs), instrumental activities of daily living (IADLs), and the activities that enrich one's life without fear of attack, accident, or imposed interference. Vulnerability to environmental risks increases as people become less physically or cognitively able to recognize or cope with real or potential hazards.

This chapter discusses the influence of changing health and disability on safety and security. Included are vulnerability to temperature extremes, effects of natural and human-generated or human-made disasters, crime, fire safety, gun and driving safety, and the role of assistive technology in enhancing independence

and the ability to live safely at home. Elder-friendly communities that foster aging in place and promote safety and security are also discussed.

HOME SAFETY

The safety of older adults at home is a worldwide concern. Identification of safety issues can assist in developing measures to help individuals stay at home for longer as they age (aging in place). Safety has been primarily studied in acute care and long-term care; few studies focus on safety at home, and the emphasis has been on physical safety. A more holistic view is recommended and includes the following dimensions: physical, social, emotional and mental, and cognitive safety (Kivimaki et al., 2019).

BOX 21.1 **Resources for Best Practice**

Disaster Management
- **American Red Cross:** Disaster and emergency preparedness for older adults. https://www.redcross.org/get-help/how-to-prepare-for-emergencies.html.
- **Centers for Disease Control and Prevention (CDC):** Interim infection prevention and control recommendations to prevent SARS-CoV-2 spread in nursing homes. https://www.cdc.gov/coronavirus/2019-ncov/hcp/long-term-care.html.
- **Federal Emergency Management Agency (FEMA):** Prepare for emergencies now: information for older adults. https://www.ready.gov/sites/default/files/2020-03/ready_prepare-now-seniors.pdf.
- **National Institute on Aging:** Hot weather safety for older adults. https://www.nia.nih.gov/health/topics/hyperthermia. Cold weather safety for older adults. https://www.nia.nih.gov/health/topics/hypothermia.

Crime Prevention and Fire Protection
- **Age Safe America:** Crime prevention tips for elderly. https://agesafeamerica.com/crime-prevention-tips-elderly/.
- **FBI.gov:** Elder fraud: Common fraud schemes and ways to protect yourself. https://www.fbi.gov/scams-and-safety/common-scams-and-crimes/elder-fraud.
- **National Crime Prevention Council:** https://www.ncpc.org/.
- **National Fire Protection Association and the CDC:** Remembering when: a fire and fall prevention program for older adults. https://www.nfpa.org/~/media/files/public-education/resources/education-programs/remembering-when/rwprogrambook.pdf?la=en.

Driving
- **AARP:** CarFit: helping mature drivers find their safety fit. https://www.aarp.org/auto/driver-safety/info-2010/carfit-exam-checklist.html.
- **Alzheimer's Association, Dementia and Driving Resource Center:** Examples of helpful communication techniques and short video role-plays of talking about driving cessation. https://www.alz.org/help-support/caregiving/safety/dementia-driving.
- **American Automobile Association:** Driver improvement courses, online defensive driving course. https://seniordriving.aaa.com/maintain-mobility-independence/driver-improvement-courses-seniors/take-online-defensive-driving-course/.

Aging in Place and Technology
- **Home Safety Self Assessment Tool (HSSAT) v.3. Aging & Technology Research Center:** Online home safety self-assessment tool (HSSAT). https://www2.tompkinscountyny.gov/files2/cofa/documents/hssat_v3.pdf
- **CDC Grand Rounds:** Technology and Health: Aging Safely and More Independently: Presentations and videos on technology for older adults. https://www.youtube.com/watch?v=XRYyGtAWXnQ.
- **National Aging in Place Council:** Information and resources for aging in place. https://www.ageinplace.org/.
- **National Shared Housing Resource Center.** https://nationalsharedhousing.org/.
- **Village to Village Network (Village Housing Model).** https://www.vtvnetwork.org/.

Actions to promote home safety must be multifaceted and individualized to the areas of identified risks. They are particularly important for older adults who are at risk for falls. Home safety assessments by occupational therapists are recommended in evidence-based protocols for fall risk reduction (Chapter 20). However, they are not widely conducted. A survey of community-living older adults found that approximately one-half reported never seeing a home safety checklist (Lach & Noimontree, 2018). Several home safety evaluation instruments can be used to increase knowledge of safety and assist older adults and their caregivers to develop home safety plans (Box 21.1). Education about home safety is an important component of care of older adults and an integral part of discharge planning.

CRIMES AGAINST OLDER ADULTS

Risks and Vulnerability

Older individuals share many of the same fears about violent crime held by the rest of the population, but they may feel more vulnerable because of ill health and disability. Living alone, being lonely, and having sensory, mobility, and memory impairments may make older adults more susceptible to crime. Property crime is the most common crime against individuals ages 65 years and older. Older adults are more likely to be victims of consumer fraud and scams that include telemarketing fraud, email scams, and undelivered services. Older adults also experience rising problems with identity theft. Cybercrime is any criminal activity in which a computer (or networked device) is targeted or used. In 2020 cybercrime complaints soared to a record high, with total losses of more than $4.2 billion and losses to those ages 50 years and older exceeding $1.8 billion. This represents a 69% jump from 2019 and is attributed to exploitation of the COVID-19 pandemic for financial gain (Skiba, 2021).

Fraudulent Schemes Against Older Adults

Every year millions of older adults fall victim to some type of financial fraud or confidence scheme. Common scams include investment fraud, tech support scams, romance scams, grandparent scams, government impersonation scams, sweepstakes or lottery scams, home repair scams, family caregiver scams, and TV or radio scams. Older adults are often targeted because they tend to be trusting and polite and usually have financial savings, own a home, and have good credit. Older adults also may be less likely to report fraud because they don't know how, may be ashamed at having been scammed, or are concerned that their relatives will lose confidence in their ability to manage their own financial affairs.

Medical fraud is another serious type of fraud that affects older adults on a national scale. Medical supplies and equipment delivered to homes by various suppliers may be grossly overpriced or charged for but never received by the client. Scams to defraud Medicare beneficiaries for the Medicare Part D benefit also have been reported. Callers ask for bank information and use the account numbers to electronically withdraw money for a Medicare card and drug plan that is not legitimate. The Centers for Medicare and Medicaid Services (CMS) has offices to inform Medicare and Medicaid beneficiaries of ways to avoid fraud

BOX 21.2   Crime-Reduction Suggestions

Walking

- Plan your route and stay alert to your surroundings. Walk confidently
- Have a companion accompany you
- Stay in well-lighted areas
- Have your key ready when approaching your front door
- Don't dangle your purse away from your body; carry only what you need

In the Car

- Always keep door locked when you are in or out of the car
- Keep the car in gear at stop signs and traffic lights
- Plan your route and travel well-lit and busy streets
- Don't leave your purse on the seat beside you; put it on the floor
- Lock bundles or bags in the trunk
- When returning to your car, check the front and back seat and floor before entering
- If your car should break down, get far enough off the road, turn on emergency flashers, raise the hood, get back in the car, lock the door, and wait for help

At Home

- Never open your door automatically; use an optical viewer or ring camera; consider a home security system
- At night, draw blinds or drapes
- Lock doors, windows, and garage door
- Don't leave notes on the door when going out; don't place keys under mats, in mailboxes, or in other receptacles outside your door
- Leave lights on when going out at night; use a timer to turn lights on and off when you are away for an extended period
- Notify neighbors and the police when going away on a trip; cancel deliveries and mail
- Be wary of unsolicited offers to make repairs to your home; deal only with reputable businesses
- Don't hesitate to report crimes or suspicious activities
- Organize a buddy system or neighborhood watch

BOX 21.3   Protection Against Fraud and Cybercrime

- Recognize scam attempts and end all communication with the perpetrator
- Search online for the contact information and the proposed offer. Other people likely have posted information online about individuals and businesses trying to run scams
- Resist the pressure to act quickly. Call the police if you feel there is danger to yourself or a loved one
- Be cautious of unsolicited phone calls, mailings, and door-to-door service offers
- Never give or send any personally identifiable information, money, jewelry, gift cards, checks, or wire information to unverified people or businesses
- Make sure all computer antivirus and security software and malware protections are up to date
- Disconnect from the internet and shut down your device if you see a pop-up message or locked screen
- Be careful what you download, never open an email attachment from someone you don't know, and be wary of email attachments forwarded to you
- Take precautions to protect your identity if a criminal gains access to your device or account. Immediately contact your financial institutions to place protections on your accounts and monitor your accounts and personal information for suspicious activity

and also provides toll-free numbers to report suspected fraud. National agencies have combined forces to bring about reform. The Federal Bureau of Investigation (FBI) also provides information on elder fraud (see Box 21.1). Suggestions for prevention of crime, fraud, and cybercrime are presented in Boxes 21.2 and 21.3. Nurses can be instrumental in reducing fear of crime and assisting older adults in exploring ways in which they may protect themselves and feel more secure.

FIRE SAFETY FOR OLDER ADULTS

Older adults are more threatened with death or injury by fire than any other age group. Fire-related death rates are three times higher in people older than 80 years than in the rest of the population (National Hispanic Council on Aging, 2017). The risk of injury during a fire is greater if medication, illness, mobility, and sensory impairments slow response time or decision making and if help is not available to contain the fire and help the person escape.

A number of factors predispose the older adult to fire injuries. In home-dwelling older adults, economic or climatic conditions may promote the use of ill-kept heating devices. Attempts to cook over an open flame while wearing loose-fitting clothing, or inability to manage spattering grease from a frying pan, can often start a fire from which the individual cannot escape. Failing vision can contribute to a person setting a cooktop burner, heating pad, or hot plate at too high a temperature, resulting in fire or thermal injury.

Individuals living in apartment dwellings are often at the mercy of inadequate repair and safety measures and the careless behaviors of others. Many individuals living in their own homes cannot afford home repairs, placing them at risk for fire. Most fires occur at home during the night, and deaths are attributed to smoke injury more often than burns. Smoking materials are the most common sources of residential fires. Plastic articles and other synthetics can produce noxious fumes that are deadly, particularly to individuals with preexisting respiratory disorders. Resources for fire prevention are presented in Box 21.1.

VULNERABILITY TO ENVIRONMENTAL TEMPERATURES

Extreme weather events such as heat waves, cold spells, floods, storms, and droughts are increasing across the globe. These extreme events are an emerging environmental health concern and potentially affect the health status of millions of people around the globe. More than one-half of older adults live in areas that disproportionately experience the effects of heat waves, forest fires, hurricanes, and coastal flooding (McDermott-Levy et al., 2019). Heat-related and cold-related deaths increase with age, particularly for those ages 75 years and over. Extreme heat is the leading cause of death related to the weather. Older adults, low-income people of color, chronically ill individuals, and those who cannot afford the cost of electricity are especially at risk of extreme heat (Moran, 2020). Many older adults do not have the physical, cognitive, social, and economic resources to avoid or mitigate the effects of exposure to these extreme weather events. Preventive measures require attentiveness to impending climate changes and protective alternatives. Early intervention in extreme temperature exposure is crucial because excessively high or low body temperatures further impair thermoregulatory function and can be lethal.

Thermoregulation

Neurosensory changes in thermoregulation delay or diminish the individual's awareness of temperature changes and may impair behavioral and thermoregulatory response to dangerously high or low environmental temperatures. These changes vary widely among individuals and are related more to general health than to age. The ability to sense heat, to sweat, and to increase skin blood flow are all reduced in healthy older adults. The risk of heat-related illnesses or injuries are increased in older adults with obesity, cardiovascular disease, respiratory disease, and diabetes, which affect normal thermoregulatory responses. In addition, many drugs affect thermoregulation by affecting the ability to vasoconstrict or vasodilate, both of which are thermoregulatory mechanisms. Other drugs inhibit neuromuscular activity (a significant source of kinetic heat production), suppress metabolic heat generation, or dull awareness (tranquilizers, pain medications). Alcohol inhibits thermoregulatory function by affecting vasomotor responses in either hot or cold weather.

Economic, behavioral, and environmental factors may combine to create a dangerous thermal environment in which older adults are subjected to temperature extremes from which they cannot escape or that they cannot change. Caregivers and family members should be aware that individuals are vulnerable to temperature extremes if they are unable to shiver, sweat, control blood supply to the skin, take in sufficient liquids, move about, add or remove clothing, adjust bedcovers, or adjust the room temperature. A temperature that may be comfortable for a young and active person may be too cold or too warm for an older adult who is frail. Economic conditions often play a role in determining whether an older adult living in the community can afford air conditioning or adequate heating. Local governments and communities must coordinate response strategies to protect older adults. Strategies may include providing fans and opportunities to spend part of the day in air-conditioned buildings and identification of high-risk individuals.

Temperature Monitoring in Older Adults

Diminished thermoregulatory responses and abnormalities in both the production and the response to endogenous pyrogens may contribute to differences in fever responses between older and younger individuals in response to an infection. Careful attention to temperature monitoring in older adults is very important, and often this technical task is not given adequate consideration by professional nurses.

Up to one-third of older adults with acute infections may present without a febrile response. In addition, baseline temperatures in frail older adults may be lower than the expected 98.6°F. If the baseline temperature is 97°F, a temperature of 98°F is a 1°F elevation and may be significant.

Temperatures reaching or exceeding 100.9°F are very serious in older adults and are more likely to be associated with serious bacterial or viral infections. Careful attention to temperature monitoring in older adults is very important and can prevent morbidity and mortality. Accurate measurement and reporting of body temperature require professional nursing supervision.

Hyperthermia

When body temperature increases above normal ranges because of environmental or metabolic heat loads, a clinical condition called heat illness, or *hyperthermia*, develops. Administration of diuretics and low intake of fluids exacerbate fluid loss and can precipitate the onset of hyperthermia in hot weather. Hyperthermia is a temperature-related illness and is classified as a medical emergency. Annually, there are numerous deaths among older adults from temperature extremes; therefore prevention and education are very important nursing responsibilities.

Although most of these problems occur in the home among individuals who do not have air conditioning to use during temperature extremes, older adults with multiple physical problems residing in institutions may be especially vulnerable to temperature changes. Individuals with cardiovascular disease, diabetes, or peripheral vascular disease and those taking certain medications (anticholinergics, antihistamines, diuretics, beta blockers, antidepressants, antiparkinsonian drugs) are at risk. The CMS requires that nursing homes have alternate sources of energy to maintain temperatures to protect resident health and safety and for the safe and sanitary storage of provisions. Interventions to prevent hyperthermia when ambient temperature exceeds 90°F (32°C) are presented in Box 21.4.

Hypothermia

More than half of all hypothermia-related deaths happen in individuals over age 65 (Johns Hopkins Medicine, 2021). Hypothermia is produced by exposure to cold environmental temperatures and is defined as a core temperature of less than 95°F (35°C). Hypothermia is a medical emergency requiring comprehensive assessment of neurological activity, oxygenation, renal

BOX 21.4 Tips for Best Practice
Preventing Hyperthermia

- Drink 2 to 3 L of cool fluid daily and eat smaller, more frequent meals.
- Minimize exertion, especially during the warmest times of the day.
- Use air conditioning or go to where air conditioning is available (malls, library); use fans.
- Wear light, loose-fitting cotton clothing and hat when outside; remove most clothing when indoors.
- Take tepid baths or showers.
- Apply cold wet compresses or immerse the hands and feet in cool water.
- Evaluate medications for risk of hyperthermia.
- Avoid alcohol.

function, and fluid and electrolyte balance. When exposed to cold temperatures, healthy individuals conserve heat by vasoconstriction of superficial vessels, shunting circulation away from the skin where most heat is lost. Heat is generated by shivering and increased muscle activity, and a rise in oxygen consumption occurs to meet aerobic muscle requirements. Under normal circumstances, heat is produced in sufficient quantities by cellular metabolism of food, friction produced by contracting muscles, and the flow of blood.

Recognizing and Analyzing Cues

Hypothermia in older adults presents with more subtle cues and occurs more easily than in younger adults. Paralyzed or immobile individuals lack the ability to generate significant heat by muscle activity and become cold even in normal room temperatures. Individuals who are emaciated and have poor nutrition lack insulation and fuel for metabolic heat-generating processes, so they may be mildly hypothermic. Circulatory, cardiac, respiratory, or musculoskeletal impairments affect either the response to or the function of thermoregulatory mechanisms. Other risk factors include excessive alcohol use; poor nutrition; inadequate housing; and the use of sedatives, anxiolytics, phenothiazines, and tricyclic antidepressants (Box 21.5).

Hypothermia also can occur when the individual with some degree of thermoregulatory impairment undergoes surgery, is injured in a fall or accident and not found right away, or is lost or left unattended in a cool place. The more severe the impairment or prolonged the exposure, the less able the thermoregulatory responses are to defend against heat loss. Unfortunately, a dulling of awareness accompanies hypothermia, and individuals experiencing the condition rarely recognize the problem or seek assistance. For the very old and frail, environmental temperatures less than 65°F (18°C) may cause a serious drop in core body temperature to 95°F (35°C).

Detecting hypothermia among community-dwelling older adults is sometimes difficult because, unlike in the clinical setting, no one is measuring body temperature. For individuals exposed to low temperatures in the home or the environment, confusion and disorientation may be the first overt signs. As judgment becomes clouded, an individual may remove clothing or fail to seek shelter, and hypothermia can progress to profound levels.

Solutions, Nursing Actions, and Outcomes

All body systems are affected by hypothermia, although the most deadly consequences involve cardiac arrhythmias and suppression of respiratory function. Correctly conducted rewarming is the key to good management, and the guiding principle is to warm the core before the periphery and raise the core temperature 0.5°C to 2°C per hour. Heating blankets and specially designed heating vests are used in addition to warm humidified air by mask, warm intravenous boluses, and other measures depending on the severity of the hypothermia.

Recognition of clinical signs and severity of hypothermia and hyperthermia is an important nursing responsibility. The potential risk of hypothermia and its associated cardiorespiratory and metabolic exertion make prevention important and early recognition vital. It is important to closely monitor body temperature and pay particular attention to lower- or higher-than-normal readings compared with the person's baseline. For individuals in hospitals or long-term care facilities, nurses are responsible for keeping older adults in appropriate temperatures for comfort and prevention of problems.

Educating older adults and their families about hypothermia and prevention and treatment is important. Nurses also must advocate for resources in the community to ensure appropriate temperatures in the homes of older adults and surveillance when temperature changes occur. Regular contact with home-dwelling older adults during cold weather is crucial. For those with preexisting alterations in thermoregulatory ability, this surveillance should include even mildly cool weather. Because heating costs are high in the United States, the Department of Health and Human Services provides funds to help low-income families pay their heating bills. Specific interventions to prevent hypothermia are outlined in Box 21.6.

VULNERABILITY TO NATURAL DISASTERS

Natural disasters such as hurricanes, tornadoes, floods, wildfires, and earthquakes claim the lives of many individuals worldwide each year. In addition, human-made or human-generated disasters include chemical, biological, radiological, and nuclear

---

BOX 21.5 Factors That Increase the Risk of Hypothermia in Older Adults

Thermoregulatory Impairment
Failure to vasoconstrict promptly or sufficiently on exposure to cold
Failure to sense cold
Failure to respond behaviorally to protect oneself against cold
Diminished or absent shivering to generate heat
Failure of metabolic rate to rise in response to cold

Conditions That Decrease Heat Production
Hypothyroidism, hypopituitarism, hypoglycemia, anemia, malnutrition, starvation
Immobility or decreased activity (e.g., stroke, paralysis, parkinsonism, dementia, arthritis, fractured hip, coma)
Thinning hair, baldness
Diabetic ketoacidosis

Conditions That Increase Heat Loss
Open wounds, generalized inflammatory skin conditions, burns

Conditions That Impair Central or Peripheral Control of Thermoregulation
Stroke, brain tumor, Wernicke's encephalopathy, subarachnoid hemorrhage
Uremia, neuropathy (e.g., diabetes, alcoholism)
Acute illnesses (e.g., pneumonia, sepsis, myocardial infarction, congestive heart failure, pulmonary embolism, pancreatitis)
Anesthesia and surgery

Drugs That Interfere With Thermoregulation
Tranquilizers (e.g., phenothiazines); sedative-hypnotics (e.g., barbiturates, benzodiazepines); antidepressants (e.g., tricyclics); vasoactive drugs (e.g., vasodilators); alcohol (causes superficial vasodilation; may interfere with carbohydrate metabolism and judgment); others (e.g., methyldopa, lithium, morphine)

BOX 21.6 Tips for Best Practice

Preventing Cold Discomfort and Development of Accidental Hypothermia in Frail Older Adults

- Maintain a comfortably warm ambient temperature no lower than 68°F. Many frail older adults will require much higher temperatures.
- Provide generous quantities of clothing and bedcovers. Layer clothing and bedcovers for best insulation. Be careful not to judge your patient's needs by how you feel working in a warm environment.
- Provide a head covering whenever possible—in bed, out of bed, and particularly outdoors.
- Cover patients well when in bed or bathing. The standard—a light bath blanket over a naked body—is not enough protection for frail older adults.
- Cover patients with heavy blankets for transfer to and from showers; dry quickly and thoroughly before leaving the shower room; cover the head with a dry towel or hood while wet. Shower rooms and bathrooms should have warming lights.
- Dry wet hair quickly with warm air from an electric dryer. Never allow the hair of frail older adults to air-dry.
- Use absorbent pads for individuals with urinary incontinence who are unable to ambulate to the toilet rather than allowing urine to wet large areas of clothing, sheets, and bedcovers.
- Provide as much exercise as possible to generate heat from muscle activity.
- Provide hot, high-protein meals and bedtime snacks to add heat and sustain heat production throughout the day and as far into the night as possible.

terrorism and food and water contamination. Older adults are at great risk during and after disasters and have the highest casualty rate during disaster events when compared with all other age groups (Malik et al., 2018). The COVID-19 pandemic has claimed the lives of more older adults around the world than those in other age groups. Although deaths in nursing homes received enormous attention, far more older adults who perished from COVID-19 lived outside of institutions (Graham, 2021).

Older adults with dementia and those with serious and chronic kidney disease, immune deficiencies, severe neurological conditions, and multiple medical conditions were especially vulnerable (Graham, 2021). Long-term care facility deaths made up over a third of all US deaths based on COVID Tracking Project (CTP) data, which include nursing homes, assisted living, and other long-term care facilities. The impact on these communities is likely higher because of missing historical deaths from both state and CMS data and inconsistent, nonstandardized reporting by states. (Long-Term-Care COVID Tracker, 2021) (Chapter 6).

Older adults may be less likely to seek formal or informal help during disasters or may be unable to do this independently. Many lack access to the technology that supplies communication during disasters. Many older adults cannot easily evacuate because they do not drive, are physically unable to evacuate, or may refuse. Older adults at most risk include but are not limited to those who depend on others for daily functioning, the medically frail, those with limited mobility, those who are socially isolated or live alone, and those who are cognitively impaired or institutionalized. The older and poorer the individual, the more likely the person is to be isolated and vulnerable.

Adopting tailored disaster preparedness plans that address the general and emergency health needs for older adults is a worldwide concern. Families caring for older adults need to have individualized emergency plans. Public health prevention planning and programs are needed to identify older adults at increased risk in the event of disasters and address their needs. Communities need to enhance preparedness and information networks among organizations and agencies that serve older adults (American Red Cross & American Academy of Nursing, 2020; Shih et al., 2018). Gerontological nurses can assist in the development of these plans and educate fellow professionals and community agencies about the special needs of older adults. Nurses also can provide educational programs and outreach on disaster preparedness to older adults. Box 21.1 presents resources for emergency and disaster preparedness.

GUN SAFETY

Gun safety among older adults is relevant to medical and public health professionals, given that older adults experience changes in memory, function, and mood that may increase risks of gun-related injuries and deaths. Older adults have the highest gun ownership in the United States, with 27% of people 65 years and older owning one or more firearms and 37% living in a home with a firearm present. Estimates are that 60% of households of individuals with a diagnosis of dementia have one or more firearms, and the presence of guns does not vary by the degree of dementia. Individuals with severe cognitive impairment are as likely to have firearms in their homes as those with mild cognitive impairment.

Older adults, particularly White males, also have high rates of suicide, and 71% of the time they use guns (Chapter 30). Evaluating gun safety and risk of injury is important in care of older adults; questions about gun ownership and gun safety should be asked as routinely as questions about driving, especially when there is a dementia diagnosis. The 5 Ls approach (Box 21.7) is recommended for assessment of firearm safety practices (Galluzi & Warner-Moran, 2018; Morgan & Rowhani-Rahbar, 2020).

BOX 21.7 5Ls Approach to Assessing Gun Safety Practices

- **Locked:** Is there a gun present? Is it locked?
- **Loaded:** Is it loaded?
- **Little children:** Are there children present in the home?
- **Feeling Low:** Does the gun owner feel low, having suicidal thoughts?
- **Learned owner:** Has the owner had formal gun safety training?

Galuzzi, K., Warner-Maron, I. (2018). Guns and older adults: The physician's role. *Journal of the American Osteopathic Association, 118*(12), 775–780. doi: 10.7556/jaoa.2018.169.

TRANSPORTATION SAFETY

Adequate, affordable, and convenient transportation services are a critical link in the ability of older adults to remain independent and functional and to age in place. The lack of accessible transportation may contribute to other problems, such as social withdrawal, poor nutrition, depressive symptoms, and health decline. A "crisis in mobility" exists for many older adults because of the lack of an automobile, an inability to drive, limited access to public transportation, health factors, geographical location, and economic considerations. Urban buses and subways can be physically hazardous and often dangerous. Rural and suburban areas may not have accessible transportation systems, making transportation by car essential. Even walking can be dangerous, and older adults are more likely to be injured or killed as pedestrians than as car drivers. Efforts to make walking safer include raised pavement markings, median islands, increased time for pedestrian crossings, and lowered speed limits.

County, state, or federally-subsidized transportation is provided in certain areas to assist individuals in reaching social services, nutrition sites, health services, emergency care, recreational centers, daycare programs, physical and vocational rehabilitation centers, grocery stores, and library services. Some senior centers and assisted living facilities also offer transportation services. Although transportation often can be found for special needs, it is virtually impossible to locate transportation for pleasure or recreation, and many of these services are restricted to individuals with serious physical or mental impairments.

Ride-sharing services such as Uber and Lyft can assist in providing more transportation options, but some older adults may not be able to afford these services or may not feel safe using them. Some of these transportation services offer special services for individuals who need more assistance, such as wheelchair-accessible vehicles or a driver trained to provide additional assistance. Assessment of older adults needs to include transportation needs. Referrals to local social service and aging organizations, such as Area Agencies on Aging, can be made to assist in obtaining information on transportation resources and financial assistance for services.

Driving

Older adults' driving is a critical public health issue. Driving is one of the IADLs for most older adults because it is essential to obtaining necessary resources. Currently, 83% of individuals ages 70 years and older have a driver's license. For many older adults, alternate transportation is not available, and consequently they may continue driving beyond the time when it is safe. Driving is a highly complex activity that requires a variety of visual, motor, and cognitive skills. Age alone is not a good indicator of driving safety, but health conditions, sensory functioning, road design and traffic, and weather conditions contribute to increasing concern with driving safety as individuals age (Edwards et al., 2017). Cognitive functions necessary for driving, such as attention and spatial orientation, are especially impaired with dementia, making this population especially vulnerable to unintentional vehicle injury and death (Davis & Owens, 2021).

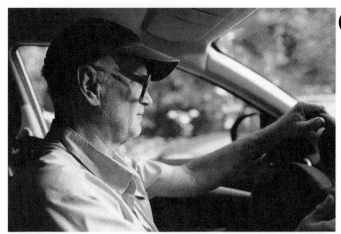

Driving is the preferred means of travel for older adults. (©iStock. com/danr13.)

Driving Safety

Older drivers typically drive fewer miles than younger drivers and tend to drive less at night, during adverse weather conditions, or in congested areas. Generally they choose familiar routes, and fewer older drivers speed or drive after drinking alcohol than drivers of other ages. However, when compared with younger age groups, older adults have more accidents per mile driven. Motor vehicle accidents are more likely to cause death in adults 65 years and older than in younger adults and are the second leading cause of unintentional death in adults over the age of 65 years (Davis & Owens, 2021). Improving the safety of cars through new design and adaptations should be considered for older drivers to enhance safety (Box 21.8).

The legal regulations regarding driver's license renewal for older drivers and the responsibility of medical practitioners to identify unsafe drivers vary among states and countries. Driver's license renewal procedures may include accelerated renewal cycles, renewal in person rather than electronically or by mail, and vision and road tests. The issues of driving in the older adult population are the subject of a great deal of public discussion.

BOX 21.8   Adaptations for Safer Driving

- Wider rear-view mirrors
- Pedal extensions
- Less complicated, larger, and legible instrument panels
- Electronic detectors in front and back that signal when the car is getting too close to other cars, drifting into another lane, or likely to hit center dividers or other highway infrastructure
- Technology that facilitates left turns by alerting drivers when it is safe to make the turn
- Better protection on doors
- Booster cushions for shorter-stature drivers
- "Smart" driving assistants (under development) that automatically plan a safe driving route based on the person's driving habits
- GPS devices

Modified from Dugan E, Lee C: Biopsychosocial risk factors for driving cessation: findings from the Health and Retirement Study, *J Aging Health* 25:1313–1328, 2013.

Many older drivers and their families struggle with issues related to continued safety in driving. Tips for driving safety are presented in Box 21.9.

Driving and Dementia

Driving is one of the largest ethical issues associated with dementia. Dementia, even in the early stages, can impair the cognitive and functional skills required for safe driving. There is at least a twofold greater risk of crashes for drivers with dementia when compared to age-matched individuals without dementia (Wiese & Wolff, 2016). Estimates are that about 33% of older adults with dementia are active drivers, and 50% continue driving for up to 3 years post diagnosis. Many individuals early in the course of dementia are still able to pass a driving performance test, so a diagnosis of dementia should not be the sole justification for revocation of a driver's license. Due to the varied rate of progression for Alzheimer's disease, there is no standardized timeline for driving cessation for this population (Davis & Owens, 2021).

However, research results suggest that declines in driving performance likely precede problems with thinking, memory, or cognition in individuals in the later stages of preclinical Alzheimer's disease (Roe et al., 2017). In innovative research, nurse researcher Ruth Tappen at Florida Atlantic University and her colleagues are testing and evaluating a readily and rapidly available, unobtrusive in-vehicle sensing system, which could provide the first step toward future widespread, low-cost early warnings of cognitive changes affecting driving. Recent research results give evidence that individuals in the early stage of Alzheimer's disease may have self-awareness of their driving ability and self-regulate their driving to enhance safety (see Research Highlights).

RESEARCH HIGHLIGHTS

Self-Regulation of Driving Behaviors in Persons With Early-Stage Alzheimer's Disease

Purpose

To determine if persons with Alzheimer's disease (AD) or mild cognitive impairment (MCI) reported awareness of driving ability and made self-regulatory changes to the same degree as older adults without AD.

Method

Driving awareness and behaviors were collected using a self-report survey. Results of the AD/MCI group were compared to a similarly aged control group.

Results

Individuals with AD/MCI reported less confidence in their driving ability and worried about getting lost more often than the control group. They also were more likely to have stopped driving than the control group. The AD/MCI group reported that they avoided driving in unfamiliar situations, drove less often, and drove with another person significantly more than the control group. In addition, they rated themselves as good or excellent drivers less often and got lost more often than those without AD/MCI. Yet, most (77%) continue to drive.

Conclusion

Results suggest that individuals with AD or MCI have some self-awareness of limitations in their driving ability and that they often self-regulate their driving behaviors. Since many continue to drive after their diagnosis, it is important to discuss driving ability and limitations they have put on their driving, as well as to ask caregivers for their insights and concerns. Individuals may continue to drive when they are not comfortable doing so because of the difficulties associated with driving cessation. Finding methods for improving safe driving practices is important.

Data from Davis R, Owens M: Self-regulation of driving behaviors in persons with early-stage Alzheimer's disease, *J Gerontol Nurs* 47(1):21–26, 2021.

BOX 21.9 Tips for Best Practice

Driving Safety

- Include the person in all discussions about driving safety.
- Encourage the individual to conduct a self-assessment of driving abilities.
- Assess vision and hearing and ensure appropriate use of corrective lenses and hearing devices.
- Evaluate medical conditions that may interfere with driving ability (arthritis, Parkinson's disease, dementia, stroke) and ensure appropriate treatment, and adaptations that may be necessary to enhance driving safety.
- Suggest vehicle adaptations and older adult driving assessment programs if indicated.
- Encourage the individual to modify driving habits, such as not driving on unfamiliar roads, during rush hour, at dusk or at night, in inclement weather, or in heavy traffic.
- Avoid risky spots like ramps and left turns.
- Advise individual to limit night driving.
- Discuss strategies to decrease the need to drive including arranging for home-delivered groceries, prescriptions, and meals; having personal services provided in the home; asking a caregiver to obtain needed supplies or act as a copilot; and exploring community resources for transportation.
- Ask the family to have the family lawyer discuss with the individual the financial and legal implications of a crash or injury.

From National Institute on Aging: *Older drivers* (website). https://www.nia.nih.gov/health/older-drivers#besafe. Accessed January 2021.

Many states have implemented the Silver Alert system. Similar to Amber Alerts for missing children, Silver Alert is designed to create a widespread lookout for older adults who have wandered from their surroundings while driving a car. Silver Alert features a public notification system to broadcast information about missing persons, especially older adults with Alzheimer's disease or other mental disabilities, in order to aid in their return. Silver Alert uses a wide array of media outlets, such as commercial radio stations, television stations, and cable television, to broadcast information about missing persons. Silver Alert also uses message signs on roadways to alert motorists to be on the lookout for missing older adults and provide the car's make, model, and license plate number.

Driving Cessation

Relinquishing the mobility and independence afforded by driving one's own car has many psychological ramifications and inconveniences. Giving up driving is a major loss for an older adult both in terms of independence and pleasure and in feelings of competence and self-worth. The health consequences of driving cessation include social isolation, health problems, institutionalization, higher mortality, and an approximately doubled risk of depression (Davis & Ohman, 2017). Women are more likely than men to stop driving for less pressing reasons than health, and at a younger age. Older men seem to place more value on the ability to drive, and on owning a car, than older women. Therefore one can expect more stress involved with the decision not to drive for older men.

Voluntarily giving up a driver's license, rather than having it revoked, is associated with more positive outcomes. Specialized driving cessation support groups aimed at the transition from driver to nondriver also may be beneficial in decreasing the negative outcomes associated with this decision. "Family members require support and education about how to give feedback on driving safety in a way that ensures the message is carefully timed, received as well as possible, and supports relationships" (Liddle et al., 2017, p. 87). Box 21.10 presents a self-evaluation of driving skills and safety.

USING CLINICAL JUDGMENT TO PROMOTE HEALTHY AGING: DRIVING SAFETY

Recognizing and Analyzing Cues

Driving ability should be included in assessment of the functional abilities of older adults. Areas to be assessed include whether an individual can drive, feels safe driving, and has a driver's license. Questions about the individual's actions to self-regulate driving by modifying driving behaviors to avoid complex driving situations and difficult road conditions should be included in assessment along with safety information (see Box 21.9). For individuals with a dementia diagnosis, discussions about driving safety should begin when dementia is diagnosed, and driving evaluations should be conducted every 6 months or as needed as the disease progresses.

Additional areas of evaluation include skills needed for safe driving, such as vision and hearing screening, cognitive assessment, medication review, assessment of range of motion, and evaluation of strength and general mobility. These evaluations help identify limitations that could affect an individual's ability

---

BOX 21.11   Safe Drive

S	Safety record	**R**	Reaction time
A	Attention skills	**I**	Intellectual impairment
F	Family report	**V**	Vision and visuospatial function
E	Ethanol use	**E**	Executive functions
D	Drugs		

---

to make driving decisions or to exit the car quickly. A mnemonic, SAFE DRIVE, addresses key components in screening older drivers (Box 21.11).

There is no gold standard for determining driving competency, but comprehensive driving evaluations are offered by driver rehabilitation specialists through local hospitals and rehabilitation centers and private or university-based driving assessment programs. Components of a thorough driving examination include a history and physical, vision and hearing evaluation, cognitive assessment, and road test (Wiese & Wolff, 2016). Some programs that evaluate driving ability may use a standardized computer driving simulation. There is a lack of resources for driving evaluations, and the evaluation is also very expensive and not covered by Medicare or insurance.

Solutions, Nursing Actions, and Outcomes

Planning for driving cessation should occur for all older adults before their mobility situations become urgent. Health care providers should encourage open discussion of issues related to driving with the older adult and the family and should identify impairments that affect safe driving, correct them when possible, and offer alternatives for transportation. Unfortunately, studies have shown that health care providers are often reluctant to discuss driving with individuals with dementia, and even fewer refer patients for formal assessment of their driving ability (Davis & Owens, 2021). Nursing education programs should include content on driving safety, functional assessment of older drivers, driving cessation programs, and community transportation resources (Wiese, 2020).

BOX 21.10   Self-Evaluation of Driving

We all age differently. For this reason, there is no way to set one age when everyone should stop driving. So, how do you know if you should stop? To help decide, ask yourself:

- Do other drivers often honk at me?
- Have I had some accidents, even if they were only "fender benders"?
- Do I get lost, even on roads I know?
- Do cars or people walking seem to appear out of nowhere?
- Do I get distracted while driving?
- Have family, friends, or my doctor said they're worried about my driving?
- Am I driving less these days because I'm not as sure about my driving as I used to be?
- Do I have trouble staying in my lane?
- Do I have trouble moving my foot between the gas and the brake pedals, or do I sometimes confuse the two?
- Have I been pulled over by a police officer about my driving?

    If you answered "yes" to any of these questions, it may be time to talk with your doctor about driving or have a driving assessment.

From National Institute on Aging: Is it time to give up driving? (website). https://www.nia.nih.gov/health/older-drivers#give-up. Accessed January 2021.

⚡ SAFETY TIPS

Nurses can empower older adult drivers by teaching them about health-promoting behaviors and safety tips that will minimize driving errors. If a family member or friend has observed a pattern of unsafe driving behaviors, the nurse can share key phrases for starting a conversation regarding driving concerns, such as "Driving on the roads today is so much more difficult than it used to be," "That was a close call today while driving to the ____; I worry about your safety," and "Did you speak with your doctor about the effects of your recent medications on driving?" Having a calm conversation is vital to protecting the older adult's dignity.

For families facing a dementia diagnosis, the Alzheimer's Association's Dementia and Driving resource center contains examples of helpful communication techniques and short video role-plays of talking about driving cessation (Box 21.1). For many older adults, giving up driving is a major loss, and the emotional and physical consequences can be significant. A key component of successful management of driving cessation is the support group, where all family members can express their frustrations and also learn about effective techniques for coping with challenges. Memory and wellness centers, including adult day programs, and senior centers may offer support groups as a component of driving cessation programs.

Despite the growing challenges associated with driving safety in older adults, there is a lack of research on the effectiveness of interventions to improve safety, address driving cessation, and educate health professionals on the issue. Nursing research can contribute to the development and testing of effective interventions (Wiese & Wolf, 2016; Wiese, 2020). Box 21.1 presents additional resources for driving safety. *Healthy People 2030* includes objectives for pedestrian, driving, and gun safety.

> ### ♥ HEALTHY PEOPLE 2030
>
> - Reduce motor vehicle crash–related deaths
> - Reduce pedestrian injuries and deaths on public roads
> - Reduce firearm-related deaths and nonfatal firearm-related injuries

Data from US Department of Health and Human Services: *Healthy People 2030* (website), 2020. https://health.gov/healthypeople.

EMERGING TECHNOLOGIES TO ENHANCE SAFETY OF OLDER ADULTS

Advancements in all types of technology hold promise for improving quality of life, decreasing the need for personal care, and enhancing independence and the ability to live safely at home and age in place (Pepito & Locsin, 2019). The costs of nursing homes and assisted living, as well as the reluctance of older adults to move to these settings, are driving sales and innovation in the technology markets. A growing concern related to the increasing number of older adults is the lack of both family and paid caregivers who can provide care in the individual's home (Chapter 32). "Existing and emerging solutions are opening the door for a new era of 'tech-enabled caregiving' with the potential to make life better for caregivers and older adults" (Andruszkiewicz & Fike, 2015–2016, p. 64).

Assistive technology is any device or system that allows a person to perform a task independently or that makes the task easier and safer to perform. Assistive technology is decreasing the number of older adults who depend on others for personal care in ADLs and presents cost-effective alternatives to human services and institutionalization. *Gerotechnology* is the term used to describe assistive technologies for older adults, and these technologies are expected to significantly influence how we live in the future.

Health care technologies, robotics, telemedicine, mobility and ADL aids, remote activity monitoring (RAM) systems, and environmental control systems (smart houses and intelligent homes) are some examples of assistive technology (Choi et al., 2019; Zmora et al., 2021). Apple has a new health feature for anyone with an iPhone that monitors walking steadiness using metrics such as walking speed, step length, and the time both feet are in contact with the ground to monitor how stable a user is. It can tell individuals if they are walking steadily and issue an alert if it thinks they are at increased risk of falling. Apple Watch has a fall detection feature that can prompt users to call emergency services or automatically make a call if the user is immobile for around a minute (Wetsman, 2021).

Telehealth

Telehealth is the use of technologies to enable clinicians to remotely diagnose, monitor, and treat patients. Telehealth offers exciting possibilities for managing medical problems in the home or other setting, reducing health care costs, and promoting self-management of illness, particularly in rural and underserved areas. Telehealth reduces health care costs, transportation, and time on the part of the patient. The COVID-19 pandemic also has highlighted additional benefits of telehealth, such as reduced infection exposures. The federal government has recognized these benefits and implemented regulatory waivers and rule changes aimed at increasing telehealth accessibility and Medicare coverage for the service. At this time, reimbursement is tied to physicians and health systems. Evidence abounds that nurse-managed programs tend to be innovative, be high quality, and reach underserved populations and should be included for reimbursement. Interdisciplinary approaches are also important and should be considered (Brody et al., 2020). Telehealth also can be effective for delivering interventions designed for family caregivers (Chi & Demiris, 2017).

Research on the effectiveness of telehealth technology, acceptance of the technology by patients and providers, and identification of barriers and ways to telehealth delivery are important. Results of a recent study of the use of telehealth among homebound older adults suggest that the majority of patients needed assistance from a family member or paid caregiver to complete the visit. Cognitive and sensory impairments and comfort with technology affect how older adults are able to manage devices used for telehealth services.

Disparities in access to broadband also present obstacles to specific demographic groups (Brody et al., 2020). About a third of Americans in rural areas cannot access sufficient internet to support video-based telehealth (Kalicki et al., 2021) (Chapter 8). Telehealth may not be an effective method for all patients, and "further study is needed to ensure that increased telehealth use does not worsen existing inequalities, hinder communication between patients and providers, or lead to missed diagnoses and worse outcomes for older patients" (Kalicki et al., 2021, p. 2409; Mallow et al., 2021).

Smart Homes

Many exciting technologies are being developed to support monitoring and management of older adults' health and homes and to support aging in place and remote caregiving (Turjamaa et al., 2019). RAM systems track activity in a home or care facility using motion detectors or other sensors and relay this information to a monitoring company, facility staff, or family caregivers. RAM systems allow caregivers to track daily behavior passively and be notified about deviations from daily routines. Newly evolving smart home systems include a combination of home-control applications (e.g., appliances, lighting, security systems) and safety, health, wellness, and social connectivity technologies. These technologies can simultaneously and continuously monitor environmental conditions, daily activity patterns, vital signs, movement patterns, sleep patterns, medication adherence, and falls.

Examples of smart home technology adaptations include smart pill dispensers with automated reminders; smart stoves that automatically shut off when left unsupervised; smart mattresses to monitor sleep duration, body movement, and sleep cycles; sensors to measure sitting time and provide notification to promote physical activity; and virtual reality social gatherings with distant family and friends (Choi et al., 2019). Motion and pressure sensors may be useful in the homes of older adults with cognitive impairment. These sensors can detect movement and the absence of movement. If there has been no movement for a period of time, a monitoring system is activated and a plan of action initiated, depending on the person's response or lack of response. Pressure sensors can be used under the mattress and can turn on bedside lights when the individual gets out of bed and activate an alarm if the individual does not return to bed in a specified period of time. Sensors placed in entry doors or GPS watches or pendants can detect if a person leaves the home, and the person's location, and can send messages to caregivers. SmartSoles, shoe insoles with an embedded GPS device, may help locate individuals with dementia who wander from their home.

Robots

Robotic technology for health care is more advanced in Europe and Japan than in the United States at this time, but we can expect to see increased development and use of robotics in nursing. Already developed are robots that can help lift both individuals and objects, remind patients to take their medicine or administer the medication, check a person's vital signs, provide help in the event of a fall, and assist with baths and meals. A child-sized therapist robot on wheels with a humanlike torso is being developed for use in homes and long-term care facilities to assist with the high level of attention that individuals with dementia require for safety and function.

Research is ongoing to develop a humanoid nurse robot with a caring function, specifically designed for the functional and practical use of older adults with dementia (Locsin et al., 2018; Miyagawa et al., 2019). Programming robots with basic skills in humanlike caring is essential because these machines are increasingly in use as health care partners-in-caring. Many ethical issues have been raised about the use of robots, and nurses will play an important role in ensuring that technological competence is balanced with caring to enhance the well-being of the individual (Beuscher et al., 2017).

Robopets and Therapeutic Interactive Pets

The benefits of animal-assisted therapy in hospitals and long-term care facilities are well documented. However, bringing in live animals presents its own challenges, such as hygiene needs, potential allergies, and brevity of the interaction. These challenges can be offset by using robopets and therapeutic interactive pets (TIPs). An example that has been extensively studied is PARO, a certified medical therapeutic robot developed in Japan (Fig. 21.1) (http://www.parorobots.com). PARO looks like a baby harp seal and weighs about as much as a human baby. In interaction with people, PARO responds as if it is alive, moving its legs and head, making sounds, and responding to touch and

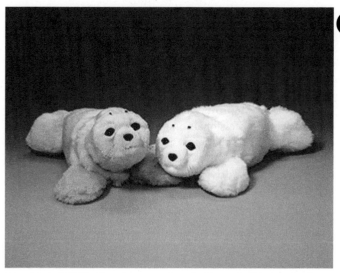

Fig. 21.1 PARO, the therapeutic robotic seal. (Used with permission from AIST JP/PARO ROBOTS US INC.)

sound. PARO can recognize the direction of voice and words such as its name, greetings, and praise with its audio sensor. Benefits of interaction with robopets include increased interaction and engagement, reduction of agitation, decreased loneliness, pleasure, and comfort (Abbott et al., 2019; Hudson et al., 2020; Moyle et al., 2017).

Dr. Bryanna Streit LaRose and Dr. Melissa Johnston, Florida Atlantic University College of Nursing, conducted quality improvement projects to evaluate the use of a TIP for individuals with neurocognitive diseases. LaRose (2019) conducted her project in an adult day center, and Johnston (2020) implemented her project virtually in the home setting due to COVID-19 restrictions. Family caregivers were involved in the implementation of the home-based project. Results of both the evidence-based and the quality improvement endeavors included improvements in mood and behavior, as evaluated by mood, emotion, depression, and cognition scales. In addition, qualitative feedback showed that participants enjoyed interacting with the TIP. Family caregivers reported that the TIP encouraged expression of feelings and a sense of comfort, similar to live companionship.

TIPs, robotic cats as well as dogs, are commercially available and less costly than others built specifically for medical use. Implementing TIPs in varied settings, such as home, adult day programs, and long-term care, is consequently more affordable (Fig. 21.2). To help combat isolation during the COVID-19 pandemic, the manufacturer of the TIPs in the projects described above, in partnership with the Florida Department of Elder Affairs and the New York Association on Aging, distributed TIPs to isolated older adults in the two states. Placement was determined by each state agency, and individuals were able to keep their robotic pets (Novotney, 2020).

Not everyone chooses to engage with robopets and TIPs. Occasionally, older adults, families, and staff may not have an affinity for robotic pets. Therefore it is important to determine participant preferences and history with pets before engaging the individual with a robopet or TIP. Robopets and TIPs are not

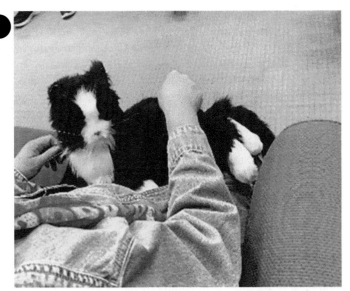

Fig. 21.2 An individual enjoying a companion animated therapy pet. (Ageless Innovation LLC, Joy for All Pets, https://joyforall. com/.)

intended to replace human interaction, but there appears to be benefit for using them as therapy for agitated or isolated individuals in adult day programs, home and community settings, and long-term care facilities. Further study of the most appropriate use of robopets and TIPs and evaluation of their effects should be conducted across settings of care. However, their use seems to be an effective nonpharmacological approach to promote positive outcomes for individuals with neurocognitive diseases across settings. Participant and caregiver input and feedback is essential in design and evaluation of programs using TIPs or robopets.

As the baby boomers and future generations age, comfort with technology will increase, and people will seek options for better, safer, and greater independence in ways not yet imagined. At this time, many of the assistive technologies can be cost prohibitive, but with advances in development they may become more accessible and affordable for more people. Issues of privacy and data sharing need consideration, and training and support

for proper use of devices and application are important. Most passive remote monitoring technologies are developed without input from older adults. Many systems are complex and difficult to use, especially for individuals with limited technology and health literacy skills.

Research is needed on assistive technologies that are user friendly, and nurses need to be aware of available technology to improve safety (Czaja, 2015). "Nurses can play essential roles in designing future research to improve the design and use of mobile and connected health technologies and researching their effects on older adults' health outcomes and ability to age in place. Nurses are also in a prime position to lead interprofessional teams of engineers, computer scientists, physicians, informaticians and other health professionals and partner with patients and their families to design, develop and implement technology in a holistic manner" (Wang, 2018, p. 4).

AGING IN PLACE

Developing elder-friendly communities and providing increasing opportunities to age in place can lead to enhanced health and well-being. Aging in place is the ability to live in one's own home and community safely, independently, and comfortably, regardless of age, income, or ability level. Many state and local governments are assessing the community and designing interventions to enhance the ability of older adults to remain in their homes and familiar environments. These interventions range from adequate transportation systems to home modifications and universal design standards for barrier-free housing.

Components of an elder-friendly community include the following: (1) addresses basic needs; (2) optimizes physical health and well-being; (3) maximizes independence for the frail and disabled; and (4) provides social and civic engagement. Fig. 21.3 presents elements of an elder-friendly community. Efforts to create physical and social urban environments that promote healthy and active aging and a good quality of life are occurring worldwide.

The World Health Organization (WHO) Global Network of Age-Friendly Cities and Communities helps cities and communities become more supportive of older adults by addressing

Addresses Basic Needs

• Provides appropriate and
  affordable housing
• Promotes safety at home and
  in the neighborhood
• Ensures no one goes hungry
• Provides useful information about
  available services

**Optimizes Physical and Mental
Health and Well-Being**

• Promotes healthy behaviors
• Supports community activities
  that enhance well-being
• Provides ready access to
  preventive health services
• Provides access to medical,
  social, and palliative services

Promotes Social and Civic Engagement

• Fosters meaningful connections
  with family, neighbors, and friends
• Promotes active engagement
  in community life
• Provides opportunities for meaningful
  paid and voluntary work
• Makes aging issues a community-wide priority

**Maximizes Independence for
Frail and Disabled**

• Mobilizes resources to
  facilitate "living at home"
• Provides accessible transportation
• Supports family and other caregivers

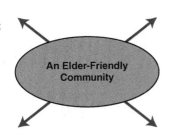

An Elder-Friendly
Community

Fig. 21.3 Essential elements of an elder-friendly community. (From AdvantAge Initiative, Center for Home Care Policy and Research, Visiting Nurse Service of New York.)

their needs across eight dimensions: the built environment; transportation; housing; social participation; respect and social inclusion; civic participation and employment; communication; and community support and health services (WHO, 2018).

A majority of older-midlife and older adults want to age in place and stay in their own homes or, if that is not possible, stay in their communities as they grow older. Only 3.1% of older adults live in institutions (Lach, 2021). However, for many older adults, the ability to find affordable, physically accessible, and well-located homes in their community is a significant challenge. There is also a lack of affordable and accessible rental units and federally subsidized housing for older renters. The racial and ethnic diversity of the growing number of older adults in the United States also has significant implications. "Faced with lifelong discrimination, many minority groups have lower rates of home ownership, lower median incomes, and fewer assets—factors that significantly constrain their housing choices in old age" (Gonyea & Melekis, 2017– 2018, p. 50).

Only 1% of US housing units have all five components of what are known as "universal design" features: no-step entry, single-floor living, extra-wide doorways and halls, accessible electric controls and switches, and level-style doors and faucet handles. Remodeling an existing home to install these accessibility features is expensive, and many cannot afford to remodel. An interesting concept is the "granny pod," a stand-alone housing structure that the family puts in their backyard for an aging relative. These tiny homes, or granny flats, are gaining popularity as viable alternatives to expensive long-term care facilities and enhance the ability of older adults to age in place.

Aging in Community Models

Naturally occurring retirement communities (NORCs) are neighborhoods or buildings in which a large segment of the residents are older adults. They are not purpose-built senior housing or retirement communities but are places where community residents have aged in place and where they intend to spend the rest of their lives. NORCs provide a range of health and social services for the residents as well as individual assessments of risk, coordination of nonprofessional services, and referrals and follow-up.

The village model is another community program that aids in successful aging in neighborhoods. An individual can join an existing village in their area or create their own village with neighbors. The prototype village is Beacon Hill in Boston. Beacon Hill is an independent, self-governing, not-for-profit organization run by volunteers and paid staff who coordinate access to affordable services for older adults in their communities. Services include transportation, health and wellness programs, home repair, social and education activities and trips, and discounts on goods and services.

Cohousing communities, a concept that originated in Denmark, are another growing option that older adults may find appealing. Most of the cohousing projects are intergenerational, but some also are designed specifically for individuals 50 years of age and older. Cohousing is a type of intentional, collaborative housing in which residents actively participate in the design and operation of their neighborhoods. Communities usually are designed as attached or single-family homes along one or more pedestrian streets or clustered around a central courtyard. There is a common house where residents can gather and share a common meal or socialize. Community members work together to care for the common property. In most cases, cohousing communities are started by prospective residents, who often partner with a developer to design and finance the project. Some are started by architects and developers who then organize a group of future residents to buy into the project.

Shared housing among adult children and their older relatives has become a choice for many because of cultural preferences or need. The sharing may relieve the economic burdens of maintaining a home after widowhood or retirement on a fixed income. Chapter 32 discusses multigenerational housing. Another model of shared housing is that of opening up one's personal home to others. Older adults often live in houses that were purchased in their young adult years and find that as they age, much of the space may be underused. Sharing a house can be easily implemented by locating, screening, and matching older adults looking for houses to share with those who have them. The National Shared Housing Resource Center has established subgroups nationally to assist individuals interested in home sharing.

As the baby boomers age, we can expect to see more innovative housing movements that create successful opportunities for healthy aging in the community and provide a range of options for older adults beyond what is available now. Box 21.1 presents some resources for aging in the community.

▮ KEY CONCEPTS

- Recognizing and analyzing cues to older adults' vulnerability during disasters and taking action to develop preventive and supportive responses to enhance safety are important nursing responsibilities
- Thermoregulatory changes, chronic illness, and medications may predispose the older adult to hypothermia and hyperthermia. Careful attention must be paid to temperature monitoring and provision of adequate heating and cooling in weather extremes.
- Older adults are often targets of crime and fraud.
- Reducing fire hazards is essential to feelings of security.
- Driving safety for older adults is an important issue, and health care professionals must be knowledgeable about assessment, safety interventions, and transportation resources.

- Technology advances hold promise for improving quality of life, decreasing the need for personal care assistance, and enhancing independence and the ability to live safely.
- Nurses can play essential roles in research to improve the design and use of mobile and connected health technologies and evaluate the effects on health outcomes and ability to age in place.
- Efforts to make communities more elder-friendly are underway across the globe. New and innovative ideas for aging in the community will continue to change living options for older adults.

NEXT-GENERATION NCLEX® (NGN) EXAMINATION–STYLE QUESTIONS

Mrs. Walters, an 82-year-old female, resides in a secure dementia unit. She has a history of peripheral vascular disease, hypertension, asthma, hypothyroidism, osteoarthritis, and vascular dementia. She is no longer ambulatory and spends most days sitting in her wheelchair in the atrium looking at the birds and flowers. She is 5′8″ and weighs 110 pounds (body mass index [BMI] 16.72). Her hemoglobin is 10.8 g/dL, hematocrit is 32%, albumin is 3.2 g/dL, blood urea nitrogen (BUN) is 26 mg/dL, creatinine is 1.5 mg/dL, and thyroid stimulating hormone (TSH) is 4.12 mU/L. Mrs. Walters' blood pressure is 145/86 mm Hg, pulse is 88 beats/minute, respirations are 16 breaths/minute, oral temperature is 97.3°F, and oxygen saturation is 95%. Her medications include aspirin 81 mg daily, valsartan 160 mg daily, levothyroxine 150 μg daily, acetaminophen 750 mg every 8 hours, and citalopram 20 mg daily.

Use an X to identify the nursing actions listed below that are Indicated, Contraindicated, or Non-Essential for the client's care at this time.

Intervention	Indicated	Contraindicated	Non-Essential
Monitor body temperature			
Keep environmental temperature at 65°F			
Cover with thick blanket when transporting to shower			
Allow hair to air-dry			
Provide high-protein meals and snacks			
Minimize exertion			
Drink 2 L fluid a day			

NURSING STUDY

Changing Life Situations and Environmental Vulnerability

Ethel had lived in one home for all of her married life, but when her husband died, her children worried about her safety, being alone in a big home. They feared she could fall and lie undiscovered to die of hypothermia. As well, the deteriorating neighborhood was no longer considered safe, and she could no longer drive and was limited in her ability to get around. They convinced her to move to a community in Phoenix near them.

They were able to find a suitable apartment that she could afford. For a while they visited her each week, but each visit became more depressing for them, as she continually talked about her old home, old friends, old furniture, old priest—everything old. Their visits became less frequent. She called them faithfully each morning but detected their urge to get off the phone and get on with their lives.

One morning she called her daughter Gladys and said, "I'm so sick! Yesterday I walked outside, and I swear I saw my friend Rose from the old neighborhood getting on the bus, but she didn't see me. I was so disappointed but managed to make it home, then couldn't find the key to my apartment so finally had to call 911 for help. They were really irritated with me when I said I had lost my key. I want to go back to Detroit. I know how things work there." After a family conclave, Ethel's children found a nice place in assisted living for Ethel and they were relieved. Ethel said, "I don't know where I am anymore. Seems I bounce around like a rubber ball." She seldom left her room except for meals, and soon she needed meals brought to her. Last week she wandered out and, when found, had suffered a serious case of heat stroke.

CLINICAL JUDGMENT QUESTIONS AND ACTIVITIES

Questions 1 and 2 refer to the Nursing Study.

1. What alternatives could you suggest to Ethel's family as they decide on the best living situation for her?
2. How could Ethel's family have involved her in the decision making about her living situations?
3. Locate low-cost housing in your area and assess it for convenience and safety.
4. What type of support does your community provide to assist older adults to safely age in place?
5. What crimes against older adults are of concern in your community?
6. What are your city's and state's plans for disaster preparedness for older adults living in the community or in institutions?
7. Compare your community to the characteristics of an elder-friendly community described in the chapter.
8. Survey the homes of older adults you are serving in your clinical practice for the presence or absence of safety features.

RESEARCH QUESTIONS

1. What criminal activities are of most concern to older adults?
2. What home safety factors are the most frequent causes of concern for older adults?
3. What are the most frequent causes of fires among older adults?
4. What do older adults fear most in their environment?
5. What is the impact of new "driver assist" features (e.g., warning systems, forward collision, lane departures) on reducing the number of accidents in older adults?
6. What are the most effective ways to therapeutically communicate concerns about unsafe driving and driving cessation to decrease emotional upset?
7. What are the barriers to the use of assistive technology in institutions and personal homes?

REFERENCES

Abbott R, Orr N, McGill P, et al.: How do "robopets" impact the health and well-being on residents in care homes? A systematic review of qualitative and quantitative evidence, *Int J Older People Nurs* 14(3):e12239, 2019.

American Red Cross & American Academy of Nursing: *Closing the gaps: advancing disaster preparedness, response and recovery for older adults* (website), 2020. https://www.redcross.org/content/dam/redcross/training-services/scientific-advisory-council/253901-03%20BRCR-Older%20Adults%20Whitepaper%20FINAL%201.23.2020.pdf.

Andruszkiewicz G, Fike K: Emerging technology trends and products: how tech innovations are easing the burden of family caregiving, *Generations* 39(4):64–68, 2015 –16.

Beuscher L, Fan J, Sarkar N, et al.: Socially assistive robots: measuring older adults' perceptions, *J Gerontol Nurs* 43(12):35–43, 2017.

Brody A, Sadarangani T, Jones T, et al.: Family-and-person centered interdisciplinary telehealth: policy and practice implications following onset of the COVID-19 pandemic, *J Gerontol Nurs* 46(9):9–12, 2020.

Chi N, Demiris G: The roles of telehealth tools in supporting family caregivers, *J Gerontol Nurs* 43(2):3–5, 2017.

Choi Y, Lazar A, Demiris G, et al.: Emerging smart home technologies to facilitate engaging with aging, *J Gerontol Nurs* 45(12):41–48, 2019.

Czaja SJ: Can technology empower older adults to manage their health?, *Generations J Am Soc Aging* 39(1):46–51, 2015.

Davis R, Ohman J: Driving in early-stage Alzheimer's disease: an integrative review of the literature, *Res Gerontol Nurs* 10(2):86–100, 2017.

Davis R, Owens M: Self-regulation of driving behaviors in persons with early-stage Alzheimer's disease, *J Gerontol Nurs* 47(1):21–26, 2021.

Edwards J, Lister J, Lin FR, et al.: Association of hearing impairment and subsequent driving mobility in older adults, *Gerontologist* 57(4):767–775, 2017.

Galuzzi K, Warner-Maron I: Guns and older adults: the physician's role, *J Am Osteopath Assoc* 118(12):775–780, 2018. doi:10.7556/jaoa.2018.169.

Gonyea J, Melekis K: Women's housing challenges in later life: the importance of a gender lens, *Generations J Am Soc Aging* 41(4):45–52, 2017 –18.

Graham J: *Clarity on COVID count: pandemic's toll on seniors extended well beyond nursing homes* (website), 2021. https://khn.org/news/article/covid-death-toll-seniors-new-research-beyond-nursing-homes-dementia-risk/. Accessed August 2021.

Hudson J, Ungar R, Albright L, et al.: Robotic pet use among community-dwelling older adults, *J Gerontol B Psychol Sci Soc Sci* 75(9):2018–2028, 2020.

Johns Hopkins Medicine: *What is hypothermia* (website), 2021. https://www.hopkinsmedicine.org/health/conditions-and-diseases/hypothermia#:~:text=Hypothermia%20is%20an%20abnormally%20low,to%20heart%20failure%20and%20death.

Johnston M: *Evaluating a virtual program of therapeutic interactive pets to improve behavioral and psychological symptoms and cognitive status among older adults experiencing Alzheimer's disease and related dementias*, Boca Raton, FL, 2020, Unpublished DNP project paper, Florida Atlantic University, Christine E. Lynn College of Nursing.

Kalicki A, Moody K, Franzosa E, et al.: Barriers to telehealth access among homebound older adults, *J Am Geriatric Soc* 69(9):2404–2411, 2021 https://doi.org/10.1111/jgs.17163.

Kivimaki T, Stolt M, Charalambous A, et al.: Safety of older people at home: an integrative literature review, *Int J Older People Nurs* 15(1):e12285, 2019. doi:10.1111/opn.12285.

Lach H: Home sweet home: resources for promoting mobility for aging in place across settings, *J Gerontol Nurs* 47(5):3–6, 2021.

Lach H, Noimontree W: Fall prevention among community-dwelling older adults: current guidelines and older adult responses, *J Gerontol Nurs* 44(9):21–29, 2018.

LaRose BS: *Improving behavioral and psychological symptoms and cognitive status of participants with dementia through the use of therapeutic interactive pets*, Boca Raton, FL, 2019, Unpublished DNP project paper Florida Atlantic University, Christine E. Lynn College of Nursing.

Liddle J, Gustafsson L, Mitchell F, et al.: A difficult journey: reflections on driving and driving cessation from a team of clinical researchers, *Gerontologist* 57(1):82–88, 2017.

Locsin R, Tanioka T, Yashura Y, et al.: Humanoid nurse robots as caring entities: a revolutionary probability?, *Int J Nurs Studies* 3(2):146, 2018.

Long-Term-Care COVID Tracker: *About 8% of people who live in US long-term-care facilities have died of COVID-19—nearly 1 in 12. For nursing homes alone, the figure is nearly 1 in 10* (website), 2021. https://covidtracking.com/nursing-homes-long-term-care-facilities. Accessed May 2021.

Malik S, Lee D, Doran K, et al.: Vulnerability of older adults in disasters: emergency department utilization by geriatric patients after Hurricane Sandy, *Disaster Med Public Health Prep* 12(2):184–193, 2018. doi:10.1017/dmp.2017.44.

Mallow J, Davis S, Herczyk J, et al.: Dose of telehealth to improve community-based care for adults living with multiple chronic conditions: a systematic review, *Scientific Research*, 2021 10(1) https://doi.org/10.4236/etsn.2021.101002.

McDermott-Levy R, Kolanowski A, Fick D, et al.: Addressing the health risks of climate change in older adults, *Our Gerontol Nurs* 45(11):21–29, 2019.

Miyagawa M, Yasuhara Y, Tanoika T, et al.: The optimization of humanoid robot's dialog in improving communication between humanoid robot and older adults, *Intelligent Control and Automation* 10(3):118–127, 2019.

Moran G: Nursing homes aren't equipped to provide life-saving A/C in the event of a power outage, *Popular Science*, July 30, 2020 https://www.popsci.com/story/environment/hurricanes-nursing-homes-power-heat/. Accessed May 2021.

Morgan E, Rowhani-Rahbar A: Firearm safety in an aging United States, *JAMA Netw Open*, 2020 3(7):e2011182.

Moyle W, Jones CJ, Murfield JE, et al.: Use of a robotic seal as a therapeutic tool to improve dementia symptoms: a cluster-randomized controlled trial, *J Am Med Dir Assoc* 18(9):766–773, 2017.

National Hispanic Council on Aging: *Home fire safety for older adults* (website), 2017. http://www.nhcoa.org/home-fire-safety-for-older-adults/. Accessed May 2021.

Novotney A: *Robotic pets helping to curb loneliness amid pandemic* (website), 2020. https://www.mcknights.com/print-news/robotic-pets-helping-to-curb-loneliness-amid-pandemic/. Accessed June 2021.

Pepito J, Locsin R: Constantino: caring for older persons in a technologically advanced nursing future, *Health* 11(5), 2019. https://m.scirp.org/papers/92368.

Roe C, Babulal G, Head D, et al.: Preclinical Alzheimer's disease and longitudinal driving decline, *Alzheimers Dement (NY)* 3(1):74–82, 2017.

Shih R, Acosta J, Chen E, et al.: *Improving disaster resilience among older adults*, Santa Monica, CA, 2018, Rand Corporation.

Skiba K: *How cybercriminals stole $1.8 billion from unsuspecting older Americans in 2020* (website), 2021. https://www.aarp.org/money/scams-fraud/info-2021/fbi-cybercrime-report.html.

Turjamaa R, Pehkonen A, Kangasniemi M: How smart homes are used to support older people: an integrative review, *Int J Older People Nurs* 14:e12260, 2019 https://doi.org/10.1111/opn.12260.

Wang J: Mobile and connected health technologies for older adults aging in place, *J Gerontol Nurs* 44(6):3–5, 2018.

Wetsman N: *Apple's new health features bring new focus to elder care technology* (website), 2021. https://newstral.com/en/article/en/1196132626/apple-s-new-health-features-bring-new-focus-to-elder-care-technology. Accessed June 2021.

Wiese L: Research highlights. In Touhy T, Jett K, editors: *Toward healthy aging*, ed 10, St Louis, 2020, Elsevier, pp 269–270.

Wiese LK, Wolff L: Supporting safety in the older adult driver: a public health nursing opportunity, *Public Health Nurs* 33(5):460–471, 2016.

World Health Organization (WHO): *Global network for age-friendly cities and communities, 2018* (website), 2018. https://extranet.who.int/agefriendlyworld/who-network/. Accessed May 2021.

Zmora R, Mitchell L, Finlay J, et al.: Dementia caregivers' experiences and reactions to remote activity monitoring system alerts, *J Gerontol Nurs* 47(1):13–19, 2021.

22 CHAPTER

Living Well With Chronic Illness

Kathleen Jett

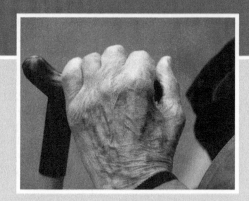

http://evolve.elsevier.com/Touhy/TwdHlthAging

AN OLDER ADULT SPEAKS

If I'd known I was going to live this long, I'd have taken better care of myself.

Eubie Blake, on his 100th birthday

A STUDENT SPEAKS

I thought that people just got sicker as they got older. I didn't realize that some level of health was possible even if one is chronically ill.

Nursing student, age 18

LEARNING OBJECTIVES

On completion of this chapter, the reader will be able to:
1. Identify the most common chronic disorders of late life.
2. Describe the concept of frailty and explain how it applies to chronic disease.
3. Recognize and analyze the cues that indicate that a person is at risk for frailty or has become frail.
4. Describe a conceptual model that may be useful for guiding the nurse in the development of solutions to promote healthy aging regardless of limitations in function.
5. Construct nursing solutions and actions that are consistent with the chronic illness trajectory.

Chronic illnesses are those that are persistent regardless of treatment. Their onset may be insidious and only recognized during a comprehensive health screening (Chapter 9). The most common chronic diseases in the United States are hypertension, heart disease, and cancer or diabetes, depending on ethnicity or race (Fig. 22.1) (Federal Interagency Forum on Aging Related Statistics, 2020). Heart disease, cancer, and diabetes have been the leading causes of death and disability and the leading drivers of health care cost in the United States. The top causes of death in low-income countries have been pneumonia, heart disease, diarrhea, HIV/AIDS, and stroke (World Health Organization [WHO], 2021b). The ranking of death due to COVID-19 in the United States ranged from first (January), to seventh (July), to third (November) during 2021 (Ortaliza et al., 2021).

Among persons at least age 65 without a subjective report of a cognitive impairment, 52.4% report no chronic disease, 35.8% at least one, 22% at least two, and 16.1% three or more comorbid

chronic conditions. Persons with subjective reports of some amount of cognitive impairment report many more chronic diseases: only 13.2% reported none, 29.9% report one, 24.9% report two, and 32% report at least three (Centers for Disease Control and Prevention [CDC], 2021). There are notable racial and ethnic differences in subjective reports of both cognitive decline and number of diagnosed chronic conditions (Table 22.1).

In a younger adult, the initial symptoms of a potential disease may be identified early enough to prevent chronicity. For example, when hypertension is recognized early, interventions can decrease the risk of later heart disease (Chapter 23). However, too often a disease may not be recognized in older adults until end-organ damage has already occurred. Diabetic retinopathy may be found during an annual eye exam, indicating that diabetes has been present long enough to have already caused permanent, irreversible damage.

When a diagnosis does not occur until late in the disease process, the solutions can only remediate and prevent further

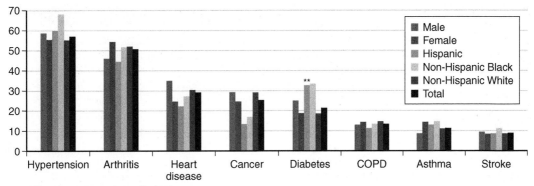

* Most recent data, released in 2020
** highly variable by country of origin

Fig. 22.1 Percentage of people age 65 and over who report having selected chronic health conditions, by sex, race, and Hispanic origin, 2018.* *COPD,* Chronic obstructive pulmonary disease. (From Federal Interagency Forum on Aging Related Statistics: *Older Americans 2020: key indicators of well-being. Indicator 16: chronic health conditions,* Washington, DC, 2020, US Government Printing Office, p 101.)

TABLE 22.1   Percentage of Adults at Least 45 Years Old, Subjective Report of Cognitive Decline and Chronic Disease

	SUBJECTIVE COGNITIVE DECLINE		WITHOUT SUBJECTIVE COGNITIVE DECLINE	
	No Chronic Disease	At Least One Chronic Disease	No Chronic Disease	At Least One Chronic Disease
Age				
45-64	22.6	77.4	59.9	47.1
65+	13.7	86.3	26.5	73.5
Sex				
Female 45+	16.2	83.8	40.1	59.9
Male	22.2	77.8	46.4	53.6
Race or ethnicity				
Non-Hispanic White	18.5	81.5	42.2	57.8
Non-Hispanic Black	13.6	86.4	39.9	60.1
American Indian and Alaskan Native	11.6	88.4	32.6	67.4
Asian and Pacific Islander	50.4	49.6	50.2	49.8
Hispanic, any race	23.8	76.2	50.6	49.4

From Centers for Disease Control and Prevention: *Chronic disease and cognitive decline—a public health issue* (website), 2020. https://www.cdc.gov/aging/publications/chronic-diseases-brief.html.

damage rather than provide a cure. The desired outcomes include minimizing complications, delaying the associated mortality, and optimizing health-related quality of life (Chapter 2). Desired outcomes are based on a balance of personal preferences, prognosis, interactions between conditions, and the feasibility of treatment and care (risk:benefit ratio) (Reuben et al., 2020).

The relationship between chronic disease, aging, and lifestyle is complex. Some chronic diseases occur so often in later life that they referred to as "age-related," but they are not normal parts of aging. We know now that many chronic diseases could be avoided through preventive strategies, especially when started at a young age. A number of risk factors are within control of the individual and, if eliminated, a significant amount of disease could be prevented (Box 22.1). Understanding which preventive solutions are the most effective is becoming clearer as the National Institutes of Health and the WHO provide leadership and investment in outcomes research.

For today's older adult with a preexisting chronic disease, the importance is its effect on function. The effect may be as little as an inconvenience or as great as an impairment of one's ability to live independently. When superimposed on the normal changes with aging, the likelihood of the person developing frailty and needing assistance in daily living increases over time.

BOX 22.1   Major Risk Factors for the Development of Chronic Disease

Tobacco use and exposure to secondhand smoke or pollutants
Poor nutrition
Physical inactivity
Excessive alcohol use
Obesity

Data from Centers for Disease Control and Prevention (CDC): *How you can prevent chronic diseases* (website), 2020. https://www.cdc.gov/chronicdisease/about/prevent/index.htm; CDC: *About chronic diseases* (website), 2021. https://www.cdc.gov/chronicdisease/about/index.htm.

TABLE 22.2   Chronic Illness Trajectory

Phase	Description
1. Pre-trajectory	Before the illness course occurs, the preventive phase, no symptoms are recognizable.
2. Trajectory onset	Initial cues to a chronic disease are present. Includes the diagnostic period.
3. Stable	Controlled illness course and symptoms. Stable disease.
4. Unstable	Illness course or symptoms not controlled by regimen but not requiring or desiring hospitalization. Cues suggesting deterioration can be recognized.
5. Acute	Active illness or complications that require hospitalization for management. Observation of cues indicates prompt response is necessary for the person to restabilize and survive.
6. Crisis	Life-threatening situation; acute threat to self-identity. If frail, death is nearing.
7. Comeback	A period of remission from the crisis. May be temporary. May not occur in those who are frail.
8. Downward	Progressive decline in physical or mental status characterized by increasing disability or symptoms. Very rapid deterioration in those who are frail.
9. Dying	Immediate hours, days, and weeks preceding death. Signs of death easily recognized.

As discussed in Chapter 2, the US Department of Health and Human Services (USDHHS, n.d.) puts forth and updates the document *Healthy People* regarding the health of the public. Solutions to achieve healthier outcomes have included increasing regular physical activity; reducing obesity; smoking cessation or avoidance; managing stress; and taking effective, safe, and appropriate medications. The WHO (2021a) has developed a global action plan identifying multiple targets and indicators that assist countries to set national goals and policies addressing the prevention and optimal management of chronic diseases. These cover a wide range of topics and are like many found in *Healthy People 2030*.

Any consideration of chronic disease in later life leads to multiple questions. Why do some persons develop many of the "chronic diseases of old age" and others do not? As the understanding of genomics develops, will the line between aging and chronic conditions become more blurred or clearer? We have learned that most lung diseases in late life are the result of life choices earlier in life, such as smoking, yet as one ages, susceptibility to pneumonia increases, even for the nonsmoker. With the introduction of antiretroviral therapy in the 1990s, persons with human immunodeficiency virus (HIV) are living longer than they ever had before. An HIV diagnosis no longer means imminent death; it has become another chronic disease. Some survivors of the COVID-19 infection have developed new chronic conditions, the duration of which is still unknown. How will this new "collection" of chronic diseases affect the morbidity and mortality of aging persons and society?

THE CHRONIC ILLNESS TRAJECTORY

Although there are many conceptual models from which chronic illness can be viewed, the trajectory model has long helped health care providers understand the realities of chronic illness and its effect on individuals (Corbin & Strauss, 1992; Lubkin & Larsen, 2012; Strauss & Glaser, 1975). Using this model, chronic illness is viewed from a life course perspective or along a trajectory—on a health and wellness continuum (Chapter 2).

The chronic illness trajectory (Table 22.2) represents nine phases along which a person moves up and down. These are (1) pre-trajectory, (2) trajectory onset, (3) stable, (4) unstable, (5) acute, (6) crisis, (7) comeback, (8) downward, and (9) dying. During the pre-trajectory phase (#1), preventive practices are used to prevent the development of a chronic disease to the extent possible; for example, eating a heart-healthy diet to prevent hypertension.

At the beginning of the trajectory phase (#2), early symptoms of illnesses are recognizable, but health outcomes still can be optimized. In the stable phase (#3), the chronic condition is present, and while not curable, it can be *controlled* so that few if any symptoms are recognizable complications are minimized, and a high quality of life can be maintained. This stability is due in large part to secondary prevention, including the receipt of high-quality medical care provided by nurse practitioners and high-quality nursing from the gerontological nurse and staff. For those with more complex chronic diseases, achieving the highest outcome possible requires coordination between members of the health care team, often with the nurse coordinating this care.

During periods of unstable disease exacerbations (#4), one or more of the dimensions that define the individual are compromised. In the aging adult this is a particularly precarious stage because the uncontrolled chronic disease is superimposed on reduced physiological reserve and other normal changes of aging (Chapter 3). In some cases, the chronic diseases lead to frailty, at which time further deterioration of health is likely. For those who are already frail, a previously controlled health condition can rapidly become acute or life-threatening. The nurse is instrumental in ensuring that prompt action is delivered in a manner that maximizes the chances that the person can return to the highest level of wellness possible. If care and action are delayed for those who are frail, it may not be possible to stop the overall downward trend.

In the acute phase (#5), severe and unrelieved symptoms associated with disease complications are present. Should this phase be reached, the nurse may be the one to inform the person and the family that a complete return to the trajectory phase

(#2) may not be possible, but every effort will be made to control any distressing symptoms and keep the person comfortable. For those who are very ill with multiple comorbidities, this phase may be bypassed, and the person may proceed directly from the unstable phase (#4) to the crisis phase (#6).

In the crisis phase (#6), major complications of a chronic disease become critical and life-threatening, such as an acute myocardial infarction (AMI) in a person with heart disease. The nurse provides or facilitates immediate emergency care but only to the point that was expressed by the person in an advance directive or by a health care proxy at the time of the event. Nurses caring for ill and frail patients need to know the content of their advance directives and understand their wishes in order to respond appropriately in a life-threatening situation.

Although less likely in frail older adults, the person may be able to restore equilibrium (#7) or a somewhat steady state for a period of time. The older one becomes, the more chronic diseases accumulate and the less likely the person will ever return to a period when cues of symptoms are not recognizable. This is important in conversations about resuscitative efforts in frail persons or those with multiple chronic conditions. The downward phase (#8) is that which ends in death (Lubkin & Larsen, 2012). During this phase the nurse has a significant opportunity, responsibility, and privilege to provide comfort at the end of life, to reassure those who are dying, to ensure that the dying patient continues to receive the highest quality of nursing and medical care possible, and to provide the patient's significant others with the support they may need (Chapter 34).

During acute exacerbations of chronic diseases, hospitalization may be necessary, followed by active rehabilitation at home or at designated rehabilitation centers or skilled nursing facilities found in high-income countries. Once the disease has stabilized, the person may return to full function or to partial function. If the limitations become chronic, physical, functional, or cognitive assistance will be needed. Informal help may be available with a move to the home of a friend or family member. Others may have the resources to hire the formal help of professional caregivers. Still others move to institutional settings such as assisted living facilities, nursing homes, or group homes. Unfortunately, options in the United States are dependent on personal financial resources; there are solutions for the very poor and the wealthy, but solutions are tenuous at best for near-poor and middle-income individuals and families.

The shape and stability of the trajectory are influenced by the combined efforts, attitudes, and beliefs held by the person, family members, and significant others. Gerontological nurses have the opportunity to promote healthy aging at any point on the trajectory. The person's perceptions of both needs met and functional limitations are paramount to predicting movement along the illness trajectory (Corbin & Strauss, 1992).

FRAILTY

The association between age, chronic disease, and the development of frailty remains unclear. However, there is an international consensus that the meaning of frailty is a multidimensional syndrome characterized by decreased reserves and diminished

---

BOX 22.2 Cues That Indicate the Frailty Phenotype

- Recorded unintentional weight loss of >5% or 10 pounds in the last year
- Self-report of exhaustion/fatigue (inability to walk several hundred yards or >3–4 week without exhaustion)
- Low activity level (<383 kcal/wk in men and <270 kcal/wk in women)
- Low grip strength (dynamometer): <18 kg in women and <30 kg in men; dominant hand, 3 tries
- Slow gait speed: inability to walk 6 meters in ≤ 30 seconds

  Analysis: Three of five cues recognized = Frail and further analysis is urgent; One or two cues are recognized = risk for frailty and preventive actions needed.

From Bond SM: The frail hospitalized older adult. In Boltz M, editor: *Evidence-based geriatric nursing protocols for best practice*, ed 6, New York, 2021, Springer, pp 563–576.

---

resistance to stressors. Evidence of the chronic inflammation of aging and poor metabolic repair are present (Chapter 3) (Bond, 2021). Frailty indicates an increased vulnerability to adverse outcomes, including the development of geriatric syndromes, hospitalization, postoperative complications, and death (see Chapter 9, Box 9.7). When any of the geriatric syndromes are present with frailty, the vulnerability to any challenge to physical, cognitive, or emotional health is significantly increased. Age-related decreases in reserve capacity are exacerbated, sometimes to the point that compensation is not possible. Once one is frail, preventive strategies for underlying chronic conditions are not likely to be effective (Pilotto et al., 2018).

The phenotype of frailty has been described by Fried et al. (2001) and includes distinct cues that can be recognized by direct observation or self-reported (Reuben et al., 2020) (Box 22.2). If all five cues are present and cannot be attributed to another cause, this is a billable International Classification of Diseases (ICD)–10 diagnosis code, R54 "age-related debility." In the past this was conceptualized as "failure to thrive." This model may not be applicable to hospitalized older adults due to impact of the acute illness or injury (Bond, 2021).

The Frailty Index for Elders (FIFE) was designed to identify cues that can be found in an existing dataset (such as the Minimum Data Set [MDS]; see Chapter 9). Ten cues are potentially recognized, and analysis is based on scoring: 0 = no frailty, 1 to 3 = risk for frailty, and 4+ = frailty. The FIFE has been found useful in the identification of those who are frail and as a means to track changes in condition (Tocchi, 2016).

An alternate model is that of cumulative deficits (Rockwood & Mitnitski, 2007). Frailty is defined in terms of recognizable signs coupled with abnormal laboratory results, specific disease states, disabilities, overall reduced homeostatic reserve, altered cognition, and mood. There are a number of these multidimensional indices; most are very long but have a greater ability to identify the cues associated with moderate and severe frailty (Bond, 2021; Tocchi, 2016).

The frailer one is, the faster one proceeds along the chronic illness trajectory, the less likely one can maintain or regain stability, and the greater the risk for death at any time one becomes unstable. Medical and social diagnoses leading to frailty may never be found (primary frailty). At other times frailty is related to the deterioration of a specific chronic disease (secondary frailty) consistent with the downward slope of the trajectory. Those with secondary frailty may have worse prognoses than those with primary frailty. Attention to increasing exercise tolerance, correcting protein-calorie malnutrition, reducing polypharmacy, and optimal management of underlying chronic diseases may have positive effects, but this is not yet known, especially with regard to the latter (Bond, 2021; Reuben et al., 2020).

The number of older adults recognized as frail varies widely from 4% to 60%, depending in part on how frailty is measured (Bond, 2021; Reuben et al., 2020). The rate increases with age, especially in women over 85 years of lower socioeconomic status. The number is expected to increase rapidly in the near future, consistent with the burgeoning population, especially those at least 80 years of age.

Working with older adults who are either frail or living with chronic illnesses means that the gerontological nurse has an opportunity to improve health outcomes and quality of life (Box 22.3). The next several chapters provide basic information on the most common chronic conditions the gerontological

---

BOX 22.3   Nurses' Role in Caring for Persons With Chronic Diseases

- Assessing the older person's and the family's strengths and challenges
- Teaching related to healthy lifestyle modifications, preservation of energy, and self-care strategies
- Encouraging the reduction of modifiable risk factors
- Counseling the individual in the development of reasonable expectations of self
- Providing access to resources when possible
- Referring appropriately and when needed
- Organizing and leading interdisciplinary case conferences and team meetings
- Facilitating advance care planning and palliative care when appropriate

---

nurse will encounter in persons as they age today and merit special attention. However, we neither cover all possible conditions nor provide a comprehensive medical management of these disorders. Solutions and actions will be proposed to promote healthy aging regardless of a person's place on the chronic illness trajectory.

KEY CONCEPTS

- The effects of chronic illness range from mild to life limiting, with each person responding to unique circumstances in a highly individualized manner.
- Coping with chronic illness is a physical, psychological, and spiritual challenge.
- The chronic illness trajectory is a useful framework to facilitate understanding changes in function and designing solutions and actions to promote healthy aging.
- The desired outcomes related to healthy aging include minimizing risk for disease and frailty and, in the presence of either, alleviating symptoms, delaying or avoiding the development of complications including end-organ damage, and maximizing function and quality of life. It also includes providing comfort to the dying.
- The gerontological nurse has the potential to serve as a leader in the promotion of health and the prevention of disease at all phases along the trajectory.

REFERENCES

Bond SM: The frail hospitalized older adult. In Boltz M, editor: *Evidence-based geriatric nursing protocols for best practice*, ed 6, New York, 2021, Springer, pp 563–576.

Centers for Disease Control and Prevention (CDC): *About chronic diseases* (website), 2021. https://www.cdc.gov/chronicdisease/about/index.htm.

Corbin JM, Strauss A: A nursing model for chronic illness management based upon the trajectory framework. In Woog P, editor: *The chronic illness framework: the Corbin and Strauss nursing model*, New York, 1992, Springer.

Federal Interagency Forum on Aging Related Statistics: *Older Americans 2020: key indicators of well-being*, Washington, DC, 2020, US Government Printing Office.

Fried LP, Tangen CM, Walston J, et al.: Frailty in older adults: evidence for a phenotype, *J Gerontol A Biol Sci Med Sci* 56(3):M146–M156, 2001.

Gundlapalli AV, Lavery AM, Boehmer TK, et al.: Death certificate–based ICD-10 diagnosis codes for COVID-19 mortality surveillance—United States, January–December 2020, *MMWR* 70(14):523–527, 2021.

Lubkin I, Larsen PD: *Chronic illness: impact and intervention*, ed 8, Burlington, MA, 2012, Jones & Bartlett.

Ortaliza J, Orgera K, Amin K, et al: *COVID-19 preventable mortality and leading cause of death ranking* (website),Dec 10, 2021, CO-VID-19 preventable mortality and leading cause of death ranking | KFF

Pilotto A, Daragjati J, Veronese N: CGA and clinical decision-making: the multidimensional prognostic index. In Pilotto A, Martin FC, editors: *Comprehensive geriatric assessment*, London, 2018, Springer, pp 79–92.

Reuben DB, Herr KA, Pacala JT, et al.: *Geriatrics at your fingertips*, ed 22, New York, 2020, American Geriatric Society.

Rockwood K, Mitnitski A: Frailty in relation to the accumulation of deficits, *J Gerontol A Biol Sci Med Sci* 62:722–727, 2007.

Strauss A, Glaser B: *Chronic illness and the quality of life*, St Louis, 1975, Mosby.

Tocchi C: *Try this: the Frailty Index for Elders (FIFE)* (website), 2016. https://hign.org/consultgeri/try-this-series/try-this-frailty-index-elders-fife.

US Department of Health and Human Services (USDHHS): *Healthy People 2030: building a healthier future for all* (website), n.d. https://health.gov/healthypeople.

World Health Organization (WHO): *Health promotion* (website), 2021a. https://www.who.int/health-topics/health-promotion#tab=tab_1.

World Health Organization (WHO): New study presents state of world's health (website), 2021b. https://www.who.int/news/item/27-10-2008-new-study-presents-state-of-the-world-s-health.

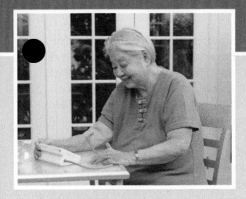

CHAPTER 23

Vascular Disorders

Kathleen Jett

http://evolve.elsevier.com/Touhy/TwdHlthAging

A STUDENT SPEAKS

I thought all hearts sounded the same, but after gaining a little more experience I started hearing all sorts of differences.

Helen, a 19-year-old nursing student

AN OLDER ADULT SPEAKS

I had always been very active and healthy, and then slowly I started feeling more and more tired. I just thought it was due to growing older but found out that my heart was no longer beating as it should.

Isabelle, age 86

LEARNING OBJECTIVES

On completion of this chapter, the reader will be able to:

1. Describe the cues suggestive of age-related changes in the vascular systems.
2. Identify the most common vascular disorders occurring in later life.
3. Describe how the signs and symptoms of vascular disorders in older adults differ from those recognized in younger adults.
4. Suggest solutions that promote healthy aging in the face of cardiovascular and cerebrovascular disease regardless of the stage of illness.

THE AGING CARDIOVASCULAR SYSTEM

The cardiovascular system, composed of the heart and blood vessels, is the vehicle through which oxygenated, nutrient-rich blood is transported throughout the body and metabolic waste is carried to the excretory organs. The association between cardiovascular functioning and morbidity, mortality, and longevity is well established. Blood pressure (BP), blood flow, and cardiac function must all be maintained within a homeostatic range for survival. Yet as the person ages, homeostatic maintenance becomes more difficult, and age alone is a major risk factor for cardiovascular illness independent of age, race, or ethnicity (Bilder, 2016).

The major change to the aging heart muscle is the progressive decline in cardiac reserve. It takes longer for the heart to accelerate to meet a sudden demand for oxygen and longer to return to its resting state. This has little effect on the day-to-day lives of healthy older adults but becomes quite significant when an increased cardiac response is needed due to a physical or mental challenge such as exercise, acute emotional distress, infection, fluid or blood loss, surgery, or hypoxia.

The resting heart rate decreases approximately 0.6 to 0.8 beats/min/year and cannot increase as easily in older adults compared to younger adults, and clinical recognition of a psychological or physiological crisis may be delayed. Even a person with a presumably healthy heart may not be able to maintain heart function during stress, and failure can occur quickly. In the presence of preexisting disease, this age-related change has the potential to increase both morbidity and mortality when it is not possible for the already damaged heart to suddenly work harder.

Lipid deposits and increases in collagen replace elastin, and cross-linking thickens and stiffens the valves separating the heart chambers, especially in women (Bilder, 2016). In some cases, the valves no longer close completely, allowing the blood to backflow, and a murmur can be recognized as a cue to the incompetent value. Murmurs are "graded" by sound intensity and documented as such (Table 23.1). In older adults, murmurs are most often heard in the aortic area and less so in pulmonic area. An occasional extra (ectopic) beat may be heard and is usually insignificant.

A *mild systolic murmur* (between S1 and S2) is an expected finding in the older adult. If the nurse auscultates a systolic murmur in an asymptomatic older adult, unlike a younger adult, most older adults will say, "I've had that for years." It is a medical emergency if it is a new finding and is accompanied by

Grade or Intensity	Description
I/VI	Barely audible
II/VI	Audible, soft
III/VI	Easily audible
IV/VI	Easily audible with a thrill
V/VI	Easily audible with a thrill, stethoscope lightly on chest
VI/VI	Easily audible with a thrill, stethoscope not on chest

TABLE 23.1   Grading the Intensity of Heart Murmurs

any signs or symptoms of cardiovascular distress. *Diastolic murmurs* (heard between S_2 and S_1) are always indicative of a serious problem in cardiac hemodynamics, and these persons should be followed closely by a cardiologist if possible. The gerontological nurse's ability to monitor this fragile condition is an essential skill.

Due to the high rate of heart disease in today's older population, the gerontological nurse must be alert to signs of rapid decompensation of both the well and the fragile older adult. The escalating potential of any heart disease as one ages increases the responsibility of the gerontological nurse to ensure that the person's wishes regarding resuscitation in such circumstances are known.

CARDIOVASCULAR DISEASE

By the time one is in later life, the lifestyle choices made earlier, coupled with age-related changes, influence the very high rate of cardiovascular disease (CVD). Both the prevalence and the incidence of CVD are so high that they are often mistaken as normal parts of aging and referred to as "disease of old age," but they do not have to be inevitable.

One in every four non-infectious deaths in the United States is related to heart disease; about 655,000 die each year, one person every 36 seconds. Research has found that the risk factors for overall CVD are universal. They include those that the person cannot control, those in full control of the person, and those suspected to have an influence (Table 23.2). Smoking, exposure to smoke, and uncontrolled hypertension are particularly important risk factors for all CVDs (Centers for Disease Control and Prevention [CDC], 2021a).

TABLE 23.2   Risk Factors for Cardiovascular Disease

Unmodifiable	Treatable	Modifiable
Age	Diabetes	Smoking
Male	Elevated blood	Overweight and obesity
Family history and	pressure	Unhealthy diet
genetics	Hyperlipidemia	Physical inactivity
Race	Sleep apnea	Substance misuse: alcohol, cocaine
		Excess stress

The most serious complication of CVD is an acute myocardial infarction (AMI) from a sudden occlusion of an artery by a blood clot or plaque. As blood attempts to pass through a narrowed vessel, either acute or long-term cardiac anoxia occurs. An AMI may be triggered anytime there is a sudden need for myocardial oxygen and the aging heart cannot respond adequately.

A definitive diagnosis of an AMI requires the documentation of changes in biochemical markers within 24 to 72 hours of the event (Baik & Dhruva, 2021) (Chapter 10). In many cases, lifesaving measures can be initiated if they are consistent with the person's expressed or preexpressed wishes.

The most common CVD seen in older adults—hypertension (HTN), chronic heart disease (CHD), heart failure (HF), and atrial fibrillation (AF)—are summarized in this chapter. For more detailed examinations of these conditions, the reader is referred to geriatric medicine and nursing texts that are disease based.

Hypertension

Hypertension (HTN) is the most common chronic disease encountered by the gerontological nurse. It significantly increases one's risk for heart disease, stroke, and death, yet only 1 in 4 persons has it under control. Men have HTN slightly more often than women (47% vs 43%), and the rate increases with age; up to 75% in those at least 75 years old have HTN, with prevalence varying by race (CDC, 2021b; Saxena et al., 2021) (Fig. 23.1). The most common pattern for older adults is referred to as "isolated systolic HTN" when only the systolic pressure is elevated (Aronow, 2017). Most persons over 65 years of age have or will develop HTN, but half of these are among those whose BP is not controlled (Kulkarni et al., 2017).

The normal changes in the aging arterial system (thickening, increased inflammation) coupled with lifelong habits (e.g., smoking) are the factors most likely to account for the increased incidence of HTN with aging. If the exact cause of HTN cannot

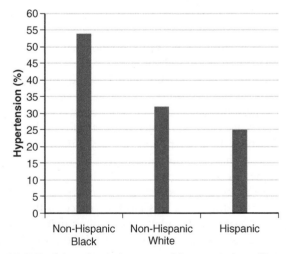

Fig. 23.1 Racial and ethnic rates of hypertension. (From National Heart, Lung, and Blood Institute: *High blood pressure* (website), 2020. https://www.nhlbi.nih.gov/health-topics/high-blood-pressure.)

HEALTHY PEOPLE 2030

Hypertension

- Goal: Increase the proportion of adults with hypertension whose blood pressure is under control
- Baseline: 47.8% of adults at least 18 years old with hypertension had it under control 2013–2016.
- Target: 60.8%

From Office of Disease Prevention and Health Promotion: *Increase control of high blood pressure in adults* (website), 2020. https://health.gov/healthypeople/objectives-and-data/browse-objectives/heart-disease-and-stroke/increase-control-high-blood-pressure-adults-hds-05.

be determined, it is referred to as primary. Secondary HTN can result from several conditions, including chronic kidney disease and obstructive sleep apnea, or medications such as nonsteroidal antiinflammatories, decongestants, caffeine, some supplements (e.g., saw palmetto, St. John's wort), and nicotine (Saxena et al., 2021).

Recognizing and Analyzing Cues

Most older adults with HTN do not have recognizable cues, and a diagnosis is not made until the BP is found to be elevated during a routine health screening or when end-organ damage has already occurred (Table 23.3). It is recommended that all adults at least 40 years of age are screened for HTN at least once a year. Consideration of more frequent screenings should be made for those at higher risk (i.e., smokers, those who are obese, and those of African American descent) (US Prevention Services Task Force [USPSTF], 2021).

Some people report dizziness, headache, "bad blood," light-headedness, a "swimmy head," or a "full head." When any of these subjective reports are made, the nurse asks if an elevated or lowered BP is suspected. Upon BP measurement, the person may be normotensive, hypotensive, or hypertensive.

The recognition of any cardiac risk factors will inform potential solutions, including information about the recognition and

prevention of adverse events through lifestyle changes. A diagnosis of HTN cannot be made unless elevations are found on at least two separate occasions; more than two readings may be necessary in older adults due to the variability of age-related vasculature stiffening.

Tips for Best Practice

Measures should be made only after 5 minutes of rest, in both arms, both sitting and standing, and with the correctly sized cuff at heart level. The highest reading is used and documented. If the readings are more than 10 mm Hg different, this is a cue to additional underlying cardiovascular problems.

Older adults already will know if they have "white coat effect," wherein an office reading is elevated but normal when done outside of the clinical setting. It is recommended that ambulatory blood pressure monitoring (ABPM) or home blood pressure monitoring (HBPM) be used to confirm a diagnosis of hypertension (USPSTF, 2021). Home monitoring also may identify "masked hypertension," wherein the readings are normal in the office but otherwise high. When untreated, the risk for an adverse cardiovascular event such as an AMI or stroke is high (Saxena et al., 2021). ABPM is recommended for both diagnosis and decision making about medication use and dosage changes. Frail elders are more likely to show a greater variability in readings, and multiple readings are required. It is very important that any home device used is reliable and the person's technique is accurate (Box 23.1). Routine laboratory testing and an electrocardiogram (ECG) are done to establish baseline information, including the presence or absence of other CVD and end-organ damage (Box 23.2).

Both the definition of and the overall guidelines for treatment of HTN are provided through the collaborative efforts of

BOX 23.1 Tips for Best Practice

Evaluation of Ambulatory Home Blood Pressure Monitoring

- Observe the technique that the person uses in the measurement of blood pressure (BP) using a personal home device.
- Duplicate the measurement using the same device but with the nurse conducting the measurement.
- Measure the BP using either a reliable and tested automated BP cuff or a cuff and a stethoscope.
- If there is a discrepancy, even with a person using good technique, counsel the person regarding the replacement of the home device.

TABLE 23.3 Looking for Signs of End-Organ Damage From Hypertension

Physical	Laboratory Abnormalities	Electrocardiogram
Ophthalmological vascular changes	CBC	Evidence of past AMI
Carotid bruits	CMP	Cardiac arrhythmia
Distended neck veins	Lipid panel	
Third or fourth heart sound	TSH	
Pulmonary rales	Urinalysis	
Reduced peripheral pulses		
Cardiac arrhythmia		
Cognitive impairment		

AMI, Acute myocardial infarction; *CBC,* complete blood count; *CMP,* comprehensive metabolic panel; *TSH,* thyroid-stimulating hormone.

BOX 23.2 Routine Laboratory Tests in the Evaluation of Elevated Blood Pressure

Complete blood count
Urinanalysis
Complete metabolic panel (includes electrolytes and creatinine)
Hemoglobin A_{1c}
Lipid panel
Thyroid panel

BOX 23.3   Blood Pressure Levels

Normotensive (<120/80)
  Elevated (SBP 120–129 mm Hg and DBP <80 mm Hg)
  Stage 1 hypertension (SBP 130–139 mm Hg or DBP 80–89 mm Hg)
  Stage 2 hypertension (SBP ≥140 mm Hg or DBP ≥90 mm Hg)

DBP, Diastolic blood pressure; *SBP*, systolic blood pressure.
From American Heart Association: *Understanding blood pressure readings* (website), 2021. https://www.heart.org/en/health-topics/high-blood-pressure/understanding-blood-pressure-readings.

BOX 23.4   Prohibitive Medication Expense

Ms. Snyder was a newly retired 67-year-old nurse. Her retirement income was adequate to meet her basic needs. When she was diagnosed with hypertension, her health care provider gave her samples of the beta blocker Bystolic to try. It worked well with no notable side effects, but to continue using it would increase her monthly drug costs by $125, almost 100%, which she felt was prohibitive in the long run.

SAFETY TIP

The angiotensin-converting enzyme inhibitors and the angiotensin II receptor blockers are both potassium-sparing medications and cannot be used together or with a potassium supplement or high-potassium foods due to the risk of hyperkalemia (Chapter 10).

---

the American College of Cardiology (ACC) and the American Heart Association (Box 23.3). The guidelines were last updated in 2020 with the recommendation that the BP goal for most older adults at least 65 years of age is lower than 130/80 mm Hg. However, the final report of the SPRINT research trial included data indicating that those at increased risk for CVD who maintained a systolic BP lower than 120 had significantly fewer AMIs, strokes, heart failures, or deaths from cardiac causes than those with the previously recommended goal of systolic BP lower than 140 (SPRINT Research Group, 2021). Both the ACC and its European counterpart advise cautious treatment and close monitoring, especially in those over 80 years of age. Treatment goal decisions are individually determined based on a combination of clinical judgment, patient preference, and life expectancy, especially in those with multiple comorbidities (Agarwala et al., 2020).

Pharmacological Interventions

Pharmacological interventions are often necessary to reach an acceptable BP in older adults. The decision is based on the level of HTN and a calculated 10-year risk of developing atherosclerotic CVD (http://tools.acc.org/ASCVD-Risk-Estimator-Plus/#!/calculate/estimate/). Other considerations are the status of concurrent diseases, the risk of polypharmacy, side effect profile, and cost or insurance coverage. It is not uncommon that several different types of antihypertensives are tried or needed to obtain control, and the costs can become prohibitive (Box 23.4).

The current guidelines recommend angiotensin-converting enzyme (ACE) inhibitors, angiotensin II receptor blockers (ARBs), calcium channel blockers (CCBs), or thiazide diuretics as first-line therapy due to the evidence that they all can potentially prevent heart disease. As the goals to BP control are individualized, so is the choice of pharmacological therapy. The first-line agent for some Black older adults or those who are salt sensitive with uncomplicated HTN is a diuretic or a CCB, as these appear to be most effective for them.

CCBs have been found useful and safe in older adults, especially the newer class of dihydropyridines (e.g., amlodipine) (Reuben et al., 2020). However, these have been associated with ankle edema, flushing, headache, and gingival hypertrophy. CCBs are heterogeneous as a group, and the risks and benefits of one are not the same as with another. Bradycardia can occur, and the nurse must take the person's pulse before administering a CCB. Older adults in the community must be taught how to do this reliably and what to do with the result.

Beta blockers are frequently prescribed to older adults when heart disease is already present. Potential side effects include fatigue, elevation in blood sugar in diabetics, and impotence. The nurse must watch for bradycardia with this group of medications.

Although no longer considered first-line therapy, many older adults take furosemide (Lasix) when the first-line medications alone are not adequate. This and other loop diuretics are potassium wasting, so they must be given either with a potassium-sparing medication such as an ACE inhibitor or ARB or with a potassium supplement.

A prescribing provider, such as a nurse practitioner, should do everything possible to minimize the number of medications taken by older adults and to keep the regimen as simple as possible (e.g., once-daily dosing) (Chapter 11). Due to the high risk for treatment-related orthostatic hypotension and related falls, initially the lowest dose is prescribed and the gerontological nurse checks the person's BP frequently to assess for medication side effects and the need for a dose adjustment. By reducing or eliminating modifiable risk factors, HTN often can be controlled or prevented, leading to healthier aging (see Table 23.1).

There is now good evidence that older adults who can maintain a blood pressure lower than 130/80 mm Hg will have the best outcomes (i.e., fewer AMIs, strokes, episodes of heart failure, and deaths). Improving outcomes also will reduce the risk for vascular dementia and the development of or worsening of renal insufficiency. At the same time, excessive lowering (<110/60 mm Hg) has been associated with higher mortality (Saxena et al., 2021).

Coronary Heart Disease

Although not a normal change of aging, the incidence of coronary heart disease (CHD) (most often of arterial origin or CAD) rises significantly with age and is the most common form of heart disease. It is caused by stiffening of the vessels, narrowing of the lumen, and increased inflammation in the coronary arteries through a process called atherosclerosis. Blood vessels become partially or completely blocked by plaques of cholesterol and other products that adhere to the vessel walls. Once this occurs, the heart is deprived of oxygen and nutrients and ischemia results, leading to tissue death. When risk factors are present (Table 23.2), the changes in the blood vessels occur earlier.

Heart disease, specifically an AMI, is the primary cause of noncommunicable mortality for older men from all racial and ethnic groups and White women over 65 years of age in the United States. For women who are from the Pacific Islands, Asian American, American Indian, Alaskan Native, or Hispanic, heart disease is second to cancer (2017 data) (CDC, 2021a). However, an excess number of deaths from cardiac arrests were seen during the COVID-19 pandemic (Baldi et al., 2020).

A noninvasive diagnostic measure such as a stress test and laboratory tests for cardiac serum markers are necessary for diagnosis (Chapter 10). Invasive tests such as a cardiac catheterization are not always appropriate, especially for those who are very frail or have limited life expectancies, or when the priority is optimizing quality rather than length of life (Chapter 34).

Recognizing and Analyzing Cues

In older adults, the first cue to CHD may be an AMI or death. One in five of these AMIs in older adults are referred to as "silent MIs." They are asymptomatic and only discovered when a resting ECG is done during the evaluation of another problem (CDC, 2021a). The classic cues recognized in younger adults, such as sudden, gripping chest pain with radiation to arm and chin, may not be present in older adults, or the signs may be completely atypical, such as an unexplained fall or a sudden change in mental status (Table 23.4).

Angina (chest pain) from ischemia in later life is usually less severe, shorter in duration, and described as postprandial epigastric pain, or as pain in the back or shoulders rather than the jaw or chest (Aronow, 2017). These symptoms may be misdiagnosed as arthritis, muscular back pain, or reflux. However, cues that they are anginal include worsening over time; increasing in frequency, intensity, or duration; and occurring with less and less provocation (i.e., unstable angina). Unstable angina is associated with arrhythmias, tachycardia, and ventricular fibrillation. Cues of worsening of CHD are identical to those symptoms that are seen in many other chronic diseases common in late life, making analysis and prioritization difficult.

TABLE 23.4   Key Differences in the Cues of Cardiac-Related Chest Pain, Classic/Younger and Atypical/Older Adults

Cue	Classic/ Younger	Atypical/Older Adult
Chest pain	Present	Absent
Radiations of pain to arm or jaw	Often present	Absent
Sweating	Often present	Absent
Dyspnea	Often present	May be only symptom
Fatigue	Often present	May be only symptom

Adapted from Taffet GF: Coronary artery disease and atrial fibrillation. In Ham RJ, Sloane PD, Warshaw GA, et al, editors: *Primary care geriatrics: a case-based approach*, Philadelphia, 2014, Elsevier, pp 395–405.

If the person's heart is markedly enlarged, pulsations may be visible and there will be a left shift of the point of maximum impact. Although assessment for jugular venous pressure is standard in a complete assessment, this is not always possible or appropriate in the older adult due to difficulty in assuming the needed recumbent position and to changes of the neck tissue that lead to inaccurate readings.

Tips for Best Practice

Veterans with ischemic heart disease that served in and around Korea, Vietnam, or at several bases in the United States may be eligible for disability related to Agent Orange exposure.

From US Department of Veterans Affairs: *Agent Orange exposure and VA disability compensation* (website), 2021. https://www.va.gov/disability/eligibility/hazardous-materials-exposure/agent-orange/

Pharmacological Interventions

Pharmacological interventions will always be necessary and used in conjunction with nonpharmacological solutions. Medications include a combination of aspirin, clopidogrel (Plavix), and nitrates (isosorbide). The antihypertensive agents in the beta blockers (e.g., metoprolol, atenolol) and ACE inhibitor groups have been found to prolong life after an AMI. Nondihydropyridines CCBs (e.g., verapamil, diltiazem) only can be used with caution due to the risk for worsening of systolic dysfunction with them (Reuben et al., 2020). During an ischemic event, additional treatment is needed, usually sublingual or aerosol nitroglycerin.

Atrial Fibrillation

Atrial fibrillation (AF) is the most common type of cardiac dysrhythmia in late life. The pulse is rapid and irregular when disorganized electrical impulses from the atrioventricular (AV) node are sent to the atria. As a result, blood pools in the atria, leading to a heightened risk of blood clot formation. The condition is not fatal, but left untreated, AF is associated with cognitive impairment; increased mortality, especially from strokes and HF; or sudden death from tachycardia-induced heart damage (National Heart, Lung, and Blood Institute [NHLBI], n.d. a). An estimated 12.1 million Americans are expected to have a diagnosis of AF by 2030. While it may occur in younger adults, it is found most often in older White men, with the incidence increasing each decade until it affects approximately 10% of those over 80 years of age (CDC, 2021c; Nguyen et al., 2021).

Although HTN is the most important of the risk factors, AF also may be the end result of multiple conditions and disorders. These include obesity; diabetes; sleep apnea; hyperthyroidism; acute or chronic pulmonary disease; chronic renal disease; heavy alcohol use; several cardiomyopathies, including CHD; HF; and valvular abnormalities (NHLBI, n.d. a). AF may be associated with worsening HF or end-stage renal disease. Prevention or appropriate treatment of any of these will reduce the risk for the development or worsening of AF (Sudharshan et al., 2021).

BOX 23.5   Sometimes I Can Feel the Palpitations

Ruth is a 75-year-old active and energetic woman with paroxysmal atrial fibrillation. Because of this condition, she takes anticoagulants—that is, she takes medication to prevent her blood from clotting to decrease her risk of having a stroke. Most of the time Ruth's heart beats regularly, and at other times it does not. When it does not, she has a sense of "chest palpitations" but they have never given her "problems." One day Ruth's heart seemed to be beating much more than usual. She checked it, and it was at least 180 beats per minute, it was highly irregular, and she was not feeling well. She called for an ambulance and was taken immediately to the hospital, where she was stabilized and then sent home.

Recognizing and Analyzing Cues

In many cases AF itself is completely asymptomatic, and cues are recognized only at the time of a stroke or by the nurse or other practitioner as part of a thorough auscultation of the heart. The pulse may be irregularly irregular (IRIR) or regularly irregularly (RIR) and documented as such.

If symptoms are reported, they are vague, such as fatigue, recurrent falls, episodes of syncope, and "dizzy spells," and mistakenly attributed to "old age" or the onset of frailty. Since other underlying chronic diseases are always present, the diagnosis of AF may be elusive. When it is finally recognized, the pulse rate is rapid and the rhythm is irregular. The irregularity may have a pattern or be completely random (paroxysmal); it may be acute and occur only once (lasting <48 hours), intermittent, or persistent. Occasionally people report the sensation of "palpations" and intermittent shortness of breath or nonspecific chest pain, especially if the fibrillation is paroxysmal (Box 23.5). An ECG or a 24-hour Holter monitor may confirm persistent AF but may miss that which is intermittent. Measurement of serum electrolytes and thyroid function are done to rule out a reversible cause.

Pharmacological Interventions

Sometimes AF resolves on its own. A normal heart rhythm may be restored by AV node radiofrequency ablation or mechanical or medication cardioversion in younger adults but less often in older adults. It also may resolve when the underlying cause is treated successfully. However, when it becomes persistent, pharmacological interventions are required to treat the irregularity, slow the pulse rate, reduce the risk of complications, and promote comfort. Beta blockers are the drugs of choice for rate control, but bradycardia is a potential side effect. For those who are otherwise asymptomatic and have a normal ejection fraction, the target resting pulse is less than 110 bpm and less than 80 bpm for those who are symptomatic or have a reduced ejection fraction. Amiodarone is used to restore a normal rhythm but interacts with several other medications (including warfarin) and has several serious side effects. Rhythm control will reduce symptoms but does not reduce mortality or incidence of stroke.

Decisions about the use of antithrombotic agents is individualized to balance reduced stroke risk with increased risk

TABLE 23.5 CHA_2DS_2-VASc Instrument to Determine Risk for Stroke

Score	0	1	$\geq 2^a$
1 point each for HF, HTN, DM, vascular disease, age ≥ 65, female			
2 points for age ≥ 75, history of stroke	ASA or no treatment	ASA, no treatment, or anticoagulant	Anticoagulant

[a]AHA and ACC recommend anticoagulation for score ≥ 1 in men and ≥ 2 in women and for all persons age ≥ 75 with AF.
ACC, American College of Cardiology; *AF,* atrial fibrillation; *AHA,* American Heart Association; *ASA,* acetylsalicylic acid; *DM,* diabetes mellitus; *HF,* heart failure; *HTN,* hypertension.

TABLE 23.6   HAS-BLED Instrument to Determine Risk for Bleeding With Anticoagulant Therapy

Score	Analysis
1 point for each HTN, abnormal renal function, abnormal liver function, prior stroke, prior major bleed, labile INR, age ≥ 65, alcohol use, drug use	If CHA_2DS_2-VASc score is 1 and HAS-BLED score is ≥ 2, risk of bleeding may outweigh the risk of stroke. If CHA_2DS_2-VASc is ≥ 2 and HAS-BLED exceeds the score, the risk of bleeding may outweigh the risk of stroke.

HTN, Hypertension; *INR,* international normalized ratio.

for bleeding. Instruments to assist in this determination are the CHA_2DS_2-VASc tool for determining stroke risk (Table 23.5) and the HAS-BLED for bleeding risk (Table 23.6) (Li et al., 2018). Although warfarin has been the gold standard for anticoagulation in older adults, the newer direct-acting anticoagulant (DOAC) dabigatran (Pradaxa) and the factor Xa inhibitors (e.g., Xarelto, Eliquis) are now recommended for use in most persons with AF and nonvalvular heart disease. They have been found to have lower rates of all-cause mortality, stroke, and bleeding. They have fewer drug-drug and drug-food interactions than warfarin but may be cost prohibitive. Warfarin must be used for persons with an artificial heart valve (Kumbhani et al., 2020).

Warfarin has a very narrow therapeutic window and must be monitored closely to ensure that the anticoagulation level is within an appropriate range (via international normalized ratio [INR]) (Chapter 10). There is a heightened risk of bleeding. Vitamin K is the antidote and can quickly inactivate the effects of warfarin. Warfarin interacts with most antibiotics and many dietary supplements and herbal products (Chapter 9); when these are taken, even closer monitoring is necessary, and temporary reductions in the dose of warfarin may be necessary.

The DOACs and factor Xa inhibitors do not require monitoring, and there is less risk for bleeding (Sudharshan et al., 2021). Several reversal agents have been developed or are in development but must be administered in an emergency department. A person who is taking any of the DOACs should be directed to promptly seek emergency support with any obvious bleeding or the potential of bleeding (e.g., following a fall) (Cuker et al., 2019).

For those at high risk for a traumatic injury or at low risk for a stroke or when anticoagulants are not tolerated, aspirin and/or clopidogrel may be used for persons under 75 years of age. This combination has not been found to be effective in persons over 75 years of age (Reuben et al., 2020). Those with persistent AF are at a high risk for stroke, and lifelong anticoagulation therapy remains the gold standard.

Heart Failure

Heart failure (HF) is the loss of the ability of the cardiac muscle to pump enough blood to support the organs in the body (CDC, 2020). Age-related decreases in cardiac reserve combined with heart damage causes ventricles to enlarge, dilate, and weaken. They may not be able to relax enough to fill adequately (right-sided failure) or pump strongly enough to empty fully (left-sided failure), or both. Failure can occur quickly, often within the first few hours or days after the damage from an AMI, or more slowly when associated with long-standing diseases, especially HTN, diabetes, and obesity.

About 6 million people in the United States have HF at any one time, 60% of whom are at least 65 years old. It is the most common cause of hospitalization for those receiving Medicare (Chapter 5). The incidence and prevalence increase dramatically with age and the accumulation of chronic diseases. It occurs most often in men, but the prevalence is slightly greater in women primarily because their prognoses are better and therefore they live longer with the disease.

Although a tentative medical diagnosis is often made empirically (based on signs and symptoms), several other tests and measurements are done to support or refute the gross observations (Box 23.6). Measurement of brain natriuretic peptide (BNP) and N-terminal pro-B-type natriuretic peptide (NT-proBNP) are potentially useful in differentiating shortness of breath due to HF from that caused by other conditions such as pneumonia or chronic pulmonary disease (Sudharshan et al., 2021). An echocardiogram is necessary to determine the extent of heart damage as demonstrated by the ejection fraction (EF)—that is, the percentage of blood that leaves the ventricle with each pulsation.

In diastolic dysfunction, the EF is less than 40% (HFrEF) and persons are always symptomatic, may be very ill, and have limitations in both function and day-to-day quality of life. The typical illness trajectory is one of steady decline. The overall prognosis is very poor, with a 5-year survival rate of about 25% in those over 65 years of age and a median survival of less than 2 years for those over 85 years of age (Sudharshan et al., 2021).

Those with preserved EF (>40%; HFpEF) have systolic disease and initially will have asymptomatic periods or periods with few or mild symptoms, interspersed with acute exacerbations often leading to hospitalization for stabilization. However, the heart damage will progress over time, symptoms will increase, function will decline as EF is lost, and ultimately only palliative care will be possible.

Recognizing and Analyzing Cues

The recognition of HF may appear straightforward in persons with signs of severe cardiac damage, especially dyspnea on exertion or edema of the ankles and lower legs, but be more difficult in older adults with less severe disease. Like most of the chronic diseases in later life, HF may become evident only when there is a need for the heart to increase its pumping capacity such as during exertion or following blood loss (including repeated venipucture). If the signs or symptoms are atypical, they may be mistakenly attributed to another condition (Box 23.7).

The classic sign of left-sided heart failure is dyspnea on exertion. Other cues include orthopnea, coughing, and paroxysmal nocturnal dyspnea. Dyspnea at rest eventually will develop. The classic sign of right-sided failure is edema. It is not uncommon to have both sides affected at the same time in older adults.

Many people will rationalize declining function without realizing it. For example, persons slowly reduce their activity level, saying they are "not so fit anymore" or "just a little more tired" or "not putting my feet up enough," which they attribute to "old age." It is much more likely that these are signs of HF (Box 23.8). People with HFrEF have breathlessness, fatigue, disordered sleep, and dependent edema. Changes in edema are recognized by changes in weight.

As the EF drops, the pulse pressure narrows, and signs of impaired tissue perfusion develop, such as cool skin and central or peripheral cyanosis. Diminished cognition, perhaps to the point of delirium, is common. An episode of syncope, ventricular

---

BOX 23.6 Routine Initial Assessment Components When Heart Failure Is Suspected

Orthostatic BPs
Height/weight measurements with BMI calculation
Chest Xray
Functional Status
Laboratory: CBC, UA, electrolytes, magnesium, Creatinine, BUN, Lipid panel, Fasting glucose, Liver function, Thyroid Panel, BNP, NT-pro BNP

BMI, Body mass index; *BNP*, brain natriuretic peptide; *BP*, blood pressure; *BUN*, blood urea nitrogen; *CBC*, complete blood count; *NT-pro BNP*, N-terminal pro-B-type natriuretic peptide; *UA*, urinalysis.

From Reuben DB, Herr KA, Pacala JT, et al: *Geriatrics at your fingertips*, ed 22, New York, 2020, American Geriatrics Society.

BOX 23.7 Other Conditions Common in Later Life That May Mask the Cues of Heart Failure

Pulmonary disease[a]
Obstructive sleep apnea[a]
Obesity[a]
Anemia[a]
Hypoithroidism[a]
Depression[a]
Poor physical conditioning[a]
Venous insufficiency[b]
Renal or hepatic disease[b]
Protein or calorie malnutrition[b]
Medications (especially calcium channel blockers)[b]

[a]Especially dyspnea, [b]Especially edema

BOX 23.8   Classic and Atypical Signs of Heart Failure in Older Adults

Classic	Atypical	Atypical (Cerebral)
Dyspnea	Chronic cough	Falls
Orthopnea	Insomnia	Anorexia
Paroxysmal nocturnal dyspnea	Weight loss/anorexia	Behavioral disturbances/irritability
Peripheral edema	Abdominal discomfort/nausea	Decreased functional status
Unexplained weight gain	Nocturia	Confusion/delirium
Weakness	Syncope	
Poor exercise tolerance	Cool/clammy skin	
Abdominal pain		
Fatigue/lethargy		

From Sudharshan S, Sandvall B, Rich MW: Heart failure and rhythm disorders. In Walter LC, Chang A, editors: *CURRENT diagnosis and treatment: geriatrics*, ed 3, New York, 2021, McGraw Hill, pp 303–316.

TABLE 23.7   Standard Medications Used to Treat Heart Failure With Nursing Actions

Systolic Heart Failure	Potential Effects	Nursing Actions
ACE inhibitors and ARBs	Improved QOL, fewer symptoms and hospitalizations	Watch for worsening of renal function, hyperkalemia, hypotension, cough. Monitor renal function and BP
Beta blockers	Reduced mortality and hospitalizations	Teach to monitor resting heart rate (<45 bpm), cues to hypotension (<SBP), bronchospasm
Spironolactone	Reduces mortality up to 30% (when EF ≤35%)	Monitor renal function, cues to gynecomastia
Diuretics	Not recommended except for relief of congestion and edema, maintain euvolemia	Teaching regarding daily weight (report >3 pound/day), sodium and fluid intake control, monitor electrolytes
Nitrates	Promote diuresis and lower BP	Watch for hypotension and unexplained falling

ACE, Angiotensin-converting enzyme; *ARB,* angiotensin II receptor blocker; *BP,* blood pressure; *EF,* ejection fraction; *QOL,* quality of life; *SBP,* systolic blood pressure.

---

tachycardia, or uncontrolled fibrillation in someone with pre-existing HF should be regarded as a harbinger of sudden death.

Pharmacological Interventions

Medical and pharmacological solutions are geared toward stabilization and prevention and in response to acute events. Pharmacological interventions are always necessary for the person with HF and are based on EF and the presence or absence of symptoms and volume overload (Table 23.7). For those with HFpEF without symptoms, the focus is on controlling the underlying cause, such as HTN or AF. Digoxin should be avoided. At any time that volume overload is present, diuretics (e.g., furosemide) are used.

In the acute care setting, nursing actions initially focus on balancing fluid load and assuring effective oxygenation. Medications are administered to provide safe diuresis, IV fluids are used very judiciously, and there is careful measurement of intake and output to monitor effectiveness of interventions. The person is likely to be very ill and at high risk for rapid decline physically, cognitively, and emotionally. Pharmacological interventions for those with HF are also based on the level of symptoms and their effect on function and activity.

Diuretics are also used to address fluid overload in persons with HFrEF but must be used with caution in persons with any renal insufficiency. ARBs have been shown to improve outcomes in older adults, and ACE inhibitors have been effective in persons under 75 years of age but not over 75 years of age. Beta blockers usually are added when fluid volume is stable. Efficacy and dosage vary in some cases between races (Reuben et al., 2020).

USING CLINICAL JUDGMENT TO PROMOTE HEALTHY AGING: CARDIOVASCULAR DISEASE

Both nonpharmacological and pharmacological solutions are usually necessary to optimize outcomes. Solutions are usually generated by the combined efforts of a multidisciplinary team within the context of the person's resources, preferences, and prognosis. Expert coordination of care is necessary, often lead by a nurse.

Solutions, Nursing Actions, and Outcomes

The most desirable outcome of healthy cardiovascular aging is to prevent HTN and thereby greatly reduce the risk for the development of vascular disorders and their associated morbidity and mortality. Those with elevated BP without HTN may be able to prevent its progression to a chronic state through proactive solutions.

Nonpharmacological solutions emphasize addressing all applicable reversible factors (see Table 23.2). Lifestyle changes have been found to be highly effective in reducing BP and therefore in reducing the risk of subsequent complications, especially AMIs and stroke (Turco et al., 2018).

Assessment of teaching and learning needs and the social determinants of a person's health will inform the specific nursing actions. Information and instruction may be needed related to home medication use, diet (especially fluid and sodium guidance), continence issues related to diuretic use and disability, advance care planning, preservation of energy, sexual activity, exercise and activity, anticipatory guidance regarding progression of symptoms, and signs of exacerbations and what to do about these (e.g., weight gain or loss).

Healthy Eating and Optimal Weight

Weight loss and exercise are recommended for all who are obese (body mass index >30 kg/m²). Weight loss of as little as 10% has been found to reduce BP. However, data now suggest that being underweight poses as great a risk for premature mortality as does being overweight (Saxena et al., 2021). Healthy eating is now the priority. Decreasing intake of sodium and cholesterol; increasing intake of fruits, vegetables, whole grains, and lean animal or plant protein; and minimizing intake of trans fat, processed red meat, refined carbohydrates, and sweetened beverages are fundamentals of "heart-healthy" eating. Guidance is available via the DASH (Dietary Approaches to Stop Hypertension) and Mediterranean diets. Both have been found to reduce CVD-associated deaths. If the person can read, teaching a person how to read food labels is an important part of preventive health education (Chapter 15).

Exercise and Physical Activity

Staying physically active will help the person control weight and improve the heart and may lower BP (Chapter 19). Walking 30 minutes a day at least five times a week or 150 accumulated minutes of moderate-intensity activity has shown to be beneficial to older adults for whom this activity is not contraindicated. A structured, individualized exercise program is a key component of cardiac rehabilitation and found to improve exercise tolerance and quality of life for those with heart disease. However, for those with advanced heart disease it does not reduce hospitalizations or mortality.

Smoking Cessation and Prevention

Smoking increases BP by causing vasoconstriction. The consequences of this are seen across vascular diseases and significantly increase the risk for poor outcomes. Nurses can help people find ways to stop smoking and avoid secondhand smoke and other pollutants.

Self-Care

The nurse works with the person to find ways to safely follow a medical treatment plan (Chapter 11), including when and how to take what. If taking an anticoagulant, this includes helping patients understand the dangers and benefits of the therapy the impact of medication, food, herb, and nutritional supplement interactions; the need for strict adherence; and the effect of high and low vitamin K. Nurses often perform point-of-care warfarin monitoring, and advanced practice nurses adjust doses as needed. Nurses often are involved in conversations regarding the risk-benefit ratio of continuing anticoagulation therapy for the person at risk for falling or has a history of falling (Chapter 20).

The nurse can help the person with CVD learn to minimize fatigue and maintain independence for as long as possible. This includes home modifications to reduce effort and reducing fall risk (Chapter 20). Educational nursing actions include the recognition of signs and symptoms indicating an early or pending crisis (Box 23.9). For someone with HF, a gain of 3 to 5 pounds in a day may be an indicator of cardiac compromise and the need to seek medical help or hospitalization. The nurse serves as a resource person for those willing to take steps to reduce their stress or improve their stress management. This may be through individual counseling or community programs. Mental health care is now available via telehealth as a covered service under Medicare (albeit with limited reimbursement to the provider). The nurse refers persons for rehabilitation for substance overuse

---

BOX 23.9 Cues to Potential Exacerbation of Illness in an Older Adult With Cardiovascular Disease

- Lightheadedness or dizziness
- Disturbances in gait and balance
- Loss of appetite or unexplained loss of weight
- Inability to concentrate or shortened attention span
- Changes in personality or mood
- Changes in grooming habits
- Unusual patterns in urination or defecation
- Vague discomfort, frequent bouts of anxiety
- Excessive fatigue, vague pain
- Withdrawal from usual sources of pleasure

---

when needed (Chapter 30). The nurse supports and encourages older adults to participate in all possible preventive activities and to obtain expert care to maintain their health and wellness to the extent possible. Special attention is given to controlling diabetes due to its close association with heart disease and death and hypertension as a precursor to other CVDs. The nurse promotes healthy aging by awareness and use of the multiple resources available to help persons live the healthiest lives possible.

Resources for Best Practice

American Heart Association: http://www.heart.org
Center for Disease Control: http://www.cdc.gov
Million Hearts® 2022: http://www.millionhearts.hhs.gov
Indian Health Service: http://www.ihs.gov
Dietary Approaches to Stop Hypertension (DASH) Diet: https://www.nhlbi.nih.gov/health-topics/dash-eating-plan

---

If a CVD is first recognized on a routine or incidental ECG, prioritization of care and needs can begin immediately based on the extent of apparent damage, the person's wishes, and resources. In some cases, the faster solutions are developed, the more the damage can be minimized. However, the achievement of these is complicated by the presence of comorbid conditions that strongly influence the prioritization of needs (Table 23.8).

The desired outcomes for persons with CVD are optimal wellness in the presence of illness through disease stabilization

---

TABLE 23.8 Impact of Concurrent Chronic Conditions on Person With Heart Failure

Condition	Impact
Cognitive Limitations	Difficulty adhering to care plan
Depression	Worsens prognosis
Falls	Aggravated by needed medications
Urinary Incontinence	Aggravated by needed medications
Frailty	Aggravated by hospitalizations

From Sudharshan S, Sandvall B, Rich MW: Heart failure and rhythm disorders. In Walter LC, Chang A, editors: *CURRENT diagnosis and treatment: geriatrics,* ed 3, New York, 2021, McGraw Hill, pp. 303–316.

and symptom control and the maintenance of the highest quality of life possible. Maintaining optimal function for as long as possible and the receipt of palliative care when appropriate are priority nursing actions. These require very prompt response to any signs of a new problem, worsening of a chronic condition, or a sudden event such as an AMI or acute HF (see Box 23.9).

Maximizing the outcome of a witnessed AMI is paramount to prevent further tissue damage. Most health care professionals are required to stay current in at least Basic Life Support resuscitation skills and be prepared to perform cardiopulmonary resuscitation (CPR) and use an automatic electronic defibrillator (AED) whenever and wherever it is needed. Bystander resuscitation efforts will improve survival and neurological outcomes, but there are multiple barriers to this occurring, especially fear of causing injury and fear of lack of skills (Becker et al., 2019).

Nurses work with persons and their significant others to determine their wishes related to medical crises and their desire for aggressive measures, such as hospitalization, intubation, and resuscitation (NHLBI, n.d. b). In discussions with older adults and their significant others the nurse must be very clear that even if CPR is desired, it is not always recommended and, perhaps more importantly, the person's illnesses will not be improved afterward and the need for intubation is possible. Even if resuscitation efforts are successful in an acute care setting, those who are even moderately frail are unlikely to survive to discharge. For those who are nearing the end of their lives, the desired outcome in older adults is comfort (Chapter 34).

THE AGING PERIPHERAL VASCULAR SYSTEM

The younger heart propels oxygen-rich blood through highly elastic and flexible arteries that expand and contract depending on the body's need for oxygen. The BP is regulated in part by the size of the arterial lumen and its ability to contract and relax as needed (Fig 23.2). The baroreceptors found in the larger arteries reflexively respond to increases in BP by causing vasodilation and reducing the heart rate, thus lowering the BP. Deoxygenated blood returns to the heart by way of the veins, propelled by contractions of the surrounding muscles. The blood is prevented from moving backward (by the pull of gravity) by a series of valves.

Several of the same age-related changes seen in the skin and muscles affect the blood vessels. The elastin fibers in the vessel walls fray, split, straighten, and fragment. With reduced elasticity, the lumen narrows, and there is underlying inflammation. Baroreceptors become less sensitive, increasing the risk for HTN, especially in women. The risk for peripheral vascular disease is directly related to thickening of the vessel wall (Bilder, 2016). When the blood flow to the organs is compromised, end-organ damage occurs. For those without CVD or diabetes, there is little change in blood flow to the coronary arteries or brain. However, perfusion of other tissues and organs is reduced and has implications for medication metabolism and excretion, as well as fluid and electrolyte balance (Chapter 9). The veins become stretched and the valves less efficient. Pooling of the blood leads to increased venous pressure, and edema develops more quickly.

PERIPHERAL VASCULAR DISEASE

Peripheral vascular disease (PVD) is a general term indicating any of the diseases of arterial or venous systems. The two major types are peripheral arterial disease (PAD) and chronic venous insufficiency (CVI). Venous thromboembolism (VTE) is closely linked to CVI both as a causative factor and as a consequence.

PAD is an atherosclerotic ischemic disease with reduced or blocked arterial circulation into the extremities. It is the result of end-organ damage from long-standing HTN and CHD. Consequently, prevention and treatment are tied to addressing the modifiable risk factors of the original disorders. The prevalence is more than 10% in those over 60 years old and more than 25% in those over 75 years old. When ischemia is present long enough, the surrounding tissue deteriorates, and skin ulcers develop with or without trauma. If an ulcer is not recognized and treated early enough, infection may develop to the point of gangrene, necessitating amputation to save the part of the limb above the lesion. When the ischemia is severe, there is a mortality rate of 25% in the first year, a 30% amputation rate, and a 5-year survival rate of less than 40% (Ang & Iannuzzi, 2021).

CVI is a global term used to describe anatomical or functional changes to the venous system. Normal venous function depends on vein patency, intact valves, and a functioning calf muscle to pump the blood from the periphery back to the right side of the heart. When any of these are impaired or compromised, venous hypertension and sustained venous pressure result in edema. Up to 80% of the general population will have CVI at some time, increasing in incidence with age. Once it occurs, 30% to 50% of the time it is progressive. Risk factors include age, obesity, smoking, prolonged standing or dependency, and history of lower extremity injury or trauma (Ghaniwala & Carman, 2021).

VTE includes deep vein thrombosis (DVT) and pulmonary embolism (PE), which together are the third leading cause of cardiovascular-related death in the United States. The risk increases with age, and 60% of such events occur to older adults. Risk factors include CVI, obesity, long-distance travel, immobilization, surgery, and trauma. The reverse blood flow through the incompetent valves results in increased hydrostatic pressure and pain when the extremity is dependent and during ambulation. Up to 50% of all cases of DVT are asymptomatic (Ang & Iannuzzi, 2021).

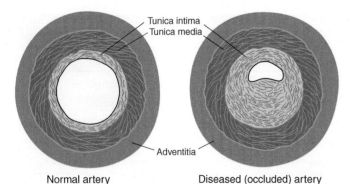

Tunica intima
Tunica media

Adventitia

Normal artery   Diseased (occluded) artery

Fig. 23.2 Arteriosclerosis. (From Huether SE, McCance KL: *Understanding pathophysiology*, ed 5, St Louis, 2012, Mosby.)

Recognizing and Analyzing Cues

Most older adults with PAD are asymptomatic or will have non-specific symptoms of cramping, numbness or tingling of the extremity, or muscle weakness and fatigue. Some will have the classic symptoms of intermittent claudication. Lower extremity pain increases with exertion as the tissue demand for oxygen increases and is instantly relieved by rest. When elevated, the extremity may be pale and cool, consistent with ischemia, and red or purple with dependency as gravity pulls the blood into the ischemic limb (Reuben et al., 2020). The person will report that they sleep with legs in a dependent position or alter their activity to avoid the symptoms or attribute the pain to arthritis or the aging process, and diagnosis is delayed. A few people will not be diagnosed until there is severe limb ischemia, ulcerations, loss of tissue, and/or infection. If any of these cues are recognized or PAD is suspected, urgent solutions are required to avoid limb loss (Ang & Iannuzzi, 2021).

A walking history is key to assessment in PAD. Determining how far the person can walk or how long the leg can be elevated before the pain starts establishes baseline data that can be used in the measurement of outcomes. The presence of foot ulcerations, especially between the toes and those associated with ill-fitting shoes, are cues to advanced disease and inform the prioritization of hypotheses. An abnormal ankle-brachial index (ABI) is the final diagnostic indicator of the presence and extent of disease (Ang & Iannuzzi, 2021).

Like PAD, CVI initially may be asymptomatic and not diagnosed until trophic skin changes or venous statis ulcers are recognized. Symptoms may be nonspecific: extremity heaviness, pain or aching, late-day fatigue, burning, itching, or throbbing. There is pooling of blood from venous stasis and edema of the ankle and lower leg, initially soft and pitting and later firm and resistant to pressure. As a progressive disease, it leads to persistent pain, stasis dermatitis, and skin ulcerations that can lead to amputation. Over time, long-standing stasis of blood leads to the deposition of hemosiderin in the subcutaneous tissue. The lower calf appears dark or speckled brown in lightly pigmented skin and a dull gray in more darkly pigmented tissue.

Venous thromboembolism (PE or DVT) is the most dangerous complication of CVI in older adults. The signs and symptoms are also often nonspecific, making diagnosis difficult and delaying treatment in these life- and limb-threatening events. A person may report nonspecific symptoms of not feeling well or limb pain. Cues of a DVT include swelling, erythema, increased warmth, and varicosities of the superficial veins. Although the absence of lower extremity hair is important in a younger adult, this is not a significant finding in later life due to the loss of body hair in the normal course of aging. If a DVT is suspected, the assessment of a comparative measurement of calf circumference is necessary. A duplex ultrasound is required for diagnosis and an ABI is necessary to determine the co-condition of PAD (Ghaniwala & Carman, 2021; Reuben et al., 2020). A positive Homan's sign (calf pain with foot flexion) has long been thought to be a useful assessment measure, but it has been found to be unreliable.

Careful palpation for the presence or absence of pulses and auscultation of the carotid and femoral pulses for bruits provide additional information about the quality of peripheral circulation. There are several reasons that a pulse may not be easily palpable, especially in the presence of edema. Unless the limb is pale and cool, it cannot be assumed that there is no pulse, only that the pulse is not palpable and measurement of capillary refill time (should be <3 seconds) is more useful. Unless the skin is broken, the nurse must make a judgment whether to wear gloves, especially for the assessment of temperature.

The symptoms of a PE are not as straightforward as has been thought. In older adults only tachycardia and tachypnea may be observed, without the classic chest pain and shortness of breath. Even when pleuritic chest pain, dyspnea, or cough is present, a PE is often overlooked in older adults. An ECG is required to differentiate a PE from an AMI, HF, musculoskeletal injury, or infection, such as pneumonia or COVID-19.

A PE will be confirmed with a chest x-ray or magnetic resonance imaging (MRI), but even the suspicion of one should be treated as a medical emergency. Both DVT and PE require hospitalization to resolve the thromboembolism. A PE should be suspected anytime the person has recently had a DVT, or is at risk for one, and complains of sudden shortness of breath and has a low oxygen saturation rate.

Pharmacological Interventions

Pharmacological interventions specific to PVD are associated with management of edema and pain. Either chronic or intermittent diuretics may be necessary. Antiplatelet agents (e.g., aspirin) usually are prescribed for persons with PAD preventatively. If diabetes mellitus is present, tight glycemic control may be necessary (Chapter 27). Topical, oral, and/or intravenous antibiotics may be needed.

Once a DVT or a PE has occurred, it will be treated medically with anticoagulants. Once the acute clot is resolved, the risk for another DVT is permanent, and lifetime anticoagulation may be necessary (Ghaniwala & Carman, 2021). If the person is taking an anticoagulant such as heparin, Lovenox (enoxaparin), or warfarin, the nurse may be responsible for laboratory interpretation and dosage adjustment (Chapter 10).

The desired outcomes for persons with PVD are the prevention or prompt treatment of complications. In working toward this, quality of life is increased and unnecessary mortality minimized. Outcomes can be measured by patient-reported mobility, pain relief, degree of edema, and rate of wound healing or stabilization, while recognizing that once a wound develops it may never heal completely.

USING CLINICAL JUDGMENT TO PROMOTE HEALTHY AGING: PERIPHERAL VASCULAR DISEASE

Pain relief, edema management, and skin care are the priorities of care for persons with PVD. Solutions are directed toward comfort and prevention of complications and prompt nursing action when they occur. Pain relief usually requires both pharmacological and nonpharmacological interventions, often through the efforts of a multidisciplinary team.

Solutions, Nursing Actions, and Outcomes

Skin care and pain relief are interconnected, as the development of wounds can result in chronic pain, and pain alone is a harbinger of an ulcer. Nursing actions for either PAD or CVI include instructing people about the importance of expert skin and foot care, supportive and correctly fitting footwear, prompt recognition of even the slightest injury or a minor wound, and prompt reporting of any changes to a health care provider. Daily skin inspection and protection against the effects of pressure, friction, shear, and maceration are essential actions by both the nurse and the individual. If the person has diabetes or peripheral neuropathy for any reason, regular and careful inspection could prevent an amputation. For those with visual limitations, assistance is required. If someone is not available to check the bottom of the foot, a nonbreakable mirror placed on the floor may help those with adequate vision.

Special care must be taken to ensure that venous stasis ulcers and arterial ulcers are differentiated and treated appropriately (Table 23.9). They are always potentially limb-threatening, and it is recommended that the nurse consult with colleagues who are wound care specialists to develop the most appropriate nursing actions. The nurse is usually the leader in planning and implementing patient education related to skin care (Table 23.10) (Chapter 14).

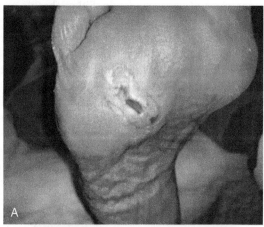

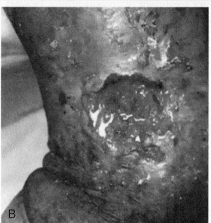

(A) Arterial ulcer. **(B)** Venous stasis ulcer. (Adapted from Mattox KL, Townsend CM, Beauchamp RD, et al: *Sabiston textbook of surgery: the biological basis of modern surgical practice*, ed 21, St Louis, 2022, Elsevier.)

TABLE 23.9   Comparison of Arterial and Venous Insufficiency of the Lower Extremities

Characteristics	Arterial	Venous
Pain	Pain with elevation of lower extremities Pain initially relieved when legs become dependent Pain returns when walking short distances (claudication) but is relieved by rest (legs still dependent)	Deep ache, relieved by elevation Deep muscle pain with acute deep vein thrombosis
Pulses	Absent or weak	Normal
Skin	Thin, shiny, dry skin Thickened toenails Absence of hair growth Cool Pallor with elevation Rubor with dependency	Firm ("brawny") edema Reddish brown discoloration (hyperpigmentation) Evidence of healed ulcers Presence of varicose veins Progressive edema Dark erythema with acute deep vein thrombosis
Ulcer location	Between toes or at tips of toes Metatarsal or phalangeal heads Heels, sides, or soles of feet Lateral malleolus Pretibial area	Medial malleolus
Ulcer characteristics	Well-defined edges Necrotic tissue Deep, pale base Nonbleeding	Uneven edges Ruddy granulation tissue Superficial Bleeding

Because PAD is an ischemic condition, nothing should be done to restrict circulation to the affected limb. Sitting with legs crossed, wearing restrictive clothing, and using compression stockings or dressings (e.g., Unna boot) are usually contraindicated. The disease will progress rapidly if the person smokes or is exposed to tobacco smoke or other pollutants that cause vasoconstriction. A dedicated walking program designed by a physical therapist with progressive ambulation may help reduce pain for those with PAD. Some improvement should be felt in 4 to 8 weeks and significant improvement in 12 to 26 weeks. If not, surgical angioplasty or the insertion of a stent may be necessary (Reuben et al., 2020).

With CVI, oxygenated blood enters the arteries, but its movement out of the extremities through the veins and back to the heart is limited or obstructed. Elevation, compression devices, and ankle and foot exercises are the major interventions. Elevation of the legs above the heart for 30 minutes three to four

TABLE 23.10 Promoting Healthy Aging for the Person With Peripheral Vascular Disease

Give Legs a Rest	Take Care of the Skin
Elevate the feet above heart level while sleeping, while sitting, and several times a day.	Examine feet daily, including the soles, sides, and between the toes.
Change Positions Frequently	Wash lower legs and feet regularly with mild soap and water.
Avoid activities that require standing or sitting with feet dangling for long periods.	Use moisturizing cream and emollients after washing.
Give Legs Support (as Directed Only)	Do **not** use lanolin or petroleum-based creams when wearing support hose made with latex.
As directed (chronic venous insufficiency [CVI] only), wear professionally made graduated compression from ankles to knees.	Avoid activities that can injure the legs or feet.
Replace hose as needed to maintain usefulness.	Monitor legs for skin changes: Persistent edema Discoloration
Hose on in a.m. and off in p.m.	Dryness and/or itching

times a day can reduce edema and improve skin microcirculation. The foot of the bed can be elevated with blocks or books. Customized, fitted, below-the-knee compression stockings (not TED hose) or pneumatic compression pumps are helpful but difficult to use when living alone, and costs are not covered by Medicare unless ulcers are already present. Velcro compression devices are easier to use. The compression replaces or enhances that provided by the muscles and facilitates wound healing, reduces venous dermatitis and sclerotic changes, and counteracts excessive venous pressure. The nurse can work with the person with obesity on a plan for weight reduction to decrease the pressure on the veins.

Multiple conditions common in late life can have some of the same signs and symptoms of PVD. For example, heart failure and many medications such as calcium channel blockers, beta blockers, and nonsteroidal antiinflammatories can cause edema, and diabetes results in numbness, tingling, and nonhealing wounds on the extremities. The gerontological nurse may be the first one to recognize the cues that indicate a potential PVD. The development of hypotheses related to the care of a person with a vascular disorder discussed here begin with a good history, physical examination, and review of symptoms (Chapter 9). While the type of problem may appear evident, confirmatory testing is required to develop the appropriate nursing interventions.

CEREBROVASCULAR DISORDERS

The cerebrovascular disorders discussed here include the ischemic stroke, transient ischemic attack (TIA), and hemorrhagic stroke. All are characterized by acute-onset neurological changes resulting from anoxic damage to the brain. Both morbidity and mortality are dependent on the type of event and the time between onset and treatment. Some of the immediate neurological deficits may be the same or similar, but the treatment and prognoses of ischemic and hemorrhagic events are dramatically different, and an urgent and accurate diagnosis is essential. All strokes are medical emergencies. Without treatment, 10% to 15% of those who have had a TIA will have a major stroke within 3 months, with the greatest risk being in the first week (CDC, 2021d).

Although the total number of deaths from stroke has declined in the United States, there has been an increase in stroke-related deaths among persons who identify as Hispanic (CDC, 2021d). The US death rates are highest in the "stroke belt" of the southeastern section of the country and lowest in the Northeast and Southwest. Stroke primarily affects older adults, and the rate doubles for both men and women every 10 years after the age of 55 (Nguyen et al., 2021). Black men have twice the risk of having a stroke as White men. In addition to age and race or ethnicity, other risk factors include diabetes, uncontrolled HTN, obesity, and smoking. Stroke is a leading cause of disability: over half who survive never regain independence (CDC, 2021e). One of the goals of *Healthy People 2030* is to reduce stroke-related mortality from the baseline of 37.1 deaths per 100,000 persons in 2018 to 33.4 by 2030 (ODPHP, 2021).

Eighty-seven percent of all strokes are ischemic; blood clots or other particles suddenly block cerebral blood flow and therefore oxygenation. Brain tissues deprived of oxygen die quickly. *One minute of brain ischemia can kill 2 million nerve cells and 14 billion synapses!* A TIA causes a temporary blockage, usually for less than 5 minutes.

Ischemic strokes also can be caused by hematological disorders, hypoperfusion, and arteriosclerosis (see Fig. 23.2). Hematological disorders include those that result in hypercoagulability and hyperviscosity syndromes. Hypoperfusion can be a result of dehydration, cardiac arrest, syncope, or hypotension, including overtreatment of HTN.

A hemorrhagic stroke occurs when a blood vessel in the brain leaks or ruptures. A subdural hematoma (SDH) is the result of hemorrhage from torn veins and bleeding into the dura and the arachnoid membranes. Head trauma is the most common cause and is highest among older adults due to the combination of age-related brain atrophy, falls, and use of antithrombotic agents. If acute, neurological deficits are found with an altered mental state. If the SDH is chronic ("a slow bleed"), the cues may be somnolence, cognitive impairment, reports of headaches, and occasionally seizures (Nguyen et al., 2021). Blood floods the surrounding brain tissue with an intracerebral hemorrhage (ICH). The most important contributing factors for a spontaneous ICH in older adults are HTN, the use of anticoagulants, acute inflammatory illness, and accidental injury (e.g., from falls). Anticoagulants increase the risk for an ICH, worsen the severity, and double the mortality rate (Nguyen et al., 2021).

The subarachnoid hemorrhage (SAH) causes bleeding into the deep areas in the brain. The rupture is usually at the site of an aneurysm. If the person is also receiving anticoagulant medications, the bleeding will be rapid (Nguyen et al., 2021).

When the classic signs of a potential stroke are present, one is presumed until proven otherwise (Box 23.10). Diagnosis requires both neurological dysfunction and a computed

BOX 23.10 Cues of a Stroke

If you think someone may be having a stroke, act FAST and do the following simple test:

F Face: Ask the person to smile. Does one side of the face droop?
A Arms: Ask the person to raise both arms. Does one arm drift downward?
S Speech: Ask the person to repeat a simple phrase. Is the person's speech slurred or strange?
T Time: If you observe any of these signs, call 9-1-1 immediately.

TABLE 23.11 Effects of Left-Sided and Right-Sided Strokes

Left	Right
Weakness or paralysis on right side of body	Weakness or paralysis on left side of body
Speech or language problems	Visual problems (bilateral left field deficit)
Slow, cautious behavior	Quick, overly curious behavior
Impairment of organizational skills	Poor decision making
Facial weakness or swallowing problems	Facial weakness or swallowing problems
Memory loss	Memory loss

tomography (CT) scan or an MRI to differentiate the type of stroke. All are life-threatening and require prompt diagnosis and treatment to increase the chance of survival and decrease the risk for disability.

Recognizing and Analyzing Cues

The specific neurological deficit reflects the area of the brain affected (Table 23.11). Sudden unilateral weakness can be recognized 80% of the time, and speech or motor deficits 90% of the time. Changes in sensation, cognition, balance, and vision may occur (Nguyen et al., 2021). When the signs and symptoms resolve quickly and without treatment, a TIA is suspected. About one-third of those with TIA symptoms do not seek health care and only later report: "I think I had a mini-stroke last week."

A person having a hemorrhagic stroke may have a decreasing level of consciousness and report a sudden and severe headache with no known cause ("the worst headache of my life"). Nausea and vomiting suggest increased cerebral edema. There is a potential for seizures, and death can occur quickly. Loss of consciousness indicates a very poor prognosis (Moran et al., 2017).

Whenever paralysis occurs, spasticity leading to contractures in the affected limb or limbs is a risk. Other complications include DVT in a flaccid lower limb, aspiration pneumonia, or urinary tract infections.

Pharmacological Interventions

It is imperative that the type of stroke be determined immediately so that the appropriate medical treatment can be initiated.

When an ischemic stroke has been verified, the nurse will administer recombinant tissue plasminogen activator (rtPA). It has been found that those who receive rtPA within 3 hours of the event are more likely to recover fully without disability and less likely to need skilled rehabilitation in a nursing facility (CDC, 2021d).

Medical treatment of a hemorrhagic stroke begins with stopping the bleeding. If a person with a hemorrhagic stroke were to accidentally receive rtPA, rapid death would occur. A very small intracerebral hemorrhage may resolve on its own. If caught early enough, an endovascular or surgical treatment may be attempted for a SDH. No medical or surgical treatment is available for a subarachnoid hemorrhage, and the prognosis is very poor. If the person survives the first several hours, the goal is palliative care for the patient and support for the family.

Pharmacological treatment following the acute event for both a TIA and a nonhemorrhagic stroke is an antiplatelet agent such as daily low-dose aspirin or clopidogrel for persons under 70 years of age (American Stroke Association, 2020). For those who cannot dependably swallow pills, chewable aspirin is available. Aggressive control of HTN, lipids, and diabetes is necessary to lower the risk for another stroke. Antiplatelet therapy has not been found to prevent a COVID-19 related stroke (Keller, 2021).

USING CLINICAL JUDGMENT TO PROMOTE HEALTHY AGING: CEREBROVASCULAR DISORDERS

The gerontological nursing actions when caring for those with cerebrovascular illnesses are like those for other acute and chronic conditions. Interventions are based on the prioritized hypothesis during an acute event followed by actions to prevent recurrence or complications.

Solutions, Nursing Actions, and Outcomes

Prompt recognition of cues that indicate a possible stroke has occurred is the priority. If consistent with the wishes of the patient, the nurse mobilizes an emergency response and works in tandem with medical providers during the acute phase. Assessment of airway, breathing, and circulation is continuous, with expansion to the other areas identified by FANCAPES as soon as possible (Chapter 9).

After the acute period, the priority is preventing another stroke by addressing the underlying cause such as HTN. Due to the life-threatening nature of a stroke, other priorities are to review end-of-life issues, the presence or absence of a health care proxy, and teaching the person and family or significant others what to expect after a stroke. This includes the plans for restorative and rehabilitative interventions either at home or in a long-term care facility.

To have the best outcome in the poststroke period, the nursing priority is to complete a comprehensive assessment to identify the most relevant lifestyle risk factors and prevention needs, prevent unnecessary hospitalization and complications, and ensure home safety (Chapter 21).

KEY CONCEPTS

- Vascular diseases are the leading cause of death and disability in the older adult.
- The priority in the promotion of healthy aging is minimizing risk for disease.
- The presentation of many CVDs or nuances of these in older adults differ from those in younger adults (e.g., the "silent MI").
- Ischemic and hemorrhagic strokes must be differentiated before treatment can be initiated.

- Desired outcomes for all persons with vascular diseases are alleviating symptoms, delaying or avoiding the development of complications including end-organ damage, and maximizing function and quality of life.
- The gerontological nurse has the potential to serve as a leader in the promotion of health, the prevention of vascular disease, and the improvement of the lives of those with vascular disease.

NEXT-GENERATION NCLEX® (NGN) EXAMINATION-STYLE QUESTIONS

Mrs. Lewis is an 85-year-old widowed woman with three sons and a daughter. Although her husband was not of the Jewish faith, she raised her children in the practices and traditions in which she was raised. None of her children live nearby, but she does have a very close friend from her synagogue who has been at her side during a long and difficult battle with heart failure. She has been admitted to the subacute unit in the skilled nursing home where you are employed. Her prognosis is very poor, and death is imminent. She has a do-not-resuscitate (DNR) order in place and a living will designating her friend as her decision maker. Between breaths she tells you that most of the time in the last 2 months she has been in the hospital and has been told there was nothing left to do but to allow a natural death. She is adamant that under no circumstances should she be returned to the hospital. Her pulse is rapid, and she is diaphoretic.

Highlight the cues that will help you determine the priorities of care for Mrs. Lewis. Underline the cue that is the top priority at this time.

CLINICAL JUDGMENT QUESTIONS AND ACTIVITIES

1. After you have thought about Mrs. Lewis's situation, discuss with a classmate how you would feel about caring for her. Could you care for her and respect her wishes?
2. What symptoms do you expect she will develop in the hours or days between her admission to the subacute unit

and her death? What are your responsibilities related to them?
3. In a discussion with other students, describe your personal feelings about caring for someone who declines treatment.

RESEARCH QUESTIONS

1. Are there any expected rituals or customs when nearing death or at the time of death in the Jewish faith?

2. Is a person with heart disease ever considered eligible for hospice services, and if so, under what circumstance?

REFERENCES

Agarwala A, Mehta A, Yang E, et al: Older adults and hypertension: beyond the 2017 guideline for the prevention, detection, evaluation, and management of high blood pressure in adults (website), 2020. https://www.acc.org/latest-in-cardiology/articles/2020/02/26/06/24/older-adults-and-hypertension.

American Stroke Association: Aspirin and stroke (website), 2020. https://www.stroke.org/en/life-after-stroke/preventing-another-stroke/aspirin-and-stroke.

Ang SK, Iannuzzi JC: Peripheral arterial disease and venous thromboembolism. In Walter LC, Chang A, editors: *CURRENT diagnosis and treatment: geriatrics*, ed 3, New York, 2021, McGraw Hill, pp 345–354.

Aronow WS: Diagnosis and management of coronary artery disease. In Fillit H, Rockwood K, Young J, editors: *Brocklehurst's textbook of geriatric medicine*, ed 8, Philadelphia, 2017, Elsevier, pp 278–287.

Baik AH, Dhruva SS: Coronary artery disease. In Walter LC, Chang A, editors: *CURRENT diagnosis and treatment: geriatrics*, ed 3, New York, 2021, McGraw Hill, pp 287–302.

Baldi E, Sechi GM, Mare C, et al.: COVID-19 kills at home: the close relationship between the epidemic and the incidence of out-of-hospital cardiac arrests, *Eur Heart J* 41(32):3045–3054, 2020.

Becker TK, Gul SS, Cohen SA, et al.: Public perception toward bystander cardiopulmonary resuscitation, *Emerg Med J* 36(11):660–665, 2019.

Bilder GE: *Human biological aging*, Hoboken, NJ, 2016, Wiley.

Centers for Disease Control and Prevention (CDC): Heart failure (website), 2020. https://www.cdc.gov/heartdisease/heart_failure.htm.

Centers for Disease Control and Prevention (CDC): Heart disease facts (website), 2021a. https://www.cdc.gov/heartdisease/facts.htm

Centers for Disease Control and Prevention (CDC): Facts about hypertension (website), 2021b. https://www.cdc.gov/bloodpressure/facts.htm.

Centers for Disease Control and Prevention (CDC): Stroke treatment (website), 2019b. https://www.cdc.gov/stroke/treatments.htm.

Centers for Disease Control and Prevention (CDC): Atrial fibrillation (website), 2021c. https://www.cdc.gov/heartdisease/atrial_fibrillation.htm.

Centers for Disease Control and Prevention (CDC): Types of strokes (website), 2021d. https://www.cdc.gov/stroke/types_of_stroke.htm.

Centers for Disease Control and Prevention (CDC): Family history and other characteristics that increase risk for stroke (website), 2021e. https://www.cdc.gov/stroke/family_history.htm.

Cuker A, Burnett A, Triller D, et al.: Reversal of direct anticoagulants: guidance from the Anticoagulation Forum, *Am J Hematol* 94(6):697–709, 2019.

Ghaniwala S, Carman TL: Chronic venous insufficiency. In Walter LC, Chang A, editors: *CURRENT diagnosis and treatment: geriatrics*, ed 3, New York, 2021, McGraw Hill, pp 367–372.

Keller DM: Antithrombotic therapy fails to prevent stroke in COVID-19 (website), 2021. *Medscape* Oct 21, 2021.

Kulkarni A, Mehta A, Yang E, et al: Older adults and hypertension: Beyond the 2017 guidelines for prevention, detection, evaluation, and management of high blood pressure in adults (website), American College of Cardiology Feb 26, 2020. Older Adults and Hypertension: Beyond the 2017 Guideline for Prevention, Detection, Evaluation, and Management of High Blood Pressure in Adults - American College of Cardiology (acc.org)

Kumbhani DJ, Cannon CP, Beavers CJ, et al.: 2020 ACC expert consensus pathway for anticoagulant and antiplatelet therapy in patients with atrial fibrillation or venous thromboembolism, *J Am Coll Cardiol* 77(5):629–658, 2020.

Li Y, Wang J, Lv L, et al.: Usefulness of the CHADS2 and R2CHADS2 scores for prognostic stratification in patients with coronary artery disease, *Clin Interv Aging* 13:565–571, 2018.

Moran C, Phan TG, Srikanth VK: Stroke: clinical presentation, management, and organization of services. In Fillit HM, Rockwood K, Young J, editors: *Brocklehurst's textbook of geriatric medicine and gerontology*, ed 8, Philadelphia, 2017, Elsevier, pp 483–490.

National Heart, Lung, and Blood Institute (NHLBI): *Atrial fibrillation* (website), n.d. a. https://www.nhlbi.nih.gov/health-topics/atrial-fibrillation.

National Heart, Lung, and Blood Institute (NHLBI): *Heart failure* (website), n.d b. https://www.nhlbi.nih.gov/health-topics/heart-failure.

Nguyen I, Fabiny A, Ovbiagele B: Cerebrovascular disease. In Walter LC, Chang A, editors: *CURRENT diagnosis and treatment: geriatrics*, ed 3, New York, 2021, McGraw Hill, pp 280–286.

Office of Disease Prevention and Health Promotion (ODPHP): Reduce stroke deaths—HDS-03 (website), 2021 https://health.gov/healthypeople/objectives-and-data/browse-objectives/heart-disease-and-stroke/reduce-stroke-deaths-hds-03.

Reuben DB, Herr KA, Pacala JT, et al.: *Geriatrics at your fingertips*, ed 22, New York, 2020, American Geriatrics Society.

Saxena S, Ayers G, Factora RM: Hypertension. In Walter LC, Chang A, editors: *CURRENT diagnosis and treatment: geriatrics*, ed 3, New York, 2021, McGraw Hill, pp 317–328.

SPRINT Research Group: Final report of a trial of intensive versus standard blood-pressure control, *NEJM* 384:1921–1930, 2021.

Sudharshan S, Sandvall B, Rich MW: Heart failure and rhythm disorders. In Walter LC, Chang A, editors: *CURRENT diagnosis and treatment: geriatrics*, ed 3, New York, 2021, McGraw Hill, pp 303–316.

Turco JV, Inal-Veith A, Fuster V: Cardiovascular health promotion: an issue that can no longer wait, *JACC* 72(8):908–913, 2018.

US Prevention Services Task Force (USPSTF): Screening for hypertension in adults: US Prevention Services Task Force reaffirmation recommendation statement, *JAMA* 325(16):1650–1656, 2021.

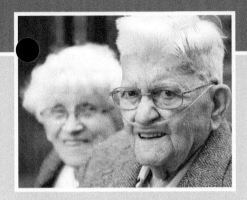

CHAPTER 24

Respiratory Disorders

Kathleen Jett

http://evolve.elsevier.com/Touhy/TwdHlthAging

A STUDENT SPEAKS

Sometimes I must take care of someone who smokes. When they return from the smoking area the smell is so strong I can hardly stand getting close to them.

La'Shawn, age 18

AN OLDER ADULT SPEAKS

I have smoked since I was 12 or 13. I started coughing a little now and then when I was in my 40s. Now that I am in my 60s, it seems like I can't ever catch my breath. They say it is something called COPD. I don't quite understand that and what it has to do with my cigarettes. I certainly could not give them up after all these years!

Helen, age 68

LEARNING OBJECTIVES

On completion of this chapter, the reader will be able to:

1. Recognize the normal changes with aging that affect the respiratory system.
2. Recognize cues to respiratory illness in late life.
3. Recognize and analyze the cues that indicate pneumonia and describe how these are different than those in younger adults.
4. Develop solutions to prioritized needs that promote respiratory health.

The respiratory system is the vehicle for gas exchange, especially the transfer of oxygen into and the release of carbon dioxide out of the blood. Respiration is dependent on functioning pulmonary, cardiac, musculoskeletal, and autonomic nervous systems. Respiratory function peaks at about 20 years of age, after which there is a steady decline over time. The rate of decline is influenced by many factors, including nutrition, level of activity, and exposure to smoke and other pollutants. The decline is two to five times faster among smokers than nonsmokers (Salzman et al., 2021). The most common chronic respiratory diseases seen late in life are chronic obstructive pulmonary disease (COPD) and asthma. Pneumonia is a life-threatening acute respiratory illness for older adults.

THE AGING RESPIRATORY SYSTEM

Although there are multiple age-related changes in the respiratory system, they are insignificant when one is well and free of illness or comorbid conditions. Like all other systems, there is a reduced capacity to respond to sudden changes, and when confronted with a sudden demand for increased oxygen with exercise or when exposed to noxious or infectious agents, a previously unknown respiratory deficit may become evident and quickly become life-threatening. These include loss of elastic recoil and increased chest wall stiffening and resistance to air exchange. Normal changes with aging include redistributed lung capacity and reduced sensitivity to anoxia (Table 24.1). Diminished inspiratory and expiratory muscle strength of the thorax results in reduced residual capacity, shallower respirations, and increased respiratory effort (Fig. 24.1). If kyphosis is present or the costovertebral joints are affected by arthritis, expansion of the chest cavity is further reduced. The most significant changes are lowered efficiency of gas exchange and reduced ability to handle thickened secretions. The cilia, which normally act as brushes to repel foreign substances or propel mucus out of the trachea, thicken and become less responsive and less effective. Compounded by a diminished chemoreceptor sensitivity, blunted cough reflex, and reduced immune response, there is

TABLE 24.1 Normal Changes With Aging and Potentially Serious Consequences at the Time of Respiratory Illness

Change	Potential Consequence
Ossification of the costal cartilage, less compliant rib cage	Potential for less expansion, such as when exercising or when increased respirations are needed
Loss of elastin attachment in the alveolar walls	Collapse of the small airways and uneven alveolar ventilation, trapping air and increasing dead space, decreasing vital capacity, and decreasing expiratory flow
Chemoreceptor function is altered or blunted at the peripheral and central chemoreceptor sites	Compensatory responses to hypercapnia and hypoxia are decreased while perception of dyspnea is intact or even enhanced. This response is independent of mechanical lung changes and is attributed to alterations in the neuromuscular drive to breathe. Compensatory responses may be significantly hindered in situations of stress

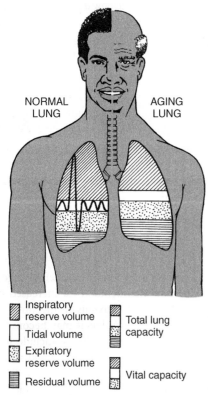

NORMAL LUNG   AGING LUNG

Inspiratory reserve volume

Tidal volume

Total lung capacity

Expiratory reserve volume

Residual volume

Vital capacity

Fig. 24.1 Changes in lung volume with aging. (From McCance KL, Huether SE: *Pathophysiology: the biologic basis for disease in adults and children*, ed 7, St Louis, 2014, Mosby.)

a higher risk for infection and a decreased ability to respond to anoxia. Overall, age-related changes are especially dangerous for those who have limited mobility, impaired oropharyngeal muscle movement (dysarthria or dysphagia) due to injury or stroke, or chronic disease such as Parkinson's disease or preexisting pulmonary disorders.

Viral infections are very common in older adults, especially in those with respiratory compromise. The viral infection can rapidly become acute bacterial bronchitis or pneumonia. Age-related decrease in immune response may delay diagnosis and hence treatment.

RESPIRATORY DISORDERS

Respiratory disorders occur significantly more often with age, as do associated hospitalizations and deaths. Both COPD and lung cancer are increasingly common. Respiratory infections are the most life-threatening complications, especially COVID-19 and influenza-related pneumonia.

Chronic Obstructive Pulmonary Disease

COPD is an inflammatory condition, characterized by a persistent and irreversible airway obstruction and/or alveolar abnormalities, usually caused by inhalation of toxins and pollutants earlier in life, such as dust, chemicals, and especially tobacco smoke, directly or indirectly from secondhand smoke (Global Initiative for Chronic Obstructive Lung Disease [GOLD], 2021). Eighty to ninety percent of all COPD is the result of cigarette smoking, and smokers are 13 times more likely to die of the disease than nonsmokers (Salzman et al., 2021). COPD significantly increases the risk for COVID-19–related hospitalization and mortality (Meza et al, 2021). In 2017, tobacco was attributed to 3.3 million deaths worldwide: 1.5 million from COPD, 1.2 million from cancer, and 600,000 from respiratory infections and tuberculosis. COPD is the third leading cause of death (excluding COVID-19) worldwide, causing 3.23 million deaths in 2019. The majority of these deaths occur in low and middle income countries (World Health Organization [WHO], 2021).

Over 15 million adult Americans and 10% of those at least 65 years of age have COPD, and approximately 50% of those with low pulmonary function are not aware that they already have COPD (Centers for Disease Control and Prevention [CDC], 2021a). There are significant geographic variations in prevalence, from 15.3 per 100,000 in Hawaii to 61.4 per 100,000 in Kentucky; the associated death rate is highest in the Mississippi and Ohio River Valleys (CDC, 2021b). It is the one noninfectious chronic disease that is decreasing.

The diagnosis is primarily made based on a careful analysis of signs and symptoms, frequency of exacerbations (acute worsening), associated hospitalizations, and presence or absence of risk factors (Box 24.1). Spirometry after bronchodilation may be used to confirm and quantify airflow obstruction (GOLD, 2021). Whereas younger adults are likely to respond to a "bronchodilator challenge" with temporarily improved airflow, this is not always seen in older adults due to the age-related changes noted above (Salzman et al., 2021). Spirometry is not always available and cannot be done in persons with cognitive impairments if they are unable to follow directions.

COPD is the umbrella term for the clinical conditions of emphysema and chronic bronchitis. When airflow obstruction is combined with thickening and inflammation of bronchial walls, hypertrophy of mucous glands, constriction of smooth muscle, and production of excess mucus, it is referred

BOX 24.1 Risk Factors for Chronic Obstructive Pulmonary Disease

Exposure or history of exposure to tobacco smoke
Exposure to indoor pollutants such as heating fuels
Exposure to occupational pollutants such as dust or chemicals
Exposure to outdoor pollutants such as biomass emissions
Age
History of asthma, reactive airway disease, or recurrent respiratory infections
Female
Low socioeconomic status
Genetic: alpha-1 antitrypsin deficiency or MMP12 and glutathione S-transferase encoding

Data from Global Initiative for Chronic Obstructive Lung Disease: *Pocket guide to COPD diagnosis, management, and prevention* (website), 2021. https://goldcopd.org/wp-content/uploads/2020/11/GOLD-2021-POCKET-GUIDE-v1.0-16Nov20_WMV.pdf.

BOX 24.2 Living With COPD

Mobility limitations
Early disability/inability to work
Depression
Need for special equipment such as supplemental oxygen
Increased health-related expenses
Limitations in social activities
Increased risk for memory loss or confusion
Increased number of comorbid chronic conditions (e.g., heart disease, arthritis, diabetes, stroke)
Frequent emergency room visits and hospitalizations

From Centers for Disease Control and Prevention (CDC): *Basics about COPD* (website), 2021a. https://www.cdc.gov/copd/basics-about.html

to as chronic bronchitis. Acute episodes of bronchitis are stimulated by new exposure to toxins, including pollution, viruses, and bacteria. It is diagnosed clinically by a productive cough for 3 months in 2 consecutive years or 6 months in 1 year (Salzman et al., 2021). When there is destruction of the alveoli where air exchange should be occurring and enlargement of the distal airspace, it is referred to as emphysema (Fig. 24.2). Measurement of the diffusing capacity for carbon monoxide may help differentiate between these two subtypes (Reuben et al., 2020). Cancer as a cause for the symptoms can be identified on a chest x-ray.

Changes in medications or hospitalization with respiratory support is frequently needed when COPD suddenly worsens. Invasive endotracheal intubation may be needed for those with respiratory acidosis that progresses despite therapy or for those with impaired consciousness. In the older adult, sudden altered mental status may indicate acute hypoxemia or hypercapnia.

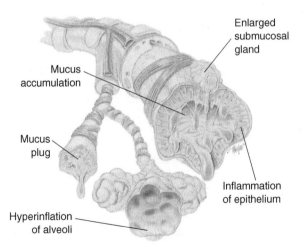

Fig. 24.2 Inflammation and thickening of mucous membrane with accumulation of mucus and pus leading to obstruction characterized by productive cough. (From McCance KL, Huether SE: *Pathophysiology: the biologic basis for disease in adults and children,* ed 7, St Louis, 2014, Mosby. Modified from Des Jardins T, Burton GG: *Clinical manifestations and assessment of respiratory disease,* ed 3, St Louis, 1995, Mosby.)

Although the acute phase (Chapter 22) is usually resolved in 10 days to 2 weeks, lung function may take 4 to 6 weeks to return to baseline, if ever. In the advanced stages the prognosis is very poor. COPD significantly impairs the person's quality of life in multiple ways (Box 24.2).

Recognizing and Analyzing Cues

COPD has a long asymptomatic stage; overt symptoms may not appear until partial lung function already has been irretrievably lost. The most common cues are wheezing; persistent, progressive dyspnea on exertion; and a chronic cough with or without mucus production (Salzman et al., 2021; Reuben et al., 2020). Later signs include prolonged expiration with pursed-lip breathing, a barrel chest, hyperresonance on percussion, fingernail clubbing, use of accessory muscles for breathing, and either pink (emphysema dominant) or pale lips and nail beds (bronchitis dominant). In older adults, weight loss accompanies fatigue and subsequent declines in functional status. Persons with emphysema have little sputum production and appear flushed because they are able to get enough oxygen into the lungs, but it becomes trapped, and exhalation is labored. Persons with chronic bronchitis have chronic thick sputum production, have a frequent cough, and are pale and somewhat cyanotic, due to the hypoxia associated with difficulty getting oxygen into the lungs and reduced air exchange.

COPD is a progressively debilitating condition characterized by periods of worsening of symptoms and functioning between periods of control. Exacerbations are recognized when baseline signs, symptoms, and functional status worsen; they may be insidious or acute, and cues of increasing dyspnea and changes in the volume or color of sputum color are recognizable. It is not unusual for older adults with a history of COPD to have oxygen saturation rates between 90% and 95%; when it drops below this, there is always cause for urgent concern. Rates below 88% are almost always respiratory emergencies, and the person may be advancing to a state of respiratory failure. Worsening orthopnea, paroxysmal nocturnal dyspnea (PND), and respiration rate greater than 30 breaths/min signal an emergent acute illness.

The analysis of cues and prioritization of solutions requires detailed information related to the history of the current illness, especially pertinent to a cough and shortness of breath (SOB). When did it start? How long are the episodes of coughing? Is

TABLE 24.2   The Modified Medical Research Council Dyspnea Scale

Score	Subjective Report of Dyspnea
0	I only get breathless with strenuous exercise.
1	I get short of breath when hurrying on the level or walking up a slight hill.
2	I walk slower than people of the same age on the level because of breathlessness, or I have to stop for breath after walking at my own pace on the level.
3	I stop for breath after walking about 100 yards or after a few minutes on the level.
4	I am too breathless to leave the house or I am breathless when dressing or undressing

From Global Initiative for Chronic Obstructive Lung Disease: *Pocket guide to COPD diagnosis, management, and prevention* (website), 2021. https://goldcopd.org/wp-content/uploads/2020/11/GOLD-2021-POCKET-GUIDE-v1.0-16Nov20_WMV.pdf; Reuben DB, Herr KA, Pacala JT, et al: *Geriatrics at your fingertips*, New York, 2020, American Geriatrics Society.

BOX 24.3   Cues Found in the Physical Assessment of the Older Adult With Chronic Obstructive Pulmonary Disease Used to Prioritize Needs

Presence or absence of cough, dyspnea, sputum production
Diminished or distant breath sounds
Hyperresonance on percussion
Prolonged expiratory phase of respirations
Expiratory wheeze
Barrel chest
Use of accessory muscles while breathing
Pale lips or nail beds

Pharmacological Interventions

There are no pharmacological interventions that can reverse the course of COPD, but medications are available to reduce symptoms and therefore improve health-related quality of life. The choices are based on the presence and intensity of dyspnea, sputum volume and color, airflow limitations, and frequency of exacerbations or hospitalizations. No medical interventions are recommended for persons who are asymptomatic.

When symptoms are present, a stepped approach is used; when any treatment is ineffective it should be discontinued to reduce the risks associated with polypharmacy (Chapter 11). When symptoms are only present intermittently (e.g., when exposed to a toxin), a short-acting beta agonist (e.g., albuterol) and/or antimuscarinic (e.g., Atrovent) is used. A long-acting beta agonist (e.g., Serevent) or an antimuscarinic (e.g., Spiriva) is used when symptoms are persistent. During acute exacerbations, a short course of IV, oral, or inhaled corticosteroids (e.g., Flovent) is used, and an antibiotic such as azithromycin is added if the person is not a current smoker. A mucolytic agent such as guaifenesin can be tried if a chronic, productive cough is present.

Asthma

Asthma is either long term (beginning before 12 years of age) or late onset (beginning after age 40). Long-term asthma is associated with an allergic mechanism and airflow obstruction and is more severe with less reversibility than late-onset asthma, the latter often being related to obesity, tobacco use, and chronic exposure to pollutants. Asthma may be chronic or intermittent following exposure to triggers (Box 24.4). It is characterized by variable and recurring airway hyperresponsiveness, bronchoconstriction, and inflammation (Salzman et al., 2021). Approximately 5% to 10% of older adults have asthma but account for 50% of the associated deaths. Older persons of color with with moderate to severe asthma or uncontrolled asthma are more likely to be hospitalized with COVID-19 (CDC, 2021c). Those

there any associated pain? What seems to make it better, and what makes it worse? Is the person using anything to treat the cough? Is the person smoking (and how much) or exposed to smoke or other respiratory irritants, including those of environmental sources? If the cough is productive, what is the color, texture, and odor of the mucus? Has the color changed? Purulent (green) sputum is a cue suggestive of infection. Does the color change according to the time of day? A darker color in the morning with later clearing is typical of many persons with chronic bronchitis. If the person says, "I don't know what the color is—I swallow it," asking about any change in taste of the sputum is also an indication of worsening from baseline. The Modified Medical Research Council Dyspnea Scale is used to qualify the level of breathlessness, dyspnea, or SOB (Table 24.2).

Early in the disease there may not be any cues apparent in the physical assessment, but these develop as the disease advances (Box 24.3). It is important to be able to clearly differentiate normal age-related changes and those that may be pathological in order to prioritize needs.

BOX 24.4   Triggers for the Development or Worsening of Asthma in Older Adults

Tobacco smoke (cigarettes, pipes, cigars, secondhand smoke)
Cannabis smoke
Outdoor air pollution or allergens
Organic or inorganic occupational dust
Cockroach or dust mites
Pets
Mold
Chemical irritants: smoke from burning grass or wood
Upper respiratory tract infections
Strong odors
Cold air
Gastroesophageal reflux disease (GERD)
Nonsteroidal antiinflammatory drugs (NSAIDs; e.g., Advil)
Beta blockers

Adapted from Centers for Disease Control (CDC): *Common asthma triggers* (website), 2020. www.cdc.gov/asthma/triggers.html

with obstructive sleep apnea (OSA) are at increased risk for asthma, and in turn, those with asthma are at increased risk for OSA (Kong et al., 2017). Those with asthma are at significantly higher risk for lower respiratory tract infections (e.g., pneumonia), prolonged debility, reduced quality of life, and depression.

The development of asthma is influenced by genetics, environment, and lifestyle. The strongest risk factor is exposure to inhaled substances that triggers bronchoconstriction and airway inflammation (Reuben et al., 2020). When long-standing, untreated, or undertreated, the airway walls thicken, and bronchial fibrosis can occur. Repeated exposure to the antigen either desensitizes the person or potentiates a chronic inflammatory response.

Asthma is both underdiagnosed and undertreated in older adults when the symptoms are attributed to normal changes with aging, cardiovascular disease, or are simply labeled "COPD." The person with asthma may have developed a tolerance to the bronchoconstriction and minimizes the reports of symptoms despite the respiratory compromise that is present. Acute or severe exacerbations are closely linked to allergic mechanisms, viral or bacterial infections, with repeated hospitalizations. Those older than age 65 are nine times more likely to die from asthma than the general population. Reducing the number of related deaths from 9.4 per million persons to 8.9 per million is part of the US plan to improve the public's health by 2030 (Office of Disease Prevention and Health Promotion [ODPHP], n.d. a).

The diagnosis of asthma is suspected any time symptoms vary over time and intensity and airflow limitations are measured on spirometry or peak flow meter. Reversibility of the limitation may be demonstrated when symptoms improve following administration of a bronchodilator. About 95% of those with asthma also have allergic rhinitis and subjectively improve with treatment of this (Reuben et al., 2020). More than 50% of those with reversible airway obstruction have both COPD and asthma (Salzman et al., 2021)

Recognizing and Analyzing Cues

The classic signs of asthma are recurrent episodes of wheezing, shortness of breath, and chest tightness brought on by triggers or an infection. Cough is most often the initial symptom in older adults. A dry cough may be dominant in older adults and confused with heart failure, COPD, gastroesophageal reflux disease (GERD), or chronic aspiration (Reuben et al., 2020). The cough may sound identical to that caused by nonsteroidal antiinflammatories, angiotensin-converting enzyme (ACE) inhibitors, or beta blockers. The wheezing is characteristically limited to the expiratory phase of respiration and may increase in intensity during cold weather, exercise, and sleep.

The tolerance of symptoms varies greatly from one person to another. For those with mild to moderate disease, symptoms may be intermittent. In younger adults and children, symptoms are usually worse at night or in the early morning, but this diurnal variation occurs less often in older adults. The frequency of symptoms provides a reliable measure of a person's need for and response to therapy. Day-to-day variations of respiratory function can be measured by home peak flow meters (PFMs) in younger adults, but the readings are less reliable in older

adults due to normal age-related decreases in vital capacity (Reuben et al., 2020).

Pharmacological Interventions

As with COPD, a stepped approach to pharmacological interventions is used and based on the number of symptoms in the previous 4 weeks. When symptoms are only occasionally present, a short-acting beta agonist (SABA; e.g., albuterol) may be all that is needed; alternatively, routine use of an inhaled corticosteroid (ICS) due to the inflammatory nature of the disease may be needed. When this is not adequate and symptoms return with any regularity, a long-acting beta agonist (LABA; e.g., Serevent) or long-acting leukotriene modifier (e.g., Montelukast) with a routine ICS may be needed. A SABA should always be available to use as needed. A LABA cannot be used for acute events. When this regimen is still not adequate (with nonpharmacological interventions—discussed later), a person should be treated by a pulmonologist if at all possible.

Pneumonia

Pneumonia is a fungal, bacterial, or viral lower respiratory tract infection that causes the lung tissue to become inflamed, mucus to thicken, and gas exchange at the alveoli to become difficult or impossible (Table 24.3). Pneumonia is one of the 10 leading causes of death for persons older than age 65 for all racial and ethnic groups and is approximately five times higher in persons at least 65 years old compared to younger adults; 90% of pneumonia-related deaths occur to older adults (Salzman et al., 2021). It is most often associated with COPD exacerbation, influenza or COVID-19, or aspiration of oropharyngeal or gastrointestinal substances.

TABLE 24.3	Symptoms of Pneumonia
Bacterial	**Viral**
Moist cough[a]	Dry cough
Fever[a]	Fever[a]
Sweating	
Shivering	
Loss of appetite	
Headache	Headache
General aches and pains	Muscle pain
Colored sputum (yellow/green, blood-tinged)	
Breathlessness	
Tachypnea	
Chest tightness	
Pleuritic pain (especially on inspiration)	
Weakness	Weakness (high risk of developing bacterial pneumonia)

[a]Not always present in older adults. Data from Saltzman B, Snyderman D, Weissberger M, et al: Chronic lung disease. In Walter LC, Chang A: *CURRENT diagnosis and treatment: geriatrics*, ed 3, New York, 2021, McGraw Hill, pp 373–388.

Pneumonia is classified either as a *community-acquired disease* (CAD) or a *hospital-acquired condition* (HAC) (nosocomial), beginning while a patient is in a hospital or other institutional setting such as a nursing home. The most common cause of nosocomial pneumonia is aspiration of colonized oral secretions or reflux of stomach contents from enteral or oral feeding.

Factors that increase risk for pneumonia include the normal changes of aging and the comorbid conditions of alcoholism, asthma, COPD, or heart disease. Those who live in communal settings or are homeless are particularly susceptible. Dental caries and periodontal disease are common in late life and predispose one to develop pneumonia as a secondary infection. However, many cases of pneumonia either can be prevented or have their lethality lessened by receipt of the two pneumonia immunizations, the COVID-19 immunizations, and annual influenza immunization. Mortality is further reduced by effective, appropriate, and prompt interventions. Decreasing the number of hospital admissions for pneumonia among older adults from 713.9 per 100,000 in 2016 to 645.5 per 100,000 by 2030 is part of the US plan to improve the public's health (ODPDP, n.d. b).

Recognizing and Analyzing Cues

The cues to pneumonia are often incorrectly initially attributed to something else, such as underlying COPD or medications (Table 24.4). The older adult with pneumonia "looks sick" and may have body aches, a fever ($\geq$100°F), rapid respirations (>25 breaths/min), and lower blood pressure (BP). The person is unlikely to have rhinorrhea or a sore throat (Kaysin & Viera, 2016). Atypical signs in later life may include falling, mental status changes or signs of confusion, and general deterioration and may be incorrectly attributed to the appearance of a geriatric syndrome (Chapter 22). An abnormal chest x-ray, fever, and elevated white blood cell count would be expected when bacterial pneumonia is diagnosed, but these signs may be delayed in an older adult. A drop in oxygen saturation, the development of new or purulent sputum, a sudden increase in the volume of expectorant, or unusual dyspnea suddenly can become life-threatening, and if treatment is not started promptly, it may be too late, and death from sepsis can occur. For the best possibility of survival of a frail elder, very prompt intervention is necessary as soon as an infection is determined to be a reasonable explanation for changes (Hope-Gill & Pink, 2017). Detailed algorithms for pneumonia severity are available. Antibiotics usually are indicated in older adults when the *strong possibility* of pneumonia or an acute exacerbation of COPD-associated bronchitis is suspected; to wait for the appearance of the signs and symptoms seen in younger adults puts older adults at unnecessary risk.

USING CLINICAL JUDGMENT TO PROMOTE HEALTHY AGING

As with most chronic conditions, a team approach is needed to maximize the quality of life and functional capacity for persons with respiratory disorders and illnesses. The core team includes the nurses, physician, respiratory therapist, and pharmacist. It also may include a pulmonologist, spiritual advisor, and cultural healer. The team works together with the person and significant others to develop solutions that:

- Maximize independence and minimize disability
- Improve function to the extent possible
- Minimize hospitalizations
- Increase exercise and activity tolerance
- Increase self-esteem and self-care skills
- Maximize quality of life and comfort

The analysis of needs of the older adult with a respiratory disorder is often complicated by the presence of other chronic disorders and side effects from the necessary medications. For those who are very frail or cognitively impaired, actions related to respiratory health are the responsibility of the nurse and other caregivers.

Episodes of acute respiratory illness must be differentiated from congestive heart failure, arrhythmias, pulmonary embolism, or cor pulmonale, so that needs can be prioritized. Caring requires multiple solutions and nursing actions (Box 24.5).

Solutions, Nursing Actions, and Outcomes

Solutions and actions to promote healthy outcomes for the older adult with respiratory disorders include both pharmacological and nonpharmacological approaches, including lifestyle change (see Box 24.5). The critical gerontological nursing actions are to prevent illness and recognize the earliest cues of respiratory infection, worsening of any underlying heart disease, and changes in cognition or functional status.

Prevention

Nurses actively promote healthy aging through prevention of respiratory problems. First and foremost, the person with a respiratory disorder or infection who is a smoker must stop smoking and avoid environments in which there may be exposure to tobacco smoke or other pollutants. For older adults who have smoked for many years, this will be particularly difficult; for those who live in impoverished communities where

TABLE 24.4 **Differentiating Chronic Obstructive Pulmonary Disease (COPD) and Asthma**	
COPD	**Asthma**
Apparent at midlife or later	Most onset <12 years of age
Symptoms slowly progressive	Symptoms vary by day
History of smoking or other exposure	Symptoms worse at night and early morning
	Allergy, rhinitis, and/or eczema common (young life onset)
	Family history
	Obesity (late life onset)

Data from Global Initiative for Chronic Obstructive Lung Disease: *Pocket guide to COPD diagnosis, management, and prevention* (website), 2021. https://goldcopd.org/wp-content/uploads/2020/11/GOLD-2021-POCKET-GUIDE-v1.0-16Nov20_WMV.pdf.

BOX 24.5 Tips for Best Practice

Caring for the Person With Chronic Obstructive Pulmonary Disease

Emotional Support

Accept and encourage expression of emotions.

Be an active listener.

Be cognizant of conversational dyspnea; do not interrupt or cut off conversations.

Education

Teach breathing techniques:

- Pursed-lip breathing
- Diaphragmatic breathing
- Cascade coughing (series)

Teach postural drainage.

Teach about medications: what, why, frequency, amount, side effects, and what to do if side effects occur.

Teach use and care of inhalers, spacers, and equipment.

Teach signs and symptoms of respiratory tract infection.

Teach about sexual activity:

- Sexual function improves with rest.
- Schedule sex around best breathing time of day.
- Use prescribed bronchodilators 20 to 30 minutes before sex.
- Use positions that do not require pressure on the chest or support of the arms.

pollution is common, this may be impossible. Yet without smoking cessation, any treatment will be of limited use and life will be shortened. Nurses may promote or conduct smoking cessation programs. The effectiveness and safety of the use of e-cigarettes as a tool for smoking cessation are unknown (GOLD, 2021).

Nurses participate in community efforts to administer immunizations, especially those against influenza (annual), pneumonia (PCV13 Prevnar and PPSV23 Pneumovax), and COVID-19 There are no Medicare copays or deductibles for these immunizations (Chapter 5). Nurses participate in social activism to reduce health disparities and political activism working with industry leaders and environmental agencies to advocate for clean air. In occupational settings, the nurse can contribute to the health of coworkers by promoting healthy work environments and, in some cases, monitoring patients, residents, and employees for exposure to and adequate treatment of any of the respiratory disorders, especially infections. In doing so, the nurse can decrease the prevalence of respiratory diseases and their associated morbidity and mortality in older adults.

Self-Care

The gerontological nurse works with older adults and their significant others to understand their illnesses and both pharmacological and nonpharmacological self-management strategies. For the person with intermittent symptoms, only a "rescue inhaler" may be necessary: short-acting bronchodilator or beta agonist to enable air to move in and out of the lungs easily. The person should be taught that rescue medications can never be used regularly and that long-acting medications can never be used in acute situations. If rescue medications are needed

regularly, a reevaluation of the nursing actions and medical plan of care is needed to improve control of chronic symptoms, especially activity tolerance.

Inhaled medications may be taken several ways, including via handheld metered-dose inhalers (MDIs), dry-powder inhalers, and electric nebulizers. Correct technique is necessary to derive benefit. Several devices, such as spacers for those with limited manual dexterity or limited ability to hold the breath, are available to facilitate effective drug delivery. All self-administration requires the cognitive ability to follow directions and recognize respiratory distress. For those with limited cognition, nebulizers are usually preferable if tolerated. The nurse helps determine which of these devices has the greatest chance of being used successfully and works with the caregivers (when needed) to help the person who would benefit from their use. In the outpatient setting nurses should review a person's skill and knowledge at each meeting. In the long-term case setting the nurse directly oversees the use of all inhalers and nebulizers. Users must rinse their mouths out thoroughly after inhaling steroids and carefully clean and dry spacers monthly to minimize the risk of a *Candida* infection. Long-acting oral medications, such as Singulair, may be an effective alternative for some.

Frequent hand-washing, avoiding crowded locations, and using a mask when around others with potential infections are highly recommended strategies to reduce risk for infection of any kind.

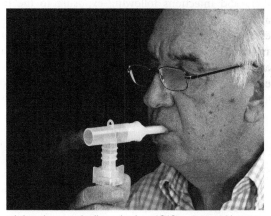

Older adult using a nebulizer device. (©iStock.com/Juanmonino.)

Monitoring respiratory function with a handheld peak flow meter may be somewhat helpful for the person with asthma but is not recommended for those with COPD. Self-care includes knowing about the condition, what triggers exacerbations and how to avoid these, and the urgency of promptly seeking help if any signs of infection develop.

Supplemental Oxygen

For persons with severe resting chronic hypoxemia (≤88% saturation rate), their quality of life and longtime survival are improved with supplemental oxygen. Use of oxygen for 15 hours a day is usually sufficient. Routine oxygen should not be used by persons with stable disease or with only moderate, intermittent desaturation (GOLD, 2021). Persons using oxygen require instruction in equipment use and safety. There are very specific and somewhat complicated Medicare rules regarding insurance coverage (payment) for home oxygen use (Centers for Medicare and Medicaid Services [CMS], 1993). Monitoring oxygen saturation can now be done in the home setting due to the wide availability of devices without a prescription, but their home use is controversial and cannot take the place of professional measures (US Food and Drug Administration [FDA], 2021).

Pulmonary Rehabilitation

Pulmonary rehabilitation programs have been found to improve exercise tolerance and quality of life and to decrease the number of hospitalizations. A multidisciplinary team provides self-care education and support to the patient and significant others. This may include physical and occupational therapy and home health care provided by registered nurses (RNs), advanced practice registered nurses (APRNs), physicians, and hospice team members.

Advance Care Planning

Many chronic respiratory diseases in late life cannot be cured. The nurse is instrumental in facilitating palliative care services when appropriate. Both acutely and chronically ill patients with frequent exacerbations or significantly deteriorated function benefit from advance care planning when culturally permissible (Chapter 4). This planning should include a discussion of how long readmission to acute care hospitals is to be continued and the conditions under which intubation is desired, especially for the patient with end-stage COPD or COVID-19. Nursing actions are based on palliative goals, namely stabilizing the disease, reducing the risk of exacerbations and hospitalizations, promoting maximal functional capacity, and preventing premature disability and death.

KEY CONCEPTS

- Normal age-related changes in the respiratory system include decreased effectiveness of gas exchange and the reduced ability to handle secretions.
- COPD is almost exclusively the result of long-term exposure to tobacco smoke.
- Respiratory diseases are usually worsened by exposure to triggers and infections following exposure to the fungal, viral, or bacterial illness of others.
- The number of infections can be reduced through attention to hand-washing and oral hygiene, avoiding crowds, mask-wearing, and receipt of immunizations.
- The nurse can have a large impact on the quality of life of the older adult with respiratory problems and family members.

- The nurse helps the person learn to promptly recognize cues indicating disease worsening and prioritize the response to them.
- Nursing actions include educating older adults and their caregivers (as needed) about the appropriate use of medications, oxygen, and exercise; the avoidance of triggers; and when to see a health care provider.
- The nurse encourages the person with respiratory disorders to remain as active as possible for as long as possible and to function as fully as possible within the limitations of the disease.

NEXT-GENERATION NCLEX® (NGN) EXAMINATION–STYLE QUESTIONS

One of your assigned patients in the acute care hospital is being prepared for an elective hip replacement due to long-standing arthritis. In your assessment, you recognize that 69-year-old Mrs. Chu seems to become slightly short of breath when she is speaking. This had been attributed to her advanced age and heart disease, even though her heart disease is well controlled. As you gently proceed in your assessment, she admits that she has a cough that seems to "come and go a lot" and that she is no longer doing many of the things she used to do because she is easily fatigued. When you inquire, she tells you that she was a heavy smoker "but that was many years ago."

- Highlight the cues in the paragraph above that can be used to prioritize care for Mrs. Chu.
- Using the table below, identify the highest priority in care for Mrs. Chu prior to her scheduled surgery.

- Using the table below, select three nursing actions that will address the nursing priorities.

Priority in Care	Nursing Actions
Preoperative assessment	Respiratory physical assessment
Determine respiratory status and oxygen needs	History of respiratory health
History of smoking	Inform health care team of findings and analysis
Reduced activity tolerance	Monitor oxygen status

CLINICAL JUDGMENT QUESTIONS AND ACTIVITIES

1. When is it appropriate to discuss end-of-life issues with someone with a respiratory illness?
2. Think about the last place you either worked as a nurse or were assigned to as part of your nursing studies. Discuss any nursing actions that were used in the facility to minimize the development of respiratory infections among patients.

RESEARCH QUESTIONS

1. What are three key reasons that asthma is undiagnosed in older adults?
2. Explore reliable sources to determine if older adults are subject to the development of iatrogenic respiratory tract infections while in an acute care setting. (Hint: The Agency for Healthcare Research and Quality [AHRQ] and CDC websites might be good places to start.) If so, to what extent are older adults affected?

REFERENCES

Centers for Disease Control and Prevention (CDC): *Basics about COPD* (website), 2021a. https://www.cdc.gov/copd/basics-about.html.

Centers for Disease Control and Prevention (CDC): *Data and statistics. COPD death rates in the United States* (website), 2021b. www.cdc.gov/copd/data.html

Centers for Disease Control and Prevention (CDC): *People with moderate to severe asthma* (website), 2021c, www.cdc.gov/coronavirus/2019-ncov/need-extra-precautions/asthma.html

Centers for Medicare and Medicaid Services (CMS): *National coverage determination (NCD) for home use of oxygen (240.2)* (website), 1993. https://www.cms.gov/medicare-coverage-database/view/ncd.aspx?NCDId=169.

Hope-Gill B, Pink K: Nonobstructive lung disease and thoracic tumors. In Fillit HM, Rockwood K, Young J, editors: *Brocklhurst's textbook of geriatric medicine and gerontology*, ed 8, Philadelphia, 2017, Elsevier, pp 371–380.

Global Initiative for Chronic Obstructive Lung Disease (GOLD): *Pocket guide to COPD diagnosis, management, and prevention* (website), 2021. https://goldcopd.org/wp-content/uploads/2020/11/GOLD-2021-POCKET-GUIDE-v1.0-16Nov20_WMV.pdf.

Kaysin A, Viera AJ: Community-acquired pneumonia in adults: diagnosis and management, *AFP* 94(9):698–706, 2016.

Kong DL, Qin Z, Shen H, et al.: Association of obstructive sleep apnea with asthma: a meta-analysis, *Sci Rep* 7(1):4088, 2017.

Meza D, Khuder B, Bailey JI, et al.: Mortality from COVID-19 in patients with COPD: A US study in the N3C data enclave, *Int J Chron Obstruct Pulmon Dis* 16:2323–2326, 2021.

Office of Disease Prevention and Health Promotion (ODPHP): *Reduce asthma deaths—RD-01* (website), n.d. a. https://health.gov/healthypeople/objectives-and-data/browse-objectives/respiratory-disease/reduce-asthma-deaths-rd-01.

Office of Disease Prevention and Health Promotion (ODPHP): Reduce the rate of hospital admissions for pneumonia among older adults—OA-06 (website), n.d. b. https://health.gov/healthypeople/objectives-and-data/browse-objectives/respiratory-disease/reduce-rate-hospital-admissions-pneumonia-among-older-adults-oa-06.

Reuben DB, Herr KA, Pacala JT, et al.: *Geriatrics at your fingertips*, New York, 2020, American Geriatrics Society.

Salzman B, Snyderman D, Weissberger M, et al.: Chronic lung disease. In Walter LC, Chang A, editors: *CURRENT diagnosis and treatment: geriatrics*, ed 3, New York, 2021, McGraw Hill, pp 373–388.

US Food and Drug Administration (FDA): *Pulse oximeter accuracy and limitations: FDA safety communication* (website), 2021. https://www.fda.gov/medical-devices/safety-communications/pulse-oximeter-accuracy-and-limitations-fda-safety-communication.

World Health Organization (WHO): Chronic obstructive pulmonary disease (COPD) (website), 2021. Chronic obstructive pulmonary disease (COPD) (who.int)

Neurocognitive Disorders

Kathleen Jett

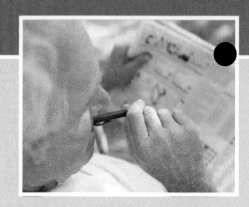

http://evolve.elsevier.com/Touhy/TwdHlthAging

A STUDENT SPEAKS

It is so frustrating taking care of someone who has Parkinson's disease. Some of them just never smile and seem so depressed. I try to be extra cheerful, but it just doesn't seem to make any difference!

Helen, age 20

AN OLDER ADULT SPEAKS

People come up to me and talk to me like they know me. I know I should, but I just can't remember who they are. I think I am losing my mind.

Bob, age 89

LEARNING OBJECTIVES

On completion of this chapter, the reader will be able to:

1. Differentiate Parkinson's disease from Alzheimer's disease and dementia with Lewy bodies.
2. Recognize the cues that indicate the need for neurocognitive testing.
3. Identify the key aspects of the assessment of those with signs of cognitive decline.
4. Describe the recent genomic advances in understanding the mechanisms of neurocognitive disorders.
5. Differentiate the key pharmacological interventions used for persons with neurocognitive disorders.
6. Describe nursing actions to promote healthy aging in persons with neurodegenerative disorders.

Neurocognitive disorders affect older adults more than any other age group. Several are neurodegenerative terminal conditions characterized by progressive declines in physical and neurological functioning. The declines may be barely noticeable in the beginning, with slight exacerbations and remissions, but the ultimate trajectory is always a downward slope. Eventually the impairments become so severe that basic self-care needs cannot be met independently. However, as the disease progresses, interventions are still available to promote the healthiest aging possible for both older adults and their significant others. The three neurocognitive disorders addressed in this chapter are Parkinson's disease (PD), Alzheimer's disease (AD), and dementia with Lewy bodies (DLB); and are neurodegenerative. There are several other neurocognitive disorders (NCDs) of importance that are not necessarily terminal conditions; they are beyond the scope of this chapter but are discussed in Chapter 26 (Box 25.1).

In the fifth edition of the *Diagnostic and Statistical Manual of Mental Disorders,* the term *dementia* was replaced with the phrase *major or minor neurocognitive disorder (NCD)* (American Psychiatric Association [APA], 2013). However, "dementia" is still heard most often in clinical settings and situations, therefore the terms are used interchangeably in this chapter.

Although they rarely occur to persons younger than the age of 60, neurodegenerative disorders are not normal parts of aging. The most common forms are AD, PD, and DLB. AD and DLB are characterized by progressive impairments in memory, thinking, language, judgment, and behavior. Those with DLB begin with cognitive changes and later develop parkinsonian-type symptoms. PD begins with physical changes and most often dementia develops later in the illness.

These three disorders (AD, DLB, PD) are among the major causes of disability and dependence worldwide. According to the World Health Organization (WHO), about 50 million people worldwide are affected by dementia, with nearly 10 million more affected each year, most at least 65 years of age. It is expected that the number will increase to 82 million by 2030 and to 152 million by 2050. Sixty percent to 70% of the persons with dementia have AD, and about 50% of the persons diagnosed with AD have evidence of at least one other NCD as well (Alzheimer's Association [AA], 2021; WHO, 2020). It

---

BOX 25.1   Examples of Other Types of Neurocognitive Disorders

Vascular neurocognitive disorder (also has been referred to as multi-infarct or poststroke dementia)
Mixed dementia
Creutzfeldt-Jakob disease
Frontotemporal disorders
Huntington's disease
Limbic-predominant age-related TDP-43 encephalopathy (LATE)

BOX 25.3   Reversible Conditions Associated With Dementia-Like Symptoms

Depression
Delirium
Side effects of medications
Thyroid disorders
Vitamin deficiencies, especially vitamin D
Excessive alcohol use
Infection

BOX 25.2   Potential Complications of Neurodegenerative Disorders

Pneumonia
Pressure injuries
Abuse or neglect from excess burden to caregiver
Untreated pain
Inability to report symptoms of another health problem
Inability to follow any prescribed treatment plan
Injuries from falls
Untreated depression
Malnutrition or dehydration

---

is estimated that nearly 1 million people in the United States, among all racial and ethnic groups, are affected by PD, 1% at age 60 and 4% at age 80 (National Institute of Environmental Health Sciences [NIEHS], 2021).

For patients in the late stages of a neurodegenerative disease, complications are consistent with any person in later life who is medically fragile (Box 25.2). These include all of the geriatric syndromes, dysphagia, and aspiration. Undernutrition and weight loss that occur even with adequate caloric consumption are indications that the terminal stage is approaching (Chapter 22). Behavioral disturbances are frightening and at times dangerous to the person affected and to those in the immediate environment. These are brought about by both brain damage caused by the illness' and side effects of medications.

The evaluation leading to a diagnosis of a presumed NCD is initiated by the person, significant other, or a health care provider when changes are noted in comparison to a prior state, especially memory loss, physical instability, or bradykinesia (slowed movements). All signs are insidious in onset, delaying diagnosis. People with an undiagnosed cognitive disorder may remark that they are having a "senior moment," when it may be something far more serious than the very slight memory loss of normal aging. Those with undiagnosed PD begin falling or may remark that they are just "slowing down." Those with undiagnosed DLB may report terrifying nightmares.

The diagnostic process begins with the assessment of all potentially reversible causes for the changes (Box 25.3). If one is not found or if the signs remain after treatment, a more expanded comprehensive exam is necessary. This will include all components described in Chapter 9, tests of gait and balance (Chapter 20), and a detailed neurological and psychological

examination using evidence-based instruments (see https://www.alz.org/health-care-professionals/cognitive-tests-patient-assessment.asp#cognitive_screening). It may include imaging or analysis of cerebrospinal fluids and a computed tomography (CT) scan or magnetic resonance imaging (MRI). It is essential that DLB and PD are differentiated from each other due to striking differences in their pharmacological therapy. Nonpharmacological solutions and nursing actions are very similar for each disorder and are addressed in detail in Chapter 26.

The evaluation of people with signs or symptoms of neurodegenerative disorders increases in complexity when the person has other confounding chronic diseases, is very frail, or has sensory limitations. An accurate diagnosis is further complicated if the person is a survivor of a COVID-19 infection with the "brain fog" associated with long-term recovery (Apple et al, 2022; Morley, 2020). A referral to a neuropsychiatrist or memory disorder center may be helpful if there is a question regarding diagnosis. For those with low incomes, in communities with few resources, or living in low- or middle-income countries, expert care, including treatment of reversible conditions, may not be possible.

ALZHEIMER'S DISEASE

First described by Dr. Alois Alzheimer in 1906, persons with neurocognitive dementia due to AD have an increased number of beta-amyloid proteins (plaques) outside the neurons and an accumulation of abnormal tau proteins inside the neurons (neurofibrillary tangles) in the brain, especially the cortical area. As a result, the number of synapses that normally connect the neurons decreases, and the neurons are deprived of nutrients, malfunction, and die. There is progressive brain damage and cell death as the number of beta-amyloid and tau proteins increase. The initial memory loss seen in all persons with AD is the result of damage to the part of the brain where memories are stored. Other brain changes include inflammation, atrophy, and a reduced capacity to metabolize glucose (AA, 2021).

In 2021, an estimated 6.2 million Americans at least 65 years old had been diagnosed with AD, and 72% were at least 75 years old. By 2050, this number is expected to reach 12.7 million but is thought to be an underestimate as the growing number of baby boomers enter their 70s and 80s (Chapter 2). Although there are more women than men with the disease, this appears to be solely due to the relative number of women outliving men at every age.

BOX 25.4 Potential Risk Factors for Cognitive Decline

Nonmodifiable	Modifiable
Advancing age	Physical inactivity
Genetics and family history	Unhealthy eating
History of traumatic brain injury	Lack of cognitive stimulation
Down syndrome	Social isolation
	Poor control of chronic conditions, especially cardiovascular disease and diabetes

---

BOX 25.5 Biomarkers for Alzheimer's Disease

Abnormal levels of beta-amyloid shown on positron emission tomography (PET) scan

Abnormal levels of beta-amyloid found in cerebrospinal fluid (CSF)

Decreased metabolism of glucose shown on PET scan

The strongest risk factors for late-onset AD (recognizable after the age of 65) are age, genetics, and family history. Other risk factors are suspected, some thought to be modifiable, others not (Box 25.4). It is noted that addressing the modifiable risk factors will not prevent ultimate dementia but may delay the development of symptoms.

Age is the most important risk factor. Only 5.3% of those 65 to 74 years of age have been diagnosed with AD, but this increases to 13.8% of those between 75 and 84 years of age, and 34.6% in those 85 years of age and over (AA, 2021). Although it does occur more often the older one becomes, it is not a normal part of aging.

Research has found that genetic risk is associated with the three forms of apolipoprotein E (APOE) found on chromosome 19—APOE-e2, APOE-e3, and APOE-e4. One of the APOEs is inherited from each parent. APOE-e3 is the most common, with at least one present in 50% to 90% of all persons, believed to be a neutral factor, neither increasing nor decreasing risk. The inheritance of APOE-e2 appears to have a protective influence, decreasing risk, while APOE-e4 appears to increase the risk. In a meta-analysis of 20 published studies, 56% of those diagnosed with AD had one copy of APOE-e4 and 11% had two copies. Higher levels of education, intellectually stimulating work at midlife, leisure activities in later life, and a strong social network decreased risk, even among those with APOE-e4. Black Americans with AD are 50% more likely than White Americans to inherit either one or two APOE-e4 genes, but also twice more likely to inherit the protective APOE-e2. Hispanic and Latinx persons of any race and Asian Americans are too diverse to be able to report trends accurately at this time (AA, 2021).

A family history is not necessary for one to develop AD, but those with a parent or sibling with the disease are at higher risk than those without an affected parent or sibling, and the level of risk increases as the number of affected relatives increases. When the disease "runs in families," nongenetic factors are thought to play as important a role as genetics.

Normal age-related cognitive changes include performing timed tasks more slowly; slowed reaction time; and mild memory loss, such as having difficulty recalling a word or name, only to remember it later. A diagnosis of AD requires the following: (1) there has been a decline from a previous level of functioning; (2) the onset was insidious; and (3) there has been gradual regression in cognitive abilities. Of important note is that the changes are "greater than expected for the person's age and educational background." These cognitive changes can be documented with standardized neuropsychological testing (Sink & Yaffe, 2021).

Persons with AD slowly decline over time. In the preclinical period, biomarkers are present indicating that biological or neurological changes are underway, but the cues are unrecognizable. It is now thought that these biomarkers may have been present for 20 years or more (Box 25.5). Later, subjective, mild, and subtle changes in memory and thinking can be recognized, but they do not disturb day-to-day life. This is referred to as mild cognitive impairment (MCI), and about 15% of those with MCI will develop dementia after about 2 years and about 33% within 5 years. Others will regain normal cognitive function, especially when a reversible cause has been found and treated (AA, 2021; Sink & Yaffe, 2021). Finally, dementia due to AD is divided into mild, moderate, or severe disease, reflective of the amount of brain damage and the person's ability to carry out everyday activities (AA, 2021). The length of time spent in each phase depends on age, genetics, sex, and other factors.

Recognizing and Analyzing Cues

The early cues recognized as AD are language difficulties, such as word finding and memory loss, specifically the ability to learn and remember new information. People will say, "I just can't seem to find the right word to say" or "You know, that thing with a handle that you drink coffee out of." Subtle signs of MCI are frequent repetition of stories and questions (Sink & Yaffe, 2021).

BREAKING RESEARCH

A new "type" of AD is being suggested, one in which early in the disease memory is intact but problems in organizing and planning are found, or "progressive dysexecutive syndrome" (Townley et al., 2020).

Early in the disease social skills may be maintained but more complex tasks or decision making are difficult. The nurse may recognize apathy and irritability in up to 70% of people with AD and depression in 30% to 50%. If depression or other mental health problems are identified, treatment of this should begin promptly to prevent the dementia from worsening unnecessarily.

Additional signs and symptoms, such as visuospatial problems and language impairment severe enough to interfere with daily function, develop as other parts of the brain are damaged or destroyed. Up to 50% of those with moderate to advanced AD will develop changes in personality and behavior (behavioral and psychiatric symptoms of dementia [BPSDs]). Especially troublesome are agitation, aggression, restlessness, sleepless-ness, hallucinations, delusions, and paranoia (Boltz, 2021; Sink & Yaffe, 2021).

The progression of cognitive and functional decline is described in detail in the Global Deterioration Scale (Table 25.1) and the Functional Assessment Staging Tool (FAST Scale), both developed and tested by geriatrician Barry Reisberg et al. The FAST Scale can be found via an internet search. These scales have been tested widely and found to be correlated with tangle counts in the brain and scoring on the Mini-Mental State Exam (MMSE; Chapter 9) (Sabbagh et al., 2010). They can be used as tools to provide anticipatory guidance to both the individual and caregivers.

Pharmacological Interventions

Because cure is not possible, pharmacological therapy is aimed at *slowing* cognitive, functional, and behavioral decline and thereby maximizing quality of life for both those with AD and their loved ones. Cholinesterase inhibitors (CIs) are considered first-line treatment and are begun as soon as the person is diagnosed. The effectiveness of the medications varies from person to person, and there are multiple potential side effects. A careful cost-benefit analysis should be done before CIs are used and periodically thereafter.

The CIs work by blocking the breakdown of acetylcholine, a chemical believed to be important for memory and thinking. The most common side effects of the CIs are nausea and diarrhea. Donepezil (Aricept) can be used at all stages; galantamine (Razadyne) and rivastigmine (Exelon) are indicated for mild to moderate neurocognitive decline. The N-methyl-D-aspartate (NMDA) receptor agonist memantine (Namenda) (usually in combination with Aricept) is added as the disease advances. It is important to remind loved ones and caretakers that these medications are not curative, they do not reverse the terminal nature of the disease, and, once stopped, the decline that "would have been" develops quickly.

When there is no precipitating or reversible cause to the BPSDs, antipsychotics are frequently used but are indicated only for those who develop psychotic symptoms and are a danger to themselves or others (Box 25.6). The use of antipsychotics in the person with dementia have been associated with an increased risk for stroke and death as well as serious side effects

TABLE 25.1 The Global Deterioration Scale

Stage	Diagnosis	Signs and Symptoms
1	No dementia seen	No complaints of memory problems or clinical evidence of cognitive deficits or functional decline. Mentally healthy at any age.
2	Subjective memory loss as age-related forgetfulness; subjective cognitive decline	Reports of memory problems, such as misplacing objects or forgetting names. May not be noticeable to others. May persist up to 15 years in otherwise healthy persons.
3	Mild cognitive impairment (MCI)	Evidence of subtle impaired concentration and difficulty with executive function. Changes will eventually be noticeable to others. May be due to other, treatable conditions such as depression or delirium. If associated with advancing dementia, average duration of 7 years.
4	Moderate cognitive decline; mild dementia	Diagnosis of Alzheimer's disease can be made with considerable accuracy. Difficulty managing instrumental activities of daily living. May have difficulty remembering personal history and recent events. Reduced emotional expression (flattened affect) and withdrawal. May exhibit denial of problems. Duration approximately 2 years in otherwise healthy persons.
5	Moderately severe cognitive decline; moderate dementia	Some assistance is needed, such as deciding what clothes to wear consistent with weather or circumstances. Short-term memory loss and lack or orientation to time, place, or date. Some remote memory difficulties. Average duration: 1.5 years in otherwise healthy persons.
6	Severe cognitive decline; moderately severe dementia	Lack of awareness of recent activities and surroundings. Requires increasing assistance with activities of daily living, initially with those which are more complex, such as dressing, but eventually with more basic activities such as toileting. Incontinent of bladder and eventually bowel as well. Misidentifies close family members. Often develops personality and behavior changes in part related to fear and frustration. Average duration: 2.5 years.
7	Very severe cognitive decline; severe dementia	Significant personality and behavior changes. Loss of speech or ability to have a coherent conversation. Progressive difficulty with moving from walking to eventually holding oneself upright. Complete incontinence. Requires assistance at all times for survival. Average duration 1.5 years. If continues to survive, will lose the ability the smile and handle oral secretions. Muscles will become rigid, and contractures are common. Primitive reflexes return, such as those found in young children, e.g., sucking and grasping. This very end stage can be indefinite, until the person dies of other causes, such as pneumonia or heart disease.

Original instrument published by Reisberg B, Ferris SH, de Leon MJ, et al: The Global Deterioration Scale for assessment of primary degenerative dementia, *Am J Psychiatry* 139:1136–1139, 1982. Has now been adapted broadly including that available from the Fisher Center on Alzheimer's Research Foundation under the direction of Dr. Barry Reisberg. The 7 Stages of Alzheimer's Disease I How Alzheimer's Progresses (alzinfo.org)

TABLE 25.2 Regions of the Brain Affected in Dementia With Lewy Bodies (DLB)

Region of the Brain	Processing Affected in DLB
Cerebral Cortex	Information processing, perception, thought, language
Limbic Cortex	Emotions and behavior
Hippocampus	Formation of new memories
Midbrain and basal ganglia	Movement
Brain stem	Sleep and alertness
Parietal lobe	Senses, including smell, differentiating the self from the outside world

From National Institute on Aging: *What is Lewy body dementia?* (website), 2018. https://www.nia.nih.gov/health/what-lewy-body-dementia-causes-symptoms-and-treatments#:~:text=Lewy%20body%20dementia%20(LBD)%20is,movement%2C%20behavior%2C%20and%20mood.

such as dyskinesias (Chapter 11) (Reuben et al., 2020; Sink & Yaffe, 2021).

The antidepressant citalopram (Celexa) has been used for BPSDs; there are fewer side effects, but the effect on BPSDs is not yet conclusive (Boltz, 2021). Mood stabilizers, especially carbamazepine (Tegretol) and valproic acid (Depakote), have shown a small benefit, but these require close laboratory monitoring of dosage and liver function (Sink & Yaffe, 2021). Benzodiazepines are not recommended for any older adult due to increased risk for falls, sedation, and other effects (American Geriatrics Society [AGS], 2019). As with any medication, reevaluation of effectiveness and side effects tolerability should be done at repeated intervals.

DEMENTIA WITH LEWY BODIES

In 1912, a German neurologist discovered abnormal protein deposits that disrupted neural functioning in people with PD. These are now referred to as Lewy bodies. They are made of alpha-synuclein, which play an important role in communication between neurons. In what we refer to as dementia with Lewy bodies (DLB) or Lewy body dementia (LBD), the alpha-synuclein first aggregate (clump together) in the cerebral cortex, basal ganglia, and brainstem, areas of the brain responsible for memory, perception, motor control, and sleep. The damage from the presence of excess Lewy bodies ultimately affects several other parts of the brain and causes brain cell death. The symptoms exhibited are associated with the portion of the brain affected (Table 25.2).

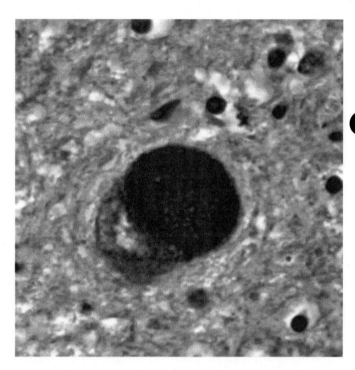

A Lewy Body in the Brain Tissue. (From National Institute on Aging: *What is Lewy body dementia?* (website), 2018. https://www.nia.nih.gov/health/what-lewy-body-dementia-causes-symptoms-and-treatments#:~:text=Lewy%20body%20dementia%20(LBD)%20is,movement%2C%20behavior%2C%20and%20mood.

About 5% of those with dementia have DLB alone; most have it in combination with other NCDs, especially AD (AA, 2021). DLB affects about 1.4 million people ages 50 and older in the United States, but that is thought to be an underestimate. It lasts an average of 5 to 8 years or from 2 to 20 years beyond the recognition of overt symptoms and is slightly more frequent in men (National Institute on Aging [NIA], 2018). It is often confused with PDD but is distinctly different in chronology of symptomatology. In DLB the cognitive changes always precede movement disorders, which *will* occur, and if someone with PD develops dementia, the movement disorders *always* precede cognitive changes should they occur. Sleep disorders and several genes have been linked to the development of DLB, but there is no known cause or cure, and only comfort measures can be offered.

The basic diagnostic evaluation is the same as for AD and PD, including an MRI or a CT scan. Potential biomarkers include reduced dopamine transport demonstrated by single-photon emission computed tomography (SPECT) or positron emission tomography (PET), abnormally low 123 iodine-MIBG myocardial scintigraphy, and a polysomnographic confirmation of rapid eye movement (REM) without atonia. If there is no other explanation for the signs and symptoms, a determination is made of "possible" or "probable" DLB based on the presentation of the core features (Box 25.7). A conclusive diagnosis can be made only through a brain autopsy (Lewy Body Dementia Association [LBDA], 2021).

BOX 25.7 Diagnosis of Dementia With Lewy Bodies

Features	Signs and Symptoms
Core features	Fluctuating cognitive ability
	Variations in attention and alertness
	Recurrent visual hallucinations, detailed
	One or more classic parkinsonian symptoms
	Disordered REM sleep
Supportive features	Significant sensitivity to first-generation antipsychotic medications
	Autonomic dysfunction
	Postural instability
	Repeated falls
	Syncope, transient, unexplained loss of consciousness
Biomarkers	Reduced dopamine transporter (DaT) uptake in basal ganglia demonstrated by SPECT or PET.
	Abnormal (low uptake) 123iodine-MIBG myocardial scintigraphy.
	Polysomnographic confirmation of REM sleep without atonia.

Interpretation:
Probable DLB: Dementia + Two or more core features alone OR one core feature with one or more biomarkers; *Possible DLB*: Dementia + One core feature and no biomarkers OR No core features with at least one biomarker.
PET, Positron emission tomography; *REM*, rapid eye movement; *SPECT*, single-photon emission computed tomography.
From Lewy Body Dementia Association: *Diagnosing and managing Lewy body dementia: a comprehensive guide for health care professionals* (website), 2021. https://www.lbda.org/wp-content/uploads/2020/09/3737-lbda-physicians-book-22dec17.pdf.

Recognizing and Analyzing Cues

Early symptoms of DLB are disordered sleep, visual hallucinations, and visuospatial impairments. The sleep problems may appear long before other signs are recognized by anyone other than the sleep partner. Often the person has a REM sleep behavior disorder (RBD) in which the person physically acts out dreams, talks, thrashes, and even falls out of bed (Chapter 18). Restless legs syndrome may occur during nighttime sleep, only relieved by walking. Insomnia and an increased need for napping are present (NIA, 2018).

Visual hallucinations occur in 80% of those with DLB and may lead to delusions and paranoia, especially with prolonged sleep deprivation (LBDA, 2021). Visuospatial impairments result in problems in judging distance or depth and misidentifying objects. Cognitive impairments with DLB include a severe loss of the ability to think, especially problem solving and using language and numerical concepts. Periods of clarity are interspersed with times when the flow of ideas is illogical (Sink & Yaffee, 2021). Unlike AD, memory problems may not appear until late in the disease.

Like those with PD, depression, apathy, anxiety, and agitation may be present. When the part of the brain controlling the autonomic nervous system is damaged, multiple signs and symptoms are present (see Box 25.8). Most people with DLB

BOX 25.8 Nonmotor Symptoms of Excessive Lewy Bodies (DLB and PD)

Neuropsychiatric
Apathy
Depression

Autonomic Nervous System
Frequent changes in body temperature
Unstable blood pressure, especially orthostatic hypotension
Dizziness
Fainting
Frequent falls
Sensitivity to heat and cold
Sexual dysfunction
Urinary incontinence
Constipation
Syncope and unexplained loss of consciousness

Sleep
Insomnia
Vivid dreams
Excessive daytime sleepiness

Sensory
Lost sense of smell
Pain
Burning
Numbness

Other
Sialorrhea (drooling)
Micrographia (small handwriting)

DLB, Dementia with Lewy bodies; *PD*, Parkinson's disease.

will develop movement disorders at some point, but these are not usually evident in the early stages and are not part of the diagnostic criteria.

Clear differentiation between cognitive declines due to PD and those due to DLB is necessary to avoid inadvertent errors in pharmacological treatment that can result in potentially life-threatening neuroleptic malignant syndrome (NMS; Chapter 11) (LBDA, 2021).

Pharmacological Interventions

Over time, persons with DLB have a wide range of symptoms, resulting in changes in the prioritization of care. CIs are often used for treatment of cognitive and behavioral changes, as they are in AD. Movement problems may be treated with levodopa, as they are in PD. Due to the significant side effects (including hallucinations), the lowest dose is always preferable and can be used only with great caution. When an irreversible cause for behavior changes with psychotic features occurs, an antipsychotic may be used. However, this drug is only indicated when the symptoms (e.g., hallucinations) are disruptive or upsetting or the person or others are in danger. An atypical antipsychotic may be used, especially quetiapine (Seroquel). Clonazepam or trazodone is sometimes used for disordered sleep but increases the risk for sedation, falling, and paradoxical agitation. No other benzodiazepines are recommended (LBDA, 2021).

⚡ SAFETY TIPS

Typical antipsychotics (e.g., Haldol) can never be used in persons with dementia with Lewy bodies because of the very high rate of irreversible adverse side effects and possible death from neuroleptic malignant syndrome (Chapter 11).

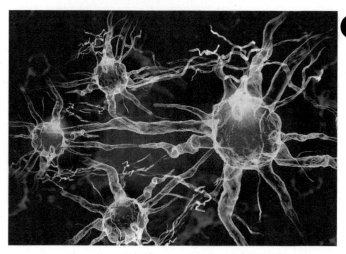

Neurons. (©iStock.com/Sergey Nivens.)

BOX 25.9   Potential Risk Factors for Parkinson's Disease

Increasing age
Exposure to pesticides (especially rotenone and paraquat)
Exposure to air pollution
Traumatic brain injury
Diet: high-temperature meat cooking
Vitamin D deficiency

Data from Chen H, Ritz B: The search for environmental causes of Parkinson's disease: moving forward. *J Parkinsons Dis* 8(Suppl 1):S9–S17, 2018; National Institute of Environmental Health Sciences: *Parkinson's disease* (website), 2021. https://www.nia.nih.gov/health/parkinsons-disease.

PARKINSON'S DISEASE

Parkinson's disease (PD) was first described by James Parkinson in 1817, but the physiological changes to the brain were not identified until 1912 (see Dementia With Lewy Bodies earlier). The accumulation of the protein alpha-synuclein, now referred to as Lewy bodies, is thought to cause damage to the nerve cells that produce the neurotransmitter dopamine and loss of nerve endings that produce norepinephrine (the chemical that controls many autonomic functions). The accumulation of Lewy bodies with PD are found deep in the brain in an area called the substantia nigra. The severity of the illness is associated with the amount of neuron loss. About 50% of the dopamine-producing neurons are lost by the time a person becomes overtly symptomatic (NIEHS, 2021).

The development of PD is thought to be caused by numerous genetic factors combined with environmental triggers and multiple potential risk factors (Box 25.9). Late-onset disease (age 60+) may take decades to develop, and by the time it is recognized, it is too late to decelerate its progression, stop it, or reverse it. Smoking, drinking caffeine, and ibuprofen use may have slight protective effects.

Due to the medical complexity of many in late life, the diagnosis of PD can be very difficult. The accuracy of a diagnosis is improved through a "challenge test"—when symptoms improve dramatically after the administration of the medication levodopa (Galifianakis & Ghazinouri, 2021). Early falls, poor response to levodopa, symmetry of motor symptoms, lack of tremor, and early autonomic dysfunction are more common in other movement disorders or as medication side effects.

Recognizing and Analyzing Cues

Nonmotor signs may develop years before recognition of the motor signs that result in a person being evaluated for PD. They are categorized as neuropsychiatric, autonomic, sleep, and sensory (see Box 25.8). The symptoms present and their intensity vary from person to person; some become severely disabled early in the disease, and others experience only minor motor disturbances until much later. However, the number of symptoms and the degree to which they will affect a person's life and function will always increase over time.

The signs and symptoms that initiate an evaluation for PD are often asymmetrical resting tremor, especially in the arm or hand, and unexplained falls. The classic signs of PD are *resting tremor* (hands, arms, legs, jaw, face), *muscular rigidity, slowed movements* (bradykinesia*), and *impaired balance and coordination*. A resting tremor is the first cue recognizable to others 70%

of the time. It is asymmetrical and rhythmic, is very slight (low amplitude), and disappears briefly during voluntary movement. The arm and hand are most often affected and less often the leg, foot, or head. The tremors are not present during sleep but increase with stress and anxiety.

Muscular rigidity is assessed with passive range of motion of an extremity. Instead of smooth movement, it is "cogwheel" in nature; movement alternates with resistance. Severe muscle cramps may occur in the toes or hands due to lack of free and regular movement. Bradykinesia affects the person's ability to perform fine motor tasks. This early sign may have the most effect on the person's ability to independently perform day-to-day self-care activities. As rigidity and bradykinesia worsen, all the striated muscles in the extremities, trunk, and ocular areas ultimately will be affected, including the muscles of mastication (chewing), deglutition (swallowing), and articulation (speaking). In the later stages, the person blinks infrequently and the face shows little animation, including that of emotion (masked facies).

There are multiple signs of impaired balance and coordination. Downward gaze becomes more difficult, and there is an involuntary flexion of the head and neck, a stooped posture, and postural instability. The characteristic gait consists of very short steps and minimal arm movements (festination). Later in the disease initiating and restarting movement is difficult and referred to as freezing. But once the person moves forward, it is with small steps and a forward lean. Turning is difficult and requires many small steps. If the person becomes unbalanced, correction is very slow and the risk for falling is high (Chapter 20).

Pharmacological Interventions

Currently there is no cure for PD, but when the symptoms interfere with the person's functioning, pharmacological interventions are initiated, and many temporarily provide dramatic relief. Nonpharmacological interventions begin as soon as the person is diagnosed.

Drug therapy is designed to control nonmotor symptoms and replace, mimic, or slow the breakdown of dopamine. Levodopa is the first-line medication and is especially effective in reducing bradykinesia and rigidity. Crossing the blood-brain barrier, it is converted to dopamine in the basal ganglia and therefore increases the amount of dopamine in the brain and inhibits hyperactive cholinergic activity. Carbidopa is usually added to minimize side effects and reduce peripheral breakdown of the levodopa.

⚡ SAFETY TIPS

To maximize effectiveness, levodopa/carbidopa must be taken on an empty stomach (30 to 60 minutes before or 45 to 60 minutes after a meal) and must be given at the same time every day.

Although it can be rapidly effective, levodopa/carbidopa has a number of drug interactions and side effects. Efficacy decreases with long-term use and higher doses are needed more often, increasing the potential for side effects, especially hallucinations. Dopamine agonists such as pramipexole and ropinirole

are sometimes used early in the disease or concurrently with levodopa/carbidopa. These are usually prescribed and monitored by a neurologist.

When medications no longer provide relief from disabling symptoms, some persons elect surgical interventions. A new treatment involves inserting a small tube directly into the small intestine so that a formulation of carbidopa/levodopa can be instilled directly. In deep brain stimulation (DBS), small electrodes are implanted in the brain and stimulate it in such a way that many of the movement-related symptoms stop. The latter is only appropriate in the severest of cases in adults younger than 70 in otherwise good health (Hales, 2016). It is unlikely that these invasive procedures would be appropriate for older adults with multiple comorbidities.

USING CLINICAL JUDGMENTS TO PROMOTE HEALTHY AGING

Everyone, especially those with strong family histories of NCDs, would like to find ways to prevent them. Unfortunately, this is currently not possible. For those with PD and the NCDs due to AD, DLB, and PDD, factors that may somewhat decrease the risk have been proposed (Box 25.10). It is of special note that research related to the effect of preventive strategies is still inconclusive.

BOX 25.10 Tips for Best Practice

Decreasing Potential Risk for Neurocognitive Disorders

Nonmodifiable
Age
Genetics
Family history
History of traumatic brain injury
Down syndrome

Modifiable
Remaining physically and cognitively active
Healthy eating
Higher levels of education
Remaining socially active
Maintaining optimal control of chronic conditions, especially cardiovascular disease and diabetes
Maintaining a blood pressure <120/80 mm Hg
No smoking or smoking cessation
Structural racism
Depression
Medications (especially antiemetics and antipsychotics)

Potential Risk Factors
Excessive alcohol use
Exposure to pollutants or heavy metal intoxication
Critical illness and short-term confusion as seen in COVID-19

Data from Alzheimer's Association: *2021 Alzheimer's disease facts and figures* (website), 2021. https://www.alz.org/media/documents/alzheimers-facts-and-figures.pdf.

Solutions, Nursing Actions, and Outcomes

Most of the potentially preventive strategies and nonpharmacological interventions to promote healthy aging in persons with neurodegenerative disorders involve the nurse working with the individual and those who are either already providing care or will be doing so. To prepare those with PD for anticipated changes in muscular flexibility and balance, tai chi has been found to increase balance skills (Huang et al., 2021). Early comprehensive health assessments, including fall and safety risk, are important to help the caregivers and nursing staff provide the highest quality and most empowering care possible (Chapter 26). The assessments are repeated periodically to monitor changes and make modifications to the nursing actions as needed. In the skilled nursing setting, periodic reassessments are done through the Resident Assessment Instrument (RAI) process (Chapter 9); however, it is just as important in the outpatient setting. This information guides the discussions around end-of-life care, including advance planning for when the point of cognitive incapacity is reached (Chapter 31). This planning includes the creation of a durable power of attorney and a living will.

At any time that the analysis of cues indicates the potential presence of a change, the nurse's priority is to quickly determine if a potentially reversible health problem has developed and ensure that this is addressed. The nurse helps the individual receive the best care possible for any comorbid chronic conditions and in doing so delays premature declines in cognition and function. For example, recent findings from the SPRINT trials indicate that maintaining systemic blood pressure lower than 120 can significantly reduce or delay the onset of MCI (SPRINT MIND Investigators for the SPRINT Research Group, 2019).

Persons with neurodegenerative disorders eventually experience changes in roles and may avoid social situations due to the accompanying signs and symptoms. For those with PD, tremors may produce embarrassing movements such as spilling food when eating in public. Drooling, a common problem with those with PD, is a socially unacceptable "behavior" in some societies. The expressionless face, slowed movement, and soft, monotone speech or aphasias may give the impression of apathy, depression, and disinterest, and therefore others are discouraged from continuing long-time relationships. A sensitive nurse is aware that the visible symptoms produce an undesired façade that may hide an alert and responsive individual who wishes to interact but is trapped in a body or brain that no longer cooperates (Chapter 26).

Nowhere in the care of others is a skilled and caring interprofessional team more essential. It includes a nurse; a neurologist; a physiatrist; speech, occupational, and physical therapists; an ophthalmologist; a rehabilitation specialist; a psychologist; a movement disorders specialist; and the hospice team. It also may include a spiritual advisor or indigenous healer. It always includes the person's significant others, who will be involved in day-to-day care at some point. Ideally it includes a physician and a nurse practitioner working as a primary care team.

Occupational therapists can assist with teaching the person how to use adaptive equipment, such as weighted utensils, nonslip dinnerware, and other self-care aids. Speech therapy is beneficial for dysarthria and dysphagia; patients can be taught facial exercises and swallowing techniques to lower the risk for aspiration-related pneumonia and weight loss.

The nurse has an active role in prevention of complications. The nurse works to prevent skin breakdown and falls and identifies exacerbation of confusion or function, which may indicate the development of a treatable condition such as an infection. As the disease progresses, the nurse is alert for problems with sleep and depression. The nurse helps older adults maintain physical and functional well-being by preventing complications such as weight loss from poor nutrition worsened by swallowing and choking difficulties, skin breakdown and impaired self-esteem from fecal and / or urinary incontinence or immobility, untreated or undertreated pain, infection, and unnecessary fatigue.

When working with persons with neurodegenerative disorders, nursing solutions and actions focus on relieving symptoms, increasing functional ability and decreasing the risk of injury, maximizing quality of life, promoting self-esteem, and preventing excess disability by maintaining independent function for as long as possible. In caring for persons with neurodegenerative disorders, regular pain assessments and appropriate pain management are essential, especially for those with rigidity, contractures, and dystonia (Chapter 29). Persons with any of the NCDs may not be able to express their pain verbally but nonetheless experience it as anyone else would under the same circumstances. The nurse is aware of this and uses alternative means to observe for potential pain (Chapter 29).

The desired outcomes in the care of those with neurodegenerative disorders are (1) appropriate use of available nonpharmacological and pharmacological interventions, (2) prompt treatment of all reversible conditions (e.g., infections), and (3) coordination between all care providers, including family members or partners. The nurse works toward solutions to decrease disparities in dementia care (Box 25.11)

Persons with neurodegenerative disorders watch their own decline over time, which challenges self-esteem. The nurse can direct the person and care partners to formal programs in stress management or group support and urge them to attempt to maintain former relationships (Chapters 32 and 33). The desired outcomes include timely referral for palliative interventions and hospice services to promote quality of life in the face of end-of-life symptoms.

BOX 25.11 Potential Causes of Race and Ethnic Disparities in Dementia Care

Stigma
Awareness and understanding of disease
Ability to obtain a diagnosis, manage disease
Access to care and support services
Uneven representation in research
Cultural beliefs (dementia as a normal part of aging)
Discrimination when care received
Lack of culturally/racially/ethnically congruent providers

From Alzheimer's Association: *2021 Alzheimer's disease facts and figures* (website), 2021. https://www.alz.org/media/documents/alzheimers-facts-and-figures.pdf.

KEY CONCEPTS

- Neurodegenerative conditions are those that have a downward trajectory and for which there is no cure.
- The diagnostic process for any of these conditions is extensive and complex.
- Some of the genes associated with AD have been identified.
- Many persons with PD also develop late-stage dementia.
- A key difference between DLB and PD is the timing of symptoms. DLB begins with cognitive declines, and movement disorders develop later. PD is a movement disorder that may

or may not lead to cognitive declines. Both are classified as Lewy body disorders.
- The core cues to PD include a resting tremor and bradykinesia.
- Treatment of each condition must be individually tailored and will change over time.
- The nurse has a key role in monitoring changes that indicate increased risk for poor outcomes and in developing interventions to maximize quality of life and healthy aging at all points along the wellness continuum.

NEXT-GENERATION NCLEX® (NGN) EXAMINATION–STYLE QUESTIONS

Helen's husband, Sam, had been diagnosed with Alzheimer's disease about 5 years earlier. Most of the time he was completely disoriented, and the nurses caring for him charted Sam as "disoriented × 4" (person, place, time, and situation). However, until very late in his life, he continued to recognize his wife. As the disease progressed, he began to have what the nurses called "behavioral disturbances." He alternated between aggression and affection toward those around him. This was especially painful for his wife. During brief moments of lucidity, he would kiss her and tell her how much he loved her, but moments later would physically hurt her in some way and accuse her of infidelities. After a long and steady decline in cognitive and functional ability, one day he stopped eating and drinking and began to fail rapidly. All knew that death was imminent. His wife tearfully shared that she was glad for Sam that he would soon no longer suffer and also whispered, "And it will also bring an end to my suffering, is that terrible to think that? He was lost to me so long ago."

1. **Highlight the cues that indicate Sam may have DLB instead of, or in addition to, AD.**
2. **How does the prioritization of Sam's care change over time?**

CLINICAL JUDGMENT QUESTIONS AND ACTIVITIES

1. Have a classroom discussion about resources in the community that would be particularly helpful for persons with neurodegenerative disorders and the persons who care for them.
2. Discuss or write a paper about the skills the nurse must have to be able to provide expert care to persons with NCDs of any kind.

RESEARCH QUESTIONS

1. What is the average life expectancy of someone with AD?
2. What areas of the United States have higher and lower rates of neurodegenerative conditions?
3. What might be the cause of this variation?

REFERENCES

Alzheimer's Association (AA): *2021 Alzheimer's disease facts and figures* (website), 2021. https://www.alz.org/media/documents/alzheimers-facts-and-figures.pdf.

American Geriatrics Society (AGS): American Geriatrics Society 2019 updated Beers Criteria for potentially inappropriate medication use in older adults, *J Am Geriatr Soc* 67(4):674–694, 2019 https://www.americangeriatrics.org/media-center/news/older-people-medications-are-common-updated-ags-beers-criteriar-aims-make-sure.

American Psychiatric Association (APA): *Diagnostic and statistical manual of mental disorders*, ed 5, Arlington, VA, 2013, American Psychiatric Association Publishing.

Apple A C, Oddi A, Peluso M J, et al.: Risk factors and abnormal cerebrospinal fluid associate with cognitive symptoms after mild COVID-19, *Annals of Clin and Translational Neurology*, 19 January 2022 Online prior to print.

Bolz M: Dementia: Assessment and care strategies Ex Ed. In Boltz M, editor: *Evidence-based geriatric nursing protocols for best practice*, ed 6, New York, 2021, Springer.

6. Cavazzoni P: FAD's decision to approve new treatment for Alzheimer's disease (website), 6/7/21.

Galifianakis NB, Ghazinouri A: Parkinson disease and essential tremor. In Walter LC, Chang A, editors: *CURRENT diagnosis and treatment: geriatrics*, ed 3, New York, 2021, McGraw Hill, pp 271–279.

Hales K: Who is a candidate for deep brain stimulation surgery?, *Neurology Solutions,* 2016. website https://www.neurologysolutions.com/surgical-therapies/criteria-deep-brain-stimulation-surgery/#:~:text=Criteria%20for%20Deep%20Brain%20Stimulation,those%20who%20have%20troublesome%20dyskinesias.

Huang J, Wang D, Wang J: Clinical evidence of tai chi exercise prescriptions: a systematic review, *Evid Based Complement Alternat Med:*2021, 2021 5558805.

Lewy Body Dementia Association (LBDA): *Diagnosing and managing Lewy body dementia: a comprehensive guide for health care professionals* (website), 2021. https://www.lbda.org/wp-content/uploads/2020/09/3737-lbda-physicians-book-22dec17.pdf.

Morley JE: COVID-19—the long road to recovery, *J Nutr Health Aging* 24(9):917–919, 2020.

National Institute on Aging (NIA): *What is Lewy body dementia?* (website), 2018. https://www.nia.nih.gov/health/what-lewy-body-dementia-causes-symptoms-and-treatments#:~:text=Lewy%20body%20dementia%20(LBD)%20is,movement%2C%20behavior%2C%20and%20mood

National Institute of Environmental Health Sciences (NIEHS): *Parkinson's disease* (website), 2021. https://www.niehs.nih.gov/health/topics/conditions/parkinson/index.cfm.

Reuben D B, Herr K A, Pacala J T, et al.: *Geriatrics at your fingertips*, ed 22, New York, 2020, American Geriatrics Society.

Sabbagh MN, Cooper K, DeLange J, et al.: Functional, global and cognitive decline correlates to accumulation of Alzheimer's pathology in MCI and AD, *Curr Alzheimer Res* 7(4):280–286, 2010.

Sink KM, Yaffee K: Cognitive impairment and dementia. In Walter LC, Chang A, editors: *CURRENT diagnosis and treatment: geriatrics,* ed 3, New York, 2021, McGraw Hill, pp 57–68.

SPRINT MIND Investigators for the SPRINT Research Group: Effect of intensive vs standard blood pressure control on probable dementia: a randomized clinical trial, *JAMA* 321(6):553–561, 2019.

Townley RA, Graff-Radford J, Mantyh WG, et al.: Progressive dysexecutive syndrome due to Alzheimer's disease: a description of 55 cases and comparison to other phenotypes, *Brain Commun* 2(1):1–19, 2020.

World Health Organization (WHO): *Dementia* (website), 2020. https://www.who.int/news-room/fact-sheets/detail/dementia.

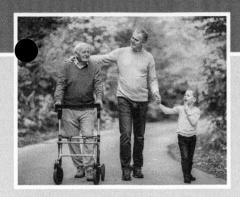

CHAPTER 26

Care of Individuals With Neurocognitive Disorders

Theris A. Touhy, Debra Hain, María Ordóñez

http://evolve.elsevier.com/Touhy/TwdHlthAging

A STUDENT SPEAKS

It is one thing to learn about neurocognitive disorders from a textbook or a lecture; it is something entirely different to care for and interact with individuals who are living with one of these disorders. My first contact as a nursing student with a person living with dementia was during a clinical experience at a skilled nursing facility (SNF) in a unit that had people with moderate to severe dementia. As students, we fed and bathed them, held their hands, and talked to them without any knowledge of whether they understood or even consciously registered any of what was said, or whether their responses were purely instinctual. Nonetheless, we had a caring approach to meeting their physical needs while preserving their dignity. Somehow, I lacked insight into their lives before the SNF and didn't even realize that I had not considered what happens in the community.

Later, as an RN-to-BSN student, I had a completely different engagement when I began my community nursing immersion experience at the Louis and Anne Green Memory and Wellness Center at Florida Atlantic University. There, older adults with concerns about their memory would come to the clinic to undergo a comprehensive geriatric evaluation of their cognitive status, be diagnosed, and obtain recommendations on how to potentially slow the progression of a neurocognitive disorder. Similarly, patients with a diagnosis of dementia would come to the day center as participants to attend cognitively stimulating and socially activating classes aimed at slowing the progression of their dementia and supporting their care partners. The caring wholeness of the center truly inspired me. I learned that there is much more to dementia than what you learn from books or hear from the news. I learned that older adults come with a history that is important to understand and respect. I embraced the concept of coming to know the person while discovering what matters most to the individual and their family. Having this inspiring experience as a student has led to my current position at the Center and my love for older adults living with neurocognitive disorders and their families.

Ismo Hujanen, BSN, RN, age 34

A NURSE SPEAKS
KNOW ME

Know who I am before you tell me what to do
I have history that makes me who I am
I am a daughter
I am a wife, mother, and grandmother, but remember,
I am not a child no matter what I do,
I have a lifetime of memories that may take time to retrieve
So just, take a few minutes to come to know me as the person I have been and will be
Take time to authentically listen and discover what matters most to me
My speech may be jumbled, so I may communicate through my behavior
So look at me; see me for who I am before you silence me with drugs
Know who I am before you care for me

Debra Hain, PhD, written with love of those with dementia whom I have cared for over many years

LEARNING OBJECTIVES

On completion of this chapter, the reader will be able to:

1. Identify the characteristics of delirium and differentiate between delirium, mild and major neurocognitive disorders (NCDs), dementia, and depressive disorders.
2. Recognize and analyze cues to delirium and implement nursing actions for prevention, early identification, and treatment.
3. Describe nursing models of care for individuals with mild and major NCDs.
4. Discuss common care concerns in the care of individuals with major NCDs (communication, behavior, personal care, safety, nutrition) and nursing actions to enhance well-being and quality of life for both individuals and their caregivers.
5. Use clinical judgment to identify and evaluate solutions and nursing actions to provide supportive relationships and environments for individuals with NCDs.

CARING FOR INDIVIDUALS WITH NEUROCOGNITIVE DISORDERS

This chapter focuses on care of older adults living with mild and major neurocognitive disorders (NCDs) and delirium, with an emphasis on nursing actions to enhance well-being. The term *dementia* has been replaced with the terms *mild* and *major neurocognitive disorders* in the fifth edition of *Diagnostic and Statistical Manual of Mental Disorders* (*DSM-5*; American Psychiatric Association [APA], 2013). Since the term *dementia* remains established in the literature, the terms *dementia* and *cognitive impairment* also may be used in this chapter to refer to NCDs. Chapter 25 presents further information about NCDs, including classification, etiology, disease-specific information, and pharmacological treatment. Cognitive functioning and aging are discussed in Chapter 8 and cognitive assessment is discussed in Chapter 9.

Person- and Family-Centered Care

It has been said that prevention is the best and most important treatment for NCDs; however, current research does not provide us with the answers or means to prevent all cases. Therefore the most important aspect of care for an individual after being diagnosed with a NCD is to take a person- and family-centered care approach (this approach is incorporated into all care activities and will be integrated throughout the chapter). Person-centered and person/family-centered care are used interchangeably; however, they always refer to the same concept: caring for the person and family as a whole. Regardless of the circumstances, a diagnosis of an NCD affects not only the person with the diagnosis but also the person's whole support system. It is imperative that the philosophy of person-centered care for individuals with mild and major NCDs guide health promotion strategies in this population, regardless of the stage of dementia.

Person-centered care looks beyond the disease and the tasks we must perform for the person to focus on the person. The focus is not on what we need to do to the person but on the person himself or herself and how to enhance well-being and quality of life. The principles of autonomy, independence, and self-determination are core to person-centered care (Lepore et al., 2017). "The person with dementia is not an object, not a vegetable, not an empty body, not a child, but an adult, who, given support, might exercise choices and respond to a respectful approach" (Woods, 1999, p. 35).

Person-centered care fosters abilities, supports limitations, ensures safety, enhances quality of life, prevents excess disability, and offers hope. The Centers for Medicare and Medicaid Services (CMS) includes person-centered care as one of the six essential themes for nursing home care, regulation, and enforcement. Person-centered care is the foundation for identifying and meeting the needs of individuals through interpersonal relationships that maintain selfhood of the person with a NCD. All older adults with NCDs are deserving of nursing actions aimed toward maintaining or achieving the highest level of physical and cognitive function possible while promoting health and well-being.

NEUROCOGNITIVE DISORDER: DELIRIUM

Although delirium is common in older adults, it often goes unrecognized, which increases the risk of functional decline, mortality, and health care costs. Nurses play a key role in early identification and implementation of interventions aimed at reducing delirium and associated risks. Depression, delirium, and the mild and major NCDs (dementia) are called the *three Ds* of cognitive impairment because they occur frequently in older adults. An estimated 50% of individuals over the age of 65 admitted to hospital settings have either delirium or dementia. These important geriatric syndromes are not a normal consequence of aging, even though the incidence and prevalence are highest in older adults.

Because cognitive and behavioral changes characterize all three Ds, it can be difficult to diagnose delirium, delirium superimposed on mild or major NCDs (dementia) (DSD), or depression (Chapter 30). Depression can cause a change in cognition in the individual with delirium, so it is important to assess for depression. If present, depression should be treated, and the individual should undergo reevaluation of cognitive status once stable. For hospitalized individuals who undergo a change in cognitive status, it is important to assess for delirium, as well as delirium superimposed on an existing cognitive disorder (DSD).

Differences Between Delirium, Dementia (Mild and Major Neurocognitive Disorder), and Depression

Delirium is characterized by an acute or subacute onset, with symptoms developing over a short period of time (usually hours

TABLE 26.1   Differentiating Delirium, Depression, and Dementia (Mild or Moderate NCD)

Characteristic	Delirium	Depression	Dementia
Onset	Sudden, abrupt	Recent, may relate to life change; can be chronic	Insidious, slow, over years and often unrecognized until deficits obvious In vascular dementia will see stair step pattern, so may see sudden change in cognitive function but should always be evaluated
Course over 24 hours	Fluctuating, often worse at night	Fairly stable, may be worse in the morning	Fairly stable, may see changes with stress; some individuals have more symptoms toward nighttime (sundowning); may see sudden change when microvascular infarct occurs in vascular dementia
Consciousness	Reduced	Clear	Clear
Alertness	Increased, decreased, or variable	Normal	Generally normal
Psychomotor activity	Increased, decreased, or mixed Sometimes increased, other times decreased	Variable, agitation or retardation	Normal, may have apraxia or agnosia
Duration	Hours to weeks	Variable and may be chronic	Years
Attention	Disordered, fluctuates	Most often no impairment; however, can see difficulty concentrating	Generally normal but may have trouble focusing
Orientation	Usually impaired, fluctuates	Usually normal; may answer "I don't know" to questions or may not try to answer	Often impaired; may make up answers or answer close to the right thing or may confabulate but try to answer
Speech	Often incoherent, slow, or rapid; may call out repeatedly or repeat the same phrase	May be slow	Difficulty finding word, perseveration
Affect	Variable but may look disturbed, frightened	Flat	Slowed response, may be labile

NCD, Neurocognitive disorder.
Modified from Sendelbach S, Guthrie PF, Schoenfelder DP: Acute confusion/delirium, *J Gerontol Nurs* 35(11):11–18, 2009.

to days). Symptoms tend to fluctuate over the course of the day, often worsening at night. People often experience reduced ability to focus, sustain, or shift attention, which leads to cognitive or perceptual disturbances. Perceptual disturbances often are accompanied by delusional (paranoid) thoughts and behavior and hallucinations. Often the hallucinations relate to seeing deceased family members—for example, the person may report talking with his or her mother.

In contrast to delirium, major and mild NCDs typically have a gradual onset and a slow, steady pattern of decline without alterations in consciousness. These disorders represent serious pathological alterations and require assessment and interventions. However, a change in cognitive function in older adults is often seen as normal and therefore is not investigated. Any change in mental status in an older adult requires a comprehensive geriatric assessment with a strong focus on cognitive function (Chapter 9). Knowledge about cognitive function in aging and appropriate assessment and evaluation are keys to differentiating these three syndromes. Table 26.1 presents the clinical features and the differences in cognitive and behavioral characteristics in delirium, mild and major NCDs, and depression. The accepted criteria for a diagnosis of delirium are presented in the *DSM-5* (APA, 2013).

Etiology

The development of delirium is a result of complex interactions among multiple causes. Delirium results from the interaction of predisposing factors (e.g., vulnerability on the part of the individual due to *predisposing* conditions such as underlying cognitive impairment, functional impairment, depression, acute illness, and sensory impairment) and *precipitating* factors or insults (e.g., medications, procedures, restraints, iatrogenic events, sleep deprivation, bladder catheterization, pain, and environmental factors). For example, an older adult with a preexisting NCD may experience delirium after receiving just a single dose of sleep medication. Although a single factor, such as an infection, can trigger an episode of delirium, several coexisting factors are also likely to be present. A highly vulnerable older individual requires a lesser amount of precipitating factors to develop delirium (Inouye, 2018).

The exact pathophysiological mechanisms involved in the development and progression of delirium remain uncertain. One single cause or mechanism is not likely, but rather emerging evidence supports the theory of complex interaction of biological factors leading to the disruption of neuronal networks (Inouye, 2018). One theory proposes that the development of delirium involves five converging pathways: neuronal aging, neuroinflammation, oxidative stress, neuroendocrine dysregulation, and circadian dysregulation. Additional research is needed to further explain this theory (Blevins, 2021; Maldonado, 2017). The causes of delirium are potentially reversible; therefore early accurate assessment and early identification are critical. Delirium is given many labels: acute confusional state, acute brain syndrome, confusion, reversible dementia, metabolic encephalopathy, and toxic psychosis.

Incidence and Prevalence

Delirium is a prevalent and serious neuropsychiatric syndrome that commonly occurs in older adults across the continuum of care. It is associated with short- and long-term consequences that can negatively influence health outcomes. Among medical inpatients, 20% to 30% of older adults develop delirium at some point during their stay. Up to 80% of patients in the intensive care unit (ICU) develop delirium. Older patients experiencing hip fracture and individuals with cognitive impairment are extremely likely to develop delirium (Blevins, 2021). Delirium may persist among older adults who developed delirium during a hospital stay. In subacute settings, delirium is highly prevalent and persistent, still present on discharge and up to 3 months after discharge (Forsberg, 2017; Shrestha & Fick, 2020). A study in a Korean nursing home found that the incidence of delirium was twice as high as that among patients in ICUs and hospitals (Moon & Park, 2018).

Delirium Superimposed on Dementia (DSD)

Older adults with mild and major NCDs are three to five times more likely to develop delirium; however, delirium is less likely to be recognized and treated as compared to delirium that occurs in those without mild and major NCD. The presence of delirium can accelerate the trajectory of cognitive decline in older adults with preexisting NCD. DSD is associated with high mortality and morbidity among hospitalized older adults. Changes in the mental status of older adults with dementia are often attributed to underlying dementia, or "sundowning," and therefore are not identified or even considered as a possible reason for changes in cognitive function. Despite its prevalence, DSD has not been well investigated, and there is a need for more research on this topic as well as development of protocols for assessment and treatment (Shrestha & Fick, 2020).

Recognition of Delirium

Delirium, one of the most significant geriatric syndromes, is considered a medical emergency. Interestingly, as previously stated, despite a high incidence and prevalence of delirium, it is underrecognized. A comprehensive review of the literature suggests that "nurses are missing key symptoms of delirium and appear to be doing superficial mental status assessments" (Steis & Fick, 2008, p. 47). Delirium in the ICU may be difficult to identify because of sedation and hypoactive disorders.

Other factors contributing to the lack of recognition of delirium among health care professionals include inadequate education about delirium, limited use of formal assessment methods, a view that delirium is not as essential to the patient's well-being in light of more serious medical problem, and ageist

---

BOX 26.1 Resources for Best Practice
Delirium and Dementia

Advance Directive for Dementia: http://www.dementia-directive.org.
American Geriatrics Society: CoCare: HELP program (formerly the Hospital Elder Life Program). https://help.agscocare.org/.
Critical Illness, Brain Dysfunction, and Survivorship (CIDS) Center: Descriptions of ICU stay, delirium experience, https://www.icudelirium.org/patients-and-families/patient-testimonials. Confusion Assessment Method for the ICU (CAM-ICU) instrument, https://www.icudelirium.org/medical-professionals/delirium/monitoring-delirium-in-the-icu.
Delirium Network.org: Family Confusion Assessment Method (FAM-CAM). https://deliriumnetwork.org/wp-content/uploads/2018/05/FAM-CAM.pdf.
Hartford Institute for Geriatric Nursing: Dementia series. https://hign.org/consultgeri/try-this/dementia.
ICU-DIARY.org: Informal network for all health care workers interested in the ICU diary. http://www.icu-diary.org/diary/start.html.
Nursing Home Toolkit: Promoting positive behavioral health. http://www.nursinghometoolkit.com/.
Society of Critical Care Medicine: Clinical practice guidelines for the management of pain, agitation, and delirium in adult patients in the ICU. https://www.sccm.org/Clinical-Resources/Guidelines/Guidelines/Guidelines-for-the-Prevention-and-Management-of-Pa.
VA.gov: Confusion Assessment Method (CAM). https://www.va.gov/covidtraining/docs/The_Confusion_Assessment_Method.pdf.

ICU, Intensive care unit.

---

attitudes. Nurses report stress and anxiety when assigned to patients with delirium, and there is often a lack of resources to support them when caring for a patient with delirium. Care for delirious patients was described by nurses as "emotionally challenging, time consuming, frustrating, and physically exhausting" (Thomas et al., 2021, p. 161).

Failure to recognize delirium, identify the underlying causes, and implement timely interventions contributes to the negative sequelae associated with the condition. Cognitive changes in older adults often are labeled as confusion, frequently accepted as part of normal aging, and rarely questioned. Confusion in a child or younger adult would be recognized as a medical emergency, but confusion in older adults may be accepted as a natural occurrence. Clearly, attitudes about care of older adults and education about delirium assessment, prevention, and treatment are essential to improve care outcomes.

Educational interventions have been shown to improve nurses' knowledge and practice of delirium care (Birge & Aydin, 2017). Nurse-led delirium prevention programs have been effective in increasing awareness of preventive care and in decreasing incident delirium in acute care patients. The delirium prevention bundle consists of an educational intervention, targeted delirium prevention strategies based on CoCare: Help program Box 26.1).

Family caregivers play an important role in the recognition and management of delirium. They often notice early changes in cognition, behavior, or physical functioning and can contrast the individual's baseline with the current status. Delirium prevention among family caregivers of older adults with dementia remains unexplored. Addressing this gap is important because

BOX 26.2   Precipitating Factors for Delirium

- Age greater than 65 years
- Cognitive impairment
- Severe illness or comorbidity burden
- Hearing or vision impairment
- Current hip fracture
- Presence of infection
- Inadequately controlled pain
- Polypharmacy and use of psychotropic medications (benzodiazepines, anticholinergics, antihistamines, antipsychotics)
- Depression
- Alcohol use
- Sleep deprivation or disturbance
- Renal insufficiency
- Aortic procedures
- Anemia
- Hypoxia or hypercarbia
- Poor nutrition
- Dehydration
- Electrolyte abnormalities
- Poor functional status
- Immobilization or limited mobility
- Risk of urinary retention or constipation
- Use of invasive equipment, restraints

From American Geriatrics Society: *Clinical practice guidelines for postoperative delirium in older adults* (website), 2014. https://geriatricscareonline.org/ProductAbstract/american-geriatrics-society-clinical-practice-guideline-for-postoperative-delirium-in-older-adults/CL018.

BOX 26.3   What Causes Delirium?[a]

D	Dementia
E	Electrolytes
L	Lungs, liver, heart, kidney, brain
I	Infection
Rx	Polypharmacy, psychotropics
I	Injury, pain, stress
U	Unfamiliar environment
M	Metabolic

[a]There is usually more than one cause.

family caregivers have valuable insight about subtle changes in cognition (Shrestha & Fick, 2020) (see Research Highlights).

Precipitating Factors for Delirium

The risk of delirium increases with the number of precipitating factors present. The more vulnerable the individual, the greater the risk. There are many predisposing and precipitating factors for delirium (Box 26.2). Identification of high-risk patients, risk factors, early and appropriate evaluation, and continued surveillance are the cornerstones of delirium prevention. Among the most predictive risk factors are immobility, functional deficits, medications, acute illness, infections, alcohol or drug abuse, sensory impairments, malnutrition, dehydration, respiratory insufficiency, surgery, and cognitive impairment. Unrelieved or inadequately treated pain significantly increases the risk of delirium (Schnitker et al., 2020). Invasive equipment, such as nasogastric tubes, intravenous (IV) lines, catheters, and restraints, also contributes to delirium by interfering with the normal feedback mechanisms of the body.

Medications can contribute to delirium, and all medications, particularly those with anticholinergic effects and any new medications, should be considered suspect. The Beers Criteria for potentially inappropriate medication use in older adults is a resource for potential problem medications (American Geriatrics Society [AGS], 2015a). The Beers Criteria list select medications that should be avoided or have the dose adjusted based on an individual's kidney function; this is critical in older adults. Baseline kidney function needs to be evaluated and monitored throughout the hospital stay. Certain high-risk medications should be avoided, if possible; however, it is equally important to start medications when needed. For example, uncontrolled pain can lead to delirium, so starting an analgesic may be the best treatment. A mnemonic representing causes of delirium can be found in Box 26.3.

RESEARCH HIGHLIGHTS

Family Caregivers' Experience of Caring for an Older Adult With Delirium: A Systematic Review

Purpose

To enhance understanding of how family caregivers perceive the experience of caring for an older adult with delirium across care settings and to identify the challenges in recognizing and managing delirium to inform future research and best practices.

Method

A systematic literature review of primary or secondary peer-reviewed articles published between 1987 and 2018 describing the experiences of family caregivers caring for older adults with delirium or delirium superimposed on dementia. A Mixed Method Appraisal Tool was used to evaluate the methodological quality, and a thematic synthesis of results was conducted to extract relevant data as per the aims of the study.

Results

Eighteen articles met the eligibility criteria, and 7 themes emerged in the process. Current challenges and gaps in knowledge of the experience were highlighted.

Data should be useful for informing best practices. A research agenda for future research is proposed. Family caregivers recognize and recall the symptoms of delirium better than the affected persons and the health care professionals caring for them. Family caregivers have limited knowledge about delirium and value information from health care professionals early in the delirium trajectory.

Conclusion

Family caregivers are important partners in the detection and management of delirium and want to be heard and involved in the management of delirium. The impact of caring for an older adult with delirium on the family caregivers should not be overlooked. More research is required to further understand the family caregivers' experience and challenges in order to support them in their caregiving role and to determine their needs and preferences of being involved in the plan of care.

Data from Shrestha P, Fick D: Family caregivers' experience of caring for an older adult with delirium: a systematic review, *Int J Older People Nurs* 15:e12321, 2020.

BOX 26.4 Clinical Subtypes of Delirium

Hypoactive Delirium
- "Quiet or pleasantly confused"
- Reduced activity
- Lack of facial expression
- Passive demeanor
- Lethargy
- Inactivity
- Withdrawn and sluggish state
- Limited, slow, and wavering vocalizations

Hyperactive Delirium
- Excessive alertness
- Easy distractibility
- Increased psychomotor activity
- Hallucinations, delusions
- Agitation and aggressive actions
- Fast or loud speech
- Wandering, nonpurposeful repetitive movement
- Verbal behaviors (yelling, calling out)
- Removing tubes
- Attempting to get out of bed
- Unpredictable fluctuations between hypoactivity and hyperactivity

---

BOX 26.5 Patient Descriptions of Delirium Experiences

Being handcuffed to a railing among criminals in the city jail, fighting to get free and guards standing by to shoot him if he escaped

Children running around without heads; kids with animal heads

Seeing helicopters evacuating patients from an impending tornado, leaving her behind

Blood seeping through holes and cracks in my skin, forming a puddle of red around me

A horror show of people trying to kill her, ants crawling on faces, finding herself on a raft, in a space pod, in the Arctic, in the desert—each with its own terrible narrative

From Amoss M: Treating the trauma of intensive care, *Johns Hopkins Magazine*, 2013, http://hub.jhu.edu/magazine/2013/summer/ptsdintensive-care. Accessed June 2018; Edmunds L: Delirium, *Johns Hopkins Medicine*, 2014, http://www.hopkinsmedicine.org/news/publications/hopkins_medicine_magazine/features/delirium. Accessed June 2018; Hoffman J: Nightmares after the ICU, *The New York Times*, July 22, 2013, http://well.blogs.nytimes.com/2013/07/22/nightmares-after-the-i-c-u. Accessed June 2018.

Clinical Subtypes of Delirium

Delirium is categorized according to the level of alertness and psychomotor activity. The clinical subtypes are hyperactive, hypoactive, and mixed (symptoms of both hypoactive and hyperactive). Box 26.4 presents the characteristics of each of hyperactive and hypoactive delirium. Because of the increased severity of illness and the use of psychoactive medications, hypoactive delirium may be more prevalent in the ICU. Although the negative consequences of hyperactive delirium are serious, the hypoactive subtype may be missed more often and is associated with a worse prognosis because of the development of complications such as aspiration, pulmonary embolism, pressure ulcers, and pneumonia.

Consequences of Delirium

Delirium is a terrifying experience for the individual, the family, and significant others, and people often think the individual is "going crazy." Delirium is associated with increased length of hospital stay and hospital readmissions; increased services after discharge; and increased morbidity, mortality, institutionalization, and illness severity (Shrestha & Fick, 2020). Posttraumatic stress disorder (PTSD) symptoms (nightmares, flashbacks, memories, and dreams that individuals were unable to comprehend), although often not recognized, may occur in adults with delirium (Battle et al., 2017) (Chapter 30) (Box 26.5). Resources on delirium, including video descriptions of delirium by patients, can be found in Box 26.1.

Although the majority of hospital inpatients recover fully from delirium, a substantial minority will never recover or recover only partially. Each episode of delirium increases the vulnerability of the brain, which further enhances the risk of dementia (Inouye, 2018). A growing body of research suggests that recovery from delirium is complex and incomplete without the timely identification in older adults with and without prior cognitive impairment. Some individuals never regain their baseline mental status and delirium increases the risk for the development of dementia as well as DSD. Further research is needed to determine the reasons for the long-term poor outcomes, whether characteristics of the delirium itself (subtype or duration) influence prognosis, and how the long-term effects might be decreased.

⚡ SAFETY TIP

Older adults with risk factors for delirium should be screened for delirium upon admission to the hospital, when transitioning from one area of care to another, and before discharge to other care settings or home. If experiencing symptoms of delirium, conduct a comprehensive geriatric assessment with a particular focus on cognitive status and potential reversible causes of delirium. Older adults who do not recover may have an underlying health condition (i.e., persistent physical illness, medication toxicity, frailty) that may affect their cognitive status.

USING CLINICAL JUDGMENT TO PROMOTE HEALTHY AGING: DELIRIUM PREVENTION AND TREATMENT

Recognizing and Analyzing Cues

Prevention of delirium is the first step in caring for vulnerable older adults who are at risk of delirium. An awareness and identification of the risk factors for delirium and a formal assessment for delirium are the first-line interventions for prevention. Delirium has been called a critical vital sign of cognitive health, and assessment should be given the same attention as other vital signs (Fick, 2018). Nurses play a pivotal role in the identification of delirium, and early intervention increases the chance for positive health outcomes.

Evaluation begins with a thorough history and identification of key diagnostic features. Several instruments can be used to assess the presence and severity of delirium. To detect changes, it is very important to determine the person's baseline cognitive status. If the person cannot tell you this, family members or other caregivers who are with the older adult can be asked to provide this information. Family members and other caregivers know the person well and will notice subtle changes in behavior. They can give information about whether these behaviors are usual for this person and, if not, when they first appeared.

If the patient is alone, the responsible party or the institution transferring the patient can provide this information by phone. Determining baseline cognitive function is essential. Do not assume that the person's current mental status represents the usual state, and do not attribute altered mental status to age alone or assume that dementia is present. All older adults, regardless of their current cognitive function, should have a formal assessment of cognition as well as screening for delirium with valid and reliable instruments to identify possible delirium when admitted to the hospital.

Several delirium-specific assessment instruments are available, such as the Confusion Assessment Method (CAM; Inouye et al., 1990) (see Box 26.1) and the Neelon and Champagne Confusion Scale (NEECHAM; Neelon et al., 1996). The CAM is the most widely used instrument and is supported by the best evidence. It identifies the key features of delirium: acute onset and fluctuating course, inattention, disorganized thinking, and altered level of consciousness. Many acute care settings have made the CAM a part of the electronic medical record.

The CAM-ICU is another instrument specifically designed to assess delirium in an intensive care population and has been validated for use in critically ill, nonverbal patients who are on mechanical ventilation (Ely et al., 2001; Rigney, 2006). The Family Confusion Assessment Method (FAM-CAM; Mailhot et al., 2020) shows qualities that are important in emergency department (ED) settings for identification of delirium. The FAM-CAM can be used as part of a systematic screening strategy in the ED in which family assessments could supplement health care professionals' assessments (see Box 26.1).

Delirium often has a fluctuating course and can be difficult to recognize, so assessment must be ongoing and include multiple data sources. Once an individual is identified as having delirium, reassessment should be conducted on every shift. Documenting specific objective indicators of alterations in mental status rather than using the global, nonspecific term *confusion* will lead to more appropriate prevention, detection, and management of delirium and its negative consequences. Findings from assessment using a validated instrument are combined with nursing observation and assessment, chart review, and physiological findings such as laboratory studies.

Solutions, Nursing Actions, and Outcomes

Because the etiology of delirium is multifactorial, interventions that are multicomponent and address more than one risk factor are more likely to be effective. There is strong evidence that multicomponent interventions can prevent delirium in both medical and surgical settings and less robust evidence that they

---

BOX 26.6   Clinical Exemplar: Delirium

Mr. M., an 81-year-old male, was admitted to an acute care facility 2 days ago because of a change in his behavior. The admitting diagnoses were dehydration and acute kidney injury. Suddenly one day he became agitated and yelled loudly. The nurse caring for him was busy with an unstable patient in the next bed, therefore her first response was to medicate Mr. M. with an antianxiety medication. The clinical practice specialist just happened to be present and recalled the risks for delirium and that nonpharmacological approaches were best. She quickly suggested to the nurse: "Let's move him out of this room to a quieter area." This simple change in environment was effective in reducing Mr. M.'s agitation, and for the next few days before discharge he remained calm. This exemplar demonstrates the importance of working together to reduce the use of pharmacological interventions in individuals with delirium.

Candice Hickman, MSN, RN, Clinical Practice Specialist

---

can reduce the severity of delirium. Early engagement of the interdisciplinary team in assessment of risk factors as soon as the patient is admitted is key to a successful delirium prevention program (Oberai et al., 2018). Continued research is necessary to evaluate what type of approach has the most beneficial effect in different clinical settings.

Nonpharmacological Approaches

A well-researched program of delirium prevention in the acute care setting, the AGS CoCare: HELP program (formerly Hospital Elder Life Program [HELP]; Inouye et al., 1999) focuses on managing six risk factors for delirium: cognitive impairment, sleep deprivation, immobility, visual impairments, hearing impairments, and dehydration. An interprofessional team of geriatric specialists, including nurses, takes a multifaceted approach to maintain cognitive and physical function for high-risk older adults, maximize independence at discharge, assist with transitions, and prevent unnecessary readmissions. Trained volunteers are also used in the program.

The Family-HELP program is an adaptation and extension of the original HELP program and educates family caregivers in selected protocols (e.g., orientation, therapeutic activities, vision, hearing). Initial research demonstrates that active engagement of family caregivers in preventive interventions for delirium is feasible and supports a culture of family-oriented care.

Most of the interventions in the HELP programs can be considered quite simple and part of good nursing care (Box 26.6). Interventions include offering herbal tea or warm milk instead of sleeping medications, keeping the ward quiet at night by using vibrating beepers instead of paging systems, removing catheters and other devices that hamper movement as soon as possible, encouraging mobilization, assessing and managing pain, and correcting hearing and vision deficits. Fall risk–reduction interventions—such as bed and chair alarms, low beds, reclining chairs, volunteers to sit with restless patients, and keeping routines as normal as possible with consistent caregivers—are other examples. Box 26.7 presents suggested nursing actions for the prevention of delirium.

The use of an intensive care diary has been shown to assist patients to make sense of their experience of delirium and

BOX 26.7   Tips for Best Practice
Prevention of Delirium

- Sensory enhancement (ensuring eyeglasses, hearing aids, listening amplifiers)
- Mobility enhancement (ambulating at least twice a day if possible)
- Bedside presence of a family member whenever possible
- Cognitive orientation and therapeutic activities (tailored to the individual)
- Pain management
- Cognitive stimulation (if possible, tailored to individual's interests and mental status)
- Simple communication standards and approaches to prevent escalation of behaviors
- Nutritional and fluid repletion enhancement
- Sleep enhancement (sleep hygiene, nonpharmacological sleep protocol)
- Medication review and appropriate medication management
- Adequate oxygenation
- Prevention of constipation
- Minimize the use of invasive medical devices, restraints, or immobilizing devices
- Pay attention to environmental noise, light, temperature
- Normalize the environment (provide familiar items, routines, clocks, calendars)
- Minimize the number of room changes and interfacility transfers

Adapted from American College of Surgeons NSQIP & American Geriatrics Society: *Optimal perioperative management of the geriatric patient* (website), 2016. https://www.facs.org/~/media/files/quality%20 programs/geriatric/acs%20nsqip%20geriatric%202016%20guidelines. ashx; American Geriatrics Society: *Clinical practice guidelines for postoperative delirium in older adults* (website), 2014. http://www. sciencedirect.com/science/article/pii/S1072751514017931.

improve communication with their families about their experiences. The practice of writing a diary has been widely used in European countries, especially those in Scandinavia, since the 1970s as a low-cost technology to improve quality of life after critical illness. ICU diaries are being implemented and evaluated in the United States, and the use of diaries may be a simple and practical nursing intervention that could reduce the level of PTSD-related symptoms for patients and relatives after critical illness (Blair et al., 2017). Entries in the diary are made by nurses and also by relatives during the patient's stay. The diary is written directly to the patient in everyday language using an empathetic and reflective style and therapeutic communication. It contains daily entries on the current status of the patient and descriptions of situations and surroundings in which the patient might find recognition. The text is often supported by photos (see Box 26.1).

Pharmacological Approaches

Pharmacological interventions to treat the symptoms of delirium may be necessary for patients who are in danger of harming themselves or others, or if nonpharmacological interventions are not effective. However, pharmacological interventions should be viewed as one approach in a multicomponent program of prevention and treatment and should not replace thoughtful and careful evaluation and management of the underlying causes of delirium. Research on the pharmacological management of delirium is limited, but with increased understanding of the neuropathogenesis of delirium, drug therapy may become more important.

Antipsychotic drugs are routinely used to treat delirium even though the US Food and Drug Administration has not approved their use for treating this condition. A systematic review and meta-analysis evaluating the effectiveness of antipsychotics for the prevention or treatment of delirium concluded that current evidence does not support the use of these medications and does not reduce delirium or improve other outcomes. Limited use of antipsychotics may be considered if the patients have hyperactive delirium that puts them or others at risk of injury or harm and all other nonpharmacological approaches have failed. If these drugs are used, they should be given for the shortest possible duration (Singu et al., 2020).

The Society of Critical Care Medicine (2018) created guidelines on clinical practice for adult patients in the ICU regarding pain, agitation, and delirium (see Box 26.1). These guidelines place great emphasis on the use of valid and reliable tools for assessment of (1) pain, agitation and sedation, and delirium in patients in the ICU; (2) the use of an interprofessional team approach; (3) avoidance of oversedation; (4) encouragement of more active participation in spontaneous awakening and breathing trials; (5) early mobilization programs; (6) pain management; and (7) environmental strategies to preserve sleep-wake cycles.

Caring for patients with delirium can be a challenging experience, since the individual has difficulty communicating and may demonstrate disturbing behaviors, such as pulling out IV lines or attempting to get out of bed, disrupt medical treatment, and compromise their own safety or that of others. It is essential that nurses realize that any behavior is an attempt to communicate something and express needs, so it is important to implement strategies to address these unmet needs while maintaining safety. Older adults experiencing delirium feel frightened and may have a sense of lost control of their lives. The calmer and more reassuring the nurse is, the safer the patient will feel.

BOX 26.8   Tips for Best Practice
Communicating With a Person Experiencing Delirium

- Know the person's past patterns.
- Look at nonverbal signs, such as tone of voice, facial expressions, and gestures.
- Speak slowly.
- Be calm and patient.
- Face the person and keep eye contact; get to the level of the person rather than standing over him or her.
- Explain all actions.
- Smile.
- Use simple, familiar words.
- Repeat as needed and allow adequate time for response.
- Reorient the person repeatedly.
- Tell the person what you want them to do rather than what you do not want them to do.
- Give one-step directions; use gestures and demonstration to augment words.
- Reassure the person's safety.
- Keep caregivers consistent.
- Assume that communication and behavior are meaningful and an attempt to tell us something or express needs.
- Do not assume that the person is unable to understand or has dementia.

Box 26.8 presents some communication strategies that are helpful in caring for individuals experiencing delirium.

CARE OF INDIVIDUALS WITH NEUROCOGNITIVE DISORDERS

Nurses provide direct care for people with NCDs in the community, hospitals, and long-term care facilities. They also work with families and staff, teaching best-practice approaches to care and providing education and support. With the rising incidence of NCDs, nurses will play an even larger role in the design and implementation of person-centered care and the provision of education, counseling, and supportive services to individuals with NCDs and their caregivers. The overriding goals in caring for older adults with NCDs are to maintain function and prevent excess disability, structure the environment and relationships to maintain stability, compensate for the losses associated with the disease, and create a therapeutic milieu that nurtures the personhood of the individual and maintains well-being and quality of life. Special skills and attitudes are required to nurse the person with dementia, and caring is paramount. It is not an area of nursing that "just anyone can do" (Splete, 2008, p. 11). The overarching principles of person-centered care of individuals with NCDs are presented in Box 26.9.

Models of Care for Individuals With NCDs

Beginning at the time of diagnosis and continuing through the course of the disease, individuals with NCDs and their caregivers require ongoing assessment and monitoring of disease progression and response to therapy. Needs change as the disease progresses, and "what matters most at any particular time in the course of the patient's experience will change as the disease progresses, the person's perspective changes, and challenges occur

that may threaten equilibrium and/or provide opportunities for growth" (Molony et al., 2018, p. S37). Assessment should occur at least every 6 to 12 months or any time there is a change in behavior or increase in the rate of decline. In long-term care facilities, frequency of assessment is guided by regulations. Medicare now provides reimbursement for a clinical visit that includes a multidimensional assessment and comprehensive care plan for individuals with a documented cognitive impairment.

The focus of assessment is to support strengths and abilities while supporting losses and limitations to enhance the ability of the individual and the caregiver to "live fully with dementia" (Molony et al., 2018, p. S36). The perspective of the individual living with a NCD should be a priority, and the individual should be involved in all discussions to the extent possible. Ongoing assessment of the individual's ability to comprehend benefits and harm of treatment options is essential when making decisions related to health care or obtaining informed consent.

Strong interprofessional collaboration is important to high-quality care of individuals with NCDs. Comprehensive nurse practitioner dementia care co-management has shown positive outcomes, including reduced ED visits, shortened hospital length of stays, increased hospice use, and delayed admission to long-term care (Jennings et al., 2019). Establishing a person/family and care provider partnership allows for shared power and shared decision making among the individual, family, and interprofessional team. In this model of care, individuals and their families are recognized as experts on their lives, wishes and preferences for care are honored, and providers are seen as experts in dementia care. Together they establish realistic and attainable goals and a plan of care that respects all parties involved.

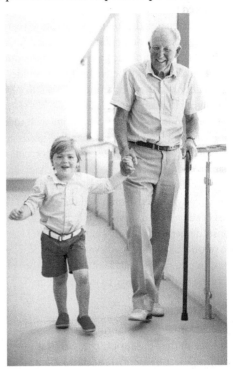

Maintaining function and preventing unnecessary decline are important. (©iStock.com/Squaredpixels.)

Differing Needs in Younger-Onset Dementia and Mild Neurocognitive Disorder

Although the focus of this chapter is on care concerns of individuals with major NCDs, it is important to note that the concerns of individuals and their caregivers living with younger-onset dementia (onset before 65 years of age), mild NCD, and early stages of major NCD are quite different. To date, the preponderance of research and intervention programs has been directed toward persons and their families living with major NCDs and has focused on preparing caregivers to cope with issues such as behavior problems, incontinence, help with activities of daily living (ADLs), and nursing home placement. Many of these issues are not relevant to those with younger-onset dementia and mild NCD, therefore they will not be of interest to them and can even be frightening and misleading.

A significant number of individuals are diagnosed with dementia earlier in their lives, even as young as in their 30s and 40s. According to the Alzheimer's Association (2021b), up to 5% of Americans living with Alzheimer's disease belong to that group. Therefore the current language guidelines suggest using the term *younger-onset dementia* instead of the previously used *early-onset dementia,* since it could be confused with early stages of symptoms of dementia at any age. Individuals with younger-onset dementia report difficulties both in the process of receiving a diagnosis and afterward. Diagnosis felt "unexpected, out of time (too young to have dementia), and led to changes in self-identity, powerlessness, social exclusion, loss of meaningful activity, and changes in relationships" (Greenwood & Smith, 2016, p. 102).

The individual diagnosed with younger-onset dementia may have dependent children at home and still be employed. The person may be forced to retire and experience a loss of income, work roles, and related benefits during prime working years. Most services for individuals with dementia are designed for older adults and do not meet the specific needs of younger individuals. Younger individuals are likely to be in better health than older adults, and meeting the safety needs of someone who is still physically able can be challenging (Sakamoto et al., 2017).

Areas of concern for caregivers of persons with mild NCD and early-stage NCD center less on personal care needs and more on communication, behavior, and relationships. Interventions that help both the person and the caregiver to deal with changing roles, stress, frustration, loss, communication difficulties, and the couple relationship are particularly needed. Continued research and development of programs of support and services for individuals with mild NCD, younger-onset dementia, and early-stage major NCD and their caregivers are a priority, as is continued evaluation of the effectiveness of interventions in practice. Research must include the voices of those experiencing the health challenge of living with an NCD.

End-of-Life Discussions

Meaningful advance care planning usually is not addressed until far too late in the course of the illness. It is not common for health care providers to inform individuals and families about end-stage dementia and the need to make wishes and preferences for care early in the disease trajectory while the individual can express desires. Health care professionals need to provide education, explore values and preferences, and facilitate end-of-life planning. The individual and the family will need information, honest communication, and ongoing support as they think about these important decisions. Although in its early stages, the palliative care movement has gained momentum as health care professionals recognize the value of palliative care in this population. Palliative care should be considered when a person is diagnosed so that there is a skilled and competent team of experts supporting the individual with NCD and the family along the disease trajectory.

Palliative care occurs on a spectrum from the beginning of a life-limiting illness where care needs may not be substantial to later in the disease trajectory where care needs are the greatest and the person meets eligibility for hospice care. Palliative care is focused on symptom management; comfort care; and psychological, social, and spiritual support. In addition, bereavement support is available for the caregivers when the individual with a NCD dies (Chapter 34). There is ample evidence that individuals with end-stage dementia receive suboptimal end-of-life care and often experience unrelieved suffering that not only deprives the patient and family of compassionate end-of-life care but also can result in overly aggressive treatments. "Health care surrogates and clinicians struggle with decision making and are often unsure whether the care they provide is what the individual would want" (Gaster et al., 2017, p. 2175).

Comprehensive dementia care management programs had high engagement in advance care planning, high rates of hospice use, and low acute care use in the last 6 months of life. However, despite the known benefits of engaging persons with dementia and their caregivers in end-of-life discussions, only a minority participate in end-of-life advance care planning or receive palliative care in community settings (Jennings et al., 2019).

Standard advance directives may not be helpful for individuals with dementia, since they typically address what the individual would want if death were imminent or there is a permanent coma state. "Dementia is a chronic, life-limiting disease with a variable trajectory. Dementia progresses slowly over many years and leaves people with a long time-frame of diminishing cognitive function and loss of ability to guide their own care" (Gaster et al., 2017, p. 2175). An advance directive for dementia that addresses the differing needs at varying stages of dementia may be a document that individuals could complete before they develop signs of dementia and could be used as a supplement to a standard advance directive form (Gaster et al., 2017) (see Box 26.1).

CARE CONCERNS FOR PATIENTS, FAMILIES, AND STAFF CARING FOR INDIVIDUALS WITH MAJOR NEUROCOGNITIVE DISORDERS

The major care concerns for patients, families, and staff caring for individuals with major NCDs include nutrition, ADLs, maintenance of health and function, safety, communication, behavioral changes, caregiver needs and support, and quality of life. Five common care concerns for individuals with a diagnosis of a major NCD and nursing actions are discussed in the remainder of this chapter: communication, behavior concerns, ADL care, wandering, and nutrition. Caregiving for persons

BOX 26.10   Patient's Descriptions of Communication Difficulties

"I forget words. Sometimes it doesn't mean much and other times it means a great deal. I have learned ways to avoid making mistakes like shaking hands when I don't remember the person's name, joking, looking at their faces for a reaction."

(Hain et al., 2014, p. 85)

"There are a range of things you want to say over and over because I think it was a word that was important to say and I'll forget . . . I hope that what I am saying makes sense."

(Hain et al., 2010, p. 165)

BOX 26.11   Tips for Best Practice

Communicating Effectively With Individuals With Neurocognitive Disorders

Envision a tennis game: The caregiver is like the tennis coach, and whenever the coach plays the ball, he or she seems to be able to put the ball where the person on the other side of the net can return it. The coach also returns the ball in such a way as to keep the rally going; he or she does not return it to score a point or win the match, but rather returns the ball so that the other player is able to reach it and, with encouragement, hit it back over the net again. Similarly, in our communication with people with dementia, our conversation and words must be put into play in such a way such that the person can respond effectively and share thoughts and feelings.

From Kitwood T: *Dementia reconsidered: the person comes first*, Bristol, 1999, Open University Press.

with NCDs is discussed in Chapter 32, and other care concerns, such as falls and incontinence, are discussed in earlier chapters of this book.

COMMUNICATION

The experience of losing cognitive and expressive abilities is both frightening and frustrating. Early in the disease, word finding is difficult (anomia), and remembering the exact facts of a conversation is challenging (Box 26.10). As the disease progresses, memory, speech, and communication also decline. NCDs affect both receptive and expressive communication components and alter the way people speak. Automatic language skills (e.g., hello) are retained for the longest time. The person may wander from the topic of conversation and bring up seemingly unrelated topics, fail to pick up on humor or sarcasm or abstract ideas in conversation, have difficulty finding the right word, easily losing a train of thought, describe familiar objects rather than calling them by name, revert to speaking in a native language, or stop paying attention during long conversations (Alzheimer's Association, 2021a).

Nonverbal and behavioral responses become especially important as a way of communicating as verbal skills become more limited. Verbal output may become less frequent, although the grammar and sounds of the language being spoken remain relatively intact. Even in the later stages of NCD, the individual may understand more than realized and still needs opportunities for interaction and caring communication, both verbal and nonverbal.

Communication is essential to person-centered care. No group of patients is more in need of supportive relationships with skilled, caring health care providers. People with cognitive and communication impairments "depend on their relationship with and trust of others to provide emotional support, solve problems, and coordinate complex activities" (Buckwalter et al., 1995, p. 15). Difficulties with communication may result in suboptimal care for individuals with NCDs. Individuals with communication difficulties show more symptoms of depression, anxiety, restlessness, agitation, and behavior problems (van Manen et al., 2020). Caregivers experience frustration and anxiety when their attempts to communicate with the person who has cognitive limitations are unsuccessful, often resulting in short interactions that are mostly task oriented. Communication with individuals experiencing NCDs requires special skills and patience.

To effectively communicate with a person experiencing a NCD, it is essential to believe that the person is trying to communicate something that is important. It is critical that nurses recognize various ways in which a person may communicate by coming to know the person. The best thing we can do is discover what the person is trying to communicate and intervene according to needs. However jumbled it may seem, the person is attempting to tell us something. It is our responsibility as professionals to understand and know how to respond. The person with an NCD cannot change his or her communication; we must change ours (Box 26.11).

Nurses can overcome barriers to communication by taking a person-centered approach. Such a framework encourages coming to know the person by taking time to find out the individual's story: "Who am I?" In some cases, people are unable to disclose a lifetime of memories, but taking the time to find out their background and making time to be present can contribute to effective communication. Research on a communication intervention in long-term care demonstrated the value of tailored communication plans based on the abilities of the residents with NCDs. The plans included how to communicate with the individual, how the resident communicates with others, and an "about me" section that gives information about the person (birthplace, work, family, interests). The results suggested that the communication intervention had positive effects on residents' quality of living and care providers' mood and perception of burden (McGilton et al., 2017).

Other factors identified as influencing a communication model for nursing staff caring for individuals with NCDs include respect for needs, identity and privacy of people with dementia, a flexible and adapted communication approach, matching language, an appealing location for communication to occur, longer duration of interaction, and music in the surroundings. Further research is needed to develop a comprehensive model of communication in care of individuals with NCDs (van Manen et al., 2020).

Research-Based Strategies for Communicating With Individuals With Neurocognitive Disorders

Classic research conducted by Ruth Tappen of Florida Atlantic University (Boca Raton, FL) et al. (1997, 1999) provided insight into communication strategies that were helpful in creating and maintaining a therapeutic relationship with people with moderate to major NCDs. In these studies, conversations between 23 participants in the middle and late stages of AD and a clinical nurse specialist were analyzed to clarify what type of communication techniques were helpful in creating and maintaining a therapeutic relationship. Findings of this study were compared with recommendations in the literature, and specific communication strategies were developed.

More than 80% of the participants' responses were relevant in the context of the conversation. The research challenged some of the commonly held beliefs about communication with persons with NCDs—for example, avoiding the use of open-ended questions and keeping communication focused only on simple topics, task-oriented topics, and questions that can be answered with yes or no responses.

Findings of the study provided suggestions for specific communication strategies that are effective in various nursing situations and hope for nurses to establish meaningful relationships that nurture the personhood of people with NCDs. Communication strategies differ depending on the purpose of communication (e.g., performing ADLs, encouraging expression of feelings). Approaches to communication must be adapted not only to the person's ability to understand but also to the purpose of the interaction. What is appropriate for assessment may be a barrier to conversation that is designed to facilitate expression of concerns and feelings (Box 26.12).

In the past, structured programs of reality orientation (orienting the person to the day, date, time, year, weather, upcoming birthdays) were often used in long-term care facilities and chronic psychiatric units as a way to stimulate memory. This intervention is still often noted as being of benefit to persons with NCDs. However, structured reality orientation (RO) may place unrealistic expectations on persons with major NCDs and may be distressing if the individual cannot remember these things. Families and professional caregivers often can be heard asking people with NCDs to name relatives, state their birth year, and remember other current facts. One can imagine how upsetting and demoralizing this might be to a person unable to remember.

This does not imply that we should not orient the person to daily activities, time of day, and other important events, but RO should be offered without the expectation that the person will remember. Caregivers can provide orienting information as part of general conversation (e.g., "It's quite warm for December 10, but it will be a beautiful day for our lunch date"). Rather than structured RO, a better approach is to go where the person is in his or her own world rather than trying to bring the person's world into yours. For example, if the individual insists that he or she needs to leave the house to meet the school bus, it is more helpful to ask the individual to talk about the times he or she did this activity rather than inform the person that his or her children are grown and no longer ride the school bus.

Validation therapy, developed by Naomi Feil in the 1980s, involves following the person's lead and responding to feelings expressed rather than interrupting to supply factual data. Communication techniques include using nonthreatening words to establish understanding, rephrasing the person's words,

---

BOX 26.12 Four Useful Strategies for Communicating With Individuals Experiencing Cognitive Impairment

Simplification Strategies

Simplification strategies are useful with activities of daily living:

- Give one-step directions.
- Speak slowly and clearly.
- Allow time for response.
- Reduce distractions.
- Have one-to-one conversations; avoid multiple caregivers interacting at the same time.
- Give clues and cues as to what you want the person to do. Use gestures or pantomime to demonstrate what it is you want the person to do (e.g., put the chair in front of the person, point to it, pat the seat, and say, "Sit here.").

Facilitation Strategies

Facilitation strategies are useful in encouraging expression of thoughts and feelings:

- Establish commonalities.
- Share self.
- Allow the person to choose subjects to discuss.
- Speak as if to an equal.
- Use broad openings, such as "How are you today?"
- Use humor appropriately.
- Follow the person's lead.

Comprehension Strategies

Comprehension strategies are useful in assisting with understanding of communication:

- Identify time confusion (in what time frame is the person operating at the moment?).
- Find the theme (what connection is there between apparently disparate topics?). Recognize an important theme, such as fear, loss, or happiness.
- Recognize the hidden meanings (what did the person mean to say?).

Supportive Strategies

Supportive strategies are useful in encouraging continued communication and supporting personhood:

- Introduce yourself and explain why you are there. Reach out to shake hands and note the response to touch.
- If the person does not want to talk, go away and return later. Do not push or force.
- Sit closely and face the person at eye level.
- Limit corrections.
- Use multiple ways of communicating (gestures, touch).
- Search for meaning in all communication.
- Know the person's past life history and daily life experiences and events.
- Recognize feelings and respond.
- Treat the person with respect and dignity.
- Show interest through body posture, facial expression, nodding, and eye contact. Assume a pleasant, relaxed attitude.
- Attend to vision and hearing losses.
- Do not try to bring the person to the present or use reality orientation. Go to where the person is and enjoy the conversation.
- When leaving, thank the person for their time and attention and information.
- Remember that the quality, not the content or quantity, of the interaction is basic to therapeutic communication.

maintaining eye contact and a gentle tone of voice, responding in general terms when meaning is unclear, and using touch if appropriate. "Although the evidence base for validation therapy is underdeveloped, the concept of honoring the feelings of the person living with dementia has face validity as part of person-centered dementia care" (Scales et al., 2018, p. S95). Helping families and caregivers understand validation therapy can assist in enhancing quality time with their loved ones.

BEHAVIOR CONCERNS AND NURSING MODELS OF CARE

One or more behavioral symptoms appear in up to 90% of individuals with dementia and become more common as the disease progresses (Piirainen et al., 2021). Compared with those who do not have behavioral and psychological symptoms of dementia (BPSDs), these individuals experiencing BPSDs are institutionalized earlier and have poorer ability to complete ADLs, greater cognitive decline, lower quality of life, and increased risk of death. In addition, their caregivers report worse quality of life than do caregivers of patients without BPSDs (Watt et al., 2019).

BPSDs occur in clusters or syndromes identified as psychosis (delusions and hallucinations), agitation, aggression, depression, anxiety, apathy, disinhibition (socially and sexually inappropriate behaviors), motor disturbances, nighttime behaviors, and appetite and eating problems. The most common symptoms are apathy, depression, and anxiety. Symptoms often co-occur, increasing their impact even more. Depression is related to BPSDs, and it is very important to screen for depression in individuals expressing BPSDs. Use of the Cornell Scale for Depression in Dementia (Chapter 9) is recommended. Lifelong psychiatric disorders (Chapter 30) and their management also may affect the development of these symptoms.

BPSDs appear to be a consequence of multiple, but sometimes modifiable, interacting factors. These factors are both external and internal and result in part from heightened vulnerability to the environment as cognitive function declines. Neurodegeneration associated with dementia also plays a role in BPSDs (Molony et al., 2018; Scales et al., 2018). The quality of the interaction between the caregiver and the person living with dementia also influences behavioral symptoms. A scoping review of the evidence on determinants of BPSDs reported the following causes as common across several behavioral symptoms: neurodegeneration, type of dementia, severity of cognitive impairments, declining functional abilities, caregiver burden, poor communication, and boredom (Kolanowski et al., 2017).

BPSDs should be viewed as a form of communication that is meaningful (rather than a problem), an expression of unmet needs, and/or a reflection of lower tolerance for stressors in the physical and psychosocial environment. They are the individual's best attempt to communicate a variety of unmet needs and an expression of distress. BPSDs cause a great deal of distress to the person and the caregivers and contribute to increased financial cost, caregiver burden, and nursing stress; poor quality of life for the person with an NCD and the caregivers; significant declines in function; and risk for physical abuse (Piirainen et al., 2021). They also often precipitate institutionalization (Austrom

---

BOX 26.13 Stressors Triggering BPSDs (PLST Model)

- Fatigue
- Change of environment, routine, or caregiver
- Misleading stimuli or inappropriate stimulus levels
- Internal or external demands to perform beyond abilities
- Physical stressors such as pain, discomfort, acute illness, and depression

BPSDs, Behavioral and psychological symptoms of dementia; *PLST,* Progressively Lowered Stress Threshold.

---

et al., 2018; Kolanowski et al., 2017). If untreated, clinically significant BPSDs are associated with faster disease progression than in the absence of such symptoms.

Several nursing models of care are helpful in recognizing and understanding the behavior of individuals with NCDs and can be used to guide practice and to assist families and staff in providing care from a more person-centered framework. The Progressively Lowered Stress Threshold (PLST) model and the Need-Driven Dementia-Compromised Behavior (NDB) model focus on the close interplay between person, context, and environment. These models propose that behavior is used to communicate or express, in the best way the person has available, unmet needs (physiological, psychosocial, disturbing environment, uncomfortable social surroundings) and/or difficulty managing stress as the disease progresses.

Progressively Lowered Stress Threshold Model

The PLST model (Hall, 1994; Hall & Buckwalter, 1987) was one of the first models used to plan and evaluate care for people with NCDs in every setting. The model suggests that environmental antecedents produce stress, which is met by a coping response that is compromised by the impact of dementia (Scales et al., 2018). Symptoms such as agitation are a result of a progressive loss of the person's ability to cope with demands and stimuli when the person's stress threshold is exceeded. An example is the person who becomes agitated in response to excess noise in the environment (loudspeaker, loud talk). Some stressors that may trigger these symptoms are presented in Box 26.13.

Using this model, care is structured to decrease the stressors and provide a safe and predictable environment. Positive outcomes from use of the model include improved sleep; decreased sedative and tranquilizer use; increased food intake and weight; increased socialization; decreased episodes of aggressive, agitated, and disruptive behaviors; increased caregiver satisfaction with care; and increased functional level (DeYoung et al., 2003; Hall & Buckwalter, 1987). Box 26.14 presents the principles of care derived from the PLST model.

Need-Driven Dementia-Compromised Behavior Model

The NDB model (Algase et al., 2003; Kolanowski, 1999; Richards et al., 2000) is a framework for the study and understanding of behavioral symptoms. All behaviors have meaning and are

---

BOX 26.14 Principles of Care Derived From the PLST Model

1. Maximize functional abilities by supporting all losses in a prosthetic manner.
2. Establish a caring relationship and provide the person with unconditional positive regard.
3. Use patient behaviors indicating anxiety and avoidance to determine appropriate limits of activity and stimuli.
4. Teach caregivers to try to find causes of behavior and to observe and evaluate verbal and nonverbal responses.
5. Identify triggers related to discomfort or stress reactions (factors in the environment, caregiver communication).
6. Modify the environment to support losses and promote safe function.
7. Evaluate care routines and responses on a 24-hour basis and adjust the plan of care accordingly.
8. Provide as much control as possible; encourage self-care, offer choices, explain all actions, do not push or force the person to do something.
9. Keep the environment stable and predictable.
10. Provide ongoing education, support, care, and problem solving for caregivers.

PLST, Progressively Lowered Stress Threshold.
Adapted from Hall GR, Buckwalter KC: Progressively Lowered Stress Threshold: a conceptual model for care of adults with Alzheimer's disease, *Arch Psychiatr Nurs* 1:399–406, 1987.

---

a form of communication, particularly as verbal communication becomes more limited. The NDB model proposes that the behavior of persons with NCDs carries a message of need that can be addressed appropriately if the person's history and habits, physiological status, and physical and social environment are carefully evaluated. Rather than behavior being viewed as disruptive, it is viewed as having meaning and expressing needs. Behavior reflects the interaction of *background* factors (cognitive changes resulting from dementia, gender, ethnicity, culture, education, personality, responses to stress) and *proximal* factors (physiological needs such as hunger or pain, mood, physical environment [e.g., light, noise, temperature]) with the social environment (e.g., staff stability and mix, presence of others).

Optimal care is provided by manipulating the proximal factors that precipitate behavior and by maximizing strengths and minimizing the limitations of the background factors. For instance, sleep disruptions are common in people with an NCD. If the person is not getting adequate sleep at night, agitated or aggressive behavior during the day may signal the need for more rest. Interventions to modify proximal factors interfering with sleep, such as noise, frequent awakenings during the night, and daytime boredom, can help meet the need for rest and sleep and decrease agitation or aggression.

USING CLINICAL JUDGMENT TO PROMOTE HEALTHY AGING: BEHAVIORAL AND PSYCHOLOGICAL SYMPTOMS OF DEMENTIA

Recognizing and Analyzing Cues

Cues to recognizing potential causes of BPSDs vary widely, and the behaviors have many potential causes. Analysis must be

done in the context of the individual's history and situation and consideration of the multiple things that could be happening. The focus must be on understanding that behavioral expressions communicate distress and that the response is to investigate the possible sources of distress and intervene appropriately.

There are many possible reasons for BPSDs. After ruling out medical problems (e.g., pneumonia, dehydration, impaction, infection or sepsis, fractures, pain, depression) as a cause of the behavior, continued evaluation is important to identify why distressing symptoms are occurring. Conditions such as constipation or urinary tract infections can cause great distress for individuals with cognitive impairment and may lead to marked changes in behavior. In a study of community-dwelling older adults with cognitive impairment, 36% had undetected illness associated with BPSDs, making adequate assessment and treatment essential. Side effects of drugs or drug-drug interactions also can contribute to the development of symptoms (Kales et al., 2015).

Pain and discomfort are associated with aggressive behaviors in individuals with NCDs. After careful evaluation of other possible causes of pain or discomfort, treatment with a trial of analgesics should be considered. Treatment of pain is challenging, especially in today's opioid epidemic where providers are often afraid to prescribe these medications. In some circumstances the person is not receiving enough medicine to control the pain and therefore may act out as a result of an inability to express symptoms verbally. It is essential for nurses to discover nonpharmacological approaches to pain and to advocate appropriate pharmacological interventions.

Understanding what triggers behavior is essential for development of interventions that address the individual's unmet need. Fear, discomfort, unfamiliar surroundings and people, illness, fatigue, depression, need for autonomy and control, caregiver approaches, communication strategies, and environmental stressors are frequent precipitants of behavioral symptoms. "For the individual with late-stage dementia, a good deal of their discomfort comes from nonphysiological sources, for example, from difficulty sorting out and negotiating everyday life activities" (Kovach, 1999, p. 412).

The need for socialization and support and stimulation to address boredom also can contribute to changes in behavior. "Lack of meaningful activity is cited by people living with dementia and family members as one of the most persistent and critical unmet needs. The provision of individualized meaningful activities may help prevent or alleviate BPSDs by enhancing quality of life through engagement, enhanced social interaction, and opportunities for self-expression and self-determination" (Scales et al., 2018, p. S96). Box 26.15 presents precipitating factors for BPSDs.

Putting yourself in the place of persons with an NCD and trying to see the world from their eyes will help you understand their behavior. Questions of what, where, why, when, who, and what now are important components of the assessment of behavior. Box 26.16 presents a framework for asking questions about the possible meanings and messages behind observed behavior. Except in late-stage NCD, when verbal communication may be problematic, the perspective of the individual should be elicited to

BOX 26.15   Conditions Precipitating Behavioral Symptoms in Individuals

- Communication deficits
- Pain or discomfort
- Acute medical problems
- Sleep disturbances
- Perceptual deficits
- Depression
- Need for social contact
- Hunger, thirst, need to toilet
- Loss of control
- Misinterpretation of the situation or environment
- Crowded conditions
- Changes in environment or people
- Noise, disruption
- Being forced to do something
- Fear
- Loneliness
- Psychotic symptoms
- Fatigue
- Environmental overstimulation or understimulation
- Depersonalized, rushed care
- Restraints
- Psychoactive drugs

BOX 26.16   Framework for Asking Questions About the Meaning of Behavior

What?

What is being sought? What is happening? Does the behavior have a physical or emotional component or both? What are the person's responses? What would be done if the person was 20 years old instead of 80 years old? What is the behavior saying? What is the emotion being expressed?

Where?

Where is the behavior occurring? What are the environmental triggers?

When?

When does the behavior most frequently occur: after activities of daily living (ADLs), family visits, mealtimes?

Who?

Who is involved? Other residents, caregivers, family?

Why?

What happened before? Poor communication? Tasks too complicated? Physical or medical problem? Person being rushed or forced to do something? Has this happened before and why?

What Now?

Approaches and interventions (physical, psychosocial).
Changes needed and by whom?
Who else might know something about the person or the behavior or approaches?
Communicate to all and include in plan of care.

BOX 26.17   Examples of Behavior and Environmental Modification Strategies for Managing BPSDs

Behavior	Strategy
Hearing voices	Evaluate hearing or adjust amplification of hearing aids.
	Assess quality and severity of symptoms.
	Determine whether the voices present an actual threat to safety or function.
	Assess noise around patient's room (e.g., staff talking in hallway).
Aggression	Determine and modify underlying causes of aggression (e.g., pain, caregiver interaction, being forced to do something).
	Teach caregiver not to confront individual, use distraction, observe facial expression and body posture, leave individual alone if safe, return later for the task (e.g., bathing).
	Create a calmer, more soothing environment.
Repetitive questioning	Respond with a calm, reassuring voice.
	Use calm touch for reassurance.
	Place warm water bottle covered with soft fleece cover on the lap or abdomen.
	Inform individual of events only as they occur.
	Structure daily routines.
	Involve person in meaningful activities.

BPSDs, Behavioral and psychological symptoms of dementia.

Use of a behavioral log or diary over a 2- to 3-day period to track when behaviors occur, the circumstances, and the responses to interventions is recommended and required in nursing facilities. The Behave-AD, the Cohen-Mansfield Agitation Inventory, and the Neuropsychiatric Inventory Nursing Home Version are examples of reliable instruments that can be used in assessment. The WeCareAdvisor (WCA) is a web-based application designed to enable family caregivers to assess, manage, and track BPSDs using nonpharmacological approaches. Testing of the tool is ongoing but use of the WCA seems to be associated with a significant decrease in caregiver stress (Kales et al., 2018). Box 26.17 presents examples of some common behaviors and possible modification strategies.

Solutions, Nursing Actions, and Outcomes

Pharmacological Approaches

All evidence-based guidelines endorse an approach that begins with comprehensive evaluation of the behavior and possible causes followed by the use of nonpharmacological interventions as a first line of treatment except in emergency situations when BPSDs could lead to imminent danger or compromise safety. Medications, including antipsychotics, may be necessary and appropriate for the palliation of patient distress when nonpharmacological interventions fail but must be used judiciously (Kerns et al., 2018).

determine what the person can describe about the situation. It is also important to understand what aspect of the behavior is most problematic or distressing for the individual and the caregiver and design individually tailored interventions (Molony et al., 2018).

Strict federal regulations monitor the use of psychotropic medications in SNFs. Prevalence rates of antipsychotic medication use has significantly declined in nursing homes as a result of several proactive measures (Chapter 6). The CMS has now expanded focus on reduction of other psychotropic medications such as antidepressant, anxiolytic, and hypnotic agents in nursing facilities. However, rates of antipsychotic use among individuals with dementia living in the community are rising. In the United States, 41.4% of adults ages 70 years and older take psychotropic medications (Basnet et al., 2020). Recommendations are to expand the efforts to curb the use of these drugs beyond nursing homes (Marselas, 2018).

Antipsychotic medication use in nursing facilities may be considered after all possible causes of behavior have been investigated; if used, these medications should be given at the lowest possible dosage for the shortest period of time, monitored closely for side effects, and be subject to gradual dose reduction and review. Pharmacological approaches may be considered, in addition to nonpharmacological approaches, if there has been a comprehensive evaluation of reversible causes of behavior, the person presents a danger to self or others, nonpharmacological interventions have not been effective, and the risk-benefit profiles of the medications have been considered. There must be documentation of all care planning related to the individual's behaviors and of use and effectiveness of nonpharmacological interventions.

⚡ SAFETY TIP

Do not use antipsychotics as a first choice to treat behavioral and psychological symptoms of dementia (BPSDs). People with dementia often exhibit aggression, resistance to care, and other challenging or disruptive behaviors. In such instances, antipsychotic medications are often prescribed, but they provide limited benefit and can cause serious harm, including stroke and premature death. Use of these drugs should be limited to cases where nonpharmacological measures have failed and patients pose an imminent threat to themselves or others. Identifying and addressing causes of behavior change can make drug treatment unnecessary (American Geriatrics Society, 2015.)

Nonpharmacological Approaches

Nonpharmacological approaches are person-centered approaches that are informed by careful investigation of the possible causes and meaning of the individual's behavioral and psychological symptoms. Nonpharmacological approaches can be grouped into three categories: (1) those targeting the individual, (2) those targeting the caregiver, and (3) those targeting the environment (Kales et al., 2015). Approaches include sensory practices (aromatherapy, massage, multisensory stimulation, bright-light therapy); psychosocial practices (validation therapy, reminiscence therapy, music therapy, animal-assisted therapy, meaningful activities); environmental design (e.g., special care units, homelike environment, gardens, safe walking areas); changes in mealtime and bathing environments; consistent staffing assignments and structured care protocols (bathing, mouth care); and support for caregivers (Scales et al., 2018).

Music therapy, personalized for the individual, has been shown to be an enjoyable and effective approach to alleviate BPSDs and enhance well-being (Scales et al., 2018). Use

---

BOX 26.18   Taking a Person-Centered Approach to BPSDs

Dr. A, a retired cardiovascular surgeon with a history of dementia, resided in a nursing home and was becoming increasingly agitated. Members of the interprofessional team expressed concerns about his behavior and the request for antipsychotic medications. Ivy, the director of nursing, knew about a new program using iPads for resident-family communication. Taking a person-centered approach, she knew that this man was a physician who was now in a medical facility where he was the one receiving care. On the recommendation from nursing, the recreational therapist downloaded cardiovascular procedure videos and placed headphones on Dr. A's head. Within a brief period, transformation took place. He became calm and appeared to enjoy the videos. Coming to know the person and recognizing his background led to nonpharmacological approaches to treat BPSDs, thus avoiding the use of antipsychotic medication.

BPSDs, Behavioral and psychological symptoms of dementia.

---

of iPads to both prevent and address agitation in individuals with dementia holds interesting possibilities. Although further research is needed related to what types of applications and programs are effective, preliminary findings suggest that even individuals with major NCDs were able to interact with the device and episodes of agitation and restlessness were reduced (Ross et al., 2015). Box 26.18 presents an exemplar on use of the iPad to calm agitation behavior.

There is a large amount of literature on nonpharmacological interventions, and these approaches are recommended in the culture change movement (Chapter 6). In general, these interventions, despite a lack of rigorous testing, have shown promise for improving quality of life for persons with dementia at home and in residential care, have no harmful side effects, and require minimal to moderate investment (Scales et al., 2018). Nonpharmacological approaches that were found to be clinically efficacious for aggression and agitation compared with usual care are multidisciplinary care, massage and touch therapy, and music combined with massage and touch therapy. Exercise, outdoor activities, and modification of ADLs also have been found to be effective for verbal aggression and physical agitation and have been shown to have greater effect than antipsychotics (Watt et al., 2019).

Continued attention to translating these interventions into real-world practice across settings in feasible and cost-effective ways is needed. Resnick et al. (2016) note that "despite regulatory requirements and availability of educational materials focused on nonpharmacological management of BPSDs, less than 2% of nursing homes consistently implement behavioral approaches" (p. 571). Identified barriers include lack of knowledge, skills, and hands-on experience with the many different approaches; belief that medication use is more effective; lack of belief in the effectiveness of nonpharmacological approaches; inadequate staffing; and lack of administrative support.

A toolkit approach that provides a variety of interventions may be useful in improving the use of nonpharmacological interventions in long-term care facilities. An online toolkit, *Promoting Positive Behavioral Health: A Nonpharmacological Toolkit for Senior Living Communities* (Kolanowski & Van Haitsma, 2013), provides many resources for nurses, other caregivers, and families, including behavior assessment tools, clinical

BOX 26.19   Practical Guidance for Nonpharmacological Approaches

- Human behaviors are a dynamic, moving target; all of us have good and bad days and what works on one day may not work the next; it can be really difficult to pinpoint "what set someone off" on any given day.
- It is all about trial and error; there is no magic bullet.
- Foster a mindset of "Let's try it and see what happens." Always have a backup approach if a given approach is not successful. One trial of an approach may not be sufficient; try again another day. Interview and observe what a "successful" direct care provider is doing and saying.
- Individualizing (tailoring) the approach to a given person is critical to success. Get to know the person's preferences, past history. Come to know the person as a unique individual.
- Relax the "rules." There is no right or wrong way to perform an activity if the individual is safe.
- Understand that behaviors are not intentional or done "in spite" but are a consequence of the person's inability to initiate or comprehend steps of a task or its purpose.

From Centers for Medicare and Medicaid Services, Center for Clinical Standards and Quality/Survey & Certification Center: *Practical guidance for nonpharmacological approaches* (website), 2013. https://www.nhqualitycampaign.org/professionalDementia.aspx#HandoutsTools. Accessed April 2019.

BOX 26.20   Understanding Behavior: Seeing Through the Eyes of the Person

You are asleep in a chair at home when suddenly you are awakened by a person you have never seen before trying to undress you. Then the person puts you naked into a hard, cold chair and wheels you down a hallway. Suddenly cold water hits you in the face, and the person is touching your private areas. You don't understand why the person is trying to do this to you. You are embarrassed, frightened, cold, and angry. You hit and scream at this person and try to get away.

decision-making algorithms, and evidence-based approaches to ameliorate or prevent BPSDs (see Box 26.1). Practical suggestions about how to prevent BPSDs that emerged from focus groups with direct care providers are presented in Box 26.19.

Despite recommendations for nonpharmacological treatment of BPSDs, antipsychotic medications are often given as the first-line response across settings without appropriate assessment of factors contributing to the behaviors (Kolanowski et al., 2017). A study of providers and families investigating factors influencing the use of medications for BPSDs despite recommendations reported the following: (1) medications were seen as safer and more effective than nonpharmacological interventions; (2) medications frequently are prescribed by physicians who are not familiar with nonpharmacological approaches; and (3) resources that facilitate and encourage alternate therapies are inadequate and underused.

Families and experienced nurses in the study recognized that there were times when even "optimally applied . . . nonmedication approaches did not work to relieve patients' distressing symptoms . . . caregivers expressed a strong need to alleviate patient distress and were uncomfortable about not intervening when symptoms affected quality of life. If medications were effective, almost all caregivers supported their use as worth the potential side effects" (Kerns et al., 2018, p. e41).

Clearly, the role of medications and nonpharmacological interventions to treat BPSDs needs further study. Health care providers and family caregivers can benefit from training, better access, and practical assistance in implementing approaches for behavioral concerns. Behavioral health programs must be better integrated with medical care for individuals with dementia. Collaborative care management programs for the treatment of AD, often led by advanced practice nurses, have been shown to increase adherence to guidelines for care of individuals with

NCDs and quality indicators, including improved health outcomes and quality of life, decreased caregiver burden, and cost savings when compared to standard-of-care models (Callahan et al., 2006; Heintz et al., 2020).

PROVIDING CARE FOR ACTIVITIES OF DAILY LIVING

The losses associated with NCDs interfere with the person's communication patterns and ability to understand and express thoughts and feelings. Perceptual disturbances and misinterpretations of reality contribute to fear and misunderstanding. Often bathing and the provision of other ADL care, such as dressing, grooming, and toileting, are the cause of much distress for both the person with dementia and the caregiver.

Bathing

Bathing is the ADL associated with the highest frequency of expressions of distress (Scales et al., 2018). Bathing is an essential aspect of everyday life that most people enjoy. However, bathing and other intimate care can be perceived as a frightening personal attack by individuals with dementia, who may respond by screaming or striking out. Being touched or bathed against a person's will violates the trust in caregiver relationships and can be considered a major affront (Rader & Barrick, 2000). In institutional settings, a rigid focus on tasks or institutional care routines, such as a shower three mornings each week, can contribute to the distress and precipitate distressing behaviors. The behaviors that may be exhibited are not deliberate attacks on caregivers by a violent person but rather a way to express self in an uncertain situation. The message is: "Please find another way to keep me clean, because the way you are doing it now is intolerable" (Rader & Barrick, 2000, p. 49) (Box 26.20).

USING CLINICAL JUDGMENT TO PROMOTE HEALTHY AGING: BATHING COMFORT

Solutions, Nursing Actions, and Outcomes

In research conducted in nursing homes, Rader and Barrick (2000) have provided comprehensive guidelines for bathing people with NCDs in ways that are pleasurable and decrease distress. Asking the question "What is the easiest, most comfortable, least

---

BOX 26.21   Tips for Best Practice

Techniques for Bathing Without a Battle

1. Rethink the bathing experience.
   - Make the experience comfortable and pleasurable.
   - Consider what makes the individual feel good.
   - Do not be in a hurry.
2. Approach techniques such as "let's get freshened up for the day" and avoiding bathing terminology (e.g., "it's time for your bath") can create a more positive environment. Tell person it is time to get freshened up and try not to ask, "do you want a bath?" because the answer may be no.
3. Have the room ready.
   - Keep the room warm and low-lit.
   - Handheld showerhead wets one area at a time.
   - Have a large towel or blanket to preserve dignity and keep person warm.
4. Begin bathing least sensitive area first.
   - Wash legs and feet first, followed by arms, trunk, perineum area, and face last.
5. Save washing hair until last or do separately.
6. Use distraction techniques.
   - Consider using music, calming sounds, or singing songs that the person likes.
   - Consider having the person hold a towel or something to provide distraction.
7. Consider a towel bath, under clothes bath, or sponge bath

From University of North Carolina Cecil G. Sheps Center for Health Services Research: *Bathing without a battle* (website), n.d. http://bathingwithoutabattle.unc.edu/.

BOX 26.22   Patient Perspectives on Wandering Behavior

"Wandering and restlessness is one of the by-products of Alzheimer's disease.... When the darkness and emptiness fill my mind, it is totally terrifying.... Thoughts increasingly haunt me. The only way I can break the cycle is to move."

(Davis, 1989, p 96)

"Very often, I wander around looking for something which I know is very pertinent, but then after a while I forget all about what it was I was looking for. When I'm wandering around, I'm trying to touch base with—anything, actually. If anything appeared, I'd probably enjoy it, or look at it or examine it and wonder how it got there. I feel very foolish when I'm wandering around not knowing what I'm doing and I'm not always quite sure how to do any better. It's not easy to figure out what the heck I'm looking for."

(Henderson, 1998)

From Davis, R. (1989). *My journey into Alzheimer's disease*. Wheaton, IL. Tyndale House
Henderson, C. (1998). *Partial view: an Alzheimer's journal*. Dallas, TX: Southern Methodist Press.

---

frightening way for me to clean the person right now?" guides the choice of interventions. *Bathing Without a Battle* is an approach that can be used to create a better bathing experience for people with dementia. These techniques show positive results in reducing BPSDs (Box 26.21).

Another innovative approach being investigated in Sweden is caregiver singing and the use of background music during ADL care in nursing homes. Caregivers play and sing familiar songs during care routines. When compared with usual care practices, this approach enhanced the expression of positive moods and emotions, increased the mutuality of communication, and reduced aggression and resistive care behaviors (Hammar et al., 2011). The provision of oral care is another ADL that often precipitates anxiety and agitation for individuals with NCDs. Person-centered oral care protocols are discussed in Chapter 16.

WANDERING

Wandering associated with NCDs is one of the most difficult concerns encountered in home and institutional settings. Wandering is a complex behavior and is not well understood. Wandering is defined as "a syndrome of dementia-related locomotion behavior having a frequent, repetitive, temporally disordered and/or spatially disoriented nature that is manifested in lapping, random and/or pacing patterns, some of which is associated with eloping, eloping attempts or getting lost unless accompanied" (Algase et al., 2007, p. 696). Risk factors for wandering include visuospatial impairments, anxiety and depression, poor

sleep patterns, unmet needs, and a more socially active and outgoing premorbid lifestyle. One in five persons with dementia wander, and wandering frequency tends to increase as cognitive function decreases (Futrell et al., 2014).

Wandering presents safety concerns in all settings. Wandering behavior affects sleeping, eating, safety, and the caregiver's ability to provide care, and it also interferes with the privacy of others. The behavior can lead to falls, elopement (leaving the home or facility), injury, and death. The stimulus for wandering arises from many internal and external sources. Wandering can be considered a rhythm, intrinsically and extrinsically driven. Box 26.22 presents insight into the behavior of wandering from the perspective of individuals with a NCD.

USING CLINICAL JUDGMENT TO PROMOTE HEALTHY AGING: WANDERING BEHAVIOR

Recognizing and Analyzing Cues

It is important to recognize and analyze cues that may trigger wandering, such as acute illness, exacerbations of chronic illness, fatigue, medication effects, and constipation. Unmet needs or pain can increase wandering (Futrell et al., 2014). The need for social interaction or to relieve boredom may be a stimulus for wandering, and research suggests that wandering is less likely to occur when the individual is involved in social interaction (Adekoya & Guse, 2019). Wandering behaviors can be predicted through careful observation and awareness of the person's patterns. For example, if a person with an NCD starts wandering or trying to leave the home in the afternoon every day, meaningful activities such as music, exercise, and refreshments can be provided at this time.

Solutions, Nursing Actions, and Outcomes

Locked units and environmental modifications are also safety measures for individuals who wander. Wandering paths such as hallways with a continuous path or circular loop (including outside walking paths) and simple visual cues or artwork and objects to support therapeutic walking should be provided. Daily supervised walks and outside time in a safe area are important interventions.

Although safety is a major concern, risks should not be the only focus. With a person-centered approach, the less wandering is seen as a problem, the more its benefits will be seen. Walking should be seen as exercise and an opportunity for socialization, and care should be structured to support safety to maintain the positive benefits for some individuals (Adekoya & Guse, 2019). There are also several instruments to determine risk for wandering, and nurse researcher May Futrell et al. (2010, 2014) developed an evidence-based protocol for wandering.

Wandering behavior also may result in people with NCDs going outside and getting lost. All people with dementia are considered capable of getting lost. Caregivers must prevent people with NCDs from leaving homes or care facilities unaccompanied, register the person in the Alzheimer's Association Safe Return program and Silver Alert if available, and have a plan of action in case the person does become lost. Protocols that include identification of individuals who may wander, a wandering prevention program to ensure safety, and an elopement response plan must be in place in care facilities. A number of assistive technology devices and programs (e.g., electronic tagging and tracking devices) can enhance the safety of persons who wander (Chapter 21).

NUTRITION

Older adults with NCDs are particularly at risk of weight loss and inadequate nutrition. Weight loss often becomes a considerable concern in later stages of NCDs, and about 90% of individuals suffer from eating problems (Ijaopo & Ijaopo, 2019). Nutritional concerns are a major source of distress for people living with NCDs and their caregivers and are identified as a top research priority. Some of the predisposing factors to nutritional inadequacy are lack of awareness of the need to eat, depression, loss of independence in self-feeding, agnosia, apraxia, vision impairments (deficient contrast sensitivity), wandering, pacing, and behavior disturbances. Weight loss increases the risk of infection, pressure injury development, poor wound healing, and hospitalization and is associated with higher mortality and morbidity. As members of interprofessional teams, nurses play a significant role in assessing nutrition in older adults with NCDs.

USING CLINICAL JUDGMENT TO PROMOTE HEALTHY AGING: NUTRITION

Solutions, Nursing Actions, and Outcomes

There has been little research on specific interventions to support food and fluid intake in individuals with NCDs, and results of a systematic review found no definitive evidence on effectiveness or lack of effectiveness of specific interventions. Further research is needed and should include individuals with different NCDs, at different stages, and in different settings. However, Abdelhamid et al. (2016) suggest that individuals and their caregivers must deal

---

BOX 26.23 Tips for Best Practice

Improving Intake for Individuals With Neurocognitive Disorders

- Serve only one dish at a time.
- Provide only one utensil at a time.
- Consider using a "spork" (combination spoon-fork).
- Serve finger foods such as fried chicken, chicken strips, pizza in bite-size pieces, fish sticks, sandwiches.
- Serve soup in a mug.
- Remove any hot items or items that should not be eaten.
- Cut up foods before serving.
- Sit next to the person at his or her level.
- Demonstrate eating motions that the person can imitate.
- Use hand-over-hand feeding technique to guide self-feeding.
- Use verbal cueing and prompting (e.g., take a bite, chew, swallow).
- Use gentle tone of voice and avoid scolding or demeaning remarks.
- Provide verbal encouragement to participate in eating by talking about food taste and smell.
- Offer small amounts of fluid between bites.
- Help person focus on the meal at hand; turn off background noise, remove clutter from the table.
- Avoid patterned dishes or table coverings.
- Use red plates, glasses, and cups; food intake may increase when food is served with high-contrast tableware.
- Use unbreakable dishes that will not slide around.
- Serve smaller, more frequent meals rather than expecting the person to complete a big meal.
- Serve family-style meals.
- Eat with carers.
- Involve in preparation of food, smelling the food cook.

Data from Dunne T, Neargarder S, Cipolloni P, et al: Visual contrast enhances food and liquid intake in advanced Alzheimer's disease, *Clin Nutr* 23(4):533–538, 2004; Spencer P: *How to solve eating problems common to people with Alzheimer's and other dementias* (website). https://www.caring.com/articles/alzheimers-eating-problems. Accessed June 2015; and *How to solve eating problems common to people with Alzheimer's and other dementias* (website). https://www.caring.com/articles/alzheimers-eating-problems. Accessed June 2018; Abdelhamid A, Bunn D, Copley M, et al: Effectiveness of interventions to directly support food and drink intake in people with dementia: a systematic review and metaanalysis, *BMC Geriatrics* 16:26, 2016.

---

with eating problems despite a lack of evidence. Some promising interventions include: (1) establishing a routine so that the individual does not have to remember time and places for eating; (2) continue to serve foods and fluids that the person likes and has always eaten; (3) provide nutrient-dense foods (e.g., peanut butter, protein bars, yogurt); (4) pay attention to mealtime ambience; (5) allow as much time as needed to eat the foods that are preferred; (6) make food available 24 hours a day; and (7) allow the person to follow the accustomed eating schedule (e.g., late breakfast, early dinner). Other suggestions to enhance food intake are presented in Box 26.23. Comprehensive nutritional assessment and nursing actions for nutritional concerns are discussed in Chapter 15.

TUBE FEEDING IN END-STAGE DEMENTIA

Increasing evidence indicates that tube feeding in the end stage of dementia does not prolong survival or improve quality of life.

BOX 26.24   Myths and Facts About PEG Tubes in Advanced Dementia and End-of-Life Care

Myths

- PEGs prevent death from inadequate intake.
- PEGs reduce aspiration pneumonia.
- PEGs improve albumin levels and nutritional status.
- PEGs assist in healing pressure injuries.
- PEGs provide enhanced comfort for people at the end of life.
- Not feeding people is a form of euthanasia, and we cannot let people starve to death.

Facts

- PEGs do not improve quality of life.
- PEGs do not reduce risk of aspiration and increase the rate of pneumonia development. In one study, the use of feeding tubes was associated with an increased risk of pressure injuries among nursing home residents with advanced cognitive impairment.
- PEGs do not prolong survival in dementia.
- Nearly 50% of patients die within 6 months following PEG tube insertion.
- PEGs cause increased discomfort from both the tube presence and the use of restraints.
- PEGs are associated with infections, gastrointestinal symptoms, and abscesses.
- PEG tube feeding deprives people of the taste of food and contact with caregivers during feeding.
- PEGs are popular because they are convenient and labor beneficial.

PEG, Percutaneous endoscopic gastrostomy.
Data from Aparanji K, Dharmarajan T: Pause before a PEG: a feeding tube may not be necessary in every candidate, *J Am Med Dir Assoc* 11:453–456, 2010; Teno J, Gozalo P, Mitchell S, et al: Feeding tubes and the prevention or healing of pressure ulcers, *Arch Intern Med* 172(9):697–701, 2012; Vitale C, Monteleoni C, Burke L, et al: Strategies for improving care for patients with advanced dementia and eating problems: optimizing care through physician and speech pathologist collaboration, *Ann Longterm Care* 17:32–39, 2009.

In fact, enteral feeding increases the risk of several complications, including aspiration and pressure injuries (Box 26.24). The proportion of nursing home residents with advanced dementia receiving feeding tubes has significantly decreased in recent years. The AGS (2015b) does not recommend feeding tubes for older adults with advanced dementia and suggests that careful hand feeding is at least as good as tube feeding for the outcomes of death, aspiration pneumonia, functional status, and patient comfort.

Food and eating are closely tied to socialization, comfort, pleasure, love, and the meeting of basic biological needs. Feeding is often equated with caring, and not providing adequate nutrition may be viewed as cruel and inhumane. Decisions about feeding tube placement are challenging and require thoughtful discussion with patients and caregivers, who should be free to make decisions without duress and with careful consideration of the patient's advance directives, if available. Many considerations factor into decisions that families and providers make about enteral feeding, including the individual's wishes in an advance directive; cultural, religious, and ethical beliefs; legal and financial concerns; and emotions.

Most feeding tube insertions occur during acute hospitalization, and decisions to place a feeding tube often are taken without completely exhausting every means to maintain a normal oral intake. Research has shown that discussions surrounding the decision often are inadequate, and health care surrogates claim they seldom have their informational needs completely met by health care providers (Teno et al., 2015). Discussion about advance directives and feeding support should begin early in the course of NCDs rather than waiting until a crisis develops. The best advice for individuals is to state preferences for the use of a feeding tube in a written advance directive. Individuals should be given information about the risks and benefits of enteral feeding in the end stages of NCDs (see Box 26.1 for reference to an advance directive).

The decision should never be understood as a question of tube feeding versus no feeding. Family members should not be made to feel that they are "starving" a loved one to death if a decision is made not to institute enteral feeding. Efforts to provide nutrition should continue, and individuals should be able to take any type of nutrition they desire at the time they desire. It is important that health care professionals provide the leadership to guide this complex decision-making process to promote true person-centered care (Gieniusz et al., 2018).

Regardless of the decision, an important nursing role is to journey with the patient's loved ones, providing support and encouraging expression of feelings. Making these decisions is very difficult, and loved ones "have to make peace with their decisions" (Teno et al., 2015). "Further research is required to establish whether tube feeding of individuals with advanced dementia provides more burdens than benefits or vice-versa and evaluate the impacts on quality of life and survival" (Ijaopo & Ijaopo, 2019, p. 1).

NURSING ROLES IN THE CARE OF PERSONS WITH NCDS

Care for someone with a NCD, whether by family members or formal caregivers, requires special skills, knowledge of evidence-based practice, and a deep understanding of the person. A major focus of nursing education and continued education of practicing nurses should be on providing in-depth information on best-practice care of individuals with NCDs. Current practice often does not reflect person-centered care and can cause great distress and poor outcomes for the individual and the caregivers.

Rader and Tornquist (1995) reflected on the knowledge required and provided a view of caregiving roles that is quite useful and understandable for all caregivers. The authors have found that nurses and family caregivers can truly relate to the practical wisdom in these words.

- **Magician role:** To understand what the person is trying to communicate both verbally and nonverbally, we must be a magician who can use our magical abilities to see the world through the eyes, the ears, and the feelings of the person. We know how to use tricks to turn an individual's behavior around or prevent it from occurring and causing distress.
- **Detective role:** The detective looks for clues and cues about what might be causing distress and how it might be changed. We have to investigate and know as much about the person as possible to be a good detective.

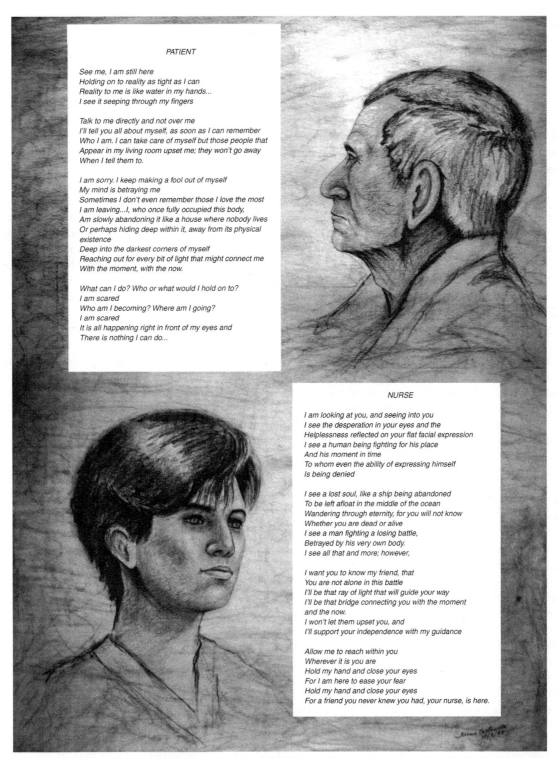

Fig. 26.1 Nurse and patient. (Copyright ©1998 by Jaime Castaneda, Lake Worth, FL.)

- **Carpenter role:** By having a wide variety of tools and selecting the right tools for the job, we build individualized plans of care for each person.
- **Jester role:** Many people with NCDs retain their sense of humor and respond well to the appropriate use of humor. This does not mean making fun of but rather sharing laughter and fun. "Those who love their work and do it well employ good doses of humor as part of the care of others, and for self-care" (Rader & Barrick, 2000, p. 42). The jester spreads joy, is creative, energizes, and lightens the burdens (Laurenhue, 2001; Rader & Barrick, 2000).

Fig. 26.1 presents a nursing situation that one nurse experienced in caring for an individual with NCDs who was being admitted to a nursing facility. Written from the perspective of the nurse and his knowledge of the patient, the story provides insight into important nursing responses, such as providing person-centered care, implementing therapeutic communication, and establishing meaningful relationships. It is a lovely example of expert gerontological nursing for individuals and a fitting way to end this chapter.

KEY CONCEPTS

- Cues to cognitive impairment are subtle, often missed, not adequately evaluated, and often attributed to aging changes. Nurses must use clinical judgment in recognizing and analyzing cues of cognitive changes and design nursing actions to prevent unnecessary decline and promote cognitive health.
- Delirium results from the interaction of *predisposing* factors (e.g., vulnerability on the part of the individual attributable to predisposing conditions such as cognitive impairment, severe illness, sensory impairment) and *precipitating* factors or insults (e.g., medications, procedures, restraints).
- Delirium is characterized by fluctuating levels of consciousness, sometimes in a diurnal pattern, and frequent misperceptions and illusions. It is often unrecognized and is attributed to age or dementia. People with dementia are more susceptible to delirium. Knowledge of risk factors, preventive measures, and treatment of underlying medical problems is essential to prevent serious consequences.
- Acute illness (e.g., urinary tract infections, respiratory tract infections), medications, and pain are frequently the causes of delirium in older adults.
- It is essential to view all behavior as meaningful and an expression of needs. The focus must be on understanding that behavioral expressions communicate distress and that the response is to investigate the possible source of distress and intervene appropriately.
- Fear, discomfort, unfamiliar surroundings and people, illness, fatigue, depression, need for autonomy and control, caregiver approaches and communication, and environmental stressors are frequent precipitants of behavioral symptoms.
- All evidence-based guidelines endorse an approach that begins with comprehensive assessment of BPSDs and possible causes followed by use of nonpharmacological interventions as a first-line treatment, except in emergency situations when symptoms could lead to imminent danger or compromise safety.
- Individuals with cognitive impairment respond best to calmness and patience, adaptations of communication techniques, and environments and relationships that enhance function, support limitations, ensure safety, and provide opportunities for a meaningful quality of life. Because individuals experiencing cognitive impairment may be unable to express their feelings and needs in ways that are easily understood, the gerontological nurse must always try to understand the world from their perspective.

NEXT-GENERATION NCLEX® (NGN) EXAMINATION–STYLE QUESTIONS

Mrs. Landers is a newly admitted long-term care resident. She is 88 years old and has late-stage dementia. In addition to Alzheimer's disease, her medical history includes hypertension, coronary artery disease, depression, and osteoporosis. The move to long-term care was planned when Mrs. Landers' dementia was mild. She participated in the selection of the facility, along with her three children. She regularly wanders in and out of other residents' rooms, picking up objects and putting them down. The assistive personnel gently guide her out of the other residents' rooms without resistance when this happens, and she smiles and repeats "yes" over and over. At 3 p.m. each day, she goes to the door and tries to leave; when assistive personnel or the nursing staff try to steer her to a diversional activity, she says, "no, no, no," pinches them, and resists redirection.

Mrs. Landers eats finger foods as she wanders. She is incontinent of bowel and bladder. Her medications include memantine 10 mg twice daily, donepezil 10 mg at bedtime, fluoxetine 20 mg daily, aspirin 81 mg daily, ezetimibe 10 mg daily, valsartan/hydrochlorothiazide 160 mg/25 mg daily, and acetaminophen 500 mg every 4 hours as needed for pain. Her admission laboratory results reveal the following:

- Hemoglobin 11 mg/dL; hematocrit 34%
- White blood cells (WBCs) 8.2 × 109/L
- Blood urea nitrogen (BUN)/creatinine 24 mg/dL and 1.4 mg/dL
- Sodium (Na)/Chloride (Cl) 144 mmol/L and 103 mmol/L
- Glucose 100 mg/dL
- Urine amber and clear, pH 5.0, nitrite negative and leukocyte esterase trace, blood negative, WBC 1/high power field (hpf), and bacteria trace

Which actions will the nurse take to address the client's most pressing needs? Select all that apply.

1. Request that the family schedule an appointment with the facility's contracted psychiatrist.
2. Put the client on a toileting program to reduce incontinence.
3. Request a dietary consult to ensure adequate intake to meet caloric needs.
4. Call the health care provider for antibiotic orders to treat a urinary tract infection.
5. Call the health care provider for as-needed lorazepam to treat agitation.
6. Call the client's children to determine previous activities that took place around 3 p.m. daily.
7. Schedule meaningful activities for the client to promote cognitive stimulation.
8. Complete a behavioral diary over a 2- to 3-day period.

NURSING STUDY

Major NCD: Behavior

Pat is an 83-year-old retired nurse who was diagnosed with major neurocognitive disorder (NCD) 3 years ago. Her other diagnoses include hypertension and osteoarthritis. She had a hip replacement 6 years ago and also has pain in her shoulders and knees from the osteoarthritis and some limitation of movement that affects her mobility. She lives with her daughter, who has brought her to the clinic for a medication check.

Her daughter tells you, the nurse, that things have not been going well. The daughter states that Pat has been verbally and physically abusive when she tries to bathe and dress her. She hits her and screams, "You're hurting me!" The daughter says that her mother was a very fastidious person and always wanted to look nice, so she cannot understand why she resists bathing and dressing. The daughter tries to give her mother a shower at least every other day, but the battles have become so bad that she has not been able to keep this schedule. The daughter tells you that her mother never took showers, preferring either a tub bath or sponge bathing at the sink. However, the shower is more convenient for the daughter, and her mother cannot get in the whirlpool tub at her house. She is concerned about her mother's appearance and also deeply hurt that her mother has been so mean to her. Her mother has been a lovely woman and never acted like this before. She asks you what she can do and if her mother needs some kind of tranquilizer.

CLINICAL JUDGMENT QUESTIONS AND ACTIVITIES

Questions 1 to 3 refer to the Nursing Study.

1. What internal and external factors could be influencing Pat's behavior?
2. What nursing framework for understanding behavior would be helpful in this situation?
3. How might you help the daughter in understanding and reacting to her mother's behavior?
4. Discuss some specific nursing actions that might be helpful in promoting comfort during bathing for persons with NCDs.
5. What type of communication techniques would be helpful in assisting with ADLs for a person with a NCD?

RESEARCH QUESTIONS

1. What barriers do nurses encounter in recognizing delirium in hospitalized older adults?
2. How does delirium influence the ability of older adults discharged from the hospital to manage their care (i.e., medications)?
3. What is the relationship between hospitalized older adults with delirium and 30-day rehospitalization?
4. What are student nurses' feelings about caring for individuals with NCDs?
5. What nonpharmacological interventions are most effective in the home setting for individuals with NCDs who wander?
6. What are the effects of an interprofessional team approach for individuals with BPSDs who reside in nursing facilities?
7. What type of dining options encourage intake in long-term care facilities?
8. Do educational programs for informal and formal caregivers of older persons with NCDs improve understanding and management of behavioral problems?
9. How do family caregivers make decisions to seek help for BPSDs in the home setting? What type of actions do they feel are most effective?

REFERENCES

Abdelhamid A, Bunn D, Copley M, et al.: Effectiveness of interventions to directly support food and drink intake in people with dementia: systematic review and meta-analysis, *BMC Geriatr* 16:26, 2016.

Adekoya A, Guse L: Wandering behavior from the perspectives of older adults with mild to moderate dementia in long-term care, *Res Gerontol Nurs* 12(5):239–247, 2019.

Algase D, Beel-Bates C, Beattie R: Wandering in long-term care, *Ann Longterm Care* 11:33–39, 2003.

Algase D, Moore D, Vandeweerd C, et al.: Mapping the maze of terms and definitions in dementia-related wandering, *Aging Ment Health* 11:686–698, 2007.

Alzheimer's Association: *Communication and Alzheimer's* (website), 2021a. https://www.alz.org/help-support/caregiving/daily-care/communications. Accessed May 2021.

Alzheimer's Association: *If you have younger-onset Alzheimer's disease* (website), 2021b. https://www.alz.org/help-support/i-have-alz/younger-onset. Accessed May 2021.

American Geriatrics Society (AGS): Beers Criteria Update Expert Panel: American Geriatrics Society 2015 updated Beers Criteria for potentially inappropriate medication use in older adults, *J Am Geriatr Soc* 63(11):2227–2246, 2015.

American Geriatrics Society (AGS): *Choosing wisely: ten things physicians and patients should question* (website), 2015b. https://www.choosingwisely.org/societies/american-geriatrics-society/. Accessed May 2021.

American Psychiatric Association: *Diagnostic and statistical manual of mental disorders,* ed 5, Washington, DC, 2013, American Psychiatric Association.

Austrom M, Boustani M, LaMantia M: Ongoing medical management to maximize health and well-being for persons living with dementia, *Gerontologist* 58(Suppl 1):S48–S57, 2018.

Basnet P, Acton G, Requeijo P: Psychotropic medication prescribing practices among residents with dementia in nursing homes: a person-centered approach, *J Gerontol Nurs* 46(2):9–15, 2020.

Battle C, James K, Bromfield T, et al.: Predictors of post-traumatic stress disorder following critical illness: a mixed methods study, *J Intensive Care Soc* 18(4):289–293, 2017.

Birge O, Aydin T: The effect of nonpharmacological training on delirium identification and intervention strategies of intensive care nurses, *Intensive Crit Care Nurs* 41:31–42, 2017.

Blair K, Eccleston S, Binder H, et al.: Improving the patient experience by implementing an ICU diary for those at risk of post-intensive care syndrome, *J Patient Exp* 4(1):4–9, 2017.

Blevins C, et al.: Delirium prevention, early recognition, and treatment. In Boltz M, Capezuti E, Zwicker D, et al, editors: *Evidence-based geriatric nursing protocols for best practice*, ed 6, New York, 2021, Springer, pp 317–329.

Buckwalter K, Gerdner L, Hall G, et al.: Shining through: the humor and individuality of persons with Alzheimer's disease, *J Gerontol Nurs* 21:11–16, 1995.

Callahan CM, Boustani MA, Unverzagt FW, et al.: Effectiveness of collaborative care for older adults with Alzheimer disease in primary care: a randomized controlled trial, *JAMA* 295:2148–2157, 2006.

Davis, R. My journey into Alzheimer's disease. Wheaton, IL. In Tyndale House, 1989.

Henderson, C. (1998). *Partial view: an Alzheimer's journal.* Dallas, TX, 1989, Southern Methodist Press.

DeYoung S, Just G, Harrison R: Decreasing aggressive, agitated, or disruptive behavior: participation in a behavior management unit, *J Gerontol Nurs* 28:22–31, 2003.

Ely E, Margolin R, Francis J, et al.: Evaluation of delirium in critically ill patients: validation of the Confusion Assessment Method for the intensive care unit (CAM-ICU), *Crit Care Med* 29:1370–1379, 2001.

Fick DM: The critical vital sign of cognitive health and delirium: whose responsibility is it? *J Gerontol Nurs* 44(8):3–5, 2018.

Forsberg M: Delirium update for postacute care and long-term care settings: a narrative review, *J Am Osteopath Assoc* 117:32–38, 2017.

Futrell M, Melillo KD, Remington R, Schoenfelder DP: Evidence-based practice guideline: wandering, *J Gerontol Nurs* 36:6–16, 2010.

Futrell M, Melillo K, Remington K, et al.: Evidence-based practice guideline: wandering, *J Gerontol Nurs* 40(11):16–23, 2014.

Gaster B, Larson E, Curtis J: Advance directives for dementia: meeting a unique challenge, *JAMA* 318(22):2175–2176, 2017.

Gieniuz M, Sinvani L, Kozikowski A, et al.: Percutaneous feeding tubes in individuals with advanced dementia: are physicians "Choosing Wisely"? *JAGS* 66:64–69, 2018.

Greenwood N, Smith N: The experiences of people with young-onset dementia: a meta-ethnographic review of the qualitative literature, *Maturitas* 92:102–109, 2016.

Hain DJ, Touhy TA, Compton Sparks D, et al.: Using narratives of individuals and couples living with early stage dementia to guide practice, *J Nurs Pract Appl Rev Res* 4:82–93, 2014.

Hain D, Touhy T, Engstrom G: What matters most to carers of people with mild to moderate dementia as evidence for transforming care, *Alzheimers Care Today* 11:162–171, 2010.

Hall G: Caring for people with Alzheimer's disease using the conceptual model of progressively lowered stress threshold in the clinical setting, *Nurs Clin North Am* 29:129–141, 1994.

Hall G, Buckwalter KC: Progressively lowered stress threshold: a conceptual model for care of adults with Alzheimer's disease, *Arch Psychiatr Nurs* 1:399–406, 1987.

Hammar L, Emami A, Engstrom G, et al.: Communicating through caregiver singing during morning care situations in dementia care, *Scand J Caring Sci* 25(1):160–168, 2011.

Heintz H, Monette P, Epstein-Lubow G, et al.: Emerging collaborative care models for dementia care in the primary care setting: a narrative review, *Am J Geriatr Psychiatry* 28(3):320–330, 2020.

Ijaopo E, Ijaopo R: Tube feeding in individuals with advanced dementia: a review of its burdens and perceived benefits, *J Aging Res*, 2019 2019:7272067 https://doi.org/10.1155/2019/7272067.

Inouye S: Delirium: a framework to improve acute care for older persons, *J Am Geriatr Soc* 66(3):446–451, 2018.

Inouye SK, Bogardus Jr ST, Charpentier PA, et al.: A multicomponent intervention to prevent delirium in hospitalized older patients, *N Engl J Med* 340:669–676, 1999.

Inouye S, van Dyck S, Alessi C, et al.: Clarifying confusion: the confusion assessment method: a new method for detection of delirium, *Ann Intern Med* 113:941–948, 1990.

Jennings L, Turner M, Keebler C, et al.: The effects of a comprehensive dementia care management program on end-of-life care, *JAGS* 00:1–6, 2019. doi:10.1111/jgs.15769.

Kales H, Gitlin L, Stanislawski B, et al.: Effect of the WeCareAdvisor on family caregiver outcomes in dementia: a randomized controlled trial, *BMC Geriatrics* 18:113, 2018.

Kales HC, Gitlin LN, Lyketsos CG: Assessment and management of behavioral and psychological symptoms of dementia, *BMJ* 350:h369, 2015.

Kerns J, Winter J, Kerns C, et al.: Caregiver perspectives about using antipsychotics and other medications for symptoms of dementia, *Gerontologist* 58(2):e35–e45, 2018.

Kolanowski A: An overview of the need-driven dementia-compromised behavior model, *J Gerontol Nurs* 25:7–9, 1999.

Kolanowski A, Boltz M, Galik E, et al.: Determinants of behavioral and psychological symptoms of dementia: a scoping review of the evidence, *Nurs Outlook* 65:515–529, 2017.

Kolanowski A, Van Haitsma K: *Promoting positive behavioral health: a non-pharmacologic toolkit for senior living communities* (website), 2013. https://www.nursinghometoolkit.com/toolkitoverview.html. Accessed May 2021.

Kovach C: Assessment and treatment of discomfort for people with late-stage dementia, *J Pain Symptom Manage* 18(6):412–419, 1999.

Ladak A: A nurse-led delirium prevention program for hospitalized older adults, *UCLA*, 2020. ProQuest ID: Ladak_ucla_0031D_18796, Merritt ID: ark:/13030/m5rg1313. Retrieved from https://escholarship.org/uc/item/3jb7v67v.

Laurenhue K: Each person's journey is unique, *Alzheimers Care Q* 2:79–83, 2001.

Lepore M, Lines LM, Wiener JM, et al.: Person-centered and person-directed dementia care, *Generations ACL Suppl*:79–81, 2017.

Mailhot T, Darling C, Ela J, et al.: Family identification of delirium in the emergency department in patient with and without dementia: validity of the Family Confusion Assessment Method (FAM-CAM), *JAGS* 68(5):983–990, 2020.

Maldonado J: Delirium pathophysiology: an updated hypothesis of the etiology of brain failure, *Int J Geriatric Psychiatry* 33(1):1428–1457, 2017.

Marselas K: *Not just a nursing home problem: antipsychotic use increasing in elderly, community-dwelling dementia patients* (website), 2018. https://www.mcknights.com/news/aarps-elizabeth-carter-efforts-to-reduce-off-label-use-need-to-be-expanded/article/760609/. Accessed July 2021.

McGilton K, Rochon E, Sidani S, et al.: Can we help care providers communicate more effectively with persons having dementia living in long-term care homes? *Am J Alzheimers Dis Other Demen* 32(1):41–50, 2017.

Molony S, Kolanowski A, Van Haitsma K, et al.: Person-centered assessment and care planning, *Gerontologist* 58(Suppl 1):S32–S47, 2018.

Moon K, Park H: Outcomes of patients with delirium in long-term care facilities: a prospective cohort study, *J Gerontol Nurs* 44(9):41–50, 2018.

Neelon V, Champagne M, Carlson J, et al.: The NEECHAM confusion scale: construction, validation, and clinical testing, *Nurs Res* 45:324–330, 1996.

Oberai T, Laver K, Crotty M, Killington M, Jaarsma R: Effectiveness of multicomponent interventions on incidence of delirium in hospitalized older patients with hip fracture: a systematic review, *Int Psychogeriatr* 30(4):481–492, 2018.

Piirainen P, Pesonene HM, Kyngas H: Challenging situations and competence of nursing staff in nursing homes for older people with dementia, *Int J of Older People Nursing*, June 2021 https://doi.org/10.1111/opn.12384.

Rader J, Barrick A: Ways that work: bathing without a battle, *Alzheimers Care Q* 1(4):35–49, 2000.

Rader J, Tornquist E: *Individualized dementia care*, New York, 1995, Springer.

Resnick B, Kolanowski A, Van Haitsma K, et al.: Pilot testing of the EIT-4-BPSD intervention, *Am J Alzheimers Dis Other Demen* 31(7):570–579, 2016.

Richards K, Lambert C, Beck C: Deriving interventions for challenging behaviors from the need-driven dementia-compromised behavior model, *Alzheimers Care Q* 1:62–72, 2000.

Rigney T: Delirium in the hospitalized elder and recommendations for practice, *Geriatr Nurs* 27(3):151–157, 2006.

Ross L, Ramirez S, Bhatt A, et al.: Tables devices (iPad) for control of behavioral symptoms in older adults with dementia. *Presented at the American Association for Geriatric Psychiatry (AAGP) 2015 Annual Meeting*, March 31, 2015.

Sakamoto ML, Moore SL, ST Johnson: I'm still here": personhood and the early-onset dementia experience, *J Gerontol Nurs* 43(5):12–17, 2017.

Scales K, Zimmerman S, Miller S: Evidence-based nonpharmacological practices to address behavioral and psychological symptoms of dementia, *Gerontologist* 58:S88–S102, 2018.

Schnitker L, Novic A, Arendt G, et al.: Prevention of delirium in older adults with dementia: a systematic literature review, *J Gerontol Nurs* 46(10):43–52, 2020.

Shrestha P, Fick D: Family caregiver's experience of caring for an older adult with delirium: a systematic review, *Int J Older People Nurs* 15:e12321, 2020.

Singu S, Koneru M, Robinson K, et al.: Are antipsychotics helpful for preventing and treating delirium, *J Gerontol Nurs* 46(4):3–5, 2020.

Society of Critical Care Medicine: Guidelines for the prevention and management of pain, agitation/sedation, delirium, immobility, and sleep disruption in adult patients in the ICU, *Crit Care Med* 46(9):e825–e873, 2018.

Splete H: Nurses have special strategies for dementia, *Caring Ages* 9:11, 2008.

Steis M, Fick D: Are nurses recognizing delirium? A systematic review, *J Gerontol Nurs* 34:40–48, 2008.

Tappen R, Williams C, Fishman S, et al.: Persistence of self in advanced Alzheimer's disease, *Image J Nurs Sch* 31:121–125, 1999.

Tappen R, Williams-Burgess C, Edelstein J, et al.: Communicating with individuals with Alzheimer's disease: examination of recommended strategies, *Arch Psychiatr Nurs* 11:249–256, 1997.

Teno J, Freedman V, Kasper J, et al.: Is care for the dying improving in the United States? *J Palliat Med* 18(8):662–666, 2015.

Thomas N, Coleman M, Terry D: Nurses' experience of caring for patients with delirium: systematic review and qualitative evidence synthesis, *Nurs Rep* 11:164–174, 2021.

Van Manen A, Aarts S, Metzelthin S, et al.: A communication model for nursing staff working in dementia care: results of a scoping review, *Int J Nurs Studies*, 2020 113:103776. doi:10.1016/j/ijnurstu.2020.103776.

Watt J, Goodarzi J, Veroniki A, et al.: Comparative efficacy of interventions for aggressive and agitated behaviors in dementia, *Ann Int Med* 171:633–642, 2019.

Woods B: Dementia challenges and assumptions about what it means to be a person, *Generations* 13:39, 1999.

27 CHAPTER

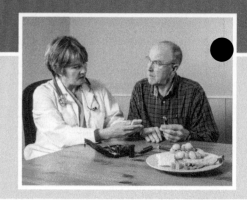

Endocrine and Immune Disorders

Kathleen Jett

http://evolve.elsevier.com/Touhy/TwdHlthAging

A STUDENT SPEAKS

The immune system is so complex and affects so many other systems, it is difficult to grasp. However, I see now how important my understanding is to provide the highest quality of care I can.

Tamara, age 30, a nurse practitioner student

AN OLDER ADULT SPEAKS

I had been wondering why I was so tired. I just could not get enough sleep. I went to my primary care provider, who did a bunch of tests and discovered I had a problem with my thyroid gland. Now that it is being treated, I cannot believe how much better I feel. Just like my old self again.

Ruth, age 72

LEARNING OBJECTIVES

On completion of this chapter, the reader will be able to:

1. Recognize the effects of the aging immune system on the body's ability to respond to potential infectious agents.
2. Recognize and analyze common conditions that may be related to changes in the aging immune system.
3. Differentiate diabetes as seen in older compared to younger adults.
4. Identify the most common pharmacological agents used to treat diabetes and explain how their use may differ in older adults.
5. Differentiate between the two major types of thyroid disorders and recognize how they differ in older adults compared to younger adults.
6. Describe the nurse's role in advancing healthy aging in persons with immune and endocrine disorders.

THE AGING IMMUNE SYSTEM

The immune system reaches its peak performance around puberty, after which it begins to lose its effectiveness and efficiency. As a result, the older one is, the less the ability to defend again an infection. Infections can occur with exposure to fewer organisms, and the cues may be atypical, be masked, be mistaken for other disease, or *appear* to be less severe (Box 27.1). For example, the symptoms of a urinary tract infection in a younger person include dysuria and frequency, but in an older adult the more common early signs are confusion and falling. Some medications can blunt an immune response, especially steroids (e.g., for pulmonary disease) and antiinflammatory drugs such as ibuprofen (e.g., for arthritis).

The immune system protects the body from toxic substances and potentially infectious and disease-causing microorganisms through (1) physical and chemical barriers, (2) innate immunity, and (3) adaptive (acquired) immunity. All three undergo significant changes with aging, resulting in dysregulation of the system, or immunosenescence, and an increased vulnerability to infection, autoimmune diseases, and chronic inflammation (Chapter 3).

The skin, mucous membranes, and pulmonary cilia provide physical and chemical barriers. Healthy, intact younger skin prevents entry of organisms into the body, and the slight acidity of sweat and oil inhibit some bacterial overgrowth. The skin becomes less acidic, allowing some bacteria to grow more rapidly on the surface, and it thins, dries, and allows bacteria to enter more easily. In adulthood the mucous membrane than lines the respiratory system produces a protective layer that can trap harmful substances as they are almost simultaneously expelled through cilia movement (coughing). Changes in later life include a reduction in the cough reflex and the cilia not being able to respond as quickly or effectively in response to an irritant or infective agent. The nasal mucosa becomes dryer and less resistant to aerosolized infective agents as well.

When the presence of a foreign substance or microorganism has breached the first barrier of defense, inflammation triggers the innate immune system. When an attack by organisms or damage is recognized, leukocytes and other proteins quickly travel to the affected area, limit the amount of effect, and destroy the "invader" through phagocytosis. Select cells communicate the presence of the foreign material to the adaptive immunity system so that it can respond as well. Innate immunity reacts to all stimuli in the same way regardless of whether it has occurred in the past; it is *nonspecific* (Rote, 2019). In normal aging, leucocyte travel slows, phagocytic activity declines, and communication for adaptive immunity is delayed or interrupted (Bilder, 2016). The impaired immunity system is thought to contribute to a chronic state of low-level inflammation and further dysregulation.

The major components of adaptive immunity are T and B lymphocytes (several different types of each). T cells are produced in the bone marrow, move to the thymus for further development, and then are stored in the lymph tissue and spleen until needed. Any substance that evokes an adaptive response is referred to as an antigen, and both T and B lymphocytes produce antibodies to help the innate response fight against it *specifically*. Once the cells have been exposed to the antigen, it is "remembered," and a much faster and more aggressive response is possible the next time the offending organism or agent is detected. New (naive) T cells are required to respond to a new antigen. By the age of 60 the thymus shrinks up to 50%, and fewer naive T cells are produced (Bilder, 2016). Elsewhere in the body there is an accumulation of old T cells, which already have a memory of a past response and are not able to react to a new antigen. Both types of T cells appear to respond more slowly to the return of a previous bacteria or virus (e.g., shingles from previous latent chickenpox) or to a new one (e.g., COVID-19) (Bilder, 2016; Soiza et al., 2021).

Although the number of B cells is stable, they produce fewer antibodies, they do not remain in the body as long, and there is an increase in the number of circulating autoantibodies and B cells becoming less sensitive to self-antigens and less able to differentiate self-cells from foreign cells. As a result, there is an increase in autoimmune responses and autoimmune disorders (Box 27.2). While the mechanism is not yet understood, it appears that the COVID-19 virus is able to induce autoimmunity in persons without a previous autoimmune disorder or inflammatory disease (Liu et al., 2021).

THE AGING ENDOCRINE SYSTEM

The endocrine glands produce hormones that exit the gland; circulate in the blood; and regulate growth, reproduction, metabolism, and response to stress. Most age-related changes are reductions: in concentration, number of receptors, sensitivity to changes, and reduced function. In contrast, the prostate gland continues to grow, producing hyperplasia and elevated concentrations of adrenal steroids. Except for the ovaries, age-related changes in the endocrine system are thought to be very mild and most likely due to the autoimmunity described in the previous section.

The complex interrelationships between the endocrine glands and the number of concurrent chronic conditions in later life make it almost impossible to specifically attribute any endocrine disease to the aging process itself. As with most other biological systems, the signs and symptoms of problems are often atypical and nonspecific in older adults. Other than menopause, an endocrine disorder may be recognized only during the evaluation for another problem such as confusion or an unexplained fall. In this chapter, the endocrine disorders of diabetes and thyroid disorders as seen in older adults are addressed.

DIABETES MELLITUS

Insulin is the hormone that regulates the metabolism of glucose to provide metabolic energy. It facilitates the uptake of glucose into the cells for immediate use and into the liver where it is converted to glycogen and stored for later use. The two main types of diabetes mellitus (DM) are type 1 (T1DM) and type 2 (T2DM). It is estimated that more than 21% of all persons at least 65 years old have been diagnosed with diabetes and more than 5% have it but have not been diagnosed (Centers for Disease Control and Prevention [CDC], 2020). In a French study, 20% of those with DM and hospitalized with COVID-19 in 2020 died within 28 days (Wargny et al., 2021).

T1DM is the result of absolute insulin deficiency due to the autoimmune destruction of beta cells in the pancreas. Historically, few people with T1DM have lived to late life. T2DM is relative insulin deficiency—the cells are not able to use the insulin produced (insulin resistance)—and is the most common type seen in older adults. There is also a very strong family association: the more family members with DM, the greater the

TABLE 27.1 Diabetes by Race/Ethnicity

Race/Ethnicity	Percentage Diagnosed With Diabetes
Non-Hispanic whites	7.5
Asian Americans	9.2
Chinese	5.6
Filipinos	10.4
Asian Indians	12.6
Other Asian Americans	9.9
Hispanics	12.5
Central and South Americans	8.3
Cubans	8.5
Mexican Americans	14.2
Puerto Ricans	12.4
Non-Hispanic blacks	11.7
American Indians/Alaskan Natives	14.7

From American Diabetes Association: *Statistics about diabetes* (website), 2021.https://www.diabetes.org/resources/statistics/statistics-about-diabetes.

BOX 27.3 Diabetes From Exposure to Toxins?

Veterans who have developed diabetes and served in and around Vietnam, near the demilitarized zone (DMZ) in Korea, and on several bases in the United States may be eligible to receive health care and disability compensation due to exposure to Agent Orange or other herbicides. Surviving spouses, children, and parents may be eligible for survivor benefits.

US Department of Veterans Affairs: Agent Orange exposure and VA disability compensation (website), 2020. https://www.va.gov/disability/eligibility/hazardous-materials-exposure/agent-orange/.

BOX 27.4 Functional Disability Associated With Diabetes

Mobility impairment	Muscle weakness
Falls	Fatigue
Incontinence	Weight loss
Cognitive impairments	

BOX 27.5 Factors Increasing the Risk for Heart Disease or Stroke Among Persons With Diabetes

Smoking
High blood pressure
Abnormal cholesterol and triglycerides levels
Central obesity (waist >40 inches for men and >35 inches for women)
Family history of heart disease
Uncontrolled diabetes

Adapted from National Institute of Diabetes and Digestive and Kidney Diseases: *Diabetes, heart disease, and stroke* (website), 2017. https://www.niddk.nih.gov/health-information/diabetes/overview/preventing-problems/heart-disease-stroke.

risk. Part of this is likely related to familial obesity, either with genetic influence or that of lifestyle and diet.

There has been a significant number of persons hospitalized with COVID-19 found to be hyperglycemic without a previous diagnosis of DM. About half of these have been found to return to a pre-infection normoglycemic state. The others were found to have high A1Cs on admission indicating previousely undiagnosed DM. These persons were most likely to be younger and less common in non-Hispanic White race or ethnicity (Cromer et al., 2022).

In 2021, the US Preventive Services Task Force (USPSTF) recommended screening for prediabetes and T2DM in asymptomatic adults 35 to 70 years old who are overweight or obese. For adults with normal blood glucose levels, screening can be done every 3 years (USPSTF, 2021). The reviewers found convincing evidence that intensive behavioral counseling for a healthful diet and regular exercise has a moderate benefit in reducing the progression of prediabetes to diabetes and reducing other cardiovascular risk factors such as hypertension and hyperlipidemia.

There is a wide variation in the prevalence of DM among ethnic and racial groups and subgroups (Table 27.1). In the United States, American Indians and Alaskan Natives have the highest rate of diabetes compared to all other groups. They are 3 times more likely than non-Hispanic Whites to be diagnosed with diabetes and 2.3 times more likely to die (2018 figures) (Office of Minority Health [OMH], 2021). Another group at high risk is older veterans who were exposed to Agent Orange during military service (US Department of Veterans Affairs [VA], 2020) (Box 27.3).

The risk for the development of complications in older adults with T2DM is compounded by the presence of multiple comorbid diseases and disorders. Persons with diabetes are at high risk for developing heart disease and have a greater chance of having a heart attack, stroke, and dementia (Amidei et al., 2021). Diabetes is associated with a high rate of depression, and those who are depressed have a higher mortality rate. Prolonged periods of hyperglycemia lead to tissue damage from the glycosylation of proteins and by-products. Functional declines are more likely unless proactive measures are taken to promote wellness (Box 27.4).

Heart disease is the most common cause of death among people with diabetes (Box 27.5) (American Diabetes Association [ADA], 2021; Cavallari et al., 2021). Macrovascular and microvascular changes cause nerve damage resulting in several complications, including peripheral neuropathy and gastroparesis. It is the leading cause of blindness, amputation, and kidney failure. Sexual dysfunction and impotence result from reduced vascular flow, neuropathy, and uncontrolled circulating blood glucose levels; erectile dysfunction is two to five times greater in those with DM than those without. The older adult with DM should be screened regularly for the development of signs of complications that are more likely to occur in this population (Box 27.6). Several geriatric syndromes are highly associated with DM and contribute to excess morbidity, especially cognitive impairment, depression, polypharmacy, incontinence, persistent pain, and falls.

BOX 27.6 Complications of Diabetes More Common in Older Adults

Dry eyes	Anorexia
Dry mouth	Dehydration
Confusion	Delirium
Incontinence	Nausea
Weight loss	Delayed wound healing

BOX 27.7 Signs of End-Organ Damage in Diabetes

Decreased visual acuity	Heart disease
Paresthesia	Stroke
Neuropathy	Periodontal disease

BOX 27.8 Cues Indicating Possible Hypoglycemia in Older Adults

Tachycardia
Sensation of heart palpitations
Diaphoresis
Tremors
Pallor
Unexplained anxiety.
Later symptoms may include: headache, dizziness, fatigue, irritability, confusion, hunger, visual changes, seizures, and coma.

BOX 27.9 Tip for Best Practice

Any time hypoglycemia is suspected, it becomes a priority of care. Glucose is administered immediately either orally if conscious or intravenously if unconscious.

Recognizing and Analyzing Cues

The classic signs of both T1DM and T2DM are polyuria, polydipsia, and polyphagia (the three Ps). As with most other conditions, the signs and symptoms are atypical in older adults. Polyuria occurs less frequently due to age-related increases in the renal tolerance for elevated glucose. Instead, the older adult may develop urinary incontinence or find that it has worsened. Polydipsia (excessive thirst) is not present as often due to age-related reduced thirst reflex. Polyphagia (excessive hunger) is reduced by age-related decreased appetite. Unplanned weight loss instead of weight gain may occur. Fatigue is common. The first sign in women may be recurrent vulvovaginal candidiasis (yeast infections). Due to the atypical, absent, or delayed signs and symptoms, the person may be found obtunded in a hyperglycemic-hyperosmolar nonketotic coma before an initial diagnosis is made (ADA, 2021). Too often a diagnosis is not made until evidence of end-organ damage becomes visible (Box 27.7).

Problems in the lower extremities are common and can have a considerable impact on function. Warning signs include cold feet, neuropathic burning, tingling, and both hypersensitivity and numbness. "Diabetic foot ulcers" can easily occur with unrecognized injury. Injury and infections are common and difficult to treat. Both the infections and the necessary antibiotics often result in unstable glucose control.

Hypoglycemia (blood glucose level <60 mg/dL) can occur from many causes, such as unusually intense exercise, alcohol intake, or medication mismanagement. Multiple cues of low blood sugar are potentially recognizable and require rapid prioritization of hypotheses and urgent solutions to address the immediate problems (Boxes 27.8 and 27.9).

Hyperglycemia in older adults is harder to detect than in younger adults because there is a higher tolerance for elevated levels of circulating glucose. It is not uncommon to find persons with fasting glucose levels of 200 to 600 mg/dL or higher. This level of unrecognized hyperglycemia increases the risk for hyperosmolar hyperglycemic nonketotic coma. This is life-threatening to persons who are medically fragile and should be considered at any time an older adult with DM is difficult to arouse. This is always a medical emergency.

Pharmacological Interventions

Care of the older adult with DM requires that the bedside or community nurse develop a knowledge base of the commonly used pharmacological interventions. These include preventive (cardiac) adjuvant therapy, such as angiotensin-converting enzyme (ACE) inhibitors, lipid-lowering agents, and aspirin. All have demonstrated to improve outcomes for those with diabetes by reducing complications and premature death. The primary care advanced practice nurse is expected to have expertise in the spectrum of pharmacological approaches to assist persons in the appropriate management of their disease and its complications.

Several medications have implications for safe use in older adults. Metformin (Glucophage) is commonly prescribed as preventive or first-line therapy; it does not cause hypoglycemia or weight gain. It is contraindicated in persons with advanced renal disease (glomerular filtrate rate <30 mL/min/1.73 m^2) and used with caution in those with reduced hepatic function or congestive heart failure. Thiazolidinediones can be used only with great caution, especially in those with heart failure or at risk for falls. Due to the very high risk for hypoglycemia, sulfonylureas (e.g., Glynase, Diabinese, Glipizide) are not recommended for use by older adults (American Geriatrics Society [AGS], 2019). Incretin-based therapies can be very expensive and, if injectable, require the same skills as insulin (discussed next).

Insulin is used when all other strategies have failed to maintain the specific glycemic goals for that person. There are long-acting preparations (e.g., Lantus), but they cannot be used until the required daily total dose is determined. This is done using shorter-acting preparations until this is known. "Sliding-scale" adjustments are not recommended (AGS, 2019). The use of insulin requires that the person or caregiver have manual dexterity to ensure that glucose levels are monitored and doses are administered or taken correctly. Visual acuity is required to fill syringes with the correct dose. Syringe magnifiers are available and may be helpful to some, but not all, with impaired vision. Prefilled syringes can be obtained and therefore could be used by someone with visual limitations; however, the cost of these is often prohibitive.

USING CLINICAL JUDGMENT TO PROMOTE HEALTHY AGING: DIABETES

The gerontological nurse has a major role in promoting healthy aging in older adults with diabetes. Ideally the nurse helps the person move toward the goals of *Healthy People 2030* and ensures that the medical diabetic care received is consistent with the standard of care established by the ADA (ADA, 2021). The focus is on prevention, early identification of disease, and delay of complications for as long as possible. Prevention includes identifying those persons at greatest risk (e.g., obese or with a positive family history), encouraging regular exercise, and maintaining excellent control of other chronic conditions.

 HEALTHY PEOPLE 2030

National Objectives Related to Diabetes

Reduce the number of diabetes cases diagnosed each year
Increase the proportion of adults with diabetes who have a yearly eye exam
Increase the proportion of people with diabetes who get formal diabetes education
Reduce the rate of death from any cause in adults with diabetes

From US Department of Health and Human Services, Office of Disease Prevention and Health Promotion: *Healthy People 2030: diabetes* (website), n.d. https://health.gov/healthypeople/objectives-and-data/browse-objectives/diabetes. Accessed June 2021.

BOX 27.10   Minimizing Cardiovascular Risk in Persons With Diabetes

Maintain a healthy diet
Exercise regularly
Maintain target blood pressure (<130/80 to 140/90 mm Hg)[a]
No smoking or exposure to smoke
Maintain target hemoglobin A_{1C}
Manage stress
Get adequate and restful sleep
Regular dental visits
Attain and maintain acceptable cholesterol and triglyceride levels

[a]Identified goal varies by organization at this time.

Although glycemic control is important, in late life the prevention and treatment of cardiovascular disease is now emphasized. Research has indicated that it may take 8 years of glycemic control before benefits are seen, wheras the benefits of better control of blood pressure and lipid levels are seen as early as in 2 to 3 years. Promoting cardiovascular health has the potential to be most efficacious in the minimization of complications in persons with DM (Box 27.10). At all times, interventions must be considered in the context of concurrent comorbid conditions, risk factors, the life expectancy and an individual cost-benefit ratio (ADA, 2021).

Solutions, Nursing Actions, and Outcomes

Screening for DM is important for early identification of prediabetes or unrecognized diabetes. Nurses participate in screenings at community health fairs and in clinical settings and conduct educational programs about the need for early diagnosis,

glycemic control, and prompt identification and treatment of complications. Some nurses choose to develop an expertise in working with those who have diabetes and become certified diabetes educators and clinicians.

Health promotion for older adults with DM begins with a comprehensive geriatric assessment (Chapter 9) with a focus on the recognition of cues that indicate the potential for or the presence of complications, including changes in cognition. A careful neurological examination includes the assessment of neuropathy and changes in sensation; a Semmes-Weinstein–type monofilament test can be used for this. The measurements of height, weight, and waist circumference can be used to calculate the body mass index (BMI), but this measure is less useful in older adults because of the age-related replacement of muscle mass with adipose tissue. Physical assessment includes a careful inspection of the feet, skin, and mouth for signs of injury or the presence of lesions.

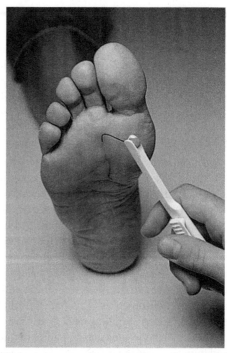

Semmes-Weinstein monofilament. (From Seidel HM: Mosby's physical examination handbook, ed 6, St Louis, 2006, Mosby.)

The use of herbal products and nutritional supplements, over-the-counter and prescription medications, "street" drugs, alcohol, and tobacco should be included in the assessment of someone with diabetes. All have a direct or indirect effect on renal, circulatory, neurological, and nutritional health and influence the risk for complications.

Due to the high prevalence of depression, the assessment includes a screen for this at the time of diagnosis, at intervals thereafter, or at any time depression is suspected by the health care provider (e.g., nurse) or reported by the patient (Chapters 9 and 30).

Expert care for older adults with diabetes requires an array of interventions and a multiprofessional team working in collaboration with the patient and the family or significant others. The nurse often serves as team leader, educator, care provider, supporter, and guide. If the person's disease is difficult to control, endocrinologists are involved, and as complications develop, more specialists are utilized, such as nephrologists, cardiologists, and wound care specialists. Nurses are expected to advocate for older adults and encourage them to expect and receive quality care to prevent the devastating end results of poor management of diabetes.

Although the goals of minimizing both hypoglycemia and hyperglycemia and controlling risk factors are potentially the same at any age, life expectancy and comorbid conditions can change the focus of care. If the person is frail, prevention of hypoglycemia, hypotension, and drug interactions is especially important. If there is not a consistent caregiver or one who has obtained the necessary diabetes education on behalf of or with the older adult, diabetes control may be impossible.

The glycated hemoglobin test (Hgb A_{1C}) has been considered the best measure of ongoing glycemic control. However, its use may either overdiagnose or underdiagnose persons with African ancestry, even over multiple generations. Due to the significant heterogeneity of those who identify as Black or mixed race, it is recommended that two different tests be conducted (e.g., a glucose tolerance test and a Hgb A_{1C} test) before a diagnosis of DM is made. This may be especially important for anyone who is near either the upper or the lower limits of the established range (5.7% to 6.5%). The Hgb A_{1C} test is known to be inaccurate in persons with nutritional deficiencies, anemia, or genetic conditions like sickle cell disease (Briker et al., 2019; Khosla et al., 2021). When used, the ADA recommends that older adults who are otherwise healthy, with few chronic illnesses and intact cognitive and functional abilities, have a goal of less than 7% to 7.5%. For those with multiple impairments, an Hgb A_{1C} goal of 8% to 8.5% is more reasonable (ADA, 2021).

The cornerstones of nonpharmacological management of DM are nutrition, exercise, and self-care.

Nutrition

Adequate and appropriate nutrition is key to healthy living and aging with DM. An initial nutrition assessment with a 24-hour recall will provide some clues to the patient's dietary habits and style of eating (Chapter 15). It is part of the nurse's responsibility to learn whether appropriate food is accessible, including necessary funds and a means of food preparation. Meal planning with a diabetes specialist is a covered service under Medicare (Table 27.2). If the person is overweight or obese, a loss of as little as 5% to 10% through healthy eating and exercise may decrease Hgb A_{1C}, improve function, lower blood pressure, and improve lipid management.

Helping people who have developed eating patterns over a lifetime is always challenging. If the older adult is from an ethnic group different from that of the nurses, they will need to learn more about the usual ingredients and methods of food preparation to be able to give reasonable instructions related to adjustments for diets optimal for living with DM. The nurse works with the individual to identify culturally specific foods that can be translated into a "diabetic diet."

TABLE 27.2 Medicare Coverage for Supplies and Services for Those With Diabetes

Supply or Service	Frequency	Cost
Screening (laboratory)	Twice a year for those at risk	No cost
Diabetes prevention program (1 time)	If laboratory tests are negative and BMI is ≥25 (≥23 if Asian) and has never been diagnosed with DM or ESRD	No cost
Diabetes Self-Management Training (DSMT)	Up to 10 hours of initial DSMT (1 individual and 9 group) and 2 hours follow-up each subsequent year (including telehealth)	20% of Medicare-approved amount after deductible met
Equipment needed for home glucose monitoring	Some restrictions to number of quarterly supplies	20% of Medicare-approved amount after annual deductible
Foot exams	Yearly for those with peripheral neuropathy	20% of Medicare-approved amount after annual deductible
Eye exam for diabetic retinopathy	Annually	20% of Medicare-approved amount after deductible met
Insulin	Monthly	Maximum of $35/month from participating plans
Medical nutrition services	Initial assessment and follow-up	No cost
Therapeutic shoes and inserts	For those with severe diabetic foot disease, annually	20% of Medicare-approved amount after deductible met

BMI, Body mass index; *DM,* diabetes mellitus; *ESRD,* end-stage renal disease.
For more information and details, see Centers for Medicare and Medicaid Services: *Is your test, item, or service covered?* https://www.medicare.gov/coverage/is-your-test-item-or-service-covered.

Exercise

Exercise improves tissue sensitivity to insulin and promotes cardiac health. Walking is an inexpensive and beneficial way to exercise; however, it needs to be done in a safe location, which cannot be assumed to be in the person's neighborhood. A more intensive exercise program, such as aerobics, cannot be started without consulting a health care provider. Those who have limited mobility can do chair exercises or, if possible, use exercise machines that enable sitting or support while standing. If the person is using insulin, exercise must be done regularly rather than erratically, and blood glucose level must be checked before and after to avoid or respond promptly to hypoglycemia.

BOX 27.11 Self-Care Skills Needed for the Person With Diabetes

Glucose Self-Monitoring
Obtaining a blood sample correctly
Using the glucose monitoring equipment correctly
Troubleshooting when results indicate an error
Recording the values from the machine
Understanding the timing and frequency of self-monitoring
Understanding what to do with the results

Medication Self-Administration: Insulin
Selecting appropriate injection site
Using correct technique for injections
Disposing of used needles and syringes correctly
Storing and transporting insulin correctly

Oral Medication Use
Knowing drug, dose, timing, and side effects
Knowing drug-drug and drug-food interactions
Recognizing side effects and knowing when to report

Foot Care and Examination
Selecting and using appropriate and safe footwear

Handling Sick Days
Recognizing the signs and symptoms of both hyperglycemia and hypoglycemia
Knowing what to do in response to symptoms

Self-Care

Due to the complexity of DM in late life, maximum wellness is difficult to achieve without considerable self-care skills. The nurse or diabetic nurse educator is often the professional who is responsible for working with the older adult in developing such skills (Box 27.11).

Self-management essentials for diabetes include knowing the signs of hypoglycemia and hyperglycemia and the actions to take if these complications arise. An identification bracelet is recommended because delirium may be a manifestation of low blood glucose level and misinterpreted as dementia, delaying prompt life-saving treatment. Self-care also includes preventive care practices for the heart, eyes, kidneys, and feet. Annual diabetes self-management training and several other diabetes-specific services are available through Medicare (see Table 27.2). Many resources are available on the websites of the National Institute of Diabetes and Digestive and Kidney Diseases (NIDDK; https://www.niddk.nih.gov/health-information/diabetes) and the CDC (https://www.cdc.gov/diabetes/managing/index.html). The resources provide links to a multitude of other sites, including those specific to ethnic and racial groups and in a variety of languages.

Implications for the Frail and Those Living in Residential Care Settings

Many of those who are frail also have DM and are dependent on others for care. This may include meal preparation, assistance with exercise, or even help with movement. In a residential care setting such as a nursing home or assisted living facility, nurses and aides are usually the ones who recognize cues of hypoglycemia and hyperglycemia and implement emergency responses. The nurse ensures that the diabetic standards of care are met and monitors the effect and side effects of diet and exercise. The nurse administers or supervises the safe administration of medications and monitors their effect.

In the home care setting the nurse works with the individual if the person is capable; if not, the nurse identifies the caregivers who are providing support and care. When needed, the caregiver is the day-to-day *de facto* nurse acting with the support of professionals in provider or home health offices.

THYROID DISEASE

The thyroid hormone is part of the body's system that controls metabolism. A fully functioning thyroid gland (or its replacement) is necessary to maintain life. Progressive fibrosis and atrophy are normal age-related changes. It is more difficult to palpate the thyroid in an older neck, but the changes are not usually clinically significant. However, thyroid disorders increase with age, especially in women. Screening should be done for all older adults with cardiovascular disease, depression, anxiety, or cognitive impairments.

The signs and symptoms are often attributed to normal aging, another disorder, a geriatric syndrome, or side effects of medications, delaying diagnosis. Thyroid diseases are diagnosed by the clinical presentation combined with laboratory findings of the total and free triiodothyronine (T3) levels, the free thyroxine (T4) levels, and the concentration of thyroid-stimulating hormone (TSH). However, the accuracy of the laboratory findings is easily affected by laboratory errors, acute illness and frailty, concurrent environmental conditions, and drug intake, making an accurate diagnosis difficult at times (Table 27.3).

Hypothyroidism

Hypothyroidism occurs when the thyroid gland fails to produce an adequate amount of free T_4, and T_3. The change in the levels of T_3 and T_4 stimulates the pituitary gland to produces excess TSH to stimulate the thyroid, but the stimulation in ineffective.

TABLE 27.3 Examples of Factors Affecting Laboratory Testing of Thyroid Functioning

Test	Increased Result	Depressed Result
TSH	Potassium iodide and lithium, laboratory error, autoimmune disease, strenuous exercise, acute sleep deprivation	Severe illness, aspirin, dopamine, heparin, and steroids
T_3	Estrogen and methadone	Anabolic steroids, androgens, phenytoin, naproxen, propranolol, reserpine, and salicylates
T_4	Estrogen, methadone, and clofibrate	Anabolic steroids, androgens, lithium, phenytoin, and propranolol (see T3)

T_3, Triiodothyronine; T_4, thyroxine, *TSH*, thyroid-stimulating hormone.
From Connor GJ: *Lab values interpretation: the ultimate laboratory tests manual of reference ranges and what they mean*, Berlin, 2020, GD Publishing Ltd.

It is thought to be caused most often by chronic autoimmune thyroiditis when the immune system attacks the thyroid gland (Hashimoto's disease). It also occurs when hyperthyroidism is overtreated, as a result of hypothalamic disorders, or due to the use of some medications, especially amiodarone and lithium (Reuben et al., 2020).

Hypothyroidism is initially diagnosed by the measurement of the TSH, free T_4, and T_3. Myxedema coma is a serious complication of untreated hypothyroidism in older adults. Rapid replacement of the missing hormones is not possible due to the risk for drug toxicity. Even with the best treatment, death may ensue. Many of those who are very ill and hospitalized may have an elevation in TSH level that is transient. When the illness resolves, so does the hypothyroidism.

> ⚡ **SAFETY TIPS**
>
> The medication amiodarone has many contraindications but is still in use for those with heart disease. It is associated with multiple toxicities, including thyroid disease. Thyroid function in all persons taking amiodarone must be monitored regularly.

Recognizing and Analyzing Cues

It is important to always note that while there are several cues that indicate possible hypothyroidism, they are easily misinterpreted; they are more subtle or vague in older adults and very different from those seen in younger adults (Box 27.12). Most experts recommend treating a TSH of 10 units/mL or higher (>7.5 units/mL in persons over age 80), but it is not clear if subclinical hypothyroidism should be treated in asymptomatic persons. Such persons who receive thyroid replacement do not have improved quality of life, muscle strength, or cognitive function and may have increased mortality (American Family Physician [AFP], 2020).

Thyroid hormone replacement is usually in the form of the medication levothyroxine. Treatment with levothyroxine is not innocuous, especially for women. Side effects include decreased bone mass and increased risk of heart disease. The older adult is very sensitive to exogenous thyroid hormones. Oral replacement should begin with 25 mcg of levothyroxine, or 12.5 mcg in persons with preexisting heart disease. The dose is adjusted every 4 to 6 weeks until stabilized and then in most cases is monitored annually (Reuben et al., 2020).

Hyperthyroidism

Hyperthyroidism it is an overproduction of thyroid hormones (and need for less stimulation). It is much less common than hypothyroidism but is associated with a high cardiac mortality and morbidity. It is most often caused by the autoimmune disorder Graves' disease but also can be caused by a toxic nodule, a multinodular goiter, or several medications, especially the iodine-containing amiodarone (Reuben et al., 2020). The onset of hyperthyroidism may be quite abrupt.

Diagnosis is made through a physical exam and laboratory testing. Primary hyperthyroidism is indicated by a low TSH and an elevated T_4. Subclinical disease is diagnosed with a low TSH and T_4 and T_3 that are slightly elevated or within normal limits. Persons with symptoms of heart disease are usually treated. Treatment includes antithyroid medications or ablative therapy.

Recognizing and Analyzing Cues

The manifestations of hyperthyroidism are often atypical in later life. Instead of heat intolerance, tremor, or nervousness, the older adult is more likely to have depression, weight loss, dyspnea, unexplained atrial fibrillation, heart failure, or confusion. The presence of any of the geriatric syndromes, such as constipation, anorexia, or muscle weakness, and other vague symptoms also may be noted. However, on further examination the causative factor may be hyperthyroidism. In later life, a condition known as apathetic thyrotoxicosis, rarely seen in younger persons, may occur, in which usual hyperkinetic activity is replaced with slowed movement and depressed affect.

USING CLINICAL JUDGMENT TO PROMOTE HEALTH AGING: THYROID DISEASE

Although the nurse may understand that little can be done to prevent thyroid disturbances in late life, organizations such as the Monterey Bay Aquarium have launched campaigns to inform consumers of the iodine and mercury levels found in seafood because of their association with thyroid diseases (http://www.seafoodwatch.org).

Solutions, Nursing Actions, and Outcomes

As advocates, nurses can ensure that a thyroid screening test be done anytime there is a possible concern. The nurse caring for frail older adults can be attentive to the possibility that the person who is diagnosed with anxiety, dementia, or depression may instead have a thyroid disturbance.

The nurse is instrumental in helping the person and family understand both the seriousness of the problem and the need for very careful adherence to the prescribed regimen (Box 27.13). If the older adult is hospitalized for acute management, the

---

BOX 27.12 Symptoms of Hypothyroidism in Older Adults

• Fatigue	• Mental slowness
• Weakness	• Drowsiness
• Depression	• Constipation
• Dry skin	

BOX 27.13 Tips for Best Practice

Levothyroxine: Specific Instructions for Administration

Levothyroxine always must be taken on an empty stomach—early in the morning, at least 30 to 60 minutes before a meal, or 4 hours after the last meal—but at the same time each day. It must be taken with a full glass of water to ensure that it does not begin to dissolve in the esophagus. It cannot be taken within 4 hours of anything containing a mineral, such as calcium (including fortified orange juice), antacids, or iron supplements. It is always dosed in micrograms, and care must be taken that micrograms are not confused with milligrams.

life-threatening nature of both the disorder and the treatment is explained so that advance planning can be done that will account for all possible outcomes.

The medical management of hypothyroidism is one of careful pharmacological replacement and, in the case of hyperthyroidism, one of surgical or chemical ablation followed by hormone replacement—both with the medication levothyroxine. The alternative Armour thyroid is not recommended for use in older adults (AGS, 2019). The nurse works with the person and significant others in the correct self-administration of medications and in the appropriate timing of monitoring blood levels.

KEY CONCEPTS

- The age-related changes in the immune system result in a decreased ability to mount a defense against antigens and increases the risk for infections in late life.
- With aging, there is an increase in autoimmunity leading to an increase in autoimmune disorders. This is also suspected to be associated with the higher number of fatalities in older persons with COVID-19.
- The most common diabetes in late life is T2DM, a combination of inadequate insulin to meet the needs of the body and insulin resistance.
- The prevalence of diabetes increases with age.
- Although the incidence of hyperthyroidism in late life is rare, hypothyroidism is seen with increasing frequency, especially among older women.

- There is a strong association between thyroid disease and heart disease. A person with either should be screened for the other on a regular basis.
- Undiagnosed or inadequately treated and monitored thyroid disorders can be life-threatening.
- The nurse plays an active role in the early recognition of cues of autoimmune disorders and infections.
- The nurse facilitates the person's receipt of evidence-based standards of care and the use of benefits available to the person to help control and treat endocrine diseases.

NEXT-GENERATION NCLEX® (NGN) EXAMINATION–STYLE QUESTIONS

Ms. P., an 82-year-old single woman, lives in a life-care community in her own apartment and has the reassurance of knowing that her medical and functional needs will be taken care of, regardless of the extent of these needs. She is at present independent. She has been gaining weight steadily since she moved into the community and attributes that to the fact that she eats much better now that she joins others in the congregate dining room for meals. She has heart failure, mild arthritis, and diabetes, which she manages with diet, exercise, and oral medications. Although she says she feels fine, lately she has noticed some increased fatigue and that her toes are cold and somewhat numb. The great toe on her left foot seems to be discolored. Because of the lack of feeling, she often walks around her apartment barefoot because she feels it increases the sensation in her feet. She has not needed to use the health care center and goes to the clinic only to pick up her medication. Her niece stopped by last week to see her and called the clinic and spoke with the nurse. The niece reported that her aunt seemed a little confused and lethargic. The niece accompanied Ms. P. to the clinic, where the nurses checked her blood pressure and blood sugar and found them to be 170/80 mm Hg and 280 mg/dL, respectively. Ms. P. said, "Oh, I don't think it is anything to worry about! I am just a little tired."

Highlight the cues and data that are not normal changes with aging but could indicate a potential complication of at least one of her chronic conditions. Of the cues identified, what are the top three priorities?

CLINICAL JUDGMENT QUESTIONS AND ACTIVITIES

1. What commonly held beliefs about aging would lead older persons to believe that the changes in their health do not warrant seeking health care?
2. You are assigned to teach a patient the basics of diabetes care. You have 1 day to do this before the person is discharged home. When you walk in the room and begin talking with

the person, you find out that she is from a culture completely different from yours. How will you begin?
3. Expanding on question 2 above, discuss with a classmate how you would approach the same situation when you find out that your patient is responsible for cooking for her whole family.

RESEARCH QUESTIONS

1. Is there any information that explains the differences in the incidence and prevalence of diabetes in various ethnic groups?

2. What types of nutritional food supplements are used by persons with diabetes?

REFERENCES

American Diabetes Association (ADA): Standard of medical care in diabetes—2021, *Diabetes Care* 44 (Suppl 1):S168–S179, 2021.

American Family Physician (AFP): Practice guideline: treatment of subclinical hypothyroidism: BMJ rapid recommendation, *Am Fam Physician* 105(2):316–317, 2020.

American Geriatrics Society (AGS): American Geriatrics Society 2019 updated Beers Criteria for potentially inappropriate medication use in older adults, *J Am Geriatr Soc* 67(4):674–694, 2019.

Amidei CB, Fayossee A, Dumurgier J, et al.: Association between age at diabetes onset and subsequent risk of dementia, *JAMA* 325(16):1640–1649, 2021.

Bilder GE: *Human biological aging*, Hoboken, NJ, 2016, Wiley-Blackwell.

Briker SM, Aduwo JY, Mugeni R, et al.: A_{1C} underperforms as a diagnostic test in Africans even in the absence of nutritional deficiencies, anemia and hemoglobinopathies: insight from the Africans in America Study, *Front Endocrinol (Lausanne)* 10:533, 2019. https://www.frontiersin.org/articles/10.3389/fendo.2019.00533/full.

Cavallari I, Bhatt DL, Steg G, et al.: Causes and risk factors for death in diabetes: a competing risk analysis from the SAVOR-TIMI 53 Trial, *J Am Coll Cardio* 77(14):1837–1840, 2021.

Centers for Disease Control and Prevention (CDC): Prevalence of both diagnosed and undiagnosed diabetes (website), 2020. https://www.cdc.gov/diabetes/data/statistics-report/diagnosed-undiagnosed-diabetes.html.

Cromer SJ, Colling C, Schatoff D, et al.: Newly diagnosed diabetes vs. pre-existing diabetes upon admission for COVID-19: Associated factors, short-term outcomes, and long-term glycemic phenotypes. *J DIabetes Complications*. Available online Feb 4, 2022.

Khosla L, Bhat S, Fullington LA, et al.: HbA1c performance in African descent populations in the United States with normal glucose tolerance, prediabetes, or diabetes: a scoping review, *Prev Chronic Dis* 18:E22, 2021.

Liu Y, Sawalha AR, Lu Q: COVID-19 and autoimmune diseases, *Curr Opin Rheumatol* 33(2):155–162, 2021.

Office of Minority Health (OMH): Diabetes and American Indians/Alaska Natives (website), 2021. https://minorityhealth.hhs.gov/omh/browse.aspx?lvl=4&lvlid=33.

Reuben DB, Herr KA, Pacala JT, et al.: *Geriatrics at your fingertips*, ed 22, New York, 2020, American Geriatrics Society.

Rote NS: Innate immunity: inflammation and wound healing. In McCance KL, Huether SE, editors:. *Pathophysiology: the biological basis for disease in adults and children*, 8, St Louis, 2019, Elsevier, pp 190–219.

Soiza RL, Scicluna C, Thomson EC: Efficacy and safety of COVID-19 vaccines in older people, *Age Ageing* 50(2):279–283, 2021.

US Department of Veterans Affairs (VA): Agent Orange exposure and VA disability compensation (website), 2020. https://www.va.gov/disability/eligibility/hazardous-materials-exposure/agent-orange/.

US Preventive Services Task Force (USPSTF): *Prediabetes and type 2 diabetes: Screening* (website), 2021. Recommendation: Prediabetes and Type 2 Diabetes: Screening | United States Preventive Services Taskforce (uspreventiveservicestaskforce.org)

Wargny M, Potier L, Gourdy P, et al.: Predictors of hospital discharge and mortality in patients with diabetes and COVID-19: updated results from the nationwide CORONADO study, *Diabetologia* 64:778–791, 2021.

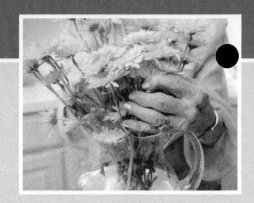

Common Musculoskeletal Disorders

Kathleen Jett

A STUDENT SPEAKS

I thought that if you were 75 years old, you would be all crippled up and could not do anything anymore, but some of the older people I have gotten to know are still playing tennis and hiking. They say their hands and feet hurt afterward, but that is not going to keep them down!

Rebecca, 19-year-old nurse

AN OLDER ADULT SPEAKS

These old bones just aren't what they used to be. I sound like a rocker just a-creakin' away.

Jesse, age 92

LEARNING OBJECTIVES

On completion of this chapter, the reader will be able to:

1. Recognize the normal changes in the aging musculoskeletal system that have the potential to affect functional status.
2. Describe a "fragility fracture" and explain its relationship to osteoporosis.
3. Differentiate the signs and symptoms of osteoarthritis, rheumatoid arthritis, and gout as manifested in older adults.
4. Select nursing actions that promote musculoskeletal health in later life.

THE AGING MUSCULOSKELETAL SYSTEM

A functioning musculoskeletal system is necessary for the body's movement in space, responses to environmental forces, maintenance of posture and activity level, and regulation of body temperature. Some level of functioning is needed to independently meet one's activities of daily living (ADLs) (Chapter 9). Although none of the age-related musculoskeletal changes are life-threatening, any can affect quality of life and the ability to remain independent and comfortable. As the changes become visible to others, they have the potential to negatively affect self-esteem.

Changes in stature and posture are two of the obvious outward signs of aging (Fig. 28.1). They occur gradually and affect skeletal, muscular, and subcutaneous and fat tissue. Vertebral discs become thinner as a result of gravity and dehydration. A stooped, slightly forward-bent posture is common and may be accompanied by slightly flexed hips and knees. To maintain eye contact, it may be necessary to extend the head slightly, which makes it appear that the person is jutting forward. These changes occur primarily because of age-related bone calcium loss and atrophic cartilage and muscle.

Bones

Bones are composed of organic tissue and inorganic products, especially minerals. The minerals, especially calcium, are in a constant state of flux. They are released into the blood and then resorbed again for new bone growth. The quality and density of the bones (bone mineral density, or BMD) peaks at about the age of 30, after which it declines by about 0.5% a year. The rate of loss is significantly influenced by nutritional, hormonal, and genetic factors and by weight-bearing exercises (Bellantoni & Gilliam, 2021; Bilder, 2016).

Eventually bone renewal cannot keep pace with resorption and the bones become brittle and fracture more easily. Reduced BMD is four times more common in older women than in older men but is present in all persons as they age, regardless of ethnicity or race. Women may lose up to 50% of their cortical bone mass by the time they are 70 years old, the extent of which depends on multiple factors (Hopkins et al., 2019). In

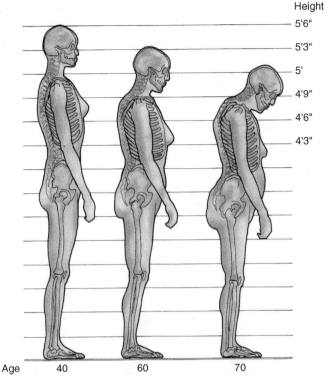

Fig. 28.1 Age-related changes in the spine as a result of bone loss. (From Ignatavicius DD, Workman ML: *Medical-surgical nursing: patient-centered collaborative care,* ed 8, Philadelphia, 2016, Elsevier.)

men, reduced BMD occurs primarily due to prolonged steroid use. Excessive loss of BMD leads to *osteopenia* or *osteoporosis.*

Joints, Tendons, and Ligaments

The tendons and ligaments in and around joints are bands of connective tissue that bind the bones to each other and make movement possible. Cartilage is a fibrous tissue that lines the joints and supports specific body parts, such as the ears and nose. While the cartilage in the ears and nose enlarges (especially in men), age-related deterioration in *articular* cartilage results from biochemical changes and increases in the levels of transglutaminase and calcium pyrophosphates. As joints dry, movement is less fluid. Pain may result if these changes progress to the extent where bone rubs on bone, as in arthritis. Cellular cross-linkage causes stiffening of the cartilage, ligaments, and tendons.

Muscles

The three types of muscles are smooth, skeletal, and cardiac. Smooth muscles are responsible for the contractibility of hollow organs such as the blood vessels. Skeletal muscles, primarily under voluntary control, are essential for movement, posture, and heat production. After the age of 50 there is a gradual loss of muscle bulk and strength. These changes are referred to as *sarcopenia* and are seen almost exclusively in the skeletal muscle. Accelerated loss occurs with inactivity and deconditioning, such as seen with increased frequency during the pandemic-induced

quarantine beginning in 2020. Sarcopenia also has been found to be increased in older adults who have had a COVID-19 infection (Welch et al., 2020).

MUSCULOSKELETAL DISORDERS

The most common musculoskeletal disorders in later life are osteoporosis, osteoarthritis, rheumatoid arthritis, and gout. Chronic pain and problems with function associated with these and other musculoskeletal problems affect more than 1.7 billion people worldwide; associated low back pain is the single most common cause of disability in 160 countries (World Health Organization [WHO], 2021). Giant cell arteritis and polymyalgia rheumatica occur less often. In this chapter we address osteoporosis, osteoarthritis, rheumatoid arthritis, and gout.

Osteoporosis

Although osteoporosis (OP) is not a normal part of aging, it is the most common metabolic bone disease and the characterized result of a gradual loss of cortical (outer shell) and trabecular bone (inner spongy meshwork) and microarchitectural deterioration. This loss of BMD excelerates rapidly in women after menopause and in anyone who takes steroids for an extended period of time. The most serious health consequences of OP are a fracture and a heightened risk for postfracture morbidity and mortality. Many people suffer multiple fractures, require long-term care, or never walk unassisted again (Chapter 20). Wrist fractures can result in severe self-care limitations.

The most common sites for such fractures are hips, vertebrae, wrist, and pelvis. Vertebral compression fractures are common in older women. They can occur from anything from a sneeze to a fall. While most are asymptomatic, they also can result in intense pain, disability, or immobility-related pneumonia. The person may attribute the pain to "normal aging" rather than a potential fracture.

Although the incidence and prevalence of OP varies by race and ethnicity, it can affect persons at all ages and in all ethnic and racial groups; those at highest risk are thin, postmenopausal, White women who do not take hormone replacement therapy (Table 28.1). Chinese Americans have low BMD but fewer fractures than other groups, and Hispanic women have been found to be least likely to use preventive measures (Richens, 2020). It is estimated that 52 million people in the United States have

TABLE 28.1	Percentage With Low Bone Mass and Osteoporosis by Race and Ethnicity	
Race	Low Bone Mass	Osteoporosis
White Americans	9	42.9
Mexican Americans	13.1	42.2
Black Americans	4.2	29.7

From Richens M: *Ten things to know about racial differences in bone health* (website), 2020. https://americanbonehealth.org/races-ethnicities/10-things-to-know-about-racial-differences-in-bone-health/.

BOX 28.1   Fragility Fractures

Fragility fractures are those resulting from forces that would not normally cause a fracture, such as from a fall from standing height or from activities such as coughing, sneezing, or abrupt movement. The spine, hip, and distal forearm are the most common sites.

---

reduced bone mass, including about 25% of women over 65 years of age and 5% of all men (Bellantoni & Gilliam, 2021).

OP is diagnosed either following a fragility fracture (Box 28.1) or by a dual-energy x-ray absorptiometry (DXA) scan of the femoral neck and spine (Fig. 28.2). The result of the scan yields a score indicating the individual's BMD in comparison to a healthy (young) reference group. *Osteopenia,* or a moderate amount of decreased BMD, is diagnosed with a "T-score" between −1 and −2.5 standard deviations from the norm, and *osteoporosis,* or a significant amount of loss of bone density, is diagnosed with a T-score greater than −2.5 standard deviations from the norm (Reuben et al., 2020). In the most recent analysis by the United States Prevention Task Force (USPTF, 2018), it was determined that there was convincing evidence that a DXA scan was an accurate predictor of hip fractures and a means to determine the appropriateness of drug therapy to stabilize or improve BMD and therefore reduce the risk of fracture.

It is recommended that all women at least 65 years old be screened for OP, but screening is not recommended for men without risk factors for secondary osteoporosis. It is also recommended for women younger than 65 years old if they are at increased risk based on an evidence-based measure such as the Fracture Risk Assessment Tool (FRAX; Chapter 20) (USPSTF, 2018) (Box 28.2). Without a diagnosis, the person does not have full access to the available treatments.

Medicare covers the cost of an initial screening and repeat scans at 24-month intervals if the person is diagnosed with OP or osteopenia *and* is receiving treatment or otherwise at increased risk. There is no deductible or copay for this service (Medicare, n.d.).

BOX 28.2   Major Risk Factors for Osteoporosis

Small body frame
Race and gender: White women
Broken bone before 50 years of age
Family history of osteoporosis
Estrogen deficiency
Inadequate calcium and vitamin D intake
Lack of weight-bearing activities
Excess alcohol use (>1 drink/day for women and >2 drinks/day for men)
Smoking or exposure to tobacco smoke
Eating disorders
Chronic use of glucocorticoids

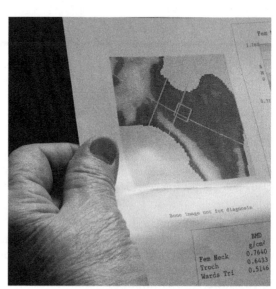

A dual-energy x-ray absorptiometry (DXA) scan of the upper femur and acetabulum (right "hip"). (©iStock.com/kgerakis.)

Recognizing and Analyzing Cues

OP is a silent condition, and a person may have neither symptoms nor a diagnosis until a fracture occurs. A sign suggestive of reduced spinal BMD is the loss of height of more than 3 cm (see Fig. 28.1; Box 28.3). The nurse may be the one to recognize changes, palpate back or joint tenderness, or learn of unexplained pain and may be the first to suspect a fracture (Box 28.4).

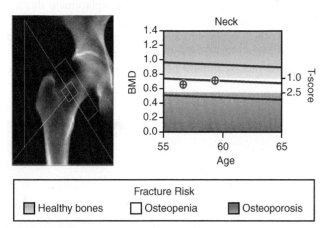

Fig. 28.2 DXA scan: determining the presence of reduced bone mineral density *(BMD).* T-score = −1.4 = osteopenia. (Radiograph from Colledge NR, Walker BR, Ralston SH: *Davidson's principles and practice of medicine,* ed 21, London, 2010, Elsevier.)

BOX 28.3   Cues That Indicate Possible Osteoporosis

Inability to stand straight or with head against a wall
Kyphosis
Fewer than 20 teeth
Rib-pelvis distance ≤2 finger-widths
Loss of >3 inches height from highest

From Bellantoni M, Gilliam M: Osteoporosis and hip fracture. In Walter LC, Chang A, editors: *CURRENT diagnosis and treatment: geriatrics,* ed 3, New York, 2021, McGraw Hill, pp 253–262.

BOX 28.4 Recognizing the Cues of a Hip Fracture and Prioritizing Nursing Actions

I knocked on Mrs. Martin's door to enroll her in a research study. I heard a loud thud followed by moaning. I was able to see a large White woman lying on the floor of the room behind the window. We were in a rural area with no cell phone service. I identified myself and was able to pry the window open with my bandage scissors and climb through. Mrs. Martin had tripped on the carpet and landed on her side, her leg in an awkward position, and cried that her hip hurt very much. I called for an ambulance, realizing that it would take some time before it could get to us. I made her as comfortable and safe as I could, being careful not to touch her hip. I was fairly certain that it was broken. It was.

BOX 28.5 Health Disparities in Prevention and Treatment of Osteoporosis: Black and White Americans[a]

Only 8.4% of Black women receive a medication to treat or prevent osteoporosis, compared to 13.6% of White women.

Black women are 18% less likely to receive a medication following a fracture.

[a]Almost universal health care available to American older adults after the age of 65 through Medicare.

From Richens M: *Ten things to know about racial differences in bone health* (website), 2020. https://americanbonehealth.org/races-ethnicities/10-things-to-know-about-racial-differences-in-bone-health/.

Pharmacological Interventions

For those at risk for OP or with existing disease, pharmacological interventions are recommended. Currently available medications include antiresorptive agents—bisphosphonates (e.g., alendronate [Fosamax]), hormone replacement, selective estrogen reception modifiers (SERMs) (e.g., raloxifene), denosumab, and calcitonin—and the anabolic agent PTH (parathyroid hormone) derivatives. Bisphosphonates are the first line of therapy but are contraindicated in person with renal failure. They can be taken orally once a day or weekly or intravenously every 3 or 6 months, depending on the medication. Calcitonin has also been found to reduce vertebral fracture pain. An adequate amount of vitamin D and calcium must be taken to avoid hypocalcemia. It is important to know that the supplements alone have *not* been found to prevent fractures (USPSTF, 2018). There are significant Black-White disparities in both the prevention and treatment of osteoporosis (Box 28.5).

⚡ SAFETY TIPS

Oral bisphosphonates for the treatment of osteopenia and osteoporosis must be taken on an empty stomach (when first awake) with a full glass of water, and the person must remain in an upright position for at least 30 minutes and nothing else can be taken by mouth for at least 30 minutes due to the risk for necrosis of the mandible, esophageal erosions, ulceration, or possible rupture, especially when taken. It must be at least 2 hours before a proton pump inhibitor (PPI) is taken.

A vertebral fracture can be exquisitely painful. Treatment usually includes aggressive pain management to allow early mobilization. If not contraindicated (e.g., hypertension, anticoagulant use),

TABLE 28.2 Age-Adjusted Prevalence (%) of Arthritis and Related Functional Limitations by Race and Ethnicity

Race/Ethnicity	Diagnosed Arthritis	Associated Activity Limitation
Asian/Pacific Islander	11.8	37.6
Hispanic/Latinx	15.4	44.3
Non-Hispanic Black	22.2	48.6
Non-Hispanic White	22.6	40.1
American Indian/ Alaskan Native	24.4	51.6
Multiracial/Other	25.2	50.5

From Centers for Disease Control and Prevention: *Arthritis: health disparities statistics* (website), 2018. https://www.cdc.gov/arthritis/data_statistics/disparities.htm.

nonsteroidal antiinflammatory drugs (NSAIDs) may provide the analgesia needed, but due to the intensity of pain, the short-term use of narcotics is usually necessary. Epidural injections, bracing, and physical therapy may be helpful. When pain is still uncontrolled, surgical procedures may be attempted (Bellantoni & Gilliam, 2021).

ARTHRITIS

Arthritis is an umbrella term for more than 100 diseases and conditions affecting the joints and surrounding tissues. More than 25% of those over 70 years of age self-report arthritis, and an estimated 14 million people in the United States have documented osteoarthritis of the knee, the majority of whom are women and/or obese (Vina & Kwoh, 2021). The prevalence of arthritis and the associated functional limitations vary by race and ethnicity but always increase with age (Table 28.2). Many of those with arthritis also have other chronic conditions. Still others are at higher risk for the development of chronic conditions if they have arthritis (Vennu et al., 2020).

Osteoarthritis

Osteoarthritis (OA) is a degenerative condition in which the normally soft and resilient cartilaginous lining of a joint becomes thin and damaged. The surrounding tissue develops inflammation, the joint space narrows, the bones rub together, and the joint itself starts to deteriorate, especially the knees, hips, hands, and spine (Figs. 28.3 and 28.4)

The cause of OA is believed to be a combination of mechanical forces (e.g., trauma, obesity) and complex molecular events affecting the entire joint. Both modifiable and nonmodifiable risk factors have been identified (Box 28.6). Social determinants that increase the risk for OA also have been identified (Vennu et al., 2020) (Box 28.7). There is no known cure; no proven treatments are available to stop its progression and, if present, OA increases the risk of death by 10% to 20% (Vina & Kwoh, 2021).

OA is most frequently diagnosed empirically, that is, based on signs and symptoms. A difficulty of diagnosis or presumed diagnosis is differentiating the signs and symptoms from atypical manifestations of other conditions common in late

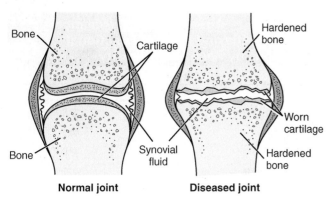

Fig 28.3 Normal joint and arthritic joint.

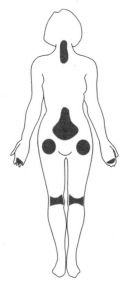

Fig. 28.4 Common locations for osteoarthritis.

life—for example, attributing shoulder pain to an acute myocardial infarction (AMI) rather than to OA. The onset is insidious, and there is no pattern to the affected joints.

Complications of OA all relate to associated pain and the effect of the degenerative changes on function and quality of life. Fortunately, for advanced disease and significant pain,

---

BOX 28.6 Risk Factors for Osteoarthritis

Modifiable
- Obesity
- Joint injury
- Infection
- Joint overuse in activities or occupation
- Muscle weakness

Nonmodifiable
- Sex (female)
- Age (50–75 years old)
- Race
- Familial predisposition

From Osteoarthritis Workgroup: *A national public agenda for osteoarthritis* (website), 2020. https://www.cdc.gov/arthritis/docs/oaagenda2020.pdf.

BOX 28.7 Social Determinants of Increased Risk for Osteoart-hritis

Income <$50,000 year
Education <High school
Unemployed
Unmarried/widowed/separated

From Vennu V, Abdulrahman TA, Alenazi AM, et al: Associations between social determinants and the presence of chronic diseases: data from the Osteoarthritis Initiative, *BMC Public Health* 20:1323, 2020.

replacements are available for some joints, and in many cases these are very successful.

Recognizing and Analyzing Cues

The classic signs of OA are stiffness with inactivity and pain with activity relieved by rest. The stiffness is greatest after extended periods of immobility such as sleep but usually resolves within 20 to 30 minutes after movement begins. Difficulty initiating joint movement and the associated immobility result in the loss of range of motion (ROM). On exam, subluxation, joint instability, swelling, and crepitus are common, all indicators of synovial deterioration. Joint narrowing is visible on x-rays.

As the joint breakdown advances, pain and duration of stiffness increases; spinal stenosis may develop in the lumbar region. Osteophytes in the joints of the fingers develop; in the distal joints they are referred to as Heberden's nodes and in the proximal joints are referred to as Bouchard's nodes (Fig. 28.5). Heberden's nodes are thought to have a hereditary component.

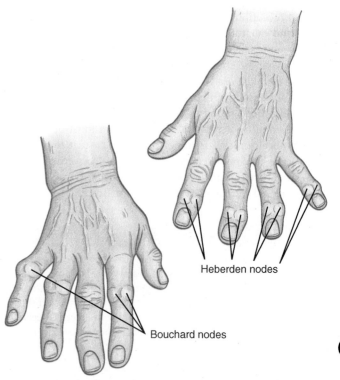

Fig. 28.5 Arthritic nodes of the fingers. (From McCance KL, Huether SE: *Pathophysiology: the biologic basis for disease in adults and children,* ed 7, St Louis, 2014, Elsevier.)

Pharmacological Interventions

The outcome of pharmacological interventions for persons with osteoarthritis is maximizing function and increasing quality of life through pain relief and joint protection. In older adults this is complicated by the frequency of co-current morbidities and medication use. Nonpharmacological nursing actions are the cornerstones for achieving these outcomes.

If the arthritis pain is mild to moderate, a 3-day course of Tylenol may be effective with minimal side effects. For moderate to severe pain, an NSAID may be effective, but this drug may present considerable risk and is contradicted in those with hypertension or taking anticoagulants. For intractable joint pain, injections with either steroids or intraarticular hyaluronans (knees only) may be attempted. A number of other products are available (e.g., topicals, Cymbalta, tramadol). In some cases, opioids are necessary to enable the person to fully function with the least amount of pain possible (Reuben et al., 2020).

⚡ RESEARCH NOTE

Glucosamine and Chondroitin for Arthritis Pain

Glucosamine and chondroitin are popular dietary supplements taken by persons attempting to obtain relief from the pain of osteoarthritis, especially of the knee and hip. Many major studies of both of these have been conducted, with conflicting results. Of the two, chondroitin may be more consistently effective (National Center for Complementary and Integrative Health, 2020).

Rheumatoid Arthritis

Rheumatoid arthritis (RA) is a systemic inflammatory autoimmune disorder affecting primarily the joints, causing pain, swelling, stiffness, and loss of function. Inflammation of the synovium (joint lining) causes destruction of the surrounding cartilage and bone. Although the onset of OA is always insidious, the onset of RA may be acute, especially in older adults (Table 28.3).

A diagnosis is made through the identification of the number, location, and types of joints involved (must include one small joint) and laboratory testing (Box 28.8). Rapid diagnosis is necessary so that treatment can begin as early as possible and therefore provide the greatest chance of joint preservation. The exact cause of RA is unknown but is now believed to be the result of interaction between environmental exposures, genetic factors (*HLA-DRB1*), and age-related increased autoimmunity

---

BOX 28.8 Serological Testing for Rheumatoid Arthritis (RA)

Erythrocyte sedimentation rate (ESR; sed rate) and C-reactive protein are markers for inflammation but are nonspecific for RA

Rheumatoid factor is present at some time in 80% of those with RA

Antibodies to cyclic citrullinated peptide (CCP) are present in 60% to 70% of those with RA

Data from Arthritis Foundation: *Rheumatoid arthritis: causes, symptoms, treatment and more* (website), n.d. https://www.arthritis.org/diseases/rheumatoid-arthritis.

(American College of Rheumatology [ACR], 2018). The associated chronic inflammation can affect organs and systems throughout the body. Those with RA have a greater risk for a serious cardiovascular event such as an AMI or a stroke, and their mortality rate is higher than those without the disease (Arthritis Foundation, n.d.; Løppenthin et al., 2019; Urman et al., 2018).

Recognizing and Analyzing Cues

There are three types of RA: monocyclic, polycyclic, and progressive. In monocyclic RA the person has one symptomatic episode limited to 3 to 5 years, but in polycyclic RA the symptoms are continuous but the intensity varies. In progressive RA symptoms increase in severity and are continuous.

RA usually affects several joints and is symmetrical, most often in both hands or feet, but also affects the large joints such as the knees. It can be initially confused with OA, but as a systemic disease it affects joints bilaterally and the body as a whole (Box 28.9). Older adults who have had RA for many years develop very painful joint deformities, especially of the hands and feet. The most common orthopedic deformity in RA is the boutonnière deformity or hyperextension of the distal interphalangeal (DIP) joint with flexion of the proximal interphalangeal (PIP) joint and extension of the DIP joint with a "swan neck" deformity (Fig. 28.6). Palliative joint replacement or repair surgeries may be needed.

Pharmacological Interventions

The disease-modifying antirheumatic drugs (DMARDs) are specific for the treatment of RA. They take several weeks to months to provide relief but are used specifically to stop the progression

---

TABLE 28.3 Comparison of Osteoarthritis, Rheumatoid Arthritis, and Gout

	Osteoarthritis	Rheumatoid Arthritis	Gout
Onset	Insidious	More acute in older adults than in younger adults	Sudden/acute
Classic symptoms	Stiffness of joint after rest resolved in <20 minutes of activity	Stiffening following rest lasting more than 20–30 minutes of activity	Acute pain
Classic cues	Affects distal interphalangeal joints, knees, hips, shoulders, and vertebrae	Affects proximal joints, may be systemic	Inflammation, especially at the base of the great toe
Key interventions	Initial treatment may be nonpharmacological such as heat and exercise, joint protection, physical therapy; later acetaminophen and nonsteroidal antiinflammatory drugs (NSAIDs)	Use of disease-modifying antirheumatic drugs (DMARDs) as soon as diagnosis is made. Joint protections, smoking cessation, physical therapy to maximize function	NSAIDs/colchicine

BOX 28.9 Signs and Symptoms of Rheumatoid Arthritis

- Tender, warm, swollen joints
- Symmetrical pattern of affected joints
- Joint inflammation often affecting the wrist and finger joints closest to the hand
- Joint inflammation sometimes affecting other joints, including the neck, shoulders, elbows, hips, knees, ankles, and feet
- Fatigue, occasional fevers, loss of energy
- Pain and stiffness lasting for more than 30 minutes in the morning or after a long rest
- Symptoms that last for many years
- Variability of symptoms among people with the disease

From Strano-Paul L, Patnaik A: Common rheumatologic disorders. In Walter LC, Chang A, editors: *CURRENT diagnosis and treatment: geriatrics*, ed 3, New York, 2021, McGraw Hill, pp 510–515.

BOX 28.10 Potential Side Effects of Methotrexate Therapy

Hepatic cirrhosis
Interstitial pneumonitis
Severe myelosuppression (rare)
Stomatitis and oral ulcers
Mild alopecia and hair thinning
Headache
Fatigue
Nausea or diarrhea

From Johns Hopkins Arthritis Center: *Rheumatoid arthritis treatment* (website), 2022. www.hopkinsarthritis.org/arthritis-info/rheumatoid-arthritis/ra-treatment.

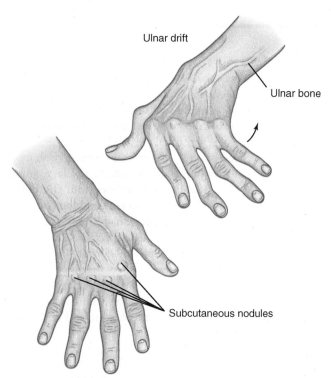

Fig. 28.6 Rheumatoid arthritis deformities. (From McCance KL, Huether SE: *Pathophysiology: the biologic basis for disease in adults and children*, ed 7, St Louis, 2014, Elsevier.)

of the disease and resultant cartilage damage and bone loss. Although a number of DMARDs are now available (e.g., tumor necrosis factor [TNF]–alpha inhibitors), methotrexate is considered first-line treatment. People who cannot be treated with methotrexate alone may be prescribed a Janus kinase (JAK) inhibitor such as Xeljanz. All are potentially toxic, and the nurse must work closely with the patient and family to be aware of early signs of potentially dangerous side effects (Box 28.10).

Those with more advanced disease may need medications called biological response modifiers or "biologic agents" (e.g., Enbrel, Humira), which block the immune system's ability to cause inflammation of the joints. Most often patients take these drugs with methotrexate, as the mix of medicines is more helpful (ACR, 2019a). However, since the effectiveness of the immune system is already reduced in later life (immunosenescence), adding a biological agent may decrease the effectiveness of preventive immunizations such as that for COVID-19 (Bajaj et al., 2021).

GOUT

Gout affects more than 3 million Americans, more often in men, women after menopause, and people with kidney disease. It is strongly linked to obesity, hypertension (high blood pressure), hyperlipidemia (high cholesterol and triglycerides), and diabetes (ACR, 2019b). Unlike RA, it is not an autoimmune disorder but an inflammatory response to the accumulation of uric acid crystals in the blood and other body fluids, especially the synovial fluid of joints. If they collect in the kidneys, they can form urate renal stones and cause renal failure.

The accumulation of uric acid crystals is the result of either overproduction of uric acid or inadequate excretion, especially the latter. It may be a one-time, acute attack, but 60% of those with one episode will have another one within 1 year and 84% in 3 years if crystals remain in the joint (Strano-Paul & Patnaik, 2021).

Recognizing and Analyzing Cues

Gout typically starts with an acute attack with sudden, intense pain in a joint, often in the middle of the night. People may report that "even the sheet hurts." The joint is bright red, hot, and too painful to touch. It occurs most often in the first metatarsal joint of the great toe but also may occur in the ankle, knee, wrist, or elbow. Fever, malaise, and chills may be present. A laboratory test finding of elevated uric acid is likely, but uric acid also may be within normal limits. Prolonged presence of uric acid crystals form painful insoluble, white nodules (tophi) in subcutaneous tissue. Many are visible and palpable. An acute attack will resolve in 3 to 14 days even without treatment.

Pharmacological Interventions

The first goal of treatment during an acute attack of gout is to stop it as promptly as possible and thereby achieve pain relief. The pain of gout may be very responsive to oral antiinflammatories such as NSAIDs and short courses of steroids or colchicine

(ACR, 2019b). If gastrointestinal irritation or bleeding is a risk, a proton pump inhibitor can be given with the NSAID; aspirin should not be used. Unfortunately, persons who also take anticoagulants cannot take NSAIDs, and those with high blood pressure should not. If not contraindicated, the nurse ensures that the person drinks an adequate amount of fluids (about 2 L/day) to help flush the uric acid through the kidneys. If pain persists, an injection of long-acting steroids into the joint may be attempted.

After the acute attack, the goal is to prevent another attack, systemic spread of the disease, and the development of chronic gout and tophi. This may be done by avoiding specific drugs (e.g., thiazide diuretics), foods that are high in purines, and alcohol, all of which increase uric acid levels. Medications are prescribed to either decrease uric acid production, such as xanthine oxidase inhibitors (e.g., allopurinol, febuxostat), or increase its excretion (e.g., probenecid) (Strano-Paul & Patnaik, 2021).

USING CLINICAL JUDGMENT TO PROMOTE HEALTHY AGING

Gerontological nurses have a direct impact on promoting musculoskeletal health in a number of ways. They are active at all levels of health promotion and disease prevention.

❤ HEALTHY PEOPLE 2030

Goals for Musculoskeletal Wellness

- Reduce the proportion of adults with arthritis who have moderate to severe joint pain.
- Reduce the proportion of adults with arthritis whose arthritis limits their work or activities.
- Reduce the proportion of adults with osteoporosis.
- Increase the proportion of older adults who get treated for osteoporosis after a fracture.

Data from the Office of Disease Prevention and Health Promotion: *Healthy People 2030* (website), n.d. https://health.gov/healthypeople/objectives-and-data/browse-objectives/older-adults.

Using clinical judgment in the application of evidence-based actions has the potential to prevent the development of osteoporosis and gout by working with older adults to reduce risk factors whenever possible. Potential outcomes of nursing solutions and actions include maximizing function and quality of life while minimizing risks and complications. The nurse working at the bedside or clinic needs to be aware of the correct techniques when administering medications, especially the bisphosphonates.

Solutions, Nursing Actions, and Outcomes

Preventive solutions include promoting healthy diets and appropriate supplementation, physical activity and exercise, protecting muscles and joints from injury, and achieving pain control. Nursing actions includes education and monitoring the effectiveness of intervention.

Nutrition

Calcium. A lifetime of adequate intake of calcium is necessary to achieve and maintain optimal bone health. The total recommended dietary allowance (RDA) for males and females

TABLE 28.4 Examples of Interactions Between Calcium and Medications or Food

Product	Interacts With	Solution
Calcium carbonate	H2 blocker (Zantac, Pepcid, Axid)[a]	Use calcium citrate form
Levothyroxine	Any calcium	At least 1 hour apart
Any calcium	Excess alcohol, protein, salt	Avoid (inhibits calcium absorption)
Any calcium	Caffeine, excess fiber, phosphorus[b]	Avoid (causes excess calcium excretion)
Calcium supplements or foods (e.g., milk)	Iron supplements	At least 2 hours in between
Any calcium supplement or food	Multivitamin/ magnesium	At least 30 minutes apart

[a]Not recommended for use in older adults for more than 6 weeks.
[b]Found in processed meats, sodas, and preserved foods.

between 51 and 70 years old is 1000 mg and 1200 mg, respectively. For those over 70 years old, the recommendation is 1200 mg daily for both men and women (Office of Dietary Supplement [ODS], 2021). Although food is the best source of calcium, supplementation is always recommended in late life. The most common forms of calcium are carbonate and citrate. Citrate is absorbed better on an empty stomach and carbonate with food. Very little calcium is absorbed into the bloodstream from the elemental formulations such as "oyster shell," and these supplements are not recommended. A careful consideration of when the calcium supplement is taken in relation to other medications and foods is very important (Table 28.4). Many find calcium supplements very constipating and may need to be taken with routine stool softeners. Calcium supplements are necessary even if someone is being treated for OP (see Pharmacological Interventions earlier).

Vitamin D. Vitamin D is essential for calcium uptake into the bones. Ultraviolet light from sunshine on the skin stimulates the production of fat-soluble vitamin D. However, older skin is less efficient in producing vitamin D, and supplements generally are recommended for all older women and anyone with a documented deficiency. The minimum dose is 600 to 800 IU per day, with adjustments based on a goal of between about 20 ng/mL and 150 ng/mL on the 1,25-dihydroxyvitamin D laboratory measurement (Chapter 10). Too much vitamin D can result in hypercalcemia. It is both prescribed and available over the counter. The vitamin D_3 formulation (cholecalciferol) is the most widely used and researched.

Although there is no way to prevent the development of gout, the risk of recurrences is influenced by diet. Avoiding nondiet soda and alcohol, restricting food high in purines, and increasing intake of water and foods that may reduce uric acid may be helpful (Table 28.5). The nurse's role includes teaching the person how to decrease the likelihood of another gout attack by using preventive measures.

Exercise

Exercise is essential for the maintenance of muscle strength and joint function and therefore independence. A skilled physical

TABLE 28.5 Gout, Uric Acid, and Food Products

Products That Increase Uric Acid Levels (High in Purine)	Product That May Lower Uric Acid Levels
Herring, mackerel, sardines, scallops, mussels, anchovies	Oranges
Asparagus, mushrooms	Strawberries
Animal organs	Bell peppers
Dried peas and beans	Pineapples
Gravy	Water
Foods sweetened with high-fructose corn syrup	

therapist, occupational therapist, or rehabilitation nurse specialist can provide an individualized therapeutic exercise plan to maintain and maximize function, reduce pain, and prevent falls. Weight-bearing activity is important to maintain bone strength for persons with OP. This may include walking, tai chi, stair climbing, dancing, and tennis. Yoga and Pilates programs have been designed especially for those who are frail. Many people have access to guided classes in local senior centers, YMCAs, an through on-line programs. They also can be prescribed and supervised by physical therapists. Tai chi and qigong have the added benefit of improving balance.

For many years it was thought that people with arthritis, especially RA, should rest their joints to protect them from damage; however, both rest and exercise are necessary. Non–weight-bearing exercise for those with RA will help keep joints supple, improve range of motion, and help maintain function. Water exercise is recommended as a gentle way to exercise joints and muscles. Even a warm, inflamed joint can be given ROM exercises to maintain movement in the joint. A physical or occupational therapist should be consulted to develop a program of rest and exercise.

Pain Relief

In caring for those with musculoskeletal disorders, the goals are to minimize disability by preventing chronic gout and further joint damage and ensuring adequate pain relief. Adequate pain relief will allow the person to function at as high a level as possible for as long as possible. The use of heat and cold is well known for management of arthritic pain. Heat will provide temporary relief in OA, but ice will reduce inflammation. Paraffin baths for the hands have been found to be very soothing. These can be individually purchased or part of the physical therapist's plan of care.

If pain is not adequately controlled, the person will decrease activity, become deconditioned rapidly, and gain weight. The weight puts more stress on the joints, leading to more pain, less activity, and more debility. A dietitian and nurse work with the person to identify weight and caloric goals and develop meal plans that are culturally acceptable but still balanced and healthy.

Joint Protection

Devices and techniques that relieve some of the pressure to the joints, and in doing so may decrease pain and improve balance, are available. For example, canes and walkers relieve hip stress. A shoe lift can improve lumbar pain. A brace is useful for knees, especially if there is lateral instability (the knee "gives out"). Persons who are no longer able to ambulate may qualify for mobility assistive devices, including electric wheelchairs and other personal mobility devices. When hands are affected, persons should avoid carrying packages by the fingers, using a cart instead, and use adaptive devices on utensils and household equipment to create a larger grip surface. A variety of adaptive equipment is available to make daily activities less problematic and less traumatic to the joints and to enhance independence and consequently self-esteem.

The simplest approaches may make big differences in helping persons to remain independent. This may include easy-to-use zipper pulls, extension devices to pick up things from a distance (e.g., the floor), or devices to slide on shoes from a sitting position. Velcro closures on clothing are useful for those whose hands are no longer fully functional. Book holders, chairs to sit on while preparing foods, larger light switches, and secure stair railings, or even moving heavier objects or those used frequently, to lower cabinet shelves, all may be very effective measures. Velcro support devices can be used for individual joints in all types of arthritis. Hip protectors can be considered for frail older adults with osteoporosis.

KEY CONCEPTS

- Although several changes occur in the musculoskeletal system, none are life-threatening, but they do affect overall function, mobility, and independence and may affect self-esteem.
- OP is diagnosed through a DXA scan or presence of a fragility fracture.
- The most important reason to be concerned about OP and osteopenia is their association with the risk for fractures and subsequent increased mortality and morbidity.
- The majority of persons with OA will have significant limitations at some point, including the inability to care for themselves.

- A major nursing concern in caring for someone with arthritis is helping the person manage pain and thereby preserve function as long as possible.
- One of the differences between OA and RA is the relationship of time to the development of joint stiffening.
- The differentiation between OA and another common and potentially serious conditions is often difficult.
- Both RA and gout are systemic, inflammatory conditions that have both joint and systemic effects; only RA is an autoimmune condition.
- Gout is the result of the deposition of uric acid crystals in a joint or joints. The onset is most often acute.

NEXT-GENERATION NCLEX® (NGN) EXAMINATION–STYLE QUESTIONS

Mrs. Svöld is an 80-year-old White woman of Scandinavian descent. She is a very petite woman who moved to a nursing home several years ago. She is dependent on others for her mobility. She is only able to get outside at the rare times her sister visits. As you review her medication list, you notice that she is not taking any supplements, including neither calcium nor vitamin D. She does, however, take the bisphosphate Fosamax.

Underline the cues that indicate potential compromise to bone health and risk for fracture. Select the top two priority educational needs from the table for persons taking bisphosphates.

Priority Educational Information for Persons Taking Bisphosphates
Take supplemental calcium and vitamin D
Remain upright for at least 30 minutes after taking medication
Take medication on an empty stomach with a full glass of water
Drink at least three glasses of water following medication to flush kidneys
Remove dentures prior to swallowing medication

CLINICAL JUDGMENT ACTIVITY

1. Analyze your own diet and activities and determine your relative risk for osteoporosis.

RESEARCH QUESTIONS

1. When should women begin to have DXA scans done?
2. Under what circumstances are DXA scans appropriate for men?

REFERENCES

American College of Rheumatology (ACR): *Genetics and rheumatic disease* (website), 2018. https://www.rheumatology.org/I-Am-A/Patient-Caregiver/Diseases-Conditions/Living-Well-with-Rheumatic-Disease/Genetics-and-Rheumatic-Disease.

American College of Rheumatology (ACR): *Rheumatoid arthritis* (website), 2019a. https://www.rheumatology.org/I-Am-A/Patient-Caregiver/Diseases-Conditions/Rheumatoid-Arthritis.

American College of Rheumatology (ACR): *Gout* (website), 2019b. https://www.rheumatology.org/I-Am-A/Patient-Caregiver/Diseases-Conditions/Gout.

Arthritis Foundation: *Rheumatoid arthritis and heart disease* (website), n.d. https://www.arthritis.org/health-wellness/about-arthritis/related-conditions/other-diseases/rheumatoid-arthritis-heart-disease. Accessed June 2021.

Bajaj V, Gadi N, Spihlman AP, et al: Aging, immunity, and COVID-19: how age influences the host immune response to coronavirus infections, *Front Physiol* 11:571416, 2021.

Bellantoni M, Gilliam M: Osteoporosis and hip fracture. In Walter LC, Chang A, editors: *CURRENT diagnosis and treatment: geriatrics*, ed 3, New York, 2021, McGraw Hill, pp 253–262.

Bilder GE: *Human biological aging*, Hoboken, NJ, 2016, Wiley Blackwell.

Hopkins LW, Smallheer BA, McCance KL: Alterations of musculoskeletal function. In McCance KL, Huether SE, editors: *Pathophysiology: the biological basis for disease in adults and children*, ed 8, St Louis, 2019, Elsevier, pp 1423–1471.

Løppenthin K, Esbensen BA, Østergaard M, et al.: Morbidity and mortality in patients with rheumatoid arthritis compared with an age- and sex-matched control population: a nationwide register study, *JOC* 9:1–7, 2019.

Medicare: *Bone mass measurement* (website), n.d. https://www.medicare.gov/coverage/bone-mass-measurements. Accessed 5/5/21.

National Center for Complementary and Integrative Health (NCCIH): Arthritis and complementary health approaches: what the science says (website), 2020. https://www.nccih.nih.gov/health/providers/digest/complementary-health-approaches-for-chronic-pain-science.

Office of Dietary Supplement, National Institutes of Health: *Calcium: fact sheet for health professionals* (website), 2021. https://ods.od.nih.gov/factsheets/Calcium-HealthProfessional/.

Reuben DB, Herr KA, Pacala JT, et al: *Geriatrics at your fingertips*, ed 22, New York, 2020, American Geriatric Society.

Richens M: Ten things to know about racial differences in bone health (website), 2020. https://americanbonehealth.org/races-ethnicities/10-things-to-know-about-racial-differences-in-bone-health/.

Strano-Paul L, Patnaik A: Common rheumatologic disorders. In Walter LC, Chang A, editors: *CURRENT diagnosis and treatment: geriatrics*, ed 3, New York, 2021, McGraw Hill, pp 510–515.

Urman A, Taklalsingh N, Sorrento C, et al: Inflammation beyond the joints: rheumatoid arthritis and cardiovascular disease, *Scifed J Cardiol* 2(3):1000019, 2018.

US Prevention Services Task Force (USPSTF): Screening for osteoporosis to prevent fracture: recommendation statement, *JAMA* 319(24):2521–2531, 2018.

Vina ER, Kwoh CK: Osteoarthritis. In Walter LC, Chang A, editors: *CURRENT diagnosis and treatment: geriatrics*, ed 3, New York, 2021, McGraw Hill, pp 245–252.

Vennu V, Abdulrahman TA, Alenazi AM, et al: Associations between social determinants and the presence of chronic diseases: data from the Osteoarthritis Initiative, *BMC Public Health* 20:1323, 2020.

Welch C, Greig C, Masud T, et al: COVID-19 and acute sarcopenia, *Aging Dis* 11(6):1345–1351, 2020.

World Health Organization (WHO): *Musculoskeletal conditions* (website), 2021. https://www.who.int/news-room/fact-sheets/detail/musculoskeletal-conditions.

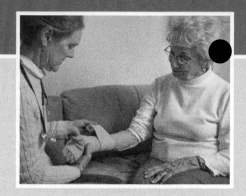

Pain and Comfort

Kathleen Jett

http://evolve.elsevier.com/Touhy/TwdHlthAging

A STUDENT SPEAKS

I know she has pain all of the time, but if I give her too many pills she will get addicted and that would be a bad thing, right?

Ana, RN, age 23

AN OLDER ADULT SPEAKS

It seems to have crept up on me—first one joint, now the other. I wouldn't call it pain really, just an ache that never goes away and keeps me from dancing like I used to.

Gloria, age 78

LEARNING OBJECTIVES

On completion of this chapter, the reader will be able to:
1. Define the concept of pain.
2. Identify factors that affect the pain experience.
3. Recognize the barriers to achieving outcomes related to pain relief for older adults.
4. Recognize the cues suggestive of pain in older persons with and without cognitive impairments.
5. Describe pharmacological and nonpharmacological interventions that provide comfort to those in pain.

The International Association for the Study of Pain (IASP, 2020) defines pain as "an unpleasant sensory and emotional experience associated with or resembling that associated with actual or potential tissue damage." All pain is multidimensional, with sensory, psychosocial, emotional, personal, and spiritual components.

The most common types of pain encountered in late life are neuropathic and nociceptive pain. Neuropathic pain is caused by a lesion or disease of the central or peripheral somatosensory nervous system (Box 29.1). It is characterized by tingling, stabbing, and burning sensations as well as abnormal sensations (dysesthesia) or pain from typically nonpainful stimuli (allodynia). Nociceptive pain arises from actual or threatened damage to nonneural tissue from somatic sources, such as osteoarthritis (Box 29.2). Persons in later life often experience both types of pain at the same time.

How we respond to pain is part of who we are. Even the words used to describe it are personal—an *ache*, a *burn*, a *pester*, or *despair*—with the language and the willingness to express it a manifestation of the cultural heritage and relationship with whom it is being discussed (Chapter 4). It can be a fleeting discomfort or something so pervasive that it wears heavily on the spirit.

The experience of physical pain is either acute or persistent (chronic). Acute pain has a distinct and sudden onset, is of short duration, and is self-limiting. The cause is clear (e.g., fracture, infection), and the pain is expected to end when the problem is resolved. It is expected by the circumstances, temporary, and usually controllable. For example, the acute pain of cardiac ischemia is temporarily relieved with nitroglycerin and permanently resolved when oxygen is restored to the myocardium. It is often accompanied by autonomic overactivity, such as diaphoresis and tachycardia. Everyone experiences acute physical pain at some point in their lives including those with verbal incapacity or cognitive limitations. However, providing comfort to those in late life becomes more complex due to the frequency of preexisting polypharmacy and concurrent conditions, including psychological pain such as depression. Acute pain is often superimposed on preexisting persistent pain. Acute pain may insidiously become chronic when treatment is inadequate.

Persistent pain is that which lasts beyond the time it would be expected and is present at least half of the time in the previous

---

BOX 29.1 Common Conditions That Produce Neuropathic Pain

Central Pain
Post-stroke
Parkinson's disease
Spinal cord injury
COVID-19

Peripheral Pain
Diabetes
Peripheral vascular disease
Herpes zoster (shingles)
Degenerative disc disease or nerve compression

BOX 29.2 Common Conditions That Produce Nociceptive Pain

Arthritis
Tumor
Peptic Ulcer
Bruises
Fractures

BOX 29.3 Tips for Best Practice

Setting Pain Goals

Mrs. Smith is a 92-year-old widow who lives alone. Her 74-year-old son lives next door and makes sure she has everything she needs. She has had stomach cancer for the past year. As her tumor enlarged, her pain increased, and eventually around-the-clock morphine was needed for her to continue her usual activities, including baking cakes for the hospice staff. The associated constipation was controlled with a stool softener, but she also had dose-related visual hallucinations. Despite efforts to lower the dose to rid her of these side effects, it was not possible to do so and maintain her pain relief. She finally declared, "I guess I will just have to learn to live with these puppies running around at my feet, better that than hurting. As least I know they are not real!"

BOX 29.4 Consequences of Untreated Pain

Falls and other accidents
Functional impairment
Slowed rehabilitation
Mood changes: depression, anxiety, fear
Caregiver strain: increased dependency
Sleep disturbance
Anorexia
Impaired cognition
Decline in social and recreational activities
Increased health care use and costs
Loss or worsening of physical function and fitness
Potential for drug or alcohol abuse or misuse

BOX 29.5 Barriers to Pain Management in Older Adults

Health Care Provider
Lack of education regarding pain assessment and management
Concern regarding regulatory scrutiny
Fears of opioid-related side effects and addiction
Belief that pain is a normal part of aging
Belief that cognitively impaired older adults have less pain
Personal beliefs and experiences with pain
Failure to accept self-report without "objective" signs
Polypharmacy

Personal
Lack of ability to assess pain by those with cognitive impairments
Fear of medication side effects and addiction
Personal and societal belief that pain is a normal part of aging
Belief that nothing can be done for pain in "old people"
Fear of being a "bad patient" if complaining
Fear of what pain may signify

System
Cost
Time
Systemic racism
Regulatory control

---

6 months (Reuben et al., 2020). It is most often associated with progressive disease (e.g., arthritis) or a known syndrome (e.g., stroke). Although persistent pain may vary in intensity over time, some level of discomfort is always present and requires consistent treatment. If the cause is something for which there is little control, such as one of the pain syndromes, a "comfort goal" is set (Box 29.3). With this information the nurse can help the older adult identify a tolerable level of pain even if it cannot be fully relieved.

PAIN IN THE OLDER ADULT

The perception of pain is altered by many factors, including the type of pain; the person's prior experience and expressions of pain; and the person's cultural, cognitive, functional, and psychological status, especially depression and anxiety. Inadequate treatment of pain leads to impaired functional status and in some cases transient cognitive impairment that can become permanent (Box 29.4). Yet the barriers to adequate pain management in older adults are significant for individual, provider, and system reasons (Box 29.5).

As one ages, the likelihood of experiencing pain increases. Approximately 50% of older adults living in the community have reported "bothersome" pain in the preceding month. Approximately 83% to 93% of those living in nursing facilities are thought to have pain on a regular basis (Horgas et al., 2021). These numbers are likely to increase as more older adults survive severe COVID-19 infections. Depending on the study, anywhere from 12% to 75% describe pain while being treated in and recovering from a stay in the intensive care unit (ICU); it is unknown how long COVID-19-related pain syndrome persists (Kemp et al., 2021) (Table 29.1).

There has been consistent evidence that pain in older adults is either unrecognized or undertreated. The gerontological nurse

TABLE 29.1 Factors Affecting the Potential COVID-19-Related Pain Syndrome

Initial Acute Pain	Infections	Procedural	Comfort as a Lower Priority for Providers
ICU specific pain	Prolonged ventilation	Prolonged immobility with muscular atrophy, contractures	Iatrogenic: pressure trauma, repeated procedures, frequent re-positioning
Neurological	Painful neurological sequalae e.g. stroke	Neuroimmune response to infection	Virus neurotropism
Psychiatric	Depression and anxiety; social isolation	Pandemic psychological burden	Risk of PTSD
During rehabilitation	New multi-morbidity	Fatigue	Lack of staff knowledge regarding COVID-19 specific rehabilitation
Typical post-infections conditions	Myalgia and arthralgia	Abdominal and chest pain	Headache; exercise intolerance

ICU, Intensive care unit; *PTSD*, posttraumatic stress disorder.
From Kemp HI, Corner E, Colvin LA: Chronic pain after COVID-19: implications for rehabilitation, *Br J Anaesth* 125(4):436–440, 2021.

BOX 29.6 Age-Related Changes in Pain Sensation: Implications for Safety

The normal age-related delay of the sensation of pain from the periphery to the brain has significant implications for safety. For example, if older skin comes in contact with a hot surface, the ever-so-slight increased exposure can result in a significantly more serious burn than in a younger adult.

may hear the comment that older adults "feel less pain" than younger adults, especially when referring to those with dementia. However, the amount of pain is the same but there are age-related differences in both its perception and tolerance. With aging there is a decrease in the density of both myelinated and unmyelinated nerve fibers that slightly *delay* the transmission of the sensation of pain from the periphery to the brain (Box 29.6). At the same time, the sensation is slower to resolve, and relief is delayed once pain is triggered.

Pain in Older Adults With Cognitive or Communication Limitations

There is no convincing evidence that persons with dementia have less pain than someone else, although there may be central nervous system changes that influence the *interpretation* of pain. If the person is unable to cognitively process the sensation in the context of prior pain experience, affective responses to

pain will differ. Multiple studies have shown that older adults who are cognitively impaired receive less pain medication, even when they experience the same acutely painful events, such as fractures or postherpetic neuralgia, that would cause pain in others. Persistent pain from sources such as arthritis do not resolve with the development of dementia.

The situation is similar for the person with communication limitations. There is no evidence that those who cannot express themselves—for whatever reason—do not experience pain in the same way as a person without this limitation. Nursing actions to promote comfort are expected regardless of the person's cognitive status or verbal abilities.

Recognizing and Analyzing Cues

It is reasonable to assess the potential for pain at each nurse-patient interaction. Older adults may be reluctant to volunteer that they are uncomfortable but often may do so when the topic is addressed directly and when acceptable language is used (e.g., "discomfort" may be more acceptable than "pain"). Whenever pain is suspected (e.g., arthritis, depression) or expected (e.g., after an injury, following a significant loss), a complex assessment is especially important, including whenever an older adult with a cognitive impairment has a change in behavior. In skilled nursing facilities the assessment of pain is a required component of the Resident Assessment Instrument (RAI) completed at the time of admission and at intervals thereafter (Chapter 9). A multidisciplinary approach is optimal but not always possible.

Assessment

The nurse is often the first one to hear the person's call for comfort of any kind, regardless of the setting, the type of nursing practice, or the means of expression. The assessment provides the information required to prioritize needs and nursing actions that are effective and culturally acceptable. Awareness of the individual's health and wellness paradigm is especially important in pain assessment (Chapter 4). What does the pain mean? Is the pain believed to be the result of imbalance, a form of punishment, or an infection? Due to the complexities of pain in the lives of older adults, certain areas require special emphasis (Box 29.7).

BOX 29.7 Tips for Best Practice
Additional Factors to Consider When Assessing Pain

Function: How is the pain affecting the person's ability to participate in usual activities and perform both activities of daily living and instrumental activities of daily living?

Alternative expression of pain: Have there been recent changes in cognitive ability or behavior, such as increased pacing, grimacing, or irritability? Is there an increase in the number of complaints? Are they vague and difficult to respond to? Has there been a change in sleep-wake patterns? Is the person resisting certain activities, movements, or positions?

Social support: What resources are available to the person in pain? What is the person's role in his or her social system, and how is pain affecting this role? How is pain affecting the person's relationship with others?

Pain history: How has the person managed previous experiences with pain? What is the perceived meaning of the past and present pain? What cultural factors affect the person's ability to express pain and receive relief?

TABLE 29.2 Example of Use of the OLD CART Mnemonic in Pain Assessment and Analysis

	Patient Report of Cues	Further Exploration by Nurse	Beginning Analysis
Onset	I first noticed it last week	Does anyone around you have this? Have you had this in the past? When?	Determine if new problem or repeat.
Location	Across the right side of my body....No, it is only on the right	Can you describe exactly where the pain is? Does it feel like it is on the inside or on the surface? Has it crossed over to the other side of the body at all?	If does not cross the body's midline, more likely to be neuropathic pain or associated with a specific organ.
Duration	Has been continuous	Do you have any thoughts if this will go away by itself or will just keep going?	Information used in negotiation of solutions later.
Characteristics	Started itching, then burning, intense	Does it keep you awake at night? What is the best and worst it has been? (see intensity measures)	These cues reinforce your analysis that it is neuropathic pain. If intensity is high most of the time, comfort is a high priority.
Aggravating factors	My clothes touching the area seems to make it worse, but I am not sure	How has this affected your day-to day life? Is it keeping you from doing anything you need or want to do?	Useful in teaching and reinforcing—to encourage self-care by listening to the body.
Relieving factors	At first a cold compress seemed to help. But now there are blisters....Tylenol seems to help a little, but it does not last long	Have others made any suggestions about what this may be or what you can do for it?	This information supports a hunch that this is shingles. Additional question: Have you had chickenpox in the past? Have you had a zoster vaccination? Not getting adequate relief. Work with prescribing provider to find curative and more lasting relief measures.
Treatments attempted	I have not tried anything yet except the Tylenol	I have some suggestions for what might help...are these things you can do now or do you have other commitments that you have to take care of first?	Seeking understanding of individual's priorities. Negotiate solutions that can accommodate these.

It is of utmost importance that the language and synonyms (e.g., pain, discomfort, ache) used by the nurse are consistent with those used by the patient. Because pain is subjective, only the person experiencing it can describe it or express it and can never be judged by another; individual report is the most reliable. Pain is whatever the person says it is. When asked about pain, the person must be given enough time to process the question, especially for older adults with cognitive impairments or with a long history of persistent pain.

The health history component of a pain assessment always begins with documentation of the person's qualitative self-report and, when possible, the quantification of both current and desired levels of comfort. Cues are sought to determine underlying cause and type of pain, characteristics, and impact on physical and psychosocial function and quality of life. If present, cues of depression, anxiety, and sleep disturbances are recognized.

The mnemonic OLD CART is a useful guide in the collection of qualitative data: Onset, Location, Duration, Characteristics, Aggravating and Relieving factors, and Treatments used in the past. Details then follow related to the factors influencing the pain experience. Analysis of the cues and information provided will indicate the type of pain, the priorities of care, and potential interventions (Table 29.2).

The most common ways to quantify the intensity of pain are by using numerical and visual rating and verbal descriptor scales. They have been found to be useful for both persons who are cognitively intact and those with mild to moderate impairments. They are not appropriate for those with severe cognitive impairments and may not be useful for those who do not speak English or for whom certain numbers have cultural meaning (e.g., lucky or unlucky numbers). The same scale must be used each time the pain is reassessed.

Rating scales. The nurse most often uses a Numerical Rating Scale (NRS) to assess the intensity of pain. The patient is asked to describe the pain on a scale of 0 to 10, with 0 being no pain and 10 being the worst pain imaginable. A Visual Rating Scale uses the same range and instructions, but the numbers are on a line, a ruler, or an image of a ladder (Fig. 29.1). This method can be used to describe pain at the present time, ever, or during a set period of time, such as "in the last week." The use of these scales requires that the person has numerical fluency, which can never be assumed.

For those without numerical skills or who express reticence, Verbal Descriptor Scales (VDSs) are more appropriate. They are considered valid, reliable, and easy to use (Horgas et al., 2021). Pain intensity is measured by asking the person to choose from a set of descriptors (i.e., worst pain imaginable, etc.). The Pain Thermometer is a diagram of a thermometer with word descriptions that show increasing pain intensities that can be read to the person if needed. There are several "Faces Pain Scales" as a useful alternative (Fig. 29.2). All are composed of a series of facial expressions, and the person is asked to select the one that best demonstrates the pain intensity. Some are in black and white, and others amplify the expressions with color. This type of scale may be effective with a person with cognitive

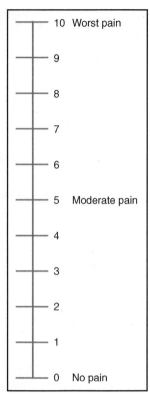

Fig. 29.1 Example of a Numerical Rating Scale (NRS). (From Pasero C, McCaffery M: *Pain assessment and pharmacologic management,* St Louis, 2011, Mosby.)

BOX 29.9 Tips for Best Practice

Assessment of Pain in Persons With Impaired Communication Skills

Attempt to obtain a self-report of pain from the patient; a yes or no response is acceptable.

Look for possible causes of pain or discomfort, such as common conditions and procedures that cause pain (e.g., arthritis, surgery, wound care, history of persistent pain, constipation, lifting or moving).

Observe and document patient behaviors that may indicate pain or distress or that are unusual from the person's normal patterns and responses. Behavioral observation scales may be used but should be used consistently and with proper training.

Medicate before performing any procedure that can cause discomfort.

Use surrogate reports (family members, caregivers) of behavior changes and the patient's usual patterns and responses to pain and discomfort. This must be from a person who knows the patient well and should be combined with the other assessment techniques.

If comfort measures and attention to basic needs (e.g., warmth, hunger, toileting) are not effective, attempt an analgesic trial based on the observed intensity of the pain and analgesic history. If behaviors improve, continue and add appropriate nonpharmacological interventions. If potential pain-related cues persist, adjust pharmacological and nonpharmacological interventions as needed until cues indicate comfort.

Observe for side effects and response.

limitations; however, it can also be perceived by the person as an affective scale (e.g., emotional distress as in depression or anxiety) and must be used with caution. A scale of any kind is not useful when working with someone whose culture prohibits either the acknowledgment or the expression of pain. There are also several multidimensional measures that combine intensity with contributing and relieving factors. The McGill Pain Questionnaire is used most often (Box 29.8).

Observational instruments. Providing comfort to those who cannot express themselves verbally for whatever reason requires an alternate approach. These pain assessment instruments are based on careful observation of behaviour, attention to caregiver reports, and knowing when subtle changes have occurred (Box 29.9). In nursing homes and other care settings, the registered nurse works with the certified nursing assistants (CNAs), who may be the ones to recognize the subtle and sometimes contradictory cues regarding the person's needs and level of comfort (Box 29.10).

The Pain Assessment Checklist for Seniors with Limited Ability to Communicate (PACSLAC) is a comprehensive behavioral assessment tool that may be used as both an initial pain screening instrument and an interval measure. There are six domains of observation: facial expression, verbalizations and vocalizations, body movement, changes in interpersonal interactions, changes in activity patterns or routines, and mental status changes when the person is engaged in an activity of some kind (e.g., walking, eating). The PACSLAC can serve as a guide for care regardless of who is providing it and can be used to assess pain in those

Fig. 29.2 Example of a Faces Pain Scale. (From Swartz MH: *Textbook of physical diagnosis,* ed 7, St Louis, 2014, Saunders.)

BOX 29.10   Pain Cues in the Person With Communication Difficulties

Changes in Behavior
Restlessness and/or agitation or reduction in movement
Repetitive movements
Physical tension such as clenching teeth or hands
Unusually cautious movements, guarding

Activities of Daily Living
Sudden resistance to help from others
Decreased appetite
Decreased sleep

Vocalizations
Person groans, moans, or cries for unknown reasons
Person increases or decreases usual vocalizations

Physical Changes
Pleading expression
Grimacing
Pallor or flushing
Diaphoresis (sweating)
Increased pulse, respirations, or blood pressure

BOX 29.11   Resources for Best Practice

Observational Tools

Critical Care Pain Observation Tool (CPOT): https://www.mdcalc.com/critical-care-pain-observation-tool-cpot.
Mobilization-Observation-Behavior-Intensity-Dementia-2 Pain Scale (MOBID-2): https://www.nccdp.org/resources/Mobid-2PainScaleenglish.pdf.
The University of Iowa: Source for the PACSLAC, the PAINED, and several other instruments and detailed information. https://geriatricpain.org/.

with cognitive impairments (Natavio et al., 2020). Although the presence of pain may be inferred, the evaluation of the intensity of the pain for these persons is not always possible.

The PAINED, MOBID-2 Pain Scale, and CPOT Pain Scale are recommended for use as observational instruments (Box 29.11).

USING CLINICAL JUDGMENT TO PROMOTE HEALTHY AGING

Working with older adults in pain and helping them achieve optimal comfort are especially challenging. There are potentially multiple sources and sites for the physical pain and confounding variables such as chronic conditions, frailty, and the emotional pain of depression. Pain always interferes with health-related quality of life. Relief of both acute and persistent pain takes commitment and the determination of all involved. It is optimal to use multimodal approaches combining pharmacological and nonpharmacological interventions.

Using clinical judgment in promoting comfort in late life requires skills in systematic assessment, the development of comprehensive and inclusive solutions, careful follow-up to determine the effectiveness and appropriateness of nursing actions, and implementation of changes as needed.

Solutions, Nursing Actions, and Outcomes

Pain management is that in which the chosen interventions work in harmony to provide comfort and maximize function. At the most basic level the nurse encourages people to use what has been effective in the past, as long as it does not cause harm. This is particularly applicable for older adults who have experience with persistent pain in themselves or others. Older adults often combine the approaches used in Western medicine and those learned through their personal and cultural experiences.

Nonpharmacological Interventions

Although pharmacological interventions have been the mainstay of the Western model of pain management, it is now well recognized that nonpharmacological measures alone, or combined with pharmacological approaches, are the most effective. Nursing interventions always begin with nonpharmacological approaches to pain management. Many have been used for dozens or even thousands of years. Only when these are not adequately effective should pharmacological approaches be *added*. Several nonpharmacological approaches are described here, acknowledging that whole chapters could be devoted to any one approach. The data to support the efficacy of any one of these vary (see http://www.nccih.nih.gov). Mind-body or mindfulness practices have been researched widely, and there is now some evidence to support their use relative to specific conditions (National Center for Complementary and Integrative Health [NCCIH], 2022a).

Mind-body practices. Physical pain is often accompanied by a strong affective component. Emotional or psychological pain is also associated with strong physical and visceral components. Physical pain is not experienced alone but with the emotions of anger, frustration, or despair. Emotional responses stimulate the sympathetic nervous system, releasing norepinephrine. The norepinephrine in turn increases the sensation of pain and stimulates physiological inflammation. Hence solutions designed to reduce associated emotional reactions lessen physiological manifestations of pain, such as muscle tension or gastrointestinal (GI) distress. Distraction, relaxation, and mindfulness meditation all enable the quieting of the mind and muscles, releasing tension and anxiety and in doing so relieving or lessening pain sensations (NCCIH, 2022b (Box 29.12). At a minimum, distraction and relaxation should be used prior to and adjunctive to all pharmacological interventions.

BOX 29.12   Using Distraction During a Painful Procedure

People often express fear of injections and venipuncture. I have found simple distraction to be immensely effective. Just as I insert the needle I ask, "What is your favorite color?" As they try to think of the answer, I am usually already done with the procedure, and many do not notice it has occurred.

Mindfulness meditation and guided imagery are used to promote deeper relaxation. Yoga, tai chi, and qigong are mind-body practices that can serve to reduce pain while increasing balance and proprioception. Imagery uses the person's imagination to focus on settings full of happiness and relaxation rather than on the current stressors . Developing skills to teach patients about each of these practices is an important component of nursing practice.

Heat and cold. Heat and cold have been used for centuries to relieve pain. Neither should have direct exposure to skin to avoid burns. Cold reduces muscle and nerve irritation and is ideal for both acute and persistent muscle pain. A product such as IcyHot can be purchased, but frozen food or ice is more accessible. Ice is the most effective when it is used 24 to 48 hours after an injury. Heat increases circulation to an area and is very comforting to areas affected by arthritis, and a warm cloth or a paraffin bath is ideal as the heat moves into the tissue. Both dry and moist heat can be use for 15 to 20 minutes at a time for those with mild pain and for 30 to 120 minutes for more severe pain.

> ⚡ **SAFETY ALERT**
>
> Heat and cold can never be used by those with diabetes, dermatitis, vascular disease, or a deep vein thrombosis.

Exercise. It is thought that the less active an individual is, the less tolerable activity becomes. Anyone who becomes inactive may feel more general discomfort than the active person. Both passive and active range of motion and stretching can be used with heat and cold. Tightened muscles can be warmed, stretched, and then cooled. Exercises can be guided by an informed nurse or, when more complex movement and stretching is needed, a physical therapist. See also Chapters 19 and 28. When combined with healthful eating, weight loss will lessen pressure on the joints and muscles. When activity or exercise have the potential to cause pain, the administration of an analgesic medication 20 to 30 minutes beforehand may lessen or eliminate discomfort and fear of discomfort during and after the activity and greatly enhance the individual's capacity and willingness to participate. The nurse should learn the patient's tolerance for activity and work within those parameters.

Transcutaneous electrical nerve stimulation. Transcutaneous electrical nerve stimulation (TENS) and transcutaneous vagal nerve stimulation have been studied for many years. Although there have been some promising results in the treatment of acute pain, especially as an adjuvant to medications, its effectiveness is still inconclusive (Abd-Elsayad et al., 2021). It is often used by physical therapists in combination with stretching and strengthening exercises. Patients often anecdotally report that at least they were doing "something." TENS units are now available commercially without a prescription.

Acupuncture and acupressure. In acupuncture tiny needles are inserted along specific meridians or pathways in the body consistent with the locations used in traditional Chinese medicine (meridians). It is thought to stimulate the body to heal in locations associated with the location of needle placement.

It should not be used by persons with a bleeding disorder or who have a pacemaker. Acupressure is pressure applied with the thumbs or tips of the index finger at the same locations. Acupuncture and acupressure have been used for thousands of years. Evidence supports the benefit of acupuncture specifically for several conditions, including low back pain, neck pain, knee pain and arthritis, and headaches (Horgas et al., 2021; NCCIH, 2022c).

Energy and touch therapies. Some say the use of touch therapy is a legacy in nursing. Over the years, different kinds of touch have been formalized to include those referred to as contact therapy (e.g., massage) and noncontact therapies (e.g., healing touch, therapeutic touch, Reiki). Like acupuncture, the goal is to stimulate the body's own healing properties. The acceptability of touch by individuals and cultures varies considerably. Some physical contact may never be acceptable, such as cross-gender touch in strict Muslim or Orthodox Jewish traditions. The culturally sensitive nurse makes no assumptions and always requests permission before touching a patient.

Assistive devices. Assistive devices are used to "offload" to reduce stress and weight on painful joints. Custom orthotics, lumbar supports, canes, and walkers are common. Nursing actions include both teaching how to use these devices and monitoring technique.

Psychological therapy and self-care education. Psychological therapy in pain management is a means of helping persons learn that self-efficacy and self-care skills are both powerful mediators of pain and that the coping skills they used in the past can be used in new ways. Cognitive behavioral therapy (CBT) has been found to be particularly effective (Horgas et al., 2021). Spiritual coping strategies may further enhance self-confidence and comfort.

Music. Music as an adjunct to pharmacological treatment of pain has been found to be especially useful postoperatively. Studies have shown a decrease in the intensity of pain and/or opioid requirements while listening to preferred music (Laframboise et al., 2021). The use of music for relief of pain in persons with dementia is promising but not yet conclusive (Moreno-Morales et al., 2020).

Pharmacological Interventions

Pharmacological interventions to promote comfort in older adults are a significant part of gerontological nursing. The approaches are based on action plans collaboratively created by persons in pain, their significant others, and other health care professionals. Achieving comfort is a process of trial and error to find a balance between potential benefits and harm and must always be at the forefront of care. Persons with persistent pain are often afraid of becoming addicted when they may need pharmacological intervention for the rest of their lives to maintain some level of independence.

The safe use of pharmacological agents requires knowledge of both the changes in the pharmacokinetics, the pharmacodynamics that accompany aging, and the potential food, disease, and drug interactions (Chapter 11). Pharmacological intervention ranges from acetaminophen (Tylenol) to opioids. While treatment regimens vary, all are guided by the same underlying

BOX 29.13   Tips for Best Practice

Principles of Pain Management

Every older adult deserves adequate pain management.

The treatment plan must be based on the person's goals.

Follow the basic guide to all pain: *"It is what the person says it is."*

Drug doses may be able to be minimized through the simultaneous use of nondrug therapies.

Prevent or manage side effects promptly.

Perform ongoing evaluation of effectiveness of interventions to know when they need to be adjusted, when goals are not reached.

Incorporate all affected members of caregivers, professional and informal, in teaching.

principles (Box 29.13). At all times, the least invasive route of delivery should be used, avoiding intramuscular administration if at all possible (Chapter 11).

To achieve the highest level of comfort, it is necessary to ease the "memory of pain," especially for those with persistent pain. This means that it is necessary to prevent the pain, not simply relieve it. The most effective way to do this is to provide doses around the clock (ATC); with the most appropriate medication and at the appropriate dosage, a more stable therapeutic plasma level can be reached and the extremes of overmedication and undermedication eliminated. Additional analgesia is prescribed on an as-needed basis (PRN) and should be used freely for pain that "breaks through" the ATC management. Current recommendations are to (1) establish comfort goals, (2) start with the lowest anticipated effective dose, (3) monitor the response frequently, and (4) increase the dose slowly to the desired effect: "Start low, go slow, but go!" Pain management in the care of older adults is hindered by a societal expectation that pain is a natural part of aging even when function and quality of life are compromised.

Nonopioid analgesics. Nonopioid drugs (e.g., acetaminophen, ibuprofen, naproxen) are considered the initial treatment for mild to moderate pain in older adults. Wheras a 24-hour maximum of 4 grams of acetaminophen may be appropriate for younger adults, a maximum 24-hour dose is 3 grams for older adults and 2 grams for those who are frail, are over age 80, drink alcohol on a regular basis, or have any renal or hepatic insufficiency. It has been found to be effective for the most common causes of pain, such as osteoarthritis and back pain. With few side effects or drug interactions, acetaminophen can be used for ATC management if this provides relief. Unfortunately, if used regularly, it will increase the risk for bleeding if the person is taking the anticoagulant warfarin.

A current problem with acetaminophen is that the marketed product comes in 500 mg "extra strength" (interpreted as extra relief) tablets, caplets, or gel caps. Extended-release 650 mg tablets are also available. Many older adults are accustomed to taking two tablets (two 325 mg tablets) every 4 hours. When two 500 mg tablets are taken every 4 hours or there are "hidden" doses in either other over-the-counter (OTC) products (e.g., cold preparations) or other prescribed products, the maximum dose may be reached quickly and inadvertently.

Nonsteroidal antiinflammatory drugs (NSAIDs) block the pain message from the site to the sensation point in the brain and reduce inflammation. They have been highly effective for inflammatory conditions such as rheumatoid arthritis and acute muscle strain. If used, they should be limited to 1 to 2 weeks at a time. NSAIDs have more side effects and drug-disease interactions than acetaminophen. They should not be taken by those with hypertension, impaired renal function, or heart failure. They have been associated with an increased incidence of cardiovascular events, such as acute myocardial infarctions. The severity of GI toxicity increases with age, especially after 75 years of age (Bruckenthal, 2017). Coadministration of a proton pump inhibitor or H2 blocker may be helpful to reduce the risk of bleeding, but it does not reduce cardiac risk.

The NSAIDs most often used are aspirin, ibuprofen (Advil), and naproxen (Aleve, Naprosyn). Many people have ibuprofen at home, or it is easily accessible to them. Naproxen appears to be safer than ibuprofen because it has fewer detrimental GI side effects (especially bleeding) but cannot be used by persons with heart disease.

Cyclooxygenase-2 (COX-2) selective inhibitors were introduced to reduce the risk of GI bleeding. However, the side effects are the same as the NSAIDs, and the American Geriatrics Society (AGS) Beers Criteria list them as "only use with caution" (Chapter 11). Celecoxib (Celebrex) inhibits cytochrome P450 and enzyme CYP2C9 and in doing so may elevate the plasma concentrations of several other drugs, such as beta blockers (Bruckenthal, 2017).

Finally, nonopioid pain-relieving topical patches, gels, and creams are available, such as lidocaine patches or nonsteroidal creams for localized pain. They have fewer systemic side effects but can produce rashes and other skin irritation (Reuben et al., 2020). According to the AGS Beers Criteria, muscle relaxants should be avoided due to their strong anticholinergic effects (Chapter 11).

Opioid analgesics. Many older adults have comorbid conditions that prevent the use of some nonopioid medications or cannot afford alternatives. For pain that has not been relieved by nonopioids or where their use has resulted in impaired function and quality of life, opioids may be needed. When carefully selected and monitored, they can be used safely and effectively in older adults with moderate to severe pain. Initially a short trial of fast-acting formulations is recommended. When the pain is persistent, ATC dosing is needed. After the 24-hour dose is determined, long-acting, extended-release formulations of the same medication can be used for ease in dosing and maintenance of comfort. A short-acting medication is used for breakthrough pain, and when this is needed regularly, the baseline long-acting dose will need adjustment. Unfortunately, too often the titration of dosing is not done, and pain relief is inadequate, especially in the long-term care setting.

⚡ SAFETY TIPS

Meperidine (Demerol), which is used in younger adults in acute pain, is always contraindicated in the older adult.

BOX 29.14   Side Effects of Opioids

Increased risk of fall with fracture
Impaired sexual performance
Increased sensitivity to other pain
Bladder dysfunction
Cognitive impairment
Depression
Dizziness

BOX 29.15   CDC Recommendations for the Use of Opioids

Begin with nonpharmacologic and non-opioid interventions
Establish goals for comfort and function levels
Discuss risks and benefits
Begin with fast acting opioids
Use lowest dose effective
Short term use for acute pain
Evaluate benefits and harms frequently
Counsel regarding risk for dependence and home safety
Review state prescription drug monitoring program data (PDMP)
Consider urine testing as appropriate
Avoid concurrent use of benzodiazepines and opioids
Provide help with opioid use disorders as needed

CDC, Centers for Disease Control and Prevention.
From CDC: *About CDC's opioid prescribing guideline* (website), 2021. https://www.cdc.gov/opioids/providers/prescribing/guideline.html.

Due to age-related physiological changes, older adults are often more sensitive to opioids, with a resultant higher peak and a longer duration of action. Sedation, respiratory depression, nausea, constipation, and impaired cognition are potential side effects when they are started or when doses are increased (Box 29.14). The risk for respiratory depression can be reduced by the use of low doses and slow increases until relief is obtained. Safety measures, such as fall precautions, are needed until the person is stabilized. Constipation is almost universal, and preventive nursing actions should be implemented at the same time as opioid use begins. A daily dose of a combination stool softener, a mild stimulant laxative, and adequate fluid intake are necessary. Prophylactic use of an antiemetic may be helpful for associated nausea until it resolves over time.

There has been a great deal of concern about the "opioid epidemic" in the United States, especially overprescribing, overuse, drug diversion, and potential decrease in overall life expectancy (Rummans et al., 2018). Although younger adults are more affected by the problems of dependence, diversion, and overdoses, they are potential problems for older adults as well (Horgas et al., 2021). Overuse and overdoses can occur when a clear goal is not identified and careful follow-up is not done to monitor effectiveness and the development of adverse events. Inadvertent diversion can occur when others have access to the medications.

The Centers for Disease Control and Prevention, several professional and licensing organizations, and most states have issued guidelines regarding opioid use (Box 29.15). Database systems are in place for the documentation and tracking of prescriptions written and filled. In many cases provider continuing education is required for license renewals. Limitations in the frequency and amount of opioids dispensed have been implemented. It is too early to know of the effects these steps will have on misuse and if they will perpetuate the problem of undertreatment of pain for many older adults.

Older adults without a history of other substance abuse are at low risk for opioid abuse when treated for pain. However, misuse does occur and is a current national public health concern; nurses at all levels of practice can play a part in reducing misuse through careful teaching, participation in monitoring, and developing strategies to decrease the risk of diversion. This may involve helping persons living at home to find ways to keep their medications safe or making sure that the narcotic count at the end of each shift is done consistently and carefully.

Adjuvant pain medications. Adjuvant pain medications are those intended for another purpose but found to have an additive effect to the analgesic, enhancing the potential pain relief, especially antidepressants and anticonvulsants. They are an essential component in treating neuropathic pain. The early antidepressants such as amitriptyline and doxepin can be effective, but the strong anticholinergic effects prohibit their use with older adults. There is not good evidence of effectiveness of the antidepressants in the selective serotonin receptor group (SSRI; e.g., Prozac), but the selective serotonin and norepinephrine reuptake inhibitors (SNRIs) have been found to be effective (Reuben et al., 2020). The SNRI duloxetine (Cymbalta) is the only one that is approved for both neuropathic and nociceptive pain (Gazelka et al., 2020).

Gamma-aminobutyric acid (GABA) analogs such as gabapentin and some antiepileptics have been found to be helpful for neuropathic pain such as herpetic neuralgia. They are sedating and need to be used at low doses.

Cannabis has been used for medical purposes for hundreds of years. It has two major components, the psychoactive tetrahydrocannabinol (THC) and the nonpsychoactive cannabidiol (CBD). Both bind with a receptor that blocks the passage of inflammation from the periphery to the brain and in doing so blocks the perception of pain (Xu, 2019). While the use of cannabis is still federally illegal, an increasing number of states are legalizing it for medical use and, in some cases, recreational use as well. A group of nurses established the American Cannabis Nurses Association in 2006 with the goal of becoming a recognized and certified nursing specialty. The association is dedicated to providing nurses with scientific and educational opportunities to increase the understanding of the use of cannabis as a therapeutic agent (https://www.cannabisnurses.org).

In a European study of 3000 persons using cannabis, most were using it for pain, 97% reported relief, and 16% were able to either reduce their dose or discontinue opioids (Abuhasira et al., 2018). However, since that time, several systemic reviews have found little to no effect on pain when used with older adults, noting a paucity of research related to cannabis and older adults (Chang et al., 2021; Minerbi et al., 2019). Another study points out that while few adverse events were found when cannabis was used alone, there were potential dangers when it was used concurrently with acetaminophen, opioids, and adjuvants such as antidepressants and antiepileptics. Whereas the analgesic effects of the opioids were enhanced, the metabolism of other medications was altered in such a way as to increase the risk of adverse effects (e.g., hepatic failure) and the need for close monitoring and dose reductions (Vázquez et al., 2020). The most common recommendation was for thorough discussions between professional health care providers and individuals who have an interest in using a cannabis product.

Pain Clinics

Pain clinics provide a specialized, often comprehensive, multi-professional approach to the management of pain that has not responded to the usual, more standard approaches described herein. Their use should be encouraged when appropriate and available. The number and types of pain clinics and programs have increased in response to continued poor pain management in general health care practice. These clinics may be inpatient, outpatient, or both. They are generally one of three types: syndrome-oriented, modality-oriented, or comprehensive. Syndrome-oriented centers focus on a specific chronic pain problem, such as headache or arthritis. Modality-oriented centers focus on a specific treatment technique, such as mindfulness, acupuncture and acupressure, or opioids. The comprehensive centers tend to be larger, include many services, and be associated with medical centers. A comprehensive treatment plan is developed by pain specialists using multiple modalities. However, it is well known that the "opioid epidemic" has been

most serious in rural areas where there are neither clinics nor pain management specialists and providers of any kind can be accessed only at long distances. Telehealth may improve the care of persons in pain, but even this is challenged by significant disparities in technology. Nurses should be familiar with the resources for pain management available in their communities and provide patients and families with the necessary information to make a knowledgeable decision in selecting reputable services.

Evaluation of Effectiveness

The effectiveness of solutions designed to relieve pain is quantitatively measured with the repeated use of the intensity scale. Supplemental qualitative indicators of comfort include physical changes such as relaxation of muscles that were tense and rigid or a relaxed position rather than one that was constricted. When pain is relieved, there is an increase in activity and expressions of self-worth. The person is better able to concentrate and focus and has an increased attention span, regardless of cognitive status. The individual is better able to rest, relax, and sleep. It may seem as if the person whose pain is finally relieved sleeps for an excessively long period, but this is in response to the exhaustion that the previous pain imposed on the body, mind, and spirit.

The nurse works to advocate for the person so that adjustments of treatment regimens and interventions are based on the reassessment findings. Pharmacological treatment always must begin with low doses and then increased until relief is obtained and combined with nonpharmacological nursing actions. In no other circumstances is it more important to adequately relieve pain and discomfort than it is in frail older adults who cannot communicate their needs.

KEY CONCEPTS

- The gerontological nurse can advocate for and work with the older adult and significant others to prevent needless suffering and achieve a high level of pain relief and health-related quality of life.
- Multiple modalities are available today to promote comfort, and when used together, in most cases pain can be relieved.
- The experience of pain is multifactorial with physical, psychological, and spiritual dimensions.
- Pain is a subjective experience that is unique to everyone.
- The pain most common in later life is that which is persistent.
- The undertreatment of pain in older adults, especially those in long-term care facilities, is well documented.
- A careful assessment of the presence or absence cues of pain is possible regardless of the person's cognitive status.
- If it is reasonable to expect that any person in a particular circumstance would experience pain, it is reasonable to expect

- that pain is being felt by the person who lacks the ability to communicate verbally.
- It is never acceptable to fail to treat pain (or the expectation of pain) to the extent possible.
- In many cases, acetaminophen is recommended as the first-line approach for the pharmacological management of mild to moderate pain.
- ATC dosing of the appropriate dose of the appropriate medication will most likely optimize persistent pain relief.
- The use of NSAIDs for pain relief in the older adult must be done with caution, with knowledge of the contraindications and awareness of the increased risk for associated cardiac events.
- In some cases, the use of opioids has been found to be very effective and has the potential to significantly restore function to persons with persistent pain.
- Optimal pain management incorporates both pharmacological and nonpharmacological solutions and actions.

NEXT-GENERATION NCLEX® (NGN) EXAMINATION–STYLE QUESTIONS

Helen Thomas, who is 97 years old, lives alone, considers herself well, and is almost always bright and cheerful. She has had osteoarthritis for the past 30 years. Her hips ache most of the time and keep her from doing everything she wants to do, but she "does pretty good for an old lady." She takes over-the-counter NSAIDs every day to take away the "sharp" pain. When walking her dog in the snow, she fell and broke a hip. She has considerable postoperative hip pain, but she does not want to "bother the nurses." She becomes less talkative and more irritable, and declares that she "just wishes they would give me that pill I take at home." When the nurse conducts a thorough assessment, she finds that Ms. Thomas is slightly confused, is getting very little sleep, and now has a pressure injury on her coccyx. She complains that her repaired hip hurts most of the time, as does her "good side" and now her "tailbone." Ms. Thomas has been prescribed Tylenol as needed, but she takes very little of it. She is not given any of the NSAIDs she was taking at home. She is resistive to rehabilitation.

Highlight the risk factors for poor pain management. Underline the cues that indicate discomfort. Highlight the priority in care that will be addressed if Ms. Thomas is made comfortable.

CLINICAL JUDGMENT QUESTIONS AND ACTIVITIES

1. Discuss the reasons for sporadic pain medication and inattention to the cues suggestive of pain in older adults.
2. In what situations do you believe addiction to pain medications is a priority concern?
3. Discuss issues of power and control related to pain management.

RESEARCH QUESTIONS

1. What type of persistent pain do older adults find most intolerable?
2. How is the pain of arthritis described?
3. What nonpharmacological means of pain control are used most frequently?
4. What nonpharmacological means of pain control are effective, and in what circumstances do they provide pain relief?
5. How effective is patient-controlled analgesia (PCA) when used by older adults?
6. For whom and under what circumstances should the various modalities of pain management be used?
7. How does culture influence pain expression and treatment?
8. What culturally based remedies for pain are used, and what is their efficacy?

REFERENCES

Abd-Elsayed A, Tang T, Karri J, et al: Neuromodulation for pain management in the inpatient setting: a narrative review, *Cureus* 13(3):e1392, 2021.

Abuhasira R, Schleider LB, Mechoulam R, et al: Epidemiological characteristics, safety and efficacy of medical cannabis in the elderly, *Eur J Intern Med* 49:44–50, 2018.

Bruckenthal P: Pain in the older adult. In Fillit HM, Rockwood K, Young J, editors: *Brocklehurst's textbook of geriatric medicine and gerontology*, ed 8, Philadelphia, 2017, Elsevier, pp 932–938.

Chang Y, Zhu M, Vannabouathong C, et al: Medical cannabis for chronic noncancer pain: a systematic review of health care recommendations, *Pain Res Manag* 2021:8857948.

Gazelka HM, Leal JC, Lapid MI, et al: Opioids in older adults: implications, prescribing, complications, and alternative therapies for primary care, *May Clin Proceeding* 95(4):793–800, 2020.

Horgas AL, Laframboise-Otto J, Aul K, et al: Pain management in the older adult editor. In Boltz M, editor: *Evidence-based geriatric nursing protocols for best practice*, ed 3, New York, 2021, Springer, pp 353–374.

International Association for the Study of Pain (IASP): IASP announces revised definition of pain (website), 2020. https://www.iasp-pain.org/publications/iasp-news/iasp-announces-revised-definition-of-pain/.

Kemp HI, Corner E, Colvin LA: Chronic pain after COVID-19: implications for rehabilitation, *Br J Anaesth* 125(4):436–440, 2021.

Laframboise-Otto JL, Horodyski MB, Parvataneni HK, et al: A randomized controlled trial of music for pain relief after arthroscopic surgery, *Pain Mang Nurs* 22(1):86–93, 2021.

Minerbi A, Häuser W, Fitzcharles MA: Medical cannabis for older patients, *Drugs Aging* 36(1):39–51, 2019.

Moreno-Morales C, Calero R, Moreno-Morales P, et al: Music therapy in the treatment of dementia: a systematic review and meta-analysis, *Front Med (Lausanne)* 7:160, 2020.

Natavio T, McQuillen E, Dietrich MS, et al: A comparison of the Pain Assessment Checklist for Seniors with Limited Ability to Communicate (PACSLAC) and Pain Assessment in Advanced Dementia Scale (PAINED), *Pain Manag Nurs* 21(2020):502–509, 2020.

National Center for Complementary and Integrative Health (NCCIH): *Mind and body practices* (website), 2022a. https://www.nccih.nih.gov/health/mind-and-body-practices.

National Center for Complementary and Integrative Health (NCCIH): *Relaxation techniques: What you need to know* (website), 2022b. www.nccih.nih.gov/relaxation-techniques-what-you-need-to-know.

National Center for Complementary and Integrative Health (NCCIH): *Acupuncture: in depth* (website), 2022c. https://www.nccih.nih.gov/health/acupuncture-in-depth.

Reuben DB, Herr KA, Pacala JT, et al: *Geriatrics at your fingertips*, ed 22, New York, 2020, American Geriatrics Society.

Rummans TA, Burton MC, Dawson NL: How good intentions contributed to bad outcomes: the opioid crisis, *May Clin Proc* 93(3):344–350, 2018.

Vázquez M, Guevara N, Maldonado C, et al: Potential pharmacokinetic drug-drug interactions between cannabinoids and drugs used for chronic pain, *BioMed Res Int* 2020:3902740, 2020.

Xu Y: Cannabinoids and glycinergic modulation of pain. Conference proceedings from Natural Products And Pain: The search for nonopioid analgesics, Bethesda, MD, February 6, 2019. https://www.nccih.nih.gov/news/events/natural-products-and-pain-the-search-for-novel-nonopioid-analgesics Accessed June 2021.

30 CHAPTER

Mental Health

Theris A. Touhy

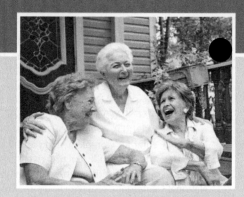

http://evolve.elsevier.com/Touhy/TwdHlthAging

A STUDENT SPEAKS

I find it a bit depressing to think about getting old. This is such a fun time in my life. But, when you think about it, older adults don't have to worry about school or a job. Some of the older adults I met at the retirement community are busier than I am and don't seem depressed. But, then there are those who are in nursing homes and I am sure they are depressed and lonely. I think it's important to enjoy each day now because you just don't know what life will bring when you're old.

Roseanna, age 23

AN OLDER ADULT SPEAKS

An older adult wrote his philosophy succinctly:
I have no idea about what would constitute happiness for anyone else, considering the differences in taste and preferences, and no spate of ideas about improving the lot of the aged. But I am sure that among other things, a calm acceptance of the facts of life is a great help. I consider serenity and peace of mind two of the greatest gifts I have, although I cannot tell you where they came from or how to get them.

(Burnside, 1975)

LEARNING OBJECTIVES

On completion of this chapter, the reader will be able to:

1. Discuss factors contributing to mental health and wellness in late life.
2. Discuss the effect of common mental health disorders on individuals as they age.
3. Recognize and analyze cues to anxiety and depression in older adults and use clinical judgment to identify solutions and nursing actions to promote mental health.
4. Recognize and analyze cues to suicidal risk and use clinical judgment to identify and evaluate solutions and nursing actions to intervene.
5. Recognize and analyze cues of substance abuse in older adults and use clinical judgment to identify and evaluate solutions and nursing actions for intervention and treatment.

MENTAL HEALTH

Mental health is not different in late life, but the level of challenge may be greater. Developmental transitions, life events, physical illness, cognitive impairment, and situations calling for psychic energy may interfere with mental health in older adults. These factors, though not unique to older adults, often influence coping skills and adaptation. However, anyone who has survived 80 or so years has been exposed to many stressors and crises and has developed tremendous resilience. The majority of older adults face life's challenges with equanimity, good humor, and courage. It is our task to discover the strengths and adaptive mechanisms that will assist them to cope with the challenges. Well-being in later life can be predicted by cognitive and affective functioning earlier in life. Thus it is very important to know the older adult's past patterns and life history (Chapter 7).

Mental, neurological, and substance use disorders are prevalent in all regions of the world and are major contributors to morbidity and premature mortality. The prevalence of mental health disorders may be even higher than reported statistics indicate because these disorders are both not always reported and not well researched. Predictions are that the number of older adults with mental illness will soon overwhelm the mental health system. In both the developed and the developing world, mental health care for older adults lags behind that for other age groups, and mental disorders have not received adequate attention in global health.

Many individuals in the baby boomer generation have experienced mental health consequences from military conflict, and the 20th century drug culture also will add to the burden of psychiatric illnesses in the future. The baby boomer generation is also more aware of mental health concerns and more comfortable seeking treatment, which will add to the challenges facing the mental health care system. The most prevalent mental health problems in late life are anxiety, severe cognitive impairment, and mood disorders. Alcohol abuse and dependence are also growing concerns among older adults, and the incidence of opioid use and misuse is also increasing. Mental health disorders are associated with increased use of health care resources and overall costs of care.

The focus of this chapter is on the differing presentation of mental health disturbances that may occur in older adults and the nursing actions important in maintaining the mental health and well-being of older adults at the optimum of their capacity. Readers should refer to a comprehensive psychiatric-mental health text for more in-depth discussion of mental health disorders. A discussion of neurocognitive disorders (NCDs) and the behavioral symptoms that may accompany these disorders is found in Chapters 25 and 26. *Healthy People 2030* includes mental health and mental health disorders as a topic area.

❤ HEALTHY PEOPLE 2030
Mental Health and Mental Disorder

- Improve mental health through prevention and by ensuring access to appropriate quality mental health services.
- Increase the proportion of primary care facilities that provide mental health treatment on-site or by paid referral.
- Increase the proportion of adults with serious mental illness who get treatment.
- Increase the proportion of homeless adults with mental health problems who receive mental health services.
- Increase the proportion of adults with depression who get treatment.
- Reduce the proportion of persons who experience major depressive episodes.
- Increase the proportion of primary care visits where adults are screened for depression.
- Reduce the suicide rate.
- Reduce the proportion of people who had alcohol use disorder in the past year.
- Increase the proportion of people with a substance use disorder who got treatment in the past year.
- Increase the proportion of people who get a referral for substance use treatment after an emergency department visit.

Data from US Department of Health and Human Services: *Healthy People 2030* (website), 2020. https://health.gov/healthypeople.

STRESS AND COPING IN LATE LIFE

Stress and Stressors

To understand mental health and mental health disorders in aging, it is important to be aware of stressors and their effect on the functioning of older adults. The experience of stress is an internal state accompanying threats to self. Healthy stress levels motivate one toward growth, whereas stress overload diminishes one's ability to cope effectively. As a person ages, many situations and conditions occur that may create disruptions in daily life and drain one's inner resources or create the need for new and unfamiliar coping strategies resulting in stress overload.

Effects of Stress

There is ongoing research about the connection between emotions and health and illness, but it is known that the mind and body are integrated and cannot be approached as separate entities. Stress may reduce one's coping ability and negatively affect neuroendocrine responses that ultimately impair immune function. Older adults show greater immunological impairments associated with distress or depression. Research on psychoneuroimmunology has explored the relationship between psychological stress and various health conditions such as cardiovascular disease, type 2 diabetes, certain cancers, Alzheimer's disease, frailty, and functional decline. The production of proinflammatory cytokines influencing these and other conditions can be stimulated directly by negative emotions and stressful experiences.

Older adults often experience multiple, simultaneous stressors (Box 30.1). Some older adults are in a chronic state of grief because new losses occur before prior ones are fully resolved; stress then becomes a constant state of being. The ability to tolerate stress varies among individuals and is influenced by current and ongoing stressors, by health, and also by coping ability. For example, if an individual has lost a significant person in the previous year, the grief may be manageable. If the individual has lost a significant person and developed painful, chronic health problems, the consequences may be quite different and

BOX 30.1 Potential Stressors in Late Life

Abrupt internal and external body changes and illnesses
Other-oriented concerns: children, grandchildren, spouse, or partner
Loss of significant people
Functional impairment
Sensory impairments
Memory impairment (or fear of)
Loss of ability to drive (particularly men)
Acute discomfort and pain
Breach in significant relationships
Retirement (lost social roles, income)
Ageist attitudes
Fires, thefts
Injuries, falls
Major unexpected drain on economic resources (house repair, illness)
Abrupt changes in living arrangements to a new location (home, apartment, room, or institution)
Identity theft and fear of scams

can cause stress overload. In the older adult, stress may appear as a cognitive impairment or behavior change that will be alleviated as the stress is reduced to the parameters of the individual's adaptability. Regardless of whether stress is physical or emotional, older adults will require more time to recover or return to prestress levels than younger people.

Any stressors that occur in the lives of older adults actually may be experienced as a crisis if the event occurs abruptly, is unanticipated, or requires skills or resources the individual does not possess. Through a lifetime of coping with stress, some individuals have developed a tremendous stress tolerance, whereas others will be thrown into crisis by changes in their lives with which they feel unable to cope. It is important to remember that there is great individual variability in the definition of a stressor. For some, the loss of a pet canary is a major stressor; others accept the loss of a good friend with grief but without personal disorganization.

Factors Affecting Stress

Researchers concerned with the effects of stress in the lives of older adults have examined many moderating variables and have concluded that cognitive style, coping strategies, social resources (social support, economic resources), personal efficacy, and personality characteristics are all significant to stress management. Social relationships and social support are particularly salient to stress management and coping. Social relationships may reduce stress and boost the immune system by providing resources (information, emotional, or tangible) that promote adaptive behavioral or neuroendocrine responses to acute and chronic stressors.

Robins et al. (2018) identified the increasing social isolation of community-dwelling older adults as a significant factor on the older adult's health and well-being, and weaker social relationships have been associated with higher hospital readmission rates and longer hospital lengths of stay (Valtorta et al., 2018). Social isolation during the COVID-19 pandemic contributed significantly to the stress of both community-living and institutionalized older adults.

Resilience is a factor that may explain the ability of some individuals to withstand stress. Resilience is defined as "flourishing despite adversity" (Hildon et al., 2009, p. 36). The process of resilience is characterized by successfully adapting to difficult and challenging life experiences, especially those that are highly stressful or traumatic. Resilient people "bend rather than break" during stressful conditions and are able to return to adequate (and sometimes better) functioning after stress (bouncing back).

Characteristics associated with resilience include positive interpersonal relationships, a willingness to extend oneself to others, optimistic or positive affect, keeping things in perspective, setting goals and taking steps to achieve these goals, high self-esteem and self-efficacy, determination, a sense of purpose in life, creativity, humor, and a sense of curiosity. Older adults may demonstrate greater resilience than younger individuals and the ability to maintain a positive emotional state under stress. Social support from the community, family, and professionals; access to care; and availability of resources can facilitate resilience. Some factors that influence one's ability to manage stress are presented in Box 30.2.

Enhancing functional status and independence, promoting a sense of control, fostering social supports and relationships,

---

BOX 30.2 Factors Influencing the Ability to Manage Stress

- Health and fitness
- A sense of control over events
- Awareness of self and others
- Patience and tolerance
- Resilience
- Hardiness
- Resourcefulness
- Social support
- A strong sense of self

---

and connecting to resources are all important nursing actions to enhance coping ability. Practices such as meditation, yoga, HeartMath, mindfulness, exercise, and spirituality and religiosity can enhance coping ability. Mind-body therapies that integrate cognitive, sensory, expressive, and physical aspects are most helpful. Reminiscence is useful in understanding the coping style of an older adult, helping the individual to remember how he or she coped successfully, suggesting how these strategies might be applied to the current situation, and enhancing self-esteem and feelings of self-worth (Chapter 7).

USING CLINICAL JUDGMENT TO PROMOTE HEALTHY AGING: MENTAL HEALTH

Recognizing and Analyzing Cues

Similar to other conditions, cues of mental health problems may be looked at as a normal consequence of aging or blamed on dementia by both older adults and health care professionals. Symptoms of mental health conditions manifest differently in older adults compared to younger individuals. In older adults, many mental health disorders present with physical complaints (e.g., body aches, insomnia, poor appetite) rather than emotional symptoms. The presence of comorbid medical conditions complicates recognition and diagnosis due to overlapping or overshadowing symptoms (Rose, 2021).

General issues in the psychosocial assessment of older adults involve distinguishing among normal, idiosyncratic, and diverse characteristics of aging and pathological conditions. Baseline data are often lacking from an individual's earlier years. Using standardized tools and functional assessment is valuable, but the data will be meaningless unless placed in the context of the individual's early life and hopes and expectations for the future. An understanding of past and present history, the person's coping ability, the degree of social support, and the effect of life events are all part of a holistic assessment. Careful listening to the person's life story, an appreciation of the person's strengths, and coming to know each person in his or her own uniqueness are the cornerstones of assessment.

Solutions, Nursing Actions, and Outcomes

Assessment of mental health includes examination of cognitive function and conditions of anxiety and adjustment reactions, paranoia, substance use, depression, and suicidal risk. Assessment of mental health also must focus on social intactness and affective responses appropriate to the situation. Attention span, concentration, intelligence, judgment, learning ability, memory, orientation, perception, problem solving, psychomotor ability, and reaction time are assessed in relation to cognitive intactness and must be considered when making a psychological assessment. Assessment includes specific processes that are intact, as well as those that are diminished or compromised. Assessment for specific mental health concerns is discussed throughout this chapter and in Chapter 9. Assessment of cognitive function is discussed in Chapter 9 and 25.

Obtaining psychosocial assessment data from older adults is best done when the individual is rested and in short sessions after some rapport has been established. Performing repeated assessments at various times of the day and in different situations will give a more complete psychological profile. It is important to be sensitive to a patient's anxiety, special needs, and disabilities and vigilant in protecting the person's privacy. The interview should be focused so that attention is given to strengths and skills and life challenges.

FACTORS INFLUENCING MENTAL HEALTH CARE

Attitudes and Beliefs

Older adults with evidence of mental health disorders, regardless of race or ethnicity, are less likely than younger people to receive needed mental health care from mental health specialists. Some of the reasons for this include reluctance on the part of older adults to seek help because of pride of independence, stoic acceptance of difficulty, unawareness of resources, and lack of adequate insurance coverage for mental health problems. Stigma about having a mental health disorder, particularly for older adults, discourages many from seeking treatment. Ageism also affects identification and treatment of mental health disorders in older adults. As well, the myth that older adults do not respond well to treatment is still prevalent (Chapter 7).

Other factors present barriers to appropriate diagnosis and treatment for mental health concerns, including the lack of knowledge on the part of health care professionals about mental health in late life; inadequate numbers of geropsychiatrists, geropsychologists, and geropsychiatric nurses; and limited availability of psychiatric care, specifically geropsychiatric services. Increased attention to the preparation of mental health professionals specializing in geriatric care is important to improve mental health care delivery to older adults.

Geropsychiatric nursing (GPN) is the master's level subspecialty within the adult-psychiatric mental health nursing field. Advanced practice registered nurses (APRNs) must be prepared to care for the growing number of older adults with mental health needs, but inclusion of GPN content continues to remain limited in graduate nursing programs. It is essential that both graduate and undergraduate nursing students receive adequate preparation to competently care for the growing numbers of older adults with mental health challenges. An initiative to prepare APRNs in the specialty is the Geropsychiatric Nursing

Initiative (GPNI), which provides guidelines and learning materials to improve the knowledge and skills of nurses in mental health care of older adults (Box 30.3).

Culture and Mental Health

Mental illness is found in all societies, but the frequencies of different types of mental illness vary, as do the social connotations. The standards that define "normal" behavior for any culture are determined by that culture itself. What may be defined as mental illness in one culture may be viewed as normal behavior in another. Different cultures and communities also exhibit and explain symptoms of mental distress in various ways (Box 30.4). Cultural beliefs also influence who makes health care decisions, help-seeking behavior, preferences for type of treatment, and provider characteristics.

In the United States, disparities in mental health service use by racial and ethnic minority groups are well documented. Mental and behavioral health is a critical and frequently unaddressed matter in racial and ethnic minority communities. Cultural variation in beliefs about the causes of mental illness and the effects of treatment; past discrimination; and the lack of mental health treatments that are congruent with preferences, values, and beliefs contribute to disparities. In all ethnic groups, the cost of services or lack of health insurance and the belief that mental health services would not help also influence access. Minority individuals may experience symptoms that are underdiagnosed, undiagnosed, or misdiagnosed for cultural, linguistic, or historical reasons (American Psychological Association, 2020).

Disparities are found in many groups. Although not well researched, sexual minority individuals, particularly older gay

---

BOX 30.3   Resources for Best Practice

American Academy of Nursing: Geropsychiatric Nursing Collaborative. https://www.aannet.org/initiatives/early-initiatives/geropsychiatric-nursing-collaborative.

American Society of Consultant Pharmacists STAMP Out Prescription Drug Misuse and Abuse Toolkit: Resource for health professionals to educate older adults and providers of senior services about prescription drug misuse and abuse. https://www.ascp.com/page/STAMPOut.

C-P.A.W.W. (Canines providing assistance to wounded warriers: health research initiative for veterans). https://nursing.fau.edu/outreach/c-paww/.

Centers for Disease Control and Prevention: PEARLS Toolkit. https://www.cdc.gov/prc/resources/tools/pearls.html.

Evidence-Based Practice Guideline: Secondary Prevention of Late-Life Suicide. https://www.ncbi.nlm.nih.gov/pubmed/30208188.

Friendship Line (managed by the Institute on Aging); National Suicide Prevention Lifeline (managed by the Institute on Aging): Available 24 hours a day, 7 days a week. Friendship Line: 1-800-971-0016; National Suicide Prevention Lifeline: 1-800-273-8255.

Hartford Institute for Geriatric Nursing: The Impact of Event Scale-Revised (IES-R). https://hign.org/sites/default/files/2020-06/Try_This_General_Assessment_19.pdf.

National Alliance on Mental Illness: Help for individuals and their families who are experiencing mental health disorders. https://www.nami.org/

National Center for PTSD: https://www.ptsd.va.gov/.

Online treatment navigator for alcohol use disorder: Step-by-step guide for finding professionally led treatment. https://alcoholtreatment.niaaa.nih.gov/.

BOX 30.4   Cultural Variations in Expressing Mental Distress

- **Ataque de nervios** (attack of nerves): A syndrome among individuals of Latin descent, characterized by symptoms of intense emotional upset, including acute anxiety, anger, grief; screaming and shouting uncontrollably; attacks of crying, trembling, heat in the chest rising into the head; and verbal and physical aggression. May include seizure-like or fainting episodes and suicidal gestures. Attacks frequently occur because of a stressful event relating to the family (e.g., death of a relative, conflict with spouse or children, witnessing an accident involving a family member). Symptoms are similar to acute anxiety or panic disorder. Related conditions are "blacking out" in southern United States and "falling out" in West Indies.

- **Susto** (fright): A cultural expression for distress and misfortune prevalent among some Latinos in the United States and among people in Mexico, Central America, and South America. Illness is attributed to a frightening event that causes the soul to leave the body and results in unhappiness, sickness, and difficulty functioning in social roles. Symptoms include appetite and sleep disturbances, feelings of sadness, low self-worth, and lack of motivation. Symptoms are similar to those of posttraumatic stress disorder (PTSD), depression, and anxiety.

- **Khyâl cap** (wind attacks): A syndrome found among Cambodians in the United States and in Cambodia. Symptoms include dizziness, palpitations, shortness of breath, and cold extremities. Concern that *khyâl* (a wind-like substance) may rise in the body, along with blood, and cause serious effects such as entering the lungs to cause shortness of breath or asphyxia or entering the brain to cause dizziness, tinnitus, and a fatal syncope. Attacks frequently brought about by worrisome thoughts. Symptoms include those of panic attacks, generalized anxiety disorder, and PTSD.

BOX 30.5   Cultural Components of the *Diagnostic and Statistical Manual of Mental Disorders (DSM-5)*

- Cross-cultural variations in presentations
- Cultural concepts of distress
- Cultural formulation interview (CFI)
- Questions that can be used during a cultural assessment of particular groups, such as older adults and immigrants

From Multicultural Mental Health Resource Centre: *Cultural formulation* (website), 2018. https://www.multiculturalmentalhealth.ca/clinical-tools/cultural%20formulation/. Accessed June 2018.

BOX 30.6   Tips for Best Practice
Cultural Interview Questions

- "Sometimes people have different ways of describing their problem to their family, friends, or others in the community. How would you describe your problem to them?"
- "What troubles you most about your problem?"
- "Why do you think this is happening to you?"
- "What do you think are the causes of your problem?"
- "What do others in your family, friends, or others in your community think are the causes of your problem?"
- "Are there aspects of your background or identity that are causing other concerns or difficulties for you?"
- "Sometimes people have various ways of dealing with problems like your problem. What have you done to cope with your problems?"
- "Often people look for help from many different sources, including different kinds of doctors, helpers, or healers. In the past what kinds of treatment, help, advice, or healing have you sought for your problem? What have others advised?"
- "What do you think would be helpful?"
- "Do you have any concerns about the therapist-patient relationship?"

Adapted from American Psychiatric Association: *Diagnostic and statistical manual of mental disorders*, ed 5, Washington, D.C., 2013, American Psychiatric Association.

---

men, demonstrate higher rates of mental disorders, substance abuse, suicidal ideation, and deliberate self-harm than heterosexual individuals (Hoy-Ellis et al., 2016). Sexual minority stress (gay-related stigma, discrimination or prejudice, concealment of sexual preferences, excessive human immunodeficiency virus [HIV] bereavements) and aging-related stress are thought to contribute to the unique mental health challenges of these individuals (Chapter 33). The effect of minority stress on health disparities in sexual minority individuals, and individuals of different races, ethnicities, and cultures, is an important area of research. Research is also needed on the effect of other stressors such as war, terrorism, displacement, and immigration on mental health.

The *Diagnostic and Statistical Manual of Mental Disorders (DSM-5)* (American Psychiatric Association, 2013) has an increased emphasis on culture and mental health, including the range of psychopathology across the globe, not just illnesses common in the United States, western Europe, and Canada. Another significant change in the *DSM-5* is the developmental approach and examination of disorders across the life span. This is particularly relevant for older adults because symptoms of mental distress may present differently than in younger individuals.

An increased understanding of the importance of cultural perspectives for individuals across the life span will facilitate more accurate assessment of mental health disorders, wellness, and illness and lead to fewer misdiagnoses. Enhancing the cultural proficiency of health care professionals will assist in structuring more culturally appropriate services, thus improving treatment outcomes and decreasing disparities. Some of the cultural components in the *DSM-5* are presented in Box 30.5. A Cultural Formulation Interview (CFI; American Psychiatric Association, 2013), including Kleinman's (1980) explanatory model, Leininger's Sunrise Enable model (Wehbe-Alamah, 2015), and Ray's (2016) *Transcultural Caring Dynamics in Nursing and Health Care*, guides health care providers in culturally relevant assessment. Box 30.6 presents best practice tips for culture assessment. Research on all aspects of culture and mental health is critical. Chapter 4 discusses culture in more depth.

Availability of Mental Health Care

Dedicated financing for older adult mental health services is limited even though about 20% of all Medicare beneficiaries experience some mental disorder each year. Medicare spends five times more on beneficiaries with severe mental illness and substance abuse disorders than on similar beneficiaries without these diagnoses. More than half of dual-eligible persons (those with both Medicare and Medicaid) have mental or cognitive impairments. The 2008 mental health parity legislation ended Medicare's discriminatory practice of imposing a 50% coinsurance requirement for outpatient mental health services. In 2014 coinsurance was reduced to 20%, bringing payments for mental health care in line with those required for all other Medicare Part B services (Center for Medicare Advocacy, 2020).

The Centers for Medicare and Medicaid Services (CMS) health risk assessment and annual wellness visit for Medicare beneficiaries includes screening for depression, questions on alcohol consumption, and detection of cognitive impairment. Medicare also covers a yearly depression screening at no cost to beneficiaries. However, coverage for follow-up care for such problems remains limited (Jeste et al., 2018). Concerns remain about the 190-day lifetime limit for care in inpatient psychiatric facilities and the high out-of-pocket costs of prescription drugs. More comprehensive and integrated mental health care is needed, especially considering the aging of the baby boomer generation.

Settings of Care

Older adults receive psychiatric services across a wide range of settings, including acute and long-term inpatient psychiatric units, primary care, and community and institutional settings. The majority of older adults treated for mental health services receive care from primary care providers. Less than 3% receive treatment from mental health professionals (American Psychological Association, 2020). It is critical to integrate mental health and substance abuse with other health services, including primary care, specialty care, home health care, and residential community-based care.

Primary care providers must routinely screen for mental health problems in older adults and develop working relationships with mental health practitioners in their area to improve access and communication. Successful models include mental health professionals in primary care offices; care managers; community-based, multidisciplinary geriatric mental health treatment teams; and use of APRNs (SAMHSA-HRSA Center for Integrated Health Solutions, 2018).

In acute care settings, nurses will encounter older adults with mental health disorders in emergency departments or in general medical-surgical units. Admissions for medical problems are often exacerbated by depression, anxiety, cognitive impairment, substance abuse, or chronic mental illness, and these conditions are often unrecognized by primary care providers. Nurses who can recognize cues of mental health problems early and seek consultation and treatment will enhance timely recovery. Advanced practice psychiatric nursing consultation is an important and effective service in acute care settings.

Long-term care facilities and, increasingly, residential care/assisted living facilities (RC/ALFs), although not licensed as psychiatric facilities, are providing the majority of care given to older adults with psychiatric conditions. The bulk of mental health services is focused on symptom management of Alzheimer's disease and other dementias. However, excluding dementia, individuals with mental health concerns account for close to 50% of all nursing facility residents. Older adults in nursing facilities are almost twice as likely to experience symptoms of depression, self-harm, or suicidal ideation as community-dwelling older adults (Rose, 2021). It is often difficult to find placement for an older adult with a mental health problem in these types of facilities, and few are structured to provide best practice mental health care. In addition, patients with mental health diagnoses had lower access to high-quality facilities as measured by the overall quality of care and by facility staffing (Temkin-Greener et al., 2018).

Some of the obstacles to mental health care in nursing facilities and RC/ALFs are (1) shortage of trained personnel; (2) limited availability and access for psychiatric services; (3) lack of staff training related to mental health and mental illness; and (4) inadequate Medicaid and Medicare reimbursement for mental health services. An insufficient number of trained personnel affects the quality of mental health care in nursing facilities and often causes great stress for staff.

New models of mental health care and services are needed for nursing facilities and RC/ALFs to address the growing needs of older adults in these settings. Psychiatric services in nursing homes, when they are available, are commonly provided by psychiatric consultants who are not full-time staff members, and their services are inadequate to meet the needs of residents and staff. Training and education of frontline staff who provide basic care to residents is essential. There is an urgent need for well-designed controlled studies to examine mental health concerns in both nursing facilities and RC/ALFs and the effectiveness of mental health services in improving clinical outcomes. Chapter 6 discusses long-term care in more depth.

MENTAL HEALTH DISORDERS

Anxiety Disorders

Prevalence and Characteristics

Epidemiological studies indicate that anxiety disorders are common in the overall population. Agoraphobia, panic disorder (PD), and generalized anxiety disorder (GAD) are the most common disorders, with women having a significantly higher rate of anxiety than men. Interestingly, anxiety rates dropped significantly after the age of 75 years (Canuto et al., 2018). Anxiety disorders are not considered part of the normal aging process, but the changes and challenges that older adults often face may contribute to the development of anxiety symptoms and disorders or reactivate prior anxiety disorders. Increasing frailty, medical illness, losses, pain, lack of social support, traumatic events, medications, poor self-rated health, the presence of another psychiatric illness, and an early-onset anxiety disorder are all risk factors for late-life anxiety disorders.

Late-life anxiety is often comorbid with major depressive disorder, cognitive decline and dementia, and substance abuse. Almost half of older adults diagnosed with major depression also meet the criteria for anxiety. Current evidence suggests that anxiety is even more common than depression in community-dwelling older adults and may precede depressive disorders. There is some evidence to suggest that anxiety may be predictive of cognitive decline, but anxiety also develops in response to cognitive decline. Symptoms of anxiety may occur in 75% of individuals diagnosed with dementia (Fung et al., 2018). Anxiety symptoms and disorders are associated with many negative consequences, including increased hospitalizations, decreased physical activity and functional status, sleep disturbances, increased health service use, substance abuse, decreased life satisfaction, and increased mortality. Further investigation is needed on all aspects of anxiety in older adults.

USING CLINICAL JUDGMENT TO PROMOTE HEALTHY AGING: ANXIETY

Recognizing and Analyzing Cues

Data suggest that approximately 70% of all primary care visits are driven by psychological factors (e.g., panic, generalized anxiety, stress, somatization) (American Psychological Association, 2020). This means that nurses often encounter anxious older adults and can identify anxiety-related symptoms and initiate assessments that will lead to appropriate treatment and management. Whether symptoms represent a diagnosable anxiety disorder is perhaps less important than the fact that the individual will suffer needlessly if assessment and treatment are not addressed. Assessment of anxiety in older adults focuses on physical, social, and environmental factors; past life history; long-standing personality; coping skills; and recent events.

The general and pervasive nature of anxiety may make diagnosis difficult in older adults. In addition, older adults tend to deny the psychological symptoms, attribute anxiety-related symptoms to physical illness, and have coexistent medical conditions that mimic symptoms of anxiety. As well, stigma associated with mental disorders is a factor for older adults. Cues to anxiety most often present in physical complaint, such as difficulty sleeping, stomach complaints, and general malaise. Avoiding previously enjoyed activities and increasing social isolation are major signs of both anxiety and depression. Often, health care providers may attribute these symptoms to "getting older," as a result of age-related stereotypes.

Some of the medical disorders that cause anxiety include cardiac arrhythmias, mitral valve prolapse, delirium, dementia, chronic obstructive pulmonary disease (COPD), heart failure, hyperthyroidism, hypoglycemia, postural hypotension, pulmonary edema, and pulmonary embolism. The presence of cognitive impairment also may make diagnosis complicated. Anxiety is also a common side effect of many drugs (Box 30.7). A review of medications, including over-the-counter (OTC) and herbal or home remedies, is essential, with elimination of those that cause anxiety if possible (Chapter 11).

It is important to investigate all possible causes of anxiety, such as medical conditions and depression. Diagnostic and laboratory tests may be ordered as indicated to rule out medical problems. Cognitive assessment is included if cognitive impairment is suspected. When comorbid conditions are present, they must be treated. Several assessment and screening tools have been developed specifically for use with older adults: Geriatric Anxiety Inventory (GAI), Adult Manifest Anxiety Scale-Elderly (AMAS-E), Geriatric Anxiety Scale (GAS), and Worry Scale (WS) (Balsamo et al., 2018). If such instruments are used, they should be weighed carefully with other data—complaints, physical exam, history, and collateral interview data.

BOX 30.7 Medications That May Cause Anxiety Symptoms

- Anticholinergics
- Digitalis
- Theophylline
- Antihypertensives
- Beta blockers
- Beta-adrenergic stimulators
- Corticosteroids
- Over-the-counter medications such as appetite suppressants and cough and cold preparations
- Caffeine
- Nicotine
- Withdrawal from alcohol, sedatives, and hypnotics

When assessing anxiety reactions in individuals who reside in nursing facilities, look for daily disturbances, such as with staff or caregiver changes, room changes, or events over which the individual feels a lack of control or influence. By themselves, these circumstances seldom provoke an anxiety reaction, but they may be "the straw that breaks the camel's back," particularly in older adults who are frail. Nurses must be alert to the cues of anxiety in older adults who are frail or those with dementia because symptoms are subtle and the individuals may be unable to tell us how they are feeling. Carefully observing behavior and searching for possible reasons for changes in behavior or patterns are important (Chapter 26).

Solutions, Nursing Actions, and Outcomes

Although further research is needed to provide evidence to guide treatment, existing studies suggest that anxiety disorders in older adults can be treated effectively. Treatment choices depend on the symptoms, the specific anxiety diagnosis, comorbid medical conditions, and any current medication regimen. Creighton et al. (2018) found that pharmacotherapy was typically the first line of treatment, even though there is growing evidence that nonpharmacological interventions such as cognitive behavioral therapy (CBT) and alternative medications are the recommended treatments. If the individual has more than one anxiety disorder or suffers from comorbid depression, substance abuse, or medical problems, treatment may be complicated. Suggested nursing actions for anxiety in older adults are presented in Box 30.8.

Pharmacological Interventions

Pharmacotherapy is a treatment option for many patients with anxiety disorders, either in combination with CBT or as standalone treatment. However, research on the effectiveness of medication in treating anxiety in older adults is limited. Age-related changes in pharmacodynamics and issues of polypharmacy make prescribing and monitoring in older adults a complex undertaking. Antidepressants in the form of selective serotonin reuptake inhibitors (SSRIs) are usually the first-line treatment. Within this class of drugs, those with sedating rather than stimulating properties are preferred. Careful monitoring of response and side effects is important.

BOX 30.8 Tips for Best Practice

Nursing Actions for Anxiety in Older Adults

- Establish a therapeutic relationship and come to know the person.
- Listen attentively to what is said and unsaid; pay attention to nonverbal behavior; use a nonjudgmental approach.
- Support the person's strengths and have faith in the person's ability to cope, drawing on past successes.
- Encourage expression of needs, concerns, and questions.
- Screen for depression.
- Evaluate medications for anxiety side effects; adjust as needed.
- Manage physical conditions.
- Accept the person's defenses; do not confront, argue, or debate.
- Help the person identify precipitants of anxiety and their reactions.
- Teach the person about anxiety, symptoms, and their effects on the body.
- If irrational thoughts are present, offer accurate information while encouraging the expression of the meaning of events contributing to anxiety; reassure of safety and your presence in supporting them.
- Intervene when possible to remove the source of anxiety.
- Encourage positive self-talk, such as "I can do this one step at a time" and "Right now I need to breathe deeply."
- Teach distraction or diversion tactics; progressive relaxation exercises; deep breathing.
- Encourage participation in physical activity, adapted to the person's capabilities.
- Encourage the use of community resources such as friends, family, churches, socialization groups, self-help and support groups, and mental health counseling.

Second-line treatment may include short-acting benzodiazepines (alprazolam, lorazepam, mirtazapine). Treatment with benzodiazepines should be used for short-term therapy only (<3 months) and relief of immediate symptoms, but they must be used carefully in older adults. The American Geriatrics Society's (2015) Beers Criteria include a strong recommendation to avoid any type of benzodiazepine for the treatment of insomnia or agitation. Use of these medications may be appropriate for only a few select indications, including severe GAD that is unresponsive to other therapies.

However, benzodiazepine use continues to increase with age, growing to use in nearly one-third of those 65 to 80 years of age (Chapter 18). In addition, only a small proportion of patients who received prescriptions for benzodiazepines were referred to or received psychotherapy or antidepressant therapy. Older adults are not receiving treatments that are both more appropriate and safer (Maust et al., 2016).

Benzodiazepines in older adults can cause cognitive impairment, falls, and other serious side effects. Fall risk is significantly increased with use of benzodiazepines, particularly among older adults with osteoporosis, sensory loss, Parkinson's disease, arthritis, polypharmacy, or orthostasis; those who use the restroom frequently at night; and those with a history of falls (Markota et al., 2016). Use of older drugs, such as diazepam or chlordiazepoxide, should be avoided because of their long half-lives and the increased risk of accumulation and toxicity in older people. Nonbenzodiazepine anxiolytic agents (buspirone) also may be used but not on an as-needed basis (prn). Buspirone has fewer side effects, but it requires a longer period of administration (up to 4 weeks) for effectiveness. See Chapters 11, 18, and 26 for discussions of the use of benzodiazepines in older adults.

Nonpharmacological Interventions

Psychosocial approaches for anxiety include CBT, exposure therapy, mindfulness-based stress reduction (MBSR), and interpersonal therapy. Increasing evidence supports the effectiveness of psychotherapy in treating anxiety in older adults, often in combination with pharmacotherapy. CBT is designed to modify thought patterns, improve skills, and alter the environmental states that contribute to anxiety. CBT may involve relaxation training and cognitive restructuring (replacing anxiety-producing thoughts with more realistic, less catastrophic ones) and education about signs and symptoms of anxiety. Telephone-delivered and internet-based CBT are increasingly available, and preliminary evaluation has shown improved patient outcomes, increased access to care, low cost, and ease of use (Kruse et al., 2017).

MBSR is a new technique that introduces the concept of mindfulness through the practice of techniques such as yoga, mindful breathing, and other forms of meditation. Exposure therapy, also used in treatment of posttraumatic stress disorder (PTSD), involves controlled exposure to events and situations that cause anxiety until anxiety lessens and the body and mind are trained to view the situation with less distress. Complementary and alternative therapies include biofeedback, progressive relaxation, acupuncture, yoga, massage therapy, art therapy, music therapy, dance therapy, meditation, prayer, and spiritual counseling. The therapeutic relationship between the patient and the health care provider is the foundation for any intervention. Support from family, referral to community resources and support groups, and provision of educational materials are other important interventions.

POSTTRAUMATIC STRESS DISORDER

Although originally considered an anxiety disorder, the *DSM-5* removed PTSD from the classification of anxiety disorders and included it in a new chapter, Trauma- and Stressor-Related Disorders. PTSD was once considered a psychological condition of combat veterans who were "shocked" by and unable to face their experiences on the battlefield. Individuals with PTSD were labeled as weak, faced rejection from their military peers and society in general, and were removed from combat zones or discharged from the military. Today we know that PTSD is a psychobiological mental disorder associated with changes in brain function and structure and can affect survivors of combat experience but also terrorist attacks, natural disasters, mass trauma events, serious accidents, assault or abuse, and even sudden and major emotional losses (National Institute of Mental Health, 2019).

The impact of various traumatic stressors related to the COVID-19 pandemic, as well as the effects of less severe types of stress exposure, has already led to diverse mental health problems, including anxiety, depression, PTSD, and other trauma- and stress-related illness. Post-COVID-19 stress disorder is recognized as another consequence of the global pandemic. Those who have experienced COVID-19, or lost loved ones to the virus, and first responders and hospital personnel are particularly vulnerable. Other stressors such as social isolation, unemployment and economic losses, and working from home while caring for children and other family members also have contributed to anxiety, depression, and substance use in the general population.

Research on these effects, as well as appropriate options for treatment, will be important (Tucker & Czapla, 2021).

Prevalence

The prevalence of current PTSD in adults over 60 years of age ranges from 1.5% to 4%, which is a lower prevalence rate than in other age categories. Data from a nationally representative sample reported that older adults experienced fewer potentially traumatic experiences than younger or middle-aged adults. Most of the research on PTSD has been conducted with male veterans of military combat. The lifetime prevalence rate for PTSD for Vietnam veterans is estimated to be 30.9% of men and 26.9% of women, for Gulf War veterans is 12.1%, and for veterans in Operation Enduring Freedom/Operation Iraqi Freedom is 13.8% (Gradus, 2017). In addition to military combat, older adults in our care now have also experienced other events that may precipitate PTSD, including the Great Depression, the Holocaust, racism, and the COVID-19 pandemic. Frequently identified by older adults as the worst or one of the worst stressful events are unexpected deaths or serious illness or injury to someone close to them; their own serious illness; and for women, sexual assault and intimate partner violence. Fourteen percent of women ages 65 years and older reported a history of physical or sexual assault during their lifetimes (Cook & Simiola, 2017).

Older adults experiencing PTSD may have managed to keep symptoms under control during their life, but if they become cognitively impaired, they may no longer be able to control thoughts, flashbacks, or images. This can be the cause of great distress that may be exhibited in aggressive or hostile behavior. Older adults who are survivors of the Holocaust may experience PTSD symptoms when they are placed in group settings in institutions. Older women with a history of physical or sexual assault also may experience symptoms of PTSD when institutionalized, particularly during the provision of intimate bodily care activities, such as bathing. Box 30.9 provides some clinical examples of PTSD.

Symptoms

The *DSM-5* includes four major symptom clusters for diagnosis of PTSD: (1) reexperiencing; (2) avoidance; (3) persistent negative alterations in cognition and mood; and (4) alterations in arousal

---

BOX 30.9   Clinical Example of Posttraumatic Stress Disorder (PTSD) in Older Adults

Jack's Story

Jack, an 80-year-old World War II (WWII) veteran with dementia, was admitted to a large Veterans Administration (VA) nursing home. Jack's wife told the staff that he had been a high school principal who was very successful in his position. He had recurring frightening dreams throughout his life related to his war experiences, and he would always turn off the radio or TV when there were programs about WWII. Now, because of his dementia, he was unable to control his thoughts and feelings. While in the nursing home, he would become very agitated and attempt to hit other residents around him when placed in the large day room. The staff recognized this as a PTSD reaction from his years as a prisoner of war. They always placed him in a smaller day room near the nursing station away from other residents, where he remained calm and pleasant. The aggression stopped without the need for medication.

---

and receptivity (including irritable or aggressive behavior and reckless or self-destructive behavior) (American Psychiatric Association, 2013). Individuals often reexperience and relive the traumatic event in episodes of fear and experience symptoms such as helplessness; flashbacks (reliving the trauma over and over, including physical symptoms like a racing heart or sweating); intrusive thoughts; bad dreams; images; avoidance of thoughts or situations that remind them of the traumatic event; poor concentration; irritability; increased startle reactions; and numbing of emotional responsiveness (detachment, flattened or absent affect). Symptoms may be present within a short period following the trauma, but a person may have a delayed response from a year to several years or longer. Although the majority of older adult trauma survivors do not develop PTSD, a significant minority do and, unless treated, appear to experience a waxing and waning of symptoms across their life span (National Institute of Mental Health, 2019).

USING CLINICAL JUDGMENT TO PROMOTE HEALTHY AGING: PTSD

Recognizing and Analyzing Cues

The care of the individual with PTSD involves awareness that certain events may trigger inappropriate reactions, and the pattern of these reactions should be identified when possible. Knowing the person's history and life experiences is essential in understanding behavior and implementing appropriate actions. Assessment of trauma and related symptoms should be routine in older adults because they may not report traumatic experiences or may minimize their importance. Similar to other mental health concerns, cues to PTSD symptoms include physical concerns, pain, sleep difficulties, or cognitive problems rather than emotional problems.

PTSD often co-occurs with physical illness, substance use disorders, and chronic pain. Reports of physical issues should be followed with questions about changes in mood and activities. Depression is present in half of individuals with PTSD, making it very important to assess routinely for depression and suicidal ideation. Cognitive screening for delirium or dementia is important. The Impact of Event Scale-Revised (IES-R) is a screening instrument for PTSD that also may be used (Christianson & Marren, 2013) (see Box 30.3).

Solutions, Nursing Actions, and Outcomes

Effective coping with traumatic events seems to be associated with secure and supportive relationships; the ability to freely express or fully suppress the experience; favorable circumstances immediately following the trauma; productive and active lifestyles; strong faith, religion, and hope; a sense of humor; biological integrity; and resilience. PTSD has a strong genetic component similar to other psychiatric disorders. Approximately 30% of the variants in PTSD are caused by genetics alone. As gene research and brain imaging technologies continue to improve, scientists are more likely to be able to pinpoint when and where in the brain PTSD begins. Other research is attempting to identify which factors determine whether someone with PTSD will respond well to one type of intervention or another, aiming to develop more personalized, effective treatment (National Institute of Mental Health, 2019; Nievergelt et al., 2019).

The understanding of how to treat PTSD among older adults is still developing. Current treatment recommendations for older adults include CBT and prolonged exposure therapy. The Warrior Wellness Study (Hall et al., 2018) examines the effects of exercise on older veterans with PTSD. Other therapies shown to improve PTSD symptoms include cognitive processing therapy, eye movement desensitization and reprocessing, and narrative exposure therapy. Cognitive therapy aims to isolate dysfunctional thoughts and assumptions about the trauma that seem to cause distress. Individuals are encouraged to challenge the truth of the beliefs and to substitute them with more balanced thoughts. Exposure therapy involves recalling distressing memories of the trauma or event via controlled exposure to reminders of the event. Exposure can be done by imagining the trauma, reading descriptions of the event, or visiting the site of the trauma until distress associated with the memory lessens and the body and mind are retrained to view the situation as less dangerous than it was perceived to be (National Institute of Mental Health, 2019).

In a very innovative holistic nonpharmacological approach, nurse researcher Cheryl Krause-Parello, Christine E. Lynn College of Nursing, Florida Atlantic University, has explored the use of service dogs with wounded military and veterans to promote healing from the effects of war. Canines Providing Assistance to Wounded Warriors (C-P.A.W.W.) focuses on biological and psychosocial stress indicators in the military veteran population and examines the relationship between human-animal interaction and stress biomarkers in vulnerable populations, including military veterans and children of sexual abuse. The long-term goal of Krause-Parello's research is to implement effective interventions to modulate the long-term effects of PTSD on returning active duty military and veterans and to identify additional populations where this intervention will be effective (Galoustian, 2018). Research on the effects of C-P.A.W.W.'s model of care has demonstrated reduction of stress, increased quality of life, and stronger social relationships when interacting with a canine such as a service dog, therapy dog, companion animal, or personal pet. Study results also demonstrated that having a service dog allowed the individual to decrease or stop psychotropic medication and reduce the undesirable side effects associated with these medications (Krause-Parello, 2018). Box 30.3 presents information on the C-P.A.W.W. program.

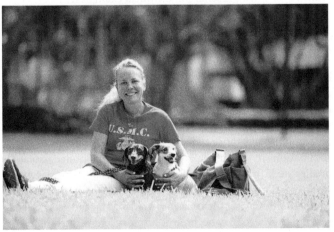

Nurse researcher Dr. Cheryl Krause-Parello. (Photograph by Alex Dolce, Florida Atlantic University.)

Evidence-based psychospiritual interventions also may be effective in the treatment of veterans with PTSD and may be more acceptable among those who have a fear of mental illness-related stigma. Individuals able to find meaning and purpose in their traumatic experiences are less likely to develop chronic PTSD. Providers should inquire about the spiritual component of PTSD and help the individual find meaning in their life (Chapter 35). Pharmacological therapy is also used, and sertraline and paroxetine have received approval by the US Food and Drug Administration (FDA) to treat PTSD. Careful monitoring of these medications is necessary in older adults (Chapter 9).

Therapies should be individualized to meet the specific concerns and needs of each unique patient and may include individual, group, and family therapy. Internet-based therapy, self-help therapy, and telephone-assisted therapy are other creative formats to make interventions more widely available, particularly for improving response to mass trauma events. Further research is necessary to understand the various presentations of PTSD in late life and validate and improve the effectiveness of available treatment approaches (Department of Veterans Affairs, 2019). Other resources for management of PTSD can be found in Box 30.3.

SCHIZOPHRENIA

Prevalence

Older adults are the fastest growing segment of the total population of individuals living with schizophrenia, and the numbers are expected to grow in the coming decades with the increased longevity of the population. The onset of schizophrenia for men is between the ages of 10 to 25 years and for women is between 25 and 35 years. Approximately 3% to 10% are diagnosed after the age of 40 years. Onset of schizophrenia after the age of 45 years is identified as late-onset; after the age of 60 years, the onset of schizophrenia is rare (American Psychiatric Association, 2013).

Symptoms

The main symptoms associated with schizophrenia can be categorized into *positive* symptoms of delusions, hallucinations, disorganized speech, and disorganized behavior; *negative* symptoms of flat or blunted affect, anhedonia, and avolition; and cognitive symptoms of poor executive functioning and limited attention span (American Psychiatric Association, 2013). By the age of 65 years, persons living with schizophrenia experience fewer delusions and hallucinations but still experience some degree of impairment. Symptoms of cognitive impairment usually do not improve as the person ages, and individuals with schizophrenia are at high risk for receiving a diagnosis of dementia. More than one-quarter had a dementia diagnosis by age 66, and by age 80, prevalence increased to 70% (Stroup et al., 2021).

Consequences

Individuals with severe persistent mental illnesses such as schizophrenia form a disenfranchised group whose access to medical care has been limited, leading to greater functional declines, morbidity, and mortality. Individuals with schizophrenia generally have a life expectancy 10 to 20 years shorter than that of the general population (World Health Organization, 2021). This reduction in years has been attributed to cardiovascular disease related to antipsychotics, poor diet, limited exercise, and smoking. Continued research is needed specifically to examine the effects of living with schizophrenia as an older adult across the globe.

Schizophrenia is a costly disease both in terms of personal challenges and with regard to medical care costs. The living situations for older adults who have schizophrenia can be challenging, with the majority living in nursing homes, assisted living, boarding houses, or on the streets. Interventions to improve independent functioning, irrespective of age and in conjunction with community services, would decrease need for institutionalization and decrease health care costs for care. The care of older adults with schizophrenia is expected to become a serious burden for our health care system, requiring the development of integrated models of care across the continuum.

USING CLINICAL JUDGMENT TO PROMOTE HEALTHY AGING: SCHIZOPHRENIA

Solutions, Nursing Actions, and Outcomes

Treatment for schizophrenia includes both pharmacological and nonpharmacological interventions. First-generation antipsychotics (e.g., haloperidol) have been effective in managing the positive symptoms of schizophrenia but are problematic in older adults and carry a high risk of disabling and persistent side effects, such as tardive dyskinesia (TD). The Abnormal Involuntary Movement Scale (AIMS) is useful for evaluating early symptoms of TD (Chapter 11). The second-generation, atypical antipsychotic medications (e.g., risperidone, olanzapine, quetiapine), given in low doses, are associated with a lower risk of extrapyramidal symptoms (EPS) and TD. Another adverse effect of antipsychotics is the potential for weight gain and diabetes. The use of weight-neutral medications is recommended, and dietary education, waist circumference, and weight should be routinely included in assessment of individuals with schizophrenia (Hjorthøj et al., 2017). Federal guidelines for the use of antipsychotic medications in nursing homes provide the indications for use of these medications in schizophrenia.

Other important interventions include a combination of support, education, physical activity, and CBT. A positive approach on the part of health care professionals, patients, and their families, combined with interventions to enhance quality of life, is important. Mushkin et al. (2018) interviewed 20 aging adults to develop an understanding of living with schizophrenia and the person's well-being. Participants reported that the decrease in positive symptoms like delusions and hallucinations enhances well-being. The participants viewed old age as a "window of opportunity" and a "chance to live a normal life" (p 980).

Families of older adults with schizophrenia experience the burden of caring for a family member with a chronic disability and dealing with their own personal aging. Community-based support services that include assistance with housing, medical care, recreation services, and services that help the family plan for the future of their relative are necessary. There are relatively few services in the community for older adults

with schizophrenia. The National Alliance on Mental Illness (NAMI) is an important resource for clients and their families (see Box 30.3).

PSYCHOTIC SYMPTOMS IN OLDER ADULTS

The onset of true psychiatric disorders is low among older adults, but psychotic manifestations may occur as a secondary syndrome in a variety of disorders, the most common being NCDs and Parkinson's disease (Chapters 25 and 26).

Paranoid Symptoms

New-onset paranoid symptoms are common among older adults and can present in a number of conditions in late life. Paranoid symptoms can signify an acute change in mental status as a result of a medical illness or delirium, or they can be caused by an underlying affective or primary psychotic mental disorder. Paranoia is also an early symptom of Alzheimer's disease, appearing approximately 20 months before diagnosis. About 30% to 40% of persons with NCDs experience paranoid or persecutory delusions (Wallace, 2019). Medications, vision and hearing loss, social isolation, alcoholism, depression, the presence of negative life events, financial strain, and PTSD also can be precipitating factors of paranoid symptoms.

Delusions

Delusions are fixed beliefs that guide one's interpretation of events and help make sense of disorder, even though they are inconsistent with reality. The delusions may be comforting or threatening, but they always form a structure for understanding situations that otherwise might seem unmanageable. A delusional disorder is one in which conceivable ideas, without foundation in fact, persist for more than 1 month. Common delusions of older adults are of being poisoned; of personal objects being stolen; of children taking their assets; of being held prisoner; or of being deceived by a spouse, partner, or lover. In older adults, delusions often incorporate significant persons as opposed to the global grandiose or persecutory delusions seen in younger individuals. It is always important to determine if what "appears" to be delusional ideation is in fact based in reality. Box 30.10 presents some clinical examples.

Hallucinations

Hallucinations are best described as sensory perceptions that occur in the absence of external stimuli and may be spurred by the internal stimulation of any of the five senses. Although not attributable to environmental stimuli, hallucinations may occur as a combined result of environmental factors. Hallucinations arising from psychotic disorders are less common among older adults, and those that are generated are thought to begin in situations in which one is feeling alone, abandoned, isolated, or alienated. To compensate for insecurity, a hallucinatory experience is stimulated, often an imaginary companion. Imagined companions may fill the immense void and provide some security, but they also may become accusatory and disturbing.

The character and stages of hallucinatory experiences in later life have not been adequately defined. Many hallucinations are

BOX 30.10 Clinical Examples of Delusions

Maggie's Story

Maggie persistently held on to the delusion that her son was a very important attorney and was coming to force the administration to discharge her from the nursing home. Her son, a factory worker, had been dead for 10 years. The events of her day, her hopes, and her status were all organized around this belief. It is clear that without her delusion she would have felt forlorn, lost, and abandoned.

Herman's Story

Herman was an 88-year-old man in a nursing home who insisted that he must go and visit his mother. His thoughts seemed clear in other respects (often the case with people who are delusional), and one of the authors (P. Ebersole) suspected that he had some unresolved conflicts about his dead mother or felt the need for comforting and caring. P.E. did not argue with Herman about his dead mother because arguing is never a useful approach to persons with delusions. Rather, she used the best techniques she could think of to assure Herman that she was interested in him as a person and recognized that he must feel very lonely sometimes. Herman continued to say that he must go and visit his mother. When P.E. could delay his leaving no longer, she walked with him to the nurses' station and found that his 104-year-old mother did indeed live in another wing of the institution and that he visited her every day.

BOX 30.11 Clinical Example: Is It a Hallucination?

One older woman in a nursing home who had Alzheimer's disease and was experiencing agnosia would look in the mirror and talk to "the nice lady I see in there." "Do you want to eat or go out for a walk with me?" she would ask. It was comforting to her, and therefore she did not need medication for her "hallucination," as some would have labeled her behavior. As is the case with many disease symptoms, frail elders do not typically manifest the cardinal signs we have been taught to associate with certain physical and mental disorders. Diagnostic criteria, and often evidence-based practice guidelines, have been developed as a result of observation and research with younger people and may not always fit the older person. Until knowledge and research on the unique aspects of aging increase, nurses and other health care professionals are urged to individualize their assessment and treatment of older people using available guidelines specific to older people.

in response to physical disorders, such as dementia, Parkinson's disease, sensory disorders, and medications. Older adults with hearing and vision deficits also may hear voices or see people and objects that are not actually present (illusions). Some have explained this as the brain's attempt to create stimulation in the absence of adequate sensory input. If the hallucinations are not disturbing to the person, they do not necessitate treatment (Box 30.11).

USING CLINICAL JUDGMENT TO PROMOTE HEALTHY AGING: PSYCHOTIC SYMPTOMS

Recognizing and Analyzing Cues

The assessment dilemma is often one of determining whether paranoia, delusions, and hallucinations are the result of medical illnesses, medications, dementia, psychoses, sensory deprivation, or overload. Depending on the precipitating factors, treatment will vary. Treatment must be based on a comprehensive assessment and on a determination of the nature of the psychotic behavior (primary or secondary psychosis) and the time of onset of first symptoms (early or late). Treating the underlying cause of a secondary psychosis caused by medical illnesses, dementia, substance abuse, or delirium is a priority.

Assessment of vision and hearing is also important because these impairments may predispose the older adult to paranoia or suspiciousness. Psychotic symptoms and/or paranoid ideation also present with depression, so depression screening also should be conducted. Assessment of suicide potential is also indicated because individuals experiencing paranoid symptoms are at significant risk for harm to self. It is never safe to conclude that someone is delusional or paranoid or experiencing hallucinations unless you have thoroughly investigated the person's claims, evaluated physical and cognitive status, and assessed the environment for contributing factors to the behaviors (see Box 30.10 and 30.11).

Solutions, Nursing Actions, and Outcomes

Frightening hallucinations or delusions, such as feeling that one is being poisoned, usually arise in response to anxiety-provoking situations and are best managed by reducing situational stress; being available to the person; providing a safe, nonjudgmental environment; and attending to the fears more than the content of the delusion or hallucination. Direct confrontation is likely to increase anxiety and agitation and the sense of vulnerability; it also may disrupt the relationship. A more useful approach is to establish a trusting relationship that is nondemanding and not too intense.

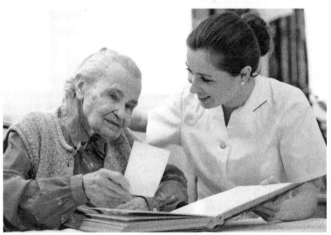

Demonstrating respect and a willingness to listen is the foundation for a caring nurse-patient relationship. (©iStock.com/AlexRaths.)

It is important to identify the individual's strengths and build on them. Demonstrating respect and a willingness to listen to concerns and fears are important. It is important that the nurse be trustworthy, give clear information, and present clear choices. Do not pretend to agree with paranoid beliefs or delusions, but rather ask what is troubling to the person and provide reassurance of safety. It is important to try to understand the person's level of distress, and how he or she is experiencing what is troubling. Other suggestions are to avoid television, which can be confusing, especially if the person awakens and finds it on or has a hearing or vision impairment. In addition, reduce clutter in the person's room and eliminate shadows that can appear threatening. Provide glasses and hearing aids to maximize sensory input and decrease misinterpretations.

If symptoms are interfering with function and interpersonal and environmental strategies are not effective, antipsychotic drugs may be used. The newer atypical antipsychotics (risperidone, olanzapine) are preferred but must be used judiciously, with careful attention to side effects and monitoring of response. None of the antipsychotic medications are approved for use in treatment of behavioral responses in individuals with NCDs. Atypical antipsychotic medications include a black box warning related to an increased risk of death when prescribed for older adults with dementia-related psychosis. See Chapter 26 for further discussion of behavior and psychological symptoms in dementia and nonpharmacological interventions.

BIPOLAR DISORDER (BD)

Bipolar I disorder involves periods of severe mood episodes from mania to depression. Bipolar II disorder is a milder form of mood elevation, involving milder episodes of hypomania that alternate with periods of severe depression. The length of the phases of depression and mania varies, lasting from days to weeks. BD is a lifelong disease that usually begins in adolescence, but 20% of adults with BD experience their first episode after 50 years of age. With the aging of the population, predictions are that there will be a drastic increase in the number of older adults with BD in the coming decades. BD often stabilizes in late life, and individuals tend to have longer periods of depression. Mania is a more frequent cause of hospitalization than depression, but depression may account for more disability. Similar to other psychiatric disorders in older adults, comorbidities often mask the presence of the disorder, and it is frequently misdiagnosed, underdiagnosed, and undertreated.

USING CLINICAL JUDGMENT TO PROMOTE HEALTHY AGING: BIPOLAR DISORDER

Recognizing and Analyzing Cues

Assessment includes a thorough physical examination and laboratory and radiological testing to exclude physical causes of the symptoms and identify comorbidities. A medication review should be conducted because symptoms can be a side effect of medications. Obtaining an accurate history from the individual and the family is important and should include assessment of symptoms associated with depression, mania, hypomania, and a family history of BD. Episodes of mania combined with depressed features and a family history of BD are highly indicative of the diagnosis (Box 30.12).

Solutions, Nursing Actions, and Outcomes
Pharmacotherapy

The pharmacological treatment of BD mostly consists of combinations of at least two drugs, including mood stabilizers (lithium

---

> **BOX 30.12   Focus on Genetics**
>
> Research on the genetic basis for mental health disorders such as depression, schizophrenia, and bipolar disorder is being conducted by the National Institute of Mental Health Center for Collaborative Genetic Studies on Mental Disorders (https://www.nimhgenetics.org/). The latest genome-wide study identified shared genetic risk factors between schizophrenia and bipolar disorder, bipolar disorder and depression, and schizophrenia and depression, the first evidence of overlap between these disorders. Continuous research on gene discovery for mental health disorders is ongoing.

and anticonvulsants), atypical antipsychotics, and antidepressants. Lithium, the most commonly used substance for individuals with BD, has neurological effects that make it difficult for older adults to tolerate. Lithium also has a long half-life (more than 36 hours), and dosing needs to be adjusted based on renal function. Medications that can affect urine production (diuretics) can alter lithium levels. Lithium levels, blood urea nitrogen (BUN) levels, and creatinine plasma levels need to be monitored closely.

Anticonvulsant medications such as valproic acid, divalproex sodium, and lamotrigine are more commonly used in BD treatment, although use of lamotrigine calls for monitoring for Stevens-Johnson syndrome. Medication levels and liver function tests must be monitored. Many of the anticonvulsant medications have an FDA warning that their use may increase suicide risk, so careful monitoring for changes in mood and behavior and signs of suicidal ideation is important.

Antidepressants such as fluoxetine, paroxetine, and venlafaxine can be used to treat depression in BD in combination with other medications. Because these medications can trigger mania, careful assessment is important. Atypical antipsychotic drugs are sometimes used, but with the same safety warnings discussed earlier, and are not to be used if NCDs are suspected. Olanzapine, aripiprazole, and quetiapine are all approved for the treatment of BD and may relieve symptoms of severe mania and psychosis (Chapter 11).

Psychosocial Approaches

Patient and family education and support are essential, and the family must understand that the individual is not able to control mania and irritating behaviors because of a chemical imbalance in the brain. Treatment with medication and intensive psychotherapy, CBT, interpersonal and rhythm therapy (improving relationships with others and managing regular daily routines), and family-focused therapy have been reported to be effective in improving recovery rates. Electroconvulsive therapy (ECT) may be useful if the individual's symptoms are severe, the risks of ECT are less than that of other treatments, the BD is refractory to an adequate trial with other treatment strategies, or when the patient prefers this treatment modality (Soreff & Xiong, 2019).

Medication regimens can be complicated, and many individuals struggle to remain adherent. An important nursing action is educating patients and families about the benefits and risks of prescribed medications, the importance of monitoring therapeutic effects, side effects, and the value of medication management systems. Individuals recognize that the drugs help and prevent hospitalizations, but they also resent that they need them. Addressing their feelings and finding ways to enhance their ability to continue with an effective regime is important (Soreff & Xiong, 2019).

Education is an important component of all psychosocial interventions, and nurses can assist patients in learning about BD and its treatment. Psychoeducation should include developing an acceptance of the disorder, becoming aware of factors influencing symptoms and signs of relapse, learning how to communicate with others, and establishing regular sleep and activity habits. Teaching patients to keep a log to monitor mood changes, activity levels, stressors, and amount of sleep is important. Collaborative care models involving the patient, the family, the support team, the health care provider, other professionals, and community resources are most effective. Developing and maintaining a therapeutic alliance with the individual and the family is most important in enhancing outcomes.

DEPRESSION

Depression is not a normal part of aging, and studies show that most older adults are satisfied with their lives. To understand depression, the nurse must understand the influence of late-life stressors and changes and the beliefs that older adults, society, and health professionals may have about depression and its treatment.

Prevalence

Depression is a significant public issue and remains underdiagnosed and undertreated in the older adult population. Some estimates of depression in older adults living in the community range from less than 1% to about 5% but rise to 13.5% in those who require home health care and to 11.5% in hospitalized individuals. Depression affects more than one-fifth of nursing home residents (Queiros et al., 2021). Depression is more common in individuals who have other illnesses or whose function becomes limited. Symptoms of depression can be triggered by other chronic conditions such as NCDs (Chapter 25), Parkinson's disease, heart disease, cancer, and arthritis, as well as other life events and stressors. One-third of widows and widowers meet the criteria for depression in the first month after the death of their spouse, and half of these individuals remain clinically depressed after 1 year (Centers for Disease Control and Prevention, 2021; Mental Health America, 2021) (Chapter 32). Depression is the leading cause of disability globally and a major factor in the burden of disease worldwide (World Health Organization, 2021). The prevalence of depressive disorders in older adults is expected to more than double by 2050 (Jeste et al., 2018).

Estimates are that 17% of older adults have symptoms of depression that do not meet the criteria for major depressive disorder (MDD); these symptoms are referred to as subsyndromal depression, dysthymic depression, and mild depression (Bruce & Sirey, 2018). The *DSM-5* uses the term *persistent* depressive disorder to describe symptoms that are long-standing (lasting 2 years or longer) but do not meet the criteria for MDD. Recognition and treatment are important because persistent depressive disorder has a negative impact on physical and social functioning

and quality of life for many older adults and is associated with an increased risk for a subsequent major depression. There is limited research about older adults with mild depressive disorders, but there is some evidence that preventive psychological interventions aimed at reducing symptoms and preventing the onset of a major depression may be of benefit (Cuijpers et al., 2019).

Prevalence rates of depression in older adults likely underestimate the extent of the problem. Only 38% of adults ages 65 and older believe that depression is a "health problem," and only 42% would seek help from a health professional (Mental Health America, 2021). Stigma associated with depression may be more prevalent among older adults and affect decisions to seek treatment. Perceived stigma may be less of a concern for the future older adult population due to increased awareness of mental health concerns and greater likelihood of seeking treatment. Many older adults, particularly those who have survived the Great Depression, both world wars, the Holocaust, and other tragedies, may see depression as shameful, evidence of a flawed character, self-centered, a spiritual weakness, and a sin or retribution.

Consequences

Depression is a common and serious medical condition second only to heart disease in causing disability and harm to an individual's health and quality of life. Depression and depressive symptomatology are associated with negative consequences such as delayed recovery from illness and surgery, excess use of health services, cognitive impairment, exacerbation of coexisting medical illnesses, malnutrition, decreased quality of life, substance abuse, and increased suicide and non-suicide-related deaths. It is highly likely that nurses will encounter a large number of older adults with depressive symptoms in all settings. Recognizing depression and enhancing access to appropriate mental health care are important nursing roles to improve outcomes for older adults.

Etiology

The causes of depression in older adults are complex and must be examined in a biopsychosocial framework. Factors of health, gender, developmental needs, socioeconomics, environment, personality, losses, and functional decline are all significant to the development of depression in late life. Biological causes, such as neurotransmitter imbalances, have a strong association with many depressive disorders in late life. This may be a factor in the high incidence of depression in individuals with neurological conditions such as stroke, Parkinson's disease, and NCDs.

Serious symptoms of depression occur in 30% to 50% of individuals with Alzheimer's disease, and depression is also a risk factor for dementia, particularly among individuals who are 45 to 64 years old. Prevention and delay of dementia can be expected through active intervention for midlife depression (Yu et al., 2020). Among individuals with Alzheimer's disease, depression is the earliest observable symptom in at least one-third of cases (Jeste et al., 2018). Depression in individuals with Alzheimer's disease may be due to an awareness of progressive decline, but research suggests that there also may be a biological connection between depression and Alzheimer's disease (Chapters 25 and 26). Medical disorders and medications also can result in depressive symptoms (Boxes 30.13 and 30.14.).

BOX 30.13 Medical Conditions and Depression

Cancers

Cardiovascular disorders

Endocrine disorders, such as thyroid problems and diabetes

Metabolic and nutritional disorders, such as vitamin B_{12} deficiency, malnutrition, and diabetes

Neurological disorders, such as Alzheimer's disease, stroke, and Parkinson's disease

Viral infections, such as herpes zoster and hepatitis

Vision and hearing impairment

BOX 30.14 Medications and Depression

Antihypertensives

Angiotensin-converting enzyme (ACE) inhibitors

Methyldopa

Reserpine

Guanethidine

Antiarrhythmics

Anticholesteremic drugs

Antibiotics

Analgesics

Corticosteroids

Digoxin

L-Dopa

BOX 30.15 Risk Factors for Depression in Older Adults

- Chronic medical illnesses, disability, functional decline
- Alzheimer's disease and other dementias
- Bereavement
- Caregiving
- Female (2:1 risk)
- Socioeconomic deprivation
- Family history of depression
- Previous episode of depression
- Admission to long-term care or other change in environment
- Medications
- Alcohol or substance abuse
- Living alone
- Widowhood

Other important factors influencing the development of depression are alcohol abuse, loss of a spouse or partner, loss of social supports, lower income level, caregiver stress (particularly caring for a person with dementia), and gender. Some common risk factors for depression are presented in Box 30.15.

USING CLINICAL JUDGMENT TO PROMOTE HEALTHY AGING: DEPRESSION

Recognizing and Analyzing Cues

Making the diagnosis of depression in older adults can be challenging, and symptoms of depression present differently in older adults. Primary care physicians accurately recognize less than one-half of

patients with depression (Mental Health America, 2021). Older adults who are depressed report more somatic complaints, such as insomnia, loss of appetite, weight loss, memory loss, and chronic pain. It is often difficult to distinguish somatic complaints from the physical symptoms associated with chronic illness. Both symptoms must be evaluated. Decreased energy and motivation, lack of ability to experience pleasure, increased dependency, poor grooming and difficulty completing activities of daily living (ADLs), withdrawal from people or activities enjoyed in the past, decreased sexual interest, and a preoccupation with death or "giving up" are also signs of depression in older adults. Feelings of guilt and worthlessness, seen in younger depressed individuals, are seen less frequently in older adults.

Individuals often present with complaints of memory problems and a cognitive impairment of recent onset that mimics dementia but subsides upon remission of depression (previously called pseudodementia). It is essential to differentiate between dementia and depression, and older adults with memory impairment should be evaluated for depression. Symptoms such as agitation, physically aggressive behavior, and repetitive verbalizations in persons with dementia may be indicators of depression (Chapter 26).

Comprehensive assessment involves a systematic and thorough evaluation using a depression screening instrument, interview, psychiatric and medical history, physical (with focused neurological exam), functional assessment, cognitive assessment, laboratory tests, medication review, determination of iatrogenic or medical causes, and family interview as indicated. Assessment for depressogenic medications, for alcohol and substance abuse, and for related comorbid physical conditions that may contribute to or complicate treatment of depression also must be included (Box 30.16). Screening of all older adults for depression should be incorporated into routine health assessments across the continuum of care. The Geriatric Depression Scale (GDS) was developed specifically for screening older adults and has been tested extensively in a number of settings. The Cornell Scale for Depression in Dementia (CSDD) is recommended for the assessment of depression in older adults with dementia (Chapter 9).

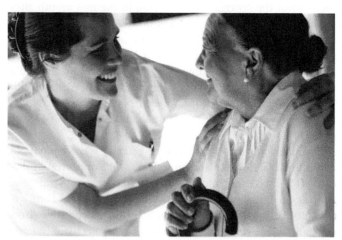

Creating hopeful environments in which meaningful activities and supportive relationships can be enjoyed is an important nursing role in the treatment of depression. (©iStock.com/Yuri.)

BOX 30.16   Tips for Best Practice

Assessment of Depression

- Use a depression screening tool (Geriatric Depression Scale or Cornell Scale for Depression in Dementia if cognitive impairment is present).
- Assess for suicide: ask a direct question—"Have you thought of killing or harming yourself?"
- Investigate somatic complaints and look for underlying acute or chronic stressful events.
- Investigate sleep patterns, changes in appetite or weight, socialization pattern, level of physical activity, and substance abuse (past and present).
- Ask direct questions about psychosocial factors that may influence depression: abuse, poor environmental conditions, and changes in the patient role after death or disability of a spouse or partner.
- Obtain psychiatric and medical histories.
- Perform a physical exam, including a focused neurological exam.
- Evaluate and treat chronic illnesses to improve outcomes and prevent exacerbations.
- Complete a functional assessment, paying close attention to changes in activities of daily living function.
- Perform a cognitive assessment; depressed patients may show little effort during examination, answer "I don't know," and have inconsistent memory loss and performance during exam.
- Conduct a medication review (assessment for medications that may cause depressive symptoms).
- Assess for psychotic symptoms (delusions, hallucinations) and symptoms of bipolar disorder.
- Perform laboratory tests as appropriate to rule out other causes of symptoms (e.g., thyroid-stimulating hormone [TSH], T_4, serum B_{12}, vitamin D, folate, complete blood count, urinalysis).
- Use family or significant others in obtaining key information to correlate patient's symptoms with others' observations; always assess and interview patient first.

Solutions, Nursing Actions, and Outcomes

The goals of depression treatment in older adults are to decrease symptoms, reduce relapse and recurrence, enhance function and quality of life, and reduce mortality and health care costs. Actions are individualized and are based on history, severity of symptoms, concomitant illnesses, and level of disability. There is a wide range of treatments for depression, and outcomes for older adults generally are similar to those observed for younger populations. However, this may not be true for older individuals who are frail or those with multiple medical comorbidities.

Health professionals often expect older adults to be depressed and may not take appropriate action to assess for and treat depression. The differing presentation of depression in older adults and the increased prevalence of medical problems that may cause depressive symptoms also contribute to inadequate recognition and treatment. Even if depression is identified, most older adults with significant depression do not receive guideline-consistent, if any, depression treatment (Bruce & Sirey, 2018). All health care professionals must receive adequate education about depression in older adults in order to provide safe, effective care. Older adults also may have limited knowledge about depression. Patient and family education about depression is an important nursing action since approximately 68% of older adults know little or almost nothing about depression, and 58%

believe that it is "normal" for people to get depressed as they grow older (Mental Health America, 2021).

Guidelines suggest that effective treatment for major depression is a combination of pharmacological therapy and psychotherapy or counseling with psychotherapy alone. The effects of psychotherapy are comparable with those of antidepressant medication in the short term and probably more effective in the longer term. Although psychotherapies are effective in the treatment of depression, the effects are still modest, as are those of antidepressant medication. Despite evidence-based guidelines calling for combined pharmacological and psychotherapeutic treatment, and the fact that older adults often prefer psychotherapy to psychiatric medications, psychological interventions often are not offered as an alternative. Reasons for this include time, reimbursement constraints, and a limited well-trained geriatric mental health workforce (Cuijpers et al., 2019).

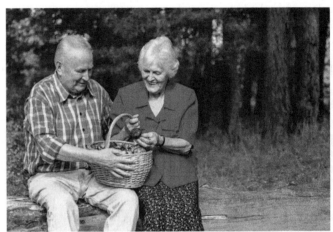

Older adults enjoying an activity together. (©iStock.com/Fred-Froese.)

Nonpharmacological Approaches

Types of nonpharmacological treatment that have been found to be helpful in depression include family and social support, education, grief management, exercise, humor, spirituality, CBT, brief psychodynamic therapy, interpersonal therapy, reminiscence and life review therapy (Chapter 7), problem-solving therapy, and complementary therapy such as tai chi (Chapter 19). Exercise also has been associated with a significant reduction in depressive symptoms (Seo & Chao, 2018). The development of effective, simplified, and accessible psychotherapeutic approaches, including internet-based programs, geared toward older adults is important. These types of programs have been shown to have comparable effects to conventional individual therapies. The quality of research on the effects of psychotherapeutic interventions is suboptimal, and further research is needed (Cuijpers et al., 2019).

There are few systematic studies testing the efficacy of behavioral interventions for mild depression in individuals with NCDs, but several interventions hold promise. Problem-adaptive therapy (PATH), a home-delivered intervention that also involves caregivers, has been found to reduce depressive symptoms. Reminiscence therapy (Chapter 7) has been reported to improve depressive symptoms in individuals with mild to moderate dementia. Another intervention, behavior therapy-positive events (BT-PE), teaches caregivers to increase the patient's engagement in pleasant activities and positive interactions (Bohlken et al., 2017; Cuijpers et al., 2019).

Integrated care. The majority of older adults prefer to be treated for depression by primary care providers rather than mental health specialists. New models of care providing both primary and behavioral care in the same setting are designed to promote collaboration between primary care providers and mental health specialists in planning and treating older adults. There is evidence that integrated care improves access, quality, and outcomes of depression treatment. The most effective models involve systematic depression screening, a depression care manager to work directly with the patients over time (often nurses), and the use of evidence-based depression treatment (Bruce & Sirey, 2018). Several collaborative interventions delivered in the home have also shown effectiveness in reducing depression symptoms, depression remission, and improved quality of life (Box 30.17).

Pharmacological Approaches

Antidepressants may effectively treat depression in older adults but have a high risk for adverse effects because of multiple medical comorbidities and drug-drug interactions from polypharmacy. Two-thirds of older adults who use antidepressants receive drugs that are either contraindicated or have the potential for moderate to major interactions (Kok & Reynolds, 2017). The most commonly prescribed antidepressants are the SSRIs. These agents work selectively on neurotransmitters in the brain to alleviate depression. The SSRIs are generally well tolerated in older adults, but anticholinergic and sedative effects may be associated with physical and cognitive impairment.

For those who do not respond to an adequate trial of SSRIs, there is another group of antidepressants that combines the inhibition of both serotonin and norepinephrine reuptake inhibitors (SNRIs) (e.g., venlafaxine [Effexor]). These also may be preferred by those who are engaged in or who anticipate sexual activity because they are less likely to have sexual side effects. One of the atypical antidepressants, such as bupropion (Wellbutrin) or trazodone, also may be used. Since the development of the SSRIs and SNRIs, the older monoamine oxidase (MAO) inhibitors and tricyclic antidepressants are no longer indicated due to their high side effect profile, including risk for falls.

All antidepressant medications must be closely monitored for side effects and therapeutic response. There are more than 20 antidepressants approved by the FDA for the treatment of depression in older adults, and several may have to be evaluated to determine the medication most effective for the individual. Similar to other medications for older adults, doses should be lower at first (50% of the target dose) and titrated as indicated until adequate treatment effect is ensured. If the patient has responded to treatment, it is not clear how long the medication should be continued, but if there is a lifetime history of depression, recommendations are that pharmacotherapy should be maintained for at least 2 years to prevent recurrence (Kok & Reynolds, 2017). (See Chapter 11 for in-depth information on pharmacological treatment for depression.)

Other Treatments

Electroconvulsive therapy (ECT) is the most effective treatment for older adults with major depression, with efficacy ranging from 60% to 80%. ECT is also indicated for patients at risk for severe harm because of psychotic depression, suicidal ideation, severe malnutrition, or a medical condition that worsens because they refuse medication (Kok & Reynolds, 2017). ECT results in a more immediate response in symptoms and is also a useful alternative for older adults who are frail with multiple comorbid conditions who are unable to tolerate antidepressant treatment. ECT is much improved, but older adults will need a careful explanation of the treatment because they may have many misconceptions about it.

Rapid transcranial magnetic stimulation (rTMS) is an FDA-approved treatment to treat major depressive disorder in adults for whom medication was not effective or tolerated. The treatment consists of administering brief magnetic pulses to the brain by passing high currents through an electromagnetic coil adjacent to the patient's scalp. The targeted magnetic pulses stimulate the circuits in the brain that are underactive in patients with depression, with the goal of restoring normal function and mood. For most patients, treatment is administered in 30- to 40-minute sessions over a period of 4 to 6 weeks. The effectiveness of the treatment is still being evaluated in older adults. TMS is contraindicated for persons who have seizures; stroke; brain injury, trauma, or surgery; pacemakers; or intracranial magnetic devices. Box 30.18 presents suggestions for families and professionals caring for older adults with depression.

BOX 30.17 Exemplar Program

PEARLS (Problem-Solving to Overcome Depression)

- Targets homebound older adults with chronic conditions to provide "house-calls" for depression, particularly in underserved communities.
- Incorporates program into existing community-based programs that deliver care and resources to clients.
- Designed to treat minor depression and persistent depressive disorder by teaching behavioral and problem-solving techniques and pleasant activities scheduling.
- Utilizes the Chronic Care and Collaborative Care Models.
- Uses a psychiatrist-led team with trained counselors to work one-on-one with participants in eight in-home sessions followed by a series of maintenance telephone session contacts.
- A supervising psychiatrist reviews cases regularly, addresses other causes of depression, and works with the individual's primary care provider to assess treatment effectiveness and need for more formal depression treatment including medications.
- Results show reduction in depression symptoms, lower rates of hospitalization, and improved function, emotional well-being, and quality of life.
- Program included in SAMSHA's National Registry of Evidence-Based Programs and Practices and Agency for Healthcare Research and Quality Innovation Exchange.

From Health Promotion Research Center: PEARLS (website), n.d. www.pearlsprogram.org. Accessed March 2019.

BOX 30.18 Tips for Best Practice

Family and Professional Support for Depression

- Provide relief from discomfort of physical illness.
- Enhance physical function (i.e., regular exercise and/or activity; physical, occupational, recreational therapies).
- Develop a daily activity schedule that includes pleasant activities.
- Increase opportunities for socialization and enhance social support.
- Provide opportunities for decision making and the exercise of control.
- Focus on spiritual renewal and rediscovery of meanings.
- Reactivate latent interests or develop new ones.
- Validate depressed feelings as aiding recovery; do not try to bolster the person's mood or deny the despair.
- Help the person become aware of the presence of depression, the nature of the symptoms, and the time limitation of depression.
- Emphasize depression as a medical, not mental, illness that must be treated like any other disorder.
- Provide easy-to-use educational materials to older adults and family members, such as those available through the National Institute of Mental Health (NIMH).
- Involve family in patient teaching, particularly younger family members who may have different life experiences related to depression and its treatment.
- Demonstrate faith in the person's strengths.
- Praise any and all efforts at recovery, no matter how small.
- Assist in expressing and dealing with anger.
- Do not stifle the grief process; grief cannot be hurried.
- Create a hopeful environment in which self-esteem is fostered and life is meaningful.

SUICIDE

Some of the highest suicide rates in the United States and globally are among older adults. Rates among older White men are higher than in any other demographic group, and older widowers are especially vulnerable (Chapter 32). Women in all countries have much lower suicide rates, possibly because of greater flexibility in coping skills based on multiple roles that women fill throughout their lives. Despite these alarming statistics, there is little research on suicide ideation and behavior among older adults. Butcher and Ingram (2018) raise the question of the effect of ageism and suicide. Older adults may internalize the negative stereotypes of aging, and health care professionals also can reflect ageism in practice (Chapter 7). "It is common for health care providers to view suicidal thinking as a normal reaction in older adults" (Butcher & Ingram, 2018, p 21). These statistics contribute to the concern about the increasing mental health problems in future generations of older adults and call for increased prevention efforts in this age group.

In most cases, depression and other mental health problems, including anxiety, contribute significantly to suicide risk. Common precipitants of suicide include physical or mental illness, death of a spouse or partner, substance abuse, chronic pain, limited social support, living alone, financial strain, and a history of suicide attempts. Adults over age 65 who have been diagnosed with an NCD are more than twice as likely to die from suicide compared to older adults who do not suffer from an NCD. The risk of suicide is particularly elevated among adults 65 to 74 years of age and in the first 90 days following a dementia diagnosis. Individuals with frontotemporal dementia are also at a higher risk of suicide death than those with other types of NCDs (Schmutte et al., 2021) (Chapters 25 and 26). One of the major differences in suicidal behavior in the old and the young is the lethality of method. Eight in 10 suicides for men older than age 65 were with firearms (Morgan & Rowhani-Rahbar, 2020) (Chapter 21).

Many older adults who die by suicide reached out for help before they took their lives. Three-fourths of older adults who commit suicide had seen their physician within 1 month before death, 40% had visited within 1 week of the suicide, and 20% had visited the physician on the day of the suicide (American Psychological Association, 2018). Depression is frequently missed, and older adults with suicide ideation or with other mental health concerns often present with somatic complaints. The statistics suggest that opportunities for assessment of suicidal risk are present but that the need for intervention is not seen as urgent or even recognized. Consequently, it is very important for providers in all settings to inquire about recent life events, implement depression screening for all older adults, evaluate for anxiety disorders, assess for suicidal thoughts and ideas based on depression assessment, and recognize warning signs and risk factors for suicide.

USING CLINICAL JUDGMENT TO PROMOTE HEALTHY AGING: SUICIDE

Recognizing and Analyzing Cues

Older adults with suicidal intent are encountered in many settings. It is our professional obligation to prevent, whenever possible, an impulsive destruction of life that may be a response to a crisis or a disintegrative reaction. The lethality potential of an older adult must always be assessed when elements of depression, disease, and spousal loss are evident. Any direct, indirect, or enigmatic references to the ending of life must be taken seriously and discussed. In the nursing home setting, the Minimum Data Set (MDS) (Chapter 9) includes screening for suicide risk and mandates that long-term care facilities have effective protocols for managing suicide risk. The Joint Commission recommends suicide risk screening in all settings.

All older adults should be screened for suicidal ideation at each primary care visit. "Suicide prevention cannot be limited to hospital, primary care, and clinic settings, but rather must reach into communities and culture" (Butcher & Ingram, 2018, p 29). Early detection is the first level of suicide prevention, and crisis intervention follows as a second level of prevention support for older adults at risk. If the older adult has personal, medical, or situational risk factors, screening should take place every 6 months or more frequently if indicated. Suicide screening should be conducted at the time of receiving a diagnosis of a NCD, particularly among older men living with chronic pain and mental health or substance abuse disorders. Safety counseling may be indicated with patients and caregivers, particularly safe storage or removal of firearms and certain medications (Schmutte et al., 2021). If there is suspicion that the older adult is suicidal, use direct and straightforward questions such as the following:

- Have you ever thought about killing yourself?
- How often have you had these thoughts?
- How would you kill yourself, if you decided to do it?

> ### ⚡ SAFETY TIPS
>
> Always ask direct questions of the patient and family about suicide risks and suicide ideation.

Assessment should include (1) identification of risk factors, medical problems, medications, functional status, nutritional status, personal and family psychiatric history, alcohol or substance drug use, and complete physical and neurological exam; (2) evaluation of cognitive function; (3) screening for depression; (4) psychological strengths, coping skills, spirituality, sexuality, suicidal ideation, past attempts at suicide; and (5) quantity and quality of social support, financial status, legal history, and potential for elder abuse (Butcher & Ingram, 2018). Assessing gun safety is important since gun access is a significant risk factor for suicide in older adults. Chapter 21 provides a protocol for gun safety assessment. The Columbia-Suicide Severity Rating Scale (C-SSRS) is an evidence-based suicide assessment tool used by many hospitals and organizations. Other resources can be found in Box 30.3.

The most important consideration for the nurse is to establish a trusting and respectful relationship with the person. Because many older adults have grown up in an era when suicide bore stigma and even criminal implications, they may not discuss their feelings in this area. It is also important to remember that among older adults, typical behavioral clues such as putting personal affairs in order, giving away possessions, and making wills and funeral plans are indications of maturity and good judgment in later life and cannot be construed as indicative of suicidal intent. Even statements such as "I won't be around long" or "I'm ready to die" may be only a realistic appraisal of the situation in old age.

Solutions, Nursing Actions, and Outcomes

It is important to have a suicide protocol in place that clearly defines how the nurse will intervene if a positive response is obtained from any of the direct questions about suicidal ideation. The person should never be left alone for any period until help arrives to assist and care for him or her. Patients at high risk should be hospitalized, especially if they have current psychological stressors and/or access to lethal means. Patients at lower risk may be treated as outpatients provided they have adequate social support and no access to lethal means. Other crisis interventions include partial hospitalization, day treatment, antidepressant medications, communicating risk to family, care management, counseling, support groups, assistance with financial stress, increased social involvement, and increased activity with faith community (Butcher & Ingram, 2018).

Suicide is a taboo topic for most of us, and there is a lingering fear that the introduction of the topic will be suggestive to the patient and may incite suicidal action. Precisely the opposite is true. By introducing the topic, we demonstrate interest in the individual and open the door to honest human interaction and connection on the deep levels of psychological need. It is the nature of our concern and our ability to connect with the alienation and desperation of the individual that will make a difference. Older adults who are isolated, depressed, and suicidal challenge the depth of nurses' ingenuity, patience, and self-knowledge.

SUBSTANCE USE DISORDERS

Substance abuse among older adults is one of the fastest growing health problems in the United States. The baby boomer generation has had more exposure to alcohol and illegal drugs in their youth and has a more lenient attitude about substance abuse. In addition, psychoactive drugs became more readily available for dealing with anxiety, pain, and stress. Although alcohol remains the most frequent reason for admission to substance abuse treatment, this proportion is declining. Cocaine- and heroin-related admissions are on the rise in older adults, and the incidence of opioid abuse and misuse is also increasing. Despite these increases, substance abuse in older adults remains an underrecognized and undertreated public health concern (Jeste et al., 2018). "Screening and prevention of unhealthy substance abuse is critical to address the potential enormous public health impact of increasing substance use by older adults" (Han & Moore, 2018, p. 117). The *Healthy People 2030* box presented earlier in the chapter includes objectives related to substance abuse.

Alcohol Use Disorder

Prevalence and Characteristics

Alcohol remains the most commonly used substance among older adults, and its use is expected to increase considerably. The most severe alcohol abuse is seen in people ages 60 to 80 years, but not in those older than 80 years. Two-thirds of older adults with alcohol abuse are early-onset drinkers (alcohol use began at 30 or 40 years of age), and one-third are late-onset drinkers (use began after 60 years of age). Late-onset drinking may be related to situational events such as illness, retirement, or death of a spouse and includes a higher number of women. Alcohol-related problems in older adults often go unrecognized, although the residual effects of alcohol abuse complicate the presentation and treatment of many chronic disorders.

Gender Issues

Although men (particularly older widowers) are four times more likely to abuse alcohol than women, the prevalence in women may be underestimated. The number and impact of older female drinkers are expected to increase over the next 20 years as the disparity between men's and women's drinking decreases. Women of all ages are significantly more vulnerable to the effects of alcohol misuse, including faster progression to dependence and earlier onset of adverse consequences. Even low-risk drinking levels (no more than one standard drink per day) can be hazardous for older women. Older women also experience unique barriers to detection of and treatment for alcohol problems.

Physiology

Older adults, especially females, develop higher blood alcohol levels because of age-related changes (increased body fat, decreased lean body mass, and total body water content) that alter absorption and distribution of alcohol. Decreases in hepatic metabolism and kidney function also slow alcohol metabolism and elimination. A decrease in the gastric enzyme alcohol dehydrogenase results in slower metabolism of alcohol and higher blood levels for a longer time. Risk of gastrointestinal ulceration and bleeding related to alcohol use may be higher in older adults because of the decrease in gastric acidity that occurs in aging.

Consequences

The health consequences of long-term alcohol use disorder include cirrhosis of the liver, cancer, immune system disorders, cardiomyopathy, cerebral atrophy, dementia, and suicide. Other effects of alcohol in older adults include urinary incontinence, which results from rapid bladder filling and diminished neuromuscular control of the bladder; gait disturbances from alcohol-induced cerebellar degeneration and peripheral neuropathy; depression; functional decline; increased risk for falls and other injuries; and sleep disturbances and insomnia. Alcohol misuse also has been implicated as a major factor in morbidity and mortality as a result of trauma, including falls, drownings, fires, motor vehicle crashes, homicide, and suicide. Alcohol use also exacerbates conditions such as osteoporosis, diabetes, hypertension, and ulcers. Many drugs that older adults use for chronic illnesses cause adverse effects when combined with alcohol (Box 30.19). All older adults should be given precise instructions regarding the interaction of alcohol with their medications.

Alcohol Guidelines for Older Adults

The possible health benefits of alcohol in moderation have been reported in the literature (reduced risk of coronary artery disease, ischemic stroke, Alzheimer's disease, and vascular dementia). As a result, older adults may not perceive alcohol use as potentially harmful. Because of the increased risk of adverse effects from alcohol use, the National Institute of Alcohol Abuse and Alcoholism defines "at-risk drinking" for men and women ages 65 years and older as more than one drink per day (Box 30.20). Health professionals must share information

---

BOX 30.19 Medications Interacting With Alcohol

Analgesics
Antibiotics
Antidepressants
Antipsychotics
Benzodiazepines
H2-receptor antagonists
Nonsteroidal antiinflammatory drugs (NSAIDs)
Herbal medications (echinacea, valerian)
Acetaminophen taken on a regular basis, when combined with alcohol, may lead to liver failure
Alcohol diminishes the effects of oral hypoglycemics, anticoagulants, and anticonvulsants

---

BOX 30.20 National Institute on Alcohol Abuse and Alcoholism Guidelines for Alcohol Use in Older Adults

Definition of a Standard Drink

- One 12-ounce can or bottle of regular beer, ale, or wine cooler
- One 8- or 9-ounce can or bottle of malt liquor
- One 5-ounce glass of red or white wine
- One 1.5-ounce shot glass of distilled spirit (gin, rum, tequila, vodka, whiskey, etc.); label on bottle will say 80 proof or less

From National Institute on Alcohol Abuse and Alcoholism: What is a standard drink? (website), n.d. https://www.niaaa.nih.gov/what-standard-drink.

---

with older adults about safe drinking limits and the deleterious effects of alcohol intake.

USING CLINICAL JUDGMENT TO PROMOTE HEALTHY AGING: ALCOHOL USE DISORDER

Recognizing and Analyzing Cues

Alcohol and other substance use-related problems among older adults are too frequently undetected by health care professionals. The challenges associated with recognizing and analyzing cues of alcohol use problems include poor symptom recognition, lack of provider training, inadequate knowledge of screening instruments, lack of time, skepticism about benefits, fear of patient reactions, and the belief that patients will not be candid about substance use (DiBartolo & Jarosinski, 2017). Alcohol-related problems may be overlooked in older adults because these problems do not drastically disrupt their lives or are not clearly linked to physical disorders. Health care providers also may be pessimistic about the ability of older adults to change long-standing problems.

The US Preventive Services Task Force (2018) recommends that adults 18 years and older in primary care should be screened by clinicians for alcohol misuse. Screening should be a part of health visits for people older than the age of 60 years in primary, acute, and long-term care settings. Although alcohol is the drug most often used among older adults, assessment should include all substances used (recreational drugs, prescription, nicotine, opioids, and OTC medications).

The Hartford Institute of Geriatric Nursing recommends that the Short Michigan Alcoholism Screening Test – Geriatric Version be used with older adults because it is more age appropriate than other instruments (Table 30.1). A single question also can be used for alcohol screening: "How many times in the past year have you had 5 or more drinks in a day (if a man), or 4 or more drinks (if you are a woman older than 65 years of age)?" If the individual acknowledges drinking that much, follow-up assessment is indicated.

Depression is often comorbid with alcohol abuse, and both alcohol and depression screenings should be offered routinely at health fairs and other sites where older adults may seek health information. A medication review should be conducted, and screening should be done both before prescribing any new medications that may interact with alcohol and as needed after

TABLE 30.1	Short Michigan Alcoholism Screening Test—Geriatric Version (S-MAST-G)[a]	Yes (1)	No (0)
1.	When talking with others, do you ever underestimate how much you drink?		
2.	After a few drinks, have you sometimes not eaten, or been able to skip a meal, because you didn't feel hungry?		
3.	Does having a few drinks help decrease your shakiness or tremors?		
4.	Does alcohol sometimes make it hard for you to remember parts of the day or night?		
5.	Do you usually take a drink to relax or calm your nerves?		
6.	Do you drink to take your mind off your problems?		
7.	Have you ever increased your drinking after experiencing a loss in your life?		
8.	Has a doctor or nurse ever said they were worried or concerned about your drinking?		
9.	Have you ever made rules to manage your drinking?		
10.	When you feel lonely, does having a drink help?		
TOTAL S-MAST-G SCORE* (1–10)			

[a]Scoring: 2 or more "Yes" responses indicate an alcohol problem.
From the Regents of the University of Michigan: *Short Michigan alcohol screening test—geriatric version (S-MAST-G)*, Ann Arbor, MI, 1991, University of Michigan Alcohol Research Center.

life-changing events. Alcohol abuse should be suspected in an older adult who presents with a history of falling, unexplained bruises, or medical problems associated with alcohol abuse problems.

Alcoholism is a disease of denial and not easy to diagnose, particularly in older adults with psychosocial and functional decline from other conditions that may mask decline caused by alcohol. Early signs such as weight loss, irritability, insomnia, and falls may not be recognized as indicators of possible alcohol problems and may be attributed to "just getting older." Box 30.21 presents signs and symptoms that may indicate the presence of alcohol problems in older adults.

Alcohol users often reject or deny the diagnosis, or they may take offense at the suggestion of an alcohol problem. Feelings of shame or disgrace may make older adults reluctant to disclose a drinking problem. Families of older adults with substance use disorders, particularly their adult children, may be ashamed of the problem and choose not to address it. Health care providers may feel helpless over alcoholism or uncomfortable with direct questioning or may approach the person in a judgmental manner. A caring and supportive approach that provides a safe and open atmosphere is the foundation for the therapeutic relationship. It is always important to search for the pain beneath the behavior.

Solutions, Nursing Actions, and Outcomes

Alcohol problems affect physical, mental, spiritual, and emotional health. Actions must address quality of life in all these spheres and be adapted to meet the unique needs of the older adult. Abstinence from alcohol is seen as the desired goal, but a focus on education, alcohol reduction, and reducing harm is also appropriate. Increasing the awareness of older adults about

BOX 30.21 Recognizing and Analyzing Cues to Potential Alcohol Problems in Older Adults

Anxiety
Irritability (feeling worried or "crabby")
Blackouts
Dizziness
Indigestion; heartburn
Sadness or depression
Chronic pain
Excessive mood swings
New problems making decisions
Lack of interest in usual activities
Social isolation
Out of touch with family or friends
Falls
Bruises, burns, or other injuries
Family conflict, abuse
Headaches
Incontinence
Memory loss
Poor hygiene
Poor nutrition
Insomnia
Unusual response to medications
Frequent physical complaints and physician visits
Financial problems

the risks and benefits of alcohol consumption in the context of their own situation is an important goal. Treatment and intervention strategies include cognitive behavioral approaches, individual and group counseling, medical and psychiatric approaches, referral to Alcoholics Anonymous, family therapy, case management and community and home care services, and formalized substance abuse treatment. Treatment outcomes for older adults have been shown to be equal to or better than those for younger people. Providing education about alcohol use to older adults and their families and referring to community resources are important nursing roles and essential to best practices.

Long-term self-help treatment programs for older adults show high rates of success, especially when social outlets are emphasized and cohort supports are available. A significant concern is the lack of programs designed specifically for older adults, particularly older women, whose concerns are very different from those of a younger population who abuse drugs or alcohol. Health status, availability of transportation, and mobility impairments may further limit access to treatment. Development of treatment sites in senior centers and ALFs and telemedicine programs would increase accessibility. Additional resources are presented in Box 30.3.

When there is significant physical dependence, withdrawal from alcohol can become a life-threatening emergency. Detoxification should be done in an inpatient setting because of the potential medical complications and because withdrawal symptoms in older adults can be prolonged. Older adults who drink are at risk of experiencing acute alcohol withdrawal if admitted to the hospital for treatment of acute illnesses or emergencies. All patients admitted to acute care settings should be screened for alcohol use and assessed for signs and symptoms of alcohol-related problems. Older adults with a long history of consuming excess alcohol, previous episodes of acute withdrawal, and/or a history of prior detoxification are at increased risk of acute alcohol withdrawal.

OTHER SUBSTANCE USE CONCERNS

Cannabis Use

The same physiological changes with aging that increase the effect of alcohol in older adults also increase the effect of other drugs including benzodiazepines, opioids, and cannabis. With changes in attitudes toward cannabis, its legalization for recreational use in several states, and its increasing use for medicinal purposes, there has been a sharp increase in cannabis use among older adults. Chronic pain and mental health management are two common uses of medical marijuana (MMJ). The most common medical reasons reported for MMJ use are anxiety, insomnia, chronic pain, and depression (Azcarate et al., 2020). Health care providers need to be aware that their older patients may be using cannabis.

A majority of older adults use cannabis medically or recreationally without problems, but there has been limited research of its effects on older adults. Dr. Lenny Chiang-Hanisko, nurse researcher at Florida Atlantic University, is conducting research on the use of cannabis by older adults with chronic pain (see the Research Highlights box). It is important to better understand both the benefits and the risks of cannabis use so that health care professionals can educate and advise patients. Co-use of alcohol and the interaction of cannabis with other drugs

---

RESEARCH HIGHLIGHTS

Effectiveness of Medical Marijuana in Older Adults With Chronic Pain

Purpose

The purpose of this study was to investigate how older adults in Florida can safely and effectively use medical marijuana (MMJ) and to identify what age-appropriate, evidence-based education is required. Approximately 178 million (41%) adults in the United States ages 18 and older suffer from at least one painful health condition. In Florida there are 327,492 MMJ card holders, and chronic nonmalignant pain was the number-one diagnosis for which patients are registered. Symptom management in older adults, including chronic pain management, can be challenging. MMJ is often recommended in the treatment of these conditions. MMJ use among older adults is rapidly growing more than in other age groups.

Method

Data were collected using online survey tools for those ages 60 and older who had an active MMJ prescription and chronic pain residing in South Florida. Sixty participants ranged from ages 60 to 90 years (mean = 69.83) and completed the questionnaires, with most participants identifying as non-Hispanic Whites, most being retired, and 72% being female.

Results

The analysis revealed the occurrence of several common side effects of MMJ use. The largest side effect reported was an increased appetite (24.1%), followed by change in mood (20.4%), lack of concentration (13%), lethargy (11.1%), and dizziness (9.3%). Eighty-five percent (n = 51) of participants reported receiving MMJ education prior to filling their prescriptions, and 43% reported that the education was less than 20 minutes. MMJ was considered effective in reduction of overall chronic pain on a visual analog scale ranging from 0 to 100, with a decrease of pain from 71.38 prior to MMJ use to 35.13 after use. This result was statistically significant [t(42) = 11.68, $P < .001$] and indicated a potentially large effect, with Cohen's d = 1.82.

Conclusion

MMJ should be considered carefully for each patient with frequent monitoring for efficacy and adverse events. There is a critical need to access the current training and advising on patients' ability to use MMJ safely and effectively.

Data from Chiang Hanisko L et al.: *Effectiveness of medical marijuana in older adults with chronic pain,* Cannabis Clinical Outcomes Research Conference (CCORC), Consortium for Medical Marijuana Clinical Research, virtual conference, April 8–9, 2021.

and prescription medications needs further study (Choi et al., 2019; Han & Palamore, 2020; Wallace, 2019).

OPIOID DRUG USE

Opioid use in older adults has become an increasingly concerning issue, but the majority of media coverage and research has centered on younger individuals due to their higher prevalence of use. Chronic pain is one of the most common reasons for opioid prescriptions, and more than 50% of older adults report pain. Long-term opioid prescriptions (≥90 days) have dramatically increased over the past decade, though the effectiveness of this therapy for chronic pain has yet to be established. Among long-term opioid users, 25% were adults ages 65 and older. Older women experience pain more frequently than do younger individuals, and men and older women have a higher prevalence of long-term opioid use.

Opioid-related negative outcomes such as addiction, misuse, and overdose deaths also have risen in older adults. High-prescription opioid quantity or dosage use can lead to adverse outcomes among older adults, including opioid addiction and health consequences such as respiratory complications, drug interaction-related problems, increased risk for falls, and drug overdose (Khan et al., 2020). The physiological changes of aging complicate opioid therapy in older adults, and the response to opioids is less predictable than in younger individuals. Older adults who use psychotropic drugs (anxiolytic, sedative, or hypnotic agents and antidepressants) are at greater risk for prescription opioid use and high dosage use. Taking anxiolytic, sedative, or hypnotic agents is significantly associated with chronic use of opioids. The use of benzodiazepine and opioids together significantly increases opioid-related adverse outcomes in older adults.

For decades, it was commonly accepted that older adults were at lower risk for addiction to opioids than younger patients. This may be because opioid use disorder is underreported, underdetected, and undertreated in older individuals. However, there is growing evidence indicating that older adults are uniquely vulnerable to risk of abuse. Although rates of abuse and misuse in older adults remain lower than for younger adults, it is a significant issue that requires further research. In addition, the stigma commonly associated with substance use disorders in the United States may make health care providers less likely to screen older adults or refer them for addiction treatment (Agency for Healthcare Research and Quality, 2020; Gazelka et al., 2020; Oh et al., 2019). Chapter 29 discusses pain in older adults in depth.

Prescription Drug Misuse

A more common concern seen among older adults is the misuse and abuse of prescription psychoactive medications. Dependence on sedative, hypnotic, or anxiolytic drugs, often prescribed for anxiety or insomnia and taken for many years with resulting dependence, is especially problematic for older women, who are more likely than men to receive prescriptions for these drugs. There have been dramatic increases in emergency department visits involving prescription misuse by adults 50 years of age and older, with pain relievers and medications for insomnia and anxiety most often involved (Han & Moore, 2018).

Some of the reasons for the abuse of psychoactive prescription medications may be inappropriate prescribing and ineffective monitoring of response and follow-up. In many instances, older adults are given prescriptions for benzodiazepines or sedatives because of complaints of insomnia or nervousness, without adequate assessment for depression, anxiety, or other conditions that may be causing the symptoms. Older adults may not be informed of the side effects of these medications, including interactions with alcohol, dependence, and withdrawal symptoms. More importantly, conditions such as anxiety and depression may not be recognized and treated appropriately. STAMP Out Prescription Drug Misuse and Abuse Toolkit is an excellent resource for health care professionals to use in education about prescription drug misuse and abuse in older adults (see Box 30.3).

KEY CONCEPTS

- The prevalence of mental health disorders is expected to increase significantly with the aging of the baby boomers.
- Older adults present with different cues of mental health problems. Somatic complaints are often the presenting symptoms of mental health disorders, making diagnosis difficult. Recognizing and analyzing cues and identification and evaluation of nursing actions to promote mental health is essential.
- The incidence of psychotic disorders with late-life onset is low among older adults, but psychotic manifestations can occur as secondary symptoms in a variety of disorders, the most common being Alzheimer's disease. Psychotic symptoms in Alzheimer's disease necessitate different assessment and treatment than do long-standing psychotic disorders.
- Anxiety disorders are common in later life, and reestablishing feelings of adequacy and control is the heart of crisis resolution and stress management.
- Depression remains underdiagnosed and undertreated in the older adult population and is considered a significant public health issue. Depression in older adults can be effectively treated. Unfortunately, it is often neglected or assumed to be a condition of aging that one must "learn to live with." Screening and identification of depression is an important nursing action.
- Suicide is a significant problem among older men, particularly widowers. Many individuals considering suicide are seen by a health care professional with physical complaints shortly before they commit suicide. Identification of depression and suicidal intent is important in health care visits across the continuum.
- Substance abuse, particularly alcohol, and misuse of psychoactive prescription drugs are often underrecognized and undertreated problems in older adults, particularly older women. Screening and appropriate identification of concerns are important in all settings.
- Treatment outcomes for substance abuse in older adults are equal to or better than those for younger people.

NEXT-GENERATION NCLEX® (NGN) EXAMINATION–STYLE QUESTIONS

The nurse on a behavioral health unit is admitting a patient who was brought to the emergency department earlier today by her partner after ingesting 15 acetaminophen tablets. The partner reports that although the patient has made no prior suicide attempts, she does often say, "I just wish I wasn't here anymore" and "Life just isn't worth living." The partner goes on to state that he and the patient have been together for more than 2 years, and a year after they became involved, the patient lost her adult child in a car accident. Since that time, the patient has difficulty driving in a car to go places, has missed an excessive amount of work, and has challenges participating in pleasurable activities such as seeing friends or going out for dinner. The partner says, "I tried to get her to go to see a therapist, but the closest one is about 45 minutes from our house, and she doesn't want to be in a car for that long." The patient says, "I don't know how to get past this. I feel like one of the biggest parts of my life is now missing and I'll never be able to feel happiness again." A SSRI was prescribed for the patient.

Which actions from the list below will the nurse include in the plan of care, once the client has been diagnosed by the health care provider with anxiety and depression? (Select all that apply.)

A. Provide assistance with ADLs

B. Administer haloperidol three times daily

C. Ask the patient why she would try to take her own life

D. Establish a caring relationship and encourage expression of feelings and provide support.

E. Explain that normal grieving doesn't last longer than 6 months

F. Share information about telehealth options for outpatient therapy

G. Allow the patient to stay in bed all day if she doesn't wish to get up

H. Discuss the use of selective serotonin reuptake inhibitors for anxiety and depression

NURSING STUDY

Bipolar Disorder

Myra is a 71-year-old White woman who was admitted to the geropsychiatry inpatient unit for alcohol abuse and noncompliance with her lithium, which had been prescribed for a diagnosed bipolar disorder. Myra's primary mode of coping with her depression and mood swings has been to drink alcohol, meet abusive men, and play bingo. However, when she stops taking her dose of lithium, she begins to have flight of ideas, argues with her daughters, and tries to pick up men in her apartment complex. After seeing her at home, you discover that she has a long history of being physically abused by her husband, now deceased for 8 years, and has been living with a daughter, who also has emotionally and physically abused her, causing Myra to be hospitalized. Myra's ability to test reality is compromised because of years of denial and low self-esteem. She says, "I used to have lots of times when I felt really good in between the depressions. Now I feel depressed most of the time." She tells you that her daughters harass her and interfere in her life. Your goals as a community-based nurse are to facilitate her independence (being able to live in her own apartment), to assist her with medication compliance, and to intervene with Myra to improve the relationships with her daughters. Home visits are approved through Medicare for 1 month after hospital discharge.

NURSING STUDY

Depressive Disorder With Suicidal Thoughts

Jake had cared for his wife, Emma, during a long and painful illness until she died 4 years ago. He found that alcohol provided a way to cope with his stress. Within a year after her death, Jake met a lady to whom he was very attracted, and a few months later she moved in with him. Jake managed to move his things around until some space was made for her personal items, but neither of them was very comfortable with this. He really did not like to move his things from their usual place and, because her allotted space was so small, she felt like an intruder. He collected guns, and she shuddered when she saw them. He was an avid fan of John Wayne movies, and she preferred going to the symphony. He liked meat and potatoes, and she was a vegetarian. She also disapproved of his increasing reliance on alcohol. The blending of two such different lifestyles proved difficult. In a few months she moved out, and Jake blamed himself. He said over and over, "I should have done more for her. I'm not good for anything anymore." His friends began to pull away from him, just when he needed them most, because he seemed to talk of nothing but his various aches, pains, and pills and his general discouragement with life.

Jake's consumption of alcohol increased markedly.

Jake had some health problems: a mild heart failure, a lack of exercise, dairy products gave him diarrhea, he was somewhat obese, and his knees were painful most of the time. He routinely visited his allergist, his internist, his orthopedist, and his cardiologist. However, it seemed that the more he went to these specialists, the worse he felt. He was taking several medications, and each time he saw one of his clinicians, he came away with another prescription. No one asked about his drinking, and he never mentioned it. He awoke one morning feeling very dizzy, so he went to his internist later that day. He began to share the litany of his discomforts, and the physician reminded him that at 76 years of age he could not expect to always feel in top shape.

When he returned from seeing the physician, Jake called his daughter and surprised her by saying that he had decided he would take a week off and go to Hawaii to see if the sun and sand would revive him. Jake was not usually impulsive. His daughter, fortunately, was a psychiatric nurse and was concerned about the change in his behavior.

CLINICAL JUDGMENT QUESTIONS AND ACTIVITIES

Questions refer to the Nursing Study: Bipolar Disorder.

1. How will you evaluate Myra's ability to live independently?
2. What particular strategies are necessary to meet the goals of the nursing care plan?
3. Given that Myra's primary coping strategy is drinking alcohol, how will you facilitate her sobriety and help her deal with stress?

4. How much involvement with Myra's daughters do you believe is necessary to assist with her transition back to her own apartment?
5. Given the limited number of visits covered by Medicare, what information does Myra need to provide self-care? In other words, the nurse must be teaching Myra how to live independently after discharge from home health care. What does Myra need to know?

CLINICAL JUDGMENT QUESTIONS AND ACTIVITIES

Questions 1 to 5 refer to the Nursing Study: Depressive Disorder With Suicidal Thoughts.

1. Given the situation in this case, discuss what your thoughts would be if you were Jake's daughter.
2. Given his daughter's background, what are her responsibilities in this case?
3. What action should be taken for Jake's protection?
4. Would you expect that Jake is still grieving over the death of his wife? What are your thoughts about this situation?
5. What are your thoughts about Jake's use of alcohol?
6. Discuss the variations in symptoms of depression in older adults and younger adults.
7. Describe some of the reasons that may make older adults vulnerable to depression.
8. Describe a time when you were depressed and the feelings you had. What did you do about it?
9. What is the responsibility of a student nurse in the case of suspected suicidal thoughts?

10. What are the cues or indications that an older adult is thinking of committing suicide?
11. What are some signs of suicidal intent in young adults? How are these signs different from those in older adults?
12. Do you think suicide is a sign of weakness or strength?
13. Do you agree or disagree with the following statements based on the evidence about depression and suicide in older adults?
    - Normally, older adults feel depressed much of the time.
    - Older adults are more likely than young people to admit to depression.
    - Most older adults talk about suicide but rarely try to kill themselves.
    - Depression in the older adult is helped by medications.
    - Depression may be the cause of forgetfulness.
    - Depression in the older adult is often linked with illness and alcoholism.

RESEARCH QUESTIONS

1. What is the prevalence of mental health disorders in community-dwelling older adults? What mental health care are nurses able to provide in the home?
2. How common is alcohol abuse as a strategy of self-care used by the older adult with emotional concerns?
3. What types of interventions are most appropriate for older adults with alcohol or drug abuse problems?
4. Is psychiatric home care a more cost-effective alternative than institutional care?
5. What are the cardinal symptoms of depression in the oldest-old?

6. How many primary care providers consider or evaluate for the presence of depression in older adults who see them for physical complaints?
7. What are the most reliable tools for identifying depression in cognitively intact and cognitively impaired older adults?
8. What is the meaning of depression in older adults of different races, cultures, and ethnicities?
9. What modifications need to be made in assessment and treatment of mental health disorders to enhance cultural appropriateness?

REFERENCES

Agency for Healthcare Research and Quality: *Prevention, diagnosis, and management of opiods, opiod misuse, and opiod use disorder in older adults* (website), 2020. https://effectivehealthcare.ahrq. gov/products/opioids-older-adults/report. Accessed June 2021.

American Geriatrics Society: 2015 Beers Criteria Update Expert Panel: American Geriatrics Society 2015 updated Beers Criteria for potentially inappropriate medication use in older adults, *J Am Geriatr Soc* 63(11):2227–2246, 2015.

American Psychiatric Association Diagnostic and statistical manual of mental disorders, ed 5, Arlington, VA, 2013, American Psychiatric Publishing.

American Psychological Association: *Growing mental and behavioral concerns facing older adults* (website), 2018. http://www.apa.org/ advocacy/health/older-americans.aspx. Accessed May 2021.

American Psychological Association: *Disparities in mental health status and mental health care* (website), 2020. https://www.apa. org/advocacy/health-disparities/health-care-reform. Accessed July 2021.

Azcarate P, Zhang A, Keyhani S, et al: Medical reasons for marijuana use, forms of use, and patient perception of physician attitudes among the U.S. population, *J Gen Intern Med* 35(7):1979–1986, 2020. doi:10.10007/SL11606-020-05800-7.

Balsamo M, Cataldi F, Carlucci L, et al: Assessment of anxiety in older adults: a review of self-report measures, *Clin Interv Aging* 13:573–593, 2018.

Bohlken J, Weber SA, Siebert A, et al: Reminiscence therapy for depression in dementia, *GeroPsych* 30(4):145–151, 2017.

Bruce ML & Sirey JA: Integrated care for depression in older primary care patients, *Can J Psychiatry* 63(7):439–446, 2018.

Butcher H & Ingram T: Evidence-based practice guideline: secondary prevention of late-life suicide, *J Gerontol Nurs* 44(11):20–32, 2018.

Canuto A, Weber K, Baertschi M, et al: Anxiety in old age: psychiatric comorbidities, quality of life, and prevalence according to age, gender, and country, *Am J Geriatr Psychiatry* 26(2):174–185, 2018.

Center for Medicare Advocacy: *Medical coverage of mental health and substance abuse services* (website), 2020. https://www.medicareadvocacy.org/medicare-info/medicare-coverage-of-mental-health-services/.

Centers for Disease Control and Prevention: *Depression is not a normal part of growing older* (website), 2021. https://www.cdc.gov/aging/mentalhealth/depression.htm.

Choi NG, DiNitto D, Arndt S: Potential harms of marijuana use among older adults, *Public Policy Aging Rep* 29(3):88–94, 2019.

Christianson S & Marren J: *Impact of Event Scale-Revised (IES-R)*, New York, 2013, Hartford Institute for Geriatric Nursing.

Cook J & Simiola V: Trauma and PTSD in older adults: prevalence, course, concomitants and clinical considerations, *Curr Opin Psychol* 14:1–4, 2017.

Creighton AS, Davison TE, Kissane DW: The prevalence, reporting, and treatment of anxiety among older adults in nursing homes and other residential aged care facilities, *J Affect Disord* 227:416–423, 2018.

Cuijpers P, Quero S, Downick C, et al: Psychological treatment of depression in primary care: recent developments, *Curr Psychiatry Rep*, 2019 21(129).

Department of Veterans Affairs: *PTSD treatment basics* (website), 2019. https://www.ptsd.va.gov/understand_tx/tx_basics.asp.

DiBartolo MC & Jarosinski JM: Alcohol use disorder in older adults: challenges in assessment and treatment, *Issues Ment Health Nurs* 38(1):25–32, 2017.

Fung AWT, Lee JSW, Lee ATC, Lam LCW: Anxiety symptoms predicted decline in episodic memory in cognitively healthy older adults: a 3-year prospective study, *Int J Geriatr Psychiatry* 33(5):748–754, 2018.

Galoustian G: *FAU now serves as home to, C-PAWW,* (website), 2018. https://www.fau.edu/newsdesk/articles/c-paww-nursing.php#:~:text=Florida%20Atlantic%20University's%20Christine,effects%20of%20animal%2Dassisted%20interventions. Accessed May 2021.

Gazelka H, Leal J, Lapid M, et al: Opiods in older adults: indications, prescribing, complications, and alternative therapies for primary care, *Mayo Clin Proc* 95(4):793–800, 2020.

Gradus JL: *Epidemiology of PTSD* (website), 2017 https://www.ptsd.va.gov/professional/treat/essentials/epidemiology.asp.

Hall KS, Morey MC, Beckham JC, et al: The Warrior Wellness study: a randomized controlled exercise trial for older veterans with PTSD, *Transl J Am Coll Sports Med* 3(6):43–51, 2018.

Han B, Palamore J: Trends in cannabis use among older adults in the United States, 2015–2018, *JAMA International Medicine*, 2020 https://doi.org/10.1001/jamainternmed.2019.7517. Published online February 24, 2020.

Han BH & Moore AA: Prevention and screening of unhealthy substance use by older adults, *Clin Geriatr Med* 34(1):117–129, 2018.

Hildon Z, Montgomery S, Blane D, et al: Examining resilience of quality of life in the face of health-related and psychosocial adversity at older ages: what is "right" about the way we age? *Gerontologist* 50:36–47, 2009.

Hjorthøj C, Stürup AE, McGrath JJ, et al: Life expectancy and years of potential life lost in schizophrenia: a systematic review and meta-analysis, *Lancet Psychiat* 4(4):295–301, 2017.

Hoy-Ellis CP, Ator M, Kerr C, et al: Innovative approaches address aging and mental health needs in LGBTQ communities, *Generations* 40(2):56–62, 2016.

Jeste DV, Peschin S, Buckwalter K, et al: Promoting wellness in older adults with mental illnesses and substance use disorders: call to action to all stakeholders, *Am J Geriatr Psychiatry* 26(6):617–630, 2018.

Khan S, Heller D, Latty L, et al: Association between psychotropic drug use and prescription opiod use among older adults, *Geriatr Nurs* 41(6):776–781, 2020.

Kleinman A: *Patient and healers in the context of culture: an exploration of the borderland between anthropology, medicine, and psychiatry,* Berkeley, CA, 1980, University of California Press.

Kok RM & Reynolds CF III: Management of depression in older adults: a review, *JAMA* 317(20):2114–2122, 2017.

Krause-Parello C: Human-animal connections and nursing science: what is the relationship? *Nurs Sci Quarterly* 31(3):239–242, 2018.

Kruse CS, Krowski N, Rodriguez B, et al: Telehealth and patient satisfaction: a systematic review and narrative analysis, *BMJ Open*, 2017 7(8):e016242.

Markota M, Rummans TA, Bostwick JM, et al: Benzodiazepine use in older adults: dangers, management, and alternative therapies, *Mayo Clin Proc* 91(11):1632–1639, 2016.

Maust DT, Kales HC, Wiechers IR, et al: No end in sight: benzodiazepine use among older adults in the United States, *J Am Geriatr Soc* 64(12):2546–2553, 2016.

Mental Health America: *Depression in older adults: more facts* (website), 2021. https://www.mhanational.org/depression-older-adults-more-facts. Accessed May 2021.

Morgan E & Rowhani-Rahbar A: Firearm safety in an aging United States, *JAMA Netw Open*, 2020 3(7):3201182.

Mushkin P, Band-Winterstein T, Avieli H: "Like every normal person?!" The paradoxical effect of aging with schizophrenia, *Qual Health Res* 28(6):977–986, 2018.

National Institute of Mental Health: *Post-traumatic stress disorder* (website), 2019. https://www.nimh.nih.gov/health/topics/post-traumatic-stress-disorder-ptsd/index.shtml. Accessed May 2021.

Nievergelt C, Maihofer A, Klengel T, et al: International meta-analysis of PTSD genome-wide association studies identifies sex- and ancestry-specific genetic risk loci, *Nat Commun* 19(1):4558, 2019.

Oh G, Abner E, Fardo D, et al: Patterns and predictors of chronic opioid use in older adults: a retrospective study, *PLos ONE*, 2019 14(1):e0210341.

Queiros M, von Gunten A, Martins M, et al: The forgotten psychopathology of depressed long-term care facility residents: a call for evidence-based practice, *Dement Geriatr Cogn Disord Extra* 1(38):38–44, 2021.

Ray M: *Transcultural caring dynamics in nursing and health care,* Philadelphia, 2016, FA Davis.

Robins LM, Hill KD, Finch CF, Clemson L, Haines T: The association between physical activity and social isolation in community dwelling older adults, *Aging Ment Health* 22(2):175–182, 2018.

Rose V: Supporting resident mental health: a comprehensive approach, *Ann Long-Term Care* 29(1):7–10, 2021.

SAMHSA-HRSA Center for Integrated Health Solutions: *Behavioral health in primary care* (website), 2018. https://www.integration.samhsa.gov/integrated-care-models/behavioral-health-in-primary-care.

Schmutte T, Olfson Donovan M, Maust Ming X, et al: Suicide risk in first year after dementia diagnosis in older adults, *Alzheimers Dement*, 2021. https://doi.org/10.1002/alz.12390.

Seo JY & Chao YY: Effects of exercise interventions on depressive symptoms among community-dwelling older adults in the United States: a systematic review, *J Gerontol Nurs* 44(3):31–38, 2018.

Soreff S & Xiong G: *Bipolar disorder treatment & management* (website), 2019. https://emedicine.medscape.com/article/286342-treatment. Accessed May 2021.

Stroup R, Olfson M, Huang C: Age-specific prevalence and incidence of dementia diagnoses among older US adults with schizophrenia, *JAMA Psychiatry* 78(6):632–641, 2021 doi:10/1001/jamapsychiatry.2021.0042.

Temkin-Greener H, Campbell L, Cai X, et al: Are post-acute patients with behavioral health disorders admitted to lower-quality nursing homes? *Am J Geriatr Psychiatry* 26(6):643–654, 2018.

Tucker P & Czapla C: Post-COVID stress disorder: another emerging consequence of the global pandemic, *Psychiatric Times*, 38(1), 2021 https://www.psychiatrictimes.com/view/post-covid-stress-disorder-emerging-consequence-global-pandemic. Accessed May 2021.

US Preventive Services Task Force, *Unhealthy alcohol use in adolescents and adults: screening and behavioral counseling interventions* (website), 2018. https://www.uspreventiveservicestaskforce.org/Page/Document/UpdateSummaryDraft/unhealthy-alcohol-use-in-adolescents-and-adults-screening-and-behavioral-counseling-interventions. Accessed February 2020.

Valtorta NK, Moore DC, Barron L, et al: Older adults' social relationships and health care utilization: a systematic review, *Am J Public Health* 108(4):e1–e10, 2018.

Wallace R: The 2017 cannabis report of the National Academy of Medicine: a summary of findings and directions for research addressing cannabis use among older people, *Public Policy Aging Rep* 29(3):85–87, 2019.

Wehbe-Alamah H: Madeleine Leininger's theory of culture care diversity and universality. In Smith MC & Parker ME, editors: *Nursing theories and nursing practice*, 4, Philadelphia, 2015, FA Davis, pp 303–319.

World Health Organization: *Mental health of older adults* (website), 2021. https://www.who.int/news-room/fact-sheets/detail/mental-health-of-older-adults. Accessed May 2021.

Yu JT, Xu W, Tan C, et al: Evidence-based prevention of Alzheimer's disease: systematic review and meta-analysis of 243 observational prospective studies and 153 randomised controlled trials, *J Neurol Neurosug Psychiatry* 91(11):1201–1209, 2020.

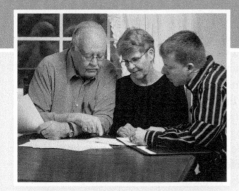

CHAPTER 31

Ethics, Decision Making, and Mistreatment

Kathleen Jett

http://evolve.elsevier.com/Touhy/TwdHlthAging

A STUDENT SPEAKS

When I was asked to go on a home visit to Mr. Jones it was obvious that he did not take care of himself. His clothes were dirty, and he smelled like urine. But he had no significant health problems and seemed undisturbed by the situation. I really did not know what to think or do.

Steffen, age 19

AN OLDER ADULT SPEAKS

I have had a feeding tube in my stomach for a long time due to cancer in my throat. I had been in the hospital recently and even though I disagreed, the social worker was concerned that I could not take care of myself at home. They sent a nurse out to check on me and, sure enough, just as she drove up I was pouring beer into my tube. I was so glad she didn't say anything about that, just asked how I was doing!

Henry, age 68

LEARNING OBJECTIVES

On completion of this chapter, the reader will be able to:

1. Differentiate the mechanisms for the protection of those who have limited decision-making capacity and discuss the advantages and disadvantages of each.
2. Identify the nurse's responsibility for the protection of those with limited capacity.
3. Differentiate between abuse and neglect.
4. Define undue influence and describe how it might be identified.
5. Recognize cultural differences in the perception and response to abuse.
6. Recognize the ethical conflicts between beneficence and autonomy in self-neglect.
7. Define the nurse's role in the prevention of mistreatment of older adults.

In the day-to-day practice of caring for older adults, gerontological nurses are asked to assist with decision making and can recognize and respond to cues to potential mistreatment and neglect. In the first section of this chapter, the ethical principles directly associated with informed decision making and older adults are discussed. This is particularly important due to the large number of those who have, or will be, asked to make decisions when their capacity to do so is limited. Several mechanisms to protect persons who lack capacity in some way are available, and these are reviewed. Finally, mistreatment of vulnerable older adults (referred to as elder mistreatment or elder abuse and neglect)

is examined relative to the nurse's role. Although gerontological nurses (unless also attorneys) cannot provide any legal advice, it is imperative that they are able to recognize several ethical and legal issues frequently encountered in their work.

ETHICS, HEALTH CARE, AND AGING

The core ethical principles in health care applicable to gerontological nursing are autonomy, beneficence, and nonmaleficence (Table 31.1). In working with older adults, nurses encounter many instances of conflict between these three principles. How

TABLE 31.1	**Ethical Principles in Nursing Practice**
Principle	**Meaning**
Autonomy	Independent decision-making capacity
Beneficence	Actions to benefit others
Nonmaleficence	No intentional harms, avoid or minimize risk of harm

can we protect those who decline health benefits or are in danger (as we perceive it) from others or themselves while respecting their choice? When someone makes a decision that, as a nurse, you do not agree is in their best interest, does that suggest the person lacks the ability to make the decision? If a decision puts the person in potential harm, what is the nurse's responsibility?

DECISION MAKING

The ethical principle of autonomy supports the concept of *self-determination* and is operationalized through *informed consent* and the *right to refuse treatment.* Consent is central to health care decision making and is expected to be an expression of the person's life goals, values, and preferences. Documented consent is required for many invasive procedures and surgeries. Consent to participate in research is a more detailed and extensive process because a treatment received may not provide benefit to the participant and the risks may not be known. Research with the very frail and those with changing levels of capacity (for any reason) has been difficult and has limited the advancement of science in some areas due to the overriding need to protect the participant consistent with the principle of nonmaleficence.

Informed consent and refusal in health care are only possible with the assumption that adults have decision-making *capacity* or, in its absence, that someone else has the legal responsibility (authority) to make decisions for them. Decisional capacity means that a person can understand a problem at hand, the risks and benefits of the decision, the consequences of the decision, and the alternative options; can decide; and is able to communicate the decision to others in some way. It is expected that the decision is consistent over time unless the circumstances surrounding it have changed. For example, a person who had consistently declined treatment for acute pain may make a different

decision if the pain becomes persistent (Chapter 29). The nurse often verifies that the information was understood and that the consent was voluntary (Box 31.1) (RegisteredNursing.org, 2021).

Until the 1980s, medical decision making in Western medicine was based on the ethical principle of paternalism. That is, patients were expected to put blind trust in physicians to make decisions that they thought were best for their patients. In 1990 the landmark case of Nancy Cruzan went to the US Supreme Court. The court determined that Ms. Cruzan had previously been clear in her desire to forgo life-extending measures if they would only serve to delay her natural death. No distinction was made between withholding and withdrawing treatment. Later, case law characterized tube feeding and intravenous feeding as medical treatments (also referred to as *artificial sustenance*), and therefore these also could be refused.

Autonomous decision making is now expected, and the Patient Self-Determination Act (PSDA), enacted in 1991, requires that patients in health care facilities are guaranteed the right to make their own decisions to accept or forgo treatment, and that these decisions are to be respected in most circumstances. This includes the right to appoint another as their decision maker. It is not uncommon to hear an older adult say, "Ask my daughter, she knows what I want." This is considered an autonomous designation of another as an extension of themselves. It is a common practice in collective cultures to delegate health care decisions to others (e.g., son, tribal elder) who will determine who is to receive health information, including that related to prognosis (Chapter 4).

Lack of capacity is *not* a question of preference or a question of the person's values or choices, but whether the person can understand the situation, options, and consequences at the level necessary for making the needed decision (Box 31.2). Capacity to consent is situational. Deciding which foods to accept is very different from deciding to undergo a surgical procedure or begin a regimen of chemotherapy or dialysis. Consent is implied in most common nursing actions, such as when the person accepts a medication that is offered or cooperates with a dressing change.

One may have full capacity for one decision but no or limited capacity for another; the greater the risk inherent in the decision, the higher the level of capacity is needed. In day-to-day gerontological practice with frail older adults, it is important to make impartial

---

BOX 31.1   **Questioning Informed Consent**
Mr. Brown is an 84-year-old African American man who was hospitalized for complications of advanced diabetes. He was scheduled for a bilateral orchiectomy the next morning. The geriatric clinical nurse specialist found him to be pleasant and in good spirits. He was also profoundly hard of hearing and had limited reading skills and poor visual acuity. A copy of his surgical consent was at the bedside with an "X" on the signature line. Mr. Brown's glasses were on his bedside table, and his hearing aids were reportedly at home. After Mr. Brown was given a stethoscope to wear, the clinical nurse specialist spoke into the bell and asked him if he had any questions about the procedure to which he had consented. He replied that it was "just something he needed for his sugar." Through the "listening device," she explained the procedure that was planned. He became noticeably upset and immediately withdrew his consent until he could find out more about his alternatives and prognosis.

BOX 31.2   **Surprising Capacity**
Ms. Henna, 85 years old, was receiving rehabilitation in a long-term care facility for a fractured hip when she unexpectedly had a stroke. She appeared to be unconscious and was receiving intravenous fluids that were triggering heart failure. Because she had not expressed her wishes in advance and had no living spokesperson, the health care staff determined that an option was to surgically insert a percutaneous endoscopic gastrostomy (PEG) feeding tube into her stomach, even though it would significantly increase her risk for pneumonia. As it may have been medically futile, it was not required. Even though Ms. Henna had not communicated in any way since the stroke, I went to her room and informed her of the problem, alternatives, and so on, and that it may be in her best interest to stop the intravenous fluids and not insert the tube. She had no response. However, as I was leaving the room, she opened her eyes and very clearly said, "Wait, if I don't have the tube, I could not eat, and I would die. I do not want to die." The tube was inserted, she never spoke again, and several months later she died from pneumonia.

BOX 31.3   Factors Affecting Nurses' Ability to Be Impartial

Skill in participatory decision making
Ability to foster a trusting relationship
Structural discrimination
   Ageism
   Racism and classism
   Sexism
   Sick-role expectations
Cultural awareness
Self-awareness
Time demands

BOX 31.4   Behavioral Triggers for Evaluation of Decision-Making Capacity

Inability to voice a decision
Blanket acceptance or refusal of care
Absence of questions about situation/treatment offered
Inconsistent reasons for accepting or refusing care
Sudden decline in functional status
Agitation, depression, or withdrawal
Hallucinations
Intoxication

From Libby C, Wojahn A, Nicolini JR, et al: *Competency and capacity* (website), 2020. https://www.ncbi.nlm.nih.gov/books/NBK532862/.

judgments regarding capacity (Box 31.3). The ability to do this may be one of the most critical skills in gerontological nursing (Box 31.4).

When capacity is questioned, it is necessary to protect the person from harm by determining who can make the best decision for them. Several mechanisms are available to increase the chance that a person's previously autonomous voice, wishes, and values are respected while needs are met and personal rights are protected. It is expected that the least restrictive mechanism is used whenever possible. The mechanisms include powers of attorney and guardianship or conservatorship and require advance care planning both within and beyond terminal conditions. It is important that nurses understand the meaning and implications of each mechanism while realizing that there are differences from state to state.

Advance Care Planning

It is not uncommon for people to prepare a "last will and testament" and appoint a person to be an executor of their estate after their death. It is less common to legally appoint a proxy or surrogate to represent their wishes by acting and speaking on their behalf if there is ever a time when they cannot do so themselves—for whatever reason.

Gerontological nurses have the responsibility to encourage their patients, neighbors, and family members to conduct advance health care planning by discussing their wishes with their significant others. It is acceptable to encourage older adults to go beyond the conversations and appoint a legal representative. At best this will include their wishes should they become incapacitated at any time, including at the end of life. This serves

as a means of "extending" some level of autonomy as health circumstances change.

Power of Attorney

A power of attorney (POA) is a person (agent) who has been legally appointed to act on behalf of another. This may be limited to a specific transaction (e.g., real estate) or asking the person to assume full responsibility for decision making regarding assets (e.g., bill paying, investments). The person named as a general POA most often represents the person in matters of business and is no longer in effect if the person becomes incapacitated. A durable POA continues after persons can no longer speak for themselves but may or may not include decision making related to health care, depending on the state where the POA was executed. As soon as the person regains abilities, the POA is no longer in effect unless requested. An important aspect of the appointment of a POA is that the person given decision-making rights is someone who has been chosen by the individual rather than appointed by a court. Designation of an agent is the least restrictive mechanism of decision-making assistance, and the individual retains all rights and responsibilities afforded by law.

Durable Power of Attorney for Health Care

The agent appointed as a durable power of attorney for health care (DPOAHC) is referred to as a *health care surrogate* or *proxy* and is responsible for making health care decisions for persons at their specific request or if they are unable to do so for themselves, and only then. Whether the surrogate can make end-of-life decisions is determined by state statutes. A *living will* is an instructive advance directive that documents a person's wishes specific to a terminal illness (discussed later). Most include the appointment of a proxy decision maker specific to the circumstances and, again, are only in effect for those who choose not to or cannot speak for themselves.

Health care proxies or surrogates are expected to use *"substituted judgment"* in making decisions based on what they believe the person would decide if able to do so and not necessarily their own choice in a similar situation (Box 31.5). As the gerontological nurse works with people who are making decisions about the selection of a surrogate, such as a POA, the nurse can encourage the person to do so with utmost care and only after in-depth discussions of wishes and values. The individual appointed as a DPOAHC, surrogate, or proxy should be willing to uphold the

BOX 31.5   Substituted Judgment

Mr. and Mrs. Jones had been married for 60 years. She had developed Alzheimer's disease a number of years earlier and reached a point where she did not always know what to do with food in her mouth. She no longer recognized her husband and was nonverbal. In almost daily distress, her husband intermittently pleaded that a "feeding tube" be placed into her so that she could "eat." However, Mrs. Jones, a registered nurse, had made it very clear to her husband and to all who knew her that she "never wanted artificial nutrition" or anything done to stop a natural death when she worsened. When Mr. Jones asked for a feeding tube, the only thing we could say was that we were very sorry, but her wishes were very clear and that is what we were bound to follow. He agreed that those indeed were her wishes and started to cry.

person's wishes or hold similar values. It is possible that a spouse may not be the best person for this task. Ongoing discussion of wishes as circumstances change over time is ideal.

Most state statutes provide a "hierarchy" of those who have the legal authority to act as an agent when preferences have not been documented and the ability to make decisions is lost, either temporarily or permanently (Reuben et al., 2020). The decision-making responsibilities begin with those at the top of the list, believed to be most likely to know the person's wishes, and proceeds down the list until a willing surrogate is found (Box 31.6).

Guardians or Conservators

Guardians or conservators are individuals, agencies, or corporations that have been legally appointed to take care, custody, and control of an incapacitated person and ensure that the person's needs are met and handled responsibly. Such appointments can be made only at court hearings in which someone demonstrates that the older adult is incapacitated in some way. In some states it is not required that the older adult be present at the hearing. If the judge agrees that this level of protection is needed, the person is declared incapacitated. Like surrogates and proxies, guardians and conservators are expected to use substituted judgment in all decision making.

In some states limits are set in the appointment of guardianship according to the degree of protection needed. Total dependency means that the person lacks all decision-making capacity and cannot meet even basic needs in any self-sustaining way. Partial dependency means that the person may be able to manage certain challenges of life, but health or cognitive abilities interfere with more complex decision making. In the latter situation, a guardian is appointed to protect the person in very specific ways.

Conservatorships and guardianships can be expensive, and dependence requiring this level of protection may deplete the person's assets, leaving little to pay for any care that may be needed. There have been many reports of exploitation and situations of "undue influence" (discussed later). The use of these mechanisms is the most restrictive, and in most cases the person loses all rights to self-determination; they should be considered only in cases of severe impairment, when decision making is needed. Nurses working with older adults and their families can encourage the use of advance care planning as an alternative that is less restrictive, noting that the definitions and rules vary from state to state. If someone is seeking to establish a guardianship

over the objection of the patient, the patient may need to hire an attorney skilled in this type of litigation.

Barriers to Completing Advance Directives

Sociodemographics, health status, literacy, experiences, cultural values, and spirituality all serve in some way as barriers to completing advance directives (Box 31.7). Those who are disadvantaged, including economically, with low health literacy levels or reduced knowledge of ACP, complete the fewest number of advance directives (Hoe and Enguidanos, 2019; Koss and Baker, 2016).

Those coming from a collectivist culture are significantly less likely to complete ACP. Instead, such decisions are left to the decision makers in the family. Those with strong beliefs in God or a higher power were much more likely to have their religious beliefs guide their end-of-life decisions than have completed ACP of any kind (Hong et al., 2018). Interpreters, used to assist the health care professional with explanations to their non-English-speaking patients, may not facilitate a clear translation of an advance directive because of cultural beliefs surrounding death or anticipation of poor health; for example, many in the Haitian culture believe that speaking of death is taboo and may cause it to occur more quickly (Coolen, 2012). See Box 31.8 for resources.

Living Wills

Since the passage of the PSDA in 1991 in the United States, any agency that is reimbursed by Medicare for services is required to provide all adult patients with information about their rights to make their own health care decisions, accept or refuse treatment, and complete an advance directive of some kind, especially living wills. In the outpatient setting, providers (e.g., physicians, nurse practitioners, physician assistants) are encouraged but not obligated to provide this information.

The PSDA recognized a living will as an advance directive that is specifically related to situations where those facing a terminal illness are unable to speak for themselves. It is a morally and, in some jurisdictions, legally binding document in which adults can express their wishes regarding end-of-life decisions for some future time when they will be unable to do so for themselves. Living wills may be as limited as decisions regarding the use of resuscitation or as detailed as decisions about dialysis, antibiotics, tube feedings, and so on. The living will includes the appointment of a proxy to uphold patients' wishes when they are no longer able to do so. Because the proxy is selected by the individual, the legal assumption is that the designated person has more authority than the next of kin (if that person is not the proxy).

A living will can be revoked only by the individual, either physically (by tearing it up), verbally, or in writing, preferably in front of witnesses. The creator of the advance directive may amend it at any time; formal language is not necessary, and one can add items in writing or cross out unwanted passages. If the person becomes incompetent, revocation is no longer possible, and the last statement of wishes stands. Nurses should know the details of living will requirements in their state, country, or other jurisdiction in which they practice. Nurses also should be familiar with the living will form or forms available in the organization at which they are employed. The exact format and signature requirements (e.g., notary) vary from state to state. See Box 31.9 for resources.

MISTREATMENT OF OLDER ADULTS

Vulnerable older persons can be harmed, or be at risk for harm, by the actions, inactions, or behaviors of others. Although states and jurisdictions define "vulnerable elder" differently, it always includes persons with dementia. Mistreatment of vulnerable older adults it is a violation of human rights and is synonymous with "elder" abuse, undue influence, exploitation, and neglect. The abuse may be physical, psychological, medical, or sexual (Box 31.10). Neglect is an act of omission or the *failure* of action by a recognized caregiver. Some abusers use their role or power over another to exploit the person in such a way that autonomy and independent decision making are relinquished. Psychological abuse can lead to undue influence and to sexual and financial abuse and exploitation. Mistreatment is classified as either intentional or unintentional. For example, a caregiver may intentionally disregard the needs of the care recipient or may lack knowledge regarding those needs or the importance of them and the mistreatment is unintentional. Should harm

---

BOX 31.10 Types of Mistreatment of Older Adults

Physical abuse: The use of physical force that results in the threat of or the infliction of bodily injury, physical pain, or impairment. It includes but is not limited to acts of violence such as striking (with or without an object), pushing, shaking, pinching, and burning. It includes the use of physical restraints, force-feeding, and physical punishment.

Sexual abuse: Nonconsensual sexual contact of any kind, including with those persons unable to give consent. It includes unwanted touching of any kind and sexual assault or battery—such as rape, sodomy, coerced nudity, and forced sexually explicit photographing. May be the result of undue influence.

Psychological abuse: The infliction of anguish, pain, or distress through verbal or nonverbal acts, including intimidation or enforced social isolation. This includes verbal assaults, insults, threats, intimidation, humiliation, belittling, and harassment. It can include forced social isolation from family, friends, or usual activities. It also includes withholding full rights to persons due specifically to their age, gender, race, ethnicity, religion, or sexual orientation (discrimination).

Medical abuse: Subjecting a person to unwanted medical treatments or procedures. Examples of this include venipuncture or the insertion of a urinary catheter (also sexual abuse) in those with dementia who refuse the procedure. It includes the use of chemical restraints (e.g., sedatives) for convenience of care rather than for protection of the person (medical neglect: failure to provide needed medical care).

Exploitation: The illegal or improper use of another's funds, property, or assets. May be the result of undue influence, such as convincing the person to sign checks or other documents, including deeds to property or wills, with the threat of withholding care or affection.

Neglect: Passive or active failure of a recognized caregiver to provide goods and services, such as food, medication, medical treatment, or personal care.

Abandonment: The desertion of a person by an individual who had assumed the responsibility of providing care or assistance.

---

occur, the abuser (or institution) can be sued for the older adult's injuries. If the abuse escalates to a criminal act or if the abuse includes theft of property or money, the abuser is subject to criminal prosecution.

Abuse and neglect in institutional settings include being physically restrained, being deprived of privacy and dignity (e.g., left in soiled clothing, personal tasks performed in the presence of others), or loss of choice in personal activities. Resident-to-resident elder mistreatment (inappropriate, disruptive, or hostile behavior among nursing home residents) is a sizable and growing problem as well. Among nursing home residents, reports are that 19.8% have experienced resident-to-resident mistreatment. Specific types of mistreatments include cursing, screaming, or yelling at another person; physical incidents such as hitting, kicking, or biting; and sexual assault. These incidents are likely to cause emotional and/or physical harm and are stressful to staff. Further research is needed to develop prevention and management interventions. All residents have the right to be protected from abuse and mistreatment, and the facility is required to ensure the safety of all residents and investigate reports of abuse. Medical abuse in this setting includes intentionally providing insufficient care (e.g., as a form of punishment), over- or undermedicating, and withholding medication (e.g., for pain) (World Health Organization [WHO], 2021).

TABLE 31.2 Prevalence of Known Cases of Elder Mistreatment, 2017

| Type of Abuse | Reported by Older Adults in the Community | INSTITUTIONAL | |
		Reported by Older Adults or Their Proxies	Reported by Staff
Psychological	11.6%	33.4%	32.5%
Physical	2.6%	13.1%	9.3%
Financial	6.8%	13.8%	Not enough data
Sexual	0.9%	1.9%	0.7%
Neglect	4.2%	11.6%	12.0%

Data from Yon Y, Mikton CR, Gassoumis ZD, et al: Elder abuse prevalence in community settings: a systematic review and meta-analysis, *Lancet Glob Health* 5(2):e147–e156, 2017; Yon Y, Ramiro-Gonzalez M, Mikton C, et al: The prevalence of elder abuse in institutional settings: a systematic review and meta-analysis, *Eur J Public Health* 29(1):58–67, 2018.

Elder mistreatment is a universal problem and occurs in all educational, racial, cultural, religious, and socioeconomic groups; in any family configuration; in every setting; and in all parts of the world. It is one of the most unrecognized and underreported social problems today. It is estimated that about 5 million older adults are abused each year in the United States (National Council on Aging [NCOA], 2021). There is emerging evidence of a significant increase in elder mistreatment that has occurred during the COVID-19 pandemic; in the United States, abuse of older adults in the community may have increased by up to 84% (Chang & Levy, 2021).

Using data from primarily high-income countries, the WHO estimates that 1 in 6 persons at least 60 years of age living in the community are abused each year. The rates in long-term care facilities are much higher, with 2 in 3 staff members admitting to having abused a resident in their care (Table 31.2) (WHO, 2021). It is thought that the number of older adults mistreated is underestimated and will increase as the population of older adults grows (Chapter 2).

Mistreatment can occur in any relationship in which there is or has been an expectation of trust. The abuser may be a caregiver but also may be any person who has contact with a vulnerable older adult. A salesperson may financially exploit an older adult through an organized scam, or a longtime formal caregiver may abuse or isolate the care receiver. Most abuse occurs in the home setting; almost 60% of abuse is perpetrated by a family member (NCOA, 2021). This may reflect a lifelong pattern that intensifies as caregiving needs develop or increase. The risk factors for one to become an abuser or to be abused are often interconnected (Box 31.11).

Unfortunately, many barriers remain in the identification of those who are mistreated. This is further complicated by varying familial, societal, and cultural perspectives on how abuse is defined and how best to respond to it (Box 31.12). Most important is the belief that what occurs inside one's home is "private" and a "family matter." Shame and embarrassment may make it

BOX 31.11 Increased Risk to Mistreat and Be Mistreated

More Likely to Mistreat
- Family member, spouse, or grown child
- One with physical or mental illnesses
- One who is abusing alcohol or other substances
- History of family violence, exposure to abuse as a child
- Cultural acceptance of interpersonal violence
- Experiencing unemployment or financial concerns
- Social isolation, lack of social support
- Impaired impulse control
- Financial or emotional dependence of the older adult
- Inability to establish or maintain positive social relationships

More Likely to Be Mistreated
- Cognitively impaired, especially with aggressive features
- Dependent on abuser
- Physically or mentally frail
- Abused the caregiver or was abused earlier in life
- Women either living alone or in a household with family members
- Exhibiting behavior that is considered aggressive, demanding, or unappreciative
- Living in an institutional setting
- Feeling deserving of abuse due to perception of personal inadequacies

Data from Nursing Home Abuse Center: *Elder abuse statistics* (website), 2021. https://www.nursinghomeabusecenter.com/elder-abuse/statistics/; Centers for Disease Control and Prevention: *Risk and protective factors* (website), 2020. https://www.cdc.gov/violenceprevention/elderabuse/riskprotectivefactors.html.

BOX 31.12 Potential Cultural Barriers to Identification of Elder Mistreatment

Latinx
- *Machismo:* Expectation of men to neglect self on behalf of others if necessary
- *Marianismo:* Role expectation of women to tolerate abuse and focus on service of others
- *Vergüenza:* Need to protect the family from shame

Asian or Pacific Islander
- Ability to endure violence as a symbol of strength and honor
- Filial duty to care for parents regardless of personal needs and responsibilities
- Unacceptability to express emotions

Japanese
- Suffering is expected to be done in a stoic manner
- Fatalism to suffering, self-blame
- Those who expose a family "shame" may be considered traitors and be sanctioned

Vietnamese
- Family problems are to be kept at home; cannot be disclosed to outsiders
- Neglect brings shame to family
- Psychological "silent treatment" most common

difficult for an older adult to report mistreatment. Older adults also may fear that the reporting will intensify the problem and that they have no alternatives for care (APA, 2020). The practitioner should be sensitive to the cultural background of the patient and family, as there are differences in how people provide care. For example, in many families caring for impaired elders is expected, even at the expense of the caregiver's needs, health, abilities, and other obligations (WHO, 2021). However, whatever the family's beliefs, the nurse is legally obligated to attempt to ensure the safety of vulnerable older adults while respecting their autonomously articulated wishes.

When several different persons are giving care, professional monitoring for mistreatment becomes especially difficult. The nurse should pay attention to the vulnerable older adult who is alone with a formal caregiver for extended periods of time and who has both lay and professional caregivers with no support or opportunities for respite for the caregiving. Circumstances increasing the risk can occur in any setting (Boxes 31.13 and 31.14).

Elder mistreatment can destroy social and family ties and lead to financial devastation. The trauma of abuse can result in the deterioration of physical, psychological, and spiritual health. Older adults who have been victims of violence have more health problems than other older adults, including increased bone or joint problems, digestive problems, depression or anxiety, chronic pain, hypertension, cardiovascular disease, hospitalizations, and nursing home placement (Houts et al., 2021).

BOX 31.13 Factors Increasing the Risk of Mistreatment of Older Adults in the Community

Poor physical or mental health (either caregiver or care recipient)
Shared living situation
Gender (women, esp. if culturally inferior social status)
Abuser dependence on the older adult
Long history of poor, conflicted, or abusive relationship
Cultural or societal tolerance of violence, especially against women
Increasing number of caregivers (usually women) needing to enter the workforce
Social isolation; migration of younger family members away from ancestral home
Unacceptability of emotional expression, especially that of fear or distress
Lack of funds to pay for care and needed supplies

From World Health Organization: *Elder abuse* (website), 2021. https://www.who.int/news-room/fact-sheets/detail/elder-abuse.

BOX 31.14 Factors Increasing Risk of Mistreatment Within Institutional Settings

Low standard of care
Staff who are poorly trained, low paid
Burnout/overworked
Poor physical condition of workplace
Policies emphasizing the institution above the residents
Drug or alcohol abuse of staff
History of criminal conduct
Inadequate supervision
Inadequate record keeping

From World Health Organization: *Elder abuse* (website), 2021. https://www.who.int/news-room/fact-sheets/detail/elder-abuse.

BOX 31.15 Factors Increasing the Risk for Exploitation Due to Undue Influence

Recent bereavement
Cognitive impairment
Dependence on others
Fearfulness
Mental or physical illness
Social isolation
Loneliness
Substance abuse

Posttraumatic stress syndrome and lowered self-efficacy even after the termination of the abusive situation may never be resolved. Those subjected to abuse are 300% more likely to die a premature death (Nursing Home Abuse Center [NHAC], 2021).

Undue Influence

According to the American Bar Association, the legal concept of *undue influence* is the result of psychological abuse of an older person for the purpose of financial or sexual *exploitation*. Most often the older adult already trusts the abuser or perpetrator, or the trust has been sought and nurtured for the purpose of influencing behavior. Although any older adult can be the victim of undue influence, some characteristics and circumstances make the risk higher (Box 31.15).

Undue influence may develop slowly as the victim is isolated from friends and family in some way, such as with the suggestion that the caregiver is the only one who cares, or the older adult meets a "new friend" who offers to provide "lifelong" care in exchange for the title to property such as the older adult's home. A person may offer false affection and even marriage to a vulnerable person *for the purpose of defrauding the person of assets*. In these cases, intervention is difficult because the victim has developed trust and reliance on the abuser and has entered the relationship voluntarily. Affection and kindness to the older adult in and of itself is not considered undue influence. It only reaches that point when the relationship leads to persuasion or coercion that limits the person's ability to make independent or informed choices and decisions (Stiegel & Quinn, 2017) (Box 31.16).

It is difficult to detect financial exploitation. Care is costly, and the person's assets may be gone before it is noticed that charges have been excessive or misappropriated. A salesperson may make an "offer you just can't refuse" or insist on an unneeded expensive repair or replacement. The use of lottery, telemarketing, and internet scams are among the many ways that older adults are financially victimized. In 2020 more than $4 billion were reported as lost by older adults (Federal Bureau of Investigation [FBI], 2020).

The forms of protection discussed above can be used both by those who are trying to prevent the influence and by those who are attempting to exert their influence unduly.

Neglect

Neglect by a caregiver requires a socially (formally or informally) recognized role and responsibility of a person to provide care to a vulnerable older adult. Neglect, most often by family

BOX 31.16   Cues of Potential Undue Influence

- Actions inconsistent with life history, previous lifelong values, and beliefs.
- Sudden changes in financial matters (e.g., life insurance policies, property titles, bank accounts, distribution of assets, will).
- Unexplained transfer of funds to someone outside of the family.
- Provision of unnecessary services.
- Unexplained changes in professional service providers (e.g., bankers, attorneys, health care providers).
- Isolated from previous family and friends.
- Person unknown to close family and friends unexpectedly moves into the person's home, or the person moves into another's home under the guise of providing better care.
- Income checks redirected without knowledge; bills not paid; multiple checks written to "cash," always in round numbers and often in large amounts.
- Sudden changes in documents when death is anticipated.
- A history of mistrust exists in the family and places unusual trust in newfound "friend."
- A power imbalance exists between the parties in matters of finances or health.
- The stronger person unduly benefits from transactions and situations.
- The older adult is never left alone with anyone, and no one is allowed to speak to the older adult without permission.
- The older adult reports meeting a "wonderful new friend who makes me feel young again," becomes suspicious of family, and begins to avoid family gatherings: "My friend is the only one who loves/understands me."

Adapted from US Department of Justice: *About elder abuse* (website), n.d. https://www.justice.gov/elderjustice/about-elder-abuse. Accessed June 2021.

BOX 31.17   Examples of Causes of Neglect by Caregivers

Caregiver personal stress and exhaustion
Multiple role demands
Lack of caregiving knowledge or skills
Unawareness of importance of the care needed
Financial burden of caregiving limiting resources available
Caregiver's own poor health, frailty, and very advanced age
Unawareness of community resources available for support and respite

members, is the most common form of mistreatment. Neglect may be a passive failure to provide goods and services, such as food, medication, medical treatment, or personal care, or the failure or inability to recognize one's responsibility to provide care (Caceres et al., 2021). Active neglect or willful deprivation occurs when needed care is withheld deliberately for malicious reasons and exposes the person to great risk of physical or emotional harm (NCOA, 2021). Neglect is most often by family caregivers and occurs for many reasons (Box 31.17). It may remain hidden until there is a medical crisis, when the person's unmet needs become visible to others.

Self-Neglect

Self-neglect is a behavior in which people fail to meet their own basic needs in the way an average person would in similar circumstances. It generally manifests itself as a refusal to or failure to provide themselves with adequate safety, food, water, clothing, shelter, personal hygiene, or health care. It may be due to diminished capacity, but it also may be the result of a long-standing lifestyle, poverty, homelessness, mental illness, or alcohol or other substance abuse. It is important for the nurse to remember that there are many people with the capacity to understand the consequences of self-neglect but nonetheless make conscious and voluntary decisions to engage in acts that threaten their health or safety as a matter of personal choice. There are both ethical and legal questions as to how much health care professionals can and should intervene in these situations. Nurses are particularly challenged by issues of self-neglect due to the potential conflict between the ethical principles of beneficence and autonomy.

In recognition of this escalating social and personal problem, countries have been working hard to understand the issue in their own countries, and many have developed proactive programs and policies to identify and provide services to persons at risk. In the United States there has been an increase in the number of training programs for persons at the "front line," such as health professionals, police officers, and first responders, and passage of more stringent laws against mistreatment. However, if the older adult maintains capacity, nothing can be done without the person's permission.

USING CLINICAL JUDGMENT TO PROMOTE HEALTHY AGING

Caring for vulnerable older adults and those with potentially diminished capacity means dealing with difficult ethical conflicts in supporting autonomy while providing benefits and protecting from harm. In many settings where gerontological nurses provide care to older adults, ethical and legal questions of capacity and decision-making authority occur quickly. At times this will include questioning the person's decision-making capacity and ability to provide informed consent. It is always necessary to determine whether the appearance of incapacity is truly one of impairment or whether it is the manifestation of choices that are inconsistent with the preferences, expectations, or values of the health care system, the nurse, caregiver, surrogate, or proxy. It is important to remember that what some might consider "poor judgment" is not the same as incapacity.

Recognizing and Analyzing Cues

Gerontological nurses are often the ones who first suspect mistreatment or find evidence of such (Box 31.18). Ethical conflicts can be and often are significant. Nurses are expected to provide safety and security to the persons under their care to the extent possible, while respecting an individual's autonomy. A unique aspect of mistreatment of older adults compared to that of children is that physically frail (and even abused or neglected) but mentally competent adults can, and often do, refuse intervention. These adults cannot be removed from harmful situations without their permission, much to the frustration of the nurse and other health care providers. How can the nurse respect autonomous decision making when, in doing so, no benefit is provided? Does this mean that the nurse is contributing to harm?

BOX 31.18 Cues of Mistreatment

Physical Abuse
- Unexplained bruising or lacerations in unusual areas in various stages of healing
- Fractures inconsistent with functional ability
- Open wounds and cuts in various stages of healing
- Sudden change in behavior, dehydration
- Reported physical abuse by the older adult

Sexual Abuse
- Bruises or scratches in the genital or breast area
- Unexplained venereal diseases or infections
- Unexplained vaginal or anal bleeding
- Fear or an unusual amount of anxiety related to either routine or necessary exam of the anogenital area
- Torn undergarments or presence of blood on sheets or linens
- Presence of pornographic material being shown to a person with diminished capacity
- Reported sexual abuse by the older adult

Medical Abuse
- Caregiver repeatedly requesting procedures that are not recommended and not desired by the care recipient
- Laboratory findings of medication overuse or underuse
- Repeated emergency department visits for no discernable reason

Psychological Abuse
- Caregiver does all the talking in a situation, even though the older adult is capable
- Caregiver appears angry, frustrated, or indifferent
- Caregiver or care recipient aggressive toward one another or the nurse
- Caregiver's refusal to allow visitors
- Changes in demeanor, such as appearing fearful of caregiver
- Being unusually emotionally withdrawn or hesitant
- Personality changes, such as repeatedly apologizing
- Reported psychological abuse by the older adult

Neglect
- Weight loss, dehydration, malnutrition
- Repeated falls
- Uncharacteristically neglected grooming
- Fecal or urine smell
- Inappropriate clothing for the situation or weather
- Insect infestation of residence
- Inadequate availability of food
- Desertion at a hospital or shopping area
- Evidence that person in need of continuous care is left alone
- Reported neglect or abandonment by the older adult

Medical Neglect
- Failure to respond or unusual delay between the beginning of a health problem and when help is sought
- Repeated missed appointments without reasonable explanations

Solutions, Nursing Actions, and Outcomes

Communication and education are the cornerstones of supporting and protecting vulnerable older adults. Health information must be presented in such a way that it is easily understood without sounding condescending. Lay language is expected unless the older adult is or was a nurse or other health care provider.

In either situation the nurse listens carefully to what is being said and not said while withholding judgments or depending on stereotyping or other forms of discrimination.

The nurse ensures that any needed communication aids are available, in working order, and used (Chapters 12 and 13). The nurse must determine when an interpreter is needed and know how to obtain one while realizing that when a child or other family member is asked to interpret, the content may be "edited" (Chapter 4). A professional, certified interpreter can act as a culture broker who will work as a bridge between the nurse and patient by explaining to the staff what is or is not appropriate to discuss and how to do so and explain to the patient why the questions are being asked or need to be asked. For example, "full disclosure" of diagnoses and prognoses is expected in the Western model of health care and forms the basis of informed consent. Yet in some cultures such a discussion may be viewed as a sign of disrespect, and any discussions of terminal conditions or prognoses are believed to shorten one's life. It is very appropriate to begin conversations with "You have a serious condition that we need to discuss. Is it best to talk with you about this, or someone else? Does anyone else need to be present during the conversation? How much would you like to know?"

Education

Education related to decision making in late life, advance planning for the protection of autonomy, and the cues to mistreatment all promote healthy aging. This includes public awareness campaigns, professional training curriculums, and continuing education programs, as well as programs where caregivers can obtain the knowledge and the skills that they need to take care of a vulnerable older adult while taking care of themselves.

Topics for educational programming can include how to protect the rights of oneself and vulnerable older adults, including the right to have the in-home supportive services needed to assist with care and the right to access government programs that support caregiving or to find the best nursing home or residential care setting as needed.

Although nurses cannot provide legal information, they do serve as resource persons ready to discuss many of the questions people have about end-of-life decision making, especially how it affects their care. The nurse must consider the factors previously discussed and must ensure that patients are informed of their rights related to the PSDA in a culturally sensitive manner. The nurse may be responsible for inquiring about the presence of an existing advance directive, offering and explaining the option, and ensuring that any existing directive still reflects the person's wishes. The nurse is also responsible for ensuring that existing or newly created advance directives are available in the appropriate locations in the medical record.

The nurse can help the person understand interventions (e.g., cardiopulmonary resuscitation [CPR], intubations, artificial nutrition) and their consequences (Box 31.19). The nurse can explain that choosing no further intervention is not "giving up" but is an active decision to allow a natural death to occur. Personal bias cannot be injected into the discussion (e.g., religious

---

BOX 31.19 Gloria's Story

They said that I got something called the COVID-19. I was sick and, in the hospital, but I recovered enough to go home. I thought I was doing pretty well but started having more and more trouble breathing. My nurse daughter-in-law Kathleen explained that my lungs had been badly damaged, and we should have a serious discussion about the "What if's," but I refused—it just didn't seem right. When the oxygen at home didn't help, I had to go back to the hospital. When Kathleen said again, "We need to talk," I knew things were bad, but I wanted to get better and go home. I just wasn't sure anymore either were possible. She told me that even the oxygen I was getting there was not helping. She asked if my heart should stop naturally, did I wanted them to use machines or medicines to get it going again. I didn't think so, but I did want something called CPR. She asked me what that was, and I told her it was just a little tap on the chest. She said, no, it is more than that and if they do it, they will probably have to put a tube in your throat to help you breathe. For sure I did not want that. The doctor asked if I wanted hospice services. Oh no—once you have hospice you can only go up or down [heaven or hell]. Kathleen explained that I could be discharged from hospice if I improved! That would be OK then, but I told them that I did not want to talk about it. They should talk to Kathleen, she knows what I want.

BOX 31.20 Tips for Best Practice

Prevention of Elder Mistreatment

- Determine (if possible) if what appears as mistreatment is lack of caregiver skills.
- Help families develop and nurture informal support systems.
- Link families with support groups.
- Teach families stress management techniques.
- Arrange comprehensive care resources.
- Provide counseling for troubled families.
- Encourage the use of respite care and daycare.
- Obtain necessary home health care services.
- Inform families of resources for meals and transportation.
- Encourage caregivers to pursue their individual interests and maintain their own health.

Box 31.21 Resources for Best Practice

Area Agencies on Aging: https://www.usaging.org/.
National Academy of Elder Law Attorneys: https://www.naela.org/findlawyer?.
National Indigenous Elder Justice Initiative: Tribal elder protection: https://www.nieji.org/codes.
Programs for Veterans: https://www.socialwork.va.gov/IPV/.
US Department of Justice: Elder Justice Initiative: https://www.justice.gov/elderjustice.

---

affiliation or otherwise) under any circumstances. The nurse is an impartial advocate for the patient regardless of decision or setting, but this is particularly important in the long-term care environment. The nurse also acts as a patient advocate by bringing together decision makers, older adults, and health care providers to discuss anything from the person's wishes to difficult issues that may arise in executing a directive.

No one can think of all possible contingencies that might require decisions regarding life-limiting conditions. The use of values assessments may help clarify what the person holds important in life and how this relates to desires for health care, quality of life, and quantity of life. Does the older adult want measures to be taken to prolong life at all costs, or does the person wish for a natural death? What are the boundaries in which suffering can be minimized? For older adults without family, the nurse may become a sounding board but must take care to not influence the outcome and may never serve as a proxy in a patient's living will or durable power of attorney.

Prevention

It is ideal to prevent mistreatment from ever occurring and for individuals to complete the advance planning that will protect their rights in the case of future incapacity. Caregiving is a daunting task, especially when caring for those with dementia. The nurse supports the caregiving dyad through referrals to support groups and respite programs. Social support and regular contact have the potential to prevent mistreatment, identify those at risk, or identify mistreatment early enough to minimize harm. This may be as simple as an educated friend, neighbor, or volunteer "checking in" with other friends and neighbors who may be isolated and vulnerable (Box 31.20). Finally, for older adults who become incapacitated, legal protection at some level may be necessary. Nurses can refer older adults and their significant others to attorneys who are certified in "elder law" and have specialized training and skills (Box 31.21).

Assessment

When working with frail and vulnerable older adults, nurses always must be vigilant and sensitive to the cues of mistreatment and evolving incapacity. Screening for mistreatment, its risk, and declining capacity should occur with each nurse-older adult or nurse-caregiver contact. Because capacity is situational, the level of orientation and understanding can be evaluated by considering the questions the person asks in relation to the decision or situation and by asking the person to describe back what is being asked, presuming that the guidelines for communication as described earlier are followed. Documentation should be as specific as possible. "Orientation × 3" is not adequate to indicate capacity. Neither is an isolated score from cognitive testing. Instead, noting specifically "Able to select from choice of foods" or "Able to determine when assistance with … is needed" is helpful. For more complex decision making, documentation such as "Unable to describe the pros and cons of the procedure after being informed of these" is needed.

Assessment always begins with determination of the person's safety. Assessment for potential mistreatment has become more refined, and many hospitals screen as part of the admission process for all of those at least 65 years old (Caceres et al., 2021). The Elder Assessment Instrument (EAI) combines both subjective and objective observations by the nurse. It has been found to be highly sensitive but less specific. A video demonstrating the use of the EAI is available (Fulmer, 2019). The Hwalek-Sengstock Elder Abuse Screening Test (H-S/EAST) is designed for use in the inpatient setting, is easily administered by the nurse, but relies heavily on subjective report by the patient (Caceres et al., 2021). However, many older adults will not self-report mistreatment for multiple reasons, including embarrassment, fear of retaliation, lack of an alternative care setting or caregiver, fear of nursing home placement, and expectations of broad familial repercussions. For the person who has full capacity and refuses assessment, it cannot be done. However, there is always a high level of suspicion when the explanation of injury is inconsistent with the medical findings, when there has been a delay in seeking needed treatment, when the older adult reports a different history of the event from the potential abuser, and when there have been repeated visits to different emergency departments and providers for similar problems. A potential abuser will not let the patient answer questions and refuses to leave during the exam but also may act angry, demeaning, oversolicitous, or indifferent. The patient will appear hesitant, nonspecific, or frightened (Houts et al., 2021).

For a person with questionable capacity and unmet needs or other signs of abuse or neglect, legal intervention will be necessary. Assessment of mistreatment cross-culturally is especially difficult and must be done in a culturally appropriate manner. When an immigrant family is undocumented, fear of being deported will override the need to report elder mistreatment. Because of the sensitive nature of such an assessment, it is recommended that all gerontological nurses and others who are in contact with older adults (e.g., emergency department staff, first responders) receive specialized training.

Early Intervention

When the cues to mistreatment are identified early, further harm may be preventable for both the older adult and the caregiver. If the abuse is triggered by the stress of caregiving (Chapter 32), nurses can be very proactive and help all involved find ways to lessen the stress. This may include finding respite services; changing the situation entirely (giving permission to the caregiver to relinquish the role); referring to support groups for expression of frustrations and peer support; teaching people how to use crisis hotlines; involving Adult Protective Services; and providing access to professional consultation, victim support groups, or victim volunteer companions. Early intervention includes formulating culturally sensitive prevention and intervention efforts, which reflects an understanding of varying roles and responsibilities within the family and their help-seeking behaviors. Most importantly, thoughtful and compassionate care is imperative for both the victim and the perpetrator.

If the abusive behavior is learned, it may be subject to change. Learned abuse theoretically can be unlearned and may respond to a close working relationship with a mentoring professional who can demonstrate positive problem solving and new ways of managing difficult situations.

Emergency Response

If the mistreatment is the result of psychopathological conditions and relationships, especially if the situation is long-standing, the nurse probably cannot prevent the abuse or it will remain hidden unless serious consequences or death occurs. Nurses can make sure that all older adults are reminded that they have inherent worth and dignity and are deserving of respect and that help is available if it is ever needed, and provide older adults with information about the resources that are available to them. The nurse can offer the same to the caregiver.

In most states, nurses are "mandatory reporters"; those who become aware or strongly suspect that abuse, neglect, or exploitation (or all) has occurred are legally required to report it to the appropriate authorities immediately. The designated authority can be found in each state's laws and also should be available in any health care setting's policy manual. Unfortunately, emergency shelters for older adults are not available in every community, especially for those with medical or psychiatric problems. Research has shown that when there are no legal consequences for the perpetrator of elder mistreatment, it is likely to continue, especially when women are the victims, those who are married, and those who live with the perpetrator (Caceres et al., 2021).

For nurses working in long-term care facilities, the state's long-term care ombudsman program can be contacted, especially when the situation is less clear. Ombudsmen are either volunteers or paid staff members who are responsible for acting as advocates for vulnerable residents in institutions (http://www.ltcombudsman.org) (Administration for Community Living, 2021). All reports, either to the state ombudsman or adult protective services, will be investigated.

Advocacy

An advocate is one who maintains or promotes a cause; defends, pleads, or acts on behalf of another; and fights for those who cannot fight for themselves. The nurse is an advocate as a member of both a profession and a community. As a professional advocate, the nurse has a responsibility to protect the patient from abuse, neglect, and exploitation from all sources, including institutions, staff, guardians, caregivers, surrogates, or proxies. Gerontological nurses can become familiar with the laws that specifically affect older adults in their state and be willing to contact the designated protective services within their institution and the community when there is evidence of mistreatment.

Nurse advocates function in various arenas: within their own profession and agency; with other professionals and other agencies; with families, neighbors, and community representatives; and with professional organizations, legislators, and courts.

Nurses act as advocates when they support people as autonomous free agents who have the right to make decisions and to be involved in all conversations about their health care needs *should they choose to do so*. In a health care setting, advocacy is acting for or on behalf of another in terms of supporting the best interests of that other person with respect to accepting and refusing health care. However, situations occur in the care of older adults when the person is either not strong enough or does not have the capacity to exert measures to protect their own interests. When this occurs, the nurse's role is to ensure that not only that older adults are protected but also that their voices are not lost even when they cannot express themselves.

As a member of a community, nurses are advocates when they volunteer as an ombudsman, for a crisis or abuse hotline, or for an international program for the protection of older adults or when they testify at the judicial appointment of a conservator or guardian or as a witness to mistreatment. Nurses are key participants in testing the effectiveness of models to prevent elder mistreatment and responding to those in need (Stoeckle & Bane, 2020).

KEY CONCEPTS

- Unless adjudicated otherwise, all adults have a presumed capacity to control their lives, including what happens to their bodies; they legally have the autonomous right to make health-related decisions to both accept and reject treatment.
- Informed consent is based on the ethical principle of autonomy, which requires the capacity to understand a situation, the choices that are available, and the consequences of a decision.
- In the health care setting, an individual may have legal competence but have diminished or varying levels of capacity to make health-related decisions.

- Varying levels of protection are available to protect a person with diminished capacity and to ensure that the person's voice is still heard.
- Elder mistreatment is an umbrella term that covers abuse, neglect, exploitation, and abandonment.
- The nurse has a legal responsibility to report mistreatment of frail or disabled older adults that is known to or responsibly believed to have occurred or is occurring.
- Advance directives and living wills provide persons with the opportunity to express wishes and appoint a proxy to act on those wishes when they are unable to do so for themselves.

NEXT-GENERATION NCLEX® (NGN) EXAMINATION–STYLE QUESTIONS

Mrs. Henry, 87 years old, is admitted to the medical/surgical floor of a community hospital with a fractured right orbit and ruptured eye globe. Her husband attends to her with apparent care and concern, trying to anticipate her needs. He is active and appears much younger than she is. The emergency department report states the cause of the injury as "fall at home." Although Mrs. Henry is alert and oriented, she appears very thin, frail, and withdrawn. Her husband also voices concern that she seems confused at times. When the gerontological clinical nurse specialist arrives to do a basic assessment, she reports to the nurses that she is concerned that Mrs. Henry has been abused. Her husband answers all questions posed to his wife, and as he does so, Mrs. Henry seems to withdraw even further from both him and the staff. Mr. Henry does not leave his wife's side for hours. Finally he leaves for a quick cup of coffee, and the nurse who had been providing care quickly goes into the room and asks Mrs. Henry what happened. She begins to cry and says that her husband hit her. She is immediately offered shelter and protection. She declines, saying that she has nowhere else to go but back home and that she will be okay. The husband returns to find the nurse talking to his wife privately and immediately gathers up her things, and they leave the hospital against medical advice.

Highlight the cues indicating or suggesting potential physical abuse. Underline the data that may support the suspicion of abuse but also may be from some other cause. What are the two most important cues to likely abuse?

CLINICAL JUDGMENT ACTIVITY

1. After reading this chapter, discuss with a classmate why you believe some older adults feel that they have no options but to endure abuse of any kind.

RESEARCH QUESTIONS

1. What are your responsibilities for reporting elder mistreatment in your state?
2. What resources are available to frail older adults in your community who are attempting to escape from mistreatment?
3. Is elder mistreatment the same as intimate partner violence?

REFERENCES

Administration for Community Living: *Long-term care ombudsman program* (website), 2021. https://acl.gov/programs/Protecting-Rights-and-Preventing-Abuse/Long-term-Care-Ombudsman-Program.

American Psychological Association: *Elder abuse and neglect: in search of solutions* (website), 2020. https://www.apa.org/pi/aging/resources/guides/elder-abuse.

Caceres BA, Kurup N, Fulmer T: Elder mistreatment detection. In Boltz M, editor: *Evidence-based geriatric nursing protocols for best practice,* ed 6, New York, 2021, Springer, pp 241–257.

Chang ES & Levy BR: High prevalence of elder abuse during the COVID-19 pandemic: risk and resilience factors, *Am J Geriatr Psychiatry* 29(11):1152–1159, 2021.

Coolen PR: *Cultural relevance in end-of-life care* (website), 2012. https://ethnomed.org/resource/cultural-relevance-in-end-of-life-care/.

Federal Bureau of Investigation (FBI): *Elder fraud report 2020* (website), 2020. https://www.ic3.gov/Media/PDF/AnnualReport/2020_IC3ElderFraudReport.pdf.

Fulmer T: *Elder mistreatment assessment* (website), 2019. https://hign.org/consultgeri/try-this-series/elder-mistreatment-assessment.

Hoe DF & Enguidanos S: So help me, God: religiosity and end-of-life choices in a nationally representative sample, *J Palliat Med* 23(4):563–567, 2019.

Hong M, Yi EH, Johnson KJ, et al: Facilitators and barriers for advance care planning among ethnic and racial minorities in the U.S.: a systematic review of the current literature, *J Immigr Minor Health* 20(5):1277–1287, 2018.

Houts AH, Sheets K, Okonkwo N, et al: Detecting, assessing & responding to elder mistreatment. In Walter LC & Chang A, editors: *CURRENT diagnosis and treatment: geriatrics,* 3, New York, 2021, McGraw Hill, pp 146–155.

Koss CS & Baker TA: Race differences in advance directive completion, *J Aging Health* 29(2):324–342, 2016.

National Council on Aging (NCOA): *Get the facts on elder abuse* (website), 2021. https://www.ncoa.org/article/get-the-facts-on-elder-abuse.

Nursing Home Abuse Center (NHAC): *Elder abuse statistics: statistics on elder and nursing home abuse* (website), 2021. https://www.nursinghomeabusecenter.com/elder-abuse/statistics/.

RegisteredNursing.org: *Informed consent: NCLEX-RN* (website), 2021. https://www.registerednursing.org/nclex/informed-consent/.

Reuben DB, Herr KA, Pacala JT, et al: *Geriatrics at your fingertips,* ed 22, New York, 2020, American Geriatrics Society.

Stiegel LA & Quinn MJ: *Elder abuse: the impact of undue influence* (website), 2017. https://ncler.acl.gov/pdf/Advanced-Elder-Abuse-The-Impact-of-Undue-Influence.pdf.

Stoeckle RJ & Bane S: The national collaboratory on elder mistreatment, *Generations* 44(1):33–37, 2020.

World Health Organization (WHO): *Elder abuse* (website), 2021. https://www.who.int/news-room/fact-sheets/detail/elder-abuse.

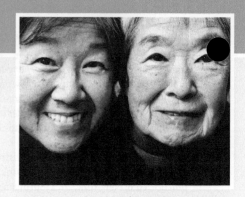

Relationships, Roles, and Life Transitions

Theris A. Touhy

http://evolve.elsevier.com/Touhy/TwdHlthAging

A STUDENT SPEAKS

I'm really worried about retirement! That is ridiculous at my age, but I keep reading and hearing about Social Security and Medicare running out of money for the baby boom generation. Those are my parents! What about me?

Joseph, age 30

AN OLDER ADULT SPEAKS

I thought when my children left home that my most important job was done. But they came home again and again, and then my mother-in-law came to live with us. Finally, the kids were really on their own and married, so now I take care of the grandchildren while they both work to make ends meet. I just pray daily that my husband will remain healthy. I don't think I could deal with one more thing.

Esther, age 64

LEARNING OBJECTIVES

On completion of this chapter, the reader will be able to:

1. Explain the issues involved in adapting to transitions and role changes in later life.
2. Discuss changes in family structure and functions in society today.
3. Examine family relationships in later life.
4. Identify the range of caregiving situations and the potential challenges and opportunities of each.
5. Use clinical judgment to identify and evaluate solutions and nursing actions to promote healthy relationships, roles, and life transitions.

This chapter examines the various relationships, roles, and life transitions that characteristically play a part in later life. Concepts of family structure and function and the transitions of retirement, widowhood, widowerhood, and caregiving are discussed. Nursing actions to support older adults in maintaining fulfilling roles and relationships and adapting to life transitions are presented.

LATE LIFE TRANSITIONS

Role transitions that occur in later life include retirement, grandparenthood, widowhood, widowerhood, and becoming a caregiver or recipient of care. The role functions of these relationships shift as societal norms and economics change. These transitions may occur predictably or may be imposed by unanticipated events. Retirement is an example of a predictable event that can and should be planned long in advance, although for some it can occur unexpectedly as a result of illness, disability, or being terminated from a job. To the degree that an event is perceived as expected and occurring at the right time, a role transition may be comfortable and even welcomed. Those persons who must retire "too early" or are widowed "too soon" will have more difficulty adapting than those who are at an age when these events are expected.

The speed and intensity of a major change may make the difference between a transitional crisis and a gradual and comfortable adaptation. Most difficult are the transitions that incorporate losses rather than gains in status, influence, and opportunity. The move from independence to dependence and becoming a care recipient is particularly difficult. Conditions that influence the outcome of transitions include personal meanings, expectations, level of knowledge, preplanning, and emotional and physical reserves. Cohort, cultural, and gender differences are inherent in all of life's major transitions. Those transitions that make use of past skills and adaptations may be less stressful. The ideal outcome occurs when gains in satisfaction and new roles offset losses.

Retirement

Issues of work and retirement for older adults are a cultural universal topic because every culture has mechanisms for retiring their older citizens. Although retirement patterns differ across the world, in industrialized nations, and in many developing nations, the expectation is that older workers will cease full-time career job employment and be entitled to economic support. However, whether that support will be adequate, or even available, is a growing concern worldwide. In the United States, many European countries, and Australia, problems are emerging as the generation born after World War II moves into retirement. Developing countries face similar issues with the growth of the older population combined with decreasing birth rates. Governments may not be able to afford retirement systems to replace the tradition of children caring for aging parents. Most countries are not ready to meet what is projected to be one of the defining challenges of the 21st century.

Retirement, as we formerly knew it, has changed. The transitions are blurring, and the numerous patterns and styles of retiring have produced more varied experiences in retirement. Retirement is no longer just a few years of rest from the rigors of work before death. It is a developmental stage that may occupy 30 or more years of one's life and involve many stages. Some individuals will be retired for longer than they worked. Retirees are living longer, and declining birth rates mean that there will be fewer workers to support them. Countries are scaling down retirement benefits and raising the age at which individuals can collect them.

People are starting to retire later as they realize the obstacles that financial challenges or obligations present to successful retirement and future independence. Sixty-nine percent of baby boomers either expect to or are already working past age 65 years. There may be financial reasons for older adults to want to keep working, or it might be that they want to stay mentally alert. The most frequently cited retirement fear across generations is outliving savings and investments (Transamerica Center for Retirement Studies, 2019).

The COVID-19 pandemic has affected retirement decisions and there has been an increase in retirement among adults ages 55 and older. As of the third quarter of 2021, 50.3% of U.S. adults 55 and older said they were out of the labor force due to retirement. It is unclear if the pandemic-induced increase in retirement among older adults will be temporary or long-lasting. The Bureau of Labor Statistics is projecting large increases in labor force participation among older adults from 2020 to 2030 with nearly 40% of individuals 65 years to 69 years of age being in the labor force by 2030, up from 33% in 2020 (Fry, 2021).

Special Considerations in Retirement

The three-legged stool for retirement (Social Security, savings, and private pensions) has become one-legged for a sizable proportion of Americans because of limited personal retirement savings and a decline in pension plans (Morley, 2017). Older adults with disabilities, those who had less access to education

or held low-paying jobs with no benefits, and those not eligible for Social Security are at increased economic risk during retirement years. Older minority women, never-married women, and divorced women are more likely to live in poverty and are less likely to receive Social Security. Prior to the legalization of same-sex marriage in the United States, individuals were denied access to Social Security survivor benefits. After legalization of same-sex marriage, married same-sex couples now have access to Social Security survivor benefits, Medicaid spend-downs, bereavement leave, and tax exemptions upon inheritance of jointly owned real estate and personal property.

Inadequate coverage for women in retirement is common because their work histories may have been sporadic and diverse. Women often retire earlier than anticipated because of family needs. Whereas most men have always worked outside the home, it is only within the past 40 years that this has been the expectation of women. Therefore large cohort differences exist. Traditionally, the variability of women's work histories, interrupted careers, the residuals of sexist pension policies, Social Security inequities, and low-paying jobs created hazards for adequacy of income in retirement. The scene is gradually changing in many respects, but the gender bias remains (Chapter 5).

Retirement Planning

Current research suggests that retirement has positive effects on life satisfaction and health, although this may vary depending on the individual's circumstances. Decisions to retire are often based on financial resources, attitudes toward work, family roles and responsibilities, the nature of the job, access to health insurance, chronological age, health, and self-perceptions of ability to adjust to retirement. Retirement planning is advisable during early adulthood and essential in middle age. However, people differ in their focus on the past, present, and future and their realistic ability to "put away something" for future needs. Retirement confidence continues to be closely related to having a retirement plan.

Retirement preparation programs are usually aimed at employees with high levels of education and occupational status, those with private pension coverage, and government employees. Thus the people most in need of planning assistance may be those least likely to have any available, let alone the resources for an adequate retirement. Individuals who are retiring in poor health, minorities, women, those in lower socioeconomic levels, and those with the least education may experience greater concerns in retirement and may need specialized counseling and targeted education efforts (Fischer, 2021).

Solutions, Nursing Actions, and Outcomes Successful retirement adjustment depends on socialization needs, energy levels, health, adequate income, variety of interests, amount of self-esteem derived from work, presence of intimate relationships, social support, and general adaptability (Box 32.1). Nurses may have the opportunity to work with people in different phases of retirement or participate in retirement education and counseling programs. Talking with clients older than age 50 about retirement plans, providing anticipatory guidance about the transition to retirement, identifying those who may be

BOX 32.1   Predictors of Retirement Satisfaction

- Good health
- Functional abilities
- Adequate income
- Suitable living environment
- Strong social support system characterized by reciprocal relationships
- Decision to retire that involved choice, autonomy, adequate preparation, higher-status job before retirement
- Retirement activities that offer an opportunity to feel useful, learn, grow, and enjoy oneself
- Positive outlook, sense of mastery, resilience, resourcefulness
- Good marital or partner relationship
- Sharing similar interests to spouse or significant other

Data from Hooyman N, Kiyak H: *Social gerontology: a multidisciplinary perspective,* ed 9, Boston, 2011, Allyn & Bacon.

BOX 32.2   Common Widower Bereavement Reactions

- Search for the lost mate
- Neglect of self
- Inability to share grief
- Loss of social contacts
- Struggle to view women as other than wife
- Erosion of self-confidence and sexuality
- Protracted grief period

at risk for lowered income and health concerns, and referring to appropriate resources for retirement planning and support are important nursing actions. In addition, the period of preretirement and retirement may be an opportune time to enhance the focus on health promotion and illness and injury prevention.

It is important to build on the strengths of the individual's life experiences and coping skills and to provide appropriate counseling and support to assist individuals to continue to grow and develop in meaningful ways during the transition from the work role. In ideal situations, retirement offers the opportunity to pursue interests that may have been neglected while fulfilling other obligations. However, for too many individuals, retirement presents challenges that affect both health and well-being, and nurses must be advocates for policies and conditions that allow all older adults to maintain quality of life in retirement.

Death of a Spouse or Life Partner

Losing a spouse or other life partner after a long, close, and satisfying relationship is the most difficult adjustment one can face, aside from the loss of a child. This loss is a stage in the life course that can be anticipated but seldom is considered. Spousal bereavement in later life is a higher probability for women due to differences in life expectancy, and while less common among men, it is still a significant event. Among those 75 years or older who had ever married, 58% of women and 28% of men had experienced the death of a spouse in their lifetime (US Census Bureau, 2021). Among individuals 75 to 84 years old, 14.7% of men and 42.9% of women are widowed; among those older than 85 years, 35.3% of men and 71.9% of women are widowed (Biddle et al., 2020).

Older women are substantially more likely to be widowed (and not remarried) than older men (37% vs. 13%), and the majority of these older widowed women live alone. The number of widows has declined, especially for women whose spouses are now living longer. The decline in widowhood in recent decades also results from the rising share of divorced older adults, particularly among those ages 65 to 74 years.

Although change in marital status is accepted as a normal life experience, the death/life partner of a spouse is a significant life event for older adults. With the loss of the intimate partner, several changes occur simultaneously in almost every domain of life and have a significant impact on well-being: physical, psychological, social, practical, and economic. Individuals who have been self-confident and resilient seem to fare best. Having frequent contact with family and friends is key to resilience in handling the loss. The transitional phase of grief, if handled appropriately, leads to the confirmation of a new identity, the end of one stage of life, and the beginning of another.

Gender differences on widowhood are found in the literature. Bereaved husbands may be more socially and emotionally vulnerable. Suicide risk is highest among men older than 80 years of age who have experienced the death of a spouse (Chapter 30). Widowers adapt more slowly than widows to the loss of a spouse and often remarry quickly. Loneliness and the need to be cared for are factors influencing widowers to pursue new partners. Having associations with family and friends, being members of a church community, and continuing to work or engage in activities can all be helpful in the adjustment period following the death of a wife. Common bereavement reactions of widowers are listed in Box 32.2 and should be discussed with male clients.

USING CLINICAL JUDGMENT TO PROMOTE HEALTHY AGING: LOSS OF SPOUSE OR LIFE PARTNER

Recognizing and Analyzing Cues

Losing a spouse or life partner can have serious physical and mental health consequences. There is an elevated risk of morbidity and mortality, particularly in the early bereavement period. The likelihood of a heart attack or stroke doubles in the critical 30-day period after a partner's death. In a sample of cognitively unimpaired widowed older adults, being widowed increased susceptibility to Alzheimer's disease clinical progression (Biddle et al., 2020). The risk seems likely to be the result of adverse physiological responses associated with acute grief. The bereavement period is also associated with an elevated risk of multiple psychiatric disorders, particularly if the death was unexpected. The risks of effects of spousal bereavement and increasing age on health, particularly chronic issues, remain elevated even among those long past the event (10+ years), so ongoing surveillance and assessment are indicated.

BOX 32.3 Patterns of Adjustment to Widowhood

Stage 1: Reactionary (First Few Weeks)

Early responses of disbelief, anger, indecision, detachment, and inability to communicate in a logical, sustained manner are common. Searching for the mate, visions, hallucinations, and depersonalization may be experienced.

Intervention: Support, validate, be available, listen to individual talk about mate, reduce expectations.

Stage 2: Withdrawal (First Few Months)

Depression, apathy, physiological vulnerability; movement and cognition are slowed; insomnia, unpredictable waves of grief, sighing, and anorexia occur.

Intervention: Protect individual against suicide, monitor health status, and involve in support groups.

Stage 3: Recuperation (Second 6 Months)

Periods of depression are interspersed with characteristic capability. Feelings of personal control begin to return.

Intervention: Support accustomed lifestyle patterns that sustain and assist individual to explore new possibilities.

Stage 4: Exploration (Second Year)

Individual begins new ventures, testing suitability of new roles; anniversaries, holidays, birthdays, and date of death may be especially difficult.

Intervention: Prepare individual for unexpected reactions during anniversaries. Encourage and support new trial roles.

Stage 5: Integration (Fifth Year)

Individual will feel fully integrated into new and satisfying roles if grief has been resolved in a healthy manner.

Intervention: Assist individual to recognize and share own pattern of growth through the trauma of loss.

Solutions, Nursing Actions, and Outcomes

Nurses interact with bereaved older adults in many settings. This is an important time for nurses to assess the health status of the individual and provide interventions to assist in coping. Knowing the stages of transition to a new role as a widow or widower will be useful in determining nursing actions, although each individual is unique in this respect. Individuals respond to losses in ways that reflect the nature and meaning of the relationships and the unique characteristics of the bereaved. Patterns of adjustment and nursing actions are presented in Box 32.3. With adequate support, reintegration can be expected in 2 to 4 years but circumstances vary. People with few familial or social supports may need professional help to get through the early months of grief in a way that will facilitate recovery. Additional information about dying, death, and grief can be found in Chapter 34.

RELATIONSHIPS IN LATER LIFE

The classic study of Lowenthal and Haven (1968) demonstrated the importance of caring relationships and the presence of a confidante as a buffer against "age-linked social losses." Maintaining a stable intimate relationship was more closely associated with good mental health and high morale than was a high level of activity or elevated role status.

Individuals seem able to manage stresses if some relationships are close and sustaining.

Increasingly evident is that a caring person may be a significant survival resource. Frequently nurses become the caring other in an older adult's life, especially among those living in nursing homes (Touhy, 2001). Social bonding increases health status through as yet undetermined physiological pathways, though studies in psychoneuroimmunology are giving us clues. Social support is related to psychological and physical well-being, and participation in meaningful social activities is also a modifying factor that may offset the risk of dementia.

Friendships

Friends are often a significant source of support in later life. The number of friends may decline, but the majority of older adults have at least one close friend with whom they maintain close contact, share confidences, and can turn to in an emergency. The social network may narrow as one ages, with intimate personal relationships being maintained and the more instrumental relationships discontinued. Research across the globe supports the value of friendship for older adults in promoting health and well-being.

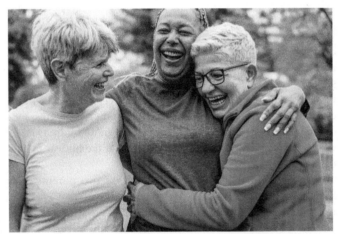

Friends play an important role in the lives of older adults. (By Michal Osmenda, Brussels, Belgium [CC BY 2.0 (http://creative-commons.org/licenses/by/2.0)], via Wikimedia Commons.)

Friendships are often sustaining in the face of overwhelming circumstances. Friends provide the critical elements of satisfactory living that families may not, providing commitment and affection without judgment. Personality characteristics between friends are compatible because the relationships are chosen and caring is shared without obligation. Trust, demonstrations of caring, and mutual problem solving are important aspects of the friendships. Friends may share a lifelong perspective or may bring a totally new intergenerational viewpoint into one's life. Late-life friendships often develop out of changing situations, such as relocation to retirement or assisted living communities, widowhood, and involvement in volunteer pursuits. As desires and pursuits change, some friendships evolve that one never would have considered in one's youth.

Considering the obvious importance of friendship, it seems to be a neglected area of exploration and a seldom considered resource for professionals working with older adults. Because close friendships have such influence on the sense of well-being of older adults, anything done to sustain them or assist in building new friendships and social networks will be helpful. Internet access and social media offer new opportunities to interact with friends or even to form new friendships. Generally, women tend to have more sustaining friendships than do men, and this factor contributes to resilience, a characteristic linked to successful aging (Chapter 30).

Nurses may include questions about the individual's friendships and their importance and availability in their assessment of older adults. Although friendships do provide much support, they are also a further source of grief in old age. The loss of friends through death occurs often, and nurses must appreciate the nature of this loss. Encouraging intergenerational friendships and linking older adults to resources for social participation and meaningful activities are important interventions.

FAMILIES

Changing Family Structure

The idea of family evokes strong impressions of whatever an individual believes the typical family should be. Because everyone comes from a family, these impressions have powerful symbolic meanings. However, in today's world, the definition of family is in a state of flux. As recently as 100 years ago, the norm was the extended family made up of parents, their grown children, and the children's children, often living together and sharing resources, strengths, and challenges. As cities grew and adult children moved in pursuit of work, parents did not always come along, and the nuclear family evolved.

The norm in the United States became two parents and their two children (nuclear family), or at least that was the norm in what has been considered mainstream America. This pattern was not as common among ethnically diverse families, where the extended family is often the norm. However, families are changing, and today the nuclear family is much less common.

Changing family patterns pose significant challenges for the future of long-term care because 80% to 90% of all long-term care services and supports are provided by spouses, adult children, and other informal caregivers. Baby boomers are more likely to live alone than previous generations, and single-person households are increasing (Vespa & Schondelmyer, 2015). Other countries are also experiencing changes in family composition, and even values, as the numbers of older adults increase and the younger members of society become more mobile and move away from their homes. In China, the extended family is disappearing, and in 2013 the country enacted a new law mandating that family members must attend to the spiritual needs of older family members and visit them frequently if they live apart. Nearly half of the country's seniors live apart from their children (Dong, 2016).

A decrease in fertility rates has reduced family size, and American families are smaller today than ever before. The high divorce and remarriage rate results in households of blended families of children from previous marriages and the new marriage. The new modern family includes single-parent families, blended families, gay and lesbian families, domestic partnerships, and childless families. Older adults without families, either by choice or by circumstance, may create their own

---

BOX 32.4 **Tips for Best Practice**

Adding an Older Adult to the Household

Questions to Ask
- What are the needs of the new member and of the family?
- Where will space be allotted for the new member?
- How will the new member be included in existing family patterns?
- How will responsibilities be shared?
- What resources in the community will assist in the adjustment phase?
- Is the environment safe for the new member?
- How will family life change with the added member, and how does the family feel about it?
- What are the differences in socialization and sleeping patterns?
- What are the older adult's needs and expectations?
- What are the older adult's skills and talents?

Modifications That May Need to Be Made
- Arrange semiprivate living quarters if possible.
- Regularly schedule visits to other relatives to give each family time for respite and privacy.
- Arrange adult day health programs and senior activities for the older adult to help keep contact with members of the adult's own generation. Consider how the older adult will feel about giving up familiar surroundings and friends.

Potential Areas of Conflict
- Space: especially if someone has given up personal space to the older relative.
- Possessions: older adults may want to move possessions into the house; others may not find them attractive or may insist on replacing them with new things.
- Entertaining: times when old and young feel the need or desire to exclude the other from social events.
- Responsibilities and chores: older adults may feel useless if they do nothing and may feel in the way if they do something.
- Expenses: increased cost of home maintenance, food, clothing, and recreation may not be shared appropriately.
- Vacations: whether to go together or alone; young persons may feel uneasy not taking the older adult out and may feel resentful if they must.
- Childrearing: disagreement over child-rearing policies.
- Childcare: finding a balance between the amount of responsibility grandparents will assume for childcare if desired and family needs and desires.

Ways to Decrease Areas of Conflict
- Respect privacy.
- Discuss space allocations.
- Discuss the older adult's furnishings before the move.
- Make it clear in advance when social events include everyone or exclude someone.
- Make clear decisions about household tasks; all should have responsibility geared to ability.
- Have the older adult pay a share of expenses if able.

"families" through communal living with siblings, friends, or others. Indeed, it is not unusual for childless older adults residing in long-term care facilities to refer to the staff as their new "family."

Multigenerational Families

The US Census Bureau defines multigenerational families as those consisting of more than two generations living under the same roof. One in four Americans live in a household with three or more generations. Multigenerational living has nearly quadrupled in the past decade, with the COVID-19 pandemic playing a strong role. However, record numbers of families were already living together in the United States before the pandemic. Multigenerational families are more common among Hispanic and Asian households but are growing among nearly all US racial groups, among all age groups, and among both men and women.

Among those living in a multigenerational household, nearly 6 in 10 say that they started or are continuing to live together because of the COVID-19 pandemic. The pandemic created challenges, especially for those cohabitating with high-risk individuals. About 7 in 10 of those currently living in multigenerational households plan to continue doing so long term. Sixty-six percent say that the economic climate was a factor in their living arrangement. Other reasons include the need for eldercare or childcare; job loss, change in job status, or underemployment; health care costs for one or more family members; cultural and family expectations; and education or retraining expenses (Generations United, 2021).

Although multigenerational living can be stressful at times, the overwhelming majority of Americans living in multigenerational homes say that their households function successfully. Benefits cited include enhanced bonds or relationships, ease of providing for care needs of one or more family members, improved finances for at least one family member, positive impacts on personal mental and/or physical health, and making it possible for at least one family member to continue school or enroll in job training (Generations United, 2021). "Multigen" remodeling or new home building to accommodate intergenerational families is an increasing trend. Box 32.4 presents tips for planning to add an older adult to the household.

Family Relationships

Family members, however they are defined, form the nucleus of relationships for the majority of older adults and their support system if they become dependent. A long-standing myth in society is that families are alienated from their older family members and abandon their care to institutions. Nothing could be further from the truth. Family relationships remain strong in old age, and most older adults have frequent contact with their families. The majority of older adults possess a large intergenerational web of significant people, including sons, daughters, stepchildren, in-laws, nieces, nephews, grandchildren, great-grandchildren, and partners and former partners of their offspring. Families provide the majority of care for older adults. Changes in family structure will have a significant impact on the availability of family members to provide care for older adults in the future.

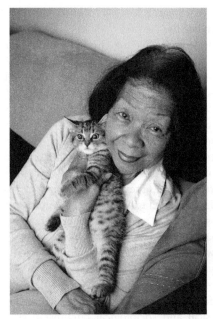

Pets are a part of the family and are particularly beneficial to older adults. They provide companionship, comfort, and caring. (©iStock.com/michellegibson.)

As families change, the roles of family members or expectations of one another also may change. Grandparents may assume parental roles for their grandchildren if their children are unable to care for them, or grandparents and older aunts and uncles may assume temporary caregiving roles while the children, nieces, and nephews work. Adult children of any age may provide limited or extensive caregiving to their own parents or aging relatives who may become ill or impaired. A spouse, sibling, or grandchild also may become a caregiver.

Close-knit families are more aware of the needs of their members and work to resolve problems and find ways to meet the needs of members, even if they are not always successful. Emotionally distant families are less available in times of need and have greater potential for conflict. If the family has never been close and supportive, it will not magically become so when members grow older. Resentments long buried may crop up and produce friction or psychological pain. Long-submerged conflicts and feelings may return if the needs of one family member exceed those of the others. In coming to know the older adult, the gerontological nurse also comes to know the family, learning of their special gifts and their life challenges. The nurse works with the older adult within the unique culture of the adult's family of origin, present family, and support networks, including friends.

Types of Families
Traditional Couples

The marital or partnered relationship in the United States is a critical source of support for older adults, and more than half of noninstitutionalized older adults live with their spouse or partner. The proportion of older adults living with their spouse decreases with age, especially for women. Almost half of women 75 years and older live alone. Men who survive their spouse into old age ordinarily have multiple opportunities to remarry if they wish. Even among the oldest-old, the majority of men are married. A woman is less likely to have an opportunity for remarriage in late life.

Often older couples live together but do not marry because of economic and inheritance reasons. An increasing number of adults age 50 years and older are in cohabitating relationships, and the rate of cohabitation has risen 75% since 2007. The rising number of cohabiters often coincides with rising divorce rates among this group. Most cohabiters age 50 and older have previously been married, including a majority who are divorced. "Older adults have a rich marital history that reflects the diverse experience of long commitment, loss via divorce or widowhood, and new partnerships as they age" (US Census Bureau, 2021).

The needs, tasks, and expectations of couples in late life differ from those in earlier years. Some couples have been married for more than 60 or 70 years. These years together may have been filled with love and companionship or abuse and resentment, or anything in between. However, in general, marital status (or the presence of a longtime partner) is positively related to health, life satisfaction, and well-being. For all couples, the normal physical and sociological circumstances in later life present challenges. Some of the issues that strain many of these relationships include (1) the deteriorating health of one or both partners; (2) limitations in income; (3) conflicts with children or other relatives; (4) incompatible sexual needs; and (5) mismatched needs for activity and socialization.

Divorce. In the past, divorce was considered a stigmatizing event. Today, however, it is so common that a person is inclined to forget the ostracizing effects of divorce from years ago. Less than 1 in 10 persons who got divorced in 1990 were age 50 or older. Since then, the gray divorce rate (divorces among older adults age 50 and older) has increased twofold (Brown & Wright, 2019). Older couples are becoming less likely to stay in an unsatisfactory marriage, and with the aging of the baby boomers, divorce rates will continue to rise. Another reason why gray divorce has increased is because a larger proportion of today's older adults are in remarriages, which have a higher risk of divorce than first marriages.

For individuals 65 to 74 years of age, the divorce rate is 39% (higher than for the general population). For adults over the age of 75 years, the divorce rate is lower at 24%. Research indicates that many late-life (gray) divorcees have grown unsatisfied with their marriages over the years and are seeking opportunities to pursue their own interests and independence for the remaining years of their lives (US Census Bureau, 2021). Health care professionals must avoid making assumptions and be alert to the possibility of marital dissatisfaction among older adults. Nurses should ask, "How would you describe your marriage?"

Long-term relationships are varied and complex, with many factors forming the glue that holds them together. Marital breakdown may be more devastating in older adults because it is often unanticipated and may occur concurrently with other significant losses. Nurses and other health care professionals must be concerned with supporting a client's decision to seek a divorce and with assisting the client in seeking counseling during the transition. Divorce initiates a grieving process similar to the death of a spouse, and a severe disruption in coping capacity may occur until the individual adjusts to a new life.

The grief may be more difficult to cope with because no socially sanctioned patterns have been established. In addition, tax and fiscal policies favor married couples, and many divorced older women are at a serious economic disadvantage in retirement.

LGBTQ+ Families

As the variations in families grow, so do the types of coupled relationships. LGBT is the most commonly known term to describe sexual and gender orientation, but as we learn more, newer descriptions have evolved to be more inclusive. LGBTQ+ is an initialism that means lesbian, gay, bisexual, transgender, queer, or questioning. The "plus" (+) is used to signify all gender identities and sexual orientations that are not specifically covered by the other five initials. The term *LGBT* also appears in this chapter, since it is a more commonly known term and more data on these identities and orientations are available at present, but nurses need to be aware of the full range of gender and sexual orientation and coupled relationships among the growing numbers of older adults.

Although the number of LGBTQ+ people of any age has remained elusive given the reluctance many have about disclosing their status, an estimated 2.7 million Americans older than 60 years of age are LGBT, with projections that this figure will increase to 10 million by 2030 (Wardecker & Matsick, 2020). It is important to recognize that there are considerable differences in the experiences of younger LGBT individuals when compared with those who are older. Older LGBT individuals did not have the benefit of antidiscrimination laws and support for same-sex partners and are more likely to have kept their relationships hidden than those who grew up in the modern-day gay liberation movement. Those LGBT older adults who came out to family members and faced the negative consequences of becoming estranged from their families of origin often created "families of choice," or chosen families. Chosen families involve individuals who are chosen to play a significant role in the life of the individual even though they are not biologically or legally related. Families of choice usually include partners, friends, coworkers, neighbors, and ex-partners—individuals who provide the same supportive functions as would be expected from one's family of origin.

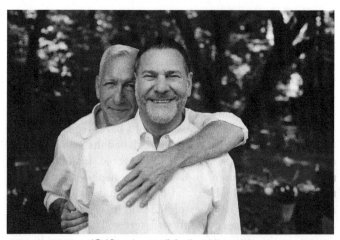

(© iStock.com/Marilyn Nieves.)

Most LGBT adults older than age 60 are single because the ability to legally marry is a recent occurrence. Many have been part of a live-in couple at some time during their life, but as they age, they are more likely to live alone. Gay and bisexual men older than age 50 are twice as likely as heterosexual men of the same age to live alone, whereas older lesbian and bisexual women are about one-third more likely to live alone. Approximately one-third of lesbian women "come out" after age 50. Many lesbian individuals married, raised children, divorced, and led double lives.

Transgender and bisexual individuals are less likely to "be out." In the case of transgender individuals, medical providers for many years required candidates for sex reassignment surgery to divorce their spouses, move to a new place, and construct a false personal history consistent with their new gender expression. These practices resulted in transgender people losing even more of their social and personal support systems than might otherwise have been the case.

Some LGBT individuals may have developed social networks of friends, members of their family of origin, and the larger community, but many lack support. Because many LGBT couples may have no or fewer children, they will have fewer caregivers as they age. However, many same-sex couples are choosing to have families, and this will necessitate greater understanding of these "new" types of families, young and old. The majority of research has involved gay and lesbian couples, and much less is known about bisexual and transgender relationships. Much more knowledge of cohort, cultural, and generational differences among age groups is needed to understand the dramatic changes in the lives of LGBT individuals in family lifestyles.

Coming to know LGBTQ+ individuals will assist nurses in providing more culturally competent, holistic care by addressing specific health issues faced by this population. "It is important for health care providers to not only understand the risk and stress associated with LGBTQ+ health disparities but also to learn more about how LGBTQ+ individuals live, socialize, and build relationships with others" (Wardecker & Matsick, 2020, p. 6). Nurse researchers are encouraged to consider study designs, methods, and procedures that support inclusion and visibility of LGBTQ+ older adults. Organizations that serve LGBTQ+ older adults in the community need to enhance outreach and support mechanisms to enable them to maintain independence and age safely and in good health. Box 32.5 includes resources for LGBTQ+ older adults.

Older Adults and Their Adult Children

In adulthood, relationships between the generations become increasingly important for most people. Older parents enjoy being told about the various activities and successes of their offspring, and these adult children begin to see aspects of themselves that have developed from their parents. At times, the relationships may become strained because the younger adults are more concerned with their own spouses, partners, and children. The parents are no longer central to their lives, though offspring may be central to the lives of their parents. The most difficult situations occur when the parents are openly

---

BOX 32.5 Resources for Best Practice
Caregiving, Family, LGBT?

Administration for Community Living: National family caregiver support program. https://acl.gov/programs/support-caregivers/national-family-caregiver-support-program.

Alzheimer's Association: Care training resources, e-learning workshops, DVDs, online care training for dementia care and certification for professionals, Respite Care Guide, Free online caregiver community. https://www.alz.org/help-support/caregiving.

Caregiver Action Network: Caregiver Help Line, Caregiver Toolkit, resources, education. https://www.caregiveraction.org/.

Diverse Elders Coalition: Caring for those who care, resources for providers: meeting the needs of diverse family caregivers. https://www.diverseelders.org/caregiving/.

Family Caregiver Alliance: Resources, education. https://www.caregiver.org/.

Grandfamilies.org: National legal resource in support of grandfamilies within and outside the child welfare system. https://grandfamilies.org/.

Lesbian and Gay Aging Issues Network (LGAIN): A constituent group of the American Society on Aging that works to raise awareness about the concerns of LGBT older adults and the unique barriers they encounter in gaining access to housing, health care, long-term care, and other needed services. https://www.asaging.org/education-topic/lgbtq-aging.

National Alliance for Caregiving: International resources and best practices in caregiving. https://www.caregiving.org/.

National Resource Center on LGBT Aging: Technical assistance resource center aimed at improving the quality of services and supports offered to LGBT older adults. https://www.lgbtagingcenter.org/.

Services and Advocacy for Gay, Lesbian, Bisexual, and Transgender Elders (SAGE). https://www.sageusa.org/your-rights-resources/health-care/.

---

critical or judgmental about the lives of their offspring. In the best of situations, adult children shift to the role of friend, companion, and confidant to the older adult, a concept known as filial maturity.

By and large, older adults and their children have relationships that are reciprocal in nature and characterized by affection and mutual support. These relationships are both the most important and potentially the most conflicted. Family resources are shared from birth and usually in some way until and after death. These resources may be tangible, such as money, belongings, and housing. Intangible resources may include advice, support, guidance, and day-to-day assistance with life. Older adults provide a family history perspective, models for growing old, assistance with grandchildren, a sense of continuity, and a philosophy of aging.

Most older adults see their children on a regular basis, and even children who do not live close to their older parents maintain close connections, so *"intimacy at a distance"* can occur. Nine in ten older adults living with others say they are in contact with their children at least weekly and about 4 in 10 say they communicate with their children on a daily basis (Stepler, 2016). New technologies, such as cell phones and the internet, make it possible for family members to be in almost constant communication with one another, regardless of their physical location.

Never-Married Older Adults

The number of adults who have never married is increasing in the United States. Older adults who have lived alone most of their lives often develop supportive networks with siblings, friends, and neighbors. Never-married older adults may demonstrate resilience to the challenges of aging as a result of their independence and may not feel lonely or isolated. Furthermore, they may have had longer lifetime employment and may enjoy greater financial security as they age. Single older adults will increase in the future because being single is increasingly more common in younger years.

Grandparents

The role of grandparenting, and increasingly great-grandparenting, is experienced by most older adults. The numbers of grandparents are at record highs and still growing at more than twice the overall population growth rate. Most Americans (83%) age 65 years and older have grandchildren. Of these grandparents, two-thirds have at least four grandchildren. Seventy-two percent think that being a grandparent is the single most important and satisfying thing in their life (American Association of Retired Persons [AARP], 2019). Great-grandparenthood will become more common in the future in light of projections of healthier aging.

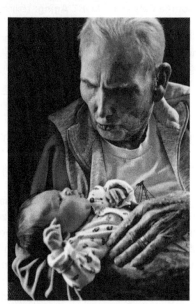

The author's grandson and his maternal great-grandfather. (Photo courtesy Ben Aronoff, Fogline Studios.)

As the term implies, the "grands" are a step beyond parents in their concerns, exposure, and responsibility. The majority of grandparents derive great emotional satisfaction from their grandchildren. Historically, the emphasis has been on the progressive aging of the grandparent as it affects the relationship with the grandchild, but little has been said about the effects of the growth and maturation of the grandchild on the relationship. Many young adults who have had close contact with their grandparents report that this relationship was very meaningful in their lives. Growing numbers of adult grandchildren are assisting in caregiving for their grandparents.

The age, vitality, and proximity of both grandchild and grandparent produce a kaleidoscope of possible activities and interactions as both progress through their aging processes. Grandparents are in frequent contact with their grandchildren, with 60% in contact on at least a weekly basis (Stepler, 2016). Geographic distance does not significantly affect the quality of the relationship between grandparents and their grandchildren. The internet is increasingly being used by distant grandparents as a way of staying involved in their grandchildren's lives and forging close bonds.

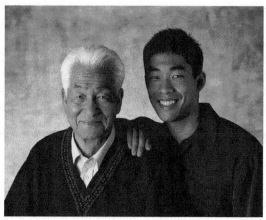

Grandparenting is an important role for older adults. (Copyright © Getty Images.)

Younger grandparents typically live closer to their grandchildren and are more involved in childcare and recreational activities (Box 32.6). Older grandparents with sufficient incomes may provide more financial assistance and other types of instrumental help. Grandparent-headed households are one of the fastest-growing US family groups, and this phenomenon is also taking place in other countries. Approximately 27 million grandparents are responsible for raising their grandchildren in the United States (Taylor et al., 2017). This phenomenon is discussed later in the chapter.

Siblings

Late-life sibling relationships are poorly understood and have been neglected by researchers. As individuals age, they often have more contact with siblings than they did in the years when family and work demands were more pressing. About 80% of older adults have at least one sibling, and they are often strong sources of support in the lives of never-married older adults, widowed persons, and those without children. For many older adults, these relationships become increasingly important

---

BOX 32.6   A Grandmother as Seen by an 8-Year-Old Child

"A grandmother is a woman who has no children of her own. That is why she loves other people's children."

"Grandmothers have nothing to do. They are just there: when they take us for a walk they go slowly, like caterpillars along beautiful leaves. They never say, 'Come on, faster, hurry up!'"

"Everyone should try to have a grandmother, especially those who don't have a TV."

because they have a long history of memories and are of the same generation and similar backgrounds. Sibling relationships become particularly important when they are part of the support system, especially among single or widowed older adults living alone.

The strongest of sibling bonds is thought to be the relationship between sisters. When blessed with survival, these relationships remain important into late old age. Service providers should inquire about sibling relationships of past and present significance. The loss of siblings has a profound effect in terms of awareness of one's own mortality, particularly when those of the same gender die. When an older adult reaches the age of the sibling who died, the reaction can be quite disruptive. Not only is grieving activated, but also rehearsal for one's own death may occur. In some cases in which an older sibling survives younger ones, there may be not only a deep grief but also pangs of guilt: "Why them and not me?" (Chapter 34).

Fictive Kin

Fictive kin are nonblood kin who serve as "genuine fake families," as expressed by noted gerontologist Virginia Satir. These nonrelatives become surrogate family and take on some of the instrumental and affectional attributes of family. Fictive kin are important in the lives of many older adults, especially those with no close or satisfying family relationships and those living alone or in institutions. Fictive kin includes both friends and often paid caregivers. Primary care providers, such as nursing assistants, nurses, or case managers, often become fictive kin. Professionals who work with older adults need to recognize the instrumental and emotional support, and the mutually satisfying relationships, that occur between friends, neighbors, and other fictive kin who assist older adults who are dependent.

CAREGIVING

There are four kinds of people in the world: those who have been caregivers, those who are currently caregivers, those who will be caregivers, and those who will need caregivers.
(Rosalyn Carter, Alzheimer's Reading Room, 2013)

Family caregiving has become a normative experience (similar to marriage, working, or retirement) for many American families. Gerontological nurses are most likely to encounter older adults with their family and friends in situations relating to caregiving of some kind. Informal caregivers (family members and other unpaid caregivers) provide the majority of care for older adults in the United States. Caregiving occurs among all generations, racial and ethnic groups, income or educational levels, family types, gender identities, and sexual orientations. The shifts we do see in caregiver demographics reflect general changes in the demographic composition of the US population.

Three in five caregivers are women (61%) and two in five are men (39%). Six in ten caregivers report being non-Hispanic White (61%); 17% are Hispanic or Latino; 14% are non-Hispanic Black; 5% are Asian American or Pacific Islander; and 3% are some other race or ethnicity, including multiracial. Thirty-two percent

of informal caregivers are caring for a parent, and 36% are caring for a spouse. Most caregivers take care of a relative (89%), whereas just 10% care for a friend, neighbor, or other nonrelative. At any given point, about 6% of adult children are providing care for a parent, but about 17% will provide care at some point in their lives.

Who is being cared for is driven greatly by the age of the caregiver, with older caregivers caring more for peers (spouse or partner, siblings, nonrelatives) and younger caregivers caring more for an older generation (parents, grandparents). There has been a shift in residence over the past 5 years, in which more caregivers report that their care recipient lives with them, the caregiver, instead of living in the recipient's own home. Many caregivers are also employed outside the home and often face great stressors in trying to manage jobs and families while caring for a parent (AARP, 2020).

> ### ♥ HEALTHY PEOPLE 2030
>
> - Help parents and caregivers improve health and well-being for their loved ones
> - Reduce anxiety and depression in family caregivers of people with disabilities
> - Reduce the proportion of unpaid caregivers of older adults who report an unmet need for caregiver support services

Data from US Department of Health and Human Services: *Healthy People 2030* (website), 2020. https://health.gov/healthypeople.

Family structures have changed, as have family caregiving networks. It is important for nurses to understand the complexity of caregiving and the many forms it may take. Defining caregiving as a dyad of a caregiver and care recipient does not reflect today's patterns of caregiving. (Family caregivers provide more than 80% of all long-term care services in the United States. Informal care provided by caregivers is universally recognized as the foundation of the long-term care system. Informal caregivers basically provide free services to care recipients. It would cost an estimated $470 billion to replace the care that family caregivers provide, more than the amount of total Medicaid spending (Family Caregiver Alliance, 2019). Without family caregivers, the present level of long-term care provision could not be sustained. Healthy People 2030 includes objectives for care-giver health.

Caregiving is considered a major public health issue across the globe, and attention to the physical and mental health of caregivers is receiving increased attention. Due to demographic changes, the demand for family caregivers of adults over the age of 65 years is increasing significantly, but we do not have an eldercare system properly equipped to support them (Eldercare Workforce Alliance, 2018). Current trends suggest that the use of paid, formal care by older adults in the community has been decreasing, while their sole reliance on family caregivers has been increasing. The need for family caregivers will increase substantially, but the number of family caregivers who are available to provide care is also decreasing substantially. The "caregiver support ratio" will start to drop when the first baby boomers begin to turn 80 years old in 2026, and by 2050 the ratio will fall to less than three potential caregivers for every

BOX 32.7   **Facts About Caregiving**

- Family caregivers are children (41.3%), spouses (38.4%), and other family and friends (20.4%).
- The average duration of a caregiver's role is 4.6 years.
- Sixty-six percent of caregivers are female, and their average age is 48. Older caregivers are more likely to care for a spouse or partner; their average age is 63 years, and one-third of them are in poor health.
- The number of male caregivers is smaller but increasing, and continued research is needed to address their unique needs. Among spousal caregivers 75 years and older, both sexes provide equal amounts of care.
- Between 12% and 18% of the total adult caregivers in the United States are estimated to be between the ages of 18 and 24, a group known as emerging adults, and they have many of the same caregiving responsibilities as older adults.
- About 43.5 million adult family caregivers care for someone who has Alzheimer's disease or other dementia. They provide care an average of 1 to 4 years more than caregivers of individuals with other illnesses.
- Almost half of lesbian, gay, bisexual, and transgender (LGBT) older adults provide caregiving assistance to families or origin or families of choice.
- More than 2.7 million grandparents are providing primary care (custodial grandparents) for grandchildren in the United States, and grandparent-headed households are one of the fastest-growing US family groups.
- Caregiving can have serious negative effects on mental and physical health. Approximately 40% to 70% of caregivers have clinically significant symptoms of depression.
- Caregiving also can present financial burdens, and women who are family caregivers are 2.5 times more likely than noncaregivers to live in poverty.

Data from American Association of Retired Persons: *Caregiving in the United States* (website), 2020. https://www.aarp.org/ppi/info-2020/caregiving-in-the-united-states.html. Accessed May 2021.

person 80 years and older (Feinberg & Levine, 2015–2016). In addition, there is a growing shortage of formal caregivers (nursing assistants, licensed practical nurses [LPNs], and registered nurses [RNs]) for long-term care services across the continuum (Chapter 1).

Some suggest that the conception of caregiving is different among the baby boomer generation. Although they recognize their responsibility to care for ill family members, they view themselves as partners in the organization of care and want to negotiate and set limits to the amount and kind of care they wish to undertake. This will require the existence of alternative resources to family care and policy and practice that no longer takes family caregiving for granted. Baby boomer caregivers and upcoming generations will expect more support and formal assistance from national and local agencies in a coordinated long-term care network (Chapter 6) (Box 32.7).

Caregiving in the LGBTQ+ Community

Caregiving in the LGBTQ+ community follows a different pattern. Nine percent of caregivers self-identify as LGBTQ+, and LGBTQ+ older adults largely care for each other. Spouses, partners, and friends provide almost 90% of the care received by LGBTQ+ older adults. The pattern reflects the importance of a "chosen family" in the lives of these older adults. However, LGBTQ+ baby boomers and millennials also take care of their aging parents at a disproportionate rate (National Resource Center on LGBT Aging, 2021). "These chosen families provide

care to the LGBTQ+ older adult, but they often go unrecognized and are not provided with adequate information to care for patients or not acknowledged as caregivers in medical settings. Nurses need to give them the support, assistance, and information they need to provide proper care to their loved one" (Wardecker & Johnston, 2018, pp. 2–3). These patterns may change for future generations of LGBTQ+ older adults who have had the benefits of marriage equality, greater social acceptance, and having children. The concern over encountering anti-LGBT bias increases the demand for informal caregiving because LGBTQ+ older adults will go to great lengths to avoid entering senior housing and are often determined to age in place at all costs. They are also less likely to access supportive in-home services because of fear of discrimination and bias. In comparison with heterosexual adults, only 20% of LGBTQ+ older adults were likely to access services such as senior centers or meal programs (Henriquez et al., 2019). Many LGBTQ+ caregivers and patients feel that their relationships with providers would be jeopardized by revealing their sexual orientation (Messecar, 2021). In a number of areas across the country, LGBTQ+ community members have launched efforts to create home care services, senior housing, and retirement communities specifically designed with their needs in mind. Many of these projects are still in development stages and are primarily designed for affluent individuals. Hopefully, as the community continues to advocate on behalf of LGBTQ+ seniors, a greater variety of housing options ultimately will be available. Local and national LGBTQ+ organizations can be a vital resource in locating community agencies that are sensitive and supportive.

Impact of Caregiving

Although caregiving is a means to "give back" to a loved one and can be a source of joy in the giving, it is also stressful. "Caregiving is a very complex issue, and assuming a caregiving role is a time of transition that requires a restructuring of one's goals, behaviors, and responsibilities. It requires taking on something new, but it is also about loss—of what was and what could have been" (Lund, 2005, p. 152). Caregivers are considered *"the hidden patient"* (Schulz & Beach, 1999, p. 2216).

Family caregiving has been associated with increased levels of depression and anxiety, poorer self-reported physical health, compromised immune function, higher rates of insomnia, increased alcohol use, and increased mortality. Caregiver burden encompasses physical, psychological, emotional, relational, social, and financial problems due to caregiving (Pristavec, 2018). Unrelieved caregiver stress increases the potential for abuse and neglect (Chapter 31).

The characteristics of ethnic minority caregivers needs further research, but studies show that these groups provide more care, provide higher-intensity care, and report worse physical health than White caregivers. In addition, formal services are not often used by ethnic minority caregivers, which puts them at further risk for negative outcomes (Messecar, 2021). Service providers need to enhance cultural competence and design programs that are culturally acceptable (Chapter 4). The Diverse Elders Coalition (2021) provides resources and online training to assist in better meeting the needs of diverse family caregivers (see Box 32.5).

Another group of caregivers who have not been studied sufficiently are younger-age caregivers. Millennials, the generation born between 1980 and 1996, represent about 10 million of the total 40 million unpaid caregivers in the United States, a number that is expected to sharply increase as the population of adults over the age of 65 doubles over the next generation. Millennials and other young caregivers are often referred to as an invisible or unrecognized group (Benjamin Rose Institute on Aging, 2019). Recent studies have found that these caregivers are more prone to depressive symptoms and burden from caregiving. Seventy-nine percent of millennial caregivers report that emotional distress is a major burden for them (Messecar, 2021). The number of younger-age caregivers is increasing, but programs to assist caregivers generally have not been designed to address their needs. Programs for caregivers and research on caregiving needs should include diverse groups of all ages.

Caregiving can be both rewarding and distressing, generating feelings of both benefit and burden for some caregivers; even with high burden, caregivers may experience high benefits. For caregivers, positive emotions often coexist with feelings of isolation, stress, or strain. Half of caregivers feel that their role as a caregiver gives them a sense of purpose or meaning in life (AARP, 2020). Caregivers experiencing benefits have better mental health and continue in the caregiving role for longer than those experiencing burden (Pristavec, 2018). Positive benefits of caregiving may include enhanced self-esteem and well-being, personal growth and satisfaction, and finding or making meaning through caregiving.

Caregiving is more likely to be perceived as rewarding if the caregiver feels needed and useful, has a close and reciprocal relationship with the care recipient, believes that the help is appreciated by the care recipient, and has an adequate support network (Monin et al., 2017). "A national sample of caregivers reported that Hispanic and Black caregivers experienced more positive rewards from caregiving, indicating that rewards are perceived or experienced quite differently by caregivers from different backgrounds or distinct demographic groups" (Messecar, 2021, p. 189). The positive benefits of caregiving have been given more attention in recent years, but further research is needed to help understand what factors influence how caregivers perceive the experience across cultures and groups and how assistance programs can focus on increasing the perception of benefits (Pristavec, 2018). Boxes 32.8 and 32.9 present further information on caregiver needs and tips for reducing stress.

Patricia Archbold et al. (1990) studied caregiving as a role and examined how the relationships between the caregiver and care recipient (mutuality) and the preparation of the caregiver for the tasks and stresses of caregiving (preparedness) influence reactions to caregiving. Most caregivers are not prepared for the many responsibilities they face and receive no formal instruction in caregiving activities. Lack of preparedness can greatly increase the caregiver's stress. Caregivers who report a high level of preparedness for caregiving experience lower levels

---

BOX 32.8 Circumstances Associated With Caregiver Stress

- Competing role responsibilities (e.g., work, home)
- Advanced age of the caregiver
- High-intensity caregiving need
- Insufficient resources
- Financial difficulty
- Poor self-reported health
- Living in the same household with the care recipient
- Dementia of the care recipient
- Length of time caregiving
- Prior relational conflicts between the caregiver and care recipient

---

BOX 32.9 Tips for Best Practice

Reducing Caregiver Stress

- Educate yourself about the disease or medical condition.
- Contact the appropriate disease-related organization to learn about resources and education and support groups to help you adapt to the challenges you encounter.
- Find a health care professional who understands the disease.
- Consult with other experts (legal, financial) to help plan for the future.
- Tap your social resources for assistance.
- Take time for relaxation and exercise.
- Use community resources.
- Maintain your sense of humor.
- Explore religious beliefs and spiritual values.
- Participate in pleasant, nurturing activities such as reading a good book or taking a warm bath.
- Seek supportive counseling when you need it.
- Identify and acknowledge your feelings; you have a right to ALL of them.
- Set realistic goals.
- Attend to your own health care needs.

Data from Mayo Clinic: *Caregiver stress: tips for taking care of yourself* (website), 2020. https://www.mayoclinic.org/healthy-lifestyle/stress-management/in-depth/caregiver-stress/art-20044784.

---

of caregiver strain after hospitalization of older adults and during cancer care and treatment (Zwicker, 2018). Further research is needed to understand the complexities of the caregiving and care-receiving role and provide a theory base for nursing actions.

Caregiving of Individuals With Neurocognitive Disorders

Caregivers of individuals with neurocognitive disorders (NCDs) provide more intensive help than caregivers of individuals without an NCD and experience greater financial, emotional, and physical challenges (Gaugler et al., 2017). Services for individuals with NCDs used to be primarily institutional, such as in nursing homes, but now more than two-thirds to three-quarters of individuals with NCD live in the community (Lepore & Wiener, 2017). Factors that increase the stress of caregiving for an individual with a NCD include grief over the multiple losses that occur, the physical demands and duration of caregiving (up to 20 years), communication difficulties,

RESEARCH HIGHLIGHTS

Maintaining Caring Relationships in Spouses Affected by Alzheimer's Disease

PERSONAL REFLECTIONS OF THE RESEARCHER

My interest in dementia developed with participation in a project to improve content on the care of older adults in nursing curricula. Later I witnessed a family member with Alzheimer's disease struggling to maintain a close marital relationship and was moved to investigate approaches to support couples. The effects of Alzheimer's disease and related dementias (AD) on marital relationships can be devastating for both partners. In individuals with dementia, communication abilities decline as the AD progresses. Without communication, marital intimacy is replaced by loneliness, frustration, and estrangement.

Purpose

The purpose of the study was to evaluate the effects of the CARE intervention (Communicating About Relationships and Emotions) on the quality of communication between spouse caregivers and their partners with AD. The sample included 15 couples living at home in South Florida. One partner had moderate-stage AD and the other self-identified as the caregiver.

Method

The researchers met with couples weekly at their homes for 10 weeks. The CARE intervention included a manual covering common AD communication challenges and coaching in applying effective communication strategies. Caregiver spouses learned to focus on valuing partners' contributions to conversation. They practiced responding to their partners' communication difficulties with empathy and facilitating participation in conversation. Spouses with AD practiced social behaviors such as making eye contact and expressing relationship-focused thoughts and feelings. At the end of each session, couples were asked to converse about a topic of their choosing, and the conversations were video recorded. Recordings were later analyzed for changes in communication behavior over time

Results

The analysis showed that caregivers' spouses learned to avoid communication that blocked further conversation. For example, they learned that questions such as "Don't you remember?" seemed like criticism and discouraged conversation, whereas questions such as "What do you think?" demonstrated caregivers' willingness to engage.

Conclusion

Nurses encounter couples like the study participants in many health care situations and can use these opportunities to assess communication quality and promote spouses' engagement with one another. Caregivers could be taught to communicate in a clear, respectful, and effective way. Some techniques include staying in the moment or talking about the past, avoiding testing their loved one's memory or arguing, and conversing patiently even if their partner was not always responsive. Both spouses improved their communication.

Williams CL, Newman D, Hammer LM: Preliminary study of a communication intervention for family caregivers and spouses with dementia, *Int J Geriatr Psychiatry* 33(2):e343–349, 2018; Williams CL: Maintaining caring relationships in spouses affected by Alzheimer's disease, *Int J Human Caring* 19(3):12–18, 2015.

The effects of NCDs on marital relationships can be devastating for both partners and lead to loneliness, frustration, and estrangement. Nursing actions to help couples strengthen their bond as a couple to maintain a sense of well-being are important (Swall et al., 2019). Enhancing communication between spousal caregivers and their loved one with a NCD has been investigated by nurse researcher Dr. Christine Williams. In the Research Highlights box, Dr. Williams discusses her innovative research. Results of the study showed that caregivers could be taught to communicate in a clear, respectful, and effective way—and the spouse with a NCD could improve. Some techniques included staying in the moment or talking about the past, avoiding testing their loved one's memory or arguing, and conversing patiently even if the partner was not always responsive.

Spousal Caregiving

Eighty percent of older adults who live with spouses with disabilities provide care for them. More wives than husbands provide care, but this is changing as the life expectancy for men increases. Caregiving spouses experience more mental and physical health problems from their caregiving; provide more intensive, time-consuming care than other family caregivers; and are less likely to receive assistance from other family members (Polenick & DePasquale, 2019). Older spouses often take on greater burden than they can reasonably handle and get by with significantly less help in the home than other types of caregivers, yet their responsibilities increase over time (Park, 2017). Spousal caregivers who perceive a great deal of strain are almost two times more likely to die than caregivers reporting some strain (Perkins et al., 2013).

Older spouses caring for partners who are ill also face many role changes. Older women may need to learn to drive, manage money, or make decisions by themselves. Male caregivers may need to learn how to cook, shop, do laundry, and provide personal care to their wives. Spousal caregivers also deal with the added responsibilities of caregiving while at the same time dealing with the anticipated loss of their spouse. Nurses should be alert to situations in which health care personnel may be able to provide supports and resources that make it possible for an individual to assume new responsibilities without being totally overwhelmed. Adult day programs, respite care services, or periodic assistance from a home health aide or homemaker may make it possible for the couple to continue to live together and ease the strain of caregiving. It is important to pay attention to the physical and mental health needs of the caregiver and those of the care recipient.

Aging Parents Caring for Adult Children With Intellectual and Developmental Disabilities

Although we tend to think of caregivers as middle-aged adults caring for older adults, an unknown number of older adults are caring for their middle-aged children with intellectual and developmental disabilities (I/DDs). In the past century, children with I/DDs were typically in institutions and usually died before reaching adulthood. Today, about 75% of adults with I/DDs

and a lack of resource availability. Demands are intensified if the care recipient demonstrates behavioral disturbances and impairments in activities of daily living (ADLs) and instrumental activities of daily living (IADLs) (Gaugler et al., 2017; Chapter 26).

now live with their parents or other family members, and more than 25% live with parents age 60 years and older (Baumbusch et al., 2017). For the first time in history, individuals with I/DDs are outliving their parents, and planning for their future is an area posing challenges for older adults and for service providers internationally.

With increased survival, adults with I/DDs are also at risk for developing chronic illnesses and will need more care and services. For example, individuals with Down syndrome are more likely to develop dementia. Often the burden of caring for a child with an I/DD has been carried by parents for their entire adult life and will end only with the death of the parent or the adult child. Parental caregivers who are aging face changes in their financial resources and health that affect their continued caregiving ability.

A majority of these caregivers worry how their child will receive care if they develop a debilitating illness or die. A study done by Baumbusch et al. (2017) reported that aging parents were increasingly aware of their own aging process and the implications for their ability to continue providing care. They were fostering connections with both informal and formal sources of care that could supplement or replace their care activities. It was important to shift their care activities from providing physical support to a focus on social and economic support and communicating their intimate knowledge of their relative with an I/DD to others who could provide care in the future. Engaging in conversations and planning for end-of-life care was a major challenge and depended to a certain extent on their relative's understanding of death and dying and their emotional readiness to live without their main care provider.

In the United States, the Planned Lifetime Assistance Network (PLAN), available in some states through the National Alliance for the Mentally Ill, provides lifetime assistance to individuals with disabilities whose parents or other family members are deceased or can no longer provide for their care. The Alzheimer's Association and other aging organizations offer education and support programs for both parents and their developmentally disabled adult children in some communities. There is a continued need for the development of both in-home and community options for developmentally disabled adults who are aging. In addition, there is a need for research exploring the experience of aging families caring for adult children with I/DDs.

Grandparents Raising Grandchildren

Over the past decade grandparents have assumed the primary caregiving responsibility for their grandchildren at an unprecedented rate. Global figures indicate that grandparents represent the majority of all kinship carers and are the largest providers of formal childcare between birth and 12 years of age (McLaughlin et al., 2017). More than 2.7 million grandparents are providing primary care (custodial grandparents) for grandchildren in the United States, and grandparent-headed households are one of the fastest-growing US family groups. A large number of grandparents provide care to multiple grandchildren simultaneously, and more than 36% have done so for more than 5 years. Grandparent caregivers are more prevalent in Latinx and Black communities, and White families have the lowest proportion of grandparent-headed families (Generations United, 2020).

The reasons why grandparents take a child into the home without the child's parents vary among countries, groups, and individuals. Many grandparents have become, by default, the primary caregivers of grandchildren because the parents are unable to provide the care needed as a result of child abuse, teen pregnancy, imprisonment, joblessness, military deployment, drug and alcohol addictions, illness, death, and other social problems. Drug addiction, especially to opioids, is behind much of the rise in the number of grandparents raising their grandchildren (Generations Now, 2020).

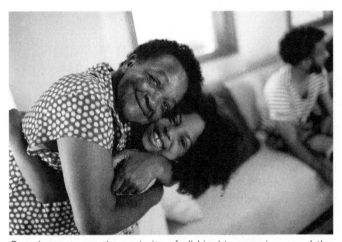

Grandparents are the majority of all kinship caregivers and the largest providers of formal childcare between birth and 12 years of age. (© iStock.com/FG Trade.)

Research related to the effect of grandparent caregiving on health status is lacking, but existing literature suggests that there are economic, health, and social challenges inherent in this role. About 25% of grandparent-headed households and more than half of grandmothers raising grandchildren live in poverty. Approximately 57% of grandparent caregivers experience depression. Often crisis situations precipitate the decision of a grandparent to assume caring for a grandchild, and time for preparation is not available. In many cases, grandparents assume care so that their grandchildren's care is not taken over by the public care system. However, many custodial grandparents are not licensed in the foster care system and are not eligible for the same services and financial support as licensed foster parents.

As with other types of caregiving, there are both blessings and burdens, and caregivers' experiences will be unique. For many grandparents, the challenges may include limited income and financial support through the welfare system, lack of informal support systems, loss of leisure activities in retirement, and shame or guilt related to their children's inability to parent (McLaughlin et al., 2017). Physical and mental stressors appear to be greater when grandparents are raising a child with a chronic illness or special needs or behavioral problems. Many of the grandchildren being cared for have a history of trauma (physical or sexual abuse, neglect, abandonment, domestic violence, exposure to violent crime and illegal activity associated with substance abuse), which complicates the challenges faced by grandparent caregivers.

Despite facing many barriers, research shows that the children in grandfamilies thrive. The benefits for the children cared for by grandparents are better than for children in non-relative care and include increased stability, greater safety, better behavioral and mental health outcomes, more positive feelings about placements, more likely to report that they "always felt loved," more likely to live with or stay connected to siblings, and greater preservation of cultural identity and community connections. Caregivers also experience benefits, such as an increased sense of purpose in life (Generations United, 2021).

USING CLINICAL JUDGMENT TO PROMOTE HEALTHY AGING: GRANDPARENT CAREGIVING

Solutions, Nursing Actions, and Outcomes

Routinely screening and monitoring the psychological distress of primary care grandparents and offering support, advice, and referral to reduce stressors are important. Currently, evidence suggests that cognitive-behavioral interventions have the most empirical support for improving grandparent caregivers' psychological well-being. Promising approaches that require further research to support their effectiveness include support groups, interdisciplinary case management, and psychoeducational interventions. Another successful service is kinship navigator programs, which provide a single point of entry for connecting to housing, household resources, physical and mental health services, and financial and legal assistance. Funding from the federal government will be used to develop, enhance, or evaluate kinship navigator programs (Administration for Children and Families, 2020). Resources to support grandparent caregivers should be available in communities and could be offered through health care institutions, schools, and churches. Web-based interventions also can be evaluated. Nurses can be instrumental in developing and conducting these types of interventions.

The Supporting Grandparents Raising Grandchildren Act, signed into law in 2018, will identify and disseminate information to help grandparents raising grandchildren address the challenges they face, such as navigating the school system, planning for their families' future, addressing mental health issues for themselves and their grandchildren, and building social and support networks. The National Family Caregiver Support Program (NFCSP), under the Older Americans Act program, provides support services, education and training, counseling, and respite care and should be encouraged in all states. Nurses can refer the grandparents to their local area agency on aging to inquire about available resources. Box 32.5 presents resources for grandparents, and suggestions for nursing actions with older

---

BOX 32.10 **Tips for Best Practice**

Nursing Actions With Grandparent Caregivers

- Early identification of at-risk grandparents
- Comprehensive assessment of physical, psychosocial, and environmental factors affecting those in the caregiving role for grandchildren
- Anticipatory guidance and counseling about child growth and development and other child-raising issues
- Referral to resources for support, counseling, and financial assistance
- Advocacy for policies supportive of grandparents who have assumed a caregiving role

---

adults who are providing primary care to their grandchildren are presented in Box 32.10.

Long-Distance Caregiving

Because of the increasing mobility of today's global society, more children move away for education or employment and do not return home. When the parent needs help, it must be provided "long distance." This is perhaps one of the most difficult situations, and it presents unique challenges. The usual impulse is to want to move the older adult into the family's home or to a more accessible location for the family, but this may not be best for the older adult or for the family (see Box 32.4).

Issues that need to be considered in long-distance caregiving include identifying a local person who will be available quickly in emergency situations; identifying reliable individuals or services that will provide daily monitoring if necessary; identifying acceptable facilities for assisted living or nursing home care if that becomes necessary; determining which family member is most likely to be free to travel to the older adult if needed; and being sure that legalities regarding advance directives, a will, and power of attorney (for health care and financial) have been established.

A profession and an industry have emerged to assist the geographically distant family member to ensure that an older relative will receive care. This profession is made up of geriatric care managers, some of whom are nurses or social workers. A care manager can be hired to do everything a family member would do if able, from being available in an emergency to helping with estate planning to making arrangements for a move to a nursing home. These services are available primarily to those who are able to pay for them because they are not covered by private insurance, Medicare, or any public agencies. Although these services are expensive, they may be far less expensive than alternative living arrangements or institutional placement (Chapter 6).

Similar services may be available for persons with very low incomes through the local Area Agency on Aging "Community Care for the Elderly" programs. When incomes are too high to qualify for Medicaid and too low to pay for private care managers, the individual and the family must do the best they can. Long-distance care then depends on the goodness of neighbors, local friends, and apartment managers and on frequent trips by the long-distance caregiver to the older adult.

USING CLINICAL JUDGMENT TO PROMOTE HEALTHY AGING: CAREGIVER HEALTH

Recognizing and Analyzing Cues

Gathering information about the family is an important component of care for older adults. Often nurses see families in times of crisis when an older family member needs care. When working with families, it is important for the nurse to be aware of their vision of what a "family" should be and what a "family" should do. Our values should not enter into the evaluation of families, and families should not be judged or labeled as dysfunctional (Feinberg & Levine, 2015–2016). It is necessary to identify the strengths within each family and to build on those strengths while recognizing the family's limitations in providing support and caregiving.

When nurses work with families from a different culture that may have unfamiliar rituals and routines, the nurses need to be particularly careful to respect these differences. Service providers need to enhance cultural competence and design programs that are culturally acceptable (Chapter 4). Thus the nurse's role is to teach, monitor, and strengthen the family system so as to maintain the health and wellness of the entire family structure.

Gathering information about a caregiving situation helps identify the specific challenges, needs, strengths, and resources of the family caregiver, and the caregiver's ability to contribute to the needs of the care recipient. Several validated caregiver assessment instruments are available, including the Preparedness for Caregiving Scale (Fig. 32.1) and the Modified Caregiver Strain Index (Fig. 32.2). The Mutuality Scale developed by Archbold et al. (1990) can be used to assess the quality of the relationship between the caregiver and the care recipient.

Although vitally important, family caregiver assessment is weak in long-term support and service programs and rare in health care settings. Caregivers report a lack of preparedness, and the majority would like more information on topics related to caregiving. Almost half of these family caregivers perform medical or nursing tasks without any preparation and few visits from home care providers (Reinhard et al., 2017). Family caregivers often perform tasks that nurses typically perform, including injections, tube feedings, operating special equipment, managing multiple medications, catheter and colostomy care, and other complex care responsibilities: "the same tasks that make nursing students tremble the first time they have to perform them" (Kennedy, 2017). Only about a third of family caregivers reported that a doctor, nurse, or social worker asked them what was needed to care for their loved one, and even fewer said that a health or social provider had asked what they needed to care for themselves (Feinberg & Levine, 2015–2016). Nurses play an important role in insuring that the family is included in plans of care for the older adult and assisted in learning to manage needed care requirements.

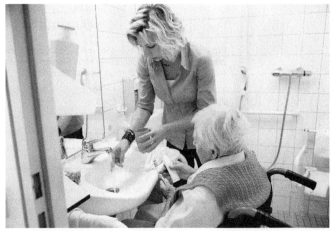
Family members provide the majority of care for older adults in the United States. Nurses play an important role in providing caregiver education and support. (© iStock.com/SilviaJansen.)

Solutions, Nursing Actions, and Outcomes

In designing actions to support caregiving, a partnership model—combining the nurse's professional expertise with the caregiver's knowledge of the family member—is recommended (Box 32.11). Given the range of caregiving situations and the uniqueness of each, interventions must be tailored to individual needs and build on the caregiver's existing strengths and resources. Actions include risk analysis, education about caregiving and stress, needed care skills, caregiver health and home safety, support groups, linkages to ongoing support, counseling, resource identification, relief or respite from daily care demands, and stress management. Education provided by nurses to help prepare the caregiver for the caregiving role, particularly at the time of discharge from the hospital or nursing home, can help prevent role strain and lessen burden. With many caregivers trying to balance caregiving responsibilities while working, educational programs offered in the workplace can be beneficial for both the caregiver and the employer (Box 32.12).

Linking caregivers to community resources, such as respite care, adult day programs, and financial support resources, is important. Respite care allows the caregiver to take a break from caregiving for various periods of time and can be one way family caregivers can take time for themselves and possibly avoid the need to relinquish their caregiving role (Roberts & Struckmeyer, 2018). Respite care may be provided in institutions, in the home, or in other community settings such as adult day service programs. However, respite care remains an important yet underused preventive resource despite it being the most commonly requested type of caregiver assistance (AARP, 2020).

Nurses should be aware of respite care resources in their communities, and the local Area Agency on Aging can provide information on respite care and other caregiver services. Some government and nonprofit agencies offer free respite help, but most respite services are paid for privately by the family. For veterans, 30 days of respite care a year is available. Respite care is covered through Medicare for individuals receiving hospice care, but Medicare allows only 5 consecutive days of benefits.

YOUR PREPARATION FOR CAREGIVING

We know that people may feel well prepared for some aspects of giving care to another person, and not as well prepared for other aspects. We would like to know how well prepared you think you are to do each of the following, even if you are not doing that type of care now.

	Not at all prepared	Not too well prepared	Somewhat well prepared	Pretty well prepared	Very well prepared
1. How well prepared do you think you are to take care of your family member's physical needs?	0	1	2	3	4
2. How well prepared do you think you are to take care of his or her emotional needs?	0	1	2	3	4
3. How well prepared do you think you are to find out about and set up services for him or her?	0	1	2	3	4
4. How well prepared do you think you are for the stress of caregiving?	0	1	2	3	4
5. How well prepared do you think you are to make caregiving activities pleasant for both you and your family member?	0	1	2	3	4
6. How well prepared do you think you are to respond to and handle emergencies that involve him or her?	0	1	2	3	4
7. How well prepared do you think you are to get the help and information you need from the health care system?	0	1	2	3	4
8. Overall, how well prepared do you think you are to care for your family member?	0	1	2	3	4

9. Is there anything specific you would like to be better prepared for? _____

_____

_____

_____

_____

MEAN SCORE of the number of items answered: _____

Fig. 32.1 Preparedness for Caregiving Scale. (From Archbold PG, Stewart BJ, Greenlick MR, et al: Mutuality and preparedness as predictors of caregiver role strain, *Res Nurs Health* 13:375–385, 1990. Reprinted with permission from John Wiley & Sons.)

These interventions, when available, can alleviate much of the stress of caregiving but are used infrequently or very late in the course of caregiving in the United States. Many countries in Europe offer generous respite care services as part of the long-term care system.

Tailored multicomponent programs designed to match a specific target population seem to have the most positive outcomes on caregiver burden and stress—for example, groups designed to assist caregivers caring for individuals with early-stage dementia or those with Parkinson's disease; programs for younger caregivers; and programs designed for specific cultural or ethnic groups. Programs that work collaboratively with care recipients and their families and are more intensive and modified to the caregiver's needs are also more successful. There are wide variations in caregiving experiences, and the needs of an adult child caring for a parent with dementia may be quite different from those of a LGBTQ+ individual caring for a friend with cancer.

A study of African American and White caregivers of individuals with Alzheimer's disease (Wilks et al., 2018) reported that spirituality was an important factor in overcoming stressful situations for both ethnic groups, but spiritual support's impact was stronger among the African American caregivers. The authors suggest that further research is needed to understand the role of spirituality in the caregiving process (Epps et al., 2020; Chapter 35). Programs for caregivers need to be culturally appropriate to reach diverse caregivers. Online training and support programs and telehealth tools seem to have great potential and need further research (Egan et al., 2018; Messecar, 2021).

Nursing actions with caregivers always must consider the great variability in family structures, resources, traditions, and history. The range of adaptations is enormous, and the goal is always to restore the balance of the system to the greatest extent possible and support caregivers in their caring. The family can be visualized as a mobile structure with many parts; when one part is touched, each part shifts to regain the

Directions: Here is a list of things that other caregivers have found to be difficult. Please put a checkmark in the columns that apply to you. We have included some examples that are common caregiver experiences to help you think about each item. Your situation may be slightly different, but the item could still apply.

	Yes, On a Regular Basis = 2	Yes, Sometimes = 1	No = 0
My sleep is disturbed (For example: the person I care for is in and out of bed or wanders around at night)	_____	_____	_____
Caregiving is inconvenient (For example: helping takes so much time or it's a long drive over to help)	_____	_____	_____
Caregiving is a physical strain (For example: lifting in or out of a chair; effort or concentration is required)	_____	_____	_____
Caregiving is confining (For example: helping restricts free time or I cannot go visiting)	_____	_____	_____
There have been family adjustments (For example: helping has disrupted my routine; there is no privacy)	_____	_____	_____
There have been changes in personal plans (For example: I had to turn down a job; I could not go on vacation)	_____	_____	_____
There have been other demands on my time (For example: other family members need me)	_____	_____	_____
There have been emotional adjustments (For example: severe arguments about caregiving)	_____	_____	_____
Some behavior is upsetting (For example: incontinence; the person cared for has trouble remembering things; or the person I care for accuses people of taking things)	_____	_____	_____
It is upsetting to find the person I care for has changed so much from his/her former self (For example: he/she is a different person than he/she used to be)	_____	_____	_____
There have been work adjustments (For example: I have to take time off for caregiving duties)	_____	_____	_____
Caregiving is a financial strain	_____	_____	_____
I feel completely overwhelmed (For example: I worry about the person I care for; I have concerns about how I will manage)	_____	_____	_____

[Sum responses for "Yes, on a regular basis" (2 pts each) and "yes, sometimes" (1 pt each)]

Total Score =

Fig. 32.2 Modified Caregiver Strain Index. (From Thornton M, Travis SS: Analysis of the reliability of the Modified Caregiver Strain Index, *J Gerontol B Psychol Sci Soc Sci* 58(2):S129, 2003. Copyright ©The Gerontological Society of America. Reproduced by permission of the publisher.)

BOX 32.11 **Tips for Best Practice**

Nursing Actions to Create and Sustain a Partnership With Caregivers

- Surveillance and ongoing monitoring
- Coaching: helping caregivers apply knowledge and develop skills
- Teaching: providing information and instruction
- Providing accurate and complete information about services; determine with the family referrals for services based on needs and preferences of caregiver and care recipient; mutually determine with the family services that are affordable, acceptable, and logistically feasible
- Fostering partnerships: fostering communication and collaboration between the caregiver and the care recipient and between them and the nurse
- Providing psychosocial support: attending to psychosocial well-being; help the caregiver and family identify effective coping strategies
- Coordinating: orchestrating the work of other health care team members and the activities of the caregiver

---

BOX 32.12 **Suggested Topics for Caregiver Education**

- Information about neurocognitive disorders and their progression
- Effective communication strategies
- Legal and financial planning, including advance care planning
- Understanding and responding to dementia-related behaviors (e.g., agitation, sleep disruption, wandering, nutrition, provision of care for activities of daily living)
- Maintaining a safe environment
- Maintaining well-being and quality of life for both the caregiver and the care recipient
- Driving issues
- Strategies to enhance caregiver resilience and positive aspects of caregiving
- Linking to support networks and resources

---

balance. The intrusion of professionals in a family system will temporarily unbalance the system and may provide an opportunity to restore the balance in a healthier manner, sometimes by adding an element or increasing the weight of one or decreasing the weight of another. Further research is needed to provide the foundation for nursing actions with family caregivers, particularly among racially and ethnically diverse families and nontraditional families. Resources for caregiving are presented in Box 32.5.

Special Considerations for Caregivers of Individuals With Neurocognitive Disorders

Therapeutic programs for both individuals with NCDs and their caregivers should be individualized to meet the varied and changing needs over the course of the illness. Interventions that are most effective are tailored to match a specific target population (e.g., spouse or adult children caregivers of individuals with an NCD) and identify their specific concerns and issues through assessment. Programs that work collaboratively with caregivers and their families and are more intensive and modified to individual needs are more successful.

Focusing on the positive aspects of caregiving and targeted interventions aimed at reducing the negative impact of caregiving, which has serious consequences on caregivers' quality of life, should be emphasized. Safety issues and challenging behaviors are associated with caregiver burden, and caregiving education programs that provide accessible, proactive advice on managing these issues may help caregivers develop greater resilience and decrease burden (Allen et al., 2019).

Although caregiver support is essential, the voice of the individual with a NCD also needs to be heard, and the individual should be included in activities and support groups. Specialized support groups for individuals with NCDs are important and should be tailored to the particular needs and level of cognitive impairment. Programs for caregivers and individuals with NCDs should be offered both in the community and in long-term care and assisted living facilities. Online psychoeducational programs for caregivers offer flexibility and can overcome the barriers of geographic distance and availability. The Alzheimer's Association is a valuable resource for both in-person and online support group formats (see Box 32.5).

Health care professionals have an important role in providing support to caregivers and linking them to programs, counseling, education, and other resources. Counseling has been shown to reduce caregiver distress, assist individuals to stay at home longer, and inform caregivers about support organizations. Research results suggest that caregiver needs are not being met by health care professionals, which leads to a decline in physical and mental health (Lindeza et al., 2020). Access to a knowledgeable provider who can follow the individual and family throughout the course of the illness is essential and leads to improved outcomes and less distress.

The current model of primary care does not adequately address the complexities of dementia care, and most caregivers do not receive adequate support to help them with dementia-related problems throughout the course of the illness. Collaborative care management programs for the treatment of AD, often led by advanced practice nurses with expertise in dementia, have been shown to improve quality of care, decrease the incidence of behavioral and psychological symptoms, and decrease caregiver stress (Chapter 26).

KEY CONCEPTS

- The ability to successfully negotiate transitions and develop new and gratifying roles in late life depends on personal and environmental supports, timing, clarity of expectations, personality, and degree of change required.
- Numerous patterns of retirement exist, and therefore retirement per se cannot be viewed categorically.
- Preretirement planning and postretirement follow-up significantly affect positive adaptation to the transition.
- Older adults and their family members carry a long history. Current family dynamics must be understood within the context of family history.
- Loss of a spouse or life partner is the role change that has the greatest potential for life disruption, and nursing support can make a significant positive difference in the transition.

- Widowers are a neglected group in the literature and in the service arena. These men are particularly vulnerable to physical and mental stress.
- Family members and other unpaid caregivers provide 80% of care for older adults in the United States.
- Grandparents are increasingly assuming primary caregiving roles with grandchildren.
- Caregiving activities are one of the major social issues of our time and a significant global public health problem.
- Nursing actions with caregivers include risk assessment, education about caregiving and stress, needed care skills, caregiver health and home safety, support groups, linkages to ongoing support, counseling, resource identification, relief or respite from daily care demands, and stress management.

NEXT-GENERATION NCLEX® (NGN) EXAMINATION–STYLE QUESTIONS

Ms. Carlyle, 73 years old, cares for her 105-year-old mother, Mrs. Stanton, who has end-stage Alzheimer's disease (AD). Ms. Carlyle has been her mother's caregiver for the past 15 years. In addition to AD, Mrs. Stanton has hypokalemia and constipation. She makes nonverbal vocalizations but no speech and has few voluntary movements of her extremities, except for banging her right wrist on her upper bedrails. She has been bedridden for the past 2 years and is incontinent of bowel and bladder. A percutaneous endoscopic gastrostomy tube was inserted 2 years ago, when dysphagia led to repeated episodes of pneumonia. She has tube feedings every 4 hours. Mrs. Stanton is 5'8" tall and weighs 125 pounds (body mass index [BMI] 19 kg/m^2). Ms. Carlyle takes meticulous care of her mother, and aside from perineal maceration and occasional yeast infections, there have been no pressure injuries.

The nurse conducts a home visit and completes a Modified Caregiver Strain Index. Ms. Carlyle scores 12 on the index, indicating that her sleep is disturbed, it is physically stressful for her to provide care for her mother, and it is distressing to her to see her mother in this state. She has also had to make adjustments with family and her personal life in order to care for her mother. The nurse sits with Ms. Carlyle, discusses the situation, and provides her with community resources to support her as a caregiver and educate her about self-care.

Which of the following indicate that the caregiver has taken steps to reduce her stress? (Select all that apply.)

1. "I joined an online Alzheimer's support group."
2. "I go for a short walk each afternoon while my mother sleeps."
3. "I arranged for respite care so that I can plan a weekend getaway."
4. "I spend time weeding my garden each day."
5. "My blood pressure is under control, so I cancelled my last two appointments."
6. "I withdrew money from my life insurance policy to care for Mom."
7. "I stopped going to my book club so that I wouldn't be away from Mom for so long."
8. "I don't go to church anymore; it's too hard to go."

NURSING STUDY

Retirement

Sandy was a professor at a small private college in a metropolitan area. Although she had taught nursing for 25 years and loved her work, it had been a demanding year, and she was very tired. A rumor had recently circulated that the college was in trouble financially. Some of the most affluent alumni could no longer be counted on for gifts and endowments because the football coach had not produced a winning team for several years. Because the tuition was becoming exorbitant, the college had recently lost some students to one of the three state college campuses within driving distance of the city. The trustees of the college, in a move to cut expenses, offered an incentive to professors who were willing to retire early; an extra year of service credit was presented for every 6 years worked. Sandy was only 55 years old but thought that the 4 years of extra credit would bring her near the minimum retirement age for Social Security (an error, of course, because her age did not change with her service credit). Rather impulsively, Sandy decided to accept the offer after telling colleagues, "Well, you know how I love to travel. Why wait until I'm too old to enjoy retirement? Why don't you think about the offer, too? This is a once-in-a-lifetime opportunity." Near the end of the academic year, the celebrations began: recognition, plaques, expressions of gratitude from students, and envy from her associates. The send-off was wonderful. In the summer, Sandy withdrew her savings and booked a cruise to the Greek islands. The journey was lovely, and she enjoyed every moment. Sandy began to feel depressed when she got off the ship but knew it was only because the elegant cruise was over. However, as fall came around, Sandy began to feel more depressed. Most of her friends were teachers, and they were all back at work. Sandy briefly thought of going to Pittsburgh to visit her sister but decided against the idea because she and her sister had never been very compatible. Then Sandy was hit with some of the realities of early retirement: she was unable to withdraw any of her considerable tax-deferred savings before she was 59½ years of age without significant penalty, her health insurance coverage was considerably less comprehensive after retirement, her colleagues were all busy, and she was very bored. Then the real blow fell. The college, in desperation, had dipped into the retirement funds to remain solvent, and the retirees' pensions were now at risk. Sandy's sister, who was a nurse, called to announce that she wanted to come and stay for a few days while she attended a conference in the city. When she arrived, Sandy overwhelmed her with the litany of woes. If you were Sandy's sister, what would you do?

CLINICAL JUDGMENT QUESTIONS AND ACTIVITIES

1. Identify several important family and social roles that older members of your family fulfill.
2. What factors should be considered in role transitions, and how can transitions be made smoother?
3. What factors must be considered in the decision to retire?
4. Discuss the differences you would expect in adaptation to retirement between an individual who retired because of ill health and one who retired because of personal choice.
5. How do you think retirement differs for men and women?
6. Describe what you think would be an ideal retirement.
7. Discuss how you think an individual can prepare for widowhood.
8. In your own family, who will provide care to an aging family member if needed? Does the family or older adult worry about being able to pay for long-term care? What provisions have been made for this possibility?
9. What do you think your role will be when you parents need help? What would you find most difficult about assisting your older parent or grandparent?

RESEARCH QUESTIONS

1. What are the challenges associated with older adults working longer?
2. What are the patterns of adaptation of widowers? How do the patterns differ for the young-old and old-old?
3. Who divorces in late life and for what reasons?
4. Are there differences in the experience of primary grandparent caregivers based on ethnicity, race, and culture?
5. How do adults who were raised by grandparents view this experience?
6. Do interventions to improve the physical health of caregivers relate to less reported stress and improved health outcomes?
7. What are the reactions of older adults to the care given by their offspring?
8. How do upcoming generations view caregiving responsibilities?

REFERENCES

Administration for Children and Families: *Kinship navigator programs to receive $19 million* (website), 2020. https://www.acf.hhs.gov/media/press/2020/kinship-navigator-programs-receive-19-million#. Accessed May 2021.

Allen A, Buckley M, Cryan J, et al: Informal caregiving for dementia patients: the contribution of patient characteristics and behaviours to caregiver burden, *Age and Ageing* 49(2):52–56, 2019.

American Association of Retired Persons (AARP): *2018 Grandparents today: national survey* (website), 2019. https://www.aarp.org/content/dam/aarp/research/surveys_statistics/life-leisure/2019/aarp-grandparenting-study. doi. 10.26419-2Fres.00289.001.pdf. Accessed July 2021.

American Association of Retired Persons (AARP): *Caregiving in the United States* (website), 2020. https://www.aarp.org/ppi/info-2020/caregiving-in-the-united-states.html. Accessed May 2021.

Archbold PG, Stewart BJ, Greenlick MR, et al: Mutuality and preparedness as predictors of caregiver role strain, *Res Nurs Health* 13:375–384, 1990.

Baumbusch J, Mayer S, Phinney A, et al: Aging together: caring relations in families of adults with intellectual disabilities, *Gerontologist* 57(2):341–347, 2017.

Benjamin Rose Institute on Aging: *Millenials, the new generation of caregivers* (website), 2019. https://www.benrose.org/-/resource-library/family-caregiving/millennials-the-new-generation-of-caregivers. Accessed May 2021.

Biddle K, Jacobs H, d'Oleire Uquillas F, et al: Associations of widowhood and β-amyloid with cognitive decline in cognitively unimpaired older adults, *JAMA Open Network* 3(2):e2001121, 2020.

Brown S, Wright M: Divorce attitudes among older adults: two decades of change, *J Fam Issues* 40(8), 2019. https://doi.org/10.1177/0192513X19832936. Accessed July 2021.

Diverse Elders Coalition: *Caring for those who care resources for providers: meeting the needs of diverse family caregivers* (website), 2021. https://www.diverseelders.org/caregiving/. Accessed July 2021.

Dong X: Elder rights in China, *JAMA Intern Med* 176(10):1429–1430, 2016.

Egan KJ, Pinto-Bruno ÁC, Bighelli I, et al: Online training and support programs designed to improve mental health and reduce burden among caregivers of people with dementia: a systematic review, *J Am Med Dir Assoc* 19:200–206.e1, 2018.

Eldercare Workforce Alliance: *Advancing a well-trained workforce to care for us as we age* (website), 2018. http://eldercareworkforce.org/. Accessed February 2021.

Epps F, Skipper A, Williams I: Broadening research and practice approaches to assessing religiosity in African American older adults, *Res Gerontol Nurs* 13(4), 2020. https://doi.org/10.3928/19404921-20200617-01.

Family Caregiver Alliance: *Caregiver statistics: demographics* (website), 2019. https://www.caregiver.org/caregiver-statistics-demographics. Accessed February 2021.

Feinberg LF, Levine C: Family caregiving: looking to the future, *Generations* 39(4):1119, 2015–2016.

Fischer M: *Black and Hispanic Americans face extra retirement planning challenges* (website), 2021. https://www.thinkadvisor.com/2021/06/11/black-and-hispanic-americans-face-extra-retirement-planning-challenges//. Accessed July 2021.

Fry, R.: Amid the pandemic, a rising share of older U.S. adults are now retired. *Pew Research Center*, 2021. November 4, 2021.

Gaugler J, Jutkowitz E, Peterson CM: An overview of dementia caregiving in the United States, *Generations* Fall (ACL Suppl.):37–42, 2017.

Generations Now: *Grandparents raising grandchildren and COVID-19: overlying risks, uncertain outcomes* (website), 2020. https://generations.asaging.org/grandparents-raising-grandchildren-covid-19. Accessed May 2021.

Generations United: *State of grandfamilies: in loving arms: the protective role of grandparents and other relatives in raising children exposed to trauma* (website), 2020. https://www.gu.org/explore-our-topics/grandfamilies/state-of-grandfamilies-in-america-annual-reports/.

Generations United: Grandfamilies (website), 2021. https://www.gu.org/explore-our-topics/grandfamilies/. Accessed May 2021.

Henriquez N, Hyndman K, Chachula K: It's complicated: undergraduate nursing students' understanding family and care of LGBTQ older adults, *J Fam Nurs* 25(4):506–532, 2019.

Kennedy M: Family caregivers need our help—and now it's the law, *Am J Nurs* 117(12):7, 2017.

Lepore M, Wiener J: Improving services for people with Alzheimer's disease and related dementias and their caregivers, *Generations* Fall (Suppl.):3–6, 2017.

Lindeza P, Rodrigues M, Costa J, et al: Impact of dementia on informal care: a systematic review of family caregivers' perceptions, *BMJ Support Palliat Care* 2020 [epub ahead of print]. doi.org/10.1136/bmjspcare-2020-002242.

Lowenthal MF, Haven C: Interaction and adaptation: intimacy as a critical variable, *Am Sociol Rev* 33:20–30, 1968.

Lund M: Caregiver, take care, *Geriatr Nurs* 26:152–153, 2005.

McLaughlin B, Ryder D, Taylor MF: Effectiveness of interventions for grandparent caregivers: a systematic review, *Marriage Fam Rev* 53(6):509–531, 2017.

Messecar D, et al: Family caregiving. In Boltz M, Capezuti E, Zwicker D, et al, editors: *Evidence-based geriatric nursing protocols for best practice*, New York, 2021, Springer, pp 191–221.

Monin JK, Brown SL, Poulin MJ, et al: Spouses' daily feelings of appreciation and self-reported well-being, *Health Psychol* 36(12):1135–1139, 2017.

Morley J: Vicissitudes: retirement with a long post-retirement future, *Gener J Am Soc Aging* 41(2):101–107, 2017.

National Resource Center on LGBT Aging: *Facts on LGBT aging* (website). 2021. https://www.lgbtagingcenter.org/resources/pdfs/SAGE%20LGBT%20Aging%20Facts%20Final%20R1.pdf. Accessed May 2021.

Park M: In sickness and in health: spousal caregivers and the correlates of caregiver outcomes, *Am J Geriatr Psychiatry* 25(10):1094–1096, 2017.

Perkins M, Howard VJ, Wadley VG, et al: Caregiving strain and all-cause mortality: evidence from the REGARDS study, *J Gerontol B Psychol Sci Soc Sci* 68(4):504–512, 2013.

Polenick CA, DePasquale N: Predictors of secondary role strains among spousal caregivers of older adults with functional disability, *Gerontologist* 59(3):486–495, 2019.

Pristavec T: The burden and benefits of caregiving: a latent class analysis, *Gerontologist* 59(6):1078–1091, 2018. doi:10.1093/geront/gny022.

Reinhard SC, Capezuti E, Bricoli B, et al-: Feasibility of a family-centered hospital intervention, *J Gerontol Nurs* 43(6):9–16, 2017.

Roberts E, Struckmeyer K: The impact of respite programming on caregiver resilience in dementia care: a qualitative examination of family caregiver perspectives, *Inquiry* 55, 2018. doi.org/10.1177/0046958017751507.

Schulz R, Beach S: Caregiving as a risk factor for mortality: the caregiver health effects study, *J Am Med Assoc* 282(23):2215–2219, 1999.

Stepler R: *Smaller share of women ages 65 and older are living alone* (website), 2016. http://www.pewsocialtrends.org/2016/02/18/smaller-share-of-women-ages-65-and-older-are-living-alone/. Accessed May 2021.

Swall A, Williams C, Hammar L: The value of "us"—expressions of togetherness in couples where one spouse has dementia, *Int J Older People Nursing* 15(2):e12299, 2019.

Taylor MF, Marquis R, Coall DA, et al: The physical health dilemmas facing custodial grandparent caregivers: policy considerations, *Cogent Med* 4(1), 2017.

Touhy TA: Nurturing hope and spirituality in the nursing home, *Holist Nurs Pract* 15:45–56, 2001.

Transamerica Center for Retirement Studies: *Retirement* (website), 2019. https://transamericacenter.org/retirement-research/19th-annual-retirement-survey.2019. Accessed May 2021.

US Census Bureau: *Marriage, divorce, widowhood remain prevalent among older populations* (website), 2021. https://www.census.gov/library/stories/2021/04/love-and-loss-among-older-adults.html#~:text=With%20marriage%20comes%20the%20risk,about%2043%25%20for%20both%20sexes. Accessed May 2021.

Vespa J, Schondelmyer E: *A gray revolution in living arrangements* (website), 2015. https://www.census.gov/newsroom/blogs/random-samplings/2015/07/a-gray-revolution-in-living-arrangements.html. Accessed May 2021.

Wardecker B, Johnston T: Seeing and supporting LGBT older adults' caregivers and families, *J Gerontol Nurs* 44(11):2–4, 2018.

Wardecker B, Matsick J: Families of choice and community connectedness: a brief guide to the social strengths of LGBTQ older adults, *Jour Gerontol Nurs* 46(2):5–8, 2020.

Wilks S, Spurlock W, Brown S, et al: Examining spiritual support among African American and Caucasian Alzheimer's caregivers: a risk and resilience study, *Geriatr Nurs* 39(6):663–668, 2018.

Zwicker D: Preparedness for caregiving scale, *Try This* (28), 2018. https://consultgeri.org/try-this/general-assessment/issue-28.pdf. Accessed May 2018.

33 CHAPTER

Intimacy and Sexual Health

Theris A. Touhy

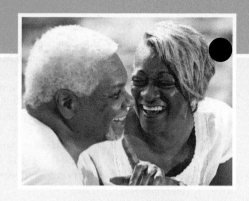

http://evolve.elsevier.com/Touhy/TwdHlthAging

A STUDENT SPEAKS

I'm sorry but I cannot imagine my grandparents having sexual intercourse or being interested in information about sexual health. I never thought much about sexuality and older adults but, I must say, I do hope that I will have a fulfilling sexual life when I am old.

Jennifer, age 21

AN OLDER ADULT SPEAKS

These early morning hours are terribly lonely … that's when I have such a longing for someone who loves me to be there just to touch and hold me … and to talk to.

Sister Marilyn Schwab
From Schwab M: A gift freely given: the personal journal of Sister Marilyn Schwab, Mt Angel, OR, 1986, Benedictine Sisters.

LEARNING OBJECTIVES

On completion of this chapter, the reader will be able to:

1. Discuss touch and intimacy as integral components of sexuality.
2. Discuss the physiological, social, and psychological factors that affect sexual function as people age.
3. Identify the effects of illness on sexual function and adaptations to enhance sexual health.
4. Discuss challenges related to intimacy and sexuality for individuals with NCDs and those residing in long-term care facilities.
5. Discuss the rising incidence of HIV/AIDS and sexually transmitted diseases among older adults and actions to promote safe practices.
6. Use clinical judgment to identify and evaluate solutions and nursing actions to promote sexual health.

TOUCH

Touch is the first of our senses to develop and provides us with our most fundamental means of contact with the external world. It is the oldest, most important, and most neglected of our senses, stronger than verbal or emotional contact. All other senses have an organ on which to focus, but touch is everywhere. Touch is unique because it frequently combines with other senses. An individual can survive without one or more of the other senses, but no one can survive and live in any degree of comfort without touch.

In the absence of touching or being touched, people of all ages can become sick and become touch starved. Touch is experienced physically as a sensation and affectively as emotion and behavior.

The interaction of touch affects the autonomic, reticular, and limbic systems, and thus profoundly affects the emotional drives. The human yearning for physical contact is embedded in our language in such figurative terms as "keep in touch," "handle with care," and "rubbed the wrong way." We will focus on touch as an overt expression of closeness, intimacy, and sexuality. We believe that an individual must recognize the power of touch and its intimacy to fully comprehend sexuality. Touch and intimacy are integral parts of sexuality, just as sexuality is expressed through intimacy and touch. Together, touch and intimacy can offer the older adult a sense of well-being. Throughout life, touch provides emotional and sensual knowledge about other individuals—an unending source of information, pleasure, and pain.

Response to Touch

The Touch Model suggests that attitudes toward touch and acceptance of touch affect the behaviors of both caregivers and patients. Two types of touch occur during the nurse-patient relationship: procedural and nonprocedural. Procedural touch (task-oriented or instrumental touch) is physical contact that occurs when a particular task is being performed. Nonprocedural touch (expressive physical touch) does not require a task and is affective and supportive in nature, such as holding a patient's hand.

People have definite feelings, opinions, and comfort with touch based on their life experience. The boundaries of tactual communication are learned culturally. Cultural and religious norms determine the appropriateness and acceptability of touch. The nurse should ask the person's permission before touching and not assume that a person likes or wants to be touched (Chapter 4). Of all health care professionals, nurses have the most frequent opportunities to provide gentle, reassuring, renewing touch. Therapeutic, caring touch by the nurse is a potent healing intervention. It is important that touching be done with respect regarding the person's comfort and with the nurse's intention of providing a comforting and healing modality within the nurse-patient relationship.

Touch Zones

Hall (1969) identifies different categories of touching—expanding or contracting zones around which every individual extends the sensory experience of touching, smelling, hearing, and seeing. The categories of touching include intimate, vulnerable, consent, and social zones (Fig. 33.1). Providing care in the zone of intimacy, which is identified generally as the area within an arm's length of the individual's body and is the space used for comforting, protecting, and lovemaking, is part of the nurse's caregiving activities. The vulnerable zone is highly sexually charged and will be protected. The most intimate area, the genitalia, is the most personally protected area of the body and causes the most stress and anxiety when approached, touched,

or viewed by the caregiver. The consent zone requires the nurse to seek out or ask permission to touch or initiate procedures to these areas. The social zone includes the areas of the body that are the least sensitive or embarrassing to be touched and that do not necessarily require permission to be handled.

Illness, confinement, and dependency seen in hospitalization and institutionalization are stresses on the intimate zone of touch. Just as caregivers enter a room without knocking, so do they often intrude into the intimate circle of touch without asking. A person's need for privacy and personal space is strongly related to acceptance and response to touch. If the need for privacy and distance is great, touch should be used judiciously.

Therapeutic Touch

Touch is a powerful healer and a therapeutic tool that nurses can use to satisfy "touch hunger" that may be present among older adults. Nursing has recognized the importance of touch and has the social sanctions to touch the body in the intimate and personal care of a person, an opportunity too often not fully used for the betterment of the older adult's adaptation to environment and location in time and space. Touch can serve as a means of providing sensory stimulation, reducing anxiety, relieving physical and psychological pain, comforting the dying, and sexual expression.

Krieger's (1975) groundbreaking experiments with therapeutic touch provided the framework for the use of therapeutic touch in nursing. Her work demonstrated physiological and psychological improvement in patients who are exposed to consistent "doses" of touch. Hands-on healing and energy-based interventions have been found in cultures throughout history, dating back at least 5000 years. "Laying on of the hands" and the power of touch to heal had largely disappeared with the scientific revolution. The phenomenon has reemerged as healing touch and therapeutic touch movements.

Many nurses have learned how to perform therapeutic and healing touch and use these modalities in their practice with people of all ages. Positive outcomes of interventions using touch in nursing homes, particularly with people with NCDs and agitated behaviors, have been reported. Further research on the use of touch with older adults is needed. Touch is a powerful tool to promote comfort and well-being when working with older adults, many of whom may not have opportunities for physical contact.

INTIMACY

Intimacy is the degree to which we express and have a need for closeness with another person. Although intimacy is often thought of in the context of sexual performance, it encompasses more than sexuality and includes five major relational components: commitment, affective intimacy, cognitive intimacy, physical intimacy, and interdependence (Youngkin, 2004). It is a warm, meaningful feeling of joy. Intimacy includes the need for close friendships; relationships with family, friends, and formal caregivers; spiritual connections; knowing that one matters in someone else's life; and the ability to form satisfying social relationships with others (Syme, 2015).

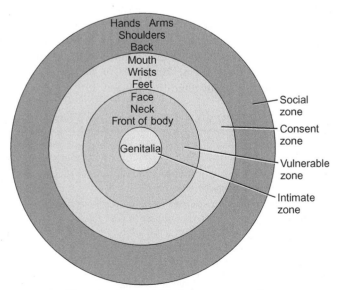

Fig. 33.1 Zones of intimacy or sexuality.

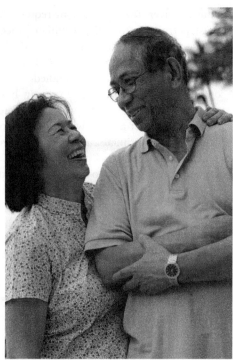

Older couples enjoy love and companionship. (©iStock.com/DanielBendjy.)

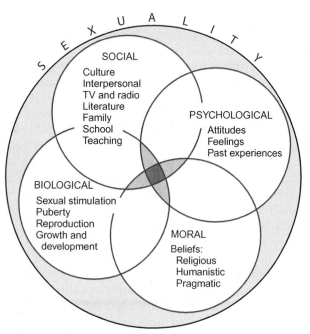

Fig. 33.2 Interrelationship of dimensions of sexuality.

Older adults may be concerned about changes in sexual intimacy, but "social relationships with people important in their lives, the ability to interact intellectually with people who share similar interests, the supportive love that grows between human beings (whether romantic or platonic), and physical nonsexual intimacy are equally—and in many instances more—important than the physical intimacy of direct sexual relations. All of these facets of intimate life are integrally woven into the fabric of aging, along with other influences that can make life rewarding" (Youngkin, 2004, p. 46). Intimacy needs change over time, but the need for intimacy and satisfying social relationships remains an important component of healthy aging.

SEXUALITY

Sexuality is a central aspect of being human throughout life and encompasses sex, gender identities and roles, sexual orientation, eroticism, pleasure, intimacy, and reproduction. Sexuality is experienced and expressed in thoughts, fantasies, desires, beliefs, attitudes, values, behaviors, practices, roles, and relationships. Although sexuality can include all of these dimensions, not all of them are always experienced or expressed. Sexuality is influenced by the interaction of biological, psychological, social, economic, political, cultural, legal, historical, religious, and spiritual factors (World Health Organization [WHO], 2020). "Sexuality begins *in utero* as we are developing as human beings and ends with our death. Sexuality is the total expression of who we are as human beings. It is the most complex human attribute and encompasses our whole psychosocial development—our values, attitudes, physical appearance, beliefs, emotions, attractions, our likes/dislikes, our spiritual selves" (Clark, 2015).

As a major aspect of intimacy, sexuality includes the physical act of intercourse and many other types of intimate activity. Enjoying and expressing one's sexuality leads to feelings of pleasure and well-being that are essential at any age to meet human needs for intimacy and belonging. Sexuality is an important marker of quality of life in older adults and is associated with mental and physical well-being, satisfactory relationships, and reduced risk of chronic diseases (Ricoy-Cano et al., 2020). Sexuality also allows a general affirmation of life (especially joy) and a continuing opportunity to search for new growth and experience. *Healthy People 2030* includes objectives related to sexual health.

Sexuality, similar to food and water, is a basic human need, yet it goes beyond the biological realm to include psychological, social, and moral dimensions (Fig. 33.2). The constant interaction among these spheres of sexuality works to produce harmony. The linkage of the four dimensions composes the holistic quality of an individual's sexuality. "Historically, sexuality has been perceived more narrowly in a biomedical context, with emphasis placed on the sexual response cycle, heteronormative behaviors (e.g., penile-vaginal intercourse), and heterosexist and ageist assumptions" (Syme, 2015, p. 36). A holistic view better reflects the philosophy of healthy aging.

♥ HEALTHY PEOPLE 2030

- Improve the health, safety, and well-being of lesbian, gay, bisexual, and transgender people.
- Reduce sexually transmitted infections (STIs) and their complications and improve access to quality STI care.
- Increase the number of nationally representative, population-based surveys that collect data on (or for) lesbian, gay, and bisexual populations.
- Increase knowledge of HIV status.
- Reduce the number of new HIV infections.
- Increase linkage to HIV medical care.

Data from US Department of Health and Human Services: *Healthy People 2030* (website), 2020. https://health.gov/healthypeople.

The social sphere of sexuality is the sum of cultural factors that influence the individual's thoughts and actions related to interpersonal relationships, and sexuality related to ideas and learned behavior. Television, radio, literature, and the more traditional sources of family, school, and religious teachings combine to influence social sexuality. The belief of that which constitutes masculine and feminine is deeply rooted in the individual's exposure to cultural factors (Chapter 4). The psychological domain of sexuality reflects a person's attitudes, feelings toward self and others, and learning from experiences. Beginning with birth, the individual is bombarded with cues and signals of how a person should act and think about the use of "dirty words" or body parts. Conversation is self-censored in the presence of or in discussion with certain people.

The moral dimension of sexuality, the "I should" or "I shouldn't," makes a difference that is based in religious beliefs or in a pragmatic or humanistic outlook. The final dimension, biological sexuality, is reflected in physiological responses to sexual stimulation, reproduction, puberty, and growth and development. Because of the interrelatedness, these dimensions affect each other directly or indirectly whenever an aspect of sexuality is out of harmony.

Sexuality validates the lifelong need to share intimacy and have that offering appreciated. Sexuality is love, warmth, sharing, and touching between people, not just the physical act of coitus. Margot Benary-Isbert, in her book *The Vintage Years* (1968), expresses the essence of sexuality in late life most eloquently (p 200):

> *Let us not forget old married couples who once shared healthy and happy days as they now share the unavoidable limitations of old age and grow even closer together in love and patience. When they exchange a smile, a glance, one can guess that they still think each other beautiful and loveable.*

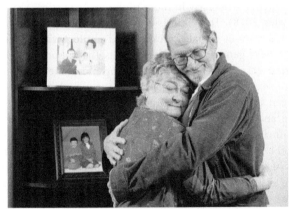

Love and affection are important to older adults. (From Sorrentino SA, Gorek B: *Mosby's textbook for long-term care assistants,* ed 5, St Louis, 2006, Mosby.)

SEXUAL HEALTH

The WHO defines sexual health as a state of physical, emotional, mental, and social well-being in relation to sexuality; it is not merely the absence of disease, dysfunction, or infirmity. Sexual health requires a positive and respectful approach to sexuality and sexual relationships and the possibility of having pleasurable and safe sexual experiences, free of coercion, discrimination, and violence. For sexual health to be attained and maintained, the sexual rights of all persons must be respected, protected, and fulfilled (WHO, 2020).

Sexual health is a realistic phenomenon that includes four components: personal and social behaviors in agreement with individual gender identity; comfort with a range of sexual role behaviors and engagement in effective interpersonal relations with both sexes in a loving relationship or long-term commitment; response to erotic stimulation that produces positive and pleasurable sexual activity; and the ability to make mature judgments about sexual behavior that is culturally and socially acceptable. These interpretations address the multifaceted nature of the biological, psychosocial, cultural, and spiritual components of sexuality and imply that sexual behavior is the capacity to enhance self and others. Sexual health is individually defined and wholesome if it leads to intimacy (not necessarily coitus) and enriches the involved parties.

Factors Influencing Sexual Health

Older adults are becoming increasingly open in their attitudes and beliefs about sexuality. A shift in views toward the end of the 20th century that emphasized the importance of sexual activity in older adulthood for a person's health and well-being has made sex in late life an indicator of "successful aging" (Sinkovic & Towler, 2018). However, a large number of cultural, biological, psychosocial, and environmental factors can influence the sexual behavior of older adults. Older adults may be confronted with barriers to the expression of their sexuality by reflected attitudes, health, culture, economics, opportunity, and historical trends. Factors affecting a person's attitudes on intimacy and sexuality include family dynamics and upbringing and cultural and religious beliefs (Chapter 4).

Older adults often internalize the broad cultural proscriptions of sexual behavior in late life that hinder the continuance of sexual expression. There remains a prevailing assumption that as we age, we become sexually undesirable, incapable of sex, or asexual. "It is erroneously believed that older adults (especially older women) are unattractive, that older sex is disgusting, risky, or 'wrong,' aging entails sexual dysfunction and sex, as a rule, should be discouraged in old age homes and other facilities" (Dhingra et al., 2016, p. 132).

Health care professionals are not immune to these stereotypes and may assume that sexual issues are of lesser concern to older adults and neglect to address this important aspect of healthy aging. It is refreshing to see more movies with older actors that incorporate more positive views of older adults enjoying intimate and satisfying sexual relationships (e.g., *The Best Exotic Marigold Hotel* and *Our Souls at Night*).

Much sexual behavior stems from incorporating other people's reactions. Older adults do not feel old until they are faced with the fact that others around them consider them old. Similarly, older adults do not feel asexual until they are continually treated as such. An often-quoted statement by Alex Comfort (1974) sums

BOX 33.1 Sexuality and Aging Women: Common Myths

- Masturbation is an immature activity of youngsters and adolescents, not older women.
- Sexual prowess and desire wane during the climacteric, and menopause is the death of a woman's sexuality.
- Hysterectomy creates a physical disability that results in the inability to function sexually.
- Sex has no role in the lives of older adults, except as perversion or remembrance of times past.
- Sexual expression in old age is taboo.
- Older adults are too old and frail to engage in sex.
- The young are considered lusty and virile; older adults are considered lecherous.
- Sex is unimportant or over in the lives of the older adults.
- Older women do not wish to discuss their sexuality with professionals.

sexual expression enhances psychological and physical well-being in older adulthood and may improve cognitive functioning (Schafer et al., 2018).

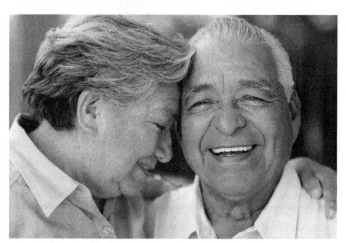

Sexuality is an important need in late life and affects pleasure, adaptation, and a general feeling of well-being. (©iStock.com/ Aldo Murillo.)

it up nicely: "In our experiences, old folks stop having sex for the same reasons they stop riding a bicycle—general infirmity, thinking it looks ridiculous, no bicycle" (p. 440). Box 33.1 presents some of the myths about sexuality in older women that may be held by older adults themselves and by society in general.

Activity Levels

For both heterosexual and lesbian, gay, bisexual, and transgender individuals, research supports that liberal and positive attitudes toward sexuality, greater sexual knowledge, satisfaction with a long-term relationship or a current intimate relationship, good social networks, psychological well-being, and a sense of self-worth are associated with greater sexual interest, activity, and satisfaction. Both early studies of sexual behavior in older adults and more recent ones indicate that older adults are continuing to enjoy active sex lives well into their 70s and 80s. In a US national poll on healthy aging, current sexual activity overall was 40%, with 46% of those ages 65 to 70, 39% of those ages 71 to 75, and 25% of those ages 76 to 80 being sexually active, with men more sexually active than women (Solway et al., 2019).

Determinants of sexual activity and functioning include the interaction of each partner's sexual capacity, physical health, motivation, conduct, and attitudes and the quality of the dyadic relationship. Having a sexual partner, frequent intercourse, good health, low level of stress, and an absence of financial worries enhanced a happy sexual relationship. Sexual activity is closely tied to overall health, and individuals with better health are more likely to be sexually active. Depression, anxiety, lack of sexual reciprocity in the couple, a monotonous and repetitive sexual relationship, and illness are some factors that may be responsible for changes in sexual behavior.

The most common reason for sexual inactivity among heterosexual couples is the male partner's health. Patterns of sexual activity in earlier years are a major predictor of sexual activity in later life, and individuals with higher levels of sexual activity in middle age show less decline as they age. Older adults with positive sexual attitudes during aging report positive sexual experiences (Ricoy-Cano et al., 2020). Regular

Cohort and Cultural Influences

The era in which a person is born and the culture one belongs to influence attitudes about sexuality. Years ago, sexuality was not openly expressed or discussed, and pleasurable sex was viewed as for men only; women engaged in sexual activity to satisfy their husbands and to make babies. Findings from qualitative research on the sexuality and sexual health of older adults noted that men's sexual satisfaction is often viewed as a woman's obligation and that women take a passive role and leave initiating sex to men, particularly in more traditional societies (Sinkovic & Towler, 2018). These kinds of experiences shape beliefs and knowledge about sexual expression and comfort with sexuality.

The next generation of older adults (baby boomers) have experienced other influences, including more liberal attitudes toward sexuality, the women's movement, a higher number of divorced adults, the human immunodeficiency virus (HIV) epidemic, and increased numbers of LGBTQ+ individuals, that will affect their views and attitudes as they age. It has been suggested that an emerging stereotype now sits alongside negative stereotypes of sex and aging: the "sexy oldie." "Sex is now being promoted as integral to physical and emotional health in older age. This new stereotype, although more positive toward the idea of active sexual lives among older adults, may create new barriers for those whose body image, physical capabilities, and partner status do not conform to the 'sexy oldie' model" (Sinkovic & Towler, 2018, p. 1239).

However, stereotypes about old age and sexuality persist despite the more liberal attitudes of newer generations toward sex and sexual behavior. It is important to come to know and understand the older adult within that person's social and cultural background and not make judgments based on one's own

TABLE 33.1 Physical Changes in Sexual Responses in Older Adults

Female	Male
Excitation Phase	
Diminished or delayed lubrication (1 to 3 minutes may be required for adequate amounts to appear)	Less intense and slower erection (but can be maintained longer without ejaculation)
Diminished flattening and separation of labia majora	Increased difficulty regaining an erection if lost
Disappearance of elevation of labia majora	Less vasocongestion of scrotal sac
Decreased vasocongestion of labia minora	Less pronounced elevation and congestion of testicles
Decreased elastic expansion of vagina (depth and breadth)	
Breasts not as engorged	
Sex flush absent	
Plateau Phase	
Slower and less prominent uterine elevation or tenting	Decreased muscle tension
Nipple erection and sexual flush less often	No color change at coronal edge of penis
Decreased capacity for vasocongestion	Slower penile erection pattern
Decreased areolar engorgement	Delayed or diminished erectile and testicular elevation
Labial color change less evident	
Less intense swelling or orgasmic platform	
Less sexual flush	
Decreased secretions of Bartholin's glands	
Orgasmic Phase	
Fewer number and less intense orgasmic contractions	Decreased or absent secretory activity (lubrication) by Cowper's gland before ejaculation
Rectal sphincter contraction with severe tension only	Fewer penile contractions
	Fewer rectal sphincter contractions
	Decreased force of ejaculation (approximately 50%) with decreased amount of semen (if ejaculation is long, seepage of semen occurs)
Resolution Phase	
Observably slower loss of nipple erection	Vasocongestion of nipples and scrotum slowly subsides
Vasocongestion of clitoris and orgasmic platform	Very rapid loss of erection and descent of testicles shortly after ejaculation
	Refractory time extended (time required before another erection ranges from several to 24 hours, occasionally longer)

belief system. Most of what is known about sexuality in aging has been gained through research with well-educated, healthy, White older adults. Further research is needed among culturally, socially, and ethnically diverse older adults; those with chronic illness; and LGBTQ+ older adults.

Biological Changes

Acknowledgment and understanding of the age changes that influence sexual physiology, anatomy, and the stages of sexual response may partially explain alteration in sexual behavior to accommodate these changes and facilitate continued pleasurable sex. Characteristic physiological changes during the sexual response cycle do occur with aging, but these vary among individuals depending on general health factors. The changes occur abruptly in women starting with menopause but more gradually in men, a phenomenon called andropause. The "use it or lose it" phenomenon applies here: the more sexually active the person is, the fewer changes that person is likely to experience in the pattern of sexual response. Changes in the appearance of the body (wrinkles, sagging skin) also may affect the older person's security about his or her sexual attractiveness. Table 33.1 summarizes physical changes in the sexual response cycle. A major nursing role is to provide information about these changes and provide appropriate assessment and counseling within the context of the individual's needs.

SEXUAL RESPONSE

The most prevalent sexual problem in men is erectile dysfunction (ED). ED is defined as the inability to achieve a full erection or the inability to maintain an erection adequate for sexual intimacy. Although most men will experience periodic episodes of ED, these episodes tend to become more frequent with advancing age. Approximately 60% of men at 60 years old and 70% of men at 70 years old have ED (Mobley et al., 2017). When discussing ED with older men, it is important to provide education about normal age-related changes. Older men require more physical penile stimulation and a longer time to achieve erection, and the duration of orgasm may be shorter and less intense.

An erection is governed by the interaction among the hormonal, vascular, and nervous systems. A problem in any of these systems can cause ED. Multiple causes can contribute to this problem in older men. Nearly one-third of ED is a complication of diabetes. Cardiovascular disease (CVD) and hypertension cause a narrowing and hardening of the arteries, leading to reduced blood flow to the corporal bodies, which is essential for achieving an erection. Recent studies have confirmed that ED also serves as a predictor of future CVD, and individuals who present with ED and CVD risk factors should be evaluated for silent CVD (Mobley et al., 2017). Alcohol abuse, smoking, medications, prostate cancer and treatment, obesity, anxiety, depression, and relationship discord are also causes of ED in older men. The new nerve-saving microsurgical techniques used for prostatectomies often spare erectile function.

The use of phosphodiesterase inhibitors such as sildenafil (Viagra), vardenafil (Levitra), and tadalafil (Cialis) has revolutionized treatment for ED, regardless of cause. Some have commented that this can be called "the Viagratization of the older population." Contraindications to the use of these medications include use of nitrate therapy, heart failure with low blood pressure, certain antihypertensive regimens, and other medications and cardiovascular conditions (Chapter 11).

Before the availability of these medications, intracavernosal injections with the drugs papaverine and phentolamine, vasoactive agents that reduce resistance of arteriolar and cavernosal smooth muscle tissue of the penis, were used. Penile implants of the semirigid, adjustable-malleable, or hinged and inflatable types are available when impotence does not respond to other treatments or is irreversible. The hinged and inflatable types, which are inserted in the testicular area, are the most popular. Another alternative is the vacuum pump device, which works by creating a vacuum that draws blood into the penis, causing an erection. Vacuum pumps are available in manual and battery-operated versions and may be covered by Medicare if deemed medically necessary.

The female response is still not well understood, and the definition and diagnostic criteria of sexual dysfunction are controversial and still under development. Difficulties reported by sexually active women related to becoming sexually aroused and achieving orgasm. Female sexual function can be influenced by factors such as culture, ethnicity, emotional state, age, previous sexual experiences, and age-related changes in sexual response. For women, frequency of intimacy depends more on the age, health, and sexual function of the partner, or the availability of a partner, rather than on their own sexual capacity.

Postmenopausal changes in the urinary or genital tract resulting from lower estrogen levels can make sexual activity less pleasurable. These changes include vaginal dryness; irritation, burning, or itching of the vulva or vagina; diminished lubrication; dyspareunia or discomfort with sexual activity; postcoital bleeding; reduced arousal, orgasm, and desire; dysuria; and urinary frequency or urgency. In a study of postmenopausal women with this syndrome, 70.7% had vaginal symptoms that may lead to avoidance of sexual relationships in order to prevent painful intercourse (Steinke, 2021). In many instances, using water-soluble lubricants such as K-Y Jelly, Astroglide, Slip, and HR lubricating jelly during foreplay or intercourse can resolve the difficulty. Topical low-dose estrogen creams, rings, or pills that are introduced into the vagina also may help to plump tissues and restore lubrication, with less absorption than oral hormones.

Women can experience arousal disorders resulting from drugs such as anticholinergics, antidepressants, and chemotherapeutic agents and from lack of lubrication from radiation, surgery, and stress. Orgasmic disorders also may result from drugs used to treat depression. Unlike ED, studies of vascular insufficiency are less clear in women. Prolapse of the uterus, rectoceles, and cystoceles can be surgically repaired to facilitate continued sexual activity. Urinary incontinence (UI) is another condition that may affect sexual activity for both men and women. Appropriate assessment and treatment of UI are important because many causes are treatable (Chapter 17).

SEXUAL HEALTH OF LGBTQ+ INDIVIDUALS

While the US census has never measured how many LGBTQ+ people live in the United States, reports estimate that there are around 3 million LGBTQ+ adults over the age of 50 in the country, and this population will increase dramatically over the next few decades given the significant aging of the population (SAGE & National Resource Center on LGBT Aging, 2021). The total number of older adults who self-identify as LGBTQ+, have engaged in same-sex behavior or romantic relationships, and/or are attracted to members of the same sex is estimated to increase to more than 20 million by 2060 (Fredriksen-Goldsen & Kim, 2017). Chapter 32 discusses LGBTQ+ relationships in more detail.

Discrimination in health and social systems affects LGBTQ+ individuals of all ages. Discrimination ranges from refusal of care to biases or incorrect assumptions to overt derogatory statements. Older adults may be even more at risk for discrimination because of lifelong experiences with marginalization and oppression. They may have been shunned by family or friends, religious organizations, and the medical community; ridiculed or physically attacked; or labeled as sinners, perverts, or criminals. In the 1950s, same-sex behaviors were typically characterized as sodomy and were criminal, and the American Psychiatric Association classified homosexuality as a psychiatric disorder (Fredriksen-Goldsen, 2016).

It was not until 1973 that homosexuality was removed from the *Diagnostic and Statistical Manual of Mental Disorders*. The baby boomer generation is the first generation of LGBTQ+ people to have lived openly gay or transgender lives in large numbers (Henriquez et al., 2019). LGBTQ+ individuals may face dual discrimination due to their age and their sexual orientation or gender identity, and older women in lesbian relationships face the triple threat of being women, being old, and having a different sexual orientation (American Psychological Association, 2018).

As a result of lifelong discrimination and negative experiences with health care agencies and personnel, LGBTQ+ older adults are much less likely than their heterosexual peers to access needed health and social services or identify themselves as gay or lesbian to health care providers. Approximately one-fifth of LGBTQ+ older adults do not disclose their sexual orientation to nurses or other kinds of providers because of fear of receiving inadequate care. As a result, they are at greater risk for poorer health than their heterosexual counterparts.

Although many LGBTQ+ adults manifest resilience and good health despite marginalization, compared to heterosexuals of similar age, gay and bisexual adults 50 years of age and older are more likely to report higher prevalence of poor general health, disabling chronic conditions, depression, high rates of substance abuse, and suicide (Burton et al., 2020; Caceres, 2019). Transgender older adults experience higher levels of discrimination compared to nontransgender lesbian, gay, or bisexual older adults and are at greater risk for disparities and poorer health outcomes (Henriquez et al., 2019).

Sexual orientation and gender identity have been identified as key gaps in health disparities research, with LGBTQ+ older adults an especially understudied population. The landmark Aging with Pride: National Health, Aging, and Sexuality/Gender Study is the first federally funded longitudinal national project designed to better understand the aging, health, and well-being of LGBTQ+ midlife and older adults and their families. With more than 2400 LGBTQ adults ranging in age from 50 to over 100, this project will deepen understanding of how various life experiences are related to changes in aging, health, and well-being over time. Most health surveys do not include sexual identity questions, so there are limited data on this population. Some population-based surveys, such as the National Health Interview Survey, have added sexual identity questions, as have some state-level efforts made through the Behavioral Risk Factor Surveillance System surveys.

The needs of LGBTQ+ older adults differ across race, ethnicity, religion, cultural beliefs, and other aspects of their identity (Caceres, 2019). There is a dearth of research addressing LGBTQ+ health. Research has been conducted primarily with middle-class White gay men and lesbians in urban areas. Even less is known about bisexual and transgender older adults. Nursing as a whole, particularly gerontological nursing, continues to remain relatively silent on LGBTQ+ issues in health and aging. Nurse researchers are encouraged to consider study designs, methods, and procedures that support inclusion and visibility of LGBTQ+ older adults.

USING CLINICAL JUDGMENT TO PROMOTE HEALTHY AGING: SEXUAL HEALTH OF LGBTQ+ INDIVIDUALS

Recognizing and Analyzing Cues

Health care providers may assume that their LGBTQ+ patients are heterosexual and neglect to obtain a sexual history, discuss sexuality, or be aware of their particular medical needs. Providers receive little education and training in the needs of this population and may lack sensitivity when caring for older LGBTQ+ individuals. Health history forms need to be inclusive and not heterosexist. Using gender-neutral terms for identification of a same-sex partner, such as *partner* or *significant other,* is much better than asking, "Are you married?" (Franc et al., 2018). This form of the question allows the nurse to look beyond the rigid category of family. You can ask individuals if they consider themselves as primarily heterosexual, homosexual, or bisexual. This question conveys recognition of sexual variety. Inquire about sexual identity, discuss sexual orientation, and ask about preferred pronouns.

Assessment should be done in a caring, nonjudgmental manner. Some individuals may choose not to answer these questions or ask how the information is relevant to their care. It is important to discuss how assessment may affect their health care (Caceres, 2019). Euphemisms are frequently used for a life partner (e.g., roommate, close friend). In a health care situation, an older woman who is lesbian may refer to herself indirectly by saying "people like us." Nurses need to become more aware of these nuances and try to understand the fear of discovery that is apparent among LGBTQ+ older adults.

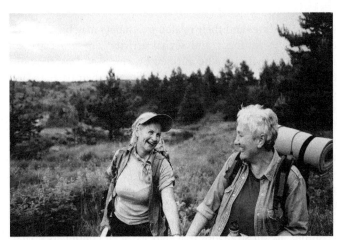

Couple enjoying hiking. (© iStock.com/Geber86.)

To treat an individual who is transgender with respect, you treat the person according to gender identity, not sex at birth. Someone who lives as a woman today is called a transgender woman and should be referred to as "she" and "her." A transgender man who lives as a man should be referred to as "he" and "him." Some transgender individuals identify as neither a man nor a woman, or as a combination of male and female, and may use terms like *nonbinary* or *genderqueer* to describe their gender identity. Those who are nonbinary often prefer to be referred to as "they" and "them." If the patient identifies as transgender, it is important to ask how the patient wishes to be addressed. Use the names that persons have asked you to call them by and the pronouns they want you to use (National Center for Transgender Equality, 2021). When caring for older adults who are transgender, it is important to use discretion and sensitivity when obtaining medical and surgical histories and performing physical examinations.

Solutions, Nursing Actions, and Outcomes

Better support and care services for LGBTQ+ individuals by care providers should include working through homophobic attitudes and discomfort when discussing sexuality, learning about special issues facing LGBTQ+ individuals, and becoming aware of resources in the community specific to this population. LGBTQ+ individuals look for indications of an inclusive and welcoming environment, which may include the display of non-discrimination policies or a rainbow flag. Environments that do not reflect a culture of inclusivity and affirmation with regard to LGBTQ+ populations may be seen as threatening (Burton et al., 2020; Franc et al., 2018).

Appropriate health teaching materials, including those that depict same-sex couples, are important, as is not making assumptions about a person's sex based on their appearance. It is important that service providers create programs that are inclusive and culturally appropriate for all individuals (Chapter 4). Programs to increase awareness of the needs of LGBTQ+ older adults and reduce discrimination are necessary, especially in light of the anticipated increase in this population.

INTIMACY AND CHRONIC ILLNESS

Chronic illnesses and their related treatments may bring many challenges to intimacy and sexual activity. Physical capacity for sexual activity may be affected by illness and psychological factors (anxiety, depression). Patients and their partners are given little or no information about the effect of illnesses on sexual activity or strategies to continue sexual activity within functional limitations. Individuals want and need information on sexual functioning, and health care professionals need to become more knowledgeable and more actively involved in sexual counseling (Byrne et al., 2017). Table 33.2 presents suggestions for individuals with chronic illness. Timing of intercourse (mornings or when energy level is highest), oral or anal sex, masturbation, appropriate pain relief, and different sexual positions are all strategies that may assist in continued sexual activity. There is no consensus on what kind of position the individual should assume for sexual activity, but a lesser amount of energy is expended by the person on the bottom during use of the missionary position.

For individuals with cardiac conditions, manual stimulation (masturbation) may be an alternative that can be used to maintain sexual function if the practice is not objectionable to the patient. Studies show that masturbation is less taxing on the heart and makes less oxygen demand. Although self-stimulation is steeped in myth and fear, masturbation is a common and healthy practice in later life. Individuals without partners or those whose spouses are ill or incapacitated find that masturbation is helpful. As children, today's older population was discouraged from practicing this pleasurable activity with stories of the evils of fondling a person's own genitals.

Attitudes have changed over the years, and recent surveys report that most men (63%) and almost half of women (47%) age 50 years and older reported masturbating in the past year. As with other sexual activities, the percentage declined with age, although a significant number of those 80 years and older indicated that they masturbated (Harvard Health Publishing, 2020). Masturbation provides an avenue for resolution of sexual tensions, keeps sexual desire alive, maintains lubrication and muscle tone of the vagina, provides mild physical exercise, and preserves sexual function in individuals who have no other outlet for sexual activity and gratification of their sexual need.

One couple, who had long sustained a satisfactory sexual relationship, was unable to imagine engaging in alternative modes of sexual expression (cunnilingus, mutual masturbation, and repositioning) that were suggested when the wife developed severe osteoarthritis. The older man brought the worn and dog-eared illustrative pamphlet back to the nurse in the health clinic: "She just won't go for it, nurse!" In such cases, the most well-meant advice may not be useful. To resolve such incompatible needs, the nurse may best counsel the most sexually active and liberal partner in ways to achieve orgasm while remaining sexually comforting for the other partner.

INTIMACY AND SEXUALITY IN LONG-TERM CARE FACILITIES

Research is needed on sexuality in residential care facilities, but surveys suggest that a significant number of older adults living in these settings might choose to be sexually active if they had privacy and a sexual partner (Syme et al., 2017). Intimacy and sexuality among residents includes the opportunity to have not only intercourse but also other forms of intimate expressions, such as touching, hugging, kissing, hand holding, and masturbation. The sexual needs of older adults in long-term care facilities should receive the same attention as nutrition, hydration, and other well-accepted needs. The older adult living in a residential care facility has the same rights as the noninstitutionalized older adult to engage in or refrain from sexual activity.

Attitudes about intimacy and sexuality among long-term care staff and often family members may reflect general societal attitudes that older adults do not have sexual needs or that sexual activity is inappropriate. Families may have difficulty understanding that their older relative may want to have a new relationship. Nursing home staff generally have limited knowledge of late life sexuality and may view residents' sexual acts as problems rather than expressions of the need for love and intimacy. Reactions may include disapproval, discomfort, and embarrassment, and caregivers may explicitly or implicitly discourage or deny intimacy needs.

LGBTQ+ older adults are particularly at risk for being discriminated against by both staff and other residents and may not receive care that is culturally safe and appropriate. In a recent survey, 60% of LGBTQ+ individuals expressed concern about verbal or physical harassment in a nursing facility setting (University of South Florida, 2020). Fears of being outed, disrespected, mistreated, and harmed are common, and these individuals often choose to stay in the closet (Steelman, 2018).

The majority of nursing facilities do not have policies addressing any aspect of resident sexuality and provide little training for staff. The evidence is clear that communication between older adults and health care professionals about sexual

TABLE 33.2 Chronic Illness and Sexual Function: Effects and Actions

Condition	Effects or Problems	Interventions
Arthritis	Pain, fatigue, limited motion Steroid therapy may decrease sexual interest or desire	Advise patient to perform sexual activity at time of day when less fatigued and most relaxed Suggest use of analgesics and other pain-relief methods before sexual activity Encourage use of relaxation techniques, such as a warm bath or shower or application of hot packs to affected joints, before sexual activity Advise patient to maintain optimal health through a balance of good nutrition, proper rest, and activity Suggest that patient experiment with different positions, use pillows for comfort and support Recommend use of a vibrator if massage ability is limited Suggest use of water-soluble jelly for vaginal lubrication
Cardiovascular disease	Most men have no change in physical effects on sexual function; one-fourth may not return to pre–heart attack function; one-fourth may not resume sexual activity Women do not experience sexual dysfunction after heart attack Fear of another heart attack or death during sex Shortness of breath	Encourage counseling on realistic restrictions that may be necessary **Post–myocardial infarction (MI):** Those able to engage in mild to moderate physical activity without symptoms generally can resume sexual activity; those with a complicated MI may need to resume sexual activity gradually over a longer period of time Avoid large meals several hours before sex Avoid anal sex Instruct patient and partner on alternative positions to avoid strain and allow for unrestricted breathing Stop and rest if chest pain is experienced, take nitroglycerin if prescribed, and seek emergency treatment for sustained chest pain **Post-CABG or pacemaker or ICD insertion:** Avoid strain or direct pressure on device and incision Individuals with poorly controlled arrhythmias should not engage in sexual activity until the condition is well managed Instruct individual that ICD could fire with sex, although uncommon; a change in device setting may be needed
Cerebrovascular accident (stroke)	Depression May or may not have sexual activity changes Often erectile disorders occur Change in role and function of partners Decreased physical endurance, fatigue Mobility and sensory deficits Perceptual and visual deficits Communication deficits Cognitive and behavioral deficits Fear of relapse or sudden death	Encourage counseling Instruct patient to use alternative positions Suggest use of a vibrator if massage ability is limited Suggest use of pillows for positioning and support Suggest use of water-soluble jelly for lubrication Suggest alternate forms of sexual expression acceptable to the individuals
Chronic obstructive pulmonary disease (COPD)	No direct impairment of sexual activity, although affected by coughing, exertional dyspnea, positions, and activity intolerance Medications may lead to erectile difficulties	Encourage patient to plan sexual activity when energy is highest Instruct patient to use alternative positions; use ample pillows for support and elevate the upper body or use a sitting upright position; avoid any pressure on the chest Advise patient to plan sexual activity at time medications are most effective Suggest use of oxygen before, during, or after sex, depending on when it provides the most benefit Teach partner to observe for breathing difficulty and allow time for change of positions and time to catch breath when needed
Diabetes	Sexual desire and interest unaffected Neuropathy and/or vascular damage may interfere with erectile ability; about 50% to 75% of men have erectile disorders; a small portion have retrograde ejaculation Some men regain function if diagnosis of diabetes is well accepted, if diabetes is well controlled, or both Women have less sexual desire and vaginal lubrication Decrease in orgasms or absence of orgasm can occur; less frequent sexual activity; local genital infections	Recommend possible candidates for penile prosthesis Suggest use of alternative forms of sexual expression Recommend immediate treatment of genital infections

Continued

TABLE 33.2	Chronic Illness and Sexual Function: Effects and Actions—cont'd	
Condition	**Effects or Problems**	**Interventions**
Cancers		
Breast	No direct physical effect; there is a strong psychological effect: loss of sexual desire, body-image change, depression or reaction of partner	Refer to support groups, sex therapists, counselors Encourage open expression of sexual concerns
Prostate	Incontinence can occur after surgery Erectile dysfunction Psychological effects Use of nerve-sparing surgery causes less dysfunction	Kegel exercises and routine toileting Use of phosphodiesterase inhibitors Provide information related to sexual functioning and continence
Most other cancers	Men and women may lose sexual desire temporarily Men may have erectile dysfunction; dry ejaculation; retrograde ejaculation Women may have vaginal dryness, dyspareunia Both men and women may experience anxiety, depression, pain, nausea from chemotherapy, radiation, hormone therapy, and nerve damage from pelvic surgery	New sexual positions may be helpful; explore alternative sexual activities

CABG, Coronary artery bypass graft; *ICD*, implantable cardioverter-defibrillator.
Data from Steinke EE: Sexuality and chronic illness, *J Gerontol Nurs* 39(11):18–27, 2013.

issues is currently poor. Privacy is a major issue in care facilities that can prevent fulfillment of intimacy and sexual needs. Suggestions for providing privacy and an atmosphere accepting of sexual activity include the availability of a private room, not interrupting when doors are closed and sexual activity is taking place, allowing residents to have sexually explicit materials in their rooms, and providing adaptive equipment, such as side rails or trapezes and double beds. In one facility where the author worked, the staff would assist one of the female residents to be freshly showered, perfumed, and in a lovely nightgown when she and her partner wanted to have sexual relations.

Staff, family, and resident education programs to promote awareness, provide education on sexuality and intimacy in later life, involve residents in discussions of sexuality, and discuss interventions to respond to residents' needs are important in long-term care settings. Staff education should include the opportunity to discuss personal feelings about sexuality, changes associated with aging, the impact of diseases and medications on sexual function, sexual expression among same-sex residents, and role-playing and skill training in sexual assessment and intervention. The facility should clearly demonstrate its acceptance of sexuality and the rights and needs of residents of all sexual orientations to have their sexual needs accepted. Information about sexuality and sexual health in informational booklets, promotional flyers, and other documents produced for current and future residents would assist in normalizing the expression of sexuality in care environments.

Sexual expression policies need to be developed with input from staff, residents, and families; displayed prominently; and reviewed with staff members. Special attention is needed to ensure that LGBTQ+ identity is respected in long-term care facilities. Issues related to sexuality and sexual health should be discussed without anxiety or discomfort so that older adults receive optimal care and treatment. The care facility should be a place where all older adults can live comfortably.

INTIMACY, SEXUALITY, AND DEMENTIA

Intimacy and sexuality remain important in the lives of persons with dementia and their partners throughout the illness. Intimacy and sexuality may serve as a nonverbal form of communication and intimacy when other cognitive skills and functions have declined. In a study by Lindau et al. (2018), the majority of partnered older men and women who experienced mild to moderate changes in cognition were sexually active, including 40% of partnered people ages 80 to 91 years. Most people, including men and women with cognitive impairment, regarded sexuality as an important part of life and reported having sex less often than they would like. Yet sexual behavior between life partners when one has dementia is not often addressed, and individuals with dementia may be viewed as asexual.

Individuals with lower cognitive scores infrequently discuss sex with a physician, and physicians rarely counsel individuals with dementia, especially women, about sexual changes that may result from dementia or other medical conditions. Nurses need to have an awareness of the sexual needs of the individual with dementia and their partner and be comfortable discussing this area with both. Communication can be encouraged by asking the question: "How has dementia affected your sexual relationship?"

As dementia progresses, particularly in individuals living in care facilities, intimacy and sexuality issues may present challenges, especially regarding cognitively impaired individuals who may lack sexual consent capacity or the ability to make one's own sexual decisions (Jones & Moyle, 2018). Inappropriate sexual behavior (exposing oneself, masturbating in public, making inappropriate sexual advances or sexual comments) also may occur in long-term care settings. These behaviors are most distressing to families, staff, and other residents. Sexual inappropriateness (sexual disinhibition) is one of the least understood aspects of dementia. Individuals with subtypes of dementia that include frontal lobe impairment (Pick's disease and alcoholic dementia) may exhibit more sexually inappropriate behavior. These kinds of behaviors may be triggered by unmet intimacy needs or may be symptoms of an underlying physical problem, such as a urinary tract or vaginal infection. The lack of privacy in care facilities may lead to sexually inappropriate behavior in public areas. Social cues such as explicit television shows also may precipitate behaviors. Bodily contact, such as in bathing residents, may be misinterpreted as a sexual act or romantic advance.

An interprofessional sexual assessment is helpful in determining the underlying need that the individual is expressing and how it might be addressed. Encouraging family and friends to touch, hug, kiss, and hold hands when visiting may help to meet touch and intimacy needs and decrease inappropriate sexual behavior. Also, allowing the person to stroke a pet or hold a stuffed animal may be helpful. Behavioral and nonpharmacological interventions are first-line treatments. Aggressive or violent behavior may require limit setting, working with the resident and family, providing for sexual expression in a nonharmful manner, and pharmacological treatment if indicated. Staff will need opportunities for discussion and assistance with interventions.

Sexuality among nursing home residents with dementia is a sensitive topic, and there are no national guidelines for determining sexual consent capacity among individuals with severe dementia. This topic is poorly understood and inadequately researched, and consensus about standard of care on this issue is limited. Determination of ability to consent for sexual activity for an individual with cognitive impairment involves concepts of voluntary participation, mental competence, and an understanding of the risks and benefits. The Hebrew Home in Riverdale, New York, initiated model sexual policies in 1995, with the most recent update in 2017. The National Institute on Aging and the Alzheimer's Association provide helpful resources on sexuality and dementia (Box 33.2).

HIV/AIDS AND OLDER ADULTS

An increasingly significant trend in the global HIV epidemic is the growing number of people age 50 years and older who are living with HIV. The latest data reported showed that in 2018, more than half (51%) of people in the United States living with HIV were over 50 years old. This trend is occurring in both developed and developing countries. While rates of HIV/AIDS have remained relatively stable and even declined a little in younger age groups, the number of older adults infected with the virus is growing. Though new HIV diagnoses are declining among people age 50 and older, 1 in 6 HIV diagnoses in 2018 were in this age group (Centers for Disease Control and Prevention [CDC], 2020).

Gay and bisexual men remain disproportionally affected by HIV, and 59% of infections among men in this older age group are attributed to male-to-male sexual contact. The number of

---

BOX 33.2   Resources for Best Practice

Benjamin Rose Institute on Aging: Sexually Transmitted Diseases in Older Adults. https://benrose.org/-/resource-library/health-and-wellness-services/sexually-transmitted-diseases-in-older-adults#:~:text=It%20may%20strike%20some%20as,B%2C%20genital%20warts%20and%20trichomoniasis.

Centers for Disease Control and Prevention (CDC): A Guide to Taking a Sexual History. https://www.cdc.gov/std/treatment/sexualhistory.pdf.

Centers for Disease Control and Prevention (CDC): Sexually Transmitted Diseases (STDs). https://www.cdc.gov/std/default.htm.

Centers for Disease Control and Prevention (CDC): Toolkit for Providing HIV Prevention Services to Transgender Women of Color. https://www.cdc.gov/hiv/effective-interventions/prevent/toolkit-transgender-women-of-color.

Hebrew Home at Riverdale: Resident sexual expression policy. https://www.riverspringliving.org/wp-content/uploads/2019/08/Sexual-Expression-Policy-1-17.pdf.

HIV-Age.org: Resources and research. https://aahivm-education.org/hiv-age.

National Center for Transgender Equality: https://transequality.org/.

National Institute on Aging: Sexuality in Later Life, changes in intimacy and sexuality in Alzheimer's disease, HIV, AIDS, and older people. https://www.nia.nih.gov/health/sexuality-later-life.

National HIV Wisdom for Older Women's Program: https://www.healthymendocino.org/promisepractice/index/view?pid=30014

National Resource Center on LGBT Aging (SAGE): Resources aimed at improving the quality of services and supports offered to lesbian, gay, bisexual, and transgender (LGBT) older adults. https://www.lgbtagingcenter.org/.

---

women living with HIV has been steadily growing in recent years, and women older than age 60 make up one of the fastest-growing risk groups; most contracted the virus from sex with infected partners (The Well Project, 2021). Transgender women are also at disproportionate risk for HIV, and transgender people of color have the highest reported rates (Human Rights Campaign, 2021). The prevalence of HIV among older adults is expected to continue to increase as more individuals become infected later in life and those who were infected in early adulthood live longer, healthier lives because of effective treatment.

The compromised immune system of older adults makes them even more susceptible to HIV or AIDS than younger adults. Older women who are sexually active are at high risk for HIV/AIDS (and other sexually transmitted infections) from an infected partner, resulting in part from normal age changes of the vaginal tissue—a thinner, drier, friable vaginal lining that makes viral entry more efficient. Studies show that sexually active older men and women do not routinely use condoms, thus increasing their risk of sexually transmitted diseases (STDs). Recently widowed or divorced individuals may not understand the need for practicing safe sex because they do not worry about an unwanted pregnancy and may not understand the risk of STDs. Older women are more likely than their younger counterparts to be in noncommitted relationships, and difficulty negotiating safe sexual relationships can contribute to

---

BOX 33.3 Guide to Risk Factors for HIV

- You are sexually active and do not use a latex or polyurethane condom.
- You do not know your partner's drug and sexual history. Questions you should ask the person: "Has your partner been tested for HIV/AIDS?" "Has your partner had a number of different sexual partners?" "Has your partner ever had unprotected sex with someone or shared needles?" "Has your partner injected drugs or shared needles with someone else?" Drug users are not the only people who might share needles. People with diabetes who inject insulin or draw blood to test glucose levels might share needles.
- You have had a blood transfusion or operation in a developing country at any time or a blood transfusion in the United States between 1978 and 1985.

---

increased HIV risk (Coleman, 2017). Box 33.3 presents some other risk factors.

USING CLINICAL JUDGMENT TO PROMOTE HEALTHY AGING: HIV

Recognizing and Analyzing Cues

Physicians, nurse practitioners, and other health professionals need to increase their knowledge of HIV in older adults and become comfortable taking a complete sexual history and talking about sex with all older adults. Sexual health issues such as sexually transmitted infections (STIs), sexual functioning, and the sexual history of adult patients should be incorporated as a routine part of the medical history throughout life. The idea that older adults are not sexually active limits health care providers' objectivity to recognize HIV/AIDS as a possible diagnosis. AIDS in older adults has been called the "Great Imitator" because many of the symptoms, such as fatigue, weakness, weight loss, and anorexia, are common to other disease conditions and may be attributed to normal aging. In addition, older adults may blame possible symptoms on aging or be reluctant to seek testing or share symptoms due to the stigma they associate with the disease.

Most US guidelines recommend HIV testing among high-risk groups regardless of age, but routine screening recommendations differ and some have a cutoff age of 65 years. The Joint Academy of HIV Medicine, the American Geriatrics Society, and the AIDS Community Research Initiative of America recommend routine opt-out screening, regardless of age. Late diagnosis of HIV can occur because health care providers may not always test older adults for HIV infection. Medicare covers annual screenings for HIV for those who are at increased risk and those who ask for the test. Also covered is annual screening for those who are at increased risk for STDs. An HIV test system is made by the Home Access Health Corporation and is the only home system approved by the US Food and Drug Administration (FDA). It is available at retail pharmacies.

Solutions, Nursing Actions, and Outcomes

Lack of awareness about HIV in older adults results in diagnosis late in the course of the disease, late start to treatment, possibly more damage to the immune system, and poorer prognoses than in younger individuals (CDC, 2020). Women tend to be diagnosed with HIV later in their disease than men, and fewer women are getting HIV treatment (The Well Project, 2021). HIV-infected older adults also may be at increased risk of geriatric syndromes that complicate their treatment and face higher rates of CVD, diabetes, hypertension, and cancer.

Estimates are that more than 30% to 50% of people with HIV have HIV-associated neurocognitive disorder (HAND), which may include deficits in attention, language, motor skills, memory, and other aspects of cognitive function that may significantly affect a person's quality of life. People who have HAND also may experience depression or psychological distress. The most severe form of HAND, called HIV-associated dementia (HAD) now occurs in less than 5% of people who have access to retroviral therapy. The more common form of HAND is mild neurocognitive disorder (MND). Researchers are studying how HIV and its treatment affect the brain, including the effects on older adults living with HIV (Family Caregiver Alliance, 2021; National Institute of Neurological Disorders and Stroke, 2021).

Highly active antiretroviral therapy (HAART) can be more complicated if there are chronic illnesses, comorbidities, and polypharmacy. Long-term effects of HAART are also not well studied. However, there is no evidence that response to therapy is different in older adults than in younger individuals, and some data suggest that older individuals may be more adherent to HAART. Presently, guidelines for care of adults 60 to 80 years of age with HIV are somewhat limited because this population has not been studied in clinical trials or pharmacokinetic trials.

Misinformation about HIV is more common among older adults, and they may know less about the disease than younger individuals. Educational materials and programs aimed at older adults need to be developed, particularly for older women. Educational materials should include information about what HIV/AIDS is and how it is (and is not) transmitted, risk-reduction counseling, symptoms of which to be aware, and the treatments that are available. For older women, including opportunities to practice communication skills with sexual partners may be helpful in sexual discussions with partners later. Small, peer-aged groups may be more successful for providing education than larger groups (Coleman, 2017). Brochures and prevention posters need to depict older adults and be designed for older learners. Jane Fowler of the National HIV Wisdom for Older Women's Program asks the question: "How often does a wrinkled face appear on a prevention poster?" (National HIV Wisdom for Older Women's Program, 2022) Box 33.2 provides additional resources.

Sexually Transmitted Infections in Older Adults

There have been significant increases in the rate of STIs (also called sexually transmitted diseases [STDs]) other than HIV/AIDS in older adults. Older adults who are sexually active may be at risk for diseases such as syphilis, chlamydia infection, gonorrhea, genital herpes, hepatitis B, genital warts, and trichomoniasis. Risk factors are similar to those for HIV/AIDS and include the increasing number of divorced and widowed older adults, unsafe sexual practices (seniors have the lowest rate of condom use compared to other age groups), access to medications to aid in sexual function, and inadequate assessment and testing for STIs in this population. Older adults are more likely to receive a diagnosis of an STI when it is too late and then are unable to benefit from the available medications in the early stages. Many STIs do not have symptoms, so many older adults do not realize that they are infected until serious and possible permanent damage has occurred. Some older adults are embarrassed to ask to be tested for STIs, and many health care providers do not assess this population for STIs. Assessment of older adults needs to include screening for STIs and sex education for prevention (CDC, 2021; Smith et al., 2020). Screening suggestions are presented in Box 33.4.

USING CLINICAL JUDGMENT TO PROMOTE HEALTHY AGING: INTIMACY AND SEXUAL HEALTH

Nurses have multiple roles in the area of sexuality and older adults. The nurse is a facilitator of a milieu that is conducive to patients asking questions and expressing their sexuality. The nurse is also an educator and provides information and guidance to those who need it. Some older adults remain or want to remain sexually active, whereas others do not see this as an important part of their lives. Nurses should open the door to discussions of sexual concerns in a nonjudgmental manner, helping those who want to continue to be sexually active and making it clear that stopping sex is an acceptable option for others.

Sexuality and intimacy are crucial to healthy aging, and the way these are expressed among older adults is changing, particularly with the aging of the baby boomers and upcoming generations. When promoting healthy aging, nurses must consider increasingly open attitudes toward sexuality, dating and developing new relationships, issues unique to LBGTQ+ older adults, the challenges of facilitating intimacy in residential settings, and the importance of promoting sexual health and safe

sex practices. Being aware of one's own feelings about sexuality and attitudes toward intimacy and sexuality in older adults of all sexual preferences is important. Only after confronting one's own attitudes, values, and beliefs can the nurse provide support without being judgmental. Discussion and assessment of the sexual health of healthy older adults and those with dementia need to be included in nursing education programs (see Research Highlights).

RESEARCH HIGHLIGHTS

Knowledge and Attitudes of Nursing Students Regarding Older Adults' Sexuality: A Cross-Sectional Study

Purpose

(1) Investigate knowledge and attitudes of nursing students regarding intimacy and sexuality of older adults; (2) examine the difference in knowledge and attitudes of nursing students in different years of study; and (3) investigate the frequency of discussing intimacy and sexuality with older adults.

Methods

The Aging Sexual Knowledge and Attitudes Scale was completed by 732 nursing students. Data were analyzed using SPSS (Statistical Package for the Social Sciences).

Results

Nursing students had moderate knowledge and positive attitudes toward the intimacy and sexuality of older adults. In contrast to attitudes, the level of knowledge differed significantly per year of nursing study, with third-year students having the highest knowledge level. Most students stated that they had never (54%) or once (13%) discussed intimacy and sexuality with older adults. Reasons to avoid talking about intimacy or sexuality were feelings of "not being the right person" and having little education on the topic.

Conclusion

Moderate knowledge and positive attitudes do not mean that intimacy and sexuality are discussed with older adults. Educational interventions should focus on continuous knowledge dissemination, role clarification, and role modeling.

Data from Wilschut V, Pianosi B, van Os-Medendorp H, et al: Knowledge and attitudes of nursing students regarding older adults' sexuality: a cross-sectional study, *Nurse Educ Today* 96:104643, 2021. doi:10.1016/j.nedt.2020.104643.

Validation of the normalcy of sexual activity and a discussion of the physiological changes that occur either with age or as a result of illness are important. Anticipation of problems in older individuals' sexual experiences can ward off anxiety, misconceptions, and an arbitrary cessation of sexual pleasure. Adaptations that will promote sexual function for individuals with chronic illness should be provided. Screening for HIV/AIDS and other STIs and education about safe sexual practices are also important.

In addition, the myth that adults do not engage in sexual activity must be put to rest. When questions about sexual issues are asked or when the older adult is examined, the nurse needs to be particularly cognizant of the era and culture in which the individual has lived to understand the factors affecting conduct.

A medication review is essential because many medications affect sexual functioning. Often medications are prescribed to both older men and women without attention to their sexual side effects. If medications that affect sexual function are necessary, adjustment of doses, use of alternative agents, and prescription of antidotes to reverse the sexual side effects are important (Chapter 11) (Box 33.5). Box 33.6 provides other suggestions for assessment, from the perspective of the older adult. The CDC provides a guide to taking a sexual history (see Box 33.2).

The PLISSIT Model (Annon, 1976) is a helpful guide for discussion of sexuality (Box 33.7).

- **Permission:** Obtain permission from the client to initiate sexual discussion. Allow the person to discuss concerns related to sexual issues and gather information about what might have changed in the person's life to affect sexual needs and response. Questions such as the following can be used: "What concerns or questions do you have about fulfilling your sexual needs?" or "In this era of HIV and other sexually transmitted infections, I ask all my patients about sexual

---

BOX 33.5 Medications That May Affect Sexual Health

Antihypertensive agents
Medications for prostate diseases
Cholesterol medications
Antidepressant agents
Other medications that affect mood
Anticholinergic agents
Pain medications (narcotics)
Osteoporosis medications
Oral hypoglycemic agents
Insulin
Chemotherapy for cancer

BOX 33.7 PLISSIT Model

P	Permission from the client to initiate sexual discussion
LI	Providing the Limited Information needed to function sexually
SS	Giving Specific Suggestions for the individual to proceed with sexual relations
IT	Providing Intensive Therapy surrounding the issues of sexuality for the clients (may mean referral to specialist)

Compiled from Annon J: The PLISSIT model: a proposed conceptual scheme for behavioral treatment of sexual problems, *J Sex Educ Ther* 2:1–15, 1976.

BOX 33.6 Tips for Best Practice

Guidelines for Health Care Providers in Talking to Older Adults About Sexual Health

Health Care Providers Should Spend Time With Older Adults
- Be available to discuss the subject.
- Give us your full attention.
- Allow time to ask questions.
- Take time to answer questions.
- Health care providers should use clear and easy-to-understand words and everyday language.

Health Care Providers Should Help Older Adults Feel Comfortable Talking About Sex
- Help us to break the ice.
- Make us feel comfortable in asking questions.
- Offer permission to express feelings and needs.
- Do not be afraid or embarrassed to discuss sexuality problems.

Health Care Providers Should Be Open-Minded and Talk Openly
- Do not assume there are no concerns.
- Be open.
- Ask direct questions about sexual activity and attitudes.
- Discuss sexual concerns freely.
- Answer questions honestly.
- Just talk about it.
- Do not evade sexual concerns.
- Be willing to discuss sexual problems.
- Probe sexual concerns if older adult wishes.

Health Care Providers Should Listen
- Listen so that we feel you are interested in our problems.
- Let us talk.

Health Care Providers Should Treat Older Adults With a Respectful and Nonjudgmental Attitude
- See us as individuals with sexual needs.
- Accept us for what we are: gay, straight, bisexual, transgender.
- Be nonjudgmental.
- Show genuine concern and respect.

Health Care Providers Should Encourage Discussion
- Make opportunities for one-to-one discussion.
- Provide privacy.
- Promote candid discussion.
- Provide discussion groups to ask questions.
- Develop support groups.

Health Care Providers Can Give Advice or Suggestions
- Provide information.
- Offer to find solutions and alternatives to given situations.
- Provide explicit pamphlets; explain sexual positions, lubrication.
- Discuss old taboos.
- Give suggestions of ways to help solve sexual problems.

Health Care Providers Need to Understand That Sex Is Not Just for the Young
- Try to eliminate the idea that sex and love are just for younger people.
- Acknowledge that sexual impulses are healthy and do not disappear as individuals age.
- Treat older adults as normal sexual beings and not as asexual people.
- Recognize that sex can improve—can become even better—when one is older.

practices and concerns. Are there any questions I can answer for you?"

- **Limited Information:** Provide the limited information to function sexually. Offer teaching about the normal age-associated changes that affect sexual performance or how illness may affect sexuality. Encourage the person to learn more about the concern from books and other sources.
- **Specific Suggestions:** Offer suggestions for dealing with problems such as lubricants for atrophic vaginitis; use of condoms to prevent sexually transmitted infections; proper use of ED medications; how to communicate sexual and other needs; ways to increase comfort with coitus or ways to be intimate without coital relations.

- **Intensive Therapy:** Refer as appropriate for complex problems that require specialist intervention.

Nursing actions will be based on coming to know the older adult and the needs identified from assessment data. Actions may center on the following categories: (1) education regarding age-associated change in sexual function; (2) compensation for age-associated changes and effects of chronic illness; (3) effective management of acute and chronic illness affecting sexual function; (4) provision of education on HIV and STDs and reduction of risk factors; (5) removal of barriers associated with fulfilling sexual needs; and (6) special interventions to promote sexual health in older adults with cognitive impairment.

KEY CONCEPTS

- Sexuality is love, sharing, trust, warmth, and physical acts. Sexuality provides an individual with self-identity and affirmation of life.
- Sexual activity continues in aging, though adaptations are needed for the age-related changes of the male and female genital systems.
- Generally speaking, medications, ill health, and lack of a partner affect sexual activity.
- Further research is needed to promote knowledge and understanding of the sexual health of LGBTQ+ older adults.

- AIDS awareness and the practice of safe sex among older adults are still lacking. Health professionals, too, do not consider older adults at risk for AIDS and STDs, even though the incidence of both in older adults is rapidly increasing.
- The major role of the nurse in enhancing the sexual health of older adults in the community or in long-term care settings is education and counseling about sexual function; adaptations for age-related changes and chronic conditions; prevention of HIV/AIDS and STDs in sexually active older adults; and the maintenance of sexuality for the older adult's health, well-being, and pleasure.

NEXT-GENERATION NCLEX® (NGN) EXAMINATION–STYLE QUESTIONS

Ms. Booth, 68 years old, comes to the senior health clinic to establish care and is accompanied by Ms. Singh, her partner of 20 years. Ms. Booth has a history of osteoarthritis in her hips and knees, coronary artery disease, chronic obstructive pulmonary disease with a 53 pack-year history of smoking, and type 2 diabetes with mild peripheral neuropathy. Her medications include meloxicam 15 mg daily, aspirin 81 mg daily, valsartan/hydrochlorothiazide 160 mg/25 mg daily, nitroglycerin sublingual (SL) 0.5 mg every 5 minutes × 3 as needed for chest pain, fluticasone/salmeterol 250 μg/50 μg inhaled twice a day, glipizide/metformin 5 mg/500 mg twice a day, and pregabalin 50 mg three times a day. Vital signs include blood pressure of 145/88 mmHg, pulse of 92 beats per minute, respiration rate of 18 breaths per minute, temperature of 97.9°F, and oxygen saturation on room air of 96%.

The nurse asks Ms. Singh to leave the room during Ms. Booth's physical examination; however, Ms. Booth asks for her partner to stay, saying that they have some sensitive questions to ask and want to ask them together. Both women appear uncomfortable. The nurse sits down, leans forward, smiles, and asks how she can help. Ms. Singh looks at Ms. Booth, then says that they are afraid to have intercourse since Ms. Booth's chest pain began 6 months ago. The nurse nods, then discusses with them ways to adapt to Ms. Booth's chronic illnesses.

Which of the following strategies should the nurse recommend to improve the client's sexual health? (Select all that apply.)

1. Engage in sexual activity at a time of day when most relaxed and less fatigued.
2. Use analgesics or other pain-relief methods, such as hot packs to affected joints, prior to sexual activity.
3. Experiment with different positions to avoid strain and allow for unrestricted breathing.
4. Use vaginal lubrication containing glycerin.
5. Treat genital infections immediately.
6. If chest pain is experienced, take nitroglycerin and then resume activities.
7. Consider alternative forms of sexual expression acceptable to both individuals.
8. Wear oxygen during sexual activity.

NURSING STUDY

Sexuality in Late Life

George was a 70-year-old man who had been widowed for 6 years. He lived alone in a lovely home in the hills of San Francisco. His many friends tried to introduce him to a lady who would be attractive to him, but they were unaware of his real concerns. Although George was attracted to young, energetic women, often barely older than his daughters, he was justifiably cautious regarding their sincere attraction to him because he had a considerable estate. In addition, his sexual desire was waning and his capacity for sexual performance was unpredictable. One thing George expressed fairly frequently was, "I don't like demands made on me." To further complicate things, George had begun to take medication to reduce his benign prostatic hypertrophy (BPH) that had become increasingly troublesome. The medication further reduced his sexual desire. In addition, George's sleep pattern was disturbed by the need to arise three or four times each night to void. George came to the clinic for follow-up evaluation of his BPH, and while talking with the nurse he began crying uncontrollably, much to his embarrassment and the nurse's surprise because George had always seemed to be a rather solid and stoic fellow who was reluctant to discuss his feelings.

CLINICAL JUDGMENT QUESTIONS AND ACTIVITIES

Questions refer to the Nursing Study.

1. How would you begin discussing sexuality with George?
2. What factors may be underlying George's sexual distress?
3. With a partner, role-play and demonstrate your interpersonal interaction with George in this situation.
4. What resources or recommendations would you suggest for George?

RESEARCH QUESTIONS

1. What do women find are the most troubling changes in their sexuality as they grow older?
2. What do men find are the most troubling changes in their sexuality as they grow older?
3. What are the differences in sexual feelings and expression in the 60-year-old, the 70-year-old, the 80-year-old, and the 90-year-old individual?
4. What chronic disorders most affect sexual performance of men and women, and how are individuals affected?
5. How many individuals older than age 60 have ever been given the opportunity to provide a thorough sexual history?
6. What strategies would be most helpful in making community resources acceptable to LGBTQ+ older adults?
7. What is the knowledge level about HIV/AIDS among people older than age 65?

REFERENCES

American Psychological Association: *Lesbian, gay, bisexual and transgender aging* (website), 2018. http://www.apa.org/pi/lgbt/resources/aging.aspx. Accessed April 2018.

Annon JS: The PLISSIT model: a proposed conceptual scheme for behavioral treatment of sexual problems, *J Sex Educ Ther* 2:1–15, 1976.

Burton C, Lee J, Waalen A, et al.: "Things are different now but": older LGBT adults experiences and unmet needs in health care, *J Transcult Nurs* 31(5):492–501, 2020.

Byrne M, Murphy P, D'Eath M, et al.: Association between sexual problems and relationship satisfaction among people with cardiovascular disease, *J Sex Med* 14(5):666–674, 2017.

Caceres B: Care of LGBTQ older adults: what geriatric nurses must know, *Geriatr Nurs* 40(3):342–343, 2019.

Centers for Disease Control and Prevention (CDC): *HIV and older Americans* (website), 2020. https://www.cdc.gov/hiv/group/age/olderamericans/index.html.

Centers for Disease Control and Prevention (CDC): *Incidence, prevalence, and cost of sexually transmitted infections in the United States* (website), 2021. https://www.cdc.gov/std/statistics/prevalence-incidence-cost-2020.htm. Accessed May 2021.

Clark T: *The circles of sexuality and aging* (website), 2015. https://www.asaging.org/blog/circles-sexuality-and-aging.

Coleman CL: Women 50 and older and HIV: prevention and implications for health care providers, *J Gerontol Nurs* 43(12):29–34, 2017.

Comfort A: Sexuality in old age, *J Am Geriatr Soc* 22:440–442, 1974.

Dhingra I, DeSousa A, Sonavane S: Sexuality in older adults: clinical and psychosocial dilemmas, *J Geriatr Ment Health* 3(2):131–139, 2016.

Family Caregiver Alliance: *HIV-associated neurocognitive disorder (HAND)* (website), 2021. https://www.caregiver.org/resource/hiv-associated-neurocognitive-disorder-hand/. Accessed May 2021.

Franc L, Moukoulou L, Scott L, et al.: LGBT inclusivity in health assessment textbooks, *J Prof Nurs* 34(6):483–487, 2018.

Fredriksen-Goldsen K: The future of LGBT + aging: a blueprint for action in services, policies, and research, *Gen J West Gerontol Soc* 40(2):6–15, 2016.

Fredriksen-Goldsen K, Kim H: The science of conducting research with LGBT older adults—an introduction to aging with pride: National Health, Aging, and Sexuality/Gender study (NHAS), *Gerontologist* 57(Suppl 1):S1–S14, 2017.

Hall ET: *The hidden dimensions*, Garden City, NY, 1969, Doubleday.

Harvard Health Publishing: *Sex in the second half* (website), 2020. https://www.health.harvard.edu/newsletter_article/sex-in-the-second-half. Accessed May 2021.

Henriquez N, Hyndman K, Chachula K: It's complicated: improving undergraduate nursing students' understanding family and care of LGBTQ older adults, *J Fam Nurs* 25(4):506–532, 2019.

Human Rights Campaign: *Transgender people and HIV: what we know* (website), 2021. https://www.hrc.org/resources/transgender-people-and-hiv-what-we-know. Accessed May 2021.

Jones C, Moyle W: Are gerontological nurses ready for the expression of sexuality by individuals with dementia? *J Gerontol Nurs* 44(5):2–4, 2018.

Krieger D: Therapeutic touch: the imprimatur of nursing, *Am J Nurs* 75:784–787, 1975.

Lindau S, Dale W, Fedmeth G, et al.: Sexuality and cognitive status: a U.S. nationally representative study of home-dwelling older adults, *J Am Geriatr Soc* 66:1902–1910, 2018.

Mobley DF, Khera M, Baum N: Recent advances in the treatment of erectile dysfunction, *Postgrad Med J* 93:679–685, 2017.

National Center for Transgender Equality: *About transgender people* (website), 2021. https://transequality.org/about-transgender. Accessed May 2021.

National Institute of Neurological Disorders and Stroke: *Clinical trials* (website), 2021. https://www.ninds.nih.gov/Disorders/Clinical-Trials/Anakinra-Recombinant-Human-IL-1-Receptor-Antagonist-Neuroinflammation-HIV.

Ricoy-Cano A, Obrero-Gaitan E, Carvaca-Sanchez F, et al.: Factors conditioning sexual behavior in older adults: a systematic review of qualitative studies (2020), *J Clin Med* 9(6):1716, 2020.

SAGE & National Resource Center on LGBT Aging: *Facts on LGBT aging* (website), 2021. https://www.lgbtagingcenter.org/resources/pdfs/SAGE%20LGBT%20Aging%20Facts%20Final%20R1.pdf. Accessed May 2021.

Schafer MH, Upenieks L, Iveniuk J: Putting sex into context in later life: environmental disorder and sexual interest among partnered seniors, *Gerontologist* 58(1):181–190, 2018.

Sinkovic M, Towler L: Sexual aging: a systematic review of qualitative research on sexuality and sexual health of older adults, *Qual Health Research* 29(9):1239–1254, 2018.

Smith M, Bergeron C, Goltz H, et al.: Sexually transmitted infection knowledge among older adults: psychometrics and test-retest reliability, *Int J Environ Res Public Health* 17(7):2462, 2020.

Solway E, Clark S, Singer D, et al: *Let's talk about sex* (website), 2019. https://www.healthyagingpoll.org/report/lets-talk-about-sex.

Steelman RE: Person-centered care for LGBT older adults, *J Gerontol Nurs* 44(2):3–5, 2018.

Steinke E, et al.: Issues regarding sexuality in older adults. In Boltz M, Capezuti E, Zwicker D, et al, editors: *Evidence-based geriatric nursing protocols for best practice,* ed. 6, New York, 2021, Springer, pp 223–240.

Syme M, Yelland E, Cornelison L, et al.: Content analysis of public opinion on sexual expression and dementia: implications for nursing home policy development, *Health Expect* 20:705–713, 2017.

Syme ML: *Sexual health in older adulthood: defining the goals,* 2015. http://asaging.org/blog/sexual-health-older-adulthood-defining-goals. Accessed April 2018.

The Well Project: *Older women: at risk for HIV* (website), 2021. https://www.thewellproject.org/hiv-information/older-women-risk-hiv#:~:text=UNAIDS%20estimates%20that%204.2%20million,live%20in%20sub%2DSaharan%20Africa. Accessed May 2021.

National HIV Wisdom for Older Women's Program, 2022. https://www.healthymendocino.org/promisepractice/index/view?pid=30014.

University of South Florida, Florida Policy Exchange Center on Aging: *Reducing unfair treatment and improving the health of lesbian, gay, bisexual, and transgender older adults* (website), 2020. https://www.usf.edu/cbcs/aging-studies/fpeca/documents/lgbtbrief.pdf. Accessed May 2021.

World Health Organization (WHO): *Defining sexual health* (website), 2020. http://www.who.int/reproductivehealth/topics/sexual_health/sh_definitions/en/. Accessed May 2021.

Youngkin EQ: The myths and truths of mature intimacy: mature guidance for nurse practitioners, *Adv Nurse Pract* 12(9):45–48, 2004.

34 | CHAPTER

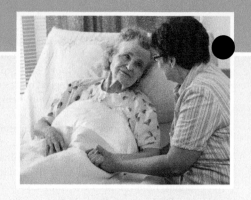

Loss, Death, and Palliative Care

Kathleen Jett

http://evolve.elsevier.com/Touhy/TwdHlthAging

A STUDENT SPEAKS

When I started nursing school, I was so afraid that I would have to take care of someone who was dying—or maybe even had died! Then I found out that to share the time before death with a person is a special privilege.

Ana, age 20

AN OLDER ADULT SPEAKS

When we were in our 60s, my friends and I met over cards, went on trips, and experienced all of the joys of retirement. We didn't have much time to worry about aches and pains. In our 70s we had less time to play because we were busy visiting one another in the hospital or in nursing homes. In our 80s we met frequently again, but it was usually at our friends' funerals, leaving little time for cards or travel. Now that I am in my 90s, hardly any of my friends are still alive; you know it gets kind of lonely.

Theresa, age 93

LEARNING OBJECTIVES

On completion of this chapter, the reader will be able to:

1. Recognize the needs of older adults in response to different types of losses.
2. Prioritize the needs of those who are grieving.
3. Recognize the aspects of palliative care where there is a special need to work within cultural boundaries.
4. Develop solutions and nursing actions that will enhance coping and the reestablishment of equilibrium within the family.
5. Discuss the attributes that are needed by the nurse to provide the highest quality of care to those experiencing loss or are dying.

LOSS AND GRIEF

Loss, grief, dying, and death are universal, incontestable events in the human experience. Some of these are associated with normal changes with aging, such as the loss of joint flexibility (Chapter 28). Other losses are related to changes in everyday life and transitions, such as moving and retirement (Chapter 32). Still others include the loss of loved ones through death or the anticipation of one's own approaching death. Some deaths are considered normative and expected, such as that of older parents. The death of adult children or grandchildren is always nonnormative and unexpected.

Loss of any kind has the potential to trigger grief, mourning, and bereavement. Grief is the *emotional response* to a loss, and mourning is a socially and culturally proscribed *behavior* following and around the time of a loss, especially from death, such as wearing black or "sitting shiva" (Box 34.1). Bereavement is the *period of time* after a loss during which grief and mourning occur. Although there are well-defined rituals in response to loss through death, no guidelines exist for many other losses, such as loss of independent functional ability, the longtime companionship of a pet, or self-concept following an amputation.

This chapter addresses grief as a response to loss and care of those who are dying and their families. The purpose of this chapter is to provide gerontological nurses with the basic information needed to promote effective grieving and safe conduct to a good death (Box 34.2). Loss is broadly considered to include anything that has meaning to the person that results in grief.

GRIEF WORK

Researchers have tried for years to understand the grieving process *(grief work)*, resulting in several models and theories to explain and predict the human response. Dr. Elisabeth Kübler-Ross was

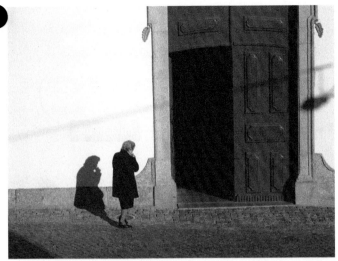

Expressions of mourning. Funeral on Friday. (©JB55, https://www.flickr.com/photos/jb55/.)

BOX 34.1   Sitting Shiva

Shiva (Hebrew word for 7) is a weeklong mourning period in Judaism expected of first-degree relatives beginning immediately following the burial and ending after the mourning service (Shacharit) 7 days later. It is designed to provide time for mourners to deal with acute grief before returning to their usual responsibilities.

BOX 34.2   Tips for Best Practice

Safe Conduct and a Good Death

The responsibility of the nurse is to provide what is referred to as *safe conduct*, helping the dying and their families navigate through unknown waters to a good death. A *good death* is one in which one's needs are met for as long as possible and life is never without meaning.

---

one of the pioneers who studied death and dying, best known for describing what became known as the five stages of death and dying (Kübler-Ross, 1969). She observed grievers who first denied their pending deaths, then were very angry, then proceeded to a process she called "bargaining," then became depressed, and finally found acceptance. Each of the early theorists described successful grieving as movement steadily through predictable stages, phases, or tasks until one eventually was able to "let go" of that which was lost or to be lost (Hall, 2011). These early models have strongly influenced how nurses, physicians, other health care professionals, and society in general view dying as a fairly linear process with the goal of reaching acceptance. Although there have been clarifications that persons may move back and forth between the stages, "reaching acceptance" has been viewed as the goal.

Newer approaches have described grief work as more of a flexible process in which a continued attachment to that which has been lost, at some level, is "normal" (Hall, 2011; Worden, 2018). Although the theories are intended to describe physical death and related grief, we propose that these same models can serve as a framework for understanding any type of meaningful loss, of which there are many in the lives of older adults.

The Loss Response Model

The Loss Response Model (LRM), developed by Jett and Jett (2014), is influenced by the systems approach of nurse theorist Dr. Betty Newman and the writing of nurse Barbara Giacquinta (1977). It can be used to improve the understanding of grieving and assist nurses in caring and comforting those who have experienced or are experiencing a loss. A framework is provided from which nursing actions can be easily developed.

In the LRM, those who are grieving are viewed as part of a system that is striving to maintain equilibrium or stability (Fig. 34.1). However, the *impact* of the loss results in *disequilibrium* or instability within the system. The impact can be the result of a sudden loss-related event, such as a death or terminal diagnosis, or the anticipation of a loss, such as a mastectomy or a move from home to a care facility. The impact causes systemic chaos during which time the grievers are emotionally and functionally compromised (*functional disruption*). As a result, those within the system have difficulty accomplishing their usual activities of daily living (Chapter 9). Common, simple activities, such as choosing what clothes to wear that normally take a few minutes may seem overwhelming. A person reports feeling distracted, restless, "at loose ends," and numb.

A system in chaos cannot survive and therefore strives to stabilize and reestablish equilibrium even while grieving. As members of the system (including nursing care staff) attempt to make sense of the event, they *search for meaning*, asking questions: "Why did this happen to us/them/me?" "How can I/we go on and how will this change my/our life?" In reacting to the loss of a child or grandchild, a common question is "Why wasn't it me?" Searching for meaning is difficult, and as it is done, *others are informed of the loss* or pending loss. Each time the story is repeated, *emotions are engaged* in ways that are consistent with

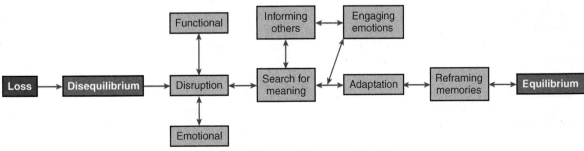

Fig. 34.1 The Loss Response Model.

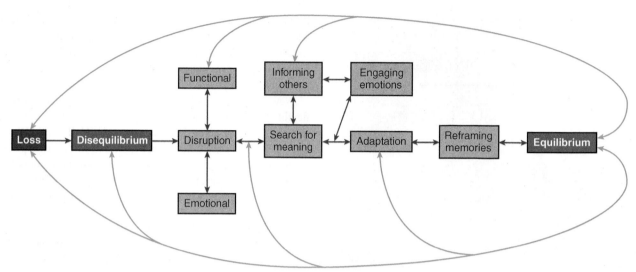

Fig. 34.2 The Loss Response Model and cyclical loss.

the griever's culture and personality; this may be with anger and lashing out at others, crying, stoicism, or silence and withdrawal. Although intense grief may be triggered at each telling, the intensity of the sorrow slowly lessens, and the duration of the renewed sadness shortens. "It has been 2 years since I lost my home and moved here. I've gotten used to it, but I still miss the place I raised my children and my independence."

As roles and situations change, *adaptation* is necessary. In the language of the LRM, adaptation is a process in which the system changes to survive, however briefly the changes last. For example, when an older adult is no longer able to assist with grandchild care, meal preparation, or decision making or to provide financial support, someone else must step in to perform the tasks and roles for the system to continue to function. In some cultures, the expectation is that the eldest son assumes his father's roles and responsibilities when the patriarch is no longer able. A caregiver may be hired, a social service agency may provide resources, disability benefits may be received, or family medical leave may become available. There is movement toward a new equilibrium as the system incorporates the loss and integrates it during bereavement. The adaptation may be an opportunity for new skills to develop or emerge or for the system to become more cohesive and function better than ever before. However, a system that was chaotic or pathological prior to the loss may not ever be able to regain or even establish equilibrium at any level and may disintegrate.

Finally, if the system is to survive after the loss, it must redefine itself. This is accomplished not by "letting go" but by *reframing memories*. In the case of a death, family portraits and reunions will still be possible but be different from how they were before as new memories are made. "Let's think of how momma would have loved to have been here, good thing Sam learned how to bake her favorite cake for us! Let us toast, 'Cheers for being together!'" If celebrations had always been held at the home of the matriarch or patriarch (eliciting the sights, smells, and memories of childhood), a move to a nursing home will prevent this custom. Adaptation leads to the development of new memories when the celebrations are held at the home of

another, such as that of a child or close friend. The system can return to a new but different steady state.

Grieving the multiple losses common in late life is not linear. As the system moves toward equilibrium, new losses often lead to new disruptions, others must be informed, and emotions must be reengaged (Fig. 34.2). One loss is often superimposed on others; no sooner has the system begun to adapt when another loss occurs, such as the loss of a home followed by a fall and the loss of independence. When the losses accumulate in quick succession, the griever may become incapacitated, a state of *bereavement overload*. Careful and skilled support and guidance may be required again and again. There has been particular concern regarding the needs of professional staff caring for dying COVID-19 patients, which also has led to the excess mortality of older COVID widows and widowers (Chapter 2).

Types of Grief

Grieving takes enormous amounts of physical and emotional energy. It is the hardest thing anyone can do and may be especially hard for those who are experiencing multiple losses at the same time, such as while aging or after a catastrophic event such as a hurricane. The most common types of grief are anticipatory, acute, shadow, and complicated. Another type the nurse should be aware of is disenfranchised or unspeakable grief.

Anticipatory Grief

Anticipatory grief is the response to a real or perceived loss before it occurs—a dress rehearsal, so to speak. One grieves in preparation for a potential loss, such as the loss of belongings, moving, or knowing that a body part or function is going to change, or in anticipation of the death of a loved one. Anticipatory grief can be therapeutic if it facilitates planning and preparation for the loss, such as purposefully distributing belongings, estate planning, or preparing for burial. For others, anticipatory grief leads to increasing sleep disturbances and declines in a caregiving spouse's self-reported health and immune health even before the death occurred, especially for those at lower socioeconomic and educational levels (Wilson et al., 2020; Wu et al., 2021).

According to Pattison (1977), anticipatory grief of an approaching death (loss) also can result in *psychological death,* a premature detachment of others from the person who is dying (e.g., has Alzheimer's), or *sociological death,* detachment of the dying person (or one facing a loss) from others, such as by cutting off relationships. In either case, the person who is facing a loss is no longer involved in the day-to-day activities of living and essentially suffers a premature loss or death.

If the loss is certain but the timing is either uncertain or not occurring as expected, anticipatory grieving may be particularly difficult, not because the loss is desired but in response to the emotional ups and downs of the waiting, with the system staying in a state of disequilibrium. Glaser and Strauss (1968) describe this as an *interruption in sentimental order;* no one knows quite how to behave. Family and friends, and nurses as professional grievers, usually deal much more easily with known losses at a known time or in a set manner.

Acute Grief

Acute grief is always a crisis, regardless of the preparation for the loss. Somatic, functional, and emotional cues of distress occur in waves of varying lengths of time during the period of impact. During acute grief, preoccupation with the loss is a normal reaction and may feel like daydreaming and a sense of unreality. Depending on the situation, feelings of self-blame or guilt may be present and manifest themselves as hostility or anger: "If only I had forced him/her to see the doctor sooner!" "You did this to me/him/her and I will never forgive you." Acute grief may lead to significant declines in the physical and mental health of all involved. It is most intense in the first 6 months and lessens over time. Many surviving spouses have been found to have significant sleep disturbances leading to impaired immune function during this time period (Wu et al., 2021).

Shadow Grief

Grieving takes time, but over the months the intense pain of the impact lessens as memories are reframed. However, the old memories never go away completely. Years later, *shadow grief* may persist (Horacek, 1991). It may temporarily inhibit some function but is considered a normal response to loss. While most often discussed in the context of perinatal death, shadow grief can occur at any age. It may be triggered by anniversary dates (birthdays, holidays, anniversaries) or by sensory stimuli, such as the smell of perfume, a color, or a sound (Carr et al., 2014) (Box 34.3).

People deal with shadow grief in many different ways. Each year, hundreds of people visit the Vietnam Veterans Memorial

in Washington, D.C., to remember and leave items that connect them to those who have died. Similarly, individuals make pilgrimages to the Wailing Wall in Jerusalem, praying and placing prayer wishes in the crevices of the wall. Throughout Latin America, especially Mexico, the annual celebration Dia de los Muertos (Day of the Dead) is a time when people visit the graves of their family members, leave food, grieve anew, and feel a renewed sense of connection with those whom they have lost.

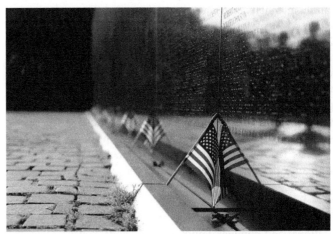

Remembering those lost. US flags at the Vietnam Veterans Memorial in Washington, D.C. (©Austin Kirk, https://www.flickr.com/photos/aukirk/.)

Complicated Grief

Shadow grief is considered healthy and restorative, and there is only a momentary disturbance in equilibrium, yet for others the shadows are debilitating. Those who are survivors of major tragedies, war, rape, abuse, the murder of a loved one, and other horrific events also are grieving, and the "shadows" are now recognized as the complicated grief of posttraumatic stress.

Complicated grief also comes in the form of acute grief that does not significantly lessen over the months and even years after the loss. Obstacles interfere with the reestablishment of equilibrium; stability is elusive. The memories resist being reframed. Issues of guilt, anger, and ambivalence toward the person who has died are factors that will impede the grieving process until these issues are resolved, and resolution is not always possible. Reactions to grief triggers are exaggerated, and memories are experienced as if they are fresh, over and over again. It may trigger a new major depressive episode or cause one to reappear (Maciejewski et al., 2016). If the depression is manifested in cognitive difficulties, it may be misinterpreted as dementia, especially in the very frail (Chapter 26). Complicated grief requires the professional intervention of a grief counselor, a psychiatric nurse practitioner, or a psychologist who is skilled in helping one cope with complicated grief.

Disenfranchised Grief

The grief of a person whose loss cannot be openly acknowledged is called *disenfranchised* or *unspeakable grief.* The grief and mourning are hidden, or expression would result in stigma; it is socially disallowed or unsupported (Mortell, 2015). The

---

BOX 34.3 Shadow Grief

I was browsing through an art show and saw several beautiful carved wooden birds. My mother collected them, and I knew she would like them. I turned to point them out to her. For that fleeting moment it felt as if she was at my side, only she had died about 10 years earlier. I stopped and thought about how much I loved and missed her and how much I wished we could share this moment. Then I moved on to the next booth, and she was gone.

survivor does not have a socially recognized right to mourn. The relationship is not recognized, the loss is not sanctioned, the griever is not recognized, and public mourning is not acceptable. The death may be one that is socially condoned, such as in capital punishment. Disenfranchised grief frequently occurs when partnerships or marriages are not acknowledged by others or the relationship is secret (e.g., extramarital), and the griever may not be able tell others of the meaning or depth of the attachment (Bristowe et al., 2016). It may follow the death of an estranged family member, death caused by suicide or AIDS, or the loss of a death row inmate (Beck & Jones, 2007–2008; Jones & Beck, 2007–2008).

The person in late life can experience disenfranchised grief when family or friends do not understand the full meaning of the loss (e.g., a person's forced retirement, the death of a pet, gradual losses caused by chronic conditions). Families coping with a member who has Alzheimer's disease also may experience disenfranchised grief when others perceive the death as a "blessing" and fail to support the griever who has struggled for years with anticipatory grief and now must cope with the actual loss.

The Family

Today's older adults are usually members of both multigenerational and complex family constellations, consisting of ex-spouses and partners, step-grandchildren, and those considered family as by affective bonds (fictive kin). Although family members may be geographically distant, in many cases some degree of filial ties exists (Chapter 32). When an older member of a family becomes seriously or terminally ill and cannot uphold the usual role or obligation within the family, the resultant functional disruption significantly alters the family balance. For example, what happens when the need for personal assistance competes with childcare needs, work demands, and other commitments of spouses, adult children, grandchildren, nieces, and nephews? When someone loses the ability to drive, who provides transportation? When a best friend or travel companion becomes frail and can no longer engage in the usual activities, who will take that person's place? Who will become the repository of both old and new memories?

Even when a loss does not create functional disruption in the family unit, friends and associates are still informed and emotions are engaged. "I feel so guilty that mom/dad had to move to a nursing home—maybe it would be better if she/he came to live with me, but I can hardly manage as it is." Dealing with the significant losses in the lives of older family members and loved ones can quickly deplete the energy of the family and system who are already burdened with their own daily living and, in many cases, raising their own children or grandchildren.

Factors Affecting Coping With Loss

To cope effectively with loss is to have the ability to move from a state of chaos to one of stability. It is to find meaning in the loss and be able to find a way to *reframe memories*. Many factors affect the ability to cope with loss and grief and help differentiate those who will do better and those who suffer (Box 34.4).

Psychiatrist Avery Weisman (1979) described those who are more likely to deal effectively with loss as "good copers"—those

---

BOX 34.4 Factors Influencing the Grieving Process

Physical
Number and status of concurrent medical conditions
Nutritional state
Quality of sleep
Physical activity
Nature of the loss or knowledge of illness
Presence or absence of related symptoms and pain
Current and projected functional abilities

Emotional
Historical coping strategies and their effectiveness
Current and past mental health, risk for decompensations
Level of maturity
Previous experience with loss or death
Immediate circumstances surrounding loss
Perception of preventability
Perceived importance of the loss
Number, type, and quality of concurrent stresses, crises, and secondary losses

Social
Social, cultural, ethnic, religious, or philosophical beliefs, rituals, and influences on expectations
Availability (and geographic proximity) of support systems and the acceptance of assistance
Education, economic resources, and occupation
Unfinished business and unresolved conflicts
Quality of communication

BOX 34.5 "I Just Need a Moment of Peace"

Mrs. Herbert was a spry 76-year-old woman and sole caregiver of her husband with Alzheimer's disease. She had just been diagnosed with metastatic breast cancer, with a terminal diagnosis. The nurses thought that she was becoming increasingly irritable and agitated after her initial calmness. I was called to assess Mrs. Herbert. We talked for a while—about her life, her plans for the future, and her usual coping strategies. She explained that she had everything under control and had already made arrangements for home care and later long-term care for her husband. As she started to cry, she said, "It's just so hard with my life disrupted here. Every morning for years I have meditated for 30 minutes. My husband respects my need for quiet, and afterward I think I can do anything! I have not been able to meditate since I have been here; the nurses and staff are always coming in my room or calling on the room's intercom—I can't find any moments of peace!"

---

who have successfully navigated crises in the past (Box 34.5). In other words, they can acknowledge the loss, understand it to the extent possible, and communicate effectively when informing others. They can maintain composure when needed and express their emotions without becoming overwhelmed. Good copers generally can use good judgment and can remain optimistic and appropriately hopeful without denying the loss. Good copers seek guidance when it is needed and use the available resources to minimize functional disruptions.

On the contrary, those who cope less effectively have few, if any, of these abilities. They tend to be more rigid, pessimistic,

BOX 34.6   "I Just Use Valium"

Mr. Jones had recently received a diagnosis of cancer, and treatment had begun. The nurses reported that "He was always on the bell," asking for help constantly and never seeming satisfied. The nurses moved him to a room across from the nurses' station, thinking this would provide more security, but it did not seem to help. When asked about the coping skills he had used for past crises he yelled: "I never cope, I just use Valium!"

and demanding (Box 34.6). They are more likely to be dogmatic and expect perfection in themselves and others, and the loss may be viewed as a failure of themselves or others. Ineffective copers are more likely to live alone; socialize little; and have few close friends, an ineffective support network, and few if any resources. They may have a history of mental illness or have guilt, anger, or ambivalence toward the person who has died or that which has been lost. The person is more likely to have unresolved past conflicts or be facing the loss at the same time as other life stressors. In some cases they will have fewer opportunities as a result of the loss. They are the persons who are most in need of sensitive gerontological nurses to recognize their need for the expert interventions of grief counselors. At the same time, nurses need support for their own frustrations when caring for poor copers.

USING CLINICAL JUDGMENT TO PROMOTE COPING WITH LOSS AND GRIEF

Loss and grief are parts of the lives of all of us and occur with increasing frequency as we age. The goal of gerontological nursing is not to prevent grief but to support those who are grieving and facilitate the return of equilibrium to the system each time a new loss occurs. Although the acute emotions associated with the impact of the loss usually will abate somewhat with time, the risk of complicated grief can be reduced.

The nurse works with those who are grieving a loss as part of the normal workday; it is both a privilege and a responsibility. It is one of the few areas in nursing in which small nursing actions can make a large difference in the lives of the persons to whom we provide care.

Recognizing and Analyzing Cues

As in any other nursing situation, the prioritization of needs and the development of solutions and nursing actions begins with assessment (Table 34.1). With the goal to facilitate the reestablishment of equilibrium to a system in chaos, it is necessary to first recognize the circumstances and meaning of that which has been or will be lost. Was the griever's identity closely tied to that which is lost, such as a lifelong athlete who is faced with never walking again? If the loss is of a partner, how was the relationship?

For those who depended on another financially, a death may leave them impoverished, significantly complicating their grief. A survivor suddenly may be homeless after the loss of a domestic partner in jurisdictions in which such relationships are not recognized. The loss of an abusive or controlling partner may liberate the survivor, who may feel guilty for not feeling the grief that others expect (Box 34.7). Knowing more about the loss and

TABLE 34.1   Recognizing and Analyzing Cues Related to Loss and Grief

Patient	Family
Historical coping strategies and effectiveness	Developmental stage of the family
Social, cultural, ethnic background	Existing subsystems
Previous experience with illness, pain, deterioration, loss, grief	Geographic proximity of support network
Mental health	Degree of flexibility or rigidity
Lifestyle	Type of communication
Fulfillment of life goals	Rules, norms, expectations
Amount of unfinished business	Values, beliefs
The nature of the illness (death trajectory, problems particular to the illness, treatment, amount of pain)	Quality of emotional relationships
	Dependence, interdependence, freedom of each member
Time passed since diagnosis	Close to or disengaged from the dying member
Response to illness	Established extrafamilial interactions
Knowledge about the illness or disease	Strengths and vulnerabilities of the family
Acceptance or rejection of the diagnosis	Style of leadership and decision making
Amount of striving for dependence or independence	Unusual methods of problem-solving crisis resolution
Feelings and fears about illness	Family resources (personal, financial, community)
Location of the patient (home, hospital, nursing home)	Current problems identified by the family
Family rules, norms, values, and past experiences that might inhibit grief or interfere with a therapeutic relationship	Quality of communication with the caregivers
	Immediate and long-range anticipated needs

BOX 34.7   "I Am Finally Free"

Sam and Hannah had been married for more than 50 years. During that time Hannah's children often encouraged her to leave Sam, since he was consistently psychologically abusive and controlling. She had been forbidden to purchase anything other than the necessities of life, even with her own money. In the last couple of years of Sam's life, the abuse had escalated before he died after a prolonged illness. Even before the elaborate funeral expected in her culture, Hannah exclaimed, "I am finally free; I can buy that blouse I have been wanting, and maybe a new couch, too!"

its effect on the person's life will enable the nurse to construct meaningful solutions and effective nursing actions.

Cues that may signal anticipatory grieving include preoccupation with the pending loss, unusually detailed planning, or a sudden change in attitude toward the thing or person to be lost. Cues indicating acute grief include crying, distress, immobility, or sadness, which may reoccur every time others are informed of the loss or the loss is acknowledged by oneself or others in the form of condolences. Cues to potential complicated grief include excessive yearning and longing, decreased interest in everyday activities, and new insomnia.

Solutions, Nursing Actions, and Outcomes

Assessment focuses on determining the presence, absence, and details related to the factors that influence grief and mourning

TABLE 34.2 **Who Is the Priority?**	
Those More Likely to Cope Better	**Those at Risk for Coping Poorly**
Avoid avoidance and acknowledge the loss	Rigid and demanding
Confront realities and take appropriate action, understand loss to extent possible	Unresolved past conflicts
Consider alternatives	Multiple concurrent stressors
Communicate effectively	Expect perfection, pessimistic
Seek and accept constructive help and support	Ineffective, if any, support systems
Maintain composure when needed	History of mental illness
Successfully navigate through crises	Guilt, ambivalence, anger toward that to be lost

Modified from Weisman A: *Coping with cancer,* New York, 1979, McGraw-Hill.

and the cues that differentiate good copers who may need fewer interventions from poor copers at high risk for requiring intensive support and care (Table 34.2).

Assessment data are obtained through therapeutic communication and clinical observation. Assessment is based on listening to the expression of spiritual or existential concerns and needs and the relationship to that which has been or will be lost. The assessment will help the nurse prioritize the potential intensity of support needed and the risk for complicated grieving.

Impact

If it is the time of *impact* (e.g., diagnosis, death, loss), nurses provide a safe environment by ensuring that basic needs, such as meals and rest, are met. At all times, active listening is preferable to giving advice. When listening, the nurse soon discovers that it is not necessarily the actual loss that is of utmost concern but rather the fear associated with the loss. The nurse does not try to answer questions and instead listens carefully to both the stated and the implied: "How will I go on?" "What will I do now?" "What will become of me?" "I don't know what to do." "How could he (she) do this to me?" Such comments may seem exaggerated or melodramatic, but to the one who is reacting to the impact of the loss it may seem that the acute pain and shock will never end. The person cannot yet look ahead or know that the despair will lessen. Those who have felt the most significant impact are the most likely to experience complicated grief and also suffer from an increase in both mortality and morbidity (O'Connor, 2019).

Functional Disruption

Nurses recognize cues to *functional disruption* and offer support and direction. The nurse helps the individual or family establish priorities and determine how to accomplish them, encouraging them to delay what they can. The nurse can either complete the task (e.g., tell them that you are going to wash the dishes; do not ask) or find a friend or other family member who is less affected and able to step in to minimize the functional disruption.

Search for Meaning

Sometimes families and individuals are looking for information about a disease or trying to understand how to find the best hospital for a treatment or the best nursing home for a long-term stay (Chapter 32). The nurse assists in finding the information whenever possible. With the availability of internet search engines and devices such as touch screens and tablets, this is often straightforward and a simple but an important action may be to suggest key search terms. While paying attention to health literacy, many sources provide reliable information in a range of languages. Active listening often helps grievers make sense of the loss and find meaning in it as they experience a change in their reality. Often this means helping the person contact a health care provider, an elder in their culture, or a spiritual leader.

Sometimes it is a spiritual search, and help is in the form of finding a resource or a place of peace, such as the chapel. Often what is needed most is someone to listen to the unanswerable questions, the "whys" and "hows," without giving answers. At other times it may be appropriate to be directive, such as suggesting that "This is not a good time to make any major decisions" (Weisman, 1979).

As grievers search for meaning, the nurse facilitates coping with loss by helping them get the information they feel they need, consider alternatives, and find ways to make their grief manageable.

Informing Others and Engaging Emotions

Sometimes nurses feel a need to help *inform others* for the grievers, thinking that this is an expression of caring. Although it appears to be, it is more therapeutic for grievers or designated cultural spokespersons to perform this task. The nurse can offer to find a phone number or just offer to "be there" when the news is being shared. In this way, the nurse provides support when the griever's emotions engage and at the same time shows respect for the person's and family's cultural values and roles. In some cultures, catharsis is expected, and in others it is the nurse who gives the griever the "permission" needed to emote.

Adaptation

As the person or family moves toward equilibrium after the impact of a loss, the nurse can help the person reorganize this new life. The nurse talks with the person who is grieving about what was most valued about that which has been lost, determines what habits and rituals were comforting related to this, and finds ways to incorporate these in a new way to the new environment. For example, if the person always had a cup of tea before bed but now does not have access to a kitchen, "cup of tea at bedtime" can become part of the individualized plan of care in the long-term care setting.

Memories Reframed and the Return of Equilibrium

For the system to return to equilibrium, however fleeting, new memories are needed. For example, the grandmother who had always hosted her eldest daughter's birthday party can still do that even if she is now a resident in a long-term care facility. The nurse can help the resident reserve a private space within the facility, send out invitations, and have the birthday party as always but reframe it as catered by the facility in the person's new "home."

The nurse collaborates with grievers by encouraging them to reminisce and share stories with others and repeat them as often as needed (Weisman, 1979). Listening to the story, endlessly repeated, is difficult to do and it is likely to change with each retelling, but this means that memories are being reframed. Reminiscence allows the reality of the loss to filter slowly into a special place in the memory. It helps the griever acknowledge that while the loss is indeed real, life can go on, even if the future is experienced in a different way. At the time when new memories are being developed, drawing out anecdotes and vignettes of the person's life before the loss will allow the person to see a different perspective.

Like good copers, good gerontological nurses must be flexible, practical, resourceful, gently realistic, and abundantly optimistic. The nurse serves as a role model who displays the behavioral qualities of responsiveness, authenticity, commitment, and competence—that is, caring. Nurses introduce themselves, establish rapport, learn the cultural rules regarding the situation, and explain their roles (e.g., nurse practitioner, charge nurse, staff nurse) and the time they will be available. The nurse fosters the griever's movement from disequilibrium and instability to a new, albeit modified, steady state, while knowing that this is highly tenuous in the lives of older adults (Box 34.8).

DYING AND DEATH

Before the 1900s, most women and men died at home, women during childbirth and men of unknown causes. During times of war, most men died in battle or from battle-associated injuries. Traditionally, people have voiced a preference to die at home, yet most often they die in acute care hospitals with wide variation in prevalence by country of residence. Early in the COVID-19 pandemic, persons over 65 years of age made up to 80% of all associated deaths. Many older adults died in long-term care facilities and hospitals; others died at home for a multitude of reasons (Powell et al, 2020).

Dying is both a challenging life experience and a private one. How people deal with their own dying is often a reflection of the way they responded to earlier losses. Most people probably die as they have lived—that is, the manner in which one faces dying is an expression of personality, circumstances, illness, and culture. Although not all older adults have had fulfilling lives or have a sense of completion (Chapter 35), many consider their deaths at the age of or after that of their parents normative. If dying occurs after a particularly prolonged or painful illness, it is sometimes rationalized as a relief. The deaths of the older community members at the time of war or through an act of violence are never considered an acceptable loss of human potential.

A major question arises when considering dying and death in late life. Since both chronic and terminal conditions often occur concurrently, the difficult question is: When is a person considered to be "dying"? During repeated acute exacerbations, with progressive health problems, or only when a terminal prognosis is predicted? Although the cues to the needs of those with terminal conditions may be recognized, they easily can be confused with those associated with frailty and exacerbations of chronic diseases.

BOX 34.8 Tips for Best Practice
Helping Grievers Move Toward Equilibrium

Impact
- Provide a safe environment
- Therapeutic listening

Functional Disruption
- Provide functional assistance

Searching for Meaning
- Provide reliable sources of information (e.g., websites)
- Inform appropriate providers of the person's need for information and make sure they receive it
- Active listening

Engaging Emotions
- "Give permission" to express emotions
- Offer physical presence
- Offer to locate usual sources of support during times of crisis (e.g., minister, tribal elder)
- Active listening

Informing Others
- Offer physical presence
- Active listening

Adaptation
- Identify meaningful events influenced by the loss
- Help find new ways of replacing that which has been lost
- Offer discussions of how the loss has affected life
- Active listening

Reframing Memories
- Offer to discuss mechanisms to develop new memories without denying connection with that or whom has been lost
- Encourage reminiscence
- Facilitate opportunities for culturally based and desired bereavement rituals
- Assure grievers that stability will return
- Active listening

The Family

Adult children often begin to see their own mortality through the death of their parents as life is reframed. Family members must separate their own identities and learn to tolerate the reality that another family member will die while they survive. A period of guilt, depression, and anxiety is common, especially when aggressive measures that prolonged the natural death were used (Young & Widera, 2021). Providing support, love, and intimacy can lead to physical and mental exhaustion, impatience, anger, and a sense of futility if the dying is prolonged. Family members likely will grieve in their own unique ways, which can hinder communication when it is needed the most. As an illness worsens, physical disability increases, and needs intensify, so may the family members' feelings of helplessness and frustration.

The family may feel pressured to provide very intimate, personal care during the final days of a relative's life. They may feel caught between experiencing the present and remembering the person as he or she was, between pushing for aggressive interventions in hopes of preventing the death or letting life take its natural course without feeling that they "have done nothing." Nurses often hear families lament that they "can't give up on them."

Despite the family's grief and pain, they are often faced with the difficult task of giving permission to die, to let the loved one know that it is all right to let go and leave them. This gesture is the last act of love and dignity that the family can offer. Occasionally, no family is available, and the task falls to the nurse to give permission to let go when the time comes.

Palliative Care

Palliative care is that which centers around comfort and coping by the family and caregivers in collaboration with the "patient." The emphasis is not on curing a life-threatening condition but facilitating quality of life by preventing or minimizing suffering. Providing such care is part of the practice of gerontological nurses who routinely care for older adults and support the caregivers who are coping with multiple losses simultaneously.

Palliative care may be elected when previously curative treatments are no longer effective, such as with end-stage cancer, heart disease, or chronic obstructive pulmonary disease (COPD). It also may be appropriate for those with irreversible degenerative diseases such as Alzheimer's disease, dementia with Lewy bodies, or Parkinson's disease (Chapter 25). This does not mean that any simple curative treatments to transient new problems are automatically withheld, such as the treatment of a urinary tract infection, unless declined or dictated in an advance directive (Chapter 31; Fig. 34.3).

The provision of palliative care requires the coordination of an interprofessional team that pools its skills and areas of expertise to help the person reach a death that is consistent with the person's values and wishes (Appendix 34.1) and symptom

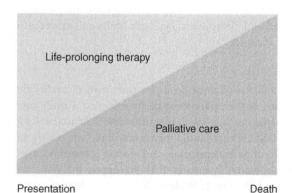

Fig. 34.3 Palliative care is offered simultaneously with life-prolonging and curative therapies for persons living with serious, complex, and advanced illness. (Adapted from Ham RJ, Sloane PD, Warshaw GA, et al: *Primary care geriatrics*, ed 6, Philadelphia, 2014, Elsevier.)

> ### BOX 34.9   Indicators of a Good Death
>
> - Timely and expert care is received when it is needed.
> - One can control one's life, environment, and death[a] to the extent that is desired and possible and in a way that is consistent with one's values and culture.
> - One can maintain composure when necessary and to the extent desired.
> - One can initiate and maintain communication with significant others for as long as possible.
> - Life continues as normally as possible while dying, with the added tasks that may be needed to deal with and adjust to the inevitable death.
> - One can always maintain *desirable* hope.
> - One can reach a sense of closure in a way that is culturally consistent with one's values and life patterns.

[a]See Appendix 34.1 for discussion of personal control of death.

free and to support loved ones both before and after the death (Box 34.9).

Whereas initially palliative care was provided primarily by specialized organizations (e.g., hospices), today it is provided regardless of setting and by anyone sharing these goals and skills. This may be in the ambulatory care clinic when the focus of the care of the person with neurodegenerative disorders is comfort (Chapter 23) or in specialized beds in an acute care or long-term care facility. A formal system of palliative care can help people understand their options, make health-related decisions that are consistent with their values, and facilitate seamless transitions from one care setting to another when needed.

Hospice

The model for the modern-day hospice is based on the medieval concept of hospitality in which a community assists the traveler at dangerous points along a journey. The dying are also travelers along the continuum of life in a community consisting of friends, family, and health care providers. However, for many years, providing comfort to those approaching death was lacking. In 1952 Englishwoman Dame Cicely Saunders, a nurse, social worker, physician, and writer, began working at St. Joseph's Hospice in London. The goal of her work and study was to reduce pain. In 1967 she established Saint Christopher's Hospice, also in London, based on the principles of teaching, clinical research, and the provision of expert and holistic pain and symptom relief (St. Christopher's, 2021). Inspired by the work of Dame Saunders, Dr. Florence Wald, the dean of the College of Nursing at Yale University, and physician Dr. Elisabeth Kübler-Ross championed the hospice concept in the United States. In 1974 Dr. Wald, two pediatricians, and a chaplain founded Connecticut Hospice in Branford, Connecticut (National Hospice and Palliative Care Organization [NHPCO], 2021).

Hospice programs in the United States started out as small, freestanding organizations supported entirely by charitable contributions and volunteer effort and provided exclusively in the person's home. The number of formal hospice programs grew rapidly, especially after the services were approved for reimbursement by Medicare, Medicaid, and many private insurers (Chapter 31). In 2018 more than 4000 hospice programs operated in the United States. Most served fewer than 50 patients at any one time, most of whom were White women. Although they were initially all nonprofit, in 2018 the majority (69.25%) of hospices were for-profit corporations (NHPCO, 2020). The variations in origins and styles reflect the style of leadership, political forces, and available resources for health and social services in the community in which they were established or continue to exist. While the care provided is palliative, it is within the specific context of a signed agreement between the individual and the organization in which the person has elected to receive only comfort care for a specific condition. Hospice services are limited to those for whom a physician has agreed that the person has a prognosis of 6 months or less if the identified illness progresses at its usual course.

At a minimum, services include medical, nursing, nursing assistant, chaplain, social work, and volunteer support. Potential services also may include massage, music, art, pet therapy, and other nonpharmacological interventions to promote comfort and quality of life. Hospices provide care not only to the dying but also to their families and friends through support groups and other bereavement services.

Most hospice care is provided in people's homes or place of residence, such as an assisted living facility. If provided at home, this becomes the primary center of care, provided by family members or friends who are taught basic care techniques as needed, including diet, exercise, and medication management, with intermittent visits from the hospice staff. Volunteers, as members of the team, are a unique aspect of care; friendship and companionship are provided.

Many hospices today have freestanding care centers where a person may go to provide caregivers with short periods of respite or when symptom management is more intense than can be provided at home. Those hospices without centers may have agreements with skilled nursing homes or acute care hospitals where the same symptom management can be achieved. When and if stabilized, the person returns home.

The unprecedented contribution of hospice continues to be the provision of comfort for those who are dying and of support for those close to them. Through both pharmacological and nonpharmacological means, symptom management often can be accomplished without denying the patient's full alertness and the ability to communicate with others. The crux of accomplishing this end is the anticipation of symptoms and actions of the caregiver before problems escalate. Both hospice and other palliative care programs support and guide the family in patient care and ensure safe passage (i.e., for the patient, that he or she will not die alone; for the family, that they will not be abandoned).

Nursing actions in hospice care incorporate solutions along the mind-body continuum. Nurses function in a variety of roles: providing direct patient care, coordinating the interprofessional team, advocating for the patient and hospice in the clinical and political arena, and working as executive officers responsible for research and educational activities (Box 34.10).

Hope

The concepts of palliative care and hospice are also about hope, a fluid concept that changes as the time of death draws near. At the beginning, the person hopes for a cure and later changes to

---

hoping for "as much time as possible." As death approaches, the hope may be for a good death.

Hope is the belief of the possible, the support of meaningful others, a sense of well-being, overall coping ability, and having had a purpose in life. Hope empowers, generates courage, motivates action and achievement, and can counter physiological, spiritual, and emotional dysfunction. Hope involves faith and trust.

Hope can be classified as desirable or expectational (Pattison, 1977). *Expectational hope* sounds like "I hope to get better" or "I hope my children get here in time." If this hope reflects unrealistic expectations, it can increase stress for the person and caregiver. However, this hope can be modified without being "taken away." With *desirable hope*, the wishes are something that would be appreciated if it were to occur but without fixed expectations. The nurse can respond to the comment "I hope I get better" from someone who is rapidly declining, with "That would be really great; in the meantime, there is so much we can do."

USING CLINICAL JUDGMENT TO PROMOTE A GOOD DEATH

The needs of the dying are like threads in a piece of cloth. Each thread is individual but necessary to the integrity and completeness of the fabric. If one thread is pulled, it touches the other threads, affecting the fabric's appearance, the thread placement, and the stability of the piece. When one need is unmet, it will affect all others because they are all interwoven. Separating the physical, psychological, spiritual, and cultural needs of the dying in late life in order to identify specific solutions and nursing actions is difficult because of this interconnection. The skill of the nurse lies in the ability to recognize, analyze, and prioritize these needs. Only then can safe and effective interventions lead to the best possible outcome, that is, a good death.

Recognizing and Analyzing Cues

Although many of the cues attributed to terminal conditions may appear obvious, they can easily be confused with frailty and exacerbations of chronic diseases (Table 34.3). However, the nurse can look for signs of an approaching death when the person begins using "coded communication," such as saying goodbye instead of the usual goodnight, giving away cherished possessions as gifts, urgently contacting friends and relatives with whom the person has not communicated for a long time, and having direct or symbolic premonitions that death is near (Box 34.11).

Cues to spiritual distress include expressions of hopelessness, meaninglessness, guilt, and despair, all of which can emerge indirectly through anxiety, depression, or anger. Agitation is frequently thought to be a manifestation of confusion or dementia but also

TABLE 34.3   Tips for Best Practice: Cues and Nursing Actions to Approaching Death

Physical Cues	Cause	Nursing Actions
Coolness	Diminished peripheral circulation to increase circulation to vital organs	Socks, light cotton blankets or warm blankets if needed; do not use electric blanket
Increased sleeping	Conservation of energy	Respect need for increased rest; inquire as to wishes regarding timing of companionship
Disorientation	Metabolic changes	Identify self by name before speaking to patient; speak clearly and truthfully
Fecal and/or urinary incontinence	Increased muscle relaxation	Change bedding as needed; use bed pads; avoid indwelling catheters if possible
Noisy respirations	Poor circulation of body fluids, immobilization, and the inability to expectorate	Elevate the head with pillows, raise the head of the bed, or both; gently turn the head to the side to drain
Restlessness	Metabolic changes and relative cerebral anoxia	Calm the patient by speech and action; reduce light; gently rub back, stroke arms, or read aloud; play soothing music; do not use restraints
Decreased intake of food and fluids	Body conservation of energy for function	Provide nutrition within limits expressed by patient or in advance directive; semisolid liquids easiest to swallow; protect mouth and lips from discomfort of dryness
Decreased urine output	Decreased fluid intake and decreased circulation to kidney	Do not push fluids
Altered breathing pattern	Metabolic and oxygen changes	Elevate the head of bed; speak gently to patient
Emotional or Spiritual Cues	**Potential Purpose**	**Nursing Actions**
Withdrawal	Prepares the patient for release, detachment, and letting go	Continue communicating in a normal manner using a normal voice tone; identify self by name; give permission to "let go"
Vision-like experiences of dead friends or family; religious vision	Preparation for death	Accept the reality of the experience for the person; reassure that the experience is normal
Restlessness	Tension, fear, unfinished business	Listen to patient express fears, sadness, and anger; facilitate completion of business if possible
Unusual communication	Signals readiness to let go	Accept without judgment; kiss, hug, cry with patient as appropriate

---

BOX 34.11   Premonitions of Death

I had been seeing Mrs. Havens at home for several months to provide palliative care. At the end of an uneventful visit, I said my usual, "See you next week!" She hugged me goodbye and whispered, "I will see you, but you won't see me. Thank you for everything." She died peacefully 3 days later with her husband at her side.

---

may be a response to the inability to express feelings of foreboding and a sense of life escaping one's grasp. Many people have said that death is not the problem; it is the dying that takes the work. This is true for all involved: the person who is dying, the loved ones, the professional caregivers such as the nurses, and the nursing assistants in care facilities, who are too often invisible grievers.

Solutions, Nursing Actions, and Outcomes

Maslow's Hierarchy of Needs (Maslow, 1943) (Fig. 34.4) can serve as a guide in the development of nursing actions, with priorities directed by the patient or, if incapacitated, by the surrogate or proxy as indicated on a living will or another advance directive (Chapter 31).

Biological and Physiological Integrity

The dying person should have the highest quality of care possible; this always means expert symptom management. The most common physical symptoms are a sense of dyspnea, nausea, fatigue, and pain and those specific to the cause of the terminal condition. They are accompanied by any other symptoms associated with underlying concurrent chronic diseases. It is never acceptable for the person's symptoms of any kind to remain either untreated or undertreated. Ensuring that the person remains comfortable is the work of the nurse and other members of the caring team.

Dyspnea is the unpleasant sensation of breathlessness. It is common among those with terminal respiratory conditions such as lung cancer, end-stage pulmonary disease and the pulmonary complications of COVID-19 but also can be present for no apparent reason at the end of life. If the decision is made to treat the direct cause of this dyspnea with antiviral medications, antibiotics, steroids, or diuretics, it is still palliative care when the goal is comfort rather than cure. There is an increasing body of evidence that opioids are effective in relieving the discomfort of "terminal" breathlessness and may be combined with an antianxiolytic such as lorazepam to alleviate the associated anxiety that opioids trigger (Young & Widera, 2021). Supplemental oxygen provides significant relief for those with hypoxia but is probably of little benefit for those who do not have hypoxia. The nurse can provide other measures, such as elevating the head of the bed, using a bedside fan blowing gently on the person's face, or minimizing the need for conversation.

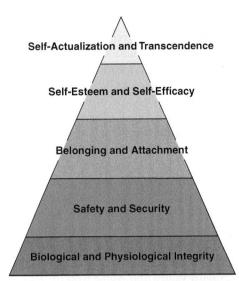

To share and come to terms with the unavoidable future
To perceive meaning in death

To maintain respect in the face of increasing weakness
To maintain independence to the extent possible
To feel like a normal person, a part of life right to the end
To preserve personal identity

To talk
To be listened to with understanding
To be loved and to share love
To be with a caring person when dying

To be given the opportunity to voice hidden fears
To trust those who care for him or her
To feel that he or she is being told the truth
To be secure

To obtain relief from physical symptoms
To conserve energy
To be free from pain

Fig. 34.4 Hierarchy of the dying person's needs, based on Maslow (1943). Modified from Beare PG, Myers JL: *Adult health nursing,* ed 3, St Louis, 1998, Mosby.)

TABLE 34.4 Examples of Common Causes of Nausea and Helpful Pharmacological Medications

Cause	Medication Class	Medication
Intestinal inflammation	Serotonin receptor antagonist	Ondansetron
Anticipatory anxiety	Benzodiazepines	Lorazepam
Constipation	Stimulant laxatives	Senna
Motion-induced labyrinthitis	Anticholinergic	Scopolamine

Adapted from Young NC, Widera EW: (2021). Geriatric palliative care. In Walter LC, Chang A, editors: *CURRENT diagnosis & treatment: geriatrics,* ed 3, New York, 2021, McGraw Hill, pp 174–180.

Nausea and sometimes vomiting are especially common as the end of life nears. This may be from disease processes or iatrogenic adverse effects, such as side effects of medications and constipation. If a cause can be found and treated, without increasing discomfort, it can be done. However, antiemetic medications and those with antiemetic effects may promote comfort (Table 34.4).

Dying requires much energy to cope with the physical assault of illness on the body and the spiritual and emotional unrest that dying initiates. Along with pain, *fatigue* is one of the most distressing symptoms but is underreported, unrecognized, and undertreated. Among the causes are adverse drug effects, hypoxia, deconditioning, and for unexplained reasons the terminal state alone. Nursing actions are directed toward helping the person conserve energy. How much can the individual do without becoming physically and emotionally taxed? What activities are the most important to do now, and must they be done independently? How much energy is needed for the patient to talk with those who are most important without becoming exhausted? Only the person who is dying can answer these questions, and the nurse can advocate for the person to be given the opportunity to do so.

The *pain* that often accompanies dying is not going to stop and usually requires a skillful combination of all the nonpharmacological and pharmacological interventions discussed in Chapter 29. The doses of medications required may be unfamiliar or uncomfortable for the administering nurse, but relief of pain is the highest priority (Box 34.12). Still, at times the person's pain may be so intense that usual solutions and interventions are unsuccessful.

In 1997 the US Supreme Court declared that while assisted suicide of any kind was illegal in the United States, pharmacological sedation for the relief of refractory pain by whatever means necessary was acceptable. The purpose of *palliative sedation* is to provide comfort but to go no further. This is based on the concept of *double effect*—that is, if the sedation provides comforts even if it is possible that death is hastened, it is considered neither assisted suicide nor euthanasia and is acceptable. The *intention* must be to relieve the suffering and not facilitate death. If intractable pain is identified, usually the administration of a 10% bolus dose of the 24-hour dose of medication is used, followed by subsequent doses every 15 minutes until pain

BOX 34.12 I Want a Hamburger and Watermelon Before I Die!

Jimmy, 55 years old, had a large, observable tumor of his large intestine with multiple metastases. All possible treatments had been unsuccessful. Initially he "did not want to starve" and was receiving total parenteral nutrition (TPN), necessitating a continuous intravenous infusion. As the TPN continued, the tumor enlarged while the rest of him shrunk, and the amount of morphine had to be increased until Jimmy was getting hundreds of milligrams a day. He had already used up his $1 million lifetime insurance coverage and had been granted permission to continue coverage. One day he told me that "it certainly seems this is not going away. If I stop the IV, I know I will die. But I really want to have a hamburger and some watermelon before then." After considerable discussion, the decision was made to turn off the TPN. In a short period of time the tumor began to shrink, and the morphine requirements lessened without any increase in symptoms. Eventually Jimmy was able to achieve his final wish, and he died shortly thereafter.

BOX 34.13   "I Just Can't Do It!"

Mr. Brown had advanced cancer with multiple bone metastases and no further treatment options. The nurse in the long-term care facility where he lived had physician orders to increase his dose of morphine per palliative care protocol as needed for comfort. On the night of his death, Mr. Brown was not fully alert but cried out, grimaced, and thrashed almost continuously. The nurse caring for him did not feel it was appropriate to give him any extra morphine because it "might affect his respirations." He screamed in apparent pain any time he was touched until he died several hours later. There was not another nurse on duty who challenged her decision.

---

is relieved (Reuban et al., 2020). The nurse who is not able to provide such relief is morally and ethically obligated to relinquish care to someone who can (Box 34.13).

By meeting the needs for freedom from pain and conservation of energy to minimize fatigue, the nurse has already begun to ensure that the person receives optimal care in order to maximize the quality of life to the extent possible for the time that remains.

Safety and Security

Dying is an emotional activity—for the dying and for those around them. In a safe and secure environment, fears and emotions can be expressed as desired and needs met. Such an environment is not intended to prevent sadness but to be able to have moments of relief. Empathetic listening and allowing those who are dying to verbalize what is on their minds are important nursing actions to promote safety and security. If tears and sadness are present, silence and touch, if acceptable, are worth more than words can convey. Physical closeness such as sitting near the person may be appropriate but not always possible, as was made clear during the care of those dying of COVID-19.

Belonging and Attachment

The need to belong is intimately tied to the need to communicate. This may be asking questions and receiving answers. Communication includes auditory, visual, and tactile stimulation to appropriately nurture and foster quality of life while dying. Verbal and nonverbal communication is necessary to convey positive messages but limited by the energy and stamina that are available at any one time. The nurse has a responsibility to ensure that the person has an opportunity for the communication desired. Nursing actions encourage openness whenever possible while respecting the patient's cultural patterns and behaviors. When the dying is openly acknowledged, the nurse may be asked, "Am I dying?" and "How and when will I die?" and "What is it going to be like?" It is essential to note that what is said and to whom is culturally determined. Talking about dying or death may be considered taboo, and speaking to the wrong person may be very inappropriate (Brown, 2017; Bryant, 2021). Hand holding, placing an arm around the shoulder, or sitting on the edge of the bed as culturally appropriate conveys to the person that the nurse or caregiver is available to listen. The counsel of the person's spiritual advisor may be needed.

The responsibility of health care professionals to assess spiritual needs during the dying process is stressed. When needs

are identified, nurses are expected to ensure that the needs are addressed. The nurse is reminded of the importance of attending to spiritual and cultural rituals that are important to the patient and family as a means of comfort and support (National Coalition for Hospice and Palliative Care, 2018).

At the specific direction of the patient, nursing actions may involve calling the patient's choice of a religious leader; sharing spiritual readings that are consistent with the patient's beliefs; reciting meditative poems and playing music of the person's choice; obtaining religious articles such as amulets, a Bible, or a rosary; or praying. *The nurse is strongly cautioned that these actions must be at the express request of the patient and may not at any time be suggested based on the nurse's own belief system.*

Loneliness may be the result of a loss of continuity with one's family life and results in existential distress. This can be soothed when the nurse asks about the person's life and those things most valued and works with the family to help the person to remain engaged in activities and past roles for as long as possible. A father who watches a certain ballgame with his son every Sunday can continue to do this regardless of the need to be in a hospital, a nursing home, or an inpatient hospice unit. A grandmother who is likely to die before a favorite grandchild's wedding can participate with planning, regardless of the age of the grandchild, if this is important to her, thereby leaving an enduring and special legacy.

Treating the person as an intelligent adult says "I care" and "You're not alone" and "You are important." The nurse can determine the personal preferences and values of the person and work toward honoring these, affirming belonging and attachment.

Self-Esteem and Self-Efficacy

As death nears, people often feel that they have less and less control over their lives and bodies. Control is the need to remain in a collaborative role relating to one's own living and dying and as active a participant in the care as desired. The person is in the process of losing everything that person has ever known or will ever know. The potential loss of identity, independence, and control over bodily functions can threaten self-esteem. The person may begin to feel ashamed, humiliated, and like a "burden." The nurse can help the person meet the need for self-efficacy by taking every opportunity to return the control to the person and helping them use any effective coping strategies used in the past and, in doing so, bolster self-esteem (Box 34.14).

Respecting one's decisions regarding end-of-life care bolsters self-esteem. This includes reviewing any previous decisions (verbal or written; e.g., in a living will—Chapter 31) when the person is able to communicate. It also includes a discussion of the preferred roles of the patient and significant other in the decision-making

---

BOX 34.14   I Need Help

For Mrs. Herbert, discussed in Box 34.5, once the nurses had the information about her daily meditation, they worked out a plan with her. Every morning between 6:00 and 6:30 a.m., she would not be disturbed. A "Do Not Disturb" sign would be placed on the intercom at the nurses' station and on her door. A noticeable change was seen in just a few days; Mrs. Herbert was calmer and coping well again. She was most appreciative to "have my life back again."

process (Chapter 4). Whenever possible, the nurse can have the person decide when to groom, eat, wake, sleep, and so on. The nurse never has the right to determine the activities of the individual, especially relating to visitors and how time is spent.

To ensure that one's end-of-life decisions transfer accurately from one care facility to another, the nurse can facilitate the completion of the POLST document (*Physicians Orders for Life-Sustaining Treatment*) whenever possible (see https://polst.org/form-patients/). It is signed by the physician (or nurse practitioner, depending on the state) after a discussion with the patient and a review of such documents as the living will. The POLST goes with the patient between settings. The POLST is not an advance directive; it is a health care provider order to emergency personnel and health care facilities and usually includes a do-not-resuscitate (DNR) order but not always (National POLST, 2021a) (Box 34.15). The POLST is not recognized in all states or organizations, yet without this or a similar document, emergency providers are required to do everything necessary to prolong life (National POLST, 2021b).

Self-Actualization and Transcendence

As discussed in detail in Chapter 35, self-actualization is individually defined but involves the presence of a sense of wholeness and belief in personal value, closely tied to self-esteem. For older adults who are facing the final steps of their journey on Earth, it may be the recognition of their own lingering continuity. The nurses can foster as normal a life as possible for those who are dying and help prevent the psychological and sociological deaths discussed earlier. Loved ones can be asked to provide life- and culture-affirming stimuli such as photographs, music, and mementos when staying at home is not possible. Self-esteem and dignity complement each other. Dignity involves the individual's ability to maintain a consistent self-concept (Box 34.16).

Reminiscence is one way of putting life in order, to evaluate the pluses and minuses of life and to think about the legacies that will be left behind (Chapter 35). It is a means of resolving conflicts if possible and making final goodbyes. Learning to say "goodbye" today leaves open the possibility of many more "hellos."

BOX 34.15 Tips for Best Practice

A do-not-resuscitate (DNR) order is a medical directive to health care professionals and first responders to refrain from initiating cardiopulmonary resuscitation in the event of a natural death. This may be found on the institutional medical record, a POLST form, or another document that is specifically recognized by a state. The nurse is often the one to facilitate this order is always available.

BOX 34.16 Transcending Nursing Home Life

I was asked to give a presentation on dying and death at a local nursing home and assumed it was for the staff. To my shock, the people waiting for me were patients, each in a wheelchair, most with their heads hung in their laps. Instead of the presentation I would have given, I walked around the room and, holding a microphone to each person, asked, "What do you want to be remembered for?" I heard, "I designed a bridge, I had a beautiful garden, I was a good mother..." As each person spoke, they lifted their heads as they could and smiled.

For some, transcendence while dying means coming to terms with the spiritual self, with the Great Spirit, Jesus, God, Allah, or Buddha—of that which has meaning to the person. If the patient has spiritual needs, arranging for pastoral care may be offered but should never be done without the person's permission. The nurse fosters transcendence by providing patients with the time and privacy for self-reflection and an opportunity to talk about whatever they need to discuss, especially about the meaning of their lives and the meaning of their deaths. Self-actualization and transcendence will not be possible unless the nursing actions include expert symptom management, care coordination, clear communication, and understanding the patients' priorities comes before all other actions.

Nurses seldom recognize the small things they do, routinely and unconsciously, to impart hope. The act of helping with grooming conveys a quiet belief that the person matters. Pain relief and comfort measures show that the individual's needs are recognized and reinforces the value of the person.

Promoting Equilibrium for the Family

The nurse is often present and supporting the family at the moment of death and in the moments both preceding and following it. Regardless of the age of the survivors, they, too, have needs, and nurses have a responsibility to care for them. Nursing actions should empower and facilitate the family to cope with the death in a manner consistent with their traditions.

Nurses can make a significant contribution to the family in fostering even momentary stability by knowing what questions to ask at the time of death, such as: What cultural or familial rituals are important right now? Is there anyone who should be called at this time? Would a spiritual advisor be a support for you right now? Have funeral arrangements already been made? If not, who can help you with this? When the death is imminent, ask: "Who needs to be notified; does this include a spiritual advisor?"

Nurses as Recipients of Care

In caring for those who are frail and dying in any setting, we are repeatedly exposed to the death of our patients; nurses are professional grievers. Some consider the death of a patient a failure—they have "lost" the person they cared for. However, when it is a good death, it can be viewed as a professional success because the nurse provided safe conduct for the dying and gentle care for the survivors. We can use the reminders of our own mortality as motivation to live the best we can with the time we have. Nurses can seek support and offer support to each other. As grievers, we too may need to tell our own story of the death to those professionals around us, in either formal or informal support groups. In addition, we need to listen to our colleagues' stories of death, over and over again if necessary.

Caring for older adults who are dying requires knowledge of the processes and skills in providing relief of symptoms or palliative care (Box 34.17). However, it is also acknowledged that working daily with the grieving or dying is an art. The development of this art necessitates inner strength. The nurse needs to have spiritual strength—strength from within. This does not mean that the nurse must have a specific religious orientation or

BOX 34.17   Nursing Skills Needed for the Practice of Palliative or End-of-Life Care

- Have ability to talk to patients and families about dying.
- Be knowledgeable about symptom control and pain-control techniques.
- Have ability to provide comfort-oriented nursing interventions.
- Recognize physical changes that precede imminent death.
- Deal with own feelings.
- Deal with angry patients and families.
- Be knowledgeable about and deal with the ethical issues in administering end-of-life palliative therapies.
- Be knowledgeable and inform patients about advance directives.
- Be knowledgeable about the legal issues in administering end-of-life palliative care.
- Be adaptable and sensitive to religious and cultural perspectives.

Modified from White KR, Coyne PJ, Patel UB: Are nurses adequately prepared for end-of-life care? *J Nurs Scholarsh* 33:147–151, 2001.

affiliation but rather that the nurse has a positive belief in self, a connection to others, and a belief that life has meaning and there is such a thing as a good death. Emotional maturity means that the nurse can reach out for help for self when needed. Finally, to provide comfort to grieving persons, nurses must be comfortable with their own lives or be able to set aside their own sadness and grief while working with that of others.

It is always important to remember that some nurses are unable to care for the dying because of their own unresolved conflicts and should not be expected to function in these roles. This may be a temporary situation associated with events in the nurse's life or something deeper, such as a traumatic experience involving the death of a loved one. Nurses should recognize their own limitations and defer care to other nurses when appropriate. In doing so, the nurse gives the most compassionate care possible.

KEY CONCEPTS

- Grief is a physical, emotional, and spiritual or existential response to loss.
- The Loss Response Model can be used to guide the development of nursing solutions and actions designed to optimize the quality of life for those who experience loss.
- Persons who are at risk for complicated grieving should receive specialized and skilled supportive care.
- The individual's response to loss and grief is similar to how that person has dealt with other stressors in life.
- An individual is living until death occurs; the nurse works with the person and significant others to maintain as high a quality of life as possible before, during, and after the loss or death.

- Hope is fluid and empowering; it can be appropriately supported during any aspect of the process of loss, grief, and mourning. Desirable hope generates courage and resilience.
- Palliative care is that which focuses on comfort rather than cure and can be provided regardless of setting.
- Hospice is a specific interdisciplinary approach to the provision of palliative care.
- Double effect is the accepted practice that permits the provision of as much medication as needed to relieve suffering, even if the amount has the potential to hasten death. It occurs in the context of palliative sedation.

NEXT-GENERATION NCLEX® (NGN) EXAMINATION–STYLE QUESTIONS

Jesse was simply unable to believe that his wife was dying. The physician told him that Jeanette was in the early stages of multiple myeloma and that she might die in less than a year or she might have remissions and live for another decade. Jesse and his wife had worked hard all their lives and raised two sons. Now they were both retired and financially secure and thought the best years of their lives were ahead of them. However, both Jesse and Jeanette were the type who approached a problem head-on. They studied all the relevant material they could find about multiple myeloma. Jeanette said that she did not want to mention her diagnosis to others because she thought that she was unable to deal with "their piteous cancer looks." She also stressed that she expected to have long remissions and to live at least 10 more years, so why trouble friends and family? As a result of her decision, Jesse was unable to share his fear and grief because he had promised to respect Jeanette's wishes. She began a series of chemotherapeutic drugs, and friends began to notice her lethargy. They began to worry about her, but she insisted, "I'm just fine." Six months passed with a steady downward course in Jeanette's condition.

Her sons began to suspect she had a malignancy, and one son, Rob, asked outright, "Are you hiding a serious illness from us?" She denied it, but Rob also noticed that Jesse was withdrawing into himself and that he was drinking more than usual. Rob knew something was wrong but was at a loss. When Rob went to the family physician for his annual checkup, the office nurse said, "Oh, Rob, how is your mother doing?" He responded, "I think there is something wrong with her. Why do you ask?"

Considering the current regulations about the protection of patient privacy, how would you respond to the son's question if you were the nurse? What is your priority in attending to the needs of Jesse? Of Jeanette? Of their children?

CLINICAL JUDGMENT QUESTIONS AND ACTIVITIES

1. Explore your likely responses to being given a terminal diagnosis. What coping strategies work for you?
2. Practice with a partner several methods that you will use to introduce the topic of dying with a patient who is critically ill and not expected to live long.
3. Discuss and strategize how you would bring up the topic of advance directives.
4. Explore with family and friends their thoughts on completing an advance directive.

RESEARCH QUESTIONS

1. What is the American Nurses Association's viewpoint on nurses' involvement in assisted suicide?
2. Is physician-assisted suicide or aid-in-death legal in your state?
3. Select a culture other than your own and explore loss, grief, and mourning rituals. How often are they used?

REFERENCES

Beck E, Jones SJ: Children of the condemned: grieving the loss of a father on death row, *Omega (Westport)* 56(2):191–215, 2007–2008.

Bristowe K, Marshall S, Harding R: The bereavement experiences of lesbian, gay, bisexual and/or trans* people who have lost a partner: a systematic review, thematic synthesis and modelling of the literature, *Palliat Med* 30(8):730–744, 2016.

Brown J: *Five death rituals to give you a new view on funerals* (website), 2017. https://www.newscientist.com/article/2152283-five-death-rituals-to-give-you-a-new-view-on-funerals/. Accessed July 2021.

Bryant S: *Death and dying: how different cultures view the end* (website), 2021. https://www.countrynavigator.com/blog/death-and-dying-how-different-cultures-view-the-end/.

Carr D, Sonnega Jn Nesse RM, et al: Do special occasions trigger psychological distress among older bereaved spouses? An empirical assessment of clinical wisdom, *J Gerontol B Psychol Sci Soc* 69(1):113–122, 2014.

Giacquinta B: Helping families face the crisis of cancer, *Am J Nurs* 77:1585–1588, 1977.

Glaser BG, Strauss AL: *Time for dying*, Chicago, 1968, Aldine.

Hall C: Beyond Kübler-Ross: recent developments in our understanding of grief and bereavement, *InPsych*, 33(6), 2011. http://www.psychology.org.au/publications/inpsych/2011, Accessed July 2018.

Horacek BJ: Toward a more viable model of grieving and consequences for older persons, *Death Stud* 15:459–472, 1991.

Jett KJ, Jett SW: The loss response model, 2014, unpublished manuscript.

Jones SJ, Beck E: Disenfranchised grief and nonfinite loss as experienced by the families of death row inmates, *Omega (Westport)* 54(4):281–299, 2007–2008.

Kübler-Ross E: *On death and dying*, New York, 1969, Macmillan.

Maciejewski PK, Maercker A, Boelen PA, et al: "Prolonged grief disorder" and "persistent complex bereavement disorder," but not "complicated grief," are one and the same diagnostic entity: an analysis of data from the Yale Bereavement Study, *World Psychiatry* 15(3):266–275, 2016.

Maslow AH: A theory of human motivation, *Psychol Rev* 50:370–396, 1943.

Mortell S: Assisting clients with disenfranchised grief: the role of the mental health nurse, *J Psychosoc Nurs Ment Health Serv* 53(4):52–57, 2015.

National Coalition for Hospice and Palliative Care: *Clinical practice guidelines for quality palliative care*, 4th edition, (available on the web) 2018. www.nationalcoalitionhpc.org/ncp.

National Hospice and Palliative Care Organization (NHPCO): *History of hospice* (website), 2021. https://www.nhpco.org/hospice-care-overview/history-of-hospice/.

National Hospice and Palliative Care Organization (NHPCO): *NHPCO facts and figures* (website), 2020. https://www.nhpco.org/wp-content/uploads/NHPCO-Facts-Figures-2020-edition.pdf.

National POLST: *What is POLST?* (website), 2021a. https://polst.org/professionals-page/.

National POLST: *Directory of POLST programs* (website), 2021b. https://polst.org/state-programs/.

O'Connor MF: Grief: a brief history of research on how body, mind, and brain adapt, *Psychosom Med* 81(8):731–738, 2019.

Pattison EM: *The experience of dying*, Englewood Cliffs, NJ, 1977, Prentice-Hall.

Powell T, Bellin E, Ehrlich AR: Older adults and COVID-19: the most vulnerable, the hardest hit, *The Hastings Center Report* 50(3):61–63, 2020.

Reuben DB, Herr KA, Pacala JT, et al: *Geriatrics at your fingertips*, ed 22, New York, 2020, American Geriatrics Society.

St. Christopher's: *Dame Cicely Saunders: her life and work* (website), 2021. https://www.stchristophers.org.uk/about/damecicelysaunders.

Weisman A: *Coping with cancer*, New York, 1979, McGraw-Hill.

Wilson SJ, Padin AC, Bailey BE, et al: Spousal bereavement after dementia caregiving: a turning point for immune health, *Psychoneuroendocrinology* 118:104717, 2020 [Epub].

Worden WJ: *Grief counseling and grief therapy: a handbook for the mental health practitioner*, ed 5, New York, 2018, Springer.

Wu EL, Brown RL, Chirinos DA, et al: Socioeconomic disparities in health: changes in sleep quality and inflammation during bereavement, *Compr Psychoneuroendocrinol* 7:100056, 2021[Epub].

Young NC, Wilders EW: Geriatric palliative care. In Walter LC, Chang A, editors: *CURRENT diagnosis & treatment: geriatrics*, ed 3, New York, 2021, McGraw Hill, pp 174–180.

The Nurse and Medical Aid in Death

Any nurse who works regularly with those who are dying will be asked at some time about what the nurse, the physician, or they can do to speed their death or ask for control over when and how this will occur. The potential for a person's ultimate control of his or her dying has risen to state and Supreme Court levels in the United States and to equivalent levels in other countries. In at least eight states and a number of countries, Physician-Assisted Dying (PAD) (also referred to as Medical Aid in Death) is legal in certain circumstances. PAD is defined as a physician providing a patient a prescription for a lethal dose of a medication, and instructions on how to use it. It can only be provided at the request of the person and under the conditions set in the "Right-To-Die" law in the state, jurisdiction, or country. In the United States the medication can never be administered by a physician, nurse, or any other health care professional. Active euthanasia, wherein a physician administers a lethal dose of a medication, is illegal in the United States, but has become legal in several countries (e.g., Netherlands; Victoria, Australia). It is usually limited to persons with "unbearable" suffering and no prospect of improvement. In most countries, active euthanasia is considered criminal homicide.

The request for aid-in-dying is an opportunity to clarify the cause of suffering, the emotional and situation factors, alternatives, and legal issues surrounding this. In 2019 the ANA advised that nurses should remain objective in discussing this issue when requested by the patient, have an ethical obligation to be knowledgeable about the issue and never abandon a patient, but also have a right to conscientiously object to being involved in the process while assuring that the person is cared for by another.

American Medical Association. (1995–2021). *Code of medical ethics: caring for patients at the end of life.* (https://www.ama-assn.org)

American Nurses Association. (2019). *ANA advises objectivity in new medical aid in dying position.* (https://www.nursingworld.org)

Srivastaca, V: Euthanasia: a regional perspective. *Ann Neurosci* 21(3):81–82, 2014.

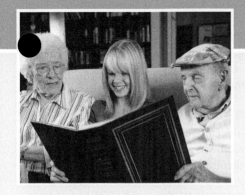

CHAPTER 35

Spiritual Health, Meaning, and Self-Actualization

Priscilla Ebersole,[a] *Theris A. Touhy*

http://evolve.elsevier.com/Touhy/TwdHlthAging

A STUDENT SPEAKS

Well, I always went to church with my parents when I was a child, but it was really boring. Now, I sometimes go with my grandmother to make her happy. I see how important it is to her, and I wonder if it will be important to me when I get really old. I'm just too busy right now.

Lori, age 22

AN OLDER ADULT SPEAKS

This is a real problem! I have three children and don't want them to squabble over my things when I'm gone. I would like it if they would each choose something special that would remind them of me, but every time I bring it up they cut me off and won't talk about it. I know there will be a big fight over the piano!

Mabel, age 84

LEARNING OBJECTIVES

On completion of this chapter, the reader will be able to:

1. Provide a comprehensive definition of self-actualization and identify several qualities of self-actualized older adults.
2. Discuss the nursing role in relation to the self-actualization of older adults.
3. Describe several examples of transcendence as experienced by older adults.
4. Specify various types of creative self-expression and describe their positive impact on health, illness, and quality of life among older adults.
5. Understand the meaning of spirituality in the lives of older adults and discuss nursing actions to facilitate spiritual health.
6. Define the concept of legacy and name several types of legacies and ways in which the nurse can facilitate their expression.

Self-actualization, spirituality, and *transcendence* are vague, ambiguous terms that mean whatever the theorist thinks. These expressions also serve as umbrella terms for other conditions and situations that are addressed throughout this chapter. These terms overlap a great deal, but we have attempted to tease out the meanings for the reader, knowing that the perception of the reader will cast a particular interpretation that we may not have thought or intended. These conditions are ineffable, within the awareness of the individual but often inexpressible. Why, if these concepts are so obscure, do we include them as the final chapter in a text for nurses working with older adults? Because these concepts are the life tasks of aging, seldom fully

approached earlier. Concerns of the young are to become established as adults; middle-aged persons are overwhelmed with the requirements of success and survival.

Older adults are more in touch with their inner psychological life than at any other point in the life cycle. Ferreting out the reason for being and the meaning of life is the concern of older adults. "As people age, confronting mortality is part of it, but as things change, they begin to recognize who they are and who they aren't, the strengths they have and haven't. They begin to think about the value and meaning of life. Tending to look more inwards rather than outwards often happens when we are 45 to 50, but there's a screaming need for it when we reach 85

---

[a]Special thanks to Dr. Priscilla Ebersole, the original author of this chapter, for her foundational and very wise contributions.

---

or 90" (Bernstein, 2009). An understanding of the developmental phases in the second half of life assists in understanding the journey toward self-actualization (Box 35.1).

Nurses likely will see numerous older adults who are apparently not seeking any of these esoteric states of existence and have never tried to cultivate their deepest inner nature. We live in a mechanistic, scientifically based culture in which cultivation of immeasurable states of being has not been necessarily regarded or regarded at all. The dramatic increase in the population of older adults has been considered a problem to be solved in an era of dwindling resources rather than a resource to enrich society.

Despite all the human efforts for the past millennia, we have not been able to completely grasp or dissect the human soul. I have many times approached this subject incorrectly by asking individuals what it is like to be old. Now that I am old, what it is like seems too concrete. What is the meaning of this stage of life? Every nurse must ask this question of older clients, friends, and parents. Do not ask on your way out the door. For many people, this notion will take some pondering. For some, it will open the door of their later lives just a crack. Others will be enlightened and will teach you a great deal.

SELF-ACTUALIZATION

Self-actualization is the highest expression of one's individual potential and implies inner motivation that has been freed to express the most unique self or the "authentic person" (Maslow, 1959, p. 3). The crux of self-actualization is defining life in such a way as to allow room for continual discovery of self. A critical consideration in developing self-actualization is an underlying sense of mastery and a sense of coherence in the life situation. This effort depends to a large extent on individual attributes and self-esteem. In this chapter, we hope to expose the nurse to the myriad evidence of self-actualization in old age and suggest

ways in which the nurse can assist older adults in seeking their own unique way of living, growing, and making meaning. The focus is on nursing actions that may encourage older adults to seek new possibilities within themselves.

Characteristics of the Self-Actualized

As we age, threats to self-esteem are strong if value is measured only by attainment, containment, power, and influence. Ethics, values, humor, courage, altruism, and integrity flourish in people who continue to grow toward self-actualization. Numerous other attributes can be mentioned. We focus only on those qualities that seem most pertinent to the older adult whom health care professionals are serving (Box 35.2).

Courage

Courage is the quality of mind or spirit that enables a person to conquer fear and despair in the face of difficulty, danger, pain, or uncertainty. Yet the person retains a positive spirit and love of life. This is courage. An older lady crippled with arthritis attends to her ailing spouse, who no longer recognizes her. This is courage. When asking older adults how they keep going day by day, various answers are given. No one has ever said to me, "It is because I am courageous." Older adults need to be told. A gold star can be given to people who have lived and survived the long battle of living many years filled with both joy and pain.

Tara Cortes, executive director of the Hartford Institute for Geriatric Nursing, shares the following quote from a 91-year-old gentleman: "It's a decision I make every morning when I wake up. I have a choice; I can spend the day in bed recounting the difficulty I have with parts of my body that no longer work, or get out of bed and be thankful for the ones that do. Each day is a gift, and as long as my eyes open, I'll focus on the new day and all the happy memories I've stored away just for this time in my life." The capacity of the spirit to find meaning in existence is often remarkable. Nurses may ask, "What sustains you in your present situation?"

Altruism

A high degree of helping behaviors is present in many older adults. The very old will remember the Great Depression and the altruism that kept people physically and spiritually alive. Neighbor helped neighbor long before the government came to the rescue. Apparently, a sense of meaning in life is strongly tied to survival and is derived from the conviction of, in some way, being needed by others. Many nurses are in the field because of altruistic motives and can understand the importance of assisting others. This idea might be discussed with the older adult.

Volunteering often involves new role development and endeavors that expand one's awareness. When volunteer services are considered as a means of personal enrichment and an expression of altruism, it is important for the individual to augment some latent interest areas and launch into pursuits perhaps unavailable earlier because of time constraints or other commitments. Nurses may question older adults about latent interests and talents that they may want to cultivate.

Humor

Metcalf (1993) explains humor: it originates in the Latin root *humour,* meaning fluid and flexible, able to flow around and wear away obstacles. In the same way that water sustains our life and well-being, humor sustains our mental well-being. Cousins (1979) and many other researchers have recognized the importance of humor in recovery from illness. The physiological effects of humor stimulate production of catecholamines and hormones and increase pain tolerance by releasing endorphins.

Older adults often initiate humor, and in our seriousness we may overlook the dry wit or, worse, perceive it as confusion. Older adults are not a humorless group and frequently laugh at themselves. Objections to jokes about old age seem to emanate from the young far more than the old. Perhaps the old, from the vantage point of a lifetime, can more clearly see human predicaments. Ego transcendence (Peck, 1955) allows one to step back and view the self and situation without the intensity and despair of the egocentric individual.

Continuous Moral Development

The moral development of mankind, on an individual and collective basis, has been of interest to philosophers and religious leaders throughout history. The driving forces of morality are love (Plato) and intellect (Aristotle). Kohlberg's refinements of his original theories have focused on the evidence, derived from autobiographies, that in maturity, transformations of moral outlook take place. Kohlberg posited old age as a seventh stage of moral development that goes beyond reasoning and reaches awareness of one's relative participation in universal morality. This stage of moral development involves identification with a more enduring moral perspective than that of one's own life span (Kohlberg & Power, 1981). This effort involves moral expansion and the exemplary impact of the fully developing older adult on the following generations, born and unborn. We have come to believe that these exemplary lives may be the most important function of older adults as we decry the honor and recognition given to individuals who seem to have little integrity or reliability. Youngsters must have models of honorable, truthful,

and honest older adults if we hope to cultivate these qualities in society and human experience.

Self-Renewal

Self-renewal is an ongoing process that ideally continues through adult life as one becomes self-actualized. According to Hudson (1999), self-renewal involves the following:

- Commitment to beliefs
- Connecting to the world
- Times of solitude
- Episodic breaks from responsibility
- Contact with the natural world
- Creative self-expression
- Adaptation to changes
- Learning from down times

Collective Self-Actualization

The collective power of self-actualized older adults has already brought about many changes in society. *Power* is a term describing the capacity of an individual or group to accomplish something, to take command, to exert authority, and to influence. The self-actualized older adult is powerful and confident. Power is the gateway to resources and recognition. The age-equality movement, older citizens returning to school, and the revolution of older adults in movements such as the Gray Panthers have produced major changes in the status and recognition of older adults. Gray Panthers recognize that issues of aging are not narrow or exclusive but rather are representative of human rights for people of all ages. Maggie Kuhn (1979), founder of the Gray Panthers, died in 1995 at the age of 89, but her beliefs and followers survive. Kuhn perceived that the issues confronting older adults are not those of self-interest. As "elders of the tribe," the old should seek "survival of the tribe" (Kuhn, 1979, p. 3).

WISDOM

Wisdom is an ancient concept that has historically been associated with the older adults of a society. Wisdom represents the pinnacle of human development and can be compared to Maslow's self-actualization or Erickson's ego integrity. In many cultures, older adults are respected for their years of experience and are awarded the role of wise older adult in political, judicial, cultural, and religious systems. In recent years, there has been renewed interest in the concept of wisdom and the capacity of the aging brain to develop unique capacities. Many skills improve with age but are not identified on standard cognitive screens, and certain testing conditions have exaggerated age-related declines in cognitive performance. The bulk of research has focused on cognitive declines and strategies to help older adults find ways to overcome cognitive failings. Because of this emphasis, research on cognitive capacities in aging and possible ways to stimulate wisdom has been limited.

Moving beyond Piaget's formal operational stage of cognitive development, adult development theories propose a more advanced cognitive stage, the postformal operational stage. In this stage, individuals develop the skills to view problems

---

BOX 35.3   Dimensions of Wisdom

- **Cognitive:** Knowledge and acceptance of the positive and negative aspects of human nature, the limits of knowledge, and of life's unpredictability and uncertainties; a desire to know the truth and comprehend the significance and deeper meaning of experiences, phenomena, and events
- **Reflective:** Being able to perceive phenomena and events from multiple perspectives; self-awareness, self-examination, self-insight; absence of subjectivity and projections (e.g., the tendency to blame other people or circumstances for one's own situation, decisions, or feelings)
- **Affective:** Sympathetic and compassionate love for others; positive emotions and behaviors toward others

From Ardelt M: Wisdom as expert knowledge system: a critical review of a contemporary operationalization of an ancient concept, *Hum Dev* 47:257–285, 2004.

---

from multiple perspectives, use reflection, and communicate thoughtfully in complex and emotionally challenging situations (Parisi et al., 2009). Recent neuroimaging research has suggested that changes in the brain, once seen only as compensation for declining skills, are now thought to indicate development of new capacities (Chapter 8).

Characteristics of Wisdom

One does not become wise simply because one grows old. Nor is wisdom achieved simply because of an accumulation of life experiences. Most agree that the achievement of wisdom is a developmental process that requires the ability to "integrate experiences across time and utilize these experiences in a reflective manner" (Parisi et al., 2009, p. 867). Maturity, integrity, generativity, the ability to overcome negative personality characteristics such as neuroticism or self-centeredness, superior judgment skills in difficult life situations, the ability to cope with difficult challenges in life, and a strong sense of the ultimate meaning and purpose of life are also associated with wisdom (Ardelt, 2004) (Box 35.3). Wisdom is a major contributor to successful aging. The renewed emphasis on wisdom and other cognitive capabilities that can develop with age provides a view of aging that reflects the history of many cultures and provides a much more hopeful view of both aging and human development.

Paths to growing older and wiser can be fostered throughout life. Viewing older adults as resources for younger people, our society places the reason for and the immense value of aging at the center of focus. This is in contrast to the view of aging as inevitable decline, personal diminishment, disengagement from life, and a drain on society. Nursing, too, must turn to the wise leaders who came before us as we chart our course for the future (Chapter 1). Priscilla Ebersole, one of the geriatric nursing pioneers, original coauthor of this textbook, and coauthor of this chapter, shares her reflections on wisdom from the perspective of her 90 years (Box 35.4). With the prospect of longer and healthier lives, older adults are looking for more meaningful and challenging ways to foster continued growth and contribute to society. Programs such as Foster Grandparents, the Experience Corps, and the Sage-ing Guild are examples of this new view.

BOX 35.4   Reflections on Wisdom: Priscilla Ebersole, Geriatric Nursing Pioneer

In thinking about wisdom, I wonder what it is and if we ever achieve anything near that in one lifetime. I now have more questions about life than I have answers.

- Where are we in the process of human evolution? We seem to be consumed with speed and technical wonders. What about the extrasensory perceptions and amazing coincidences that seemingly arise randomly? Are we still primitives?
- Dying: Doesn't it present more questions? I have become immunized as so many I love have preceded me, but it would be wonderful to know how much time I have—or would it?
- How can one develop true compassion? I have flashes of it, but find I still have many judgmental feelings about many persons and events. Is this not practical?
- How can I learn more from others? I am rather trapped in my own skin and imperfections.
- Is it true that our hormones really affect us so much? Yes, undoubtedly I have become much more aggressive with the almost total loss of estrogen. Do I care?
- Is the search for prolongevity a worthy goal? Only when one is healthy and has something to offer the world. But, really, what is healthy? Only function? Mind health?
- Does history really teach us anything? Though we seem to repeat so much of it yet pondering it and our roots remains significant for me. And what about the universe, both macro and micro of which we really still know so little? Pondering and wondering, I will never know even a bit of all I wish.

Yet, becoming old is becoming, as life seems to hold many lifetimes in one. There are so many challenges and circumstances that change one's perspective and beliefs. One begins to feel a part of and connected to every living thing. The youth and elders in one's lifetime are so significant in one's philosophy. Grandchildren and great grandchildren open new vistas of thought and opportunities to redo some of the faltering actions of parenthood.

It seems one important goal is to learn to enjoy life in spite of all the bumps one experiences along the way. Maybe learning to be content with whatever one is and whatever one can do and one's tribe, family, becomes increasingly important. One of my granddaughters said she loves to see how much I enjoy life and her ability to see that in me is something I will always treasure. That is a gift I hope to leave with her and others whom I contact. I think I have learned to really enjoy this precious gift of life. Catherine, my friend who died at 106, taught me more about aging than any experience in my life. She still giggled like a school girl as she told me of some amusing event in her life.

CREATIVITY

Creativity is a bridge between the growing self and the transcending of self. Creativity may be the transit mechanism between self-actualization (the reaching of one's highest potential) and the step beyond, to transcend the limitations of ego. "Creativity has always been at the heart of our experience as human beings . . . this need for creativity never ends" (Perlstein, 2006, p. 5). American culture has neglected to recognize the innate creativity of older adults, who are too often viewed as debilitated, dependent, burdensome, and the focus of societal problems. Promoting health in aging is more than targeting problems and developing interventions for health promotion and disease prevention. Aging encompasses potential and problems. A focus on creativity and aging and the positive impact of the arts on health, illness, and quality of life is gaining importance in our understanding of health and well-being among older adults.

The National Center for Creative Aging (https://uclartsandhealing.org/resources_pages/national-center-for-creative-aging-ncca/) is dedicated to fostering the relationship between creative expression and quality of life for older adults. The *Beautiful Minds: Finding Your Lifelong Potential* campaign is an initiative from the Center that focuses on raising awareness of people who are keeping their minds beautiful and on the actions people can take to maintain the brain. Research suggests that there are four dimensions to brain health: the nourished mind, the socially connected mind, the mentally active mind, and the physically active mind. These dimensions stress the importance of healthy diet, social engagement, cognitive stimulation, and physical activity to brain health.

Products of creativity are less important than creative attitudes. Curiosity, inquisitiveness, wonderment, puzzlement, and craving for understanding are creative attitudes. Much of the natural creative imagination of childhood is subdued by enculturation. As individuals age, some people seem able to break free of excessive enculturation and again express their free spirit when practical matters no longer demand their sole attention. Creativity is often considered in terms of the arts, literature and music, but a truly self-actualized person may express creativity in any activity.

Breaking through the habitual or traditional mode into authentic expression of self is creativity, whether it is through cooking, cleaning, planting, poetry, art, or teaching. Creative expression does not necessarily mean that the older adult has to create a work of art. Subtler ways of expressing creativity are present even in the frailest of older adults. Consider Dr. Ebersole's description of Catherine at 100 years old and living in a nursing home (Box 35.5).

Creative Arts for Older Adults

Maximizing the use of self in the later years in unique ways might be termed *creative self-actualization*. Many individuals will need the stimulus of an interested person to uncover latent interests and talents. Other adults will need encouragement to try new avenues of self-expression—some will be fitting for them and others not. Wikström suggests that art and aesthetics "help individuals know themselves, become more alive to human conditions, provide a new way of looking at themselves and the world, and offer opportunities for participation in new visual and auditory experiences" (2004, p. 30). Several ideas are presented here for nurses working with older adults to encourage creative expression (Box 35.6).

Creative arts and expression offer great value to people with dementia and hold tremendous promise to improve quality of life. Programs of dance, storytelling (Chapter 7), music, poetry, and art should be included in activities for individuals with dementia. Killick (1997, 2000, 2008) has done beautiful work

---

BOX 35.5 Catherine: Another View of Creativity

Catherine was self-actualized and creative to the best possible extent. Her physical constraints were enormous: she had no material assets, her range of activity was limited to her small cubicle in a skilled nursing facility, and her body was frail. However, her spirit was strong, and she knew and used her potential. Catherine's creativity was expressed at each meal when she rearranged, mixed, and added to her food. She carefully chopped a pickle and sprinkled it on her cottage cheese and added a little honey to her applesauce. Each meal was a small adventure. Several friends would visit regularly and bring Catherine small items she enjoyed. They could always count on being entertained with creatively embroidered tales of the past. The gifts they brought were always used in extraordinary ways. A scarf might be tied around her head. Powder, perfume, books, and other things would be bartered for favors from staff members or given as gifts. Her radio brought news of the day interspersed with classical music. Catherine created a milieu in which she enjoyed life and maintained her self-esteem. That she was self-actualized was never in doubt. Her artistry overflowed in myriad small gestures.

BOX 35.6 Ideas for Developing Creative Abilities

Art

Using oil pastels, create a drawing that represents self, or select three colors you like and three colors you dislike, using all six colors to create a self-portrait.

Draw a representation of your world.

Create a collage or mobile out of an assortment of materials and pictures that can represent subjects, such as the self, part of self you like or dislike, or the family.

In small groups, use clay to create an art piece or a statement.

Music

Play a variety of music; focus discussion on imagery and any feelings that the music evokes.

Discuss or have clients bring in music that elicits feelings of sadness, happiness, and so on.

Show a picture (can be cut from a magazine) and ask members to see if they can imagine the sounds that might go with the picture.

Express self or group through dance and movement to select music.

Movement

Create a movement to fit the way you are feeling while introducing self to group.

Have members stand and initiate a slow, swaying motion (good exercise with which to end the group session).

Have members mirror each other's movements, such as hands or the entire body, creating a duet.

Imagery

Use guided fantasies and imagery to facilitate stress reduction and relaxation, awareness, the power of one's own healing capability, and self-expression through symbols and symbolisms.

Writing

Encourage journals or diaries; set a group time available to write and share ideas.

In small groups, create a group poem.

Read selected poems or stories as a group, and then share reactions and feelings from the readings.

Create a book to be distributed to the group consisting of a collection of members' writings.

with poetry writing for persons who have dementia and has said that "people with dementia can often find a real solace and satisfaction and a creativity in speaking in this way and having it recognized as being of value because they're so used to being put down" (Killick, 2008).

At the Louis and Anne Green Memory and Wellness Center in the Christine E. Lynn College of Nursing at Florida Atlantic University, the "Artful Memories" program provides opportunities for individuals with mild to moderate dementia to learn techniques of artistic creation and expression in artistic media in a supportive and nonjudgmental environment (Chapter 26; Fig. 35.1). Works created are on display at the Center and in local art museums and also have been made into calendars (Fig. 35.2). Participants have derived a great deal of pleasure, pride, stimulation, and camaraderie from the time spent creating art.

Kagan (2020) eloquently expressed the value of the arts in care of older adults:

> The arts, as expressions of creativity, emotion, and spirit, uncover strength. For us as nurses and for our colleagues and—most critically—for older people and those who love them … imagine the possibilities of the arts. Telling our stories to glean wisdom. Hearing our poetry to learn lessons of the soul. Lis-

> tening to music for healing and harmony. Painting or sculpting our inner vision or appreciating that of another. Dancing our way to freedom, if only for the next few beats. We will find in ourselves and those in our care capacities—strength and flexibility of the soul, the mind and the body—we might never recognize without clarity brought by art. (p. 2)

RECREATION

Recreation is akin to creation. The wisdom of regularly scheduled periods of recreation and recuperation following creative acts can be traced to early Jewish writings and the creation story. If God needed time to rest and recuperate, we certainly do. Inherent in creative acts is time for renewal, time for recreation. Burnout and boredom are companions of monotony and shorten the perceived life span by emptiness and vanished time. A change of scenery or companions may be exhilarating. The opportunity to be outside or look at beautiful scenery is also renewing. Many long-term care facilities are providing opportunities for gardening and enjoying nature. Retreats from routine to periods of recreation are important, as are retreats following intensive efforts. Resources that can enhance recreational activities and programs are presented in Box 35.7.

BRINGING YOUNG AND OLD TOGETHER

Larson (2006) suggests that intergenerational programs can "help older and younger people look beyond their generational stereotypes and know each other (body, mind, and spirit)" (p. 39). Intergenerational programs can be those in which older adults assist younger people (tutoring, mentoring, childcare, foster

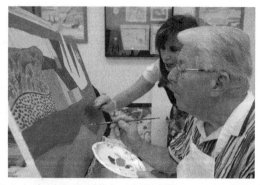

Fig. 35.1 Artful Memories program. (Courtesy Louis and Anne Green Memory and Wellness Center of the Christine E. Lynn College of Nursing at Florida Atlantic University.)

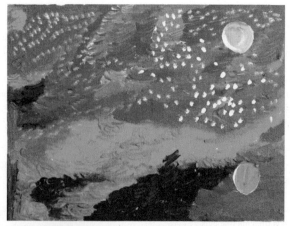

Fig. 35.2 Artwork created by Frances Hope Goldstein in the Florida Atlantic University's Louis and Anne Green Memory and Wellness Center "Artful Memories" program.

BOX 35.7 Resources to Enhance Recreational Activities and Programs

- Local florists may present a flower show or provide a flower-arranging activity.
- Police and fire departments may give safety presentations.
- Local religious leaders may lead readings and discussions of religious or philosophical works.
- Craft suppliers may give demonstrations.
- Local pharmacists may give talks on medication use.
- Nurses or nursing students may give talks on health and well-being in aging.
- Clothing stores can sponsor fashion shows.
- Bakeries may give demonstrations of pastry decoration.
- Beauty supply houses may give makeup demonstrations.
- Travel agencies may present slide shows.
- Librarians may institute great book discussions or other activities.
- Students from community colleges may provide numerous educational events and activities.
- Garden clubs or horticultural groups may provide gardening classes.
- Collectors' clubs may talk about collecting stamps, antiques, coins, or memorabilia.
- Historical societies may give tours to historic places of interest.
- Whenever possible, events should be planned as field trips to the sites of the locals involved because trips add elements of additional interest, stimulation, and involvement in the community at large.

grandparent programs); those in which younger people assist older adults (social visits, meal assistance); and those in which the young and old serve together. Benefits of intergenerational programs for younger people include increased self-esteem and self-worth, improved behavior, increased involvement and success in schoolwork, and a sense of historical and personal continuity. For older adults, contact with younger people can promote life satisfaction, decrease isolation, help develop new skills and insights, promote fulfillment, establish new and meaningful relationships, and provide a sense of meaning and purpose. Examples of such programs include Elders Share the Arts, Roots & Branches Theater company, and the Liz Lerman Dance Exchange.

Recognizing the developmental significance of contact between the generations, some long-term care facilities have included children in their milieu in various ways:

- *As residents* (children with profound developmental disabilities or severe neurological disabilities): Older adults rock, stroke, and cuddle these children, providing stimulation for both.
- *As a service to employees* (daycare centers for children of employees): Older adults sometimes assist in the care and special programs for the children, such as reading stories or teaching basic skills (tying shoes, telling time).
- *In adopt-a-grandparent programs:* One child affiliates with a resident with periodic visits, cards, and inclusion of the grandparent in some special family events.

Interesting intergenerational living programs in the Netherlands, France, and Cleveland, Ohio, offer rent-free living to college students in retirement and nursing homes. In the Netherlands, students are required to spend at least 30 hours a month acting as "good neighbors" by performing activities such as teaching new skills in use of email and social media, Skyping, walking dogs, watching sports, celebrating birthdays, and offering company. At Judson Manor in Cleveland, students from the Cleveland Institutes of Art and Music are integrated into the resident population. Students participate in the musical arts committee, assist staff therapists, volunteer at various events, and give quarterly performances to the residents (Hansman, 2015; Harris, 2016; Jansen, 2016). These innovative programs are featured in a short video (https://www.usatoday.com/videos/news/nation/2017/02/24/students-take-up-residence-retirement-homes/98342876/).

Nurses in the community may want to explore potential intergenerational experiences that might be of interest to older adults. Area Agencies on Aging can provide information on intergenerational programs available in the community. Although there are benefits to intergenerational contact when desired by the older adult, certain pitfalls must be considered. Not all older adults will enjoy contact with children. Contacts with a very young, energetic child must be brief, or the older adult is likely to become exhausted and the benefits will decrease. In intergenerational programs, young people need consistent supervision, support, and training in the developmental aspects of old age. Similarly, older adults will benefit from education and support in understanding developmental tasks of children and effective methods of intergenerational communication.

Solutions, Nursing Actions, and Outcomes: Self-Actualization and Aging

In this chapter, we have considered what aging can be and that the last years can truly actualize the most unique capacities of older adults. Our functions as nurses who value self-actualization are (1) to continually spur our clients to ask, "What is possible and suitable for me?" and (2) to assist them in finding appropriate resources and, when needed, assist in implementing activities toward self-actualization. The nature of self-actualization is self-determination and direction. Nurses are ancillary to the process but may be needed to stir the beginnings of the search. In doing so, we may move forward with our own search.

Self-actualization implies that one actualizes the potential of self through various mechanisms. We have mentioned only a few of these mechanisms in a somewhat cursory manner, knowing that these individually instituted actions have a force of their own and that once activated go far beyond the professionals' involvement. Activities such as yoga, focused meditation, the discipline of karate, and other forms of centered concentration are segued into spirituality and transcendence.

SPIRITUALITY

Spirituality is a rather indescribable need that drives individuals throughout life to seek meaning and purpose in their existence. Spirituality is difficult to define, though many people have tried. We can observe the body and we can imagine the mind in operation and measure intelligence, but there is no computed tomography (CT) scan of the spirit (Bell & Troxel, 2001). Understanding spirituality is far more elusive than learning about the pathology associated with disease and illness. Spirituality has been defined as a "quality of a person derived from the social and cultural environment that involves faith, a search for meaning, a sense of connection with others, and a transcendence of self, resulting in a sense of inner peace and well-being" (Delgado, 2007, p. 230). The spiritual aspect of people's lives transcends the physical and psychosocial to reach the deepest individual capacity for love, hope, and meaning. Spiritual health is an integral component of human well-being.

Aging as a biological process has been studied extensively. Less attention has been paid to the study of aging as a spiritual process. As people age and move closer to death, spirituality may become more important. Declining physical health, loss of loved ones, and a realization that life's end may be near often challenge older adults to reflect on the meaning of their lives. Spiritual belief and practices often play a central role in helping older adults cope with life challenges and are a source of strength in their lives. Spirituality and religious participation are highly correlated with positive successful aging, as much as are diet, exercise, mental stimulation, self-efficacy, and social connectedness.

The role of spirituality, religion, and/or belief can have numerous positive effects for older adults, including enhanced health and well-being, greater capacity to cope, social support, and opportunities to participate in society (Malone & Dadswell, 2018) (see Research Highlights box). Spirituality may be particularly important to healthy aging in "historically disadvantaged populations who display remarkable strength despite adversities in their lives" (Hooyman & Kiyak, 2005, p. 213).

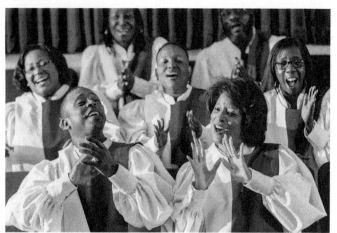

For some older adults, participating in church activities can be a source of comfort and joy. (iStock.com/kali9.)

⬚ RESEARCH HIGHLIGHTS

The Role of Religion, Spirituality, and/or Belief in Positive Aging for Older Adults

Purpose
Positive aging is gaining recognition as an approach to better understand the lives of older adults throughout the world. Positive aging encompasses the various ways in which older adults approach life challenges associated with aging and how certain approaches allow older adults to age in a more positive way. This study examines the role of religion, spirituality, and/or belief in relation to positive aging.

Method
Qualitative focus groups were conducted with 14 adults living in West London to explore the role and importance of religion, spirituality, and/or belief in their everyday lives and how this could be incorporated into the idea of positive aging. Participants ranged in age from 63 to 92 years of age. Three participants described themselves as having no religious or spiritual beliefs, 2 were Muslim, 1 was Jewish, 5 were Christian, and the remaining 3 described their religious or spiritual affiliation as a mixture of things.

Results
A thematic analysis was conducted of videotaped focus groups, and five common themes were identified: (1) changing religious landscapes in a modern world; (2) the personal and interpersonal nature of religion; (3) spirituality and/or belief; a source of strength, comfort, and hope; (4) sense of community and belonging; and (5) the need for a holistic approach.

Conclusion
Religion, spirituality, and/or belief should be included in the positive aging literature and research and be viewed as a type of support (among multiple others) that helps older adults to live positive lives despite the many challenges of aging. The participants also indicated their desire for a more personal and holistic approach to their health and well-being, where health care professionals understood more about the life of an older adult, which could include religion, spirituality, and/or belief if it is considered important for the individual.

Data from Malone J, Dadwell A: The role of religion, spirituality and/or belief in positive ageing for older adults, *Geriatrics (Basel)* 32(2):28, 2018.

Spirituality and Religion

Distinguishing between religion and spirituality is a concern for many health professionals. Religious beliefs and participation in religious obligations and rites are often the avenues of spiritual expression, but they are not necessarily interchangeable. "Religion can be described as a social institution that unites people in a faith in God, a higher power, and in common rituals and worshipful acts. Each religion involves a particular set of beliefs and a god, divinity, and/or soul is always included in the concept" (Strang & Strang, 2002, p 858). For some people, particularly older adults, formalized religion helps them feel fulfilled. Spirituality is a broader concept than religion and encompasses a person's values or beliefs, search for meaning, and relationships with a higher power, with nature, and with other people. The concept of spirituality is found in all cultures and societies.

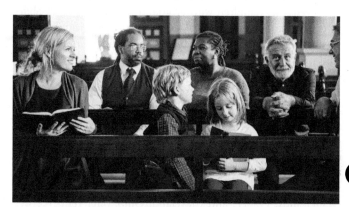

Attending formal religious services enhances meaning in life for some individuals. (© iStock.com/Rawpixel.)

For some older adults, particularly those who are frail or cognitively impaired, meeting spiritual needs may be a greater challenge than for healthier older adults. Functional decline and dependence can threaten the sense of identity and connection with others and the world, thus causing a loss of spirit. However, although aging changes can affect the body and the mind, there is no evidence that the spirit succumbs to the aging process even in the face of debilitating physical and emotional illness (Heriot, 1992). The spiritual aspect transcends the physical and psychosocial to reach the deepest individual capacity for love, hope, and meaning. The spiritual person can rise above that which is humanly expected in a situation. For example, a dying older adult in great pain who was being cared for by Dr. Ebersole (chapter coauthor) said: "This is so hard for you." That he was able to see beyond himself at that time was difficult to believe.

USING CLINICAL JUDGMENT TO PROMOTE HEALTHY AGING: SPIRITUAL HEALTH

Recognizing and Analyzing Cues

Assessment of spirituality is as important as assessment of physical, emotional, and social dimensions. A spiritual history opens the door to a conversation about the role of spirituality and religion in a person's life. People often need permission to

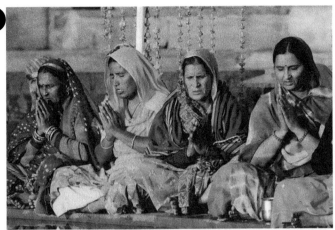

Prayer is an important spiritual practice in many cultures. (©iStock.com/kaetana_istock.)

BOX 35.8 Identifying Older Adults at Risk for Spiritual Distress

- Individuals experiencing events or conditions that affect the ability to participate in spiritual rituals
- Diagnosis and treatment of a life-threatening, chronic, or terminal illness
- Expressions of interpersonal or emotional suffering, loss of hope, lack of meaning, need to find meaning in suffering
- Evidence of depression
- Cognitive impairment
- Verbalized questioning or loss of faith
- Loss of interpersonal support

Data from Gaskamp C, Sutter R, Meraviglia M, et al: Evidence-based guideline: promoting spirituality in the older adult, *J Gerontol Nurs* 32:8–13, 2006.

talk about these issues. Without a signal from the nurse, patients may feel that such topics are not welcome. Patients welcome a discussion of spiritual matters and want health professionals to consider their spiritual needs. The older adult may have a pressing need to talk about philosophy and spiritual development. Private time for prayer, meditation, and reflection may be needed.

Nurses may neglect to explore this issue with older adults because religion and spirituality may not seem the high priority, and care focuses primarily on physical aspects. The individual should be assured that religious longings and rituals are important and that opportunities will be made available as desired. Nurses need to be knowledgeable and respectful about the rites and rituals of varying religions, cultural beliefs, and values (Chapter 4). Religious and spiritual resources, such as pastoral visits, should be available in all settings where older adults reside. It is important to avoid imposing one's own beliefs and to respect the person's privacy on matters of spirituality and religion (Touhy & Zerwekh, 2006).

An emphasis on spirituality in nursing is not new; nursing has encompassed the spiritual from its origin. The science of nursing was not seen as separate from the art and spirit of the discipline. Florence Nightingale's view of nursing was derived from her spiritual philosophy, and she considered nursing a spiritual experience, "intrinsic to human nature, our deepest and most potent resource for healing" (Macrae, 1995, p. 8). Many nursing theories address spirituality, including those of Neuman, Parse, and Watson (Martsolf & Mickley, 1998). Nursing and medicine are beginning to reclaim some of the essential healing values from their roots.

The essence of being spiritual is being whole or holistic, and attention to the spiritual needs of patients is a critical dimension of holistic nursing care. Yet surveys with practicing nurses suggest that most have had little, if any, education in spiritual care. Many nurses view spiritual nursing responses in religious terms and may feel that spirituality is a religious matter better left to clergy and religious leaders. Heriot (1992) suggested that nurses need to understand care of the human spirit both within and outside the context of religion. Goldberg (1998) asserted that the connection in the nurse-patient relationship is central to spiritual care but that most nurses are "carrying out spiritual interventions at an unconscious level" (p. 840). She called for education and research to help nurses become more aware of the importance of connection and use of self in relationships as ways of bringing the elements of spiritual care into conscious awareness.

An evidence-based guideline for promoting spirituality in the older adult (Gaskamp et al., 2006) provides a framework for spiritual assessment and interventions. The guideline identifies older adults who may be at risk for spiritual distress and who might be most likely to benefit from use of the guideline (Box 35.8). Spiritual distress or spiritual pain is "an individual's perception of hurt or suffering associated with that part of his or her person that seeks to transcend the realm of the material.

Spiritual distress is manifested by a deep sense of hurt stemming from feelings of loss or separation from one's God or deity, a sense of personal inadequacy or sinfulness before God and man, or a pervasive condition of loneliness" (Gaskamp et al., 2006, p. 9). The person experiencing spiritual distress is unable to experience the meaning of hope, connectedness, and transcendence. Spiritual distress may be manifested by anger, guilt, blame, hatred, expressions of alienation, turning away from family and friends, inability to derive pleasure, and inability to participate in religious activities that have previously provided comfort.

Spiritual Assessment Tools

There are formal spiritual assessments, but open-ended questions also can be used to begin dialogue about spiritual concerns (Box 35.9). Simply listening to older adults as they express their fears, hopes, and beliefs is important. The process of spiritual assessment is more complex than completing a standardized form and must be done within the context of the nurse-patient relationship. Spiritual assessments are intended to elicit information about the core spiritual needs and how the nurse and other members of the health care team can respond to them. These include the Faith, Importance and Influence, Community, and Address (FICA) Spiritual History (Puchalski & Romer, 2000) and the Brief Assessment of Spiritual Resources and Concerns (Koenig & Brooks, 2002; Meyer, 2003) (Box 35.10). The Joint Commission requires spiritual assessments in hospitals, nursing homes, home care organizations, and many other health care settings providing services to older adults.

BOX 35.9   Questions to Begin Dialogue About Spiritual Concerns

- Tell me more about your life.
- What has been most meaningful in your life?
- To whom do you turn when you need help?
- What brings you joy and comfort?
- What are you most proud of?
- How have you found strength throughout your life?
- What are you hopeful about?
- Is spiritual peace important to you? What would help you achieve it?
- Is your religion or God significant in your life? Can you describe how?
- Is prayer or meditation helpful?
- What spiritual or religious practices bring you comfort?
- Are there religious books or materials that you want nearby?
- What are you afraid of right now?
- What do you wish you could still do?
- What are your concerns at this time for the future?
- What matters most to you right now?

Adapted from Touhy T, Zerwekh J: Spiritual caring. In Zerwekh J, editor: *Nursing care at the end of life: palliative care for patients and families*, Philadelphia, 2006, FA Davis.

BOX 35.10   Brief Assessment of Spiritual Resources and Concerns

Instructions: Use the following questions as an interview guide with the older adult (or caregiver if the older adult is unable to communicate).
- Does your religion/spirituality provide comfort or serve as a cause of stress? (Ask to explain in what ways spirituality is a comfort or stressor.)
- Do you have any religious or spiritual beliefs that might conflict with health care or affect health care decisions? (Ask to identify any conflicts.)
- Do you belong to a supportive church, congregation, or faith community? (Ask how the faith community is supportive.)
- Do you have any practices or rituals that help you express your spiritual or religious beliefs? (Ask to identify or describe practices.)
- Do you have any spiritual needs you would like someone to address? (Ask what those needs are and if referral to a spiritual professional is desired.)
- How can we (health care providers) help you with your spiritual needs or concerns?

From Gaskamp C, Sutter R, Meraviglia M, et al: Evidence-based guideline: promoting spirituality in the older adult, *J Gerontol Nurs* 32:10, 2006. Adapted from Meyer CL: How effectively are nurse educators preparing students to provide spiritual care? *Nurse Educ* 28(4):185–190, 2003; Koenig HG, Brooks RG: Religion, health and aging: implications for practice and public policy, *Public Policy Aging Rep* 12:13–19, 2002.

For older adults with cognitive impairment, information about the importance of spirituality and religious beliefs can be obtained from family members. Nurses often see cognitive impairments as obstacles or excuses to providing spiritual care to people with dementia. Nurturing mind, body, and spirit is part of holistic nursing, and nurses must provide opportunities to all older adults, no matter how impaired, to live life with meaning, purpose, and hope (Touhy, 2001a).

Solutions, Nursing Actions, and Outcomes

The caring relationship between nurses and persons nursed is the heart of nursing that touches and supports the spirit and

BOX 35.11   Spiritual Nursing Actions

- Relief of physical discomfort, which permits focus on the spiritual
- Creating a peaceful environment
- Comforting touch, which fosters nurse-patient connection
- Authentic presence
- Attentive listening
- Knowing the patient as a person
- Listening to life stories
- Sharing fears and listening to self-doubts or guilt
- Fostering forgiveness and reconciliation
- Validating the person's life and ensuring persons they will be remembered
- Sharing caring words and love
- Encouraging family support and presence
- Fostering connections to that which is held sacred by the person
- Praying with and for the patient
- Respecting religious traditions and providing for access to religious objects and rituals
- Referring the person to a spiritual counselor

Data from Gaskamp C, Sutter R, Meraviglia M, et al: Evidence-based guideline: promoting spirituality in the older adult, *J Gerontol Nurs* 32:8, 2006; Touhy T, Brown C, Smith C: Spiritual caring: end of life in a nursing home, *J Gerontol Nurs* 31:27–35, 2005.

enhances health and well-being. Knowing persons in their complexity, responding to that which matters most to them, identifying and nurturing connections, listening with one's being, using presence and silence, and fostering connections to that which is held sacred by the person are spiritual nursing responses that arise from within the caring, connected relationship (Touhy et al., 2005). Suggestions for nursing actions to promote spiritual health are presented in Box 35.11.

Know that caring for an aging body is the least of the work with older adults. "Limiting care to the physical needs denies older adults the opportunity to live out their life with meaning, purpose, and hope" (Touhy, 2001b, p. 45). Recognizing the primacy of the spirit is essential. Some very spiritual individuals are unable to articulate their knowing. Therefore do not negate that aspect of an individual's experience because it is not expressed verbally. Realizing that biopsychosocial aspects of aging are all shards of the spirit will integrate every aspect of your work in gerontological nursing.

Nurturing the Spirit of the Nurse

"Because spiritual care occurs over time and within the context of relationship, probably the most effective tool at the nurse's disposal is the use of self" (Soeken & Carson, 1987, p. 607). Nurses' ease with their own spiritualty is vital to providing spiritual care (Wittenberg et al., 2017). Nurses should attend to their own biopsychosocial and spiritual issues in the development of compassion and empathy, attributes that serve them well in caring for others' spiritual needs. Find ways to nourish your own spirit. Thinking about what gives your own life meaning and value helps in developing your spiritual self. Examples of activities include finding quiet time for meditation and reflection, keeping your own faith traditions, being with nature, appreciating the arts, spending time with those you love, and journaling. Nurses often do not take the time to do so and become dispirited. This is especially true for nurses who work with dying patients and experience grief and loss repeatedly. Having someone to talk to about feelings is important. Practicing compassion for oneself is essential to authentic practice of compassion for others (Touhy & Zerwekh, 2006) (Box 35.12).

Faith Community Nursing

Faith community nursing (FCN) is a nursing practice specialty that focuses on the intentional care of the spirit, the promotion of an integrative model of health, and the prevention and minimization of illness within the context of a faith community (American Nurses Association, 2012). Nurses can become certified in FCN through the American Nurses Credentialing Center. FCN was originally known as *parish nursing*, but the name was changed to FCN to reflect the broader scope of the practice and the full range of faiths. FCN can assist in bridging the gaps in care in the current health care system, contribute to a reduction in acute health care costs, promote health and disease prevention, and integrate faith with health care to promote positive health outcomes. Models of care such as those implemented in FCN may be particularly relevant to meeting the health maintenance needs and spiritual needs of older adults with chronic illness living in the community.

Nurses who are involved in religious organizations also can be advocates for increasing the attention given to the health needs of older adults. Nurses may even spearhead particular services to older adults, such as peer counseling, health screening activities, daycare, home visitation programs, and respite for families. Many religious organizations reach out to homebound older adults in their community by offering visits from clergy or church members, involvement in prayer circles, and other activities to maintain connection with their faith community.

TRANSCENDENCE

Transcendence is the high-level emotional response to religious and spiritual life and finds expression in numerous rituals and modes of cosmic consciousness. Rituals provide a means of connecting with everyone through the ages who has observed similar rituals. These modes of thinking and feeling are sometimes unfamiliar to individuals who are immersed in the necessary materialistic concerns of young adulthood, yet moments do occur throughout life when one is deeply aware of being part of a larger scheme. Although some of the material in this chapter

may be obscure, it is the springboard for learning to appreciate the full life cycle. The privilege of briefly walking alongside an older adult on the last great journey can be truly inspiring.

Transcending is roused by the desire to go beyond the self as delimited by the material and the concrete aspects of living, to expand self-boundaries and life perspectives. "Transcendence involves detachment and separation from life as it has been lived to experience a reality beyond oneself and beyond what can be seen or felt" (Touhy & Zerwekh, 2006, p. 229). Creative thought and actions are vehicles of both self-actualization and self-transcendence, the bridge to universal expression and existence. Self-transcendence is generally expressed in five modes: creative work, religious beliefs, children, identification with nature, and mystical experiences (Reed, 1991). This section of the chapter deals with various mechanisms by which one transcends the purely physical limitations of existence.

Some people may use asceticism, self-denial, and rigorous rituals to reach the peaks of human experience; many others find more prosaic approaches just as effective. The thesis of Maslow's writings is that mystic, sacred, and transcendent experiences frequently arise from the ordinary elements of one's life (Maslow, 1970). Gardening, reading, holding an infant, dealing with loss, and numerous other normal events have elements of mystery. With each death of a loved one, throughout life, one is reborn to a slightly altered state. When deaths of significant others abound in the later years, older adults must be given the opportunity to express how they personally have been altered by the loss. We can speculate that with each personal loss, one moves slightly closer to the universal and away from the individual until, toward the end, one feels an affiliation with all living things—animal, plant, and mineral. Some older adults have achieved a state of existence that transcends the limits of the failing body.

Gerotranscendence

The theory of gerotranscendence (Tornstam, 1994, 1996, 2005) (Chapter 3) theorizes that human aging brings about a general potential for gerotranscendence, a shift in perspective from the material world to the cosmic and, concurrent with that, an increasing life satisfaction. Gerotranscendence is thought to be a gradual and ongoing shift that is generated by the normal processes of living, sometimes hastened by serious personal disruptions (Box 35.13). An understanding of transcendence and the unique characteristics of this transformation as one ages is important to the continued growth and development of older adults.

Achieving Transcendence

Time Transcendence

Life as experienced ordinarily involves the chronological passage of time. Some types of conscious experience alter our time perception, but the unconscious destroys time. Therefore the release of the unconscious transcends the limitations of time that conscious life experience generally imposes on us. If we conquer time, we conquer annihilation and the dimensions of time that lie within the mind. Recognizing the importance of time perception, particularly in old age, is a fertile field to

---

BOX 35.13 Characteristics of Individuals With a High Degree of Gerotranscendence

- Have high degrees of life satisfaction
- Engage in self-controlled social activity
- Experience satisfaction with self-selected social activities
- Social activities not essential to their well-being
- Midlife patterns and ideals no longer prime motivators
- Demonstrate complex and active coping patterns
- Have greater need for solitary philosophizing
- May appear withdrawn when engaged in inner development
- Have accelerated development of gerotranscendence fomented by life crises
- Feel shifts in perception of reality

---

by rote, praying, saying the rosary, practicing yoga, and playing a musical instrument are all mechanisms of release and renewal that may bring one into higher states of awareness.

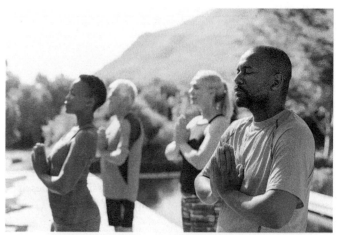

Meditation exercises. (©iStock.com/Ridofranz.)

explore more fully. Influences on time perception include age, imminent death, level of activity, emotional state, outlook on the future, and the value attached to time. Conclusions from studies of older adults generally support the view that older adults perceive time as passing quickly and favor the past over the present or the future.

Peak Experiences

A peak experience occurs when one momentarily transcends the self through love, wisdom, insight, worship, commitment, or creativity. These experiences are the extraordinary events in one's life that clearly demonstrate self-actualization and personal authenticity. Peak experience is the time when restrictive boundaries seem to vanish and one feels more aware, more complete, more ecstatic, or more concerned for others. Peak experiences include many modes of transcending one's ordinary limitations. Spiritual and paranormal experiences, creative acts, courage, and humor may all produce peak experiences. Keeping oneself open to transcendence involves finding the places in which such experiences can break through: soul-stirring concerts, sunrises, sunsets, or raging storms on mountaintops. Each individual seeks states of being in which he or she feels part of a larger whole.

Meditation

Many types and rituals of meditation have flourished in Western societies in recent years. Some methods of meditation have been used for thousands of years in Eastern cultures. Whatever the method, the goal is to quiet the mind and center oneself. When the mind slows, the body relaxes and less oxygen and nutrients are needed. Mindfulness meditation can decrease pain, improve sleep, and enhance well-being and quality of life. Meditation also may improve cognitive function.

Effective meditation requires approximately 20 minutes of focusing on a sound, a thought, or an image. Practicing two or more times daily will leave calmness, better health, and higher energy levels in its wake. Although meditation can be accomplished in any setting, a place with few distractions is helpful. People who meditate with consistency often begin to be aware of a transcendent state of being. Nurses may introduce the values of meditation to older adults and serve as guides in the beginnings of such activities. Chanting psalms, reciting poetry

Hope as a Transcendent Mechanism

Hope is the belief in the future and the expectation of fulfillment. Hope is the anchor that sustains life in the most difficult times and in the face of doubts and ennui. Some level of hope must be maintained to survive and to die in peace. Hope embodies desires and expectations and the limitless possibilities of humans in all times and places—present, past, and future. For many older adults, hope is a major means of coping, and those who lose hope lose the capacity and desire for survival. All practicing nurses have observed how a small goal or hope for the future can sustain an older adult. The grandson's graduation from college, the daughter's return from her travels, or even a birthday may keep an older adult alive until the event is safely fulfilled.

Central to the instillation of hope is the caring relationship between nurses and patients. Caring relationships characterized by unconditional positive regard, encouragement, and competence help patients feel loved and cared about, thus inspiring hope. A patient's hope for cure may change to a hope for freedom from pain, day-to-day experiences to enjoy precious moments of life, time to accomplish life goals before life is over, sharing love with family and friends, relief of suffering, death with dignity, and eternal life. Nurses may foster hope by doing the following:

1. Presenting honestly the limits of human knowledge
2. Controlling symptoms and providing comfort
3. Encouraging patient and family to become involved in positive experiences that transcend the current situation
4. Determining significant aspects of the individual's life
5. Fostering spiritual processes and finding meaning
6. Exploring beliefs and values of the older adult
7. Promoting connection and reconciliation
8. Providing opportunities for prayer, meditation, scripture reading, clergy visits, and religious rituals, if meaningful for the older adult

Other hope-promoting experiences are presented in Box 35.14.

BOX 35.14 Hope-Promoting Activities

- Feel the warmth of the sun.
- Share experiences children are having.
- See the crystal blue of the sky.
- Enjoy a garden or fresh flowers.
- Savor the richness of black coffee at breakfast.
- Feel the tartness of grapefruit to wake up the taste buds.
- Watch the activities of an animal in a tree outside the window.
- Benefit from each encounter with another person.
- Write messages to grandchildren, nieces, or nephews.
- Study a favorite painting.
- Listen to a symphony.
- Build highlights into each day such as meals, visits, Bible reading.
- Keep a journal.
- Write letters.
- Make a tape recording of your life story.
- Have hope objects or symbols nearby.
- Share hope stories.
- Focus on abilities, strengths, and past accomplishments.
- Encourage decision making about daily activities; foster a sense of control.
- Extend caring and love to others.
- Appreciate expressions of caring concern.
- Renew loving relationships.

Adapted from Jevne R: Enhancing hope in the chronically ill, *Humane Med* 9:121–130, 1993; Miller J: *Coping with chronic illness: overcoming powerlessness*, Philadelphia, 1983, FA Davis; Touhy T, Zerwekh J: Spiritual caring. In Zerwekh J, editor: *Nursing care at the end of life: palliative care for patients and families*, Philadelphia, 2006, FA Davis.

Transcendence in Illness

Serious illnesses influence how one perceives the meaning of life. A distinct shift in goals, relationships, and values often occurs among people who have survived life-threatening episodes. A heightened awareness of beauty and of caring relationships may occur, but a long period of emotional "splinting" may be necessary while recovering from the psychic wound of body betrayal. Newman (1994) contends that disease can be a manifestation of health as one confronts the crisis and as it reveals the special meanings.

Steeves and Kahn (1987) found from their work in hospice care that certain conditions facilitate the search for meaning in illness, noting the following:

- Suffering must be bearable and not all-consuming if one is to find meaning in the experience.
- A person must have access to and be capable of perceiving objects in the environment. Even a small window on the world may be sufficient to match the limited energy one has to attend.
- One must have time that is free of interruption and a place of solitude to experience meaning.
- Clean, comfortable surroundings and freedom from constant responsibility and decision making free the soul to search for meaning.
- An open, accepting atmosphere in which to discuss meanings with others is important.

Accompanying someone in grief and a quest for meaning in painful events is a privilege nurses are often given. This spiritual intimacy means being willing to suffer with another, and both

the nurse and the client will reap the benefits. One of the great rewards of working with older adults is observing and participating as they turn suffering into a spiritual event.

Sister Rosemary Donley (1991) defines the nursing role in the spiritual search of suffering individuals as compassionate accompaniment, meaning entering into another's reality and quietly, attentively sharing the experience. "Nurses need to be with people who suffer, to give meaning to the reality of suffering and, in so far as possible, to remove suffering and its causes. Here lies the spiritual dimensions of health care" (Donley, 1991, p. 180). The challenge is to find meaning and some purpose in the affliction that, unchallenged, entwines and chokes identity. (see Chapter 34)

LEGACIES

A legacy is one's tangible and intangible assets that are transferred to another and may be treasured as a symbol of immortality. The purpose of legacies is to supersede death. Courage, wisdom, and insights that we perceive in older adults become part of their legacy. The desire for meaning and immortality seems to be the basic motivation for leaving a legacy. Extending one's authentic self to others can be an important activity in the last years. Throughout life, shared experiences provide satisfaction, but in the last years this exchange allows one to gain a clearer perspective on how one's movement on earth has had an impact.

Older adults must be encouraged to identify that which they would like to leave and who they wish the recipients to be. This process has interpersonal significance and prepares one to leave the world with a sense of meaning. A legacy can provide a transcendent feeling of continuation and tangible or intangible ties with survivors. Legacies are manifold and may range from memories that will live on in the minds of others to bequeathed fortunes. Box 35.15 provides a partial list of legacies. The list is as diverse as individual contributions to humanity. Legacies are generative and are identified and shared best as one approaches the end of life. This activity reinforces integrity.

BOX 35.15 Examples of Legacies

- Oral histories
- Autobiographies
- Written or video histories
- Shared memories
- Taught skills
- Works of art and music
- Publications
- Human organ donations
- Endowments
- Objects of significance
- Tangible or intangible assets
- Personal characteristics, such as courage or integrity
- Bestowed talents
- Traditions and myths perpetuated
- Philanthropic causes
- Progeny children and grandchildren
- Methods of coping
- Unique thoughts: Darwin, Einstein, Freud, Nightingale, and others

Certain questions allow the older person to consider a legacy if ready to do so. For example:

- What is the meaning to you of your life experience right now?
- Have you ever thought of writing an autobiography?
- If you were able to leave something to the younger generation, what would it be?
- Have you ever thought of the impact your generation has had on the world?
- What has been most meaningful in your life?
- What possessions have special meaning for you? Who else is interested in them?
- Do you see some of your genetic traits emerging in your grandchildren?

Types of Legacies

Autobiographies and Life Histories

Oral histories are an approach to immortality. As long as one's story is told, one remains alive in the minds of others. Doers leave their products and live through them. Powerful figures are remembered in fame and infamy. The quiet, unobtrusive person survives in the memory of intimates and in family anecdotes. Everyone has a life story. Nurses can encourage older adults to write, talk, or express in other ways the meaning of their lives. The human experience and the poignant anecdotes bind people together and validate the uniqueness of each brief journey in this level of awareness and the assurance that one will not be forgotten.

Sharing one's personal story creates bonds of empathy, illustrates a point, conveys some of the deep wisdom that we all have, and connects us with our deepest human consciousness. "It is only when people who have loved and cared for us reach the end of life that we see the full gift we have received from them. By leaving us their reminiscences, their spirits can continue in our lives as a living memorial" (Grudzen & Soltys, 2000, p. 8). Chapter 7 provides additional discussion of storytelling, reminiscence, and life review.

Creation of Self Through Journaling

Through the personal journal, one can, in thoughtful reflection, discover meaning and patterns in daily events. The self becomes a coherent story with successive revisions as old events are reread and perceived in new contexts. The journals of older adults provide rich descriptions of the interior lives of the authors. May Sarton (1984) and Florida Scott-Maxwell (1968) are two of the best-known authors. The study of these journals and of the journals of less well-known and less articulate older adults assists nurses in understanding the inner experience of older adults and, perhaps, themselves.

Collective Legacies

Each person is a link in the chain of generations (Erikson, 1963) and as such may identify with generational accomplishments. An older adult may identify with the generation that walked on the moon or experienced World War II, the Vietnam War, or the Civil Rights Movement. The years of youthful idealism are impressed in one's memory by the political or ideological climate of the time. This time is the stage when one searches for a fit in the larger society. The importance of collective legacies to nurses lies in how they use this knowledge. For instance, the nurse may ask, "Who were the great people of your time?" "Which ones were important to you?" "What events of your generation changed the world?" "What were the most important events you experienced?" Mentioning certain historical events or asking about individual reactions is sometimes helpful. Childless individuals are becoming more prevalent with each passing generation, and they must find a way to outlive the self through a legacy. Many people choose a social legacy. Florence Nightingale would be one such person, with the grand legacy she left to nurses.

Legacies Expressed Through Other People

One's legacy can be expressed in many ways—through the development of others in a teaching or learning situation or through mentorship, patronage, shared talents, organ donations, and genetic transmission. Some creative works and research are legacies left to successive generations for continued modification and growth. In other words, one's legacy may be a product of one's own brought to fruition through someone else who also may become an intermediary to later developments. Thus people and generations are tied in sequential progress. Some examples may illustrate this type of legacy:

- An older man cried as he talked of his grandson's talent as a violinist. Both the man and his grandson shared their love for the violin, and the grandfather believed that he had genetically and personally contributed to his grandson's development as an accomplished musician.
- A professor emeritus spoke of visiting her son in a distant state and hearing him expound ideas that had been partially developed by the professor and her father before her.
- People who amass a fortune and allocate certain funds for endowment of artists, scientific projects, and intellectual exploration are counting on others to complete their legacy.

Living Legacies

Many older adults wish to donate their bodies to science or donate body parts for transplantation. This mechanism is a means to transcend death. Parts of the body keep another person alive, or in the case of certain diseases, the deceased body may provide important information leading to preventive or restorative techniques in the future. Donation of body parts in old age may not be encouraged because they are often less viable than those from younger people. Nonetheless, older bodies are welcome for use as cadavers.

The Alzheimer's Research Center operates the Dementia Brain Bank Research Program. The Brain Bank is one of the world's largest collections of brain tissue, which contributes to research on the neurochemistry, physiology, and diagnosis of dementing illnesses. People who are interested in providing such a legacy should be encouraged to call the nearest university biomedical center or Brain Bank registry and obtain more information. The nurse then has a postmortem obligation to the individual to assist in carrying out the person's wishes.

Property and Assets

Wealth may be viewed as a means toward power more often than transcendence; therefore some older adults are often reluctant to disperse material goods before their death. Some use the future legacy as a means to exert power and control over offspring. One man said, "So long as I have that bankroll, they've got to treat me with respect" (Lustbader, 1996). The power to exert influence, to punish, and to reward is often bound up in an anticipated estate distribution. Estates can be planned in certain ways that are decidedly advantageous for the planner, and the recipient, in terms of control and avoidance of lengthy probate proceedings and taxation. Because the laws are complex and ever-changing, using the services of an estate planner is advisable. The nurse's responsibility regarding wills may be limited to advising older adults to obtain legal counsel while they are healthy and competent and plan how they would like to distribute their worldly goods.

Personal Possessions

Possessions carry more meaning as time passes; individuals change, but the possession remains much the same. A possession is a way of symbolically hanging on to individuals who are gone or times that are past. For some people, keeping personal possessions is a means of hanging on to the self that is changing with time. Cherished possessions passed on through several generations may have achieved meaning through the close family member to whom they belonged. One's personally significant items become highly charged with memories and meaning, and transferring them to friends and kin can be a tender experience. Personal possessions should never be dispersed without the individual's knowledge. Because of the uncertainty of late life lucidity, these issues should be discussed early with older individuals.

People who are approaching death must be given the opportunity to distribute their important belongings appropriately to those whom they believe will also cherish them. Nurses may encourage older adults to plan the distribution of their significant items carefully. Deciding when and how best these possessions should be given is often difficult. Some people choose to distribute possessions before dying. In these cases, nurses often need to help family members accept these gifts, appreciating the meaning and recognizing the significance.

USING CLINICAL JUDGMENT TO PROMOTE HEALTHY AGING: SPIRITUAL HEALTH, MEANING, AND SELF-ACTUALIZAITON

"The responsibility of the nurse is not to make people well, or to prevent their getting sick, but to assist people to recognize the power that is within them to move to higher levels of consciousness" (Newman, 1994, p. xv). In this chapter, we have examined methods of expanding one's limited existence by developing the authentic self, transcendent self, and spiritual self and several mechanisms used to establish immortality through a legacy. These areas often become major issues in the latter part of life, and the nurse will find it a revealing, absorbing, and challenging task to be a part of this effort. An important point is that some people may avoid any such interest or concern, particularly when angry, in pain, or denying their own mortality. Nurses need not push the individual to accomplish this task but should be available to assist the person and family members. It calls for a nurse who is willing to enter into meaningful spirit-sharing relationships.

The basic mysteries of life elude scientific researchers, yet they are the essence of existence with meaning. Remembering, feeling, dreaming, worshiping, and grasping one's connection to the universe are the realities of the human spirit. Spirit synthesizes the total personality and provides integration, energizing force, and immortality. "Those of us who choose careers in aging frequently arrive to serve and to care because we see the remarkable but commonly dismissed strength in aged bodies, the beauty of human wisdom and sage judgment, and the eloquent stories of lives many decades long" (Kagan, 2020, p. 1). Such relationships have the potential to enhance inner harmony and healing. There may be no greater goal in caring for older adults than helping a person to see a life well lived and meaningful to oneself and others, thus providing hope that life's journey was not in vain. Taking advantage of these opportunities will enrich our nursing, our inner selves, and the spiritual well-being of the older adults whom we nurse.

Gerontological nursing scholar Sarah Gueldner (2007) eloquently stated:

> We must help each older adult to continue to experience and express the passions that, over a lifetime, have become who they are. Older adults should continue to make their unique and precious contributions to society, and we must not fail to take note of it in even the frailest and quietest of individuals. We must give them voice and time on the center stage of life and help them connect with each other and with society in a way that fosters appreciation of the traits, talents, and memories that still define their being. (p. 4).

The authors of this book hope that you find as much joy and fulfillment in your nursing with older adults as we have.

■ KEY CONCEPTS

- Self-actualization is a process of developing one's most authentic self. Maslow thought of self-actualization as the pinnacle of human development.
- Self-actualized individuals embody qualities of courage, humor, high moral development, and seeking to learn more about themselves and others.
- Opportunities for pursuing interests will assist individuals in developing latent talents, expressing their creativity, and rising beyond daily concerns.

- Groups working toward societal humanitarian advancement may accomplish collective actualization.
- Creativity emanates from people who are self-actualized and may be expressed in everyday activities, and the arts, music, theater, and literature.
- Transcending the material and physical limitations of existence through ritual and spiritual means is an especially important aspect of aging.

- Gerotranscendence is a theory proposed by Tornstam that implies a natural shift in concerns that occurs in the aging process. Older adults are thought to spend more time in reflection, to spend less on materialistic concerns, and to find more satisfaction in life. This effort is an attempt to define aging not by the standards of young and middle adulthood but as having distinctive characteristics of its own.
- Illnesses that occur have the potential for altering one's fundamental beliefs and hopes. Nurses must give older adults the opportunity to discuss the meaning of an illness. Some people find that these experiences bring new insights; others are angry. Empathic nurses will provide a sounding board while the individual makes sense of an illness within a satisfactory framework.
- Nurses need not neglect discussing spirituality with older adults. Older adults will respond only if it has significance for them.
- Spiritual nursing actions emanate from the caring relationship between the older adult and the nurse. The most important tool at the nurse's disposal is the use of self.

NEXT-GENERATION NCLEX® (NGN) EXAMINATION–STYLE QUESTIONS

The hospice nurse is visiting a 59-year-old patient in her home. The patient has had recurrent cancer and has been given approximately 6 months to live. The patient is well dressed and groomed and reports attempting to get her life affairs in order now that she knows she is dying. She says, "Last week I reached out to my brother after not talking for 20 years. I also started jotting down some memories from when I was a new wife and mother so that my husband and children will have them. I'm still trying to do some things I like, such as painting a little bit every day, but it's hard to stay focused when I know I will be gone soon. It's like wondering what the purpose of life is when I've worked my whole life, and now I'm going to die just when I was starting to think about retirement and grandchildren. Every time I try to pull myself together to do something good or pleasurable, that thought creeps up and depresses me. I try not to burden my family because I want them to remember me as a happy and loving person." When asked by the nurse if the patient has a faith base, the patient replies, "I've never been much for religion, and I don't belong to a church. I find my faith in enjoying peace and quiet with my family."

Drag one concept and one client finding to fill in each blank in the following sentence.

The patient is at risk for concerns with _____ due to _____.

Concept
spiritual distress
religion
wisdom
creativity
morality

Client Finding
not being a church member
questioning life's purpose
painting regularly
seeing her brother
creating a legacy

NURSING STUDY

Self-Actualization, Spirituality, and Transcendence

Melba had no children but had numerous nieces and nephews, though she did not feel particularly close to any of them. She had been a nursing instructor at a community college and had enjoyed her students but had not developed a sustained relationship with any of them after they had completed her courses. At her level of nursing education, the opportunity for mentorship was lacking, though she had occasionally taken students under her wing and arranged special experiences that they particularly desired. Because she had taught several courses each year, Melba never really developed a strong affiliation to a specialty but considered herself a pediatric nurse. She had not made any major contributions to the field in terms of research or publications; a few reviews, continuing education workshops, and some nursing newsletters had been the extent of her work outside that which was required.

Melba's husband died in 1988, and she had felt very much alone since that time, especially after her retirement 3 years ago. Before her husband's death, Melba had been too busy to think about the ultimate meaning of all her years of teaching and wifely activities. With time on her hands, she began to wonder what it all meant. Had she done anything meaningful? Had she really made a difference in anything or in anyone's life? Was anyone going to remember her in any special way? So many questions were making her morose. She had never been a religious person, though her husband had been a devout Catholic. He had believed that God had a purpose for him in life, and though he was not always able to understand what it might be, he seemed to have a sense of satisfaction. She began to wonder if she should go to church—would that make her feel less depressed?

One Sunday morning, Melba had decided to attend her neighborhood Catholic church, but on her way out she slipped on the icy walkway and sustained bilateral Colles' fractures. After a brief emergency department visit for assessment, immobilization of the wrists, and medications, Melba was sent back home with an order for home health and social service assessment on the following day. Of course, she had extreme difficulty managing the most basic self-care while keeping her wrists immobilized and was very dejected. When the home health nurse arrived the next morning, to Melba's amazement it was a former student who had graduated 4 years previously. Melba was more chagrined than pleased and greeted her with, "Oh, I hate to have you see me so helpless. I've been feeling so useless, and now with these wrists I am totally useless."

CLINICAL JUDGMENT QUESTIONS AND ACTIVITIES

1. In the nursing study, if you were the home health nurse, how would you begin working with Melba, knowing that you would be limited to just a few visits?
2. Discuss the meanings and the thoughts triggered by the student's and the older adult's viewpoints as expressed at the beginning of the chapter. How do they vary from your own experience?
3. How do nursing students learn about spirituality and spiritual nursing interventions?
4. What activities might be helpful in developing your own sense of spirituality?
5. How do cultural beliefs and traditions affect one's concept of spirituality?
6. How can nurses enhance spiritual care, self-actualization, and transcendence of self among older adults?

RESEARCH QUESTIONS

1. What aspects of intergenerational programs are enjoyed by younger and older individuals?
2. Who makes wills and when do they make them?
3. What are the motivating differences between gifts given during life and those given after one's death?
4. What is the perspective of the older adult related to spiritual assessment and spiritual care nursing actions by nurses?
5. How do nurses describe the spiritual actions they use with older adults?
6. How do nurses recognize aspects of gerotranscendence?

REFERENCES

American Nurses Association: *Faith community nursing: scope and standards of practice,* ed 2, Spring, MD, 2012.

Ardelt M: Wisdom as expert knowledge system: a critical review of a contemporary operationalization of an ancient concept, *Hum Dev* 47:257–285, 2004.

Bell V, Troxel D: Spirituality and the person with dementia: a view from the field, *Alzheimers Care Q* 2:31–45, 2001.

Bernstein A: *Spirituality and aging: looking at the big picture* (website), 2009. http://todaysgeriatricmedicine.com/news/septstory1.shtml. Accessed July 2021.

Cousins N: *Anatomy of an illness,* New York, 1979, Norton.

Delgado C: Sense of coherence, spirituality, stress and quality of life in chronic illness, *J Nurs Scholarsh* 39(3):229–234, 2007.

Donley R: Spiritual dimensions of health care: nursing's mission, *Nurs Health Care* 12:178–183, 1991.

Erikson EH: *Childhood and society,* ed 2, New York, 1963, Norton.

Gaskamp C, Sutter R, Meraviglia M, et al: Evidence-based guideline: promoting spirituality in the older adult, *J Gerontol Nurs* 32:8–13, 2006.

Goldberg B: Connection: an exploration of spirituality in nursing care, *J Adv Nurs* 27:836–842, 1998.

Grudzen M, Soltys F: Reminiscence at end of life: celebrating a living legacy, *Dimensions* 7(3):4, 5, 8, 2000.

Gueldner S: Sustaining expression on identity in older adults, *J Gerontol Nurs* 33:3–4, 2007.

Hansman H: *College students are living rent-free in a Cleveland retirement home* (website), 2015. https://www.smithsonianmag.com/innovation/college-students-are-living-rent-free-in-cleveland-retirement-home-180956930/. Accessed July 2021.

Harris J: *Students living in nursing homes—a solution to our ageing populations?* (website), 2016. https://www.weforum.org/agenda/2016/11/some-dutch-university-students-are-living-in-nursing-homes-this-is-why?utm_content=buffer07075&utm_medium=social&utm_source=twitter.com&utm_campaign=buffer. Accessed July 2021.

Heriot CS: Spirituality and aging, *Holist Nurs Pract* 7:22–23, 1992.

Hooyman N, Kiyak A: *Social gerontology: a multidisciplinary perspective,* Boston, 2005, Pearson.

Hudson F: *The adult years: mastering the art of self-renewal,* San Francisco, 1999, Jossey-Bass.

Jansen T: *The nursing home that's also a dorm* (website), 2016. https://www.citylab.com/equity/2015/10/the-nursing-home-thats-also-a-dorm/408424/. Accessed July 2021.

Kagan S: Solace and strength: ageing, the arts and nursing, *Int Jour Older People Nurs* 15(4):12357, 2020. doi:10.1111/opn.12357.

Killick J: *Dementia diary,* London, 2008, Hawker.

Killick J: *Openings,* London, 2000, Hawker.

Killick J: *You are words,* London, 1997, Hawker.

Koenig H, Brooks R: Religion, health and aging: implications for practice and public policy, *Public Policy Aging Rep* 12:13–19, 2002.

Kohlberg L, Power C: Moral development, religious thinking and the question of a seventh stage. In Kohlberg L, editor: *The philosophy of moral development,* vol 1, San Francisco, 1981, Harper & Row.

Kuhn M: Advocacy in this new age, *Aging* 3:297, 1979.

Larson R: Building intergenerational bonds through the arts, *Generations* 30:38, 2006.

Lustbader W: Conflict, emotion and power surrounding legacy, *Generations* 20:54–57, 1996.

Macrae J: Nightingale's spiritual philosophy and its significance for modern nursing, *Image J Nurs Sch* 27:8–10, 1995.

Malone J, Dadswell A: The role of religion, spirituality and/or belief in positive ageing for older adults, *Geriatrics (Basel)* 32(2):28, 2018.

Martsolf DS, Mickley JR: The concept of spirituality in nursing theories: differing world views and extent of focus, *J Adv Nurs* 27:294–303, 1998.

Maslow A: Creativity in self-actualizing people. In Anderson H, editor: *Creativity and its cultivator,* New York, 1959, Harper & Row.

Maslow A: *Religions, values and peak-experiences,* New York, 1970, Viking Press.

Metcalf CW: *Lighten up* (audiotape), Niles, IL, 1993, Nightingale Conant.

Meyer CL: How effectively are nurse educators preparing students to provide spiritual care? *Nurse Educ* 28(4):185–190, 2003.

Newman MA: *Health as expanding consciousness,* ed 2, New York, 1994, National League for Nursing Press.

Parisi J, Rebok G, Carlson M, et al: Can the wisdom of aging be activated and make a difference societally? *Educ Gerontol* 35:867–879, 2009.

Peck R: Psychological developments in the second half of life. In Anderson J, editor: *Psychological aspects of aging,* Washington, D.C., 1955, American Psychological Association.

Perlstein S: Creative expression and quality of life: a vital relationship for elders, *Generations* 30:5–6, 2006.

Puchalski C, Romer AL: Taking a spiritual history allows clinicians to understand patients more fully, *J Palliat Med* 3:129–137, 2000.

Reed PG: Toward a nursing theory of self-transcendence: deductive reformulation using developmental theories, *Adv Nurs Sci* 13:64–77, 1991.

Sarton M: *At seventy: a journal,* New York, 1984, Norton.

Scott-Maxwell F: *The measure of my days,* New York, 1968, Knopf.

Soeken K, Carson VJ: Responding to the spiritual needs of the chronically ill, *Nurs Clin North Am* 22:603–611, 1987.

Steeves RH, Kahn DL: Experience of meaning in suffering, *Image J Nurs Sch* 19:114–116, 1987.

Strang S, Strang P: Questions posed to hospital chaplains by palliative care patients, *J Palliat Med* 5:857, 2002.

Tornstam L: Gerotranscendence: a theoretical and empirical exploration. In Thomas LE, Eisenhandler SA, editors: *Aging and the religious dimension,* Westport, CT, 1994, Greenwood Publishing Group.

Tornstam L: *Gerotranscendence: a developmental theory of positive aging,* New York, 2005, Springer.

Tornstam L: Gerotranscendence: a theory about maturing into old age, *J Aging Identity* 1:37–50, 1996.

Touhy TA: Nurturing hope and spirituality in the nursing home, *Holist Nurs Pract* 15:45–56, 2001.

Touhy TA: Touching the spirit of elders in nursing homes: ordinary yet extraordinary care, *Int J Hum Caring* 6:12–17, 2001.

Touhy TA, Brown C, Smith CJ: Spiritual caring: end of life in a nursing home, *J Gerontol Nurs* 31:27–35, 2005.

Touhy T, Zerwekh J: Spiritual caring. In Zerwekh J, editor: *Nursing care at the end of life: palliative care for patients and families,* Philadelphia, 2006, FA Davis.

Wikström BM: Older adults and the arts: the importance of aesthetic forms of expression in later life, *J Gerontol Nurs* 30:30–36, 2004.

Wittenberg E, Ragan S, Ferrell B: Exploring nurse communication about spirituality, *Am J Hosp Palliat Med* 34(6):566–571, 2017.

Entry followed by *f* indicates figure, by *t* table, and by *b* box.